The Scar Book

Formation, Mitigation, Rehabilitation, and Prevention

The Scar Book

Formation, Mitigation, Rehabilitation, and Prevention

Andrew C. Krakowski, MD
Founder and Director; Scar Treatment and Revision (S.T.A.R.) Institute
Chief Medical Officer
DermOne, LLC
West Conshohocken, Pennsylvania

Peter R. Shumaker, MD
Captain, United States Navy
Chairman, Dermatology
Naval Medical Center
San Diego, California
Clinical Associate Professor of Dermatology
Uniformed Services University of the Health Sciences
Bethesda, Maryland

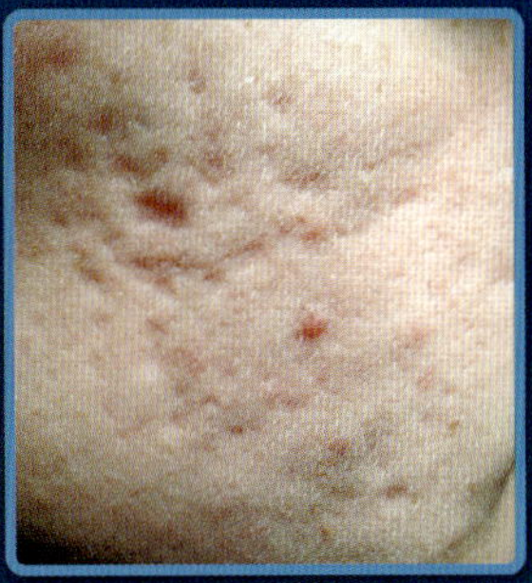

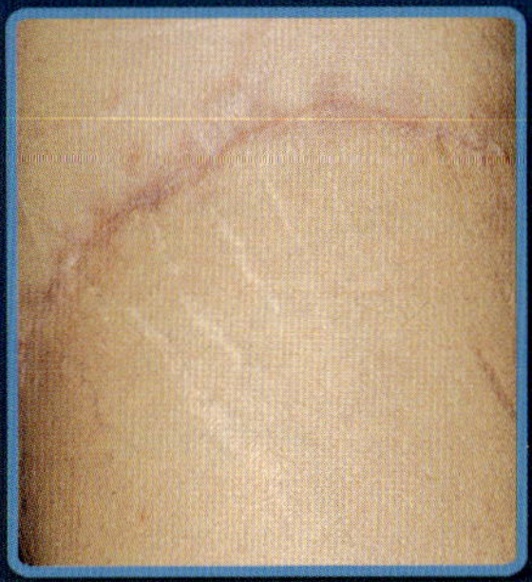

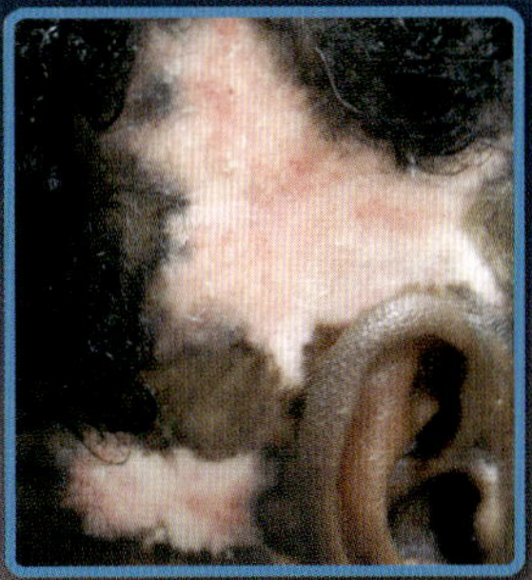

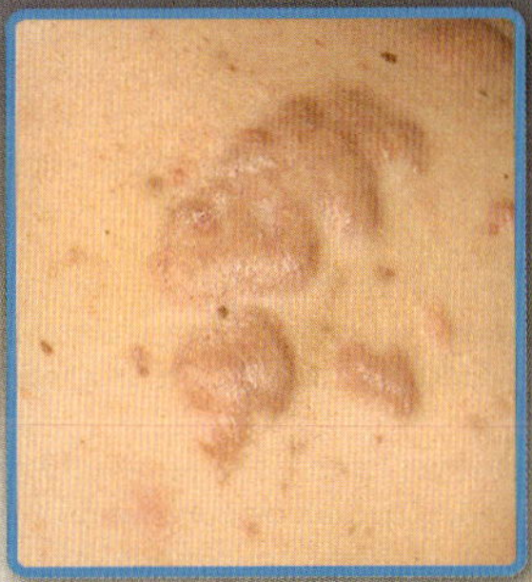

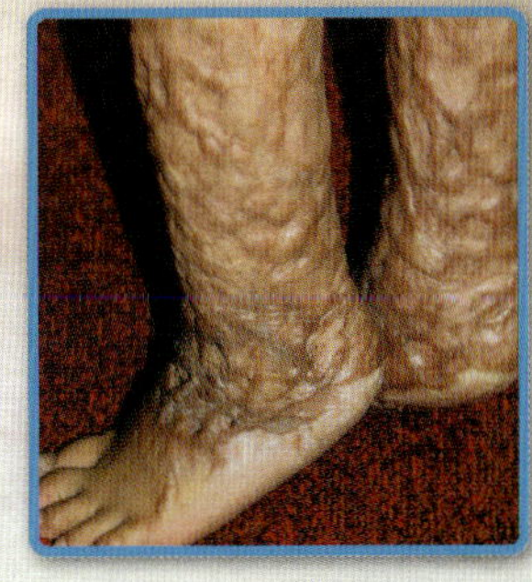

Wolters Kluwer

Philadelphia • Baltimore • New York • London
Buenos Aires • Hong Kong • Sydney • Tokyo

Executive Editor: Rebecca Gaertner
Senior Product Development Editor: Kristina Oberle
Senior Production Project Manager: Alicia Jackson
Design Coordinator: Elaine Kasmer
Senior Manufacturing Coordinator: Beth Welsh
Prepress Vendor: S4Carlisle Publishing Services

9 8 7 6 5 4 3 2 1

Printed in China

Library of Congress Cataloging-in-Publication Data

Names: Krakowski, Andrew C. | Shumaker, Peter R.
Title: The scar book : formation, mitigation, rehabilitation, and prevention / [edited by] Andrew C. Krakowski, MD, founder and director, Kids' Scar Treatment and Revision Program (S.T.A.R.), Rady Children's Hospital, assistant professor of clinical pediatrics and medicine (dermatology), University of California, San Diego School of Medicine, and Rady Children's Hospital, San Diego, California, Peter R. Shumaker, MD, Captain, United States Navy, chairman, Dermatology, Naval Medical Center San Diego, clinical associate professor of dermatology, Uniformed Services University of the Health Sciences, San Diego, California.
Description: Philadelphia : Wolters Kluwer, [2017] | Includes bibliographical references and index.
Identifiers: LCCN 2016056832 | ISBN 9781496322388 (alk. paper)
Subjects: LCSH: Scars. | Granulation tissue. | Wound healing.
Classification: LCC RD94 .S33 2017 | DDC 617.1/4—dc23 LC record available at https://lccn.loc.gov/2016056832

LWW.com

To my mother, Carol, my father, Frank, and my sister, Lauren . . . thank you for inspiring me to want to care for others and for teaching me what it means to lead by example. I am sorry for any scars I may have caused along the way.

To my greatest love, Carlisle, and to my greatest hope, Nathaniel and James . . . together, you are my life. Thank you for supporting/enduring me through this crazy endeavor. I love you more than you can possibly ever know. Yes, Nate, even bigger than the sky is blue!

To Mike Gill, my best friend in high school . . . I see you in the face of every patient I treat, and I am a better person because of it.

Andrew C. Krakowski

To my wife, Patrice, and my boys, Tim, Jack, and Garret . . . thank you for fortifying me with your love and support during this Sisyphean endeavor, and always. You are my greatest accomplishment.

To my parents, Randy and Claire . . . every trace of humility, intelligence, and compassion I can claim I owe to you (but not necessarily in that order).

To my brothers, Jeremy, Scott, and Erik . . . because you are terrific, and who knows when I will have another book.

To my grandfather, Herbert M. Giffin, MD . . . who first inspired me into a life of healing, and stirred my interest in Navy Medicine with his tales from the South Pacific.

To all the hard-chargers who have given me the privilege of caring for them, and who constantly inspire me to do more.

Peter R. Shumaker

Contributors

Murad Alam, MD, MSCI
Professor of Dermatology, Otolaryngology, and Surgery
Chief, Section of Cutaneous and Aesthetic Surgery
Northwestern University
Chicago, Illinois

Elizabeth Allen
Trustee and Principal Tutor for the Charity
The British Association of Skin Camouflage (BASC)
Chester, Cheshire, Great Britain

Saeid Amini Nik, MSc, MD, PhD
Assistant Professor
Department of Surgery
University of Toronto
Junior Scientist, Sunnybrook Research Institute
Toronto, Canada

R. Rox Anderson, MD
Director, Wellman Center for Photomedicine
Massachusetts General Hospital
Boston, Massachusetts

Peter Angelos, MD, PhD
MacLean Center for Clinical Medical Ethics
University of Chicago
Chicago, Illinois

Andrew Basnett, MD
Lieutenant Commander
United States Navy
Department of Dermatology
Naval Medical Center
San Diego, California

Thomas Beachkofsky, MD, FAAD
Major
United States Air Force
Staff Dermatologist
Wilford Hall Ambulatory Surgical Center
JBSA-Lackland, Texas
Assistant Professor of Dermatology
Uniformed Service University of the Health Sciences
Bethesda, Maryland

Joanna G. Bolton, MD, FAAD
ASDS Cosmetic Dermatologic Surgery Fellow
Cosmetic Laser Dermatology
San Diego, California

Carrick Burns, MD
Lieutenant Commander
United States Navy
Department of Dermatology
Naval Medical Center
San Diego, California

Marsha Chaffins, MD
Department of Dermatology and Pathology
Henry Ford Hospital
Detroit, Michigan

Henry Hin Lee Chan, MD, PhD, FRCP
Division of Dermatology
Department of Medicine
The University of Hong Kong
Dermatology & Laser Centre
Hong Kong, Peoples Republic of China

Sydney R. Coleman, MD
Department of Plastic Surgery
University of Pittsburgh
Pittsburgh, Pennsylvania
Department of Plastic Surgery
New York University
New York, New York
Private Practice
Tribeca Plastic Surgery
New York, New York

Dawn Cragg, MBE, CPCP
Member of the British Empire
Comite International d'Esthetique et de Cosmetologie (CIDESCO)
Confederation of International Beauty Therapy and Cosmetology (CIBTAC)
British Association of Skin Camouflage (BASC)
Nottinghamshire, Retford, United Kingdom

Paul Diegidio, MD
Division of Plastic Surgery
University of North Carolina
Chapel Hill, North Carolina

Jie Ding, MD, PhD
Division of Plastic and Reconstructive Surgery and Critical Care
Department of Surgery
University of Alberta
Edmonton, Alberta, Canada

Reinhard Dolp, MD
Sunnybrook Research Institute
Institute of Medical Science, University of Toronto
Toronto, Canada

Matthias B. Donelan, MD
Chief of Staff
Shriner's Hospital for Children
Visiting Surgeon, Massachusetts General Hospital
Associate Clinical Professor of Surgery, Harvard Medical School
Boston, Massachusetts

Dominik Duscher, MD
Division of Plastic and Reconstructive Surgery
Department of Surgery
Stanford University School of Medicine
Stanford, California

Nicole Fett, MD, MSCE
Assistant Professor of Dermatology
Center for Health and Healing
Department of Dermatology
Oregon Health and Sciences University
Portland, Oregon

Curtis Gaball, MD, FACS
Commander
United States Navy
Chairman
Department of Otolaryngology
Naval Medical Center
San Diego, California

Gerd G. Gauglitz, MD, MMS
Department of Dermatology and Allergy
Ludwig-Maximilian University
Munich, Germany

Mitchel P. Goldman, MD
Volunteer Clinical Professor of Dermatology
University of California, San Diego
Medical Director, West Dermatology
San Diego, California

Lawrence J. Gottlieb, MD
MacLean Center for Clinical Medical Ethics
University of Chicago
Chicago, Illinois

Kendra Grim, MD
Assistant Professor of Anesthesiology
The Mayo Clinic
Rochester, Minnesota

Geoffrey C. Gurtner, MD, FACS
Johnson & Johnson Professor of Surgery
Division of Plastic and Reconstructive Surgery
Department of Surgery
Stanford University School of Medicine
Stanford, California

Chad Hivnor, MD, FAAD
Colonel
United States Air Force Reserve
Staff Dermatologist
Wilford Hall Ambulatory Surgical Center
JBSA-Lackland, Texas
Assistant Professor of Dermatology
Uniformed Services University of the Health Sciences
Bethesda, Maryland

Michael Sung-Min Hu, MD, MPH, MS
Hagey Laboratory for Pediatric Regenerative Medicine
Department of Surgery
Division of Plastic and Reconstructive Surgery
Stanford University School of Medicine
Institute for Stem Cell Biology and Regenerative Medicine
Stanford University
Stanford, California
Department of Surgery
John A. Burns School of Medicine
University of Hawai'i
Honolulu, Hawai'i

C. Scott Hultman, MD, MBA, FACS
Ethel and James Valone Distinguished Professor
Chief, Division of Plastic Surgery
University of North Carolina
Chapel Hill, North Carolina

Isaac B. James, MD
Resident
Department of Plastic Surgery
University of Pittsburgh
Pittsburgh, Pennsylvania

William James, MD
Perelman School of Medicine
University of Pennsylvania Department of Dermatology
Philadelphia, Pennsylvania

J. Daniel Jensen, MD
Division of Mohs Surgery
Scripps Clinic
La Jolla, California

Marc Jeschke, MD, PhD, FACS, FCCM, FRCS(C)
Professor, University of Toronto
Department of Surgery, Division of Plastic Surgery, Department of Immunology
Director, Ross Tilley Burn Centre, Sunnybrook Health Sciences Centre
Chair in Burn Research
Senior Scientist, Sunnybrook Research Institute
Toronto, Canada

Andrew C. Krakowski, MD
Founder and Director; Scar Treatment and Revision (S.T.A.R.) Institute
Chief Medical Officer
DermOne, LLC
West Conshohocken, Pennsylvania

Tripp Leavitt, BS
Hagey Laboratory for Pediatric Regenerative Medicine
Department of Surgery
Division of Plastic and Reconstructive Surgery
Stanford University School of Medicine
Stanford, California
Boston University School of Medicine
Boston, Massachusetts

Kachiu C. Lee, MD
Wellman Center for Photomedicine
Massachusetts General Hospital
Boston, Massachusetts

Benjamin Levi, MD
Director
Burn/Wound and Regenerative Medicine Laboratory
Assistant Professor of Plastic Surgery
University of Michigan Health Systems
Ann Arbor, Michigan

Michael T. Longaker, MD, MBA, FACS
Deane P. and Louise Mitchell Professor of Surgery
Division of Plastic and Reconstructive Surgery
Department of Surgery
Stanford University School of Medicine
Hagey Laboratory for Pediatric Regenerative Medicine
Institute for Stem Cell Biology and Regenerative Medicine
Stanford University
Stanford, California

H. Peter Lorenz, MD
Hagey Laboratory for Pediatric Regenerative Medicine
Division of Plastic and Reconstructive Surgery
Department of Surgery
Stanford University School of Medicine
Stanford, California

Walter Meyer III, MD
Shriners Hospitals for Children
Galveston, Texas
Department of Psychiatry and Behavioral Sciences
University of Texas Medical Branch
Galveston, Texas

Michael E. Nemergut, MD, PhD
Assistant Professor Anesthesiology
Pediatrics and Adolescent Medicine
The Mayo Clinic
Rochester, Minnesota

Tuyet A. Nguyen, MD
Albert Einstein College of Medicine
Bronx, New York
Rady Children's Hospital
San Diego, California

Jonathan Niszczak, MS, OTR/L
Clinical Care Specialist
Burn Rehabilitation & Plastic Surgery
Bio Med Sciences, Inc.

Rei Ogawa, MD, PhD, FACS
Professor and Chief
Department of Plastic, Reconstructive and Aesthetic Surgery
Nippon Medical School Hospital
Tokyo, Japan

Keith Olsen, MD, PhD
Center for Health and Healing
Department of Dermatology
Oregon Health and Science University
Portland, Oregon

David Ozog, MD
Department of Dermatology
Henry Ford Hospital
Detroit, Michigan

Jane Petro, MD, FACS, FAACS
Professor of Surgery
New York Medical College
Valhalla, New York

Julian Poetschke, MD
Department of Dermatology and Allergy
Ludwig-Maximilian University
Munich, Germany

Bruce M. Potenza, MD, FACS, FCCM
Chief, Department of Surgery
Phoenix VA Health Care System
Phoenix, Arizona

Molly Powers, MD
Department of Dermatology
Henry Ford Hospital
Detroit, Michigan

Markus Reinholz, MD
Department of Dermatology and Allergy
Ludwig-Maximilian University
Munich, Germany

Hans-Oliver Rennenkampff, MD
Director of Plastic, Aesthetic, and Burn Surgery
Klinikum Leverkusen gGmbH
Leverkusen, Germany

Laura Rosenberg, PhD
Shriners Hospitals for Children
Galveston, Texas
Department of Psychiatry and Behavioral Sciences
University of Texas Medical Branch
Galveston, Texas

Marta Rosenberg, PhD
Shriners Hospitals for Children
Galveston, Texas
Department of Psychiatry and Behavioral Sciences
University of Texas Medical Branch
Galveston, Texas

E. Victor Ross, MD
Director
Laser and Cosmetic Dermatology
Scripps Clinic
San Diego, California

J. Peter Rubin, MD, FACS
Chair, Department of Plastic Surgery
UPMC Endowed Professor of Plastic Surgery
Professor of Bioengineering
University of Pittsburgh
Pittsburgh, Pennsylvania

Ashley Rudnick, BS
Miami Dermatology and Laser Institute
Miami, Florida

Michael A. Serghiou, OTR, MBA
Clinical Care Specialist
Burn Rehabilitation & Plastic Surgery
Bio Med Sciences, Inc.
Previously, Administrative Director
Shriners Hospital for Children
Galveston, Texas

Baddr A. Shakhsheer, MD
MacLean Center for Clinical Medical Ethics
University of Chicago
Chicago, Illinois

Peter R. Shumaker, MD, FAAD, FACMS
Captain, United States Navy
Chairman, Dermatology
Naval Medical Center
San Diego, California
Clinical Associate Professor of Dermatology
Uniformed Services University of the Health Sciences
Bethesda, Maryland

Mark Siegler, MD, MACP
Lindy Bergman Distinguished Service Professor of Medicine and Surgery
Director
MacLean Center for Clinical Medical Ethics
Executive Director
The Bucksbaum Institute for Clinical Excellence
University of Chicago
Chicago, Illinois

Puneet Singh, MD
MacLean Center for Clinical Medical Ethics
University of Chicago
Chicago, Illinois

Mayer Tenenhaus, MD, FACS
Clinical Professor, Plastic and Reconstructive Surgery
University of California at San Diego Medical Center
San Diego, California

Edward E. Tredget, MD, MSc, FRCSC
Division of Plastic and Reconstructive Surgery and Critical Care
Department of Surgery
University of Alberta
Edmonton, Alberta, Canada

Nathan Uebelhoer, DO
Commander
United States Navy (Retired)
Private Practice

Jill S. Waibel, MD
Miami Dermatology & Laser Institute
Assistant Professor (Voluntary)
Miller School of Medicine
University of Miami
Chief of Dermatology
Baptist Hospital
Miami, Florida

Fiona Wood, FRACS, AM
Director of the Burns Service of Western Australia,
Fiona Stanley and Perth New Children's Hospitals, Western Australia
Winthrop Professor of Surgery
Director of the Burn Injury Research Unit
University of Western Australia
Perth, Australia

Chi Keung Yeung, MD, FRCP
Division of Dermatology
Department of Medicine
The University of Hong Kong
Dermatology & Laser Centre
Hong Kong, Peoples Republic of China

Lisa A. Zaleski-Larsen, DO, FAAD
Cosmetic Dermatologic Surgeon
West Dermatology
San Diego, California

Preface

The roots of this book are nourished in the soil of collaboration. Few entities permeate medicine and impact as many people worldwide as scars and fibrosis, and no medical specialty is completely absolved of responsibility for the creation, or in managing the consequences, of scars. Reams of new information on scar pathophysiology and treatment are generated every year, but in our view, progress in scar management is impeded by the compartmentalization of the information by discipline and location. Thus, one of the primary objectives of the inaugural edition of *The Scar Book* is to aggregate a multitude of different perspectives into a single comprehensive source. It is an ambitious effort to help advance collective knowledge and discovery by remaining focused on the condition; a compendium of the state of the art in scar formation, treatment, and research, presented by many of the world's foremost experts.

The contributors to *The Scar Book* represent at least 10 different disciplines practicing in 7 different countries on 4 continents across the entire spectrum of care. They include thought leaders and inventors; past, present, and future Academy and Society presidents; institutional leaders and prolific authors and investigators. Many of the names will be readily recognizable to practitioners in their own respective fields, but perhaps as-yet little known in others. That is part of the point—we have much to learn from each other, and optimal care will arise from a combined approach. Whether one is helping to alleviate the burden of scars at an academic burn center or treating acne scars in the private practice setting, we hope this text offers a fresh perspective and a path forward.

We began our own earnest journey into scar management more than 8 years ago, lasers in hand. As happens so often in medicine, the observation that a judicious laser-mediated injury could help remodel a debilitating traumatic scar to a more functional and cosmetically appealing state was based largely on serendipity. It was not intuitive that reinjuring a traumatic scar in a specific way could help normalize its structure and function. Most of the lasers commonly used in scar management today were initially designed for other, often cosmetic, purposes; it required some astute observers (several of whom are contributors to this book) to turn observations into applications. Thus was the genesis of a new thread of exciting research, and the beginning of a stimulating new phase of our careers. Of course, laser treatment is just one small facet of scar management—but one that we have been eager to exchange with our colleagues for the benefit of our patients.

The textbook is divided into five sections—*Perspectives*, *Formation*, *Mitigation*, *Rehabilitation*, and *Prevention*—each highlighting a different aspect of wound healing, scar management, and research. *Perspectives*, as the name suggests, helps to introduce the current scope of the problem. Insights into the present state of trauma rehabilitation, reconstruction, and scar management are gained by learning about the past. A wide variety of medical conditions present with scars and scarlike lesions. A consideration of the similarities and differences in pathogenic pathways will undoubtedly direct future efforts in treatment and prevention. This section concludes by describing some of the ethical principles that serve to guide decision making by patients and providers in our current state of knowledge, and will help to inform future decisions fortified by new discoveries.

Formation addresses the biologic processes that begin with cutaneous injury and eventuate in normotrophic, hypertrophic, and atrophic scars. *Mitigation* introduces interventions that help to expedite wound healing after injury. *Rehabilitation* contains the largest number of chapters and reviews the current state of the art in scar management from a wide variety of perspectives. The words "mitigation" and "rehabilitation" may seem to have similar meanings. In the text, *Mitigation* is primarily dedicated to concepts that may help reduce the burden of scars as they form, and *Rehabilitation* to improving and managing the many sequelae of existing scars.

Rehabilitation includes chapters devoted to both "medical" and procedural interventions, but these divisions are indistinct. Medical management in this setting connotes primarily nonsurgical treatments (not involving "cold steel"), but actually includes a variety of minimally invasive procedures such as intralesional injections, laser, and radiation. Despite excellent new options in scar treatment, surgical scar revision remains a foundation of comprehensive care. The symptoms of pain and itch receive special attention owing to their potentially overwhelming impact on the quality of life of scar patients. Laser treatment and autologous fat grafting are highlighted given their enormous promise in scar management, and clues to future treatments may lie in further elaboration of their mechanisms of action. Since most providers employ a combination of techniques and see patients from a variety of backgrounds, a degree of overlap (and perhaps even contradiction) is expected. *Rehabilitation* includes chapters that help synthesize the information based on treatment combinations and skin type, and the nearly universal nature of atrophic scars such as striae and those that follow inflammatory acne merit a dedicated discussion.

The number and range of chapters in *Rehabilitation* should be an indication that we need not, and probably should not, attempt to go it alone in the face of physically and cosmetically debilitating scars. Additional chapters describe the enormous value of a comprehensive program of therapy (e.g., physical and occupational) and an accounting for the psychosocial aspects of recovery from traumatic injury—the hidden scars. Other contributions introduce options for scar camouflage and medical tattooing as important adjuncts to reconstruction. The editors have benefited immensely from practice environments conducive to interdisciplinary and interinstitutional cooperation and are cognizant of the potential synergy of combined efforts. Therefore, we have included chapters highlighting our own experience (and that of our colleagues) from the military and pediatric settings. The final chapter in the section elaborates on some of the practical aspects of integrating novel scar treatments into clinical practice.

As noted by multiple authors, the ultimate goal for wound healing is tissue regeneration, not the reparative processes that eventuate in a scar. Despite the section name "*Prevention*," the only way to prevent a scar in our current state of knowledge is to avoid significant injury. Equally as important as learning what to do for a scar is learning what NOT to do to avoid a scar, or to avoid exacerbating an existing scar. Selecting the name "*Prevention*" for the final section reflects optimism that a route to regenerative therapy will ultimately be found through ongoing research efforts. We all were capable of regenerative healing during early fetal development, but that capacity is sacrificed in the name of evolutionary compromise. Tantalizing clues to regenerative healing may therefore lie in the study of human fetal wound healing and in the regenerative capacity of other species. Since future advances obviously rely on ongoing discovery, scar-related research is discussed.

Embracing scar management into our own practices has been endlessly rewarding for multiple reasons. Scars, regardless of their origin or size, can be physically and emotionally devastating for the myriad patients affected by them. We currently have access to an array of effective tools and techniques that have the potential to incrementally improve the lives of our patients after virtually every encounter. It is no secret that these interventions are all too frequently imperfect, but the accelerating pace of innovation promises better treatments in the future. The ubiquitous nature of scars has also provided a vehicle for professional engagement with a wide variety of experts in other disciplines. Our common endeavor to share knowledge and better treat our patients was the inspiration for this book.

Peter R. Shumaker
Andrew C. Krakowski

Acknowledgments

One of the great joys of working in this field has been the opportunity to collaborate with a large assortment of brilliant and generous colleagues.

Thanks to a group of pioneers in laser scar revision (and often much more) including Nathan Uebelhoer, Jill Waibel, Vic Ross, Rox Anderson, Matthias Donelan, Chad Hivnor, and David Ozog for their inspiration, guidance, and friendship. Special recognition goes to Vic Ross and Lawrence Eichenfield for establishing world-class laser clinics in the Dermatology Department at the Naval Medical Center San Diego and Rady Children's Hospital, San Diego, respectively. You first taught us to heal with light, and we hope this textbook will help illuminate the way for others.

We have been fortunate to have many other talented mentors in dermatology and dermatologic surgery including Hugh Greenway, Mitch Goldman, Abel Torres, Bill James, Jim Steger, Neil Gibbs, Bruce Feldman, Moise Levy, Lucia Diaz, Sheila Friedlander, Brian Jiang, Magdalene Dohil, Kristen Kelly, and Iris Rubin.

The publication of this inaugural edition of *The Scar Book* is a huge milestone. Many thanks to the professional staff at Wolters Kluwer who helped to make sure it was not a millstone instead.

Executive Editor: Rebecca Gaertner
Development Editor: Kristina Oberle
Editorial Coordinator: John Larkin
Senior Production Project Manager: Alicia Jackson
Vendor Project Manager: Samson Premkumar Charly
Manufacturing Coordinator: Beth Welsh
Design Coordinator: Elaine Kasmer
Marketing Manager: Rachel Mante Leung
Vice President, Medicine and Advance Practice Publishing: Lisa McAllister
Vice President, Global Publishing: Jayne Marks

To our contributing authors . . . May the blood, sweat, and tears that you poured into this textbook inspire the next generation of physician-scientists and help relegate the morbidities associated with scarring to that of a distant memory.

From Andrew Krakowski:

To my East Coast mentors, Bernard Kaplan and Albert Yan . . . thank you for connecting me to the right people and for motivating me to be a lifelong "learner."

To my West Coast mentors, Larry Eichenfield and Sheila Friedlander . . . thank you for believing in me when it felt like no one else would. My clinical style is your clinical style. That is not an accident; it is a choice and one that I would make over and over again.

To my friends and colleagues, Pete Shumaker (my Co-Editor) and Nathan Uebelhoer . . . I deeply appreciate your openness to teaching new techniques when anyone else might have played their cards close to their chests. You helped create the field of "trauma dermatology" and generously invited me along for the ride.

From Peter Shumaker:

An appreciation for multidisciplinary collaboration is a gift derived from nearly 20 years of service in the United States Navy, and a major theme of this book. Although I have benefited from interactions with countless professionals in a variety of settings, for this work I am especially grateful to supportive leadership and to my colleagues in dermatology and other departments at the Naval Medical Center San Diego engaged in the rehabilitation of our wounded warriors including Facial Plastics, Plastic Surgery, Orthopedics, Physical Medicine and Rehabilitation, Physical/Occupational Therapy, Gait/Prosthetics, and C5/Project C.A.R.E. Special thanks to Lilia Levin, Doug Winstanley, John Trafeli, Mike Yablonsky, Tom Landers, Johannah Valentine, Adam Perry, Valerie Tokarz, Craig Salt, Curtis Gaball, Michelle Arnold, Trent Douglas, Kat Gallus, Eamon O'Reilly, Bob Sheu, Eric Hofmeister, Leo Kroonen, Brian Fitzgerald, Marilynn Wyatt, Jennifer Town, Marie Manuel, Tae Harris, Robin Caballa, and Trisha Buckley.

Among the most rewarding endeavors of my career has been an ongoing exchange in multidisciplinary burn scar management with our venerable counterparts in Vietnam at the National Institute of Burns in Hanoi, and Da Nang General Hospital. Cám Ón to Major General Nguyen Gia Tien, Senior Colonel Vu Quang Vinh, Captain Hoang Thanh Tuan, Captain Tong Tan Hai, Pham Tran Xuan Anh, Do Van Hung, Nguyen Quoc Viet, Nguyen Duy Khanh, their staff, leadership, and the hundreds of patients who have given our team the privilege of caring for them under the auspices of Pacific Partnership. Thanks to Lumenis for making ablative fractional laser technology available to our hosts for the exchange, and special thanks to Ms. Nguyen Phuong Hoa and the other excellent staff at the Health Affairs Attaché Office for making it look easy.

Finally, to all the people that deserved mention here, but were callously left out—Thank You!

Peter R. Shumaker
Andrew C. Krakowski

Contents

SECTION I

Perspectives

1

A Historical Perspective on Scar Management

JANE A. PETRO

KEY POINTS

- Scars are still the inevitable result of healing after tissue injury such as trauma or infection, despite new advances in wound care and injury management. Scars can also result from intentional injury as decorations or symbols of accomplishment.
- Medical care has historically made substantial gains through military attempts to protect, repair, and restore personnel who are injured.
- Due largely to the effectiveness of first aid on the battlefield, modern warfare has increased the likelihood of survival despite devastating injuries. This has presented new challenges to the treatment of wounds and the resulting scars, and in lifelong rehabilitation.
- Scars provide evidence of injury and are important forensic signs, as well as stigmatizing deformities.

All scars tell a story. A childhood fall, an adult fight, an accident, an assault—all will leave their mark. In modern times, the elective scar of a surgical incision has gone from the large *heroic* scars (the bigger the better) of general surgery, to the carefully planned, minimally invasive incisions of modern times. Once the sign of a great surgeon, the prestigious elective scar is now the nearly invisible scar. The contributions of war-related medical advances represent an important chapter in medical history. Survival from the complex blast/burn/bullet injuries of modern weapons is nearly assured and provides new challenges for recovery. Thus, the history of scars, from ancient wounds to the horrendous scars that signify survival from grievous injury, tells the story of not only human resilience, but of medical miracles.

Scars result from healing without regeneration through the deposition of collagen and fibrous connective tissue. Why the salamander can regenerate a leg and other tissue, but a human cannot, is an evolutionary conundrum. A common laboratory regeneration model is the Mexican axolotl (Fig. 1-1). This endangered species regenerates entire limbs as well as nervous tissue. Mammals are known for some specific regenerative capacities, like antlers in the deer family, which are shed and regrown annually. Humans may be able to regenerate the endometrium, liver, and kidney, but only minimal segments of fingers or toes. In general, humans heal after injury by the formation of scar tissue as a means of bridging the defect, whether it involves only skin or larger chunks of skin muscle and bone.

What is the evolutionary advantage of healing by scar versus regeneration? Energy requirements for wound healing in humans are well documented. For a simple femur fracture, the bedridden patient who normally requires 2,500 calories per day may require up to 6,000 calories per day.[1] Burns, in particular, result in high caloric requirements during recovery and are significant scar-forming injuries.[2] Burns involving less than 20% of the total body surface and wartime amputations were frequently fatal until nearly the end of the 19th century, and only slightly larger burns until well after 1950. The relative efficiency in time and energy requirements for scar healing compared to regeneration after major injury is likely an evolutionary advantage for the species, if not for the modern individual.

As the complex biology of wound healing becomes increasingly understood, greater insights into the modulation of healing and vertebrate regeneration are emerging. Genetic manipulation in one mouse species has even restored regenerative capacity. The *Lin28a* gene, silenced in maturing vertebrates, restores regenerative ability when turned on in mouse infancy, but not in maturity.[3] Another species, the African spiny mouse, can heal full-thickness skin injuries without scarring. Current intensive research on the use of stem cells for regeneration is widespread, as are clinical practices promoting their use, despite limited documentation in controlled clinical trials. The identification of the *Lin28a* and *b* genes and their role in stem cell regeneration is also being rapidly elucidated.[4] These concepts offer the promise of future transformative approaches to healing human tissues.

Scars are destined to become part of medical lore if the full potential of current research on genetic manipulation, embryonic healing, and stem cell applications is achieved.

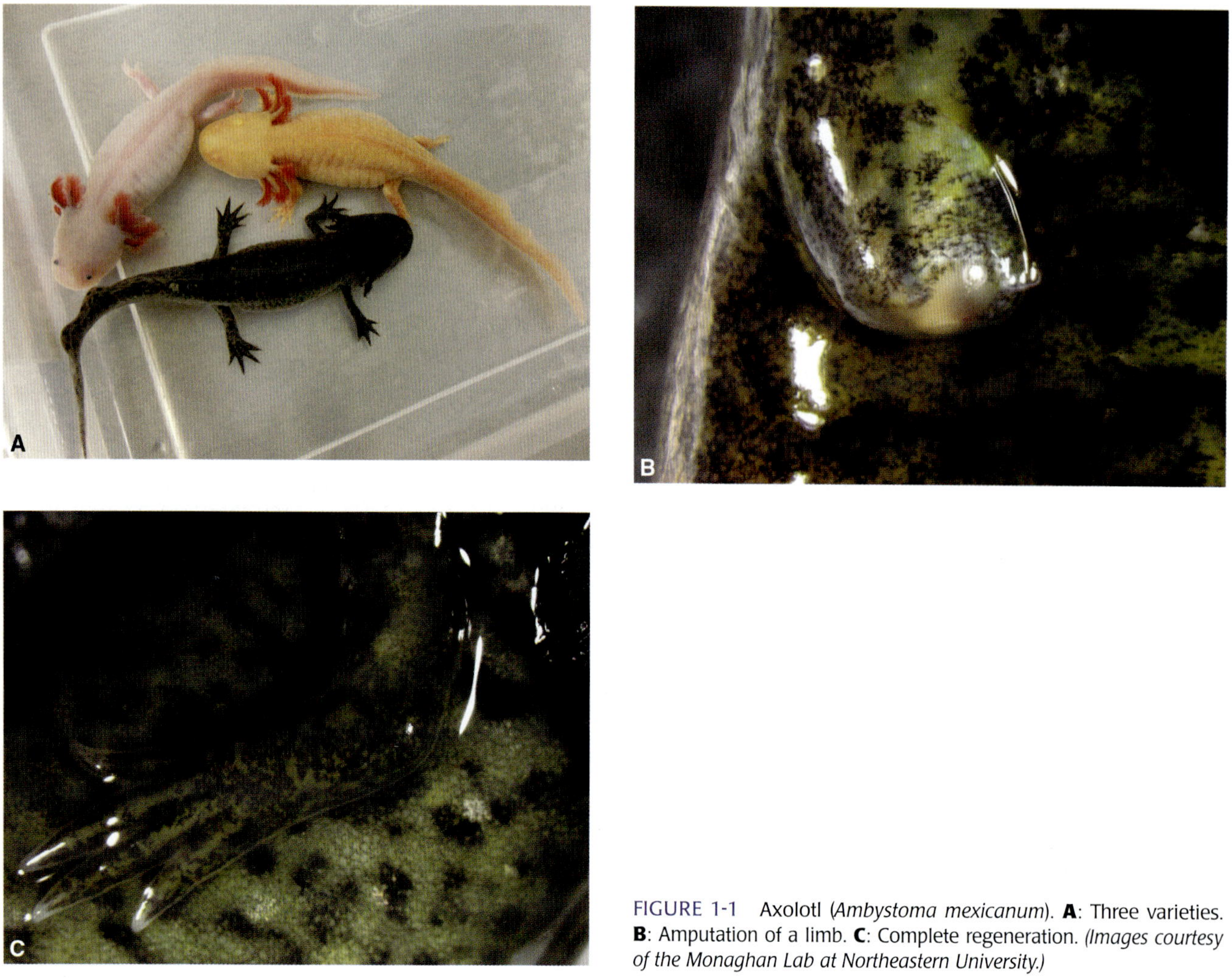

FIGURE 1-1 Axolotl (*Ambystoma mexicanum*). **A**: Three varieties. **B**: Amputation of a limb. **C**: Complete regeneration. *(Images courtesy of the Monaghan Lab at Northeastern University.)*

The management of scars to date has depended on the prevention of injury, the optimization of wound healing, and the direct treatment of scars after they have formed. This chapter will explore the progress in scar care through history, as well as the meaning scars have had in medicine, law, and literature. So many different individuals have contributed to our knowledge of wounds, their management, and the diagnosis and treatment of scars that not all of them can be introduced in this chapter. Table 1-1 provides an outline of the more important events in the years preceding the modern era of wound care and scar management. I have chosen not to focus on events of this modern era. Rather, I have offered my own view of some of the key people and events prior to the last 60 years. More recent advances are the province of other authors in their respective chapters.

Scars from Injury and for Identification

Early human history documents a variety of wounds treated in specific ways. Guido Manjo, in his encyclopedic treatment of the history of wounds, *The Healing Hand*, identified several such early nonfatal as well as fatal wounds.[5] One example involves a pre-Columbian arrowhead found in Patagonia, penetrating the sternum and assumed to be fatal. In another, a prehistoric arrowhead embedded in the tibia and sealed in place provides evidence of successful healing. Wound fatality, even in earliest times, seems a matter of chance, luck, and random fate. The fossil record has identified both a fatal injury (skull fracture) and the weapon (a humerus) in an australopithecine man. There is even evidence of healing in this skull fracture, so the injury was not immediately fatal.[6]

Manjo describes in great detail the nature of injuries and their treatment in sources as disparate as the Ebers Papyrus; ancient Chinese, Indian, and Arabic texts; as well as Greek and Roman literature. While more interested in wounds than in scars, Manjo has extracted from among the scraps of writing dating from the Egyptian-Greek period descriptions of individuals who are recognized by their scars[5]:

> Charetos, one-scar-small-finger-right-hand; Maron, eldest son of Omnephreus, aged 40, with a scar on his forehead; his brother Omnophresu, born of the same father, with no marks.

These descriptions appear in documents related to contracts, identifying the signatories at a time when last names were not used. The use of physical features including scars

Table 1-1 Historic Discoveries in Wound Healing and Scar Management

Name	Nationality	Attribution Date	Life Dates	Accomplishment
Heironimus Brunschwig	German	1497	1450–1512	Advocated careful suturing of facial wounds to minimize infection
Leonardo Botallo	Italian	1560	1519–1587	Recommended NOT using boiling oil on gunshot wounds
Ambroise Pare	French	1575	1510–1590	Strongly advocated use of wound dressings of egg yolk, turpentine, and oil of roses
				Wrote first encyclopedic text on treatment of battlefield injuries
				Collected works, "Les Oeuvers," became the cannon of military surgery
Gaspare Tagliacozzi	Italian	1597	1545–1599	Developed "distant flap" and wrote detailed textbook
Wilhelm Fabry von Hildend	German	1614	1560–1624	Classification of burns into 3 categories
				Recommended splinting to prevent contraction
Cesare Magati	Italian	1637	1579–1647	"What heals the wound is nature not the physician or his medicines"
				Advocated moist dressings only
Gentleman's Magazine	English	1794		Published description of the "Indian Flap" (forehead) of Sushruta for nasal reconstruction
Fraincois Chopart	French	1799	1743–1795	First description of a pedicle flap to reconstruct the lip
Sir Humphrey Davey	English	1799	1778–1829	Discovered nitrous oxide, but used it only as a party trick, not anesthesia
Guiseppe Baronio	Italian	1804	1758–1811	Through experimental surgery, using sheep, showed that skin grafting was effective
Dominique Jean Larrey	French	1812	1766–1842	Advanced standardized military medical care of the sick and wounded regardless of rank
				"Flying ambulances"
Jean-Louis Ailbert	French	1806	1768–1873	Clearly described keloids as a specific type of scar
Joseph C. Carpue	French	1816	1764–1846	Promoted the use of flaps, influencing von Graef, Delpech, and others
Astley Cooper	English	1817	1768–1841	First recorded description of a successful skin graft
Johann Frederick Dieffenbach	Prussian	1827	1794–1847	Wrote on tissue transplantation and regeneration
				Considered the founder of plastic surgery
Ernst Carl Friedrish Blasius	German	1833	1802–1875	Nasolabial flaps
John Mason Warren	American	1840	1811–1867	First recorded documentation of a full-thickness skin graft
William T. G. Morton	American	1846	1819–1868	Popularized the use of ether anesthesia
James Young Simpson	Scottish	1847	1811–1870	Introduced chloroform for human use first at a dinner party and then obstetrics a few days later
Oliver Wendell Holmes	American	1855	1809–1894	Incidence of Puerperal Fever reduced from 10% to 3% by careful handwashing with calcium chlorate
Louis Pasteur	French	1857	1822–1895	Discovery of the role of bacteria in fermentation and disease
Ignaz Semmelweis	Hungarian	1861	1818–1865	Recognized iatrogenic disease transmission and promoted hand washing
Karl Langer	Austrian	1861	1819–1887	First described his idea of the lines of least skin tension using cadavers
Paul Bert	French	1865	1833–1886	First description of autograft, heterograft and homograft
Joseph Lister	English	1867	1827–1912	Antisepsis, advocated carbolic acid, required staff in OR to change gowns
				Noted that chronic ulcers, when closed by skin grafts, did not contract
Jaques Louis Reverdin	French	1869	1842–1928	Partial-thickness skin grafts of very small size (pinch grafts)
JohannFriedrich von Esmarch		1870	1823–1908	Standardized military medical wound care, triage, priority by severity, not rank
George Lawson	English	1870	1831–1903	First clinical description of a full-thickness graft
Louis Zxavier Ollier	French	1872	1830–1900	Successful grafting of large sheets of skin (2–4 cm^2), successfully reducing scarring

(*continued*)

Table 1-1 Historic Discoveries in Wound Healing and Scar Management (*continued*)

Name	Nationality	Attribution Date	Life Dates	Accomplishment
Bernard Rudolph von Langenbeck	German	1874	1819–1888	Bilateral transposition flaps
John Reissberg Wolfe	Scottish	1875	1824–1904	Popularized full thickness skin grafts including dermis, but not fat
Carl Thiersch	German	1886	1822–1895	First clinical description of harvest and application of a split-thickness graft
				Recommended salicylic acid rather than carbolic acid for antisepsis
Harold Gilles	New Zealand	1917	1881–1960	Ran first medical hospital dedicated to facial injuries
				Credited as being the first modern plastic surgeon
Vilray Papin Blair	American	1920	1871–1975	Special knife for harvesting split-thickness skin grafts
Ivan Magill	Irish	1921	1888–1986	Colleague of Gilles, developed safe modern anesthesia for head and neck surgery
				Invented the endotracheal tube, Magill forceps, of laryngoscope, closed-circuit anesthesia system
Graham Humby	English	1934	1909–1970	Special knife with guard for setting thickness of skin graft harvest
Earl C. Padgett	American	1937	1893–1946	Invented the Padgett Dermatome, first equipment to harvest reliable, adjustable-thickness skin grafts
Harry M. Brown	American	1948	1914–1948	Electric power-guarded adjustable dermatome

continued throughout multiple eras. In the later 19th century, the French developed the Bertillon System of individual identification. This system applied extremely detailed anthropometric measurements, accompanied by photographs and descriptions of scars and birthmarks, as part of the means of identifying unique individuals. In the United States, the military and the penal systems adopted variations of Bertillon's System in 1887. Additionally, the Surgeon General in December 1888 required that "all soldiers be vaccinated on the outer aspect of the left leg at a point 4 inches below the head of the fibula, and that every man be so vaccinated when enlisted or reenlisted." In this manner the vaccination scar distinguished a soldier from a civilian. The use of other identifying characteristics was employed to enable ready identification of those who had been discharged dishonorably, or convicted of a crime. This was particularly directed at preventing unwanted reenlistments. The earlier system, with its careful measurement of "length of the figure, measurements of the outstretched arms, length and width of the head, of the right and left ear, left foot, middle and little finger and left forearm" was abandoned in favor of detailed descriptions of any identifying marks, their location, and only then the height of the individual. The practice of vaccination on the leg was abandoned in 1891 when it became apparent that there was a high rate of temporary disability associated with inflammation.[7] In 1889, the Army adopted a simpler method of identifying soldiers using standardized cards (Figs. 1-2 and 1-3). Note on the chart that a tattoo is also used for identification.

The last half of the 19th century saw the slow adoption of other means of identifying personnel. A military identification system using inscribed wooden tags appeared during the Chinese Taiping revolt (1851 to 1866).[8] During the American Civil War (1861 to 1865), combatants often pinned notes to their coats, or stenciled their name and address on their backpack. Not until the Franco-Prussian war of 1879 did the military issue "dog tags," so called for the "hundemarken" required of dogs in Berlin at the same time. In 1907 the British replaced their identity cards with identity discs, including name, rank, and regimental information. Dog tags continued to help reveal soldiers lost in battle during World War II, as well as Vietnam.[9] While the dog tags may still be attached on or near remains, DNA testing has been used to confirm identity since the Department of Defense began the practice in 1991 as part of the Gulf War effort.[10] Thus, the use of scars for identification is supplanted now by the use of individual genetic material.

Beyond a means of identification, in some cultures scars are used as decorative adornment. This has been recognized as a common practice in sub-Saharan Africa, and recently reviewed in the medical context.[11] The authors note the variety of techniques including the specific tools and substances applied to achieve controlled and predictable results. Figure 1-4 depicts an example of tribal scars. Kelman Cohen, in his early research on abnormal scarring, often speculated in conversation on the value of studying intentional scarification as a means of better understanding the nature of healing in accidental scars, and Cohen raised the question of how tribal scarification seemed to avoid keloid formation (Conversations with Dr. K. Cohen in 1978, 1979 at the Plastic Surgery Research Council meetings).

History of the Medical Descriptions of Scars

Scars are described in documents as ancient as the Smith Papyrus, but medical interest in scars has evolved primarily

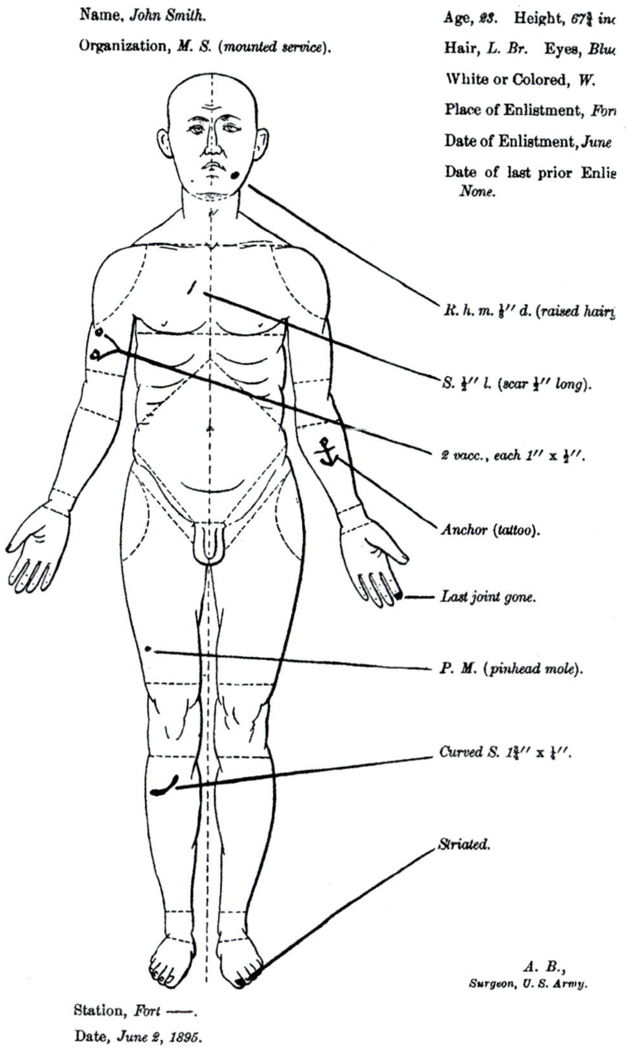

FIGURE 1-2 US Army identification card adopted in 1889 showing the frontal view with name, military organization, height, hair and eye color, etc. and indicating placement of various marks, scars, and tattoos.

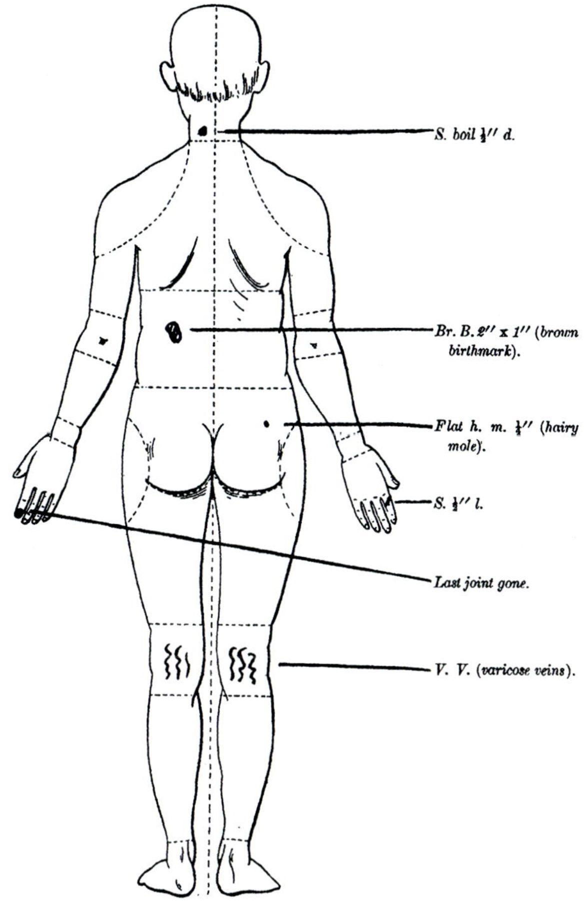

FIGURE 1-3 US Army identification card adopted in 1889 showing the posterior view indicating placement of various marks, scars, conditions, and other traumatic injuries.

during the past two centuries. "Normal" scars are those that heal under optimal conditions. This requires that the wound be clean, the wound edges are aligned properly, and that healing proceeds by primary intention. Wounds that are irregular, contaminated, and have significant tissue loss and/or heal by secondary intention often result in unsatisfactory scars. In addition, unacceptable scars may result from seemingly trivial insults (including incidental scratches or acne in some individuals) or even result during healing from well-planned and executed surgical incisions. Keloids have been considered more common in certain anatomical areas, such as the presternal or deltoid regions and have (wrongly) been considered more common among dark-skinned individuals. Pathological scars are variously described as normal, atrophic, hypertrophic, or keloidal. Several of these conditions can even be seen in the same healed scar. Pathological scars attract the most medical attention, especially those that are either keloidal or hypertrophic, and/or are causing contraction across a joint.

The earliest clear medical description of abnormal scars is attributed to a French dermatologist Jean-Louis-Marc

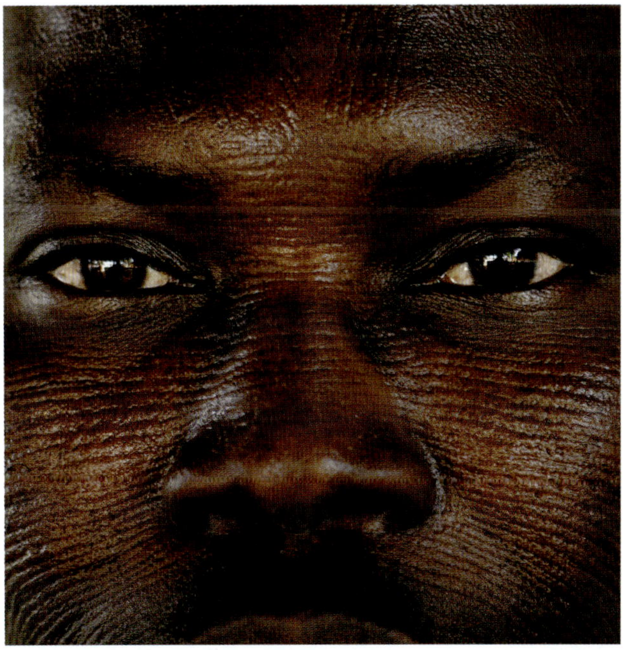

FIGURE 1-4 Benin Natitingou, April 20, 2005. Man with tribal scarification on his face. Scarification is used as a form of initiation into adulthood, beauty, and a sign of a village, tribe, and clan. *(Used with permission from Jean-Clajot Photography. http://www.jmclajot.net/. Accessed November 11, 2016.)*

Alibert. He described certain scars in 1806 in one of the first comprehensive dermatologic texts.[12] Alibert[13] was a believer in classification and ordered his dermatology descriptions along the lines of botany, dividing skin disorders into families, genera, and species. He later renamed one type of scar as a "cheloide" in a paper published in 1817 (Fig. 1-5). Scars that are heavily pigmented or reddened, and extend beyond the original boundaries of injury (keloids) seem to attract the most attention in this early literature. Hypertrophic scars, those that are red and raised but confined to the zone of injury and improve over time, have a more unclear documentation. There continues to be confusion between hypertrophic and keloid scars throughout the medical literature. Up until the end of the 19th century, most scar literature relates either dramatic surgical miracles, single case reports, or dermatologic descriptions. Not until the end of the 19th century does a true clinical science of scars begin to appear.

In addition to descriptions of scars, a literature on their correction began to appear in the 1800s. Earlier surgical procedures to correct deformities, such as Tagliacozzi and

QUELQUES RECHERCHES

SUR LA CHÉLOÏDE,

PAR J. L. ALIBERT.

CES recherches ont pour objet de faire connaître une tumeur cutanée, qui n'a été encore indiquée ni décrite par aucun observateur. C'est celle que j'avais d'abord désignée sous le nom *cancroïde*, dans les cours de clinique que je fais tous les ans à l'hôpital Saint-Louis. Mais, depuis cette époque, j'ai jugé que ce nom avait trop d'analogie avec celui de *cancer*, dont on se sert communément pour exprimer un genre d'affection tout-à-fait différent de celui qui m'occupe : ce qui pourrait entraîner de la confusion dans la science. J'ai préféré, dès-lors, signaler cette tumeur par le titre de *chéloïde*, à cause des prolongemens particuliers qu'elle projette dans ses parties latérales, et qui ressemblent assez bien aux pattes d'une écrévisse. Qu'on se représente un crâbe ou quelque autre insecte de mer, muni de plusieurs pieds, qui s'enfoncent dans la substance de la peau, on aura une idée de cette végétation aussi bizarre qu'extraordinaire. Les premiers observateurs ont agi avec sagesse, en donnant aux diverses altérations morbifiques qu'ils ont eu occasion de découvrir, des dénominations analogues aux choses qu'elles représentent : on est beaucoup mieux entendu, toutes les fois qu'on parle par images. En attendant que des faits plus nombreux nous éclairent davantage sur la nature de la chéloïde, je vais exposer ses principaux phénomènes.

Par un double rapport, la chéloïde semble se lier à la dartre et au cancer des tégumens : elle forme en quelque sorte un genre intermédiaire; ce qu'il y a de positif, c'est qu'il s'opère très-souvent, à la surface de cette tumeur, une desquammation épidermoïque, qui a la plus frappante

FIGURE 1-5 Front page of Alibert's naming of a particular scar as a keloid.

the "Indian" flaps, were not originally used for scars but to rebuild missing parts, mostly the nose. The use of skin flaps to correct the contractures and deformities of burns and other injuries had its origins in Germany and France. Edward Zeis (1807 to 1868) was a surgeon/ophthalmologist and collector of medical information. In 1813 he published *Handbuch der plastischen Chirurgie*, considered to be the first comprehensive textbook on plastic surgery. Zeis followed this with two publications collecting all the known references in the field, *Die Literatur und Geschichte der plastische Chirurgie* in Leipzig in 1863, with a supplement in 1864. This important work was made available in English by Frank McDowell with the publication of the *Zeis Index and History of Plastic Surgery 900 BC to 1863 AD.*[14]

Interest in plastic surgery, as applied to scars as well as to defects, was apparent in both France and Germany around the time of Zeis' plastic surgery text. Johann Friedrich Dieffenbach (1794 to 1847), considered one of the earliest facial plastic surgeons, wrote about the use of skin flaps on the face to repair the nose, referring to this as "sideways shifting."[15]

Hundreds of American physicians visited Europe as part of their medical training, a requirement to be considered "well educated." Thomas Mutter, a Philadelphia physician, spent a year studying medicine and surgery in Paris in 1831 and would have been aware of the work of Zeis and Dieffenbach, and possibly even that of von Langenbeck, another early expert in flaps. His principal surgical exposures were with Guillaume Dupuytren (1777 to 1835) at the Hotel-Dieu and Jacques Lisfrank de St. Martin at the Hopital de la Pitie. Both men wrote and performed surgery as public exhibitions, and it is known that Mutter paid special attention to "*les operations plastiques*." There is a disagreement between French and German scholars whether skin flaps as used in these operations were first employed by the German or the French surgeons mentioned above. Dieffenbach was known to visit and work with Lisfrank (1790 to 1847), where Mutter would have been exposed to the ideas of both the German and French surgical schools who shared their knowledge through both writing and direct teaching. Mutter returned to Philadelphia determined to practice with the same skill he had witnessed in Paris, as well as a desire for fame like those of his mentors in Europe.[16]

A decade after he returned from Paris, Mutter[17] published a successful case report of his treatment for burn scars of the neck. In this paper he describes the "monsters" (a common term at the time for any deformity, especially of the face) he encounters (Fig. 1-6), and tells how these women sustained burns from clothing catching fire while cooking. This type of severe burn is still seen in the developing world (Fig 1-7). Mutter described his own horror at these deformities and was determined to correct them using a flap of skin moved from unburned skin of the back. He goes into great detail describing the technique he uses to prepare the patient for this operation, without the use of anesthesia. This included multiple preoperative visits, educating the patient about the details of the surgery, massage of the operative sites, and establishing a mutual desire for success. The surgery was undertaken in an amphitheater with many observers, first incising the scar and releasing the contracture, then raising the skin flap from the back and rotating it into the

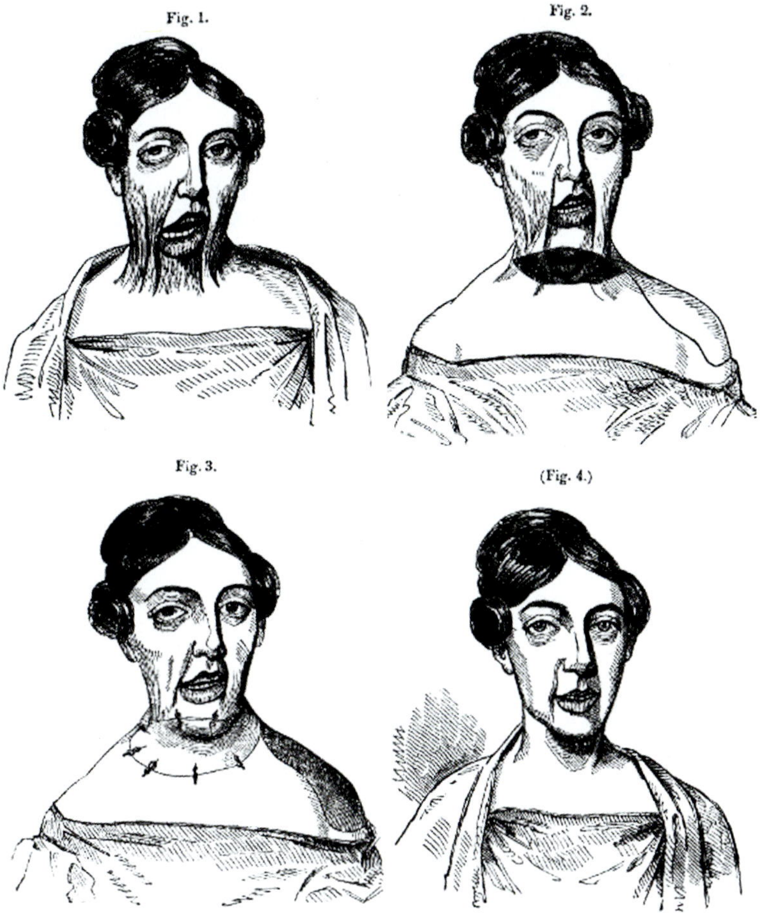

FIGURE 1-6 Mutter's case 1 showing a neck contracture treated with scar release and skin flap taken from the back. *(Published July 1843 in "Cases of Deformity From Burns Successfully Treated by Plastic Operations." Philadelphia, PA: Merrihew & Thompson Printers.)*

defect, closing both wounds with sutures. Despite a brief postoperative infection, the operation was apparently successful. His publication received wide notice, including reports in Europe,[18] and contributed to his rising fame in Philadelphia. Mutter continued to do such procedures but never published a case series. Similar procedures are sporadically reported during the rest of the 19th century, but did not become used regularly until the 20th century as surgeons such as Sir Harold Gillies began performing reconstructive surgery as part of the World War I effort.

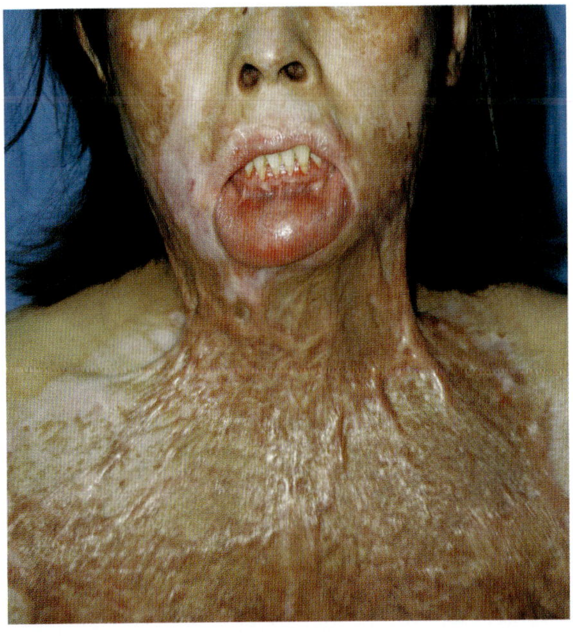

FIGURE 1-7 Contracture of the neck following a thermal burn. *(Photo courtesy of Peter R. Shumaker, MD.)*

The "Zeis Index" lists 44 unique reports related to scars in the medical literature through 1863. Volume II in this series, the "Patterson Index," extends the list of references from 1864 to 1920.[19] This work includes 227 references on keloids, 38 related to scars, 72 articles on scar cancer, and 71 on scar treatment. This relative explosion of interest includes recognition of different kinds of scars, and applications of nonsurgical (radiation, cautery, compression, electricity) and surgical treatments (skin grafts, flaps, relaxing incisions, needling).

The most comprehensive of all the papers in the Patterson Index related to scars appears in 1893, "Hypertrophies and degenerations of Cicatrices and Cicatricial Tissue."[20] Written by John Collins Warren, Jr., this work continued a tradition of Warrens in Boston as surgeons and innovators. He was the great grandson of John Warren, a Revolutionary War hero, surgeon, and one of the founders of Harvard Medical School; the grandson of John Collins Warren, also a professor of surgery at Harvard who is best remembered for his role in performing the first surgery done under general anesthesia in 1848; and the son of Jonathan Mason Warren, a surgeon who was considered to be the best cleft palate surgeon of his era, and author of a paper vastly improving the operation first described by Dieffenbach.[21] John Collins Warren, Jr. was personally acquainted with Lister and was an early advocate of surgical asepsis, becoming the first surgeon to perform intra-abdominal surgery at Massachusetts General Hospital in 1889.

Warren's paper on scars produced one of the first recognizably "modern" review articles. He describes in detail a variety of elements including the formation of scar tissue, the presence of atypical twisted fibers, changes in microscopic appearance and vascular composition over time, the differences seen between primarily and secondarily healed wounds, the differences between true and false keloids (probably hypertrophic scars), the histology of striae, scar contractures, and the way in which childhood scars develop as the patient grows. Warren then reports on three cases of painful surgical scars, and identifies neuromas within the scars. Throughout the article he refers to other authors of papers written in English, German, and French.

Warren also discusses keloids and his personal successful treatment of ear lobe keloids by surgical removal, and goes on to support the use of compression as part of scar management. He concludes his discussion with a report of the successful treatment of hypertrophic burn scars by the use of Thiersch grafts: "The subject of grafting opens up a fruitful field of research in connection with the surgical treatment of cicatrices, but the limits of this paper do not permit of more than a passing allusion to it." By the end of the 19th century, descriptions were available for scar formation, the range of scar types, and both surgical and nonsurgical treatment options, including many that are still used today.

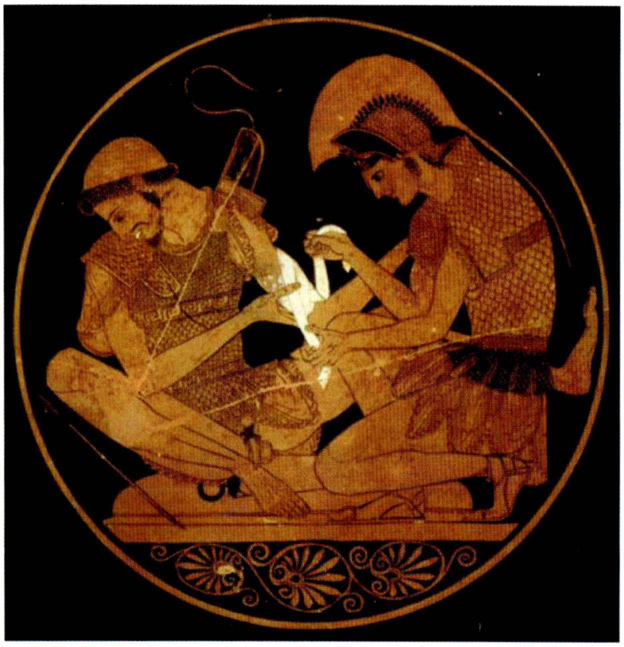

FIGURE 1-8 Date about 500 BC Achilles tending Patroclus' wounds from a red-figure kylix (drinking vessel) in the Staatliche Museum, Berlin. *(From https://upload.wikimedia.org/wikipedia/commons/b/ba/Akhilleus_Patroklos_Antikensammlung_Berlin_F2278.jpg. Accessed November 11, 2016)*

The study of the basic biology of wound healing and scar formation began in the 20th century. Research into various aspects of scar formation and mitigation including the biochemical composition of collagen and their ratios in various types of scars; the role of the myofibroblast; detailed studies of growth factors, RNA, and DNA; and the expanded role of procedures including skin grafts, flaps, and even transplantation of limbs and the face have altered our understanding of scars and improved our ability to manage them. These topics are beyond the scope of this chapter and may be covered elsewhere in the text (see Chapters 5, 6, and 12).

The Scars of War

He who desires to practice surgery must go to war.

—Hippocrates

In the Iliad, Homer describes nearly 150 distinct wounds including entrance and exit points, various weapons (sword, arrow, lance), internal injuries, and the differences between fatal and nonfatal injuries. The treatment of these wounds is well illustrated in many surviving Greek urns (Fig. 1-8). Greek and Roman generals traveled with private physicians but the troops, as illustrated in this and many other urns, treated each other. A later illustration of the wounds seen before the introduction of gunpowder is well illustrated in the "Wound Man" (Fig. 1-9).

Many variations on this image appeared in surgical texts from the 1400s to the 1600s. The introduction of gunpowder changed the nature of the injuries and scarring from war and encouraged the formal introduction of military surgeons for all troops, not just officers. Ambroise Paré (1510 to 1590) was among the first physicians to be identified as a military surgeon serving under several French kings for nearly 30 years beginning in 1536. Paré seems to have been a keen observer, noting that using boiling oil on fresh gunshot wounds was less effective than simply bandaging the wound with egg yolk, turpentine, and rose oil.[22] He also notes that his method caused less suffering as well as less damage to the tissues. He recommended ligation of arteries during amputations rather than cautery with a hot iron. His accounts of the treatment of gunshot wounds provide descriptions of the first interventions that were more likely helpful than harmful, in contravention to the standard practices of that time. Less well known, Paré is also credited with designing prostheses for both upper and lower limbs, as well as ocular prostheses that he formulated out of gold, glass, porcelain, and silver.[23,24]

Scar breakdown is one sign of scurvy, a condition that became a serious impediment to naval exploration. Vasco da Gama lost two-thirds of his crew during his 1499 voyage to India. A British expedition to the South Seas in the 1740s lost 1,300 sailors (out of the original 2,000) as well as six of their seven ships. Richard Walter, chaplain on this expedition, describes: "Skin black as ink, ulcers, difficult respiration, rictus of the limbs, teeth falling out and perhaps most revolting of all a strange plethora of gum tissue sprouting out of the mouth, which immediately rotted and lent

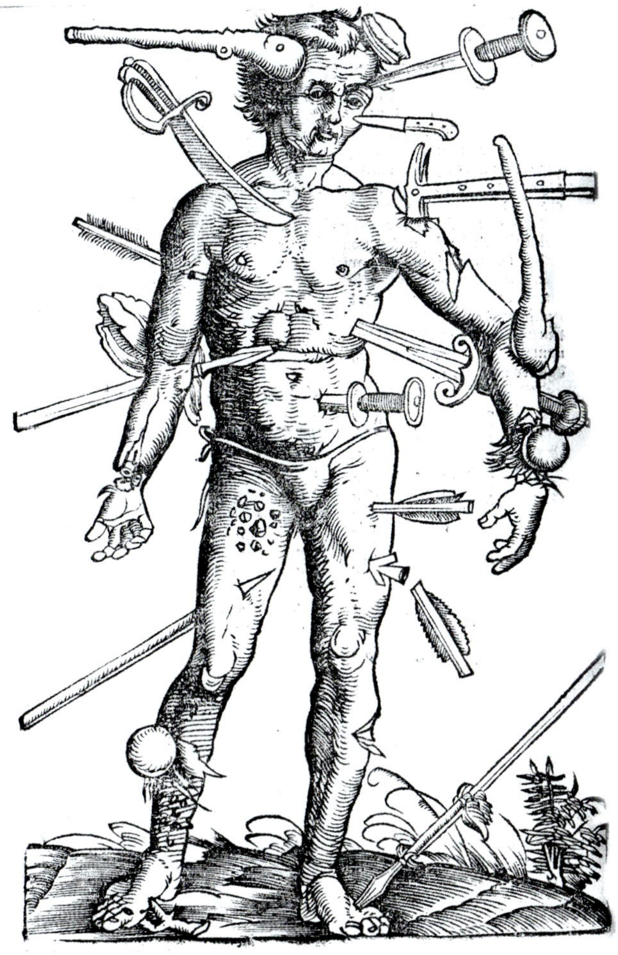

FIGURE 1-9 Hans von Gersdorff (1455 to 1529). Field book of surgery 1517. *(From https://upload.wikimedia.org/wikipedia/commons/7/73/Gersdorff_p21v.jpg. Accessed November 11, 2016.)*

the victim's breath an abominable odor."[25] It is estimated that scurvy killed nearly 2 million sailors between 1500 and 1800. There are numerous accounts of the military consequences of scurvy affecting naval forces, including that of the Spanish Armada in 1588, whose defeat by the English set the stage for British dominance in the coming centuries.[26] James Lind (1716 to 1794), a British Naval surgeon, is often described as the "discoverer" of the fact that citrus fruit prevented and cured scurvy. His famous experiment with 12 sailors who had the disease is often acclaimed the original clinical trial, first published in 1753. This myth is thoroughly debunked by Michael Bartholomew through a close reading of Lind's own work.[27] Historical research demonstrating that scurvy continued to affect middle-class Victorians and the Scott expedition at the beginning of the 20th century additionally challenges the persistent tale of how the British Navy became "Limey's."[28]

War on land in the 19th century carried high mortality, whether from direct injury or as a result of starvation, exposure, and disease. Napoleon's invasion of Russia in 1812 with 680,000 men resulted in the loss of nearly 90% of his troops in the 6 months of the campaign. Minard's chart (Fig. 1-10) is the first successful example of a graph depicting multiple types of data. It demonstrates the progress of the army into and out of Russia, the diminishing size of French military forces, geographic progress, temperature during the retreat, and sites of importance along the way. An excellent biography of Dominique Jean Larrey, the chief military surgeon to Napoleon, documents the awful conditions faced by the medical staff.[29] Delays in equipment and supplies made providing emergency care difficult. Larrey describes using his own clothing as bandages. During the Battle of Vitebsk, he personally performed 11 amputations at the shoulder over 24 hours, and he reports that nine survived and two died of dysentery. Later, at the

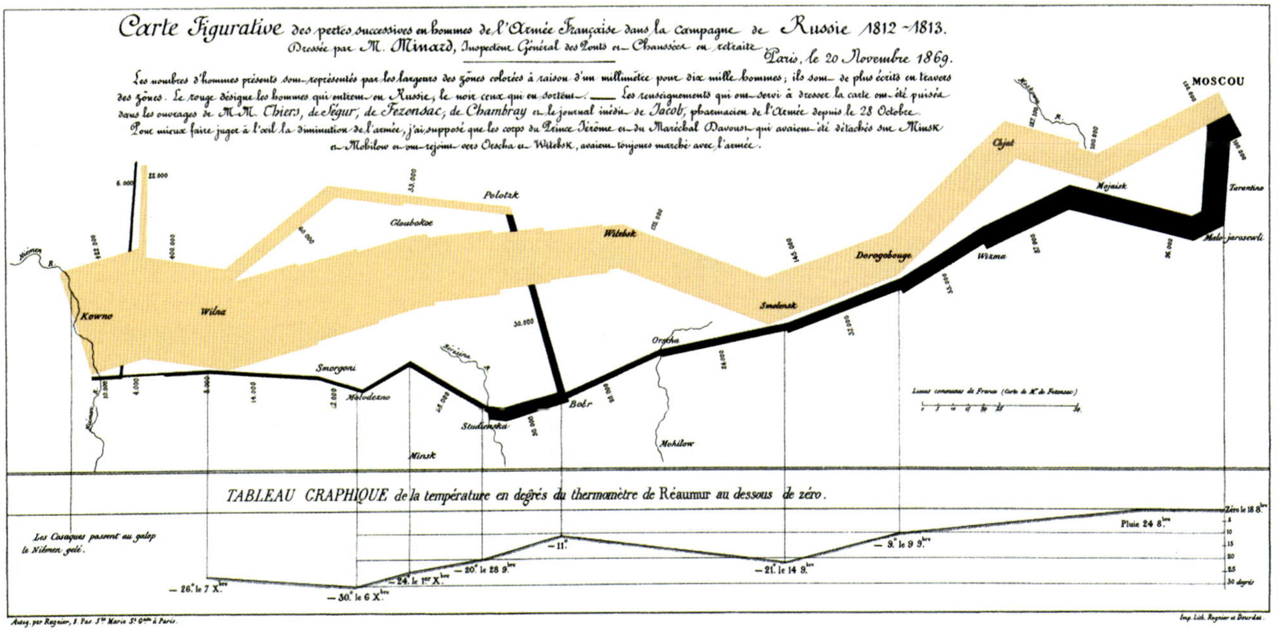

FIGURE 1-10 Charles Minard's 1869 chart showing the number of men in Napoleon's 1812 Russian campaign army, their movements, as well as the temperatures they encountered on the return path. Lithograph, 62 × 30 cm. *(From https://commons.wikimedia.org/wiki /Commons:Reusing_content_outside_Wikimedia. Accessed November 11, 2016.)*

Battle of Borodino, he is reported to have performed 200 amputations (of all types) within 24 hours. Larrey describes bureaucratic obstruction, administrative incompetence (widespread graft, theft, bribery), and other obstacles to his ability to care for the injured. Larrey further states that nearly all the wounded died of hunger. Despite the huge losses and medical disasters, the innovations Larrey brought to the war, including a new type of mobile "flying" ambulance, the deployment of a trained medical corps, and the provision of medical care at the front, all set the stage for military surgery during the coming century. Larrey is remembered for his humanity, his concern for the common soldier, his honesty, and his ability to innovate with whatever was at hand.

Among the many wars of the 19th century, the US Civil War (1861 to 1865) carried the highest mortality of any US military action with nearly 620,000 military deaths (2% of the total population), or 1 in 4 soldiers who went to war. Of those who returned, 1 in 13 had suffered the amputation of an arm or a leg.[30] The medical advancements introduced during the Civil War included the introduction of photography for documentation, the establishment and organization of a nursing corps, the use of anesthesia near the front lines, the use of morphine or whisky for pain, the establishment of standardized treatments for specific injuries, and an increased appreciation for the types of hygiene that could prevent dysentery, typhoid fever, and other contagions. William A. Hammond, the Surgeon General of the Union Army, developed a system of triage, evacuation, and the design for clean, well-ventilated buildings that decreased mortality in field hospitals from nearly 40% to 8% by the end of the war.[31] In the aftermath of the war, veteran benefits and support became a new national priority with the establishment of the Veterans Homes, a precursor to the current Veterans Administration system.

With the introduction of anesthesia, the adoption of aseptic surgical technique, and an evolving understanding of infections, the next great leap in military medicine came with preparations for World War I. Disastrous experiences during the Garza War (1891 to 1893) and the Spanish American War (1898) led to the formation of formal medical, surgical, nursing, dental, and reserve corps, as well as the formalization of medical supply sources. Field hospitals were designed, and in 1910 permanent specialized units were established. These preparations were tested in the Mexican Border conflict in 1916, and included the first use of motorized ambulances. Additional interest in field sanitation led to marked improvements later applied to the American Expeditionary Forces when the United States entered World War I. The 1916 experience also led to the consolidation of all medical and dental corps into a single Medical Department. Prominent American physicians including George Crile, Harvey Cushing, William C. Gorgas, William Welch, and William Mayo all participated in the Council of Medical Preparedness. Fifty base hospitals of 500 beds each for the Army, and 8 distinct 250 bed hospitals for the Navy were prepared in cooperation with the Red Cross.[32] Most notably, this era ushered in the reconstructive era of plastic surgery.

In 1917 the British assembled a team of physicians in Sidcup, England, headed by Sir Harold Gillies (1882 to 1960), specifically designed to treat facial injuries and disfigurements. The team at Queens Hospital provided reconstruction with skin and bone grafts, flaps and prostheses. Activity in this dedicated center resulted in numerous advances, not just in treating scars and deformities, but in anesthesia as well. Sir Gillies is considered the father of modern plastic surgery. However, his work would not have been possible without the efforts of Sir Ivan Magill (1888 to 1986), a general practitioner before the war who invented the laryngoscope, endotracheal tube, eponymous forceps, and the use of closed circuit gas delivery. Magill is considered the father of modern anesthesia. Work at the hospital included treatment for over 5,000 men during over 11,000 surgical procedures, without a single death attributed to anesthesia.

The ability to provide efficient first aid, transport the injured to secure facilities, and render appropriate medical care creates an entirely new set of challenges. Formerly fatal wounds require complex closures, reconstruction after potentially devastating tissue losses, and the restoration of function. The development of clinical uses of antibiotics during World War II and continued advances in medical and surgical services during the Korean, Vietnam, and first Gulf War led to decreasing mortality from increasingly severe wounds; these in turn led to more difficult reconstructive challenges and scar management requirements. This progression continues into the present day associated with more than a decade of conflict in Iraq and Afghanistan. Staggeringly complex and dramatic injuries have been countered with sophisticated gear (built-in tourniquets and hemostatic dressings). Rapid evacuation by helicopter to mobile hospital units and the capacity to move the injured to higher echelons of care within 24 hours have helped to increase the battlefield survival rate of those wounded from 76% during the Vietnam conflict to well over 90% today.[33]

History of Scar Interventions: Surgical and Nonsurgical

Minimizing scar formation resulting from traumatic wounds includes adherence to basic principles of wound care still practiced today: control of hemorrhage, removal of foreign bodies and cleansing, careful approximation of the wound edges, drainage (if needed), and appropriate dressings. Before the introduction of aseptic technique and anesthesia, routine elective scar interventions, while documented, were infrequent. Because scars are not clearly distinguished from other forms of skin pathology, a coherent chronology of treatment recommendations is difficult. Therefore, surgical and nonsurgical interventions will be limited to those recommended from the times of Alibert's recognition of "cheloids." Alibert in his 1816 paper[13] recommended topical treatments including sulfur, lead acetate, camphor, and opium, among others.

Linares, in a review on the history of keloids,[34] attributes the first surgical recommendations to Robert Druit (1814 to 1883). For surgery on scars caused by burns, Druit[35] discusses the need to shave the scar and keep it open using cautery, but also offers Jacques M Delpech's (1777 to 1832) view that the entire lesion be removed. No other specific operation is discussed, but removal of larger burn scars and flap closure with normal skin is mentioned. Druit's book (available online) is interesting to read and provides a comprehensive encyclopedia of standard surgical practices of the time. Though Linares suggests that Druit is referring specifically to keloids, this author's own reading of the text did not find such specificity. This reference to Druit appears regularly in later review articles without page identification.

John Da Costa (1863 to 1933) in his 1894 text *A Manual of Modern Surgery*,[36] states unequivocally that a "keloid should not be operated upon: it will only return, and will also recur in the stitch-holes. Trust to time for involution, or use pressure with flexible collodion," by which method Professor Da Costa treated a case following smallpox. Ninety years later, a paper offering a comprehensive review of the treatment of keloids and hypertrophic scars recommends, "Surgery for the treatment of keloid scar has been relegated mainly to second-line therapy for lesions unresponsive to steroids or pressure and large lesions, requiring de-bulking. Combining surgery with other therapy is usually indicated."[37]

Attention to hypertrophic scars as distinguished from keloids generally focuses on their better responses to treatment. In a 1969 review of all scars excised at Columbia Presbyterian Hospital between 1932 and 1958, 340 were clinically identified in the medical record as keloids. Cosman et al. noted a successful response to surgical excision in 83% of those lesions not histologically identified as keloids, as opposed to 53% of those confirmed as keloids.[38] This paper provides an excellent review of the various factors considered relevant to the formation of keloids as opposed to other kinds of scars, but concludes that most of the previous literature blaming hormone status, the presence of foreign bodies, heredity, race, etc., are not correct. They also review the treatment of these lesions, noting that often the diagnosis of keloid is incorrectly applied to other skin conditions. The large number of remedies recommended, and the associated poor design of clinical trials make definitive treatment protocols impossible. This continues to be a problem. Some authors suggest that keloids are not distinct entities, but represent a continuum of disordered scars.[39] The clinical distinction between keloid and hypertrophic scar is still largely based on clinical behavior. A keloid is characterized by the presence of scar tissue extending beyond the border of the original wound, while hypertrophic scars, though red, raised, and occasionally painful, remain within the borders of the original injury and often begin to resolve after approximately 2 years.

One of the most consistently recommended primary or adjuvant therapies for keloids and hypertrophic scars is the application of pressure. In 1898, an Australian named Herman Lawrence recommended scarification of the keloid followed by several months of pressure.[40] This single case report does not indicate how the pressure was applied or for how long. The use of pressure in wound healing appears in the Smith Papyrus (circa 1600 BCE), and regularly in subsequent wound care instructions. In 1924 Vilray Blair studied the benefits of mechanical pressure on wound healing.[41] James Barrett Brown and Frank McDowell, in their comprehensive 1944 paper on the healing of burn wounds of the skin, comment that without pressure dressings, skin grafts and donor sites will not heal properly. They note further that applying pressure to burn wounds may be aseptic.[42] The first clinical documentation of the utility of pressure for burn scars came from Paul Silverstein at Brooke Army Hospital in San Antonio, Texas. He noted better healing in a grafted leg being treated with compression stockings for varicose vein disease than on the opposite extremity not using the stocking. Duane Larson at the Shriner's Burn Institute in Galveston noted a similar response when using pressure splints, leading Larson to collaborate with the Jobst Institute to produce garments for postburn scar management. Their results, reported in 1971, made compression garments part of the standard of care for the prevention and treatment of scars.[43] Recent clinical studies have not found a correlation between the pressure used and efficacy,[44] and it seems that the evidence for the benefits of pressure garments is inconclusive at best; high associated cost and low compliance remain significant issues (see Chapter 19).[45]

The use of silicone topical gels and sheeting over keloids and hypertrophic scars has also been advocated for many years. In 1935, Robinson recommended topical silicone for use in nonhealing ulcers. Interest in the substance for skin lotions extended its use to dematoses and other hyperkeratotic conditions by 1954.[46] Because of its inert nature, silicone also became used in soft tissue augmentation, or in solid form as a substitute for nasal or ear cartilage. The injection of various materials to correct deformity, including depressed scars, became quite popular in the early 20th century. These materials are summarized in a review article[47] on the uses of dimethylsiloxanes, comparing them to other available synthetic materials. The list of now-unacceptable materials used in the past details celluloid, paraffin, various metals, heterograft, leather, pith wood, latex, vulcanized rubber, and gutta percha. It seems early clinicians used whatever was at hand. The clinical applications of synthetic polymers, dimethysiloxanes (silicone), halogenated carbons (Teflon), and polyvinyl alcohol compared by Brown and Ohlwiler found preferential advantages to silicone when used as a liquid, resin, or solid.[47] It replaced, in contemporary use, all the previous materials until the introduction of bovine collagen in 1981, and the array of tissue fillers now available.

Frank J. Gerow (1929 to 1993), remembered best for his role in developing and popularizing silicone breast implants, coauthored a paper in 1967 on the use of silicone in burn care. The paper recommends liquid silicone in the treatment of acute hand burns. Silicone-impregnated dressings, splints, etc., were combined with bags of liquid medical-grade silicone in which the hands were immersed during and after healing of partial thickness and deep burns. In a series of 50 hands in 29 patients, they reported supple, soft, satisfactory scars in all cases.[48]

The use of silicone gel and silicone sheets applied to scars became a recommended strategy in the 1980s, with multiple papers appearing subsequently.[49,50] Negative results are seldom reported, but a 1973 study of silicone (silastic) sheets reported that while using the sheets on fresh skin graft donor areas provided excellent pain relief, nearly all became infected with *Pseudomonas* within a few days of application.[51] This led to the recommendation for the use of silicone sheeting on healed wounds only.

The use of topical sheets or gels for prevention and treatment of scar remains commonly recommended, and there are hundreds of commercial products on the market today promoting this technique. In 1995, Reiffel noted that occluding the healing incision site with paper tape also yielded a satisfactory scar, at lower cost. He demonstrated the effectiveness of this in a series of patients, including those undergoing scar revisions.[52] This has been confirmed in subsequent clinical trials.[53] The question of whether it is pressure, occlusion, moisture, revascularization, or the related metabolic changes induced by pressure that influence scar formation and maturation remains unresolved.

Intralesional Injection and/or Radiation Therapy for Scars

A 1908 case report contains a discussion of methods available for correction of a retroauricular keloid that occurred following treatment for mastoiditis. These included: injections with thiosinamine (*Fibrinolysin*, Merck), excision, or excision with skin grafting or radiation. The consensus was that patients would prefer X-ray treatment.[54] Another case presentation in 1909 discussed the treatment of a keloid burn scar of the face (probably hypertrophic scarring) that responded to X-ray therapy, without mentioning the dose, other than "intervals of a fortnight to pastille doses of the ray." This report goes on to state that thiosinamine injections worked similarly well.[55]

The use of thiosinamine was first reported in the medical literature by Ferdinand Ritter von Hebra (1816 to 1880) for the treatment of lupus and old cicatrices by injecting in the vicinity of the lesions. At the present time, this product is commonly recommended in homeopathic therapies. Thiosinamine is extracted from mustard oil derived from black mustard (*Sinapis nigra*). There are numerous case reports in the late 1890s and early 20th century of its role in treating burn scar contractures, palmar fasciitis, elephantiasis, schistosomiasis, ringworm, and other conditions. More recently it has been used in chemistry as a weak solvent, and in photography as a reversal of light sensitivity. Medically, its use is principally homeopathic. The use of thiosinamine for contractures was first promoted by Paul Gerson Unna (1850 to 1929) who also developed the "Unna Boot," a medicated bandage used to treat venous ulcers of the lower legs. Its first use for keloids was described by Sinclair Tousey (1818 to 1887), an early advocate of medical electricity and Roentgen rays. However, in reality he was probably treating a hypertrophic burn scar rather than a keloid. Intralesional injection rather than systemic administration was recommended.[56]

The Patterson Index[19] lists 54 papers related to the treatment of keloids, 13 of which specify radium or X-ray therapy. In addition to radiation, additional treatments listed by the Patterson Index covering the literature from 1860 to 1920 include excision, electrolysis, injections of ergot, thiosinamine, thyroid extract, oil of creosote, pyrogallic acid, topical applications of dry ice (cryotherapy), or pepsin. Nearly 100 similar recommendations continue to appear in the next volume of the Index, known as the Leuz Index, covering the years 1921 to 1964.[57] Radiation, injection of pepsin-hydrochloric acid, cryotherapy, electrodessication, and even a case report of massive keloid treated by parathyroidectomy are reported.[58]

The first reports of using steroids for scars appear in 1950, with the observation that direct topical application produces thinning of the dermis.[59] Following this report, a clinical trial of adrenocorticotropic hormone administered parenterally or by direct injection into the scar showed no benefit.[60] In 1954, Merton L. Griswold (1904 to 2000) injected hypertrophic scars with hydrocortisone in 13 different cases and found that the scars did not progress, but did not regress.[61] This was contradicted in 1956 by Gustav Asboe-Hansen (1917 to 1989), a Danish dermatologist who found an 85% regression in vaccination site keloids when injected intralesionally with hydrocortisone.[62] The first report of the potential benefits of injecting corticosteroids into the wound at the time of surgical excision of scars was from Murray, in 1963.[63] However, his series was uncontrolled and he variously injected at the time of excision, applied triamcinolone topically or intralesionally, and in some cases used adjuvant radiation as well.

The introduction of intralesional triamcinolone acetonide for either hypertrophic or keloidal scars led to numerous case reports documenting successful management, as well as complications such as tissue atrophy, telangiectasia, hypopigmentation, and even Cushing's disease.[64] In one review, Ketchum and his colleagues recommend judicious intralesional injections in small doses, not to exceed 120 mg, repeated as needed no less than 4 weeks apart. The use of triamcinolone has become a standard therapy, with numerous case series reports in the following years. Contemporary review articles similarly conclude that the use of intralesional triamcinolone remains a mainstay for scar therapy.[65–68] Additional recommended topical and intralesional medical therapies include bleomycin, 5-fluorouracil, verapamil, retinoids, interferon, and calcium channel blockers, both alone or in combination with surgical treatments (see Chapters 10 and 16). These reviews also include discussion of pressure, radiation, and topical silicone gels or sheets. All note the difficulty in treating keloids, as opposed to hypertrophic scars. The most common thread among contemporary reports of medical scar therapy is the failure to identify a precise etiology, and the lack of convincing evidence-based clinical trials for the treatment of these scars despite detailed information on collagen content, biochemical composition, growth factors, etc.

One of the most promising treatments under development is the use of lasers, which will be discussed in great detail in other chapters (see Chapters 13 and 14). This contemporary innovation holds the promise of replacing or augmenting the numerous treatments of the past 100 plus years.

Scar Mitigation/Intervention

The best way to prevent a scar, of course, is to prevent injury. Automobile design has done a spectacular job of reducing injuries resulting from motor vehicle accidents. President

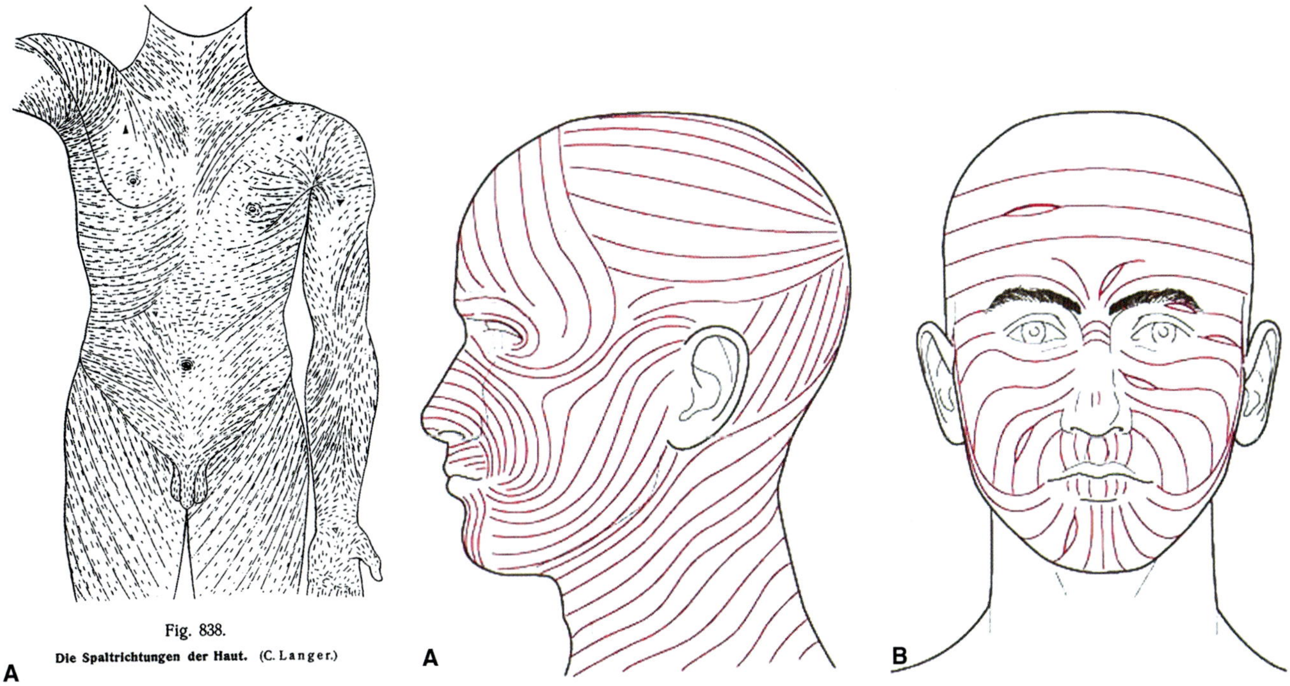

FIGURE 1-11 **A:** Langer's lines showing the axis of tension in human skin. *(From Langer C, Kopsch Fr.* Rauber's Lehrbuch der Anatomie des Menschen. *Leipzig, Germany: Georg Thieme, 1908:825.)* **B**: Kraissl's Lines *(Used with permission from iKnowlege. at http://clinicalgate.com/face-and-scalp/. Accessed November 11, 2016.)*

Lyndon Johnson signed the Motor Vehicle Safety Act of 1966, regulating various safety-related aspects of all highway motor vehicles.[69] This was the first and largest industry to be regulated by the federal government. Windshield and dashboard redesign, seatbelts, airbags, and child safety seats all followed, significantly reducing motor vehicle deaths and trauma. This has resulted in a decline by nearly 80% in deaths and injuries, while the total number of vehicles and miles driven has risen rapidly.[70] Few recognize the important role that the medical profession has played in the design changes that have contributed to these reductions, beginning with efforts in 1930 to introduce safety glass in windshields.[71] Just as evidence-based medicine drives much of our decision making, the same types of standards are applied in working to reduce motor vehicle trauma. Implementation of improved vehicular design, universal seat belt use, reduction/elimination of impaired and distracted driving, and other measures can further reduce fatality/injury rates. Similarly, burn reduction strategies such as reduced flammability in children's clothing and household fabrics,[72] hot water heater temperature regulation,[73] and mandated smoke detectors[74] have reduced burn injuries over the past 50 years. These were also physician-led initiatives.

Scar minimization after surgery emphasizes proper wound care, debridement of foreign bodies, and careful approximation of the wound edges, including the deeper layers. Wounds that become infected are more likely to result in abnormal scars, but there is no evidence that for simple, nonbite wounds, antibiotics confer any advantage in lacerations of the hand[75] or other areas.[76] The role of tension in abnormal wound healing is so widely accepted that the fact is often stated without reference (see Chapter 7). Warren, in his treatise on scars, states "The most striking peculiarity of scar tissue is its tendency to contract . . . hypertrophied cicatrices are produced when the edges of the wound retract from some cause or other. The abundant formation of new tissue is an exaggerated effort on the part of nature to supply the necessary covering for the part."[20] Warren does not reference the work of an Austrian anatomist, Karl Langer (1819 to 1887) who described his tension lines of the skin in 1861.[77] Langer used cadavers and an awl to create circular puncture wounds, delineating tension along the round shapes that changed to oval. He later modified his lines using a circular excision of skin. These direction lines have become a guide to the preferred incision lines giving the least unsatisfactory scar in elective surgery (Fig. 1-11A). Subsequent modifications have been based on studies using living skin, rather than Langer's evidence based on cadavers with rigor mortis.

In 1984, Albert Borges (1919 to 1990) provided a complete summary of the work defining optimal incision directions.[78] Borges notes that very little additional research on these principles was conducted until 1941 when Cox, in England, developed an MD thesis finding errors in Langer's lines, especially of the face and scalp; he termed these the antirelaxed skin tension lines. His principle was that "the one decision factor in the production of a fine linear scar is not so much any particular method of wound suture, but rather the relation which the direction of the incision bears to the cleavage lines. An incision that has been accurately placed in the cleavage lines . . . will leave the finest scar." Further modifications were proposed by Leonard Rubin (1912 to 2001) based on facial lines,[79] and Cornelius J Kraissl (1902 to 1999), who carefully studied the lines in the aged face and identified the role of subcutaneous muscle in determining optimum incision lines.[80] See Figure 1-11B for Kraissl's lines of the face and scalp.

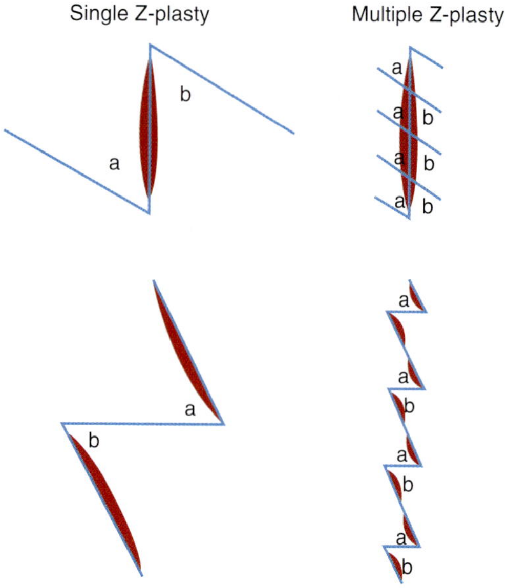

FIGURE 1-12 Single and double Z-plasty. *(From Open source, http://america.pink/images/4/8/9/1/5/8/3/en/2-z-plasty.jpg. Accessed November 11, 2016.)*

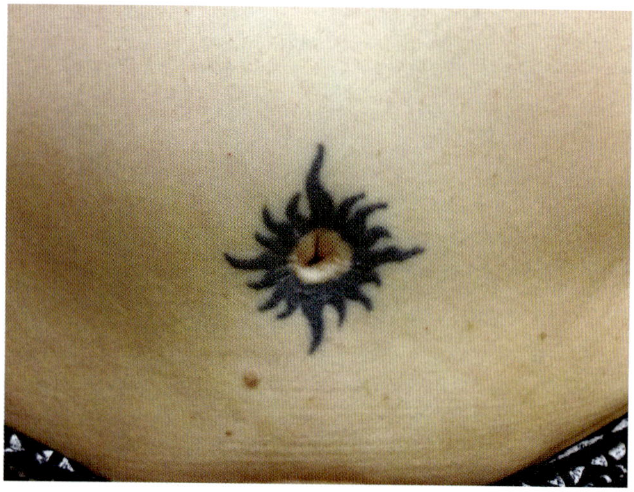

FIGURE 1-13 Periumbilical tattoo disguising abdominoplasty scar. *(Courtesy Dr. Sharon DeChiara, with permission.)*

Through an understanding of the principles of skin tension lines and their relationship to normal and abnormal scars, the concepts of the Z-plasty and W-plasty became clear. The hypertrophic (not so much the keloid) scar, if excised, may be rotated in such a way that tension along the axis of closure is interposed by adjacent skin transfer, releasing that tension during the revision. The evolution of the Z- and W-plasty is well described by Borges in his 1985 paper.[81] Many authors claim that a French ophthalmologist, Michel Serré (1799 to 1849), first described a true Z-plasty in 1842 in reporting a case he had done in 1835.[82] According to Borges, the correction of the oral commissure deformity described by Serré did not consist of a transposition of equal flaps, but an excision of tissue and rotation of the lip into the defect. The first true Z-plasty may more accurately be attributed to William E. Horner (1793 to 1853), an American anatomist and surgeon, whose Z-plasty in 1837 was designed to correct an ectropion. Variations on this operation are reported sporadically and detailed by Borges, who attributes the first true use of the term Z-plasty to Stewart Leroy McCurdy (1859 to 1931), whose paper in 1913 was titled "Z-plastic surgery: plastic operations to elongate cicatricial contractions of the neck, lips and eyelids and across joints."[83] The basic principle of the Z-plasty is straightforward, as seen in Figure 1-12, making it one of the most commonly used techniques in surgical scar revisions (see Chapter 12).

When All Else Fails, Hide the Scar

Once present a scar is unlikely to be easily erased, but strategies not involving medical interventions are available to minimize an undesirable or unsightly scar. Camouflage of scars with makeup or tattoos is certainly possible (see Chapters 20 and 21). In his memoir, George Burchett (1872 to 1953) describes working on a patient referred by Sir Harold Gillies, injecting tattoo pigment to disguise gunpowder traumatic tattoos. Burchett referred to himself as the "King of Tattooists," and he is credited with introducing cosmetic tattooing using the technique to darken eyebrows as well as cover scars. In his memoir, Burchett recounts making a tattoo that looked like a scar for a German civilian who wished to mimic the facial dueling scar that was then popular among upper class Austrian and German students during the end of the 19th and the beginning of the 20th century.[84]

Tattoos are becoming increasingly common, and are considered to be body art among young adult groups, with prevalence estimates ranging from 20% to 40% between the ages of 16 and 25.[85] Cosmetic tattooing has extended to permanent makeup, as well as nipple/areola tattoos as part of breast reconstruction. Figure 1-13 shows a tattoo designed to disguise an umbilical scar following an abdominoplasty.

The Unique History of the Individual Scar

We have already discussed the use of scars for the identification of individuals. Scars also have a distinct forensic value. Careful descriptions and even photographs are necessary in documenting domestic violence, child abuse, and torture. When evaluating an acute injury, the nature of the injury, timing, reconstruction, and impact are essential components to planning treat signi!cant improvement in inmate behaviors ment. Did healing proceed normally? Were there factors contributing to pathological scarring, or is this a normal scar? Upon evaluating a scar, a full history includes an understanding of what the exact meaning of the scar is to that individual. All recent incisions appear unsightly during normal healing. Early surgical intervention may be delayed, unless the alignment of critical features is distorted, such as along the vermillion border of the lip or the eyebrow, when early re-repair might be appropriate. Timing of the repair is as important as the methodology used. A "trivial" scar (to you) may have deep-seated repercussions, while a wholly unsatisfactory scar might have no real cause for concern by that particular patient. When the patient is requesting scar revision, the prudent physician should take into account not just the physical scar, but the emotional impact of it as well. Ultimately, it is individual judgment that determines whether the doctor chooses to undertake a scar revision, and what tools, techniques, and approach to use (see Chapter 4). The chief caveat here would be to avoid the patient with unrealistic expectations.

Scars may be a component of litigation in both civil (malpractice) and criminal cases. Who inflicted the injury? How? Why? And what comes next? In a malpractice case, there may be no interest in scar revision until AFTER the trial; in criminal litigation, the scar, as a denominator of the injury, may need to be as visible as possible. In these cases, testimony may be required to document the scar as a reasonable result of the alleged injury inflicted or the result of some other cause.

Reviews of surgical malpractice claims have shown that patient dissatisfaction with a scar is responsible for nearly 25% of claims in oculoplastic surgery[86]; it is also the most common complaint in laser tattoo removal[87] and in breast augmentation.[88] One of the earliest references in the medical literature to scar-related litigation is from 1879, in the *Boston Medical and Surgical Journal*. This report includes one physician complaining, "Under our laws I am liable to prosecution for malpractice in all these cases, as the unsightly scars of unrestored breasts and limbs and the imperfection. . . . No mortal power can resist the contraction of a scar, any more than it can control the rending and lifting power of frost."[89] Review of newspaper literature of the era indicates numerous malpractice cases starting from the 1830s, with doctors arrested and jailed for lethal and nonlethal malpractice. In today's legal climate—with minimally invasive surgery and public perceptions of medical miracles—making a scar, or trying to fix one requires not just judgment and skill but the ability to communicate clearly an informed consent that does not promise an invisible result.

Scars as Stigma

All manner of attributes have been given to individuals with scars, especially facial scars. The term "Scarface" is a nickname referring to gangsters in both the 1932 and 1983 films of the same name. Facial scarring and disfigurement are common themes in literature, theater, and film (Phantom of the Opera, Batman's the Joker, Frankenstein, The Nightmare on Elm Street, Darkman, The Lion King, etc.), with most associated with criminality and/or evil. A counterexample might be the lightning bolt scar on Harry Potter's forehead, but even this has its association being caused by the evil Voldemort. The skin and its appearance play a significant role in racial, cultural, and social identity. Thus, disruptions of this organ (the largest organ by weight in the human body) can carry enormous impact.

Literature uses the image of the facial scar as an indication of character. Scars may be a sign of past heroism (Austrian dueling scars), a sign of the divine touch (as in the "mark of Cain"), or the symbolism of the 7 P's on Dante's forehead in the "Divine Comedy," representing the seven deadly sins. Social marking of criminals and sinners also occurs, like the branding of an "A" on Hester Prynne in Hawthorne's "The Scarlet Letter," or Cervantes's note of brands marking the faces of slaves.

In 1953 Frances MacGregor and colleagues detailed four case histories of facial scarring and deformity and conducted a longitudinal analysis of the effects on the patients, their families, and their communities.[90] The authors, a psychiatric social worker, a psychiatrist, an anthropologist, and a psychologist, identified the confusing and varied reactions individuals had to both mild and severe deformity and scarring. The severity of reaction was NOT necessarily correlated with the severity of the defect seen, as a number of patients classified as having a "slight" deformity by observers instead believed themselves that their disfigurement was significant. Few psychological treatments were conclusively effective, and outcomes were generally unpredictable. MacGregor was influential in placing the social worker/psychologist/psychiatrist firmly into the burn team and patient care (see Chapter 24).

The emotional/psychological effects of scars (and other skin disorders as well) continue to be a serious problem and a subject of study. Posttraumatic stress disorder, body image issues, and disproportionate social issues must all be considered. A recent textbook of surgery includes a full chapter on the psychological consequences of facial scarring, including 56 references. [91] More recently an article on the spiritual and religious aspects of skin and skin disorders discusses the historical role faith and religious figures have played in interpreting, treating, and healing skin disorders (including scars), and the role these disorders have played in issues of identity and social/cultural acceptance.[92]

The relationship between appearance and criminality first appeared in the 19th century amid the conflict between Darwinian and Lamarckian theorists. The idea that the human species could devolve and become less human was put forward by scientists interested in concepts of ethnicity and criminality, and as a form of social commentary. Images in literature, such as the Jekyll/Hyde dichotomy, Dracula, and even Dorian Gray, were reinforced by "scientific" studies identifying criminal characteristics, including those by Benedict Morel (1809 to 1973), a French psychiatrist, and Cesare Lombroso (1835 to 1909), an Italian physician and criminologist. Characters in the novels of Charles Dickens, especially *Bleak House*, frequently reflected this view of both the best and the worst traits of humans represented by their appearance.

The theory that "degenerate" human beings can be recognized may no longer be a mainstream social or psychological science. However, contemporary research confirms that appearance has a profound effect on first impressions of such characteristics as trustworthiness, honesty, or guilt. Studies confirm that stereotypic appearances unduly influence judgment across a range of human activity including hiring practices, voting, judicial decision making, and even mating. However flawed this initial reaction may be, further information rarely alters a negative first impression.[93]

The recognition that certain features may contribute to social stigma and negatively influence behavioral outcomes led to a number of studies on the benefits of plastic or cosmetic surgery in prison populations as part of penal rehabilitation. In 1965, Edward Lewison (d. 1993) of British Columbia reported a 10-year study in which 450 patients received corrective surgery in the provincial prison system for a variety of facial deformities, including scars. He reported a significant improvement in inmate behaviors following their surgeries, but did not follow them after release.[94] In reviewing 253 inmates of the Texas state prison system who underwent corrective procedures between 1982 and 1984, the rate of recidivism 3 years following discharge in the surgically treated inmates was nearly half that of the untreated population.[95] While several studies confirmed that these programs and other "benefits" of incarceration such as job training and education result in changing attitudes toward prisons, cost cutting and privatization have led to the loss of these programs. Recent evaluation studies reviewing convictions have confirmed that ". . . physical characteristics of persons . . . have a significant impression on the trustworthiness, guilty decisions and severity of sentences. Whenever this occurs, the conceivable impression of such wrongful convictions would exonerate criminals who could pose a danger to the populace, while convict(ing) innocent people."[96]

Scars of Abuse and Torture

The role of physicians in documenting the physical evidence of abuse and torture has become a near subspecialty in establishing valid claims for civil and criminal cases, and for asylum seekers. C Henry Kempe (1922 to 1984), a pediatrician, first identified the "battered child syndrome"[97] leading to increased recognition of child abuse and the prevalence of domestic violence across all socioeconomic classes and ethnicities. Nonaccidental injuries as a cause of morbidity and mortality remain significant. One study evaluating pediatric admissions over a 4-year period identified a 7.5% incidence of abuse-related trauma, with a sixfold higher mortality in that category.[98] While most reported serious traumas involve head or intra-abdominal injury and fractures, injuries may include patterned burns from irons, cigarettes, or contact with other heated elements. Mandatory reporting requirements of suspected child abuse exist throughout North America, the European Union, Australia, South Africa, and Brazil. A high correlation exists between child abuse and domestic/spousal abuse.

Recognition of adult abuse emphasizes providing pertinent information to the victim, in the absence of the abuser, about options for safety and escape. For adults as well as children, cuts and bruises not consistent with the described source of injury, circular bruises of the wrist or ankle from grips or restraints, black eyes, repeated ER visits, and other unusual injuries including those to genital and anal areas may be indicators of abuse.

The prevalence of state-sanctioned abuse and torture is widespread despite international laws forbidding such practices. The 1948 Universal Declaration of Human Rights, the 1987 United Nations (UN) Convention against Torture, and other following agreements have not prevented an estimated 141 countries from using torture during 2015. Article 16 of this agreement requires that states may not forcibly return those seeking asylum from torture or "other acts of cruel, inhuman or degrading treatment or punishment which do not amount to torture." Evaluation of asylum seekers in the United States and Europe requires both legal and medical evaluations for evidence of and confirmation of previous torture.

Because of the legal and humanitarian obligation to evaluate asylum seekers, numerous medical human rights clinics have opened up in major cities; some within teaching programs across the United States have developed curricula for teaching appropriate evaluation techniques, documentation requirements, and referrals for care. Among those programs are those managed by Health Right International (https://healthright.org/) in several locations and numerous programs run by hospital teaching programs including Mt Sinai (https://mountsinaihumanrights.com/human-rights-clinic/), Cornell (http://www.wcchr.com/), Columbia (http://psclub.columbia.edu/clubs-organizations/human-rights-initiative), and the Social Medicine Residency Program at Montefiore in New York. International standards for such care were developed through the office of the UN High Commissioner for Human Rights. Known as the Istanbul Protocol, this *Manual on Effective Investigation and Documentation of Torture and Other Cruel, Inhuman or Degrading Treatment or Punishment* provides a template for the evaluation. The full document is available online: http://physiciansforhumanrights.org/issues/torture/international-torture.html#sthash.lWkkUifI.dpufP Accessed November 15, 2015.

Torture patterns vary by country and geographical regions. A Danish review of 154 victims identified crush injuries more commonly among refugees from Asia, including Afghanistan and Pakistan. Electrical torture was more common within the Middle East and North Africa. Overall, sexual torture occurred in 78% of women and 25% of men.[99] A similar evaluation of Swedish asylum refugees noted that 100% of the victims had been beaten with fists, sticks, or batons. Whipping with electrical cords occurred in Syria and Iran. Suspension, sharp injuries, burns, and other methods varied between regions.[100] A Bronx-based human rights clinic reported on the significant role scars played in their evaluations of 89 victims from 13 countries. Scars were documented in 87% of the cases, ranging in size from 0.1 cm to 19 cm in diameter. Sixty-eight of the 89 victims had multiple scars. Fifteen of the scars were burn marks. Nearly half of the human right clinic's clients reported that specific scars were NOT from their torture, a finding considered an indicator of credibility.[101] In another series of evaluations, scars were present around the head and neck in 69%, scars on the genitals in 10%, and burn marks in 6%.[102]

The relation between the scars and the reported mechanism of injury is important in determining credibility, regardless of the situation. The Istanbul Protocol requests that scars be rated on a 1 to 5 scale as follows:

1. Is the scar inconsistent with the reported trauma?
2. Could it have been caused by the trauma described, but is nonspecific, with other possibilities?
3. Is it highly consistent with few other possible causes?

4. Is this typical of that type of trauma, with only some other possibilities?
5. Is it diagnostic, not caused by any other mechanism than that described?

Specific scars are characteristic of known torture methods. "Tramline" or parallel strips are typical of whipping. Scars will correspond to types of impact such as blunt, sharp, or thermal, leaving distinct patterns. The size of the scars should be measured in three dimensions. Absent hair, sweat glands, or pigment changes indicate injury to deeper layers of the skin. How do the scars relate to the position of the victim and their abuser?[103] These are all important forensic issues and ought to be carefully documented.

This qualitative evaluation would equally apply to your own judgment of a patient's reliability, and may be helpful in any other medicolegal situation. High-quality properly lighted photographs of the scars, in concert with the history taken, can be conclusive to the evidence offered in a case—whether you are determining the individual's asylum qualifications or presenting evidence in a criminal case or malpractice dispute.

Conclusions

Scars are interesting things. The experienced observer can derive a great deal of information about the timing and treatment of an injury even before a history is taken. With the history, an understanding of the relationship between the patient and a scar may become clear; with this knowledge, the decision of what to do for the scar, if asked, and how to do it should become more obvious. A small scar can be a big problem, and an awful scar might not be an issue at all. If medical advances bring in an era of regeneration and scarless healing, such advances will probably not be available to everyone, so scars will continue to be living witnesses to history.

REFERENCES

1. Kakar, S, Einhorn, TA. Importance of nutrition in fracture healing. In: Holick MF, Dawson-Hughes B, eds. *Nutrition and Bone Health*. Totowa, NJ: Humana Press; 2004.
2. Machado NM, Gragnani A, Ferreira LM. Burns, metabolism and nutritional requirements. *Nair Hosp*. 2011;26:692–700.
3. Reddien PW. Lin28: time for tissue repair. *Cell*. 2013;155:738–739.
4. Shyh-Chang N, Daley GQ. Lin28: primal regulator of growth and metabolism in stem cells. *Cell Stem Cell*. 2013:12:395–406.
5. Manjo G. *The Healing Hand: Man and Wound in the Ancient World*. Cambridge, MA: Harvard University Press; 1975.
6. Ardrey, R. *African Genesis*. New York: Dell, 1967:31.
7. Alden CH. The identification of the individual with special reference to the system in use in the Office of the Surgeon General, US Army. *Am Anthropol*. 1896;9:295–301.
8. Dog tag. https://en.wikipedia.org/wiki/Dog_tag. Accessed December 15, 2015.
9. Remains of American WWII soldier reportedly found on Pacific's Northern Mariana Islands. http://www.foxnews.com/us/2013/03/26/remains-wwii-soldier-reportedly-found-on-pacifics-northern-mariana-islands.html. Accessed November 21, 2015.
10. The collection of DNA from military personnel. http://www.councilforresponsiblegenetics.org/geneticprivacy/DNA_mil.html. Accessed November 21, 2015.
11. Olubimpe AA, Olubukunola OA, Jackson, R. Observations on the procedural aspects and health effects of scarification in Sub-Saharan Africa. *J Cut Med Surg*. 2007;11:217–221.
12. *Alibert JLM. Descriptions des maladies de la peau observées a l'Hôpital Saint-Louis, et exposition des meilleures méthodes suivies pour leur traitement (in French). Paris: Barrois l'ainé*; 1806:113.
13. Alibert JLM. Quelque recherdhes sur la choloide. *Mem Soc Medicale d'Emulation*. 1817;8:744–752.
14. McDowell F, ed. The McDowell series of plastic surgery indexes volume I. In: *The Zeis Index and History of Plastic Surgery 900 BC to 1863 AD* (Complied by Edward Zeis, Translated by TJS Patterson). Baltimore, MD: Williams and Wilkins; 1977.
15. Dieffenbach JF. *Chirurgische Erfahrungen, bseonders uber die Wiederherstellung zerstorter Theile des menschlichen Korpers nach neuren Methoden. Abbildungen*. Berlin, Germany: Ensilin; 1829.
16. Aptowicz DO. *Dr. Mutter's Marvels*. New York, NY: Penguin Books; 2014.
17. Mutter TD. *Cases of Deformity from Burns Successfully Treated by Plastic Operations*. Philadelphia, PA: Merrihew & Thompson; 1843.
18. Sydenham Society Works. Bibliographical Notices. Art. 1. Cases of deformity from burns, successfully treated by plastic operations (Forbes J, ed.). *Br Foreign Med Rev*. 1844;18:525–606.
19. Patterson TJS, McDowell F. *The Patterson Index 1864–1920*. Vol. II. Baltimore, MD: Williams and Wilkins; 1978.
20. Warren, JC. Hypertrophies and degenerations of cicatrices and cicatricial tissue. *Ann Surg*. 1893;18:253–282.
21. Warren JM. Operations for fissure of soft and hard palate. *N Engl Q J Med Surg*. 1843;1:538, as reproduced in McDowell F, ed. *Silvergirls's Surgery Plastic Surgery*. Austin, TX: Silvergirl; 1977.
22. Donaldson IML. Ambroise Paré's accounts of new methods for treating gunshot wounds and burns. In: *JLL Bulletin: Commentaries on the History of Treatment Evaluation*; 2004. http://www.jameslindlibrary.org/articles/ambroise-pares-accounts-of-new-methods-for-treating-gunshot-wounds-and-burns/. Accessed November 5, 2016.
23. Thurston AJ. Paré and prosthestics: the early history of artificial limbs. *ANZ J Surg*. 2007;77:1114–1119.
24. Snyder C. Ambroise Paré and ocular prosthesis. *Arch Ophthalmol*. 1963;70:130–132.
25. Rodger NAM. *The Wooden World: An Anatomy of the Georgian Navy*. New York, NY: WW Norton; 1996.
26. Hanson N. *The Confident Hope of a Miracle: The True History of the Spanish Armada*. New York, NY: Doubleday; 2003.
27. Bartholomew, M. James Lind and scurvy: a reevaluation. *J Maritime Res*. 2002;4:1–14.
28. Carpenter KJ. *The History of Scurvy and Vitamin C*. Cambridge: Cambridge University Press; 1986.
29. Richardson R. *Larrey, Surgeon to Napoleon's Imperial Guard* (Revised Edition). Hong Kong 2000 edition.
30. Civil war causalities. http://www.civilwar.org/education/civil-war-casualties.html. Accessed November 5, 2015
31. Dixon I. Civil war medicine, modern medicine's civil war legacy. *Civil War Trust*. http://www.civilwar.org/education/history/civil-war-medicine/civil-war-medicine.html Accessed November 13, 2015.
32. http://history.amedd.army.mil/booksdocs/wwi/Jaffin/. Accessed December 1, 2015.
33. Gawande A. Casualties of war—military care for the wounded from Iraq and Afghanistan. *N Engl J Med*. 2004;351(24):2471–2475.
34. Lenares HA. Historical notes on keloids. *Burns*. 1977;3:150–152.
35. Druit R. *Principles and Practice of Modern Surgery*. Philadelphia, PA: Lea and Blanchard; 1843:427. https://books.google.com/books?id=RPwKCKRbXRMC&pg=PA54&lpg=PA54&dq=Robert+Druitt+Modern+Surgery+1844&source=bl&ots=s2NJz821JE&sig=_Pwd5WQabr0wBEYG7UlSkZY3K1k&hl=en&sa=X&ved=0ahUKEwir8eKy3bbLAhUFOD4KHfqWDjgQ6AEIODAF#v=onepage&q=Robert%20Druitt%20Modern%20Surgery%201844&f=false. Accessed November 15, 2015.
36. Da Costa J. *A Manual of Modern Surgery: General and Operative*. Philadelphia, PA: Saunders; 1894:199.
37. Rockwell WB, Cohan IK, Ehrlich HP. Keloids and hypertrophic scars: a comprehensive review. *Plast Reconstr Surg*. 1989;84:827–837.
38. Cosman B, Krikelair GF, Ju DMC, et al. The surgical treatment of keloids. *Plast Reconstr Surg*. 1961;27:335–358.
39. Huang C, Akaishi S, Hyakusoku H, et al. Are keloid and hypertrophic scar different forms of the same disorder? A fibro proliferative skin disorder hypothesis based on keloid findings. *Int Wound J*. 2012;11:517–522.
40. Lawrence, H. Keloid and intractable patches of chronic inflammation of the skin treated by scarification. *Br Med J*. 1898;2:151.
41. Blair VP. The influence of mechanical pressure on wound healing. *Ill Med J*. 1924;46:249–252.

42. Barrett-Brown J, McDowell F. Epithelial healing and the transplantation of the skin. *Ann Surg.* 1942;115:1166–1181.
43. Larson DL, Abston S, Evans EB, et al. Techniques for decreasing scar formation and contractions in the burned patient. *J Trauma.* 1971;11:807–823.
44. Macintyre L, Baird M. Pressure garments for use in the treatment of hypertrophic scars: a review of the problems associated with their use. *Burns.* 2006;32(1):10–15.
45. Esselman PC, Thombs BD, Magyar-Russell G, et al. Burn rehabilitation: state of the science. *Am J Phys Med Rehabil.* 2006;85(4):383–413.
46. LeVan P, Sternberg TH, Newcomer VD. The use of silicones in dermatology. *Calif Med.* 1954;81:210–213.
47. Barrett BJ, Ohlwiler DA, Fryer MP. Investigation of the use of dimethyl siloxanes, halogenated carbons and polyvinyl alcohol as subcutaneous prostheses. *Ann Surg.* 1960;152:534–547.
48. Spira M, Miller J, Hardy SB, et al. Silcone bag treatment of burned hands. *Plast Reconstr Surg.* 1967;39:357–265.
49. Perkins K, Carey RB, Wallis KA. Silicone gel: a new treatment for burn scars and contractures. *Burns.* 1982;9:201–204.
50. Ohmori S. Effectiveness of silastic sheet coverage in the treatment of a keloid scar. *Aesthet Plast Surg.* 1988;12:95–99.
51. Harris DR, Filarski SA, Hector RE. The effect of silastic sheet dressings on the healing of split skin graft donor sites. *Plast Reconstr Surg.* 1973;52:189–190.
52. Reiffel RS. Prevention of hypertrophic scars by long-term paper tape application. *Plast Reconstr Surg.* 1995;96:1715–1718.
53. Atkinson JM, McKenna KT, Barnett AG, et al. A randomized, controlled trial to determine the efficacy of paper tape in preventing hypertrophic scar formation in surgical incision that traverse Langer's skin tension lines. *Plast Reconstr Surg.* 2005;116:1648-1656.
54. Sequeira, JH. Case illustrating the effects of X-rays on scar-keloid. *Proc R Soc Med.* 1909;2:96–98.
55. Tilley H. Case of a keloid following operation for acute mastoid suppuration. *R Soc Med.* 1908;1:20–23.
56. Anonymous. *Merck's Archives of Materia Medica and Drug Therapy*. Vol. 3. Kenilworth, NJ: Merck; 1901:216–219. https://books.google.com/books?id=VCsTAAAAYAAJ&pg=PA218&dq=thiosinamine&hl=en&sa=X&ved=0ahUKEwiNnM-TicbLAhWIcj4KHd3vDigQ6AEIOzAG#v=onepage&q=thiosinamine&f=false. Accessed Nov 15, 2015.
57. Christopher AL. *The Leuz Index 1921 AD to 1946—The McDowell Series of Plastic Surgery Indexes* (Compiled by Christopher Leuz). Vol. III. Baltimore, MD: Williams and Wilkins; 1977.
58. Oliver G, Barasch J. Generalized keloids treated by parathyroidectomy. *Progr Med Paris.* 1946;7:292–293.
59. Baker BI, Whitaker WI. Interference with wound healing by local action of adrenocortical steroids. *Endocrinology.* 1950;46:544–551.
60. Conway H, Stark RB. ACTH in plastic surgery. *Plast Reconstr Surg.* 1951;8:354–377.
61. Griswold ML. Effects of adrenal cortical preparations on scar hypertrophy. *Plast Reconstr Surg.* 1954;13:451–161.
62. Asboe-Hansen G, Brodthagen H, Zachariae I. Treatment of keloids and topical injections of hydrocortisone acetate. *AMA Arch Derm.* 1956;73:162–165.
63. Murray RD. Kenalog and the treatment of hypertrophied scars and keloids in negroes and whites. *Plast Reconstr Surg.* 1963;31:275–280.
64. Ketchum LD, Cohen IK, Masters FW. Hypertrophic scars and keloids: a collective review. *Plast Reconstr Surg.* 1974;53:140–154.
65. Al-Atar A, Mess S, Thomassen JM, et al. Keloid pathogenesis in treatment. *Plast Reconstr Surg.* 2006;117:286–300.
66. Gauglitz GG. Management of keloids and hypertrophic scars: current and emerging options. *Clin Cosmetic and Invest Derm.* 2013; 6: 103–114.
67. Monestry S, Middelkoop E, Vranckx JJ, et al. Updated scar management practical guidelines: non-invasive and invasive measures. *J Plast Reconstr Aesthet Surg.* 2014;67:1017–1025.
68. Son D, Harijan A. Overview of surgical scar prevention and management. *J Korean Med Soc.* 2014;29:751–757.
69. Morris C. Motor vehicle safety regulation: genesis. *Law Contemp Prob.* 1968;33:36–565.
70. Historical Statistics of the United States. *Motor Vehicle Traffic Fatalities and Fatality Rates: 1900–1995*. Historical Statistics of the United States, Millennial Edition. http://hsus.cambridge.org/HSUSWeb/toc/showTable.do?id=Df184-577. Accessed November 15 2015
71. Eastman JW. "Doctors' orders": the American medical profession and the origins of the automobile design for crash protection. *Bul Hist Med.* 1981;55:407–424.
72. American Academy of Pediatrics, Communication on ACE Prevention. Report: investigation of fabrics involved in wearing apparel fires. *Pediatrics.* 1964 34:728.
73. Feldman KW, Schaller RT, Feldman JA, et al. Tap water scald burns in children. *Pediatrics.* 1978;62:1–7.
74. Reisinger KS. Smoke detectors: reducing deaths and injuries due to fire. *Pediatrics.* 1980;65:718–724.
75. Grossman JA, Adams JP, Kunec J. Prophylactic antibiotics in simple hand lacerations. *JAMA.* 1981;245:1055–1056.
76. Cummings P, Del Beccaro MA. Antibiotics to prevent infection of simple wounds: a meta-analysis of randomized studies. *Am J Emerg Med.* 1995;13:396–400.
77. Langer K. On the anatomy and physiology of the skin. *Br J Plast Surg.* 1978;31:3–8. (translated from German; Langer K. "Zur Anatomie und Physiologie der Haut. Über die Spaltbarkeit der Cutis." Sitzungsbericht der Mathematisch-naturwissenschaftlichen Classe der Wiener Kaiserlichen Academie der Wissenschaften Abt. 44 (1861).)
78. Borges AF. Relaxed skin tension lines (RSTL) versus other skin lines. *Plast Reconstr Surg.* 1984;73:144–150.
79. Rubin LR. Langer's lines and facial scars. *Plast Reconstr Surg.* 1948;3:147–155.
80. Kraissl DJ. The selection of appropriate lines for elective surgical incisions. *Plast Reconstr Surg* 1951;8:1–28.
81. Borges AF. The enigma of sere's "Z-plasty" technique. *Plast Reconstr Surg.* 1985;76:472–474.
82. Serre M. *Traité sur l'art de restaurer les difformités de la face*. Montpelier France, 1842. https://books.google.com/books?hl=en&lr=&id=6D1FAAAAcAAJ&oi=fnd&pg=PA1&dq=Serre+M++Traite+sur+l%27art+de++restaurer&ots=v6sg3CDUvz&sig=1cwQgQmgXueg3XaoVWALnqcTzSA#v=onepage&q=Serre%20M%20%20Traite%20sur%20l%27art%20de%20%20restaurer&f=false. Accessed November 5, 2016.
83. McCurdy SL. Z-plastic surgery: plastic operation s to elongate cicatricial contractions of the neck, lips and eyelids and across joints. *Surg Gynecol Obstet.* 1913;16:209–212.
84. Burchett G, Leighton P. *Memoirs of a Tattooist.* London: Oldbourne; 1958.
85. Tattooing in adolescents and young adults. http://www.uptodate.com/contents/tattooing-in-adolescents-and-adults. Accessed November 15, 2015.
86. Svider PF, Blake D, Husain Q, et al. In the eyes of the law: malpractice litigation in oculoplastic surgery. *Ophthal Plast and Reconst Surg.* 2014;30:119–123.
87. Zimmerman MC. Suits for malpractice based on alleged unsightly scars resulting from removal of tattoos. *Am Soc Derm Surg.* 1979;11:911–912.
88. Gorney M. Ten years experience in aesthetic surgery malpractice. Aesthet Surg J. 2001;21:569–571.
89. Sanger EF. Report on malpractice. Boston Med Surg J. 1879;100:41–50.
90. MacGregor FC, Abel TM, Bryt A, et al. Facial Deformities and Plastic Surgery. Springfield, IL: Charles C Thomas Publisher; 1953.
91. Price P, Tebble N. Psychological consequences of facial scarring. In: Teot L, Banwell PE, Ziegler UE, eds. Surgery in Wounds. Heidelberg: Springer-Verlag; 2004:519–526.
92. Shenefelt PD, Shenefelt DA. Spiritual and religious aspects of skin and skin disorders. Psychol Res Behav Manag. 2014;7:210–212. http://www.ncbi.nlm.nih.gov/pmc/articles/PMC4128841/. Accessed Nov 16, 2015.
93. Todorov A, Oliviola CY, Dotsch R, et al. Social attributions from faces: determinants, consequences, accuracy and functional significance. Annu Rev Psychol. 2015;66:519–545.
94. Lewison E. An experiment in facial reconstructive surgery in a prison population. Can Med Assoc J. 1965;92:251–254.
95. Freedman AM, Warren MM, Cunningham LW, et al. Cosmetic surgery and criminal rehabilitation. South Med J. 1988;81:1113–1116.
96. Anakwah N, Wiafe-Akenten B, Owusu Sarfo J, et al. Judging a book by it's cover: a legal psychological review on target's physical appearance and legal decisions. Eur J Psychol Stud. 2015;5:4–8.
97. Kempe CH, Silverman FN, Steele BF, et al. The battered child syndrome. J Am Med Assoc, 1962;181:17–24.
98. Estroff JM, Foglia RP, Fuchs JR. A comparison of accidental and non-accidental trauma: it is worse than you think. *J Emerg Med.* 2015;48:274–279.

99. Busch FR, Hansen SH, Hougen HP. Geographical distribution of torture: an epidemiological study of torture reported by asylum applicants examined at the Department of Forensic Medicine, University of Copenhagen. *Torture*. 2015;25:12–21.
100. Moisander PA, EdsonE. Torture and its sequel- a comparison between victims from 6 countries. *Forensic Sci Int*. 2003;137: 133–140.
101. Asgary RG, Metalios EE, Smith CL, et al. Evaluating asylum seekers/ torture survivors in urban primary care: a collaborative approach at the Bronx Human Rights Clinic. *Health Hum Rights*. 2006:9: 165–179.
102. Asgary R, Charpentier B, Burnett DC. Socieo-medical challenges of asylum seekers prior and after coming to the US. *J Immigr Minor Health*. 2013:15:961–968.
103. Park R, Oomen J. Context, evidence and attitude: the case for photography in medical examination of asylum seekers in the Netherlands. *Soc Sci Med*. 2010;71:228–235.

2 The Global Impact of Scars

MAYER TENENHAUS, HANS-OLIVER RENNENKAMPFF, and BRUCE POTENZA

KEY POINTS

- *Teleology of scars.* The process of scar formation is an extension of the reparative wound healing process. On one end of the spectrum, scar tissue aids in wound closure by assisting in wound contracture and reepithelialization and contributing to wound strength. There is little doubt that the ability to form a scar, the inevitable consequence of injury, directly and efficiently incurs survival benefit to the individual. The ability to rapidly and effectively close one's wounds protects the individual from further injury and insult, the importance of which cannot be overstated. From an evolutionary standpoint, delays in wound healing may have rendered an organism vulnerable. As a consequence, optimal healing represents a compromise between slower and more energy-intensive scarless healing and a quicker healing time with some degree of long-term scar sequelae.
- *Characterization and classification of scars.* There are three commonly described types of scars. They include simple, atrophic, and hypertrophic/pathologic (inclusive of hypertrophic scars [HTS] and keloids). Their histopathology, presentation, patterns of distribution, evolution, and involution are distinct.
- *Consequences globally and to the individual.* Significant consequences are associated with and result from scars. Individual, cultural, psychological, and societal influences, prejudices, and interpretations certainly play a major role in conceptualizing scars both for the individual and for society. Socioeconomic and financial challenges both as causative influences and as costs to the patient and society can similarly not be overstated.

There is little doubt that the ability to form a scar, the inevitable consequence of injury, directly and efficiently incurs survival benefit to the individual. The ability to rapidly and effectively close one's wounds protects the individual from further injury and insult, the importance of which cannot be overstated. From an evolutionary standpoint, delays in wound healing may have rendered an organism vulnerable. As a consequence, optimal healing represents a compromise between slower and more energy-intensive scarless healing and a quicker healing time, with some degree of long-term scar sequelae.

Scar formation positively impacts biologic organisms when a balance is established optimizing the functional and aesthetic result in effecting wound closure. It is perhaps here that scarring affords its greatest and most significant global and biologic impact. One can argue that pure regenerative healing represents the highest quality reparative effort. Although it remains a potential therapeutic endeavor, tragically this potential is rarely realized by higher life forms. Wound healing is a function of genetic efficiency, energy requirements, cost, benefit, and evolutionary direction.

The Global Burden of Scarring

The composite effect of the global burden of scarring as a pathologic condition remains ill defined. Reports tend to focus on subsets of patients, generally describing the complication of scarring as it relates to a specific disease entity such as burns and trauma, or scarring complicating elective surgical procedures. These reports are usually bound by single or multiple institutions and by a geopolitically similar socioeconomic area. Composite descriptions of the problems associated with scarring are estimates and at best extrapolations based on limited data. Burns represent one of the most significant contributors to trauma-related scarring. In higher income nations, data collected on the incidence of burn injuries have improved markedly with the establishment of formal databases, but middle and lower-income countries, unfortunately, can provide only limited epidemiologic data on this subject. As a result, even in this well-represented population, the true incidence of the global burden of burn injuries relies on extrapolation from limited clinical data. To further complicate matters, all burns and the associated wound care may differ greatly. Patients from higher socioeconomic countries generally receive prompt burn wound care with comparatively early excision and autografting of deep partial and full thickness injuries. Particular attention in established treatment algorithms is afforded to key areas of mobility, durability, and cosmesis for these patients. Progressive and better-funded regions generally provide adjunctive physical and occupational therapy to patients who have suffered thermal injuries, whether conservatively or surgically managed, to ensure patients have the best long-term outcome.

Patients from lower economic countries struggle with these critical care issues on many levels. Care may be delayed as the patient seeks referral from the local primary care system. They often begin a long journey up the echelons of care to a facility capable of providing care for burn injuries while awaiting safe disposition, transportation, and stabilization. Such delays and barriers to care often result in longer times for the wounds to heal, or nonoperative strategies for patients who would have benefited from an operative approach to their burn injury. This prolonged inflammatory phase of ill-treated wounds results in slow and impaired healing—both considered major contributors to the development of pathologic scar formation. In many burn patients, a nonoperative approach to deeper burns, especially over the joints, neck, and digits, may lead to scarring, contracture, and a loss of function. Scars are long-standing and tend to be a chronic problem for each patient. Unless a scar is medically modified or surgically corrected, it may leave the patient with a lifelong disability ranging from purely cosmetic to ulceration, contracture, and loss of function.

The prevalence of scarring (cumulative total of all the individuals currently affected) is a more accurate method of discussing the scope of this problem than merely the incidence of new cases of scarring. As we have seen with burn data, scar data derived from higher socioeconomic countries are reasonably reported, whereas data from middle and lower socioeconomic countries remain sparse. In the developed world, it is estimated that 100 million people develop scars resulting from surgical procedures, burns, and injury.[1] A total of 11 million patients developed cutaneous scar tissue resulting from elective operative procedures, whereas 25 million resulted from operations resulting from trauma. About 91% of postoperative patients reported a desire for improvement in the quality of wound healing along their surgical incisions,[2] and 15% experience dissatisfaction with the healing of their wound resulting from an excessive or unaesthetic scar.

Scars are a heterogeneous group of problems affecting multiple human systems. The most obvious are cutaneous scars, but there are also internal counterparts that cause a significant portion of scar-related pathologic consequences (see Chapter 3). Scar tissue that forms after abdominal surgery leads to adhesions, complications of which include bowel obstruction, infertility in women, and chronic pain. A number of important facts emerged from a large meta-analysis, by Van Goor et al.,[3] of the burden of adhesions in abdominal and pelvic surgery. The reported incidence of adhesive small bowel obstruction (SBO) was 2.4% overall, with a 4.2% incidence in pediatric patients, a 3.2% incidence in patients following lower gastrointestinal tract surgery, a 1.2% incidence following upper gastrointestinal tract surgery, a 1.5% incidence following urologic surgery, and a 1.4% incidence following laparoscopic surgery. The mean length of hospitalization for SBO was 7.8 days with a pooled hospital mortality of 2.5%. The incidence of chronic abdominal pain was 40%, with adhesions determined to be the etiologic agent of pain in 57% of the patients who underwent abdominal re-exploration.

Fibrosis adjacent to neural tissue may lead to alterations in sensory or motor function. Orthopedic joint injuries may result in scarring (arthrofibrosis), leading to decreased mobility and pain. Chronic scars may transform into a squamous cell cancer called Marjolin ulcer.[4] This may be associated with any chronic inflammatory process including burns, venous stasis, trauma, pressure sores, and pilonidal abscesses.[5] In addition to the physical problems caused by scar tissue, secondary problems may afflict the patient. These include pain, inflammation, pruritus, ulceration, and diminished range of motion. Contractures may physically limit the range of motion, or they may cause pain with motion, resulting in a decrease in the patient's voluntary efforts to perform therapy and exercise (see Chapter 19). Scars may ulcerate along tension lines and form chronic wounds. The cosmetic appearance of the scar will affect the patient to varying degrees depending on scar location and the patient's ability to cope with the scarring, the importance of which cannot be overstated.

In an ideal world, wound repair would more closely resemble a regenerative than reparative paradigm (see Chapter 27). Organisms that are able to accomplish regenerative wound healing are not hampered by scarring or even the loss of a limb; instead, they have the ability to grow new tissue that is equivalent functionally and aesthetically to the preinjured tissue. Regenerative healing is best demonstrated in lower vertebrates and early mammalian embryonic organisms. The sustained ability to maintain regenerative healing is lost with the progression to higher vertebrates. Examples of this include the salamander (tail regeneration), the newt (limb regeneration), or the zebra fish, which can heal wounds without evidence of scar tissue or loss of function.[6] In the human species, there is documented scarless fetal healing that to an extent resembles this regenerative process (see Chapter 27). Unfortunately, near the end of the second trimester, regenerative healing is lost, and normal wound healing with the potential to form a scar commences.

The process of scar formation is an extension of the reparative wound healing process. On one end of the spectrum, scar tissue aids in wound closure by assisting in wound contracture and reepithelialization and contributing to wound strength. This wound bed has the capacity to amplify the inflammatory host response to accelerate closure, but it has the downside effect of readily forming aberrant scar tissue as a consequence (see Chapter 6). Perhaps, in order to increase the speed of wound healing, we have achieved a new equilibrium between regenerative and reparative wound healing whereby the compromise for quicker healing is a less-than-normal wound matrix.

The psychosocial aspects of scarring are multifactorial and may include symptoms of anxiety, fear of socialization and stigmatization, depression, and posttraumatic stress disorder (PTSD) (see Chapter 24). These symptoms are difficult to quantify and treat, and may vary from patient to patient with similar physical manifestations of their scar tissue. Patient adaptability and coping are variables that help to mitigate psychosocial problems generated by scarring. Many consider the more highly visible scars as particularly problematic for the afflicted patient.

Wound Healing

Understanding the normal wound healing process is critical to our understanding of the development of scar tissue, and is extensively discussed in subsequent chapters. Briefly, wound healing is a complex process classically described as consisting of a continuum. Three distinct, yet overlapping, healing phases are defined by (1) *inflammation*, (2) *proliferation*, and (3) *maturation or remodeling*.[7] The inflammatory phase is characterized by two distinct processes: hemostasis and local wound debridement. Hemostasis in the wound bed is established by vasoconstriction and activation of the clotting cascade culminating in the formation of a fibrin clot. The subsequent release of cytokines and chemotactic factors recruits macrophages and neutrophils into the wound bed to phagocytize necrotic tissue, and generally occurs on days 3 to 4 postinjury.

The maturation of the wound bed to a more sterile environment is followed by the proliferative (second) phase of wound healing, which if unencumbered lasts approximately 10 days. Numerous stimulating growth factors, including vascular endothelial growth factor, platelet-derived growth factor, and transforming growth factor β, are released. As a result, there is replacement of the fibrin-based extracellular matrix (ECM) with neovascularization through angiogenesis and the establishment and deposition of granulation tissue. Migration and activation of fibroblasts facilitate the creation of new ECM composed of glycosaminoglycan, proteoglycans, and collagen in the wound bed. The ECM functions not only as a structural support but also as a critical element in cellular migration, integration, and promotion. Reepithelialization is traditionally thought to result from the migration of adjacent keratinocytes from both wound edges and adnexa such as follicular dermal buds. Normal physiologic wound contraction for closure is mediated by myofibroblasts. Wound edges of linear injuries are drawn together, while larger injuries are contracted circumferentially.

The final phase of wound healing, maturation and remodeling, is characterized by ECM alignment, remodeling of the collagen composition favoring type III, and apoptosis of senescent cells. At 4 months, the strength of a mature scar is approximately 80% of baseline, with most remodeling completed between 12 and 18 months after injury. This normal healing process is undertaken by a predominantly reparative rather than regenerative mechanism. Alterations of the wound bed may alter this process, leading to nonregulated healing, which may result in proliferative scarring. Factors such as severity of the wound, bacterial colonization counts, time to reepithelialization, and mechanical stress vectors may all play a role in the development of scarring (see Chapters 7, 8, and 9).[8]

Scar Characterization

How then to begin to objectively and comprehensively characterize the presence and effect of scar? Is it merely the histologic presence of scar that should be considered? Should one only consider visually evident scar formations—being raised and discolored—as significant? Scars can prove painful and dysaesthetic but may not be raised, tethered, or easily visualized. Certainly these all merit inclusion. Functional consequences should likely carry import: consider, for example, tendon adhesions resulting from closed fracture or infection. Certainly, scars are not merely a cutaneous manifestation or problem. One must merely consider the dire consequences of a postoperative uterine scar and its inherent risk of catastrophic rupture or ectopic pregnancy, or the formation of postmyocardial infarction scar and aneurysm formation to appreciate the holistic challenges and consequences of physiologic scar formation.

Disfigurement, or perhaps even enhancement, as characterized by the individual, culture, or the observer should be considered. How then to weigh these effects? Do certain populations figure differently in our assessment? Does one rate children more significantly? Do some cultures or individuals of a particular sex or economic status suffer more or less from deformity or functional loss? Economic, political, and social factors come into play. Access to medical, reconstructive, and rehabilitative care incurs its own cost–benefit analysis.

If we have difficulty defining what constitutes a scar and understanding when a scar is to be considered clinically, psychologically, economically, culturally, and physically relevant, then it is easy to appreciate how difficult it is to accurately assess its global impact. There is little doubt that countless individuals suffer worldwide from wounds of varied etiologic presentations. They may be related to diabetes and vascular disease; posttraumatic or surgical in origin; malignancy; radiation; associated with autoimmune disease; resulting from pressure; infection; idiopathic or genetic in origin. The costs to both society and the individual are staggering.

The history and challenge of problem scars is not a recent one (see Chapter 1). War, infection, and trauma have all tragically been experienced by all cultures and civilizations. Perhaps the earliest documentation available to us derives from Egyptian hieroglyphics with records of attempts to improve wound healing noted in both Mesopotamian and Egyptian texts. Biblical references abound with modern treatises well described by Linares, Pare, Lister, and many others.[9]

Scar Classification

The presentation of scars is highly variable, ranging from a simple, soft, flat, pale, asymptomatic linear scar seen some time after an uncomplicated laceration or surgical excision to a raised, firm, hyperpigmented, erythematous tumor associated with symptoms such as pain and itch (see Chapter 5). The simple flat linear scar in its best appearance will have the normal pigmentation of the host and represent the nearly perfect healing process from a linear cutaneous injury. If lateral tension is exerted on this wound, the scar may widen, resulting in a stretched appearance. Hyperpigmentation may occur and thinning of the scar is commonplace. Linear scars that remain in the inflammatory phase for longer periods of time may become hypertrophic.

There are three commonly described types of scars. They include simple, atrophic, and hypertrophic/pathologic (inclusive of HTS and keloids). Their histopathology, presentation, patterns of distribution, evolution, and involution are distinct. Simple scars result from cutaneous injury that heals well and within a relatively short time frame. The inflammatory process and the fibroproliferative phase of the wound healing are shortened. These scars tend to be flattened or only mildly raised, painless, and with pigmentation similar to the surrounding skin. They regress with time and fade into the surrounding tissue in the best of circumstances. A linear scar is flat and narrow and follows the path of cutaneous injury. A widespread scar is one that is stretched either longitudinally or widened, usually by mechanical forces during remodeling.

Atrophic scars occur when there is a focal loss, or loss of integrity, of the dermis and underlying subcutaneous tissue. Examples include abdominal stretch marks, or striae, that accompany trauma, obesity, or pregnancy and may occur without an epidermal injury, and depressed scars that follow significant trauma or inflammation, such as acne and varicella (chickenpox) (see Chapter 17).

HTS, as distinguished from keloids, are typically seen within the wound boundary and are associated with an accentuated or prolonged inflammatory phase. The scars are raised, widened, tender, painful, and pruritic, and follow a typical appearance pattern of erythema, violaceous, hyperpigmented, and then gradually fading toward normal color. The mean time to see the initiation of this type of scar is 4 weeks after epithelialization has occurred in the wound bed. Patients with a thermal injury have a much higher incidence of HTS than those with wounds resulting from surgery, trauma, or other etiologies. In burn patients, the mean time to initiate a HTS is 15 weeks after injury. The HTS has periods of evolution (growing and symptomatic) and periods of involution (resolution). Numerous factors act on these scars including the presence of mechanical stress, degree of inflammation, depth of injury, type of grafting and other treatment, and genetics. The final outcome of some HTS may not be known until 1.5 to 2 years after injury. HTS may become aggressive, especially if they complicate a mechanical stress line of the skin. These scars may contract and result in severe limitations of motion at specific joint areas. Efforts to control the growth of the HTS include pressure garments, silicone overlays, steroid injections, topical medication, and laser therapy (see Chapters 9, 10, and 13).[10] On the cellular level, there are theoretical approaches targeting inflammatory mediators and epithelial–mesenchymal interactions and altering the physical environment.[11]

Keloid scars are a unique form of scar tissue characterized clinically by extension of the scar outside the original boundaries of the wound. They are raised, hyperpigmented, pruritic, tender, and painful. Unlike HTS, a keloid may begin to develop as late as 12 months after injury. These lesions may wax and wane in their activity and have less of a tendency toward involution compared with HTS. Keloids may often be distinguished histologically from HTS and are characterized by disorganized collagen fibrils resulting from poor alignment of the collagen cross-links, leading to scar instability. The collagen fibrils are thicker with a higher concentration of type III collagen, chondroitin 4-sulfate, and glycosaminoglycan.[12] Keloids tend to grow more in both the horizontal and vertical dimensions compared with HTS. Mast cell production is increased in keloids, with concomitant increases in histamine production and pruritus within the scar.[13]

Literature Review

We have reviewed several published literature search engine sites in an effort to gain insights and glean objective evaluations of the global impact of scars, and found few, if any, referenced texts or studies. This deficiency is similarly noted by others.[14] We found this rather difficult to appreciate at first given its incidence, and yet perhaps not so surprising given how challenging the problem is to define. The most commonly available reviews on the topic involve pathologic scar development after burn injury. This is intuitive, as pathologic scarring is a more frequent complication after burns as compared with other types of injury or surgery.

The constellation of complaints surrounding scar formation may vary somewhat depending in part on its origin. For example, postsurgical scars often are subjectively described utilizing the parameters of pain, itching, and fragility, whereas burn scars tend to have more impact on the quality of life owing to contractures, ulcerations, and other aspects.[15] In 2003, Bombaro et al.[16] attempted to review the prevalence of HTS in their burn patient population. Whereas their initial review documented no cases of HTS in 30 Caucasian patients, a retrospective analysis of 110 patients established a prevalence of 67%. The authors then concluded that an accurate understanding of the prevalence of HTS was not known, and iterated the need for accurate studies to better define this critical data.

A recent publication from Germany by Mirastschijski et al.[17] in 2013 reviewed burn care costs associated with acute as well as subsequent early rehabilitative and reconstructive care from their largest regional health care insurance provider. In their review, the total cost of reconstructive and rehabilitative care was estimated to be 4.4 times the cost of the acute care. Of note, 96% of their costs were not hospital related but rather reflected costs for related sequelae including physical and occupational therapy, treatment adjuncts such as pressure therapy, silicone, splints, and prescriptions (see Chapter 19). Extrapolated globally using 2006 data, this cost would have amounted to 245 billion Euros, a staggering financial figure. One can only wonder what these financial costs would approximate if psychiatric care, lost productivity, and other pertinent social and societal costs were factored in (see Chapter 24).

Deitch reported on 59 children and 41 adults with injuries resulting from burns. Overall, he found 26% of the burn areas developed HTS. More importantly, burn wounds that healed within 14 to 21 days had a 33% chance of HTS, whereas the rate was 78% if the burn wound took greater than 21 days to heal.[18] In 1990, Spurr published a retrospective study looking at the incidence of HTS in children up to 5 years old, comparing outcomes in 1968 and 1984 at their burn center. He found a 50% chance of developing a HTS in both of his study groups.[19] Risk factors delineated included women, young age, burns of the neck and upper limbs, >1 surgical operation, meshed grafts, burn severity, and greater time to heal.[20] Comparison of pediatric burn survivors with a matched nonburn study group looking at body image measures demonstrated no differences in body image between the two cohorts.[21] An analysis of 703 patients with burn injuries by Gangemi et al.[22] revealed 540 (77%) developed scarring. Of these, 310 (44%) had HTS, 198 (28%) contractures with scarring, and 34 (5%) contractures without scarring. HTS induction was initially seen 23 days post-reepithelialization and lasted 15 months. Multivariate analysis revealed the following risk factors: sex (female gender), age (younger), anatomic burn site (face, neck, anterior torso, and upper extremities), number of surgical procedures, and the type of skin graft utilized (meshed). Full thickness burns were a risk factor for the development of hypertrophic contractures. Of these scars, 38% became normotrophic within 2 years, and 24% remained active for many years.

The incidence of HTS after burn injury ranges from 32% to 94%. In the United States, the cost estimate for treatment of these scars exceeded 4 billion dollars (2005).[23] A total of 1,798 patients admitted to three Dutch burn centers were followed for a 10-year period; 13% required reconstructive procedures; predictors of reconstructive surgery were burns to the arms, fire and flame burns, number of surgical interventions in the acute phase, and a larger burn size. The majority had more than one reconstruction, most often within 2 years postburn. Frequently reconstructed locations were hands, head, and neck. The most important indications for surgery were scar contractures (72%) and other scar problems such as scar instability, hypertrophy, pigmentation, contour relief, and other issues (28%). The most frequently used techniques were release/excision plus skin grafting. The mean medical cost of reconstructive surgery per patient was 8,342 Euros; the mean cost (in US dollars) was $9,273 (2014).[24]

As noted earlier, the true burden of burn injuries globally has not yet been fully realized. In 2004, there were an estimated 11 million burns severe enough to require medical attention; 300,000 of these patients died; 90% of these occurred in low-income countries where timely access to medical and surgical care is difficult.[25] As a result, prolonged inflammation and conservative management of deep partial thickness and full thickness burns often eventuates in patholog scarring. Burn injuries amounted to 17% of the disability-adjusted life years (DALYs, the loss of the equivalent of 1 year of good health) lost in adults (15 to 59 years old).

Children under 5 years of age make up 52% of the burn injuries in developing countries.[26] The etiology is similar to that in developed countries, unintentional scalding being the leading mechanism of injury. Children aged 1 to 4 were admitted to the hospital at a greater rate than older children and adults. Intentional burn injury accounts for 5% of burn admissions in the United States.[27] In India, self-immolation or burn assault accounted for 65% of the fire-related deaths in women in 2001.[28]

HTS are very dynamic in nature, further complicating the challenge of characterizing them. They are thought to undergo several stages of development and maturation, beginning with a proliferative or active growth phase, an intermediate stage where contractures may complicate the clinical presentation, and finally an involutional phase. These stages progress at different rates and extents depending upon multiple factors such as age, sex, etiology, and area of involvement. It is often quoted that pathologic scars seem to manifest with the same prevalence in both sexes, and yet (depending on which paper you review) the incidence of HTS development appears to complicate healing in women more commonly than in men. Similarly, a higher incidence of keloid presentation has been reported in women. Whether these discrepancies reflect pathophysiology or simply the increased likelihood of one seeking medical attention remains difficult to distinguish. The average age at onset of keloids is 10 to 30 years; it is often noted that individuals at the extremes of age rarely develop them. Borsini et al.[29] found that HTS occur more commonly in young patients, and that their scars evolve over longer periods of time as compared with adults. On the contrary, scarring often evolves more rapidly in elderly patients. Hypertrophy appears to be directly correlated with burn extension, infection, and delays in healing. Interestingly, HTS occur more frequently when the burn is caused by flame as compared with electrical or scald injury.

Burn injuries are only one etiologic contributor to the overall challenge of pathologic scars. Individuals of all genetic and racial backgrounds appear to have the propensity to develop them. It is, however, important to note that genetics, familial propensity, and race have long been demonstrated to be risk factors for the development of pathologic scarring. Individuals with darker pigmentation are generally considered to be at most risk for developing keloids. The incidence of keloids in persons with highly pigmented skin is often quoted as being 15 times higher than in persons with less pigmented skin.[30] Furthermore, black patients have been noted to have a twofold increase in risk for keloid development as compared with Hispanic and Asian patients.[31,32] Interestingly, a random sampling of black individuals revealed that as many as 16% had reported developing keloid scars. Caucasians and albinos are reportedly least likely to be affected.[33] Chinese individuals were noted to be more likely to develop keloids as compared with Indian or Malaysian individuals.[30]

Lim et al.[34] report that 200 million skin incisions are performed annually worldwide, and approximately 170,000 surgical scar revisions are performed in the United States alone. It has also been reported that in Hong Kong alone, 350,000 surgical procedures are performed each year for problematic scars, with more than 40% of patients suffering from pruritus and pain.[35,36] In a study by Li-Tsang et al.[35] in 2005, patients admitted to the Department of Orthopaedics and Traumatology were screened for HTS formation 30 days after nonburn-related orthopedic surgery conducted from May 2003 to December 2003.[36] In their review, the authors reported an incidence of HTS formation of 70%. The incidence of problem scar development in their burn population was felt to well exceed this value. In contradistinction to other published studies that found that the likelihood of developing HTS was very low in the elderly patient population (generally attributed to the slower metabolic rates and diminished skin tensile strength found in the mature patient[37]), Li-Tsang et al. observed a relatively high prevalence rate among their older patients. This not only implies an increased incidence, but also suggests that the problem may be more severe in the younger Chinese population. It is important to note that although the study was objectively performed and evidence based, it was undertaken rather early in the postoperative period. Longer-term follow-ups would be very helpful in elucidating the overall impact and long-term effects in this study population, as certainly the number of patients with postsurgical wounds far exceeds the number of thermally injured patients. Keloids, although not the intended study subject, can develop from 6 months to 2 years after an inciting cause. This highlights the fact that follow-up periods in most studies are inadequate.[38]

The incidence of HTS formation following cleft lip repair, although perhaps not often reported, appears to range somewhere between 1% and 50%. Cleft lip is one of the most common congenital anomalies requiring surgical correction, occurring at a rate of 79.1 per 100,000 live births.[39] A review of 186 charts of patients who underwent primary cleft lip repair by a single surgeon at Children's Hospital Los Angeles from June 1990 to June 2005 identified HTS in 25%. The incidence was elevated in patients with darker pigmentation, although no gender differences were noted.[40]

Patients who have suffered facial trauma and scarring have been noted to experience significant negative social and functional impact. A retrospective study performed at Yale included healthy 8- to 45-year-old individuals who experienced a facial laceration of 3 cm or greater and/or a fractured facial bone requiring operative intervention within 6 months to 2 years of presentation. Patients experienced a statistically significant lower satisfaction with life, more negative perceptions of body image, a higher incidence of PTSD, higher incidences of alcoholism, and an increase in depression. The authors also noted a significantly higher incidence of unemployment, marital problems, binge drinking, jail, and lower attractiveness scores.[41] These findings are, unfortunately, not unique and complement the clinical experiences of psychologist, psychiatrists, and other investigators in the field.[42–45] Interestingly, patient-rated facial scar severity was not necessarily predictive for self-esteem and depressive symptoms in patients. This observation was also noted by Hoogewerf et al.[46] in their study of thermally injured patients. The authors concluded that routine psychological screening should be performed during hospitalization in order to identify patients at risk and to optimize their treatment.

Demographically, the incidence of injuries occurring in high-income countries has been noted to be decreasing in recent years, albeit at a slower rate than the incidence of illness. This is in contradistinction to low- and middle-income countries, where both death and disability from injuries are increasing very rapidly. In this latter group, in men aged 15 to 44 years in the Americas, Europe, and the Eastern Mediterranean, more than 30% of DALYs caused either by death or disability were from injury.[47]

The Future

Over the past decades, new concepts in scar management (as depicted in other chapters of this textbook) have evolved, yet this topic is often minimally addressed in current medical school curricula. Our enhanced understanding of the pathophysiology of scarring and evolving mitigation and therapeutic strategies has changed practice for many, and provided both patients and caregivers novel opportunities and options. Much of this has been reported, discussed, and promoted at congresses round the world, from national tissue repair society meetings to global world healing conferences, and from burn meetings to internal medical society meetings focused on specific organ pathologies such as those complicating liver and kidney disease. Although generally presented in smaller focused topic sessions, this is slowly changing. Specialized meetings such as the Scar Club, the annual C.A.R.E. (Comprehensive Advanced Restorative Effort) Summit at the Naval Medical Center San Diego, and the Burn Plastic and Reconstructive Special Interest Group have addressed this dilemma and focused on encouraging specialists in this field to congregate and to deal in depth with new experimental findings and clinical results. Although few true educational platforms are currently in place, an even more global approach is sure to develop.

Decades ago unmet needs and deficiencies in wound healing led to the formation of specialized wound care providers who are certified according to evidence-based curricula. In consequence, this has resulted in improved wound care with enhanced outcomes for patients yet reduced cost. Similarly, one may consider a certified health professional in scar management favorable to improve outcomes for the scarred patient. Scar management courses could be a training platform for this specialized entity. Additional certification may not only improve care and outcomes for the patients, but may strengthen the concept of excessive or abnormal cutaneous scarring as a disease comparable to liver cirrhosis or kidney fibrosis. This strategy lays the groundwork for potentially improving financial coverage for our patients by insurance companies, leading to special scar management centers in the future, which will recruit certified specialists to further improve scar care.

Our perception of scars is multidimensional, reflecting our cultural and educational exposures. In Greek mythology, Odysseus's identity as a courageous team player, a quality essential for success in battle, is established when he suffers an injury and resultant scar while on a hunt for wild boar as a child; that scar subsequently confirms his identity on his return to Ithaca as a disguised adult. Termed bragging scars or Mensur scars, scars incurred in battle and in sport were often viewed favorably as badges of courage and honor. This was particularly true in academic centers that promoted fencing, as well as for the military.[48–50] Otto von Bismarck reportedly felt that a man's courage could be judged by the number of scars on his cheeks.[51,52]

It is interesting to note how scars are often presented in the visual world of cinema and Hollywood. Of all skin conditions seen in movies, scars have been prevalent and evident in cinema since its inception. Hypertrophic forms are generally easy to replicate, with the resultant shadowing readily visible even in classical black and white format, the results of which can prove incredibly lifelike and clinically representative, yet often exaggerated and easily distinguishable from real scars. Accordingly, scars are utilized to differentiate and establish character, reflecting, and sometimes promoting, either prejudice or pathos.

In classic black and white character depictions of old films, actors with scarred skin often represented evil, whereas the skin of the favored protagonist was depicted as smooth and unblemished. Prominent scars are often associated with violence, a criminal past, war, torture, and terror. This persists even today in modern animated features such as *The Lion King*, in which a scarred face personifies the evil antagonist named "Scar." Horror movies (e.g., *Frankenstein*) have always used severely scarred skin to frighten, alienate, and differentiate. It is interesting to note in controversy that in classical Greek and Roman times, success against evil was closely linked to scarred skin. And even today in some films (e.g., *Rocky*) the scar reflects the face of an actor who has survived trials and pain.

When depicted with scars, women, in contradistinction to men, are mostly, but not always, characterized as inferior and disfigured poignantly when the scripted characterization changes from good to evil. The breadth and cultural permeation of these arts can prove challenging for those coping with the physical manifestations and psychological effects of scars.

Our interventions as clinical care specialists will have to take these factors into account. The importance placed on artists as role models can similarly afford positive influence, depending upon provenance and intent. Fiscal, employment, and cultural sensitivities no doubt play a role. Currently, only a very few notable actors do not hide their scars; they may prove positive role models for patients with severely scared skin. Even in language, it is often impossible to dissociate the vernacular attributes of an emotional scar and physical deformity.

When to Treat?

The question of which scars to treat depends upon a number of clinical factors and patient perceptions (see Chapter 4). Basically, there are four *S*s to consider: the site of the scar, symptoms, severity of functional impairment, and the stigma perceived by the patient. Are they located in "high-visibility" areas? Are they located on joints or pressure areas such as the palms or plantar feet? What symptoms are the scars associated with (e.g., pain, pruritus, contracture "stretching," or hyperesthesia)? To what degree is there functional impairment of a joint, skin segment, neck, orifice, or digit? How does the patient perceive how "other people" view his or her scar? Lastly, what is the patient's overall concern about the scarred area?

It is reasonable to expect continued advancements in our understanding of wound healing, scar development, and amelioration to alter and improve therapeutic management. Preventive efforts including improvements in working conditions, safety, construction, and ergonomics will perhaps continue to lessen the incidence of devastating accidents and injuries. What role these future advances will play in decreasing disability and managing costs is difficult to say. Will the use of biologics and biosynthetics minimize postinjury deformity, and will this be associated with reduced cost and improved benefit to patients? Will evolving laser therapies and cellular, genetic, chemotherapeutic, stem cell, surgical, and rehabilitative efforts provide answers and strategies to improve quality of life for all? A daunting and incredibly important effort, no doubt.

REFERENCES

1. Walmsley GG, Mann ZN, Wong VW, et al. Scarless wound healing: chasing the holy. *Grail Plast Reconstr Surg*. 2015;135:907.
2. Young VL, Hutchinson J. Insights into patient and clinician concerns about scar appearance: semiquantitative structured surveys. *Plast Reconstr Surg*. 2009;124:256–265.
3. Ten Broek RP, Isssa Y, Van Santbrink E, et al. Burden of adhesions in abdominal and pelvic surgery: systematic review and met-analysis. *BMJ*. 2013;347:f5588.
4. Yu N, Long X, Lujan-Hernandez J, et al. Marjolin's ulcer: a preventable malignancy arising from scars. *World J Surg Oncol*. 2013;11:313.
5. Pekarek B, Buck S, Osher L. A comprehensive review on Marjolin's ulcers: diagnosis and treatment. *J Am Coll Certif Wound Spec*. 2011;3(3), 60–64.
6. Brockes JP, Kumar A, Velloso CP. Regeneration as an evolutionary variable. *J Anat*. 2001;199(pt 1/2):3–11.
7. Singer AJ, Clark RA. Cutaneous wound healing. *N Engl J Med*. 1999;341:738–746.
8. Berman B, Viera M, Amini S, et al. Prevention and management of hypertrophic scars and keloids. *J Craniofac Surg*. 2008;19(4):889–1005.
9. Hawkins H, Pereira C. Pathophysiology of the burn scar. In: Herndon D, ed. *Total Burn Care*. 3rd ed. Philadelphia, PA: Saunders-Elsevier; 2007:608.
10. Arno A, Gauglitz G, Barret J, et al. Up-to-date approach to manage keloids and hypertrophic scars: a useful guide. *Burns*. 2014;40(7):1255–1266.
11. Aarabi S, Longaker M, Gurtner G. Hypertophic scar formation following burns and trauma: new approaches to treatment. *PLoS Med*. 2007;4(9), e234, 1–7.
12. Wofram D, Tzankov A, Pülzl P, et al. Hypertrophic scars and keloids—a review of their pathophysiology, risk factors, and therapeutic management. *Dermatol Surg*. 2009;35:171–181.
13. Bayat A, McGrouther DA, Ferguson WJ. Skin scarring. *BMJ*. 2003;326(7380):88–92.
14. Lawrence J, Mason S, Schomer K, et al. Epidemiology and impact of scarring after burn injury: a systematic review of the literature. *J Burn Care Res*. 2012;33:136–146.
15. Brusselaers N, Pirayesh A, Hoeksema H, et al. Burn scar assessment: a systematic review of different scar scales. *J Surg Res*. 2010;164(1):e115–e123.
16. Bombaro K, Engrav L, Carrougher G, et al. What is the prevalence of hypertrophic scarring post burn? *Burns*. 2003;(29):299–302.
17. Mirastschijski U, Sander J, Weyand B, et al. Rehabilitation of burn patients: an underestimated socio-economic burden. *Burns*. 2013;39:262–268.
18. Deitch EA, Wheelahan TM, Rose MP, et al. Hypertrophic burn scars: analysis of variables. *J Trauma*. 1983;23(10):895–898.
19. Spurr ED, Shakespeare PG. Incidence of hypertrophic scarring in burn-injured children. *Burns*. 1990;3:179–181.
20. Stella M, Castagnoli C, Gangemi EN. Post burn scars: an update. *J Low Extrem Wounds*. 2008;7:176.
21. Lawrence HW, Rosenberg LE, Fauerbach JA. Comparing the body esteem of pediatric survivors of burn injury with the body esteem of an age-matched comparison group without burns. *Rehabil Psychol*. 2007;5:370–379.
22. Gangemi EN, Gregori D, Berchialla P, et al. Epidemiology and risk factors for pathologic scarring after burn wounds. *Arch Facial Plast Surg*. 2008;10(2):93–102.
23. Widgerow AD. Hypertrophic burn scar evolution and management. *Wound Heal South Afr*. 2013;6(2):79–86.
24. Hop MJ, Langengber C, Hiddingh J, et al. Reconstructive surgery after burns: a 10 year follow-up study. *Burns*. 2014;(40):1544–1551.
25. Peck M. Epidemiology of burs throughout the world. Part 1 Distribution and risk factors. *Burns*. 2011;37:1087–1100.
26. Hyder AA, Surgerman DE, Puvanachandra P, et al. Global childhood unintentional injury surveillance in four cities in developing countries: a pilot study. *Bull World Health Organ*. 2009;87:345–352.
27. Peck M. Epidemiology of burns throughout the World. Part II: Intentional burns in adults. *Burns*. 2012;38:630–637.
28. Sanghavi P, Bhalla K, Das V. Fire-related deaths in India in 2001: a retrospective analysis of data. *Lancet*. 2009;373:1282–1288.
29. Borsini M, Mandruzzato G, Lasagna G, et al. Epidemiologia della cicatrice da ustione Esperienza personale. In: Magliacani G, Teich Alasia S, eds. *XIII Congresso Nazionale SIU La cicatrice patologica*. Naples, Italy: Giuseppe De Nicola; 1998:85–88.

30. Alhady SM, Sivanantharajah K. Keloids in various races. A review of 175 cases. *Plast Reconstr Surg*. 1969;44(6):564–566.
31. Desmoulière A, Chaponnier C, Gabbiani G. Tissue repair, contraction, and the myofibroblast. *Wound Repair Regen*. 2005;13(1):7–12.
32. Deitch EA, Wheelahan TM, Paige Rose M, et al. Hypertrophic burn scars: analysis of variables. *J Trauma*. 1983;23(10):895–898.
33. Jansen D, Molnar J. Keloids. In: *Medscape*. http://emedicine.medscape.com/article/1298013-overview. Accessed June 3, 2016.
34. Lim AF, Weintraub J, Kaplan EN, et al. The embrace device significantly decreases scarring following scar revision surgery in a randomized controlled trial. *Plast Reconstr Surg*. 2014;133(2):398–405.
35. Li-Tsang C, Lau J, Chan C. Prevalence of hypertrophic scar formation and its characteristics among the Chinese population. *Burns*. 2005;31:610–616.
36. Hong Kong Hospital Authority. *Hospital Authority Statistical Report—Operation, X-ray Examination and Pathology Test Performed in Hospital Authority*. Hong Kong: Hong Kong Hospital Authority; 2003;131.
37. Oluwasanmi JO. Keloids in the Africa. *Clin Plast Surg*. 1974;1:179–86.
38. McCarty M. An evaluation of evidence regarding application of silicone gel sheeting for the management of hypertrophic scars and keloids. *J Clin Aesthet Dermatol*. 2010; 3(11): 39–43.
39. Martin JA, Hamilton BE, Sutton PD, et al. Births: final data for 2005. *Natl Vital Stat Rep*. 2007;56(6):1–103.
40. Soltani AM, Francis CS, Motamed A, et al. Hypertrophic scarring in cleft lip repair: a comparison of incidence among ethnic groups. *Clin Epidemiol*. 2012:4 187–191.
41. Levine E, Dequitis L, Pruzinsky T, et al. Quality of life and facial trauma psychological and body image effects. *Ann Plast Surg*. 2005;54:502–510.
42. Neale HW, Billmire DA, Carey JP. Reconstruction following head and neck burns. *Clin Plast Surg*. 1986;13:119–136.
43. Williams EE, Griffiths TA. Psychological consequences of burn injury. *Burns*. 1991;17:478–480.
44. Shepherd JP, Qureshi R, Preston MS, et al. Psychological distress after assaults and accidents. *BMJ*. 1990;301:849.
45. Bisson JI, Shepherd JP, Dhutia M. Psychological sequelae of facial trauma. *J Trauma*. 1997;43:495–500.
46. Hoogewerf CJ, van Baar ME, Middelkoop E, et al. Impact of facial burns: relationship between depressive symptoms, self-esteem and scar severity. *Gen Hosp Psychiatry*. 2014;(36):271–276.
47. Baker SP, O'Neill B, Ginsburg MJ, et al. *The Injury Fact Book*. 2nd ed., Lexington, Mass: Lexington Books; 1992.
48. DeMello M. *Encyclopedia of Body Adornment*. Westport, CT: Greenwood Publishing Group; 2007:237.
49. Keener C. Real Men Have Dueling Scars. *How Stuff Works*. May 4, 2009.
50. Where students fight. Scarred faces are common sights at Heidelberg. *Daily Bulletin Supplement (San Francisco)*. July 12, 1890.
51. Duelling in Berlin. *The Galveston Daily News*. November 9, 1886.
52. McAleer K. *Dueling: The Cult of Honor in Fin-de-siècle Germany*. Princeton, NJ: Princeton University Press; 1994.

3 Medical Conditions Associated with Scarring and Fibrosis

KEITH OLSEN, WILLIAM JAMES, and NICOLE FETT

KEY POINTS

- Many medical conditions present with scar-like lesions.
- These scar-like lesions often have different pathogenic pathways than scars induced by trauma.
- Understanding the similarities and differences in the pathogenic pathways of scar formation and scar-like lesion formation may help us to treat, rehabilitate, and prevent scars and scar-like lesions.

The purpose of this chapter is to familiarize you with medical conditions that mimic scars clinically, histologically, or both clinically and histologically. We have grouped these medical entities based upon the underlying pathogenic mechanisms resulting in scar-like lesions (Table 3-1). The pathogenic mechanisms include sclerosing disorders, fibrosing disorders, inflammatory diseases, acquired depositional disorders, genetic or metabolic alterations, induction via drug, toxin, or radiation, neoplastic conditions, and infectious processes. We have structured each topic to provide a brief description of the condition, basic epidemiologic data, underlying pathogenic mechanisms (when understood), how the underlying pathogenic mechanisms differ from those of normal scar formation, and treatment options. Our references will include the most recent review articles, if you desire additional information.

Sclerosing Disorders: Morphea, Lichen Sclerosus, Systemic Sclerosis

Sclerosing conditions are conditions with a histological increase in collagen fibers without an associated increase in fibroblasts.

The pathogenesis of sclerosing disorders differs from that of scar formation in the following ways. The pathogenesis of sclerosing disorders does not appear to rely upon external trauma to trigger sclerosis. Whereas normal wound healing results in vascular proliferation, blood vessels are obliterated in sclerosing disorders.[1] Although neutrophils play a prominent role in normal wound healing, they are lacking in sclerosing disorders and instead the early inflammatory infiltrate is comprised primarily of lymphocytes and plasma cells.[1] There is no epithelialization phase in the development of sclerosis; rather sclerosing disorders transition directly from inflammation to fibroplasia. Additionally, in sclerosing disorders there is a persistence of myofibroblasts, which usually undergo apoptosis in normal wound healing. There is some evidence that the fibroblasts in sclerosing disorders begin producing their own transforming growth factor (TGF)-β, which potentiates the unregulated sclerosis.[2]

Morphea

Morphea is a rare, autoimmune, clinically heterogeneous sclerosing disorder of the skin and subcutaneous structures.[3] Morphea is more common in whites and women, has an equal prevalence in children and adults, and an estimated incidence of 0.4 to 2.7 per 100,000 people.[3] Morphea presents as five clinical subtypes of disease: circumscribed (with superficial and deep variants), linear (with superficial and deep variants), generalized (defined as four or more plaques larger than 3 cm in diameter on two or more body surface regions, also with superficial and deep variants), mixed variant (combination of circumscribed and linear, or linear and generalized), and pansclerotic (sclerosis that spans the epidermis and subcutaneous tissues and involves all body surface areas other than the fingers and toes). Morphea is characterized as having an "active phase" (when patients are developing new lesions, have expansion of existing lesions, or demonstrate signs of inflammation on clinical exam) and a "damage" or "burnt-out phase" (when no new lesions are forming, lesion size is stable, and there are no clinical signs of inflammation). All subtypes of morphea present with sclerotic plaques clinically resembling scars, with varying amounts of surrounding inflammation (Fig. 3-1).

Histopathologically, early lesions of morphea reveal perivascular infiltrates composed of plasma cells and lymphocytes and increase in collagen deposition (Fig. 3-2). In late lesions of morphea, the inflammatory infiltrate remits,

Table 3-1 Scar-like conditions organized by pathogenic mechanism

Sclerosing disorders

- Morphea
- Systemic sclerosis

Fibrosing conditions

- Dupuytren's
- Peyronie's
- Nodular fasciitis
- Ledderhose
- Knuckle pads
- Pachydermodactyly
- Ainhum

Inflammatory disorders

- Eosinophilic fasciitis
- Sclerodermoid GVHD
- Lichen planopilaris/frontal fibrosing alopecia
- Malignant atrophic papulosis (perhaps should be in a "vascular" section)
- Morpheaform sarcoidosis
- Discoid lupus erythematosus
- Epidermolysis bullosa acquisita
- Lipodermatosclerosis
- Subcutaneous fat necrosis of the newborn
- Sclerema neonatorum

Acquired depositional disorders

- Scleredema
- Scleromyxedema

Genetic/metabolic

- Progerias
- Porphyrias
- Ehlers–Danlos Syndrome
- Lipoid proteinosis
- Epidermolysis bullosa–junctional, dystrophic, Kindler's
- Juvenile hyaline fibromatosis
- Werner's
- Stiff Skin Syndrome
- Pachydermoperiostosis

Drug/toxin/radiation induced

- Bleomycin
- Taxanes
- Nephrogenic systemic fibrosis
- Eosinophilia–myalgia secondary to tryptophan
- Toxic oil syndrome
- Radiodermatitis (chronic)
- Pentazocine
- Vitamin K sclerosis (Texier's)
- Oral submucous fibrosis

Neoplastic

- Morpheaform BCC
- Dermatofibroma
- DFSP
- Dermatomyofibroma
- Dermoid tumor
- Infantile fibromatosis (diffuse and digital)
- Connective tissue nevi
- Fibromatosis colli
- Angiofibroma
- Sclerotic fibroma (Cowden's associated)

Infectious

- Lobomycosis

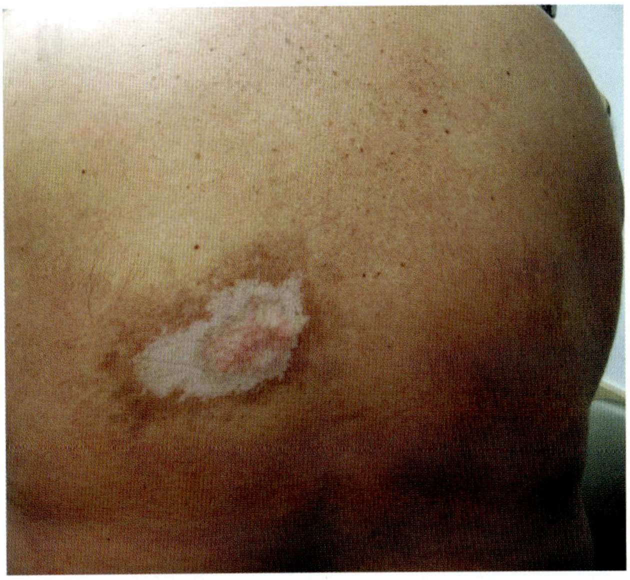

FIGURE 3-1 Morphea—white sclerotic plaque with surrounding hyperpigmentation.

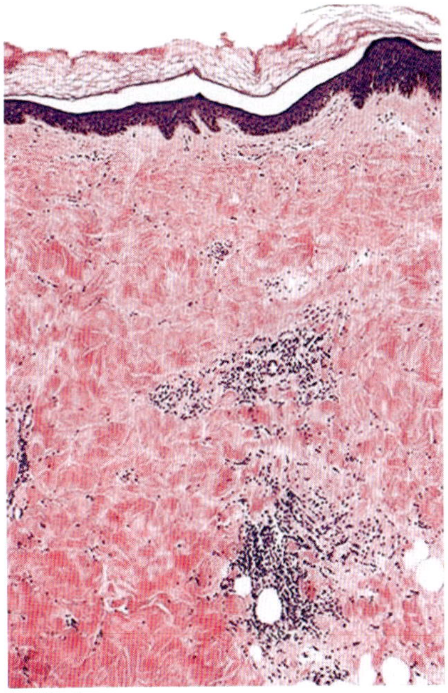

FIGURE 3-2 Morphea early histology—perivascular lymphocytic infiltrate with increased collagen deposition and loss of fat and adnexal structures.

and the dermis and subcutaneous fat are replaced by thick, pale sclerotic collagen bundles (Fig. 3-3). Dermal appendages and blood vessels are replaced by collagen.

The pathogenesis of morphea is incompletely understood at this time. Patients with morphea are likely to have an underlying genetic predisposition based on familial clustering with other autoimmune diseases and specific human leukocyte antigen (HLA) subtypes identified as predisposing factors.[4,5] Several environmental factors have been postulated to be part of the pathogenesis of disease, including Lyme disease, trauma, radiation, medications, and viral infections.[6] Autoantibodies may also be a part of the pathogenesis. Patients with morphea frequently have positive antinuclear antibodies (ANAs), single-stranded

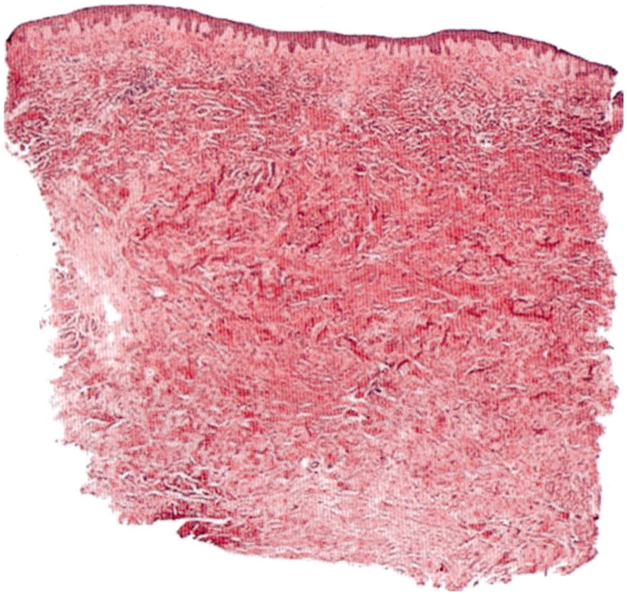

FIGURE 3-3 Morphea late histology—increased dermal collagen with loss of blood vessels, adnexa, and fat.

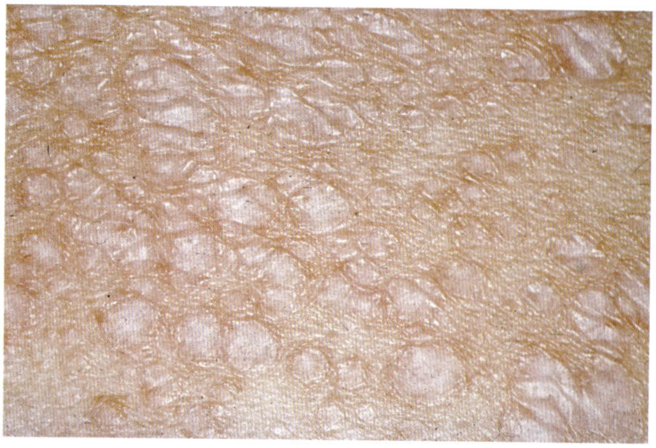

FIGURE 3-4 Lichen sclerosus et atrophicus (LSA)—white thin sclerotic macules with epidermal atrophy.

DNA antibodies, antihistone antibodies, rheumatoid factor, and anti-topoisomerase IIα antibodies.[3] The sclerosis in morphea lesions is thought to be initiated by vascular injury via environmental exposure or autoantibodies. Endothelial injury causes release of cytokines that cause increased expression of vascular cell adhesion molecule 1 (VCAM-1), intercellular adhesion molecule 1 (ICAM-1), and E-selectin.[3] The result is an initial inflammatory response characterized by T_H1^+ cells, interleukin (IL)-2, interferon gamma (IFN-γ), and tumor necrosis factor alpha (TNF-α).[7] Profibrotic cytokines such as IL-4 and -6 and TGF-β are expressed, which recruit eosinophils, $CD4^+$ T cells, and macrophages.[3] Expression of IL-6 is thought to transition the T_H1^+ environment to a T_H17 environment, and then ultimately a T_H2^+ environment characterized by IL-4 and -13.[7] This prosclerotic environment results in increases in collagen, fibronectin, and proteoglycan and a decrease in proteases.

Treatment of morphea is determined based on subtype and phase.[6] Active circumscribed morphea is typically treated with topical immunosuppressants or phototherapy. Active linear morphea is typically treated with systemic immunosuppressants. Active generalized and pansclerotic morphea are typically treated with phototherapy or systemic immunosuppressants. Treatment of the damage phase of morphea is limited by lack of data. Case reports of fillers, lasers, and fat transplants to correct contractures and disfigurement have been published.[8–18]

Lichen Sclerosus

Lichen sclerosus (LS) is a rare sclerosing disorder with a predilection for anogenital skin. LS commonly occurs in patients with morphea and may be a morphea variant. LS is much more common in women than in men and has a bimodal onset (prepubertal children and postmenopausal women).[19] Patients with LS are more likely to have a personal history of additional autoimmune diseases, such as vitiligo and autoimmune thyroiditis, and a family history of autoimmunity than healthy controls.[19] LS presents with white sclerotic plaques, typically on the anogenital skin (Fig. 3-4). The degree of sclerosis can be severe, leading to functional impairment including dysuria, constipation, and sexual dysfunction. The pathogenesis of the disease is not elucidated to date; however, genetics (particularly associations with HLAs), autoimmunity (development of anti-extracellular matrix 1 antibodies), hormones, and recurrent irritation have been proposed to serve pathogenic roles.[19] The chronic inflammation associated with LS leads to vulvar intraepithelial neoplasia (VIN), which increases the risk of development of anogenital squamous cell carcinoma (SCC). Patients with LS should be monitored closely for this potential complication.[20,21] LS is typically treated with superpotent topical steroids. Adherence to topical steroid maintenance therapy has been shown to decrease the risk of VIN and SCC.[22]

Systemic Sclerosis

Systemic Sclerosis is a rare autoimmune sclerosing disorder of the skin and internal organs with an estimated prevalence of 150 to 300 cases per million.[23] Systemic sclerosis is subdivided into two clinically distinct phenotypes: limited cutaneous systemic sclerosis (LcSScl) and diffuse cutaneous systemic sclerosis (DcSScl).[24] Both phenotypes are characterized by Raynaud's phenomenon, positive ANA, nailfold capillary changes (dilation and hemorrhage in early stages and nailfold capillary drop out and irregular arborizing vessels in later stages), sclerodactyly, and a high risk of interstitial lung disease. The patterns of skin sclerosis, autoantibodies, and additional organ involvement in the phenotypic subsets differ in the following ways. Patients with LcSScl have sclerosis that is distal to the elbows and knees, though the head and neck may also be involved. By definition, patients with DcSScl have sclerosis that extends proximal to the elbows and knees. Patients with LcSScl are more likely to have anti-centromere antibodies, whereas patients with DcSScl are more likely to express anti-Scl 70 (also called anti-topoisomerase) antibodies, and

Table 3-2 Autoantibodies and Associations

Autoantibody	Associated Diagnoses	Associated Complications
Antinuclear antibody (ANA)	Systemic lupus erythematosus (SLE) Dermatomyositis Polymyositis Sjögren's syndrome Systemic sclerosis Mixed connective tissue disease Autoimmune hepatitis	
Anticentromere antibodies	Limited cutaneous systemic sclerosis	Pulmonary artery hypertension, esophageal dysmotility, Raynaud's phenomenon
Anti-topoisomerase-1 (anti-Scl-70)	Diffuse cutaneous systemic sclerosis	Lung fibrosis
Anti-RNA polymerase III	Diffuse cutaneous systemic sclerosis	Renal crisis

anti-RNA polymerase III antibodies (Table 3-2). Patients with LcSScl are more likely to develop isolated pulmonary artery hypertension (which is sclerosis of the pulmonary artery), whereas patients with DcSScl are more likely to develop renal crisis, likely due to sclerosis of the arcuate and intralobular arteries in the glomeruli.[25] The organ sclerosis that occurs in systemic sclerosis results in high morbidity and mortality.

The pathophysiology of systemic sclerosis is exceedingly complex and incompletely understood. In broad strokes, it is felt that genetics (polymorphisms in *HLA class II* gene region, *IRF5*, *CD247*, *BANK1*, *STAT4*, *TNFSF4*, *BLK*, *C8orf13*, *IL-23R*, and *TBX21* genes)[26,27] and environmental factors (exposure to vinyl chloride, silica dust and organic solvents, medications such as bleomycin, pentazocine, cocaine, and viruses)[27] instigate an inflammatory response that is initially targeted against blood vessels. Endothelial cell damage results in upregulation of cellular adhesion molecules (VCAM, ICAM, E-selectin), chemokines (CCL 2,5,7,17,22,27, CXCL8), recruitment and activation of platelets, altered capillary permeability, and vasoconstriction (via endothelin-1).[2,28] The cellular adhesion molecules and chemokines recruit perivascular $CD3^+$ and $CD4^+$ mononuclear cells that express CD45, HLA-DR, and the IL-2 receptor and which secrete fibrogenic cytokines and chemokines (IL-1, -2, -4, -5, -6, -8, -12, -13, -17, TNF-α, and IFN-α and IFN-γ).[2,7,26,29] These lesional T cells have restricted specificities representative of oligoclonal T-cell expansion.[2] Systemic sclerosis is ultimately characterized by a shift in the T_H1 to T_H2 cytokine balance, favoring T_H2 cytokines.[2] Production of these cytokines results in inflammation, and recruitment and activation of fibroblasts and myofibroblasts, which make collagen 1, 3, 6, 7, fibronectin, and glycosaminoglycans (GAGs), resulting in fibrosis.[30] The signaling that results in overproduction of collagens, fibronectin, and GAGs in systemic sclerosis is multifaceted and involves TGF-β signaling through SMAD and SMAD-independent pathways, platelet-derived growth factor receptors (PDGFRc), canonical Wnt signaling, sonic hedgehog (SHH) signaling, aberrations in Notch signaling, microRNA signaling (particularly miR29 and miR29a), histone modifications,[30,31] and alterations in transcription factors (SP1, SMAD3, ETS1, early growth response 1, CCAAT-binding factor, SP3, CCAAT/enhancer binding protein, Y box-binding protein 1, c-KROX, and FLI-1).[2] Additionally, B-cell dysfunction may contribute to fibrosis by not only making pathogenic autoantibodies, but by secreting IL-6, which directly stimulates fibroblasts.[2]

Fibrosing Disorders: Dupuytren's, Peyronie's, Plantar Fibromatosis (Ledderhose), Knuckle Pads, Pachydermodactyly, Nodular Fasciitis, Ainhum

Fibrosing conditions are conditions with a histological increase in collagen fibers and a concomitant increase in fibroblasts.

Fibrosing conditions and scar formation share several similarities. Micro-traumas have been implicated in the development of fibrosing conditions. Both fibrosing disorders and scars have proliferation of fibroblasts and myofibroblasts and alteration in TGF-β, fibronectin, and Heat Shock Protein 47 signaling.[32] However, in fibrosing disorders alterations in pathways of fibrosis appear to be prolonged, and fibroblasts and myofibroblasts persist. Fibrosing disorders appear to be tightly tied to genetic predisposition, metabolic derangement (diabetes), and environmental exposures (tobacco and alcohol abuse). Dupuytren's disease (DP) and the knuckle pads seen in Bart–Pumphrey syndrome have both been shown to have abnormalities in connexin 26 expression compared to normal wound healing. The recent discovery of the *MYH9-USP6* fusion gene in nodular fasciitis may further inform our understanding of fibrosis in the future.

Dupuytren's

DP is a relatively common fibroproliferative disorder of the aponeurotic fascial fibers of the palm of the hand that ultimately results in flexion contractures of the fingers (Fig. 3-5). DP is most common in men of Northern European descent.[33] The development of Dupuytren's is divided into three stages (1) the proliferation phase—during which fibroblasts gather within the fascial fibers; (2) the involutional phase—during which fibroblasts align along the lines of tension and differentiate into myofibroblasts;

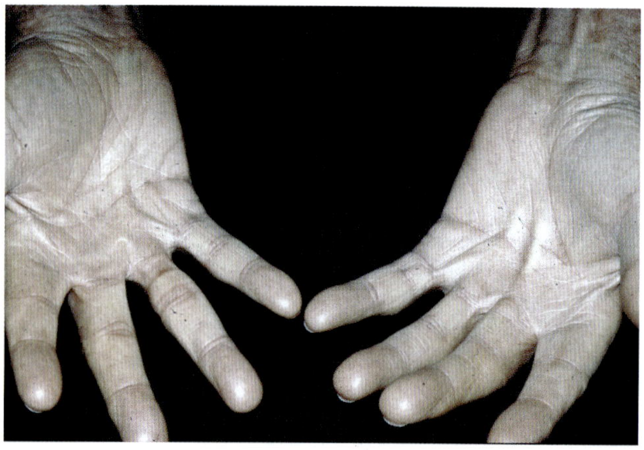

FIGURE 3-5 Dupuytren's contractures—subcutaneous palmar cords with associated finger contractions.

and (3) the residual phase—during which collagen formation predominates.[33]

The pathogenesis of DP is incompletely understood and is likely due to an interplay of genetic predisposition and environmental factors. Genetic factors are believed to play a strong role in disease development, with heritability estimated as high as 80% in the Danish population.[33,34] Genome-wide association studies have revealed relevant mutations in genes within the Wnt pathway (*WNT4*, *WNT2*, *WNT7B*, *RSPO2*).[35] HLA associations including HLADrB3, HLA A1 B8 Dr3, HLA DRB1*15[33]; changes in TGF-β signaling secondary to single nucleotide polymorphisms (SNPs) in the gene encoding transcription factor Zf9; and a heteroplasmic mutation located within the mitochondrial 16s ribosomal RNA region have been described.[33] Changes in microRNA expression that affect Wnt and β-catenin signaling have been discovered,[33,36] and a lack of downregulation of connexins 26, 30 and 43 has also been demonstrated.[32] Associated environmental factors include smoking, diabetes, and alcohol use.[33,36] Either through these genetic and environmental changes or other mechanisms that have yet to be described, changes occur in the immune system including the formation of autoantibodies to collagens 1 through 4, autoreactive T cells, and severe dysregulation of molecular pathways involved in wound healing and fibrosis including upregulation of TGF-β, IL-1, β-fibroblast growth factor (FGF), PDGF; increased production of collagen, periostin, tenascin, β-catenin, α5β1, fibronectin, and proteoglycan 4; and dysregulation of matrix metalloproteinases (MMPs).[33] DP is often treated with injection of collagenase from *Clostridium histolyticum* and surgery for recalcitrant cases.

Peyronie's

Peyronie's disease (PD) is caused by fibrosis of the tunica albuginea of the penis, resulting in penile curvature. PD is estimated to affect up to 9% men, with incidence increasing with age.[37] PD begins with an active phase, during which the patient has pain with erections, and develops progressive curvature of the penis. The quiescent phase follows a mean of 18 months later. During the quiescent phase, the penile deformity remains stable, but there is resolution of the pain.[37] The pathogenesis of PD is hypothesized to be due to abnormal wound healing induced by microbleeding within the tunica albuginea after microtrauma to the penis.[37,38] It is hypothesized that the fibrin produced with microbleeding recruits inflammatory cells and platelets, which produce inflammatory cytokines (TGF-β, PDGF, FGF, IL-1, TNF-α, plasminogen activator inhibitor-1), cause oxidative stress and ultimately excessive collagen deposition.[38] Gene expression patterns for genes regulating collagen degradation, ossification, and myofibroblast differentiation have been shown to be similar in DP and PD.[39] Overlap of DP and PD happens in 10% to 40% of patients.[38] PD is treated with injection of collagenase derived from *C. histolyticum* and surgery for refractory cases.

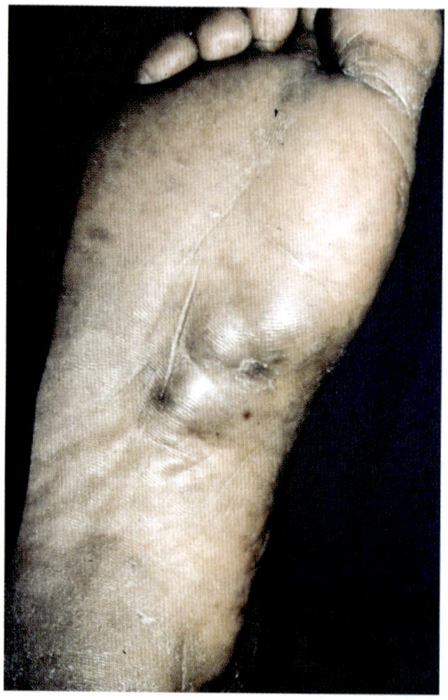

FIGURE 3-6 Plantar fibromatosis—subcutaneous plantar nodules.

Plantar Fibromatosis

Plantar fibromatosis (Ledderhose disease) is the development of superficial collagen nodules within the nonweight-bearing medial band of the plantar aponeurosis (Fig. 3-6).[40,41] Like DP it is associated with diabetes, with alcohol overuse, and in men.[40,41] Plantar fibromatosis often coexists with DP and PD. The pathogenesis of plantar fibromatosis to date has not been investigated. It is assumed that the pathogenic mechanisms of DP are similar to those causing plantar fibromatosis. Plantar fibromatosis is not treated unless patients experience pain. If the nodules are painful or limit mobility, conservative treatments include anti-inflammatories, cortisone injections, physical therapy, and orthotics. For those patients with refractory disease, radiotherapy, surgery, and extracorporeal shock wave therapy are therapeutic options, although recurrence rates are high.[40]

Knuckle Pads

Knuckle pads are asymptomatic nodules over the extensor proximal interphalangeal (PIP) joints that usually appear

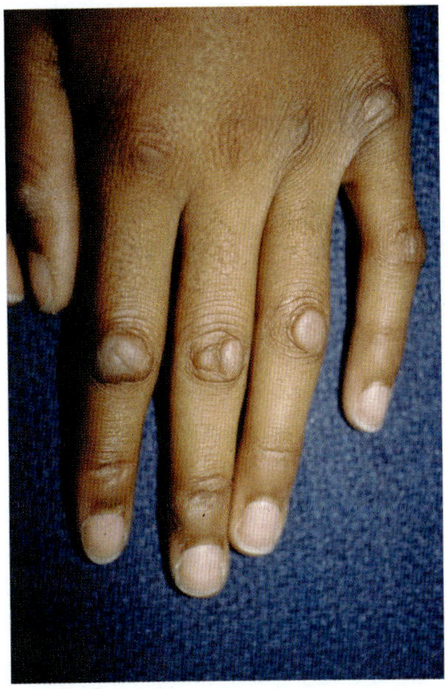

FIGURE 3-7 Knuckle pads—flesh-colored nodules over the extensor hand joints.

between the ages of 15 and 30 years (Fig. 3-7).[42] Knuckle pads have been observed to occur concomitantly with other superficial fibromatoses, although their pathogenesis has not been studied. Knuckle pads are a cutaneous finding of Bart–Pumphrey syndrome (knuckle pads, leukonychia, palmoplantar keratoderma, and deafness caused by an autosomal dominant mutation in the *GJB2* gene). Histologically, the nodules are made up of fibroblasts and collagen. Due to their asymptomatic nature and difficult-to-treat location, knuckle pads are not usually treated.

Pachydermodactyly

Pachydermodactyly (PDD) is asymptomatic thickening of the periarticular skin of the PIPs.[43] PDD is most common in adolescent men and is thought to be caused by repetitive friction to the lateral fingers due to obsessive compulsive behaviors, work, or sports. The pathogenesis is unknown. PDD may be mistaken for inflammatory arthritis. PDD should be painless and noninflammatory, and involved joints should have full range of motion.[43] Hand radiographs can distinguish PDD from pachydermoperiostosis.[43] Histopathologically, there is a thickened epidermis with increased fibroblasts and collagen deposition in the dermis. There is no reliable treatment for PDD, although avoidance of repetitive trauma may decrease disease progression.

Nodular Fasciitis

Nodular fasciitis, also referred to as pseudosarcomatous fasciitis, is a rapidly growing, painful, benign fascial tumor most commonly seen in young adults.[41,44] Nodular fasciitis typically presents on the upper extremity (usually the forearm), with trunk, head and neck, and lower extremity involvement occurring with decreasing frequency. When nodular fasciitis occurs in children, it may more commonly present on the head and neck.[45] The pathogenesis of nodular fasciitis is incompletely understood; however, a fusion gene of *MYH9-USP6* has recently been described.[46] *MYH9* is a nonmuscle myosin class II gene found in fibroblasts, endothelial cells, macrophages, and leukocytes.[46] *MYH9* encodes a protein involved in cell motility, shape, and cytokinesis.[46] *USP6* is a deubiquitinating enzyme involved in intracellular trafficking, protein turnover, cell transformation, and inflammatory signaling.[46] Histopathologically, nodular fasciitis is made up of fibroblasts and myofibroblasts, and mitotic figures are common. Nodular fasciitis may spontaneously regress. Excision results in cure, with an estimated rate of local recurrence at 2%.[41]

Ainhum

Ainhum, also referred to as dactylolysis spontanea, is the name for a fibrous band that develops around the fifth toes of patients of African descent and ultimately results in arterial narrowing, bone absorption, and finally autoamputation.[47,48] Ainhum rarely involves digits other than the fifth toe. Ainhum is most common in people of African descent, but also occurs in Asia, South and Central America, and the United States.[47,48] The highest incidence is in Nigeria.[48] The pathogenesis is unknown. No autoimmune diseases, genetic diseases, nor infectious diseases have been associated with ainhum. Histopathology reveals hyperkeratosis, acanthosis, a lymphocytic infiltration made mostly of T cells, increased fibroblasts, and collagen.[47] If diagnosed early enough, the fibrous band can be injected with steroids or resected in an effort to save the involved toe(s).

Acquired Depositional Disorders: Scleredema and Scleromyxedema

Scleredema and scleromyxedema differ from normal scarring in that the activated fibroblasts deposit excessive quantities of both collagen and GAGs.

Scleredema

Scleredema is characterized by woody induration of the skin caused by increase in collagen bundles and deposition of GAGs. Three clinical subsets of scleredema have been described: (1) scleredema secondary to diabetes mellitus, (2) scleredema secondary to infection, and (3) scleredema secondary to a monoclonal gammopathy.[49] Scleredema secondary to diabetes occurs most commonly in men with long-standing, poorly controlled diabetes with concomitant microvascular complications. The onset of the disease is slow, progressive, and chronic. The posterior neck and upper back and chest are the most commonly involved sites (Fig. 3-8). Scleredema secondary to infection can occur after any febrile illness, but most commonly after streptococcal infection. Onset is sudden and most commonly involves the head and neck, although the trunk, upper extremities, and oropharynx may be involved. Scleredema secondary to infection often self-resolves over months. Scleredema secondary to monoclonal gammopathy (usually IgG and IgA) most commonly involves the neck, upper back, and chest, although head and neck involvement has also been reported. Onset is slow, but the condition is progressive

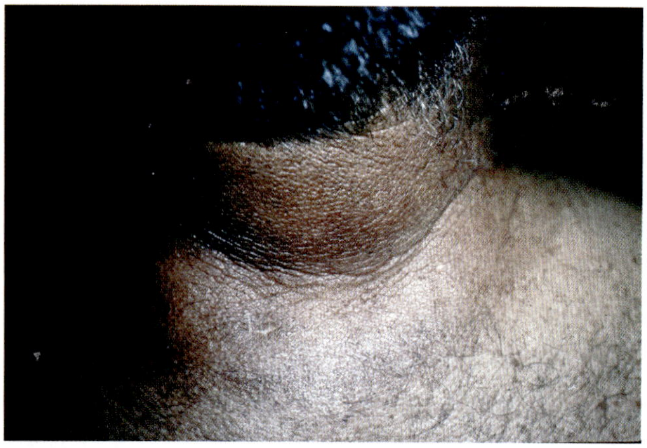

FIGURE 3-8 Scleredema—firm, thickened skin on the posterior neck and upper back.

and tends to be refractory to treatment.[49] Histopathological findings are the same in all three subsets and include a normal epidermis, a normal number of fibroblasts, and a dermis that is thickened due to an increase in collagen bundles and deposition of GAGs. The pathophysiology of scleredema is not understood and has been incompletely studied. It is postulated that in scleredema secondary to diabetes there is nonenzymatic glycosylation of dermal collagen, which potentially activates fibroblasts resulting in increased collagen production and increased GAGs.[50] It is hypothesized that the scleredema that occurs in the setting of a monoclonal gammopathy is due to paraprotein stimulation of fibroblasts.

Scleromyxedema

Scleromyxedema, also referred to as generalized lichen myxedematosus, is a rare mucinosis associated with monoclonal gammopathy, usually IgG lambda. Less than 10% of patients with scleromyxedema develop overt myeloma. Scleromyxedema presents with sheets of 2 to 3 mm firm, waxy, flesh-colored papules on the face (resulting in leonine facies), the ears, the dorsal hands, and the trunk (resulting in Shar-Pei sign) (Fig. 3-9).[51,52] Systemic involvement occurs frequently and may include dysphagia, myopathy, arthritis,

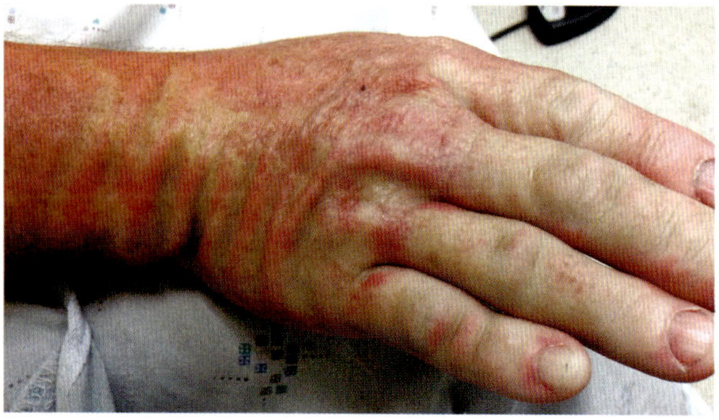

FIGURE 3-9 Scleromyxedema—erythematous edematous plaques. Bending of the skin results in increased furrowing, known as the Shar-Pei sign.

carpal tunnel syndrome, central nervous system disruption (encephalopathy, coma, stroke, seizures, psychosis), obstructive or restrictive pulmonary disease, heart block, pericardial effusions, and cardiomyopathy.[51,52] Histopathologically, the papules reveal increased numbers of fibroblasts, increased GAGs, and increased collagen. The pathogenesis of scleromyxedema remains unknown. It is assumed that monoclonal gammopathy is involved in the pathogenesis by increasing IL-1, TNF, and TGB-β, which stimulate fibroblasts to make more GAGs and collagen. However, the paraprotein itself is not enough to stimulate fibroblasts, and paraprotein levels do not correlate with disease severity. Scleromyxedema may be treated with intravenous immunoglobulin, thalidomide, or antimyeloma medications.

Inflammatory Disorders: Sclerema Neonatorum, Subcutaneous Fat Necrosis of the Newborn, Epidermolysis Bullosa Acquisita, Lichen Planopilaris, Discoid Lupus Erythematosus, Lipodermatosclerosis, Eosinophilic Fasciitis, Sclerodermoid Graft versus Host Disease, Morpheaform Sarcoidosis

While the mechanism of producing skin thickening in inflammatory disorders is unknown, a combination of the release of proteolytic enzymes or induction of fibroblast-activating intermediary molecules from cytokine pathways seems possible. There may also be overlap with the sclerosing disorders of eosinophilic fasciitis (EF) and sclerodermoid graft versus host disease (GVHD).

Sclerema Neonatorum

Sclerema neonatorum is a rare subtype of lobular panniculitis. Sclerema neonatorum presents as firm, cool to the touch, mottled and violaceous, "bound-down" plaques on the buttocks, thighs, and trunk of preterm, severely ill newborns.[53] Histologically sclerema neonatorum has a lobular inflammatory infiltrate in the subcutaneous fat with needle-shaped crystals within the adipocytes.[53] The pathogenesis of sclerema neonatorum is unknown.[53] Exchange transfusion in the setting of sclerema neonatorum and sepsis may decrease mortality. Treatment is otherwise supportive. The pathogenesis of sclerema neonatorum does not include an increase of fibroblasts or fibroblast activation but rather occurs secondary to inflammation of the subcutaneous fat.

Subcutaneous Fat Necrosis of the Newborn

Subcutaneous fat necrosis of the newborn (SCFN) is a self-limited lobular panniculitis that occurs in full-term

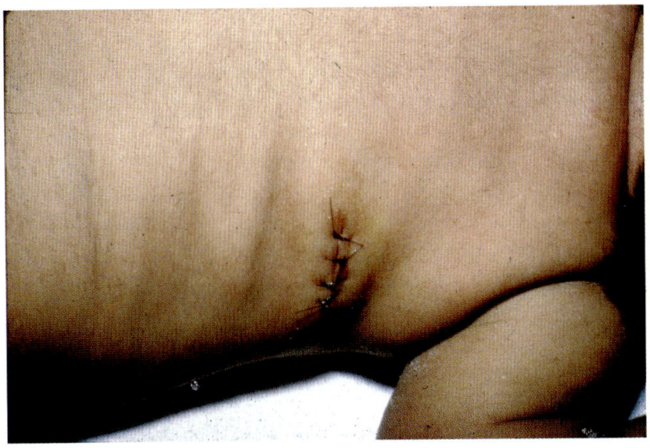

FIGURE 3-10 Subcutaneous fat necrosis of the newborn—firm subcutaneous plaques on the trunk.

infants within the first week of life.[54] SCFN presents as firm, mobile, red to violaceous nodules and plaques over the bony prominences of the trunk, buttocks, and extremities and resolves within weeks to months (Fig. 3-10).[54] Risk factors for the development of SCFN include birth asphyxia, hypothermia, preeclampsia, gestational diabetes, maternal cocaine use, and meconium aspiration. Histopathology reveals a lobular panniculitis with adipocyte necrosis and needle-shaped clefts in a radial pattern within adipocytes. SCFN incidence may be increasing due to the increased use of cooling protocols to prevent hypoxic encephalopathy. The inflammatory infiltrate in SCFN is made up of lymphocytes, histiocytes, giant cells, lipophages, and eosinophils. Neonates who develop SCFN are at risk of hypercalcemia. The pathogenesis of SCFN is unknown, but is theorized to be due to shunting of blood away from the skin in times of hypoxia, resulting in cooling of the fat, crystallization of the fat due to its higher concentration of saturated fatty acids, and granulomatous inflammation.[54]

Epidermolysis Bullosa Acquisita

Epidermolysis bullosa acquisita (EBA) is a rare autoimmune blistering disease with an estimated incidence of 0.5 cases/million/y.[55] EBA is caused by autoantibodies directed against collagen type VII, an anchoring fibril within the dermis of the basement membrane zone. Two main clinical subtypes of EBA have been described, classical (noninflammatory EBA) and inflammatory EBA (which includes bullous pemphigoid–like EBA, mucous membrane pemphigoid–like EBA, IgA bullous dermatosis–like EBA, and Brunsting–Perry pemphigoid–like EBA). The classical subtype is the most common subtype. Classical EBA presents with skin fragility, erosions, and tense blisters over areas of friction (dorsal hands, elbows, knees, low back, and buttocks) that heal with scarring and milia (Fig. 3-11). The mucosal surfaces may also be involved. EBA is diagnosed with biopsy of a tense blister stained with traditional hematoxylin and eosin (which reveals a subepidermal blister), biopsy of perilesional skin for direct immunofluorescence (which reveals linear deposition of IgG along the basement membrane zone), indirect immunofluorescence on salt split skin (which reveals linear deposition on the dermal side of the split), and ELISA for antibodies to type VII collagen. EBA has been associated with inflammatory bowel disease, likely secondary to the presence of collagen VII within the bowel wall. Patients with inflammatory bowel disease have been found to express anticollagen VII antibodies.[55] Given its noninflammatory nature, classic EBA is often recalcitrant to therapies directed against lymphocytes.[55] Rituximab, an anti-CD20 antibody, clears autoreactive antibodies and has been shown to be effective in treating recalcitrant EBA.[55]

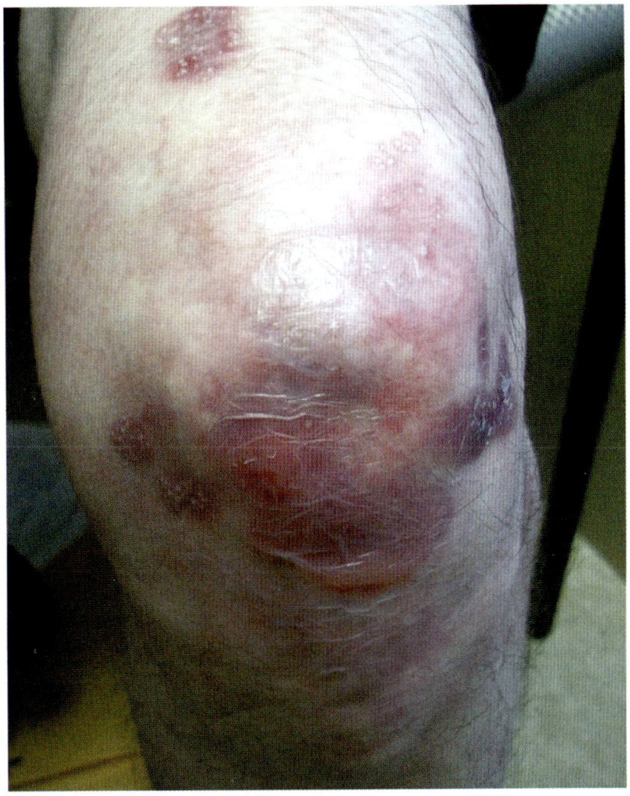

FIGURE 3-11 Epidermolysis bullosa acquisita (EBA)—tense bullae over the extensor knee in a sclerotic plaque with surrounding milia.

Scarring in EBA is thought to occur because the autoantibodies target proteins below the lamina lucida. Autoimmune blistering diseases that have antibodies directed against desmosomes and hemidesmosomes (both above the lamina lucida) do not heal with scarring. The scarring in EBA may be mediated by the abnormal functioning of collagen VII once it is bound by autoantibodies. In *Col7A1* gene knock-out animal models, wound healing has been shown to be delayed by two main mechanisms: (1) delayed reepithelialization due to altered keratinocyte migration and (2) disrupted granulation tissue maturation due to altered dermal fibroblast migration.[56] Loss of *Col7A1* results in altered laminin 332 deposition and $\alpha6\beta4$ expression, both of which play integral roles in keratinocyte migration, reassembly of the dermal–epidermal junction zone, and reformation of hemidesmosomes.[56] These findings suggest that collagen VII, laminin 332, and $\alpha6\beta4$ play integral roles in wound healing and, therefore, scarring.

Lichen Planopilaris

Lichen planopilaris (LPP) is a rare, primary lymphocytic cicatricial alopecia with three clinical phenotypes: (1) classic LPP, (2) frontal fibrosing alopecia (FFA), and (3) Graham-Little-Piccardi-Lasseur syndrome (GLPLS).[57] Classic LPP is characterized by perifollicular erythema, scale, and pustules that result in scarring hair loss (Fig. 3-12). FFA presents as a band of scarring hair loss that involves the temporal and frontal scalp and often also results in eyebrow loss. GLPLS is the combination of classic LPP features with nonscarring alopecia of the axillae and groin and follicular-based lichenoid papules on the face, trunk, or limbs. Histopathological evaluation reveals a dense lymphocytic interface band of inflammation that extends to include the follicular infundibulum and isthmus, necrotic keratinocytes, and vacuolar degeneration of the basal layer. Late stages of disease reveal perifollicular fibrosis, vertical fibrotic tracts within the dermis replacing hair follicles, and loss of sebaceous units. The pathogenesis of LPP remains unknown. LPP most commonly affects postmenopausal women, and the development of autoreactive lymphocytes has been postulated to be associated with triggers such as medications, viruses, changes in hormonal balance, topical agents, and other exposures. Treatment is targeted at preventing additional hair loss, and first-line therapies include topical and intralesional steroids.

It is postulated that cicatrial alopecias result in scarring because of the location of the inflammatory infiltrate and the loss of immune privilege of the follicular bulge.[57] Scarring alopecias have inflammation around the follicular infundibulum and isthmus—the location of the follicular bulge, which is the source of pluripotent stem cells within the follicle.[57] The inflammation is thought to deplete the pluripotent stem cells, resulting in nonreversible alopecia. Additional hypotheses include the loss of peroxisome proliferator–activated receptor γ (resulting in accumulation of lipids and a related inflammatory response within the pilosebaceous unit) and loss of CD200 (which makes the follicle more susceptible to an inflammatory response).[57]

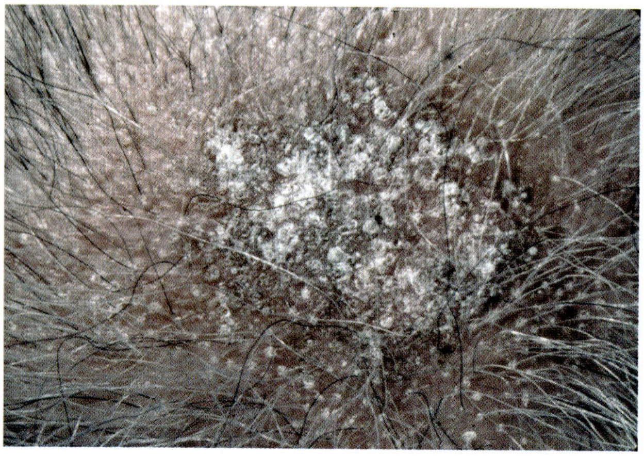

FIGURE 3-12 Lichen planopilaris—perifollicular erythema and scale with loss of follicular ostia and alopecia.

Discoid Lupus Erythematosus

Discoid lupus erythematosus (DLE), a subtype of chronic cutaneous lupus erythematosus, is the most prevalent form of cutaneous lupus erythematosus (CLE). Patients with DLE may also have concomitant systemic lupus erythematosus (SLE) and therefore should be screened for manifestations of SLE. DLE most commonly involves the head and neck. The active phase of DLE presents with erythematous scaling plaques, and the damage phase includes hypo- and hyperpigmented scarred plaques with permanent loss of pilosebaceous units (Fig. 3-13). The pathogenesis of CLE is incompletely understood and is likely due to an interplay of several factors including genetic predisposition (polymorphisms in IFN-κ, tyrosine kinase (TYK2), interferon regulatory factor 5 (IRF5), and cytotoxic T-lymphocyte–associated protein 4), ultraviolet exposure (which increases IFN-α, TNF-α, IL-6, IL-1, Ro52 and makes DNA resistant to degradation by cytosolic nucleases such as three prime repair exonuclease 1 (TREX1)), infectious agents (Epstein–Barr virus, cytomegalovirus), medications (photosensitizing drugs such as terbinafine, calcium channel blockers, hydrochlorothiazide and immunomodulators such as IFN-α and TNF-α inhibitors), hormones, regulation of cell apoptosis, and dysregulation of the immune system (increases in IFN-γ, IL-6, IL-10, chemokine ligand 9 (CXCL9), CXCL10, CXCL11, deficiencies in C1q, C1r, C1s, and deficiency in neutrophil extracellular trap degradation).[58] DLE heals with scarring, whereas other forms of CLE usually heal without scarring. This discrepancy is likely due to the cellular apoptosis within the basal layer in DLE, compared to the suprabasalar apoptosis seen in other forms of CLE. DLE is treated with sunscreens, UV light avoidance, topical steroids and immunomodulators, intralesional steroids, and, in refractory cases, systemic immunomodulators and immunosuppressants such as antimalarials, methotrexate, mycophenolate mofetil, acitretin, and thalidomide.[58]

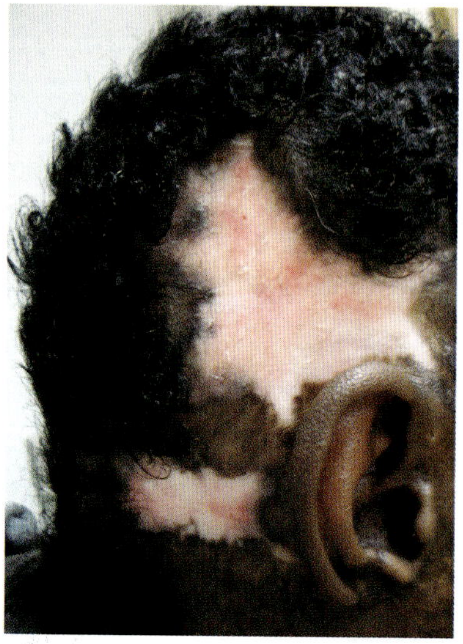

FIGURE 3-13 Discoid lupus erythematosus (DLE)—erythematous scaling sclerotic plaque with surrounding hyperpigmentation on the right parietal scalp.

Lipodermatosclerosis

Lipodermatosclerosis is a sclerosing panniculitis confined to the lower legs that is thought to be the advanced stage of chronic venous insufficiency. Lipodermatosclerosis generally occurs in middle age, is more common in women than in men, and is most prevalent in patients with obesity, hypertension, and prolonged chronic venous insufficiency.[59] Lipodermatosclerosis has an acute phase, characterized by indurated, painful erythematous to violaceous plaques, and a chronic phase, characterized by hyperpigmented bound-down firm plaques. The bound-down skin of the lower leg gives the appearance of an inverted champagne bottle (Fig. 3-14). Histopathologically, the acute phase is characterized by sparse infiltration of inflammatory cells, thickening and fibrosis of the septa within the subcutaneous fat, lipophagic changes, and adipocyte necrosis. The chronic phase reveals no inflammation, progressive fibrosis of the septa, and deposition of hyalinized, linear collagen fibers within the dermis and subcutaneous tissue.[59] The pathogenesis of lipodermatosclerosis is unknown, though dermal fibroblasts in patients with lipodermatosclerosis are more proliferative and have increased procollagen type I mRNA expression than dermal fibroblasts from normal controls.[59] Proposed pathogenic mechanisms include white blood cell trapping within incompetent veins leading to the production of tissue-degrading enzymes, endothelial cell damage and fibrin deposition, formation of microthrombi within incompetent veins resulting in tissue hypoxia and upregulation of TGF-β, and local alterations in MMPs.[59] Recently, a genetic predisposition to chronic venous disease has been suggested. SNPs in *FOXC2*, a transcription factor involved in vascular and lymphatic development, has been found to be associated with varicose veins, hemorrhoids, and venous valve failure, and polymorphisms in the *HFE* gene have been found to increase the risk of venous ulceration by sevenfold.[60] Alterations in MMPs, vascular endothelial growth factors, and collagen expression have also been suggested as pathogenic mechanisms of venous disease.[60] Lipodermatosclerosis is best treated with daily adherence to compression stockings.

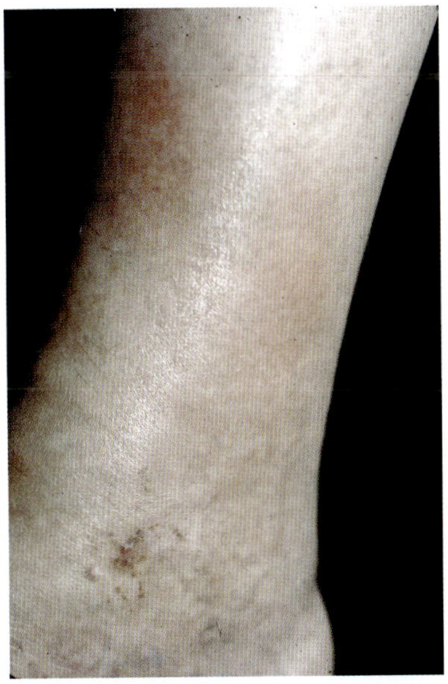

FIGURE 3-14 Lipodermatosclerosis—erythematous firm subcutaneous plaque on the left lateral lower leg.

Eosinophilic Fasciitis

EF is an exceedingly rare, autoinflammatory disorder of the lower reticular dermis, subcutaneous fat, and fascia of the trunk and extremities that is often associated with a peripheral eosinophilia, elevated inflammatory markers, and hypergammaglobulinemia.[61,62] Patients typically present with bilateral painful, nonpitting edema of the extremities with sparing of the hands and fingers, as well as feet and toes. The edema resolves into subcutaneous fibrosis. The fascial fibrosis may dramatically limit range of motion of the hands and feet. EF is differentiated from systemic sclerosis by the lack of sclerodactyly, facial involvement, and Raynaud's phenomenon. Because the inflammation and fibrosis of EF is found in the deep dermis, subcutaneous tissues, and fascia, a wedge biopsy to muscle is required to see the characteristic histological features. The epidermis and superficial dermis in EF is usually spared, but the dermis and subcutaneous fat may be replaced by hyalinized collagen. The fascia is thickened and infiltrated by mononuclear cells and frequently eosinophils. The pathogenesis of EF is incompletely understood. EF fibroblasts are activated, presumably by TGF-β, and produce increased collagen.[62] Patients with EF have been found to have decreased levels of MMP-13 (which typically degrades collagen), increased levels of tissue inhibitor of metalloproteinases 1 (TIMP1, which inhibits MMP-1), and increased IL-5.[62,63] EF is distinguished from normal wound healing in that the vast majority of cases are not due to trauma, the fibrosis is deep and does not involve the epidermis, a preceding edematous phase occurs, and a peripheral eosinophilia is common. The mainstay of EF treatment is glucocorticoids. Recent data suggest that patients treated early (within 6 months) with systemic glucocorticoids, particularly methylprednisolone pulses, and immunosuppressants have the best outcomes.[61]

Chronic Graft versus Host Disease

Chronic graft versus host disease (cGVHD) is a common and frequently fatal sequela of allogeneic hematopoietic stem cell transplantations (allo-HSCT). cGVHD is estimated to occur in 30% to 65% of allo-HSCT recipients, with a 5-year mortality rate approaching 50%.[64] cGVHD is a polymorphic condition that can affect the skin, nails, mucosa, gastrointestinal tract, liver, lungs, muscles, fascia, and bone marrow. Sclerotic GVHD is a subset of cGVHD. Patients with sclerotic GVHD present with skin features clinically and histologically similar to morphea, systemic sclerosis, or EF. Risk factors for the development of cGVHD include previous acute GVHD (aGVHD), HLA disparities, increased age of donor and recipient, use of peripheral blood stem cells for transplant, lack of T-cell depletion of the graft, men receiving graft from women, viral infections, and higher intensity conditioning regimens.[65] Of these risk factors, the use of peripheral blood stem cells for transplant and the lack of T-cell depletion of the graft are most associated with the risk of developing sclerotic GVHD.[66] The pathogenesis of the development of cGVHD is less well understood than the pathogenesis of aGVHD. cGVHD is thought to occur from thymic injury (due to aGVHD or the conditioning regimen), which results in a decrease of T-regulatory cells (Tregs) and an increase in allo-reactive $CD4^+$ T cells.[64] The increase in allo-reactive $CD4^+$ T cells shifts the immune response to a T_H2 cytokine signature (increase in IL-4, IL-5, IL-11), increases profibrotic cytokines (IL-2, IL-10, and TGF-β), and activates macrophages which produce PDGF and TGF-β.[64] Fibroblasts are activated by the profibrotic cytokines and macrophages and overproduce collagen. cGVHD pathogenesis also includes B-cell dysregulation, a hallmark of which is autoreactive B cells.[64,65] Patients with cGVHD have increased levels of B-cell activation factor, deficiencies in memory B cells and delayed reconstitution of naive B cells.[64,65] GVHD preventative regimens continue to be studied. The most commonly used prophylaxis regimen includes methotrexate with a calcineurin inhibitor. Although this regimen has been shown to decrease aGVHD, it unfortunately has not been shown to decrease the occurrence of cGVHD.[65] Treatment of cGVHD includes continuation of the calcineurin inhibitor and addition of systemic glucocorticoids.[65]

Drug- and Toxin-Induced Fibrosis and Scarring

In addition to the idiopathic systemic diseases leading to scarring, there are numerous drugs and toxins that can cause skin sclerosis or fibrosis.

Bleomycin

Bleomycin is capable of inducing pulmonary fibrosis and skin sclerosis. Bleomycin is a chemotherapeutic agent that was initially isolated from the fungus *Streptomyces verticillus*.[67] It has antitumor, antiviral, and antibacterial activities through its ability to bind to double- and single-stranded DNA and cause strand breaks.[67] Systemically, bleomycin is used to treat Hodgkin's lymphoma, testicular cancer, and SCCs. In dermatology, bleomycin is used locally to treat plantar warts and, paradoxically, has also been used to treat keloids.[68] One of the most concerning systemic side effects of bleomycin treatment is the development of pulmonary fibrosis. In the skin, bleomycin can cause various drug rashes, but in rare cases it can cause the development of an LcSScl-like disease.[69] Of the 12 reported patients with bleomycin-induced systemic sclerosis–like illness, 10 were men. All patients with bleomycin-induced systemic sclerosis–like disease developed sclerodactyly and distal sclerotic changes of their extremities, but lacked the nailfold capillary changes, telangiectasias, and calcinosis common in systemic sclerosis. Some patients developed positive ANA titers but none developed anticentromere or anti-topoisomerase autoantibodies. The majority of the reported patients improved upon cessation of treatment with bleomycin.[69]

The mechanism by which bleomycin leads to fibrosis is not fully understood. The lungs and the skin have relatively lower levels of the enzyme bleomycin hydrolase that inactivates the drug. This is one possible explanation for side effects targeting these organs.[69] As in most of the scarring diseases, TGF-β appears to play a central role in the development of fibrosis. In cultured fibroblasts, bleomycin has been shown to directly increase levels of TGF-β mRNA, leading to increased production of extracellular matrix proteins.[67] Due to its ability to cause fibrosis, the mechanism of bleomycin-induced fibrosis has been studied extensively in mouse models of pulmonary fibrosis and systemic sclerosis.[70] In skin lesions of the murine bleomycin systemic sclerosis model, TGF-β levels are increased as well as levels of phosphorylation of SMAD2/3, the intracellular pathway activated by TGF-β.[70] Bleomycin also causes a profibrotic T_H2 skewed inflammatory response. Mice treated with bleomycin show increased levels of the T_H2 cytokines IL-4 and IL-13 both in lesional areas of the skin and in the serum.[67] Bleomycin can also promote sclerosis by causing direct damage to endothelial cells through generation of reactive oxidative species. Endothelial damage then leads to increased adhesion molecules and increased inflammation.[70] Like many of the systemic scarring diseases, there is a complex interplay of factors leading to the ultimate outcome of fibrosis.

Taxanes

The taxane chemotherapy drugs, docetaxel and paclitaxel, have also been linked to a scleroderma-like skin condition. These two chemotherapeutics are derived from the European and Pacific Yew trees.[71] Their chemotherapeutic mechanism of action occurs through the stabilization of microtubules, which prevents microtubule depolymerization. This leads to cell cycle arrest and eventually apoptosis.[72] The taxanes are currently used in the treatment of breast, stomach, lung, and ovarian cancers. Taxanes have been infrequently reported to cause skin sclerosis in a dose-related manner with predominance in women; this predominance may be due to the fact that taxanes are primarily used for the treatment of breast and ovarian cancer.[71–73] The skin sclerosis occurs 6 to 12 months following treatment with taxanes, generally after an edematous phase. The sclerosis seen in taxane-induced scleroderma appears to affect the lower extremities more consistently, but can also affect the trunk and the upper extremities. Unlike systemic sclerosis, patients with taxane-induced sclerosis do not exhibit Raynaud's phenomenon, do not have nailfold capillary changes, do not have autoantibodies, and do not have internal organ involvement.[71–73]

Little is currently known about the pathogenesis of the sclerosis caused by the taxanes. Histologically, a similar inflammatory infiltrate around dermal vessels is seen in classic systemic sclerosis and taxane-induced sclerosis.[71] It is hypothesized that similar cytokines may play a role in both disorders.[71] Interestingly, anticentromere antibodies are often found in systemic sclerosis, and centromeres are the primary target of taxanes; however, this link needs to be further investigated.[71] One case report of taxane-induced sclerosis examined the expression of the friend leukemia integration 1 (Fli1) protein by immunohistochemistry.[73] The authors found that Fli1 levels were reduced or absent in both dermal fibroblasts and endothelial cells in systemic sclerosis, whereas endothelial cells retained a high expression of Fli1 in the case of taxane-induced sclerosis. This suggests a direct effect of the taxanes on fibroblasts and highlights a difference between systemic sclerosis and taxane-induced sclerosis.[73] Due to the small number of cases, treatment of taxane-induced sclerosis remains unclear. Cases have been treated by stopping the suspected offending drug and with topical or systemic steroids. These treatments have resulted in varying improvement of symptoms.[71,72]

Nephrogenic Systemic Fibrosis

Nephrogenic systemic fibrosis (NSF) was first described in 2000 in a case series of 15 patients with end-stage renal disease (ESRD).[74] NSF is characterized by fibrosis and hyperpigmentation, often first occurring on the extremities.[75] It can range in involvement from a small plaque to extensive areas of the body, though it usually spares the face (Fig. 3-15).[76] Patients can also develop red to violaceous, polygonal or retiform, fixed plaques in addition to flexion contractures. Systemic fibrosis may develop in multiple organ systems including the musculature, lymphatics, liver, lungs, heart, and gastrointestinal tract.[75] Biopsy of affected skin in NSF demonstrates a hypercellular dermis with a paucity of inflammation and collections of spindle cells that are CD45RO and CD34 positive, indicating that they originate from circulating bone marrow–derived cells.[75] Increased collagen and mucin and preserved elastin are also present in the dermis.[77] CD68, Factor XIIIa positive multinucleated giant cells, and dendritic cells can also be seen.[75]

In 2006 a link was made between gadolinium-based MRI contrast and the development of NSF. In patients with ESRD, gadolinium is not cleared as quickly as in patients with normal kidney function.[75] Certain formulations of gadolinium contrast—especially those with linear chelation of gadolinium—become unstable over time, resulting in dissociation of the gadolinium from the chelation. Free gadolinium is deposited in the interstitial space and in tissues by an unknown mechanism.[77] In vitro gadolinium has been shown to activate human monocytes and macrophages through the toll-like receptors 4 and 7. These activated macrophages then produce a number of important profibrotic cytokines and chemokines including IL-4, IL-6, IL-13, TGF-β, vascular endothelial growth factor, and many nuclear factor κB–dependent chemokines.[75,77] Fibroblasts *in vitro* can be affected by gadolinium contrast both directly and indirectly. Exposure to cultured media from gadolinium-treated monocytes as well as exposure to gadolinium directly causes dermal fibroblasts to differentiate into myofibroblasts and increase collagen Ia mRNA production.[75] Therefore, it is hypothesized that free gadolinium may propagate fibrosis both directly and indirectly.

The link between gadolinium-based contrast and the development of NSF has been further strengthened by the dramatic decrease in new cases of NSF following guidelines for the use of gadolinium-based contrast in patients with ESRD.[75] The best treatment is prevention by avoiding high-dose contrast, avoiding nonionic linear chelators in patients with ESRD, dialyzing quickly after contrast administration, and avoiding gadolinium contrast in patients with acute renal failure.[76]

For patients with NSF, many different treatments have been attempted with limited success. Oral and topical corticosteroids, cyclosporine, histamine (H2) blockers, and thalidomide appear to have done little to halt or improve the disease.[75] Some variable efficacy has been seen with renal transplant, plasmapheresis, photopheresis, ultraviolet A phototherapy, sodium thiosulfate, and sirolimus.[75] There are reports of improvement of skin symptoms following treatment with the tyrosine kinase inhibitor imatinib, which can decrease signaling through the TGF-β and PDGF pathway.[78]

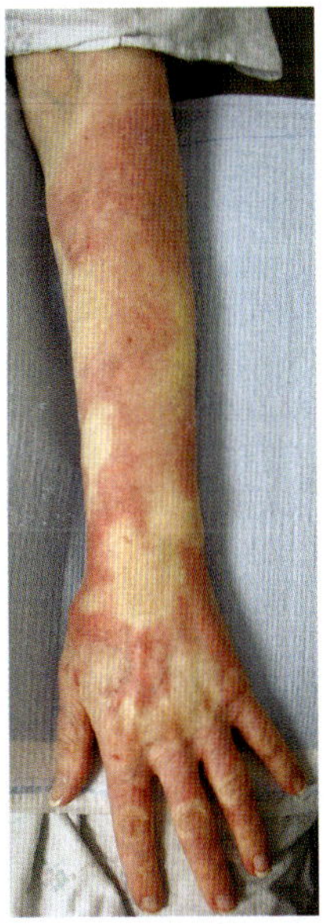

FIGURE 3-15 Nephrogenic systemic fibrosis (NSF)—firm erythematous plaques with characteristic islands of sparing.

Drug-Induced Gingival Hyperplasia

Drug-induced gingival hyperplasia (DIGH) is most commonly caused by phenytoin, nifedipine, and cyclosporine. The incidence of DIGH for patients on these medications has been estimated to be upward of 50%.[79] Interestingly, the mechanism of gingival hyperplasia appears to be different for each of these medications. Phenytoin is postulated to cause enlargement mainly through fibrosis mediated through the TGF-β pathway. Cyclosporine-induced GH occurs secondary to inflammation and not fibrosis. It is postulated that cyclosporine-induced GH occurs due to a disruption in the adaptive immune response and inhibition of hydroxylation of collagen. Nifedipine-induced GH appears to rely both on fibrotic pathways (through TGF-β and periostin) and to date undefined inflammatory pathways. All three mechanisms result in an increase in gingival mesenchymal cells and a decrease in apoptosis, thought to be mediated by TGF-β-induced expression of connective tissue growth factor (CCN2). Lastly, gingival fibroblasts are regulated by different pathways than fibroblasts found in other tissues. Gingival fibroblasts are less responsive to prostaglandin E (PGE); have a unique receptor, PGE receptor 3 (EP3R), that enhances TGF-pto signaling; and are paradoxically inhibited by the canonical Wnt signaling pathway.[79]

Radiation

Radiation is used to treat many different types of cancers including head and neck, skin, anogenital, and breast.[80] Toxic effects of radiation on the skin are well known and are often separated into acute and chronic toxicity. Acute radiation exposure can lead to erythema and wet or dry desquamation.[81] Chronic radiation changes include telangiectasias, dermal atrophy, ulceration, development of malignancies, and fibrosis. The chronic side effects of radiation on the skin typically develop months to years following radiation treatment and typically occur at doses greater than 25 Gy in a single dose, or 70 Gy in fractionated doses.[81] With the increased use of minimally invasive techniques requiring fluoroscopy, more patients are being exposed to the potential side effects of radiation.[82] Histologically, chronic radiation can lead to epidermal atrophy, telangiectatic vessels, dermal sclerosis, atypical stellate fibroblasts, and adnexal structure atrophy and loss.[80,82]

The pathogenesis of radiation fibrosis shares many features with other fibrosing disorders. Radiation causes damage to cellular DNA and RNA through the development of reactive oxygen species (ROS). This damage can lead to injury to parenchymal and endothelial cells.[83] Damage to the endothelial cells can lead to hypoxia and further induction of ROS and cellular damage. Immediately following irradiation, there is also a strong inflammatory response with production of cytokines and chemokines. Elevated TGF-β can be detected hours following irradiation, which suggests this cytokine may have a central role in the development of radiation fibrosis.[81] Increased levels of IL-1, IL-6, TNF-α, and many chemokines that are involved in the recruitment of bone marrow–derived cells are also found in affected areas in the days to weeks following the initial radiation insult.[83] Bone marrow–derived cells that are recruited following radiation injury include mesenchymal stem cells, epithelial progenitor cells, and myelomonocytic cells. These cells are important for repair of damaged tissue, angiogenesis, and vasculogenesis but also can contribute to persistent inflammation and the development of fibrosis.[80] Like most fibrosing disorders, there appears to be a complex interplay between inflammation, cell injury, and the development of fibrosis.

Since radiation has been in clinical use for many years, multiple options have been investigated to both prevent and treat the acute and chronic toxicity of radiation. Therapies have attempted to reduce the production of ROS, inhibit the development of inflammation, and block the downstream effects of major cytokines and chemokines in both preventive and treatment measures. While there has been some promising data in animal models and small clinical case series and trials, there still is no compelling evidence on the use of therapeutics to prevent or treat the development of radiation fibrosis. There have been some small positive reports using pentoxifylline and vitamin E, but larger studies are necessary.[80] Currently, the best method to prevent radiation-induced fibrosis remains to limit the amount of radiation delivered to the greatest extent possible.

Toxic Oil Syndrome and Eosinophilia–Myalgia Syndrome

Systemic fibrosis can also be caused by inadvertent exposure to toxic substances, such as in the case of the two similar diseases: toxic oil syndrome and eosinophila–myalgia syndrome. The toxic oil syndrome epidemic occurred in Spain beginning in 1981.[84] This syndrome was characterized by three clinical phases that included a wide variety of symptoms. The first phase is characterized by shortness of breath and pulmonary edema. The second phase presents with sensory neuropathy, myalgias, and muscle weakness. Skin involvement often begins during this phase and can range from localized plaques similar to morphea to more widespread involvement with changes similar to EF or Lc-SScl. The primary and secondary phases each last roughly 2 months. Around 60% of patients then progress to the third phase with development of permanent neuropathy, involuntary muscle activity, and skin sclerosis. Lab abnormalities seen during the disease include elevated peripheral eosinophils, elevated triglycerides, elevated cholesterol, and hyperglycemia. The disease affected over 20,000 people and caused more than 300 deaths. Careful epidemiologic studies traced the disease to denatured rapeseed oil from a single company that was incorrectly sold as olive oil. This oil was not intended for human consumption and was found to be contaminated with multiple chemicals including 3-(*N*-phenylamino)-1,2-propanediol (PAP), which is currently thought to have caused the disease. While the complete pathogenic mechanism is not understood, it is believed that this chemical causes diffuse apoptosis and an exaggerated T_H2 immune response leading to the development of widespread fibrosis.[85]

A very similar disease, eosinophilic–myalgia syndrome, was described in the United States in 1989. This disease shares many of the clinical characteristics of toxic oil syndrome including eosinophilia and myalgias.[86] It affected over 1500 patients and led to over 30 deaths.[87] Eventually the disease was traced to L-tryptophan dietary supplements from a single source. These supplements were found to contain 3-(phenylamino)alanine, which is chemically similar to the PAP that was linked to toxic oil syndrome. The pathogenesis of eosinophilic–myalgia syndrome likewise is thought to be similar where the toxic chemical causes acute inflammation and eosinophil activation, leading to a persistent fibrotic response characterized by production of TGF-β and IL-4.[87]

Oral Submucous Fibrosis

Oral submucous fibrosis is considered a premalignant disorder of the oropharynx. Clinically it begins with inflammation of the oral mucosa. Over time it develops into hypovascular and fibrotic plaques and nodules. In severe cases, a fibrous band can develop that restricts mouth opening. Fibrosis can also spread to the soft palate, the uvula, the tongue, and the upper esophagus. The spreading fibrosis leads to much of the morbidity including difficulty in swallowing and speaking and hearing loss due to Eustachian tube dysfunction. The development of oral submucous fibrosis has been closely linked to the habit of betel chewing. This is a common habit in South East Asia that involves chewing a combination of areca nut, betel pepper leaves, spices, and calcium hydroxide. Recently chewing tobacco has also been added to betel by many users. With the addition of tobacco, the incidence of SCC has been increasing.[88] The pathogenesis of oral submucous fibrosis is thought to occur from the chronic inflammation from various compounds found in the betel nut. Increased levels of IL-6, IL-8, TNF-β, PDGF, and FGF are found in the lesions of oral submucosal fibrosis. Treatment of early oral submucous fibrosis involves topical and intralesional corticosteroids. Many different treatments have been attempted for the later fibrotic stages, though no consistently positive results have been achieved.[88,89]

Tumor-Associated Fibrosis

Tumors, both benign and malignant, can induce local fibrosis or are caused by fibroblasts or fibroblast-like cells. The prototypical and most common of these tumors is the dermatofibroma.

Dermatofibroma

Dermatofibromas are very common dermal nodules ranging in color from white to pink to brown, with a predilection for the extremities of middle-aged women.[90] They are typically small with sizes in millimeters, but can present as nodules up to a few centimeters.[91] As they are so common and benign in behavior, their true prevalence is unknown. There are many different patterns seen histologically for dermatofibromas, but all contain variable numbers of fibroblasts, histiocytes, and blood vessels.[90] A distinguishing histological feature of dermatofibromas is that many stain positive for Factor XIIIa, which can help to differentiate dermatofibromas from the malignant neoplasm dermatofibrosarcoma protuberans (DFSP). There is still some debate as to whether dermatofibromas represent a reactive fibrotic tissue pattern or are benign fibrohistiocytic neoplasms.[91] TGF-β, PDGF, and IL-1 appear to be involved in the development of dermatofibromas, yet they are overexpressed in a very localized area compared to other types of fibrosis.[91] Multiple eruptive dermatofibromas have been reported to occur with increased frequency in patients with SLE and HIV, which suggests that immune dysregulation may also be a component of their pathogenesis.[92]

Dermatofibrosarcoma Protuberans

DFSP is a relatively rare cutaneous sarcoma of fibroblast-like cells that usually affects the trunk and proximal extremities (Fig. 3-16). The incidence of DFSP is estimated to be between 0.8 and 4.5 cases per million. The tumors tend to be slow growing and locally invasive, but do not typically metastasize. Histologically, DFSP is characterized by poorly circumscribed collections of dense spindled cells with varying amounts of collagen. About 90% of DFSPs are positive for CD34, and a large proportion of the tumors also show a characteristic t(17;22)(q22;q13) translocation. This translocation creates a fusion protein of type I collagen and PDGF-β, resulting in an increased expression of the PDGF-β gene. Surgical excision remains the treatment of choice for DFSP. Recent data show a lower recurrence rate with Mohs surgery.[93] Treatment for unresectable tumors has been attempted with the tyrosine kinase inhibitor imatinib and with local radiation therapy.[93]

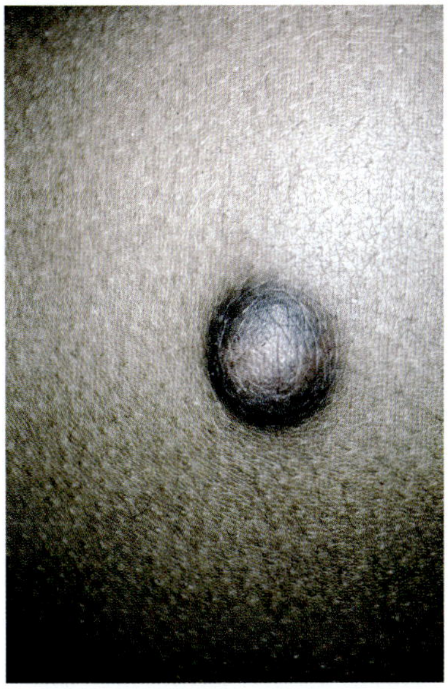

FIGURE 3-16 Dermatofibroma sarcoma protuberans (DFSP)—2 cm firm nodule on the left upper back.

Sclerotic Fibroma

Sclerotic fibroma is another rare fibrocytic tumor that can occur as a benign solitary lesion or can occur in association with Cowden's disease (multiple hamartoma syndrome). Cowden's disease is caused by an autosomal dominant mutation in the *PTEN* gene that leads to the development of many benign and malignant tumors. Clinically, sclerotic fibromas present as solitary skin-colored waxy papule, most frequently on the head and neck. Under the microscope they are well-circumscribed hypocellular dermal nodules with a characteristic appearance of thickened collagen, described as a "plywood" pattern. When they appear as a solitary lesion, they are benign and do not require treatment.[94,95]

Infantile Digital Fibromatosis

Infantile digital fibromas, also known as recurring digital fibrous tumor of childhood or inclusion body fibromatosis, are most often benign pink- to skin-colored nodules that occur on the fingers and toes of young children.[96] These tumors can grow up to a few centimeters and, interestingly, typically spare the thumb and great toe.[96] While primarily a tumor of infants, there have been rare case reports of adult presentations. The natural progression of the tumors is one of slow growth for a few months followed by more rapid growth for 10 to 14 months. This growth is then usually followed by regression. Infantile digital fibromas are composed of ill-defined fascicles of spindle cells throughout the dermis and subcutis.[97] The cells contain eosinophilic cytoplasmic inclusion bodies, which are pathognomonic for the tumor. These inclusions contain bundles of actin and vimentin filaments. The pathogenesis of these tumors is incompletely understood; however, as they are composed of myofibroblasts, it likely involves pathways related to the propagation of this cell line. Myofibroblasts can differentiate from fibroblasts through a number of triggers including TGF-β and mechanical stress. Myofibroblasts provide contractile strength during wound healing and then die by apoptosis during wound maturation. As these tumors seem to follow an exaggerated myofibroblast life cycle, a better understanding of the triggers of myofibroblast apoptosis may lead to better treatments for the tumors. Current treatments include observation, Mohs surgery, or intralesional 5-fluorouracil treatment. As these tumors are benign and regress on their own, it is difficult to assess the success rates of various treatments. Treatment is most often directed at symptom control.[97]

Dermatomyofibroma

Dermatomyofibromas are a newly described benign proliferation of myofibroblasts. These tumors present as well-circumscribed, skin-colored to red-brown plaques found most frequently on the shoulder, axilla, upper arm, and neck. They appear to affect young women predominantly but can occur in children and in men. Histologically, these tumors are well-defined fascicles of uniform spindle cells arranged most often parallel to the epidermis. The cells appear to be myofibroblasts and stain positive for vimentin, and roughly 50% of the tumors stain positive for the myoblast marker α-smooth muscle actin. The tumors stain negative for desmin, Factor XIIIa, and CD34 to help differentiate them from dermatofibromas or DFSP. As they are slow-growing benign tumors, excision is curative with low recurrence.[98,99]

Angiofibroma

Cutaneous angiofibromas, also known as fibrous papules and pearly penile papules, are benign neoplasms that are found stereotypically as solitary lesions on the nose and clustered on the glans penis. Clinically they appear as small skin-colored domed papules. On the glans penis, they typically cluster around the corona. Histologically they show a collection of fibroblasts in the dermis that can appear stellate and form multinucleated cells. The dermis contains increased collagen and decreased elastin. There are also increased collections of thin-walled vessels in the dermis. Interestingly, multiple angiofibromas can occur in the genetic syndromes tuberous sclerosis, multiple endocrine neoplasia type 1, and Birt–Hogg–Dubé syndrome. When they occur in these syndromes they typically occur as multiple lesions and can be present on the cheeks. In tuberous sclerosis, patients can also develop periungual angiofibromas that appear similar histologically to the angiofibromas on the face. These neoplasms are benign but are frequently biopsied out of concern for basal cell carcinoma (BCC) on the nose or verruca vulgaris on the penis. They only require treatment for cosmesis.[96,100]

Fibromatosis Colli

Fibromatosis colli is a rare benign condition of newborns, also called sternocleidomastoid (SCM) pseudotumor of infancy. It typically presents from birth to 4 weeks of age and is associated with traumatic birth. A slow-growing mass on the neck closely associated with the SCM muscle is the usual presentation. There can be associated torticollis in up to 20% of affected infants.[101] Occasionally, fibromatosis colli occurs in conjunction with other congenital deformities such as clubfoot or hip dislocation. Diagnosis can be made most often by clinical exam and ultrasound of the mass. If there is doubt about the diagnosis, fine needle aspiration can be performed which shows spindled fibroblasts and muscle giant cells.[102] The etiology of fibromatosis colli is thought to begin with damage to the shortened SCM muscle during birth. This damage leads to hematoma formation and subsequent migration of fibroblasts, causing atrophy of the muscle fibers. Other theories include malpositioning in the uterus, venous occlusion, and intramuscular hematoma as the initial insult leading to the damage and fibrotic repair response. The condition is benign and 95% of infants see improvements in motion after 4 weeks of physical therapy. In severe cases unresponsive to physical therapy, surgical intervention may be necessary to prevent permanent musculoskeletal damage.[101]

Connective Tissue Nevus

Connective tissue nevi are not true nevi, but are more accurately described as connective tissue hamartomas. They can be divided into three types—collagenomas, elastomas, and proteoglycanomas—based on the most prominent type of connective tissue substance seen on biopsy. Each entity can exist as a solitary lesion or as part of a genetic syndrome. Collagenomas are most commonly seen in the genetic disease tuberous sclerosis and are termed "shagreen patches." Histologically they show an ill-defined increase in collagen density and fiber thickness without a concomitant increase in fibroblast density. Elastomas can be seen in the disorders Buschke–Ollendorff syndrome and pseudoxanthoma elasticum. Increased elastic fibers in the dermis are the characteristic histological feature of elastomas. Hamartomas of proteoglycans, also known as mucin, can be seen in the genetic mucopolysaccharidosis Hunter's syndrome.[103] The genetic basis of these connective tissue nevi can be linked to the defective gene if they are syndromic, but the etiology of sporadic lesions remains unknown. Treatment is typically not necessary as the lesions are benign.[104]

Basal Cell Carcinoma

BCCs are the most common keratinocyte malignancy. They typically present as dome-shaped pearly papules, often with central ulceration. The most common histological type shows nodular collections of basaloid tumor cells in the dermis. A less common subtype of BCC is the morpheaform or sclerotic BCC. These tumors present as ill-defined pink scar–like plaques. Histologically, they show small nests and strands of tumor cells without the typical nodules and retraction artifact. They are more often deeply infiltrative and have a higher recurrence rate than nodular BCCs.[105] An interesting molecular feature of BCC is that almost all tumors show an abnormality in the SHH signaling pathway. Most commonly, mutations in the patched (*PTCH*) gene lead to constitutive activation of the hedgehog signaling pathway. Interestingly, BCCs—even the more aggressive morpheaform variant—show very stable genomes in comparison to other tumors and have almost no malignant potential. It is unknown if there is a different molecular signature of the morpheaform variant of BCC. First-line treatment for morpheaform BCC is surgical excision with Mohs surgery. Recently an inhibitor of the SHH pathway has been developed that is currently approved for treatment of inoperable BCC.[96,105,106]

Genetic Diseases with Increased Fibrosis

Premature Aging Syndromes

A group of genetic diseases called the premature aging syndromes share similar physical features including increased fibrosis and tight, thinned skin. The prototypical disorder in this group is Hutchinson-Gilford progeria syndrome (HGPS). This disorder occurs in 1 in 8 million to 1 in 4 million live births, with an estimated prevalence of 350 children worldwide.[107] Patients with HGPS are born with normal features but then start to develop symptoms during their first year, which typically begins with a decreased growth rate. This is then followed by the loss of subcutaneous fat, the onset of scleroderma-like skin changes, and the development of the characteristic facial features of beaked nose, micrognathia, prominent eyes, and protruding ears.[108] The underlying genetic defect of HGPS was identified in 2003 as a sporadic autosomal dominant mutation in the nuclear protein Lamin A.[107] Lamins are critical nuclear intermediate filaments that support the structure of the nucleolus, anchor chromatin, and tether nuclear pore complexes.[109] The mutation in most cases of HGPS leads to a dominant negative protein called progerin. Many different abnormalities have been seen in nuclear and genomic structures and regulatory proteins in cells from patients with HGPS. Fibroblasts are particularly affected by the changes and have impaired proliferation and differentiation leading to fibrosis.[110] Despite great interest in the development of treatments for progeria, none have succeeded, and the condition is invariably fatal in the early teens.[107]

Another premature aging syndrome in which skin fibrosis is a feature is Werner syndrome. Werner syndrome affects approximately 1:100,000 people in Japan, and approximately 1:1,000,000 to 1:10,000,000 people outside of Japan. Unlike HGPS, Werner syndrome patients do not typically begin to show features of the disease until their second decade. The first clinical sign is often a lack of growth during puberty. Other clinical features such as graying hair, alopecia, premature facial aging and beaked nose, and skin atrophy with scleroderma-like tightening develop in their teens and twenties. Patients also develop many diseases related to aging such as cardiovascular disease, type II diabetes, cataracts, and osteoporosis at a relatively young age. Skin changes are most common on the face and distal extremities and include atrophy, hyperpigmentation, and skin tightness similar to scleroderma. In addition, patients with Werner syndrome are prone to develop thick keratoses over pressure points and ulcers at the sites where these keratoses have been removed.[108] Patients are also at increased risk for specific malignancies including soft tissue sarcomas, osteosarcomas, and meningiomas. Werner syndrome is caused by defects in the WRN gene *(RECQL2)*, a DNA helicase. The WRN protein is involved in DNA replication, DNA recombination, telomere maintenance, and DNA repair. Cells defective in WRN have increased chromosomal abnormalities, accelerated telomere shortening, and early growth arrest. Fibroblasts appear to be severely affected by the loss of the WRN with early senescence. This could explain the dermal atrophy and skin thinning these patients experience.[111] There are currently no effective treatments for Werner syndrome.

Lipoid Proteinosis

Lipoid proteinosis is an autosomal recessive genetic disease due to a mutation in the *ECM1* gene. It is a very rare disease with approximately 250 case reports in the literature. The first clinical sign of the disease is a hoarse cry in infancy. This is due to the deposition of hyaline material in the vocal cords.[112] Other clinical features include infiltration of structures of the oropharynx, beaded eyelid papules, and skin changes including ice pick scarring of the face and neck, skin fragility, and generalized skin thickening. Variable central nervous system involvement can result in epilepsy, memory problems, and schizophrenic behavior.[113] Histologically an increase in types IV and VII collagen is seen, with a decrease in types I and III collagen. Fibroblasts have decreased procollagen I expression and develop characteristic vacuole formation in the cytoplasm. Throughout the dermis there is accumulation of hyaline material.[112] The exact function of the ECM1 protein is unknown but it encodes a secreted glycoprotein that can bind to collagen IV and laminin 332. It is hypothesized that decreased binding of ECMI to the collagen leads to increased type IV collagen production.[114] Lipoid proteinosis does not necessarily lead to increased mortality. However, morbidity from the disease is often caused by infiltration of the oropharynx, at times necessitating tracheostomy.[112]

Pachydermoperiostosis

Pachydermoperiostosis, also known as primary hypertrophic osteoarthropathy (PHO), is a rare genodermatosis with unknown prevalence. Approximately 200 cases have been reported in the literature. The disease appears to occur more frequently and more severely in men. Clinical features of the disease include thickening of the skin on the scalp, resulting in cutis verticis gyrata, digital clubbing, and periostosis. Fibroblasts from the bone marrow and skin of patients with PHO show increased proliferation. The genetic basis of the disease is unknown but has been reported as autosomal recessive, X-linked recessive, and autosomal dominant with incomplete penetrance.[115] Some cases appear to be associated with defects in the gene 15-hydroxyprostaglandin dehydrogenase, resulting in increased levels of circulating PGE2.[116]

Stiff Skin Syndrome

Stiff skin syndrome is a rare disease that presents in childhood with hardening of the skin and frequently hypertrichosis over the affected areas. The most commonly affected areas are the buttocks, thighs, and trunk. It rarely affects the hands, feet, and face. There is a lack of systemic involvement, but there can be joint contractures resulting in limited mobility. The histology of affected areas has shown increased mucin in the dermis, increased sclerotic collagen in the deep dermis, and thickened underlying fascia. Increased levels of type VI collagen and the number of myofibroblasts have also been seen in the fascia of affected patients. There is typically minimal inflammatory infiltrate in biopsies of stiff skin syndrome.[117] The pathogenesis of the disease is unknown; however, some familial occurrences have been reported, suggesting a possible genetic basis. Treatment with intense immunosuppression has led to little improvement. Current treatment is limited to physical therapy to prevent joint contractures.[117,118]

Infantile Systemic Hyalinosis

Infantile systemic hyalinosis and juvenile hyaline fibromatoses are rare autosomal recessive genetic diseases. They share many similar clinical features, differing mostly in severity. As both diseases share similar phenotypes it has been proposed that they be grouped together under the diagnosis of hyaline fibromatosis syndrome.[119] Both conditions occur due to mutations in capillary morphogenesis protein 2 (CMG2).[119] This protein is involved in cell adhesion to the basement membrane through its binding of laminins and type IV collagen. Fibroblasts grown from patients with both conditions have difficulty adhering to plates coated with laminins in culture, pointing toward a key role for this protein in cell adhesion.[120] Clinically, both diseases present with gingival hypertrophy, osteolysis, joint contractures, osteoporosis, and multiple types of skin lesions. The cutaneous lesions include papules and hyperpigmentation found on the face, neck, nostrils, and ears; nodules and plaques in the perianal region; and the development of subcutaneous tumors (most commonly around the head).[121] Histologically, accumulation of amorphous hyaline material is seen in the dermis and in the visceral organs. This material is thought to be composed of collagen VI.[120] Currently treatment of both conditions is supportive and targeted to pain control and improvement of joint contractures.[120]

Ehlers–Danlos Syndrome

Ehlers–Danlos syndrome (EDS) is a group of disorders that share the clinical features of joint hypermobility and skin laxity. These disorders are all caused by defects in the collagen I, III, or V genes, or in enzymes that are involved in the biosynthesis of collagen.[122] Other clinical symptoms vary based on which collagen is affected. There are currently 11 accepted types of EDS based on both clinical features and genetic defects. Another feature that most types share is poor wound healing and increased skin fragility. As collagen is a major component of the dermis and important in wound healing, defects in collagen impair the integrity of the dermis and slow wound healing. Patients often develop widened and thin atrophic scars (referred to as "fish mouth scars") due to deficiencies in collagen.[122,123] Treatment of EDS is targeted at symptoms and surveillance for systemic complications. Avoidance of contact sports and even the use of padding and protection on trauma-prone areas are recommended based on the severity of the disease.[124]

Infections

Lobomycosis

Lobomycosis is caused by infection with the fungus *Lacazia loboi*, a fungus endemic to the Amazon basin.[125] Infection requires traumatic inoculation. Once within the dermis, *L. loboi* is phagocytosed by macrophages, which then produce TGF-β and IL-10. The result is a subcutaneous granulomatous reaction that clinically mimics keloids. Keloidal lesions occur years after initial inoculation and are most common on the ears, arms, and legs. Histologically there is dense lymphohistiocytic inflammation within the dermis, and sheets of round yeast structures. The preferred treatment is wide local excision.[125]

REFERENCES

1. Elder DE. *Lever's Histopathology of the Skin*. 10th ed. Philadelphia, PA: Lippincott Williams and Wilkins; 2009.
2. Varga J, Abraham D. Systemic sclerosis: a prototypic multisystem fibrotic disorder. *J Clin Invest*. 2007;117:557–567.
3. Fett N, Werth VP. Update on morphea: part I. Epidemiology, clinical presentation, and pathogenesis. *J Am Acad Dermatol*. 2011;64:217–228; quiz 229–230.
4. Leitenberger JJ, Cayce RL, Haley RW, et al. Distinct autoimmune syndromes in morphea: a review of 245 adult and pediatric cases. *Arch Dermatol*. 2009;145:545–550.
5. Jacobe H, Ahn C, Arnett FC, et al. Major histocompatibility complex class I and class II alleles may confer susceptibility to or protection against morphea: findings from the Morphea in Adults and Children cohort. *Arthritis Rheumatol*. 2014;66:3170–3177.
6. Fett N, Werth VP. Update on morphea: part II. Outcome measures and treatment. *J Am Acad Dermatol*. 2011;64:231–242; quiz 243–244.
7. Kurzinski K, Torok KS. Cytokine profiles in localized scleroderma and relationship to clinical features. *Cytokine*. 2011;55:157–164.
8. Choksi AN, Orringer JS. Linear morphea-induced atrophy treated with hyaluronic acid filler injections. *Dermatol Surg*. 2011;37:880–883.
9. Consorti G, Tieghi R, Clauser LC. Frontal linear scleroderma: long-term result in volumetric restoration of the fronto-orbital area by structural fat grafting. *J Craniofac Surg*. 2012;23:e263–e265.
10. Eisen D, Alster TS. Use of a 585 nm pulsed dye laser for the treatment of morphea. *Dermatol Surg*. 2002;28:615–616.
11. Hanson AH, Fivenson DP, Schapiro B. Linear scleroderma in an adolescent woman treated with methotrexate and excimer laser. *Dermatol Ther*. 2014;27:203–205.
12. Ibler KS, Gramkow C, Siemssen PA. Autologous fat transplantation for the treatment of linear scleroderma en coup de sabre. *Skinmed*. 2015;13:74–76.
13. Kineston D, Kwan JM, Uebelhoer NS, et al. Use of a fractional ablative 10.6-mum carbon dioxide laser in the treatment of a morphea-related contracture. *Arch Dermatol*. 2011;147:1148–1150.
14. Roh MR, Jung JY, Chung KY. Autologous fat transplantation for depressed linear scleroderma-induced facial atrophic scars. *Dermatol Surg*. 2008;34:1659–1665.
15. Sivek R, Emer J. Use of a blunt-tipped microcannula for soft tissue filler injection in the treatment of linear scleroderma (en coup de sabre). *Dermatol Surg*. 2014;40:1439–1441.
16. Tawfik AA, Shokir H, Soliman M, et al. Pulsed dye laser in the treatment of localized scleroderma and its effects on CD34+ and factor XIIIa+ cells: an immunohistochemical study. *Am J Clin Dermatol*. 2013;14:235–241.
17. Thareja SK, Sadhwani D, Alan Fenske N. En coup de sabre morphea treated with hyaluronic acid filler. Report of a case and review of the literature. *Int J Dermatol*. 2013;54(7):823–826.
18. Zanelato TP, Marquesini G, Colpas PT, et al. Implantation of autologous fat globules in localized scleroderma and idiopathic lipoatrophy—report of five patients. *An Bras Dermatol*. 2013;88:120–123.
19. Fistarol SK, Itin PH. Diagnosis and treatment of lichen sclerosus: an update. *Am J Clin Dermatol*. 2013;14:27–47.

20. Carli P, Cattaneo A, De Magnis A, et al. Squamous cell carcinoma arising in vulval lichen sclerosus: a longitudinal cohort study. *Eur J Cancer Prevent*. 1995;4:491–495.
21. Leibowitch M, Neill S, Pelisse M, et al. The epithelial changes associated with squamous cell carcinoma of the vulva: a review of the clinical, histological and viral findings in 78 women. *Br J Obstet Gynaecol*. 1990;97:1135–1139.
22. Lee A, Bradford J, Fischer G. Long-term Management of Adult Vulvar Lichen Sclerosus: A Prospective Cohort Study of 507 Women. *JAMA Dermatol*. 2015;151:1061–1067.
23. Barnes J, Mayes MD. Epidemiology of systemic sclerosis: incidence, prevalence, survival, risk factors, malignancy, and environmental triggers. *Curr Opin Rheumatol*. 2012;24:165–170.
24. Fett N. Scleroderma: nomenclature, etiology, pathogenesis, prognosis, and treatments: facts and controversies. *Clin Dermatol*. 2013;31:432–437.
25. Donohoe JF. Scleroderma and the kidney. *Kidney Int*. 1992;41:462–477.
26. Katsumoto TR, Whitfield ML, Connolly MK. The pathogenesis of systemic sclerosis. *Annu Rev Pathol*. 2011;6:509–537.
27. Romano E, Manetti M, Guiducci S, et al. The genetics of systemic sclerosis: an update. *Clin Exp Rheumatol*. 2011;29:S75–S86.
28. Yamamoto T. Chemokines and chemokine receptors in scleroderma. *Int Arch Allergy Immunol*. 2006;140:345–356.
29. Badea I, Taylor M, Rosenberg A, et al. Pathogenesis and therapeutic approaches for improved topical treatment in localized scleroderma and systemic sclerosis. *Rheumatology (Oxf)*. 2009;48:213–221.
30. Beyer C, Dees C, Distler JH. Morphogen pathways as molecular targets for the treatment of fibrosis in systemic sclerosis. *Arch Dermatol Res*. 2013;305:1–8.
31. Ciechomska M, van Laar J, O'Reilly S. Current frontiers in systemic sclerosis pathogenesis. *Exp Dermatol*. 2015;24(6):401–406.
32. Holzer LA, Cor A, Holzer G. Expression of gap junction proteins connexins 26, 30, and 43 in Dupuytren's disease. *Acta Orthop*. 2014;85:97–101.
33. Shih B, Bayat A. Scientific understanding and clinical management of Dupuytren disease. *Nat Rev Rheumatol*. 2010;6:715–726.
34. Larsen S, Krogsgaard DG, Aagaard Larsen L, et al. Genetic and environmental influences in Dupuytren's disease: a study of 30,330 Danish twin pairs. *J Hand Surg, Eur Vol*. 2015;40:171–176.
35. Dolmans GH, de Bock GH, Werker PM. Dupuytren diathesis and genetic risk. *J Hand Surg*. 2012;37:2106–2111.
36. Mosakhani N, Guled M, Lahti L, et al. Unique microRNA profile in Dupuytren's contracture supports deregulation of beta-catenin pathway. *Modern Pathol*. 2010;23:1544–1552.
37. Langston JP, Carson CC 3rd. Peyronie's disease: review and recent advances. *Maturitas*. 2014;78:341–343.
38. Paulis G, Brancato T. Inflammatory mechanisms and oxidative stress in Peyronie's disease: therapeutic "rationale" and related emerging treatment strategies. *Inflamm Allergy Drug Targets*. 2012;11:48–57.
39. Qian A, Meals RA, Rajfer J, et al. Comparison of gene expression profiles between Peyronie's disease and Dupuytren's contracture. *Urology*. 2004;64:399–404.
40. Veith NT, Tschernig T, Histing T, et al. Plantar fibromatosis—topical review. *Foot Ankle Int*. 2013;34:1742–1746.
41. Ng E, Tandon AA, Ho BC, et al. Characterizing benign fibrous soft-tissue tumours in adults: why is it so difficult and what do we need to know? *Clin Radiol*. 2015;70(7):684–697.
42. Hyman CH, Cohen PR. Report of a family with idiopathic knuckle pads and review of idiopathic and disease-associated knuckle pads. *Dermatol Online J*. 2013;19:18177.
43. Dallos T, Oppl B, Kovacs L, et al. Pachydermodactyly: a review. *Curr Rheumatol Rep*. 2014;16:442.
44. Nishio J. Updates on the cytogenetics and molecular cytogenetics of benign and intermediate soft tissue tumors. *Oncol Lett*. 2013;5:12–18.
45. Hseu A, Watters K, Perez-Atayde A, et al. Pediatric nodular fasciitis in the head and neck: evaluation and management. *JAMA Otolaryngol—Head Neck Surg*. 2015;141:54–59.
46. Erickson-Johnson MR, Chou MM, Evers BR, et al. Nodular fasciitis: a novel model of transient neoplasia induced by MYH9-USP6 gene fusion. *Lab Invest*. 2011;91:1427–1433.
47. de Araujo DB, Lima SM, Giorgi RD, et al. Ainhum (dactylolysis spontanea): a case with hands and feet involvement. *J Clin Rheumatol*. 2013;19:277–279.
48. Olivieri I, Piccirillo A, Scarano E, et al. Dactylolysis spontanea or ainhum involving the big toe. *J Rheumatol*. 2005;32:2437–2439.
49. Nashel J, Steen V. Scleroderma mimics. *Curr Rheumatol Rep*. 2012;14:39–46.
50. Haustein UF. Scleroderma-like lesions in insulin-dependent diabetes mellitus. *J Eur Acad Dermatol Venereol*. 1999;13:50–53.
51. Cokonis Georgakis CD, Falasca G, Georgakis A, et al. Scleromyxedema. *Clin Dermatol*. 2006;24:493–497.
52. Rongioletti F, Merlo G, Cinotti E, et al. Scleromyxedema: a multicenter study of characteristics, comorbidities, course, and therapy in 30 patients. *J Am Acad Dermatol*. 2013;69:66–72.
53. Zeb A, Darmstadt GL. Sclerema neonatorum: a review of nomenclature, clinical presentation, histological features, differential diagnoses and management. *J Perinatol*. 2008;28:453–460.
54. Oza V, Treat J, Cook N, et al. Subcutaneous fat necrosis as a complication of whole-body cooling for birth asphyxia. *Arch Dermatol*. 2010;146:882–885.
55. Ludwig RJ. Clinical presentation, pathogenesis, diagnosis, and treatment of epidermolysis bullosa acquisita. *ISRN Dermatol*. 2013;2013:812029.
56. Nystrom A, Velati D, Mittapalli VR, et al. Collagen VII plays a dual role in wound healing. *J Clin Invest*. 2013;123:3498–3509.
57. Rongioletti F, Christana K. Cicatricial (scarring) alopecias: an overview of pathogenesis, classification, diagnosis, and treatment. *Am J Clin Dermatol*. 2012;13:247–260.
58. Kirchhof MG, Dutz JP. The immunopathology of cutaneous lupus erythematosus. *Rheum Dis Clin N Am*. 2014;40:455–474, viii.
59. Miteva M, Romanelli P, Kirsner RS. Lipodermatosclerosis. *Dermatol Ther*. 2010;23:375–388.
60. Bharath V, Kahn SR, Lazo-Langner A. Genetic polymorphisms of vein wall remodeling in chronic venous disease: a narrative and systematic review. *Blood*. 2014;124:1242–1250.
61. Lebeaux D, Frances C, Barete S, et al. Eosinophilic fasciitis (Shulman disease): new insights into the therapeutic management from a series of 34 patients. *Rheumatology (Oxf)*. 2012;51:557–561.
62. Canady J, Karrer S, Fleck M, et al. Fibrosing connective tissue disorders of the skin: molecular similarities and distinctions. *J Dermatol Sci*. 2013;70:151–158.
63. Asano Y, Ihn H, Jinnin M, et al. Serum levels of matrix metalloproteinase-13 in patients with eosinophilic fasciitis. *J Dermatol*. 2014;41:746–748.
64. Blazar BR, Murphy WJ, Abedi M. Advances in graft-versus-host disease biology and therapy. *Nat Rev Immunol*. 2012;12:443–458.
65. Socie G, Ritz J. Current issues in chronic graft-versus-host disease. *Blood*. 2014;124:374–384.
66. Uhm J, Hamad N, Shin EM, et al. Incidence, risk factors, and long-term outcomes of sclerotic graft-versus-host disease after allogeneic hematopoietic cell transplantation. *Biol Blood Marrow Transplant*. 2014;20:1751–1757.
67. Yamamoto T. Animal model of systemic sclerosis. *J Dermatol*. 2010;37:26–41.
68. Rabello FB, Souza CD, Farina Junior JA. Update on hypertrophic scar treatment. *Clinics (Sao Paulo)*. 2014;69:565–573.
69. Inaoki M, Kawabata C, Nishijima C, et al. Case of bleomycin-induced scleroderma. *J Dermatol*. 2012;39:482–484.
70. Batteux F, Kavian N, Servettaz A. New insights on chemically induced animal models of systemic sclerosis. *Curr Opin Rheumatol*. 2011;23:511–518.
71. Itoh M, Yanaba K, Kobayashi T, et al. Taxane-induced scleroderma. *Br J Dermatol*. 2007;156:363–367.
72. Farrant PB, Mortimer PS, Gore M. Scleroderma and the taxanes. Is there really a link? *Clin Exp Dermatol*. 2004;29:360–362.
73. Takahashi T, Asano Y, Ichimura Y, et al. A case of taxane-induced scleroderma: a different expression profile of Fli1 proteins in dermal fibroblasts and microvascular endothelial cells compared with systemic sclerosis. *Br J Dermatol*. 2011;164:1393–1395.
74. Cowper SE, Robin HS, Steinberg SM, et al. Scleromyxoedema-like cutaneous diseases in renal-dialysis patients. *Lancet*. 2000;356:1000–1001.
75. Bernstein EJ, Schmidt-Lauber C, Kay J. Nephrogenic systemic fibrosis: a systemic fibrosing disease resulting from gadolinium exposure. *Best Pract Res Clin Rheumatol*. 2012;26:489–503.
76. Zou Z, Zhang HL, Roditi GH, et al. Nephrogenic systemic fibrosis: review of 370 biopsy-confirmed cases. *JACC Cardiovasc Imag*. 2011;4:1206–1216.
77. Daftari Besheli L, Aran S, Shaqdan K, et al. Current status of nephrogenic systemic fibrosis. *Clin Radiol*. 2014;69:661–668.
78. Elmholdt TR, Buus NH, Ramsing M, et al. Antifibrotic effect after low-dose imatinib mesylate treatment in patients with nephrogenic systemic fibrosis: an open-label non-randomized, uncontrolled clinical trial. *J Eur Acad Dermatol Venereol*. 2013;27:779–784.
79. Trackman PC, Kantarci A. Molecular and clinical aspects of drug-induced gingival overgrowth. *J Dental Res*. 2015;94:540–546.

80. Kim JH, Kolozsvary AJ, Jenrow KA, et al. Mechanisms of radiation-induced skin injury and implications for future clinical trials. *Int J Radiat Biol.* 2013;89:311–318.
81. Martin M, Lefaix J, Delanian S. TGF-beta1 and radiation fibrosis: a master switch and a specific therapeutic target? *Int J Radiat Oncol Biol Phys.* 2000;47:277–290.
82. Boncher J, Bergfeld WF. Fluoroscopy-induced chronic radiation dermatitis: a report of two additional cases and a brief review of the literature. *J Cutan Pathol.* 2012;39:63–67.
83. Yarnold J, Brotons MC. Pathogenetic mechanisms in radiation fibrosis. *Radiother Oncol.* 2010;97:149–161.
84. Alonso-Ruiz A, Zea-Mendoza AC, Salazar-Vallinas JM, et al. Toxic oil syndrome: a syndrome with features overlapping those of various forms of scleroderma. *Semin Arthritis Rheum.* 1986;15:200–212.
85. World Health Organization, Regional Office for Europe. *Toxic oil syndrome: 10 Years of Progress.* Copenhagen: World Health Organization, Regional Office for Europe; 2004.
86. Centers for Disease Control and Prevention. Eosinophilia-myalgia syndrome and L-tryptophan-containing products—New Mexico, Minnesota, Oregon, and New York, 1989. *MMWR Morb Mortal Wkly Rep.* 1989;38:785–788.
87. Allen JA, Peterson A, Sufit R, et al. Post-epidemic eosinophilia-myalgia syndrome associated with L-tryptophan. *Arthritis Rheum.* 2011;63:3633–3639.
88. Wollina U, Verma SB, Ali FM, et al. Oral submucous fibrosis: an update. *Clin Cosmet Invest Dermatol.* 2015;8:193–204.
89. Khan S, Chatra L, Prashanth SK, et al. Pathogenesis of oral submucous fibrosis. *J Cancer Res Ther.* 2012;8:199–203.
90. Han TY, Chang HS, Lee JH, et al. A clinical and histopathological study of 122 cases of dermatofibroma (benign fibrous histiocytoma). *Ann Dermatol.* 2011;23:185–192.
91. Yamamoto T. Dermatofibroma: a possible model of local fibrosis with epithelial/mesenchymal cell interaction. *J Eur Acad Dermatol Venereol.* 2009;23:371–375.
92. Niiyama S, Katsuoka K, Happle R, et al. Multiple eruptive dermatofibromas: a review of the literature. *Acta Dermato-Venereol.* 2002;82:241–244.
93. Llombart B, Serra-Guillen C, Monteagudo C, et al. Dermatofibrosarcoma protuberans: a comprehensive review and update on diagnosis and management. *Semin Diagn Pathol.* 2013;30:13–28.
94. Rapini RP, Golitz LE. Sclerotic fibromas of the skin. *J Am Acad Dermatol.* 1989;20:266–71.
95. Bhambri A, Del Rosso JQ. Solitary sclerotic fibroma. *J Clin Aesthet Dermatol.* 2009;2:36–38.
96. Bolognia JL, Jorizzo J, Schaffer JV. *Dermatology.* 3rd ed. New York: Elsevier; 2012.
97. Heymann WR. Infantile digital fibromatosis. *J Am Acad Dermatol.* 2008;59:122–123.
98. Rose C, Brocker EB. Dermatomyofibroma: case report and review. *Pediatr Dermatol.* 1999;16:456–459.
99. Fisher C. Myofibroblastic malignancies. *Adv Anat Pathol.* 2004;11:190–201.
100. Meigel WN, Ackerman AB. Fibrous papule of the face. *Am J Dermatopathol.* 1979;1:339–340.
101. Skelton E, Howlett D. Fibromatosis colli: the sternocleidomastoid pseudotumour of infancy. *J Paediatr Child Health.* 2014;50:833–835.
102. Khan S, Jetley S, Jairajpuri Z, et al. Fibromatosis colli—a rare cytological diagnosis in infantile neck swellings. *J Clin Diagn Res.* 2014;8:FD08–FD09.
103. Uitto J, Santa Cruz DJ, Eisen AZ. Connective tissue nevi of the skin. Clinical, genetic, and histopathologic classification of hamartomas of the collagen, elastin, and proteoglycan type. *J Am Acad Dermatol.* 1980;3:441–461.
104. de Feraudy S, Fletcher CD. Fibroblastic connective tissue nevus: a rare cutaneous lesion analyzed in a series of 25 cases. *Am J Surg Pathol.* 2012;36:1509–1515.
105. Kraft S, Granter SR. Molecular pathology of skin neoplasms of the head and neck. *Arch Pathol Lab Med.* 2014;138:759–787.
106. Rodon J, Tawbi HA, Thomas AL, et al. A phase I, multicenter, open-label, first-in-human, dose-escalation study of the oral smoothened inhibitor Sonidegib (LDE225) in patients with advanced solid tumors. *Clin Cancer Res.* 2014;20:1900–1909.
107. Gordon LB, Rothman FG, Lopez-Otin C, et al. Progeria: a paradigm for translational medicine. *Cell.* 2014;156:400–407.
108. Bolognia J, Schaffer JV, Duncan KO, et al. *Dermatology Essentials.* St. Lousi: Saunders; 2014.
109. Ghosh S, Zhou Z. Genetics of aging, progeria and lamin disorders. *Curr Opin Genet Dev.* 2014;26:41–46.
110. Prokocimer M, Barkan R, Gruenbaum Y. Hutchinson-Gilford progeria syndrome through the lens of transcription. *Aging Cell.* 2013;12:533–543.
111. Ostler EL, Wallis CV, Sheerin AN, et al. A model for the phenotypic presentation of Werner's syndrome. *Exp Gerontol.* 2002;37:285–292.
112. Hamada T. Lipoid proteinosis. *Clin Exp Dermatol.* 2002;27:624–629.
113. Nanda A, Alsaleh QA, Al-Sabah H, et al. Lipoid proteinosis: report of four siblings and brief review of the literature. *Pediatr Dermatol.* 2001;18:21–26.
114. Sercu S, Zhang M, Oyama N, et al. Interaction of extracellular matrix protein 1 with extracellular matrix components: ECM1 is a basement membrane protein of the skin. *J Invest Dermatol.* 2008;128:1397–1408.
115. Castori M, Sinibaldi L, Mingarelli R, et al. Pachydermoperiostosis: an update. *Clin Genet.* 2005;68:477–486.
116. Uppal S, Diggle CP, Carr IM, et al. Mutations in 15-hydroxyprostaglandin dehydrogenase cause primary hypertrophic osteoarthropathy. *Nat Genet.* 2008;40:789–793.
117. Liu T, McCalmont TH, Frieden IJ, et al. The stiff skin syndrome: case series, differential diagnosis of the stiff skin phenotype, and review of the literature. *Arch Dermatol.* 2008;144:1351–1359.
118. Geng S, Lei X, Toyohara JP, et al. Stiff skin syndrome. *J Eur Acad Dermatol Venereol.* 2006;20:729–732.
119. El-Kamah GY, Fong K, El-Ruby M, et al. Spectrum of mutations in the ANTXR2 (CMG2) gene in infantile systemic hyalinosis and juvenile hyaline fibromatosis. *Br J Dermatol.* 2010;163:213–215.
120. Lindvall LE, Kormeili T, Chen E, et al. Infantile systemic hyalinosis: case report and review of the literature. *J Am Acad Dermatol.* 2008;58:303–307.
121. Ribeiro SL, Guedes EL, Botan V, et al. Juvenile hyaline fibromatosis: a case report and review of literature. *Acta Reumatol Port.* 2009;34:128–133.
122. Byers PH, Murray ML. Heritable collagen disorders: the paradigm of the Ehlers-Danlos syndrome. *J Invest Dermatol.* 2012;132:E6–E11.
123. De Paepe A, Malfait F. The Ehlers–Danlos syndrome, a disorder with many faces. *Clin Genet.* 2012;82:1–11.
124. Malfait F, De Paepe A. The Ehlers–Danlos syndrome. *Adv Exp Med Biol.* 2014;802:129–143.
125. Francesconi VA, Klein AP, Santos AP, et al. Lobomycosis: epidemiology, clinical presentation, and management options. *Ther Clin Risk Manag.* 2014;10:851–860.

4 Scars and Scar Management: Ethical Considerations

BADDR A. SHAKHSHEER, PUNEET SINGH, LAWRENCE J. GOTTLIEB, PETER ANGELOS, and MARK SIEGLER

KEY POINTS

- The patient perspective directs the management of scars.
- Expectations of patient and surgeon need to be concordant before any intervention to improve a scar is initiated.
- Decisions about scar management require a shared decision-making approach in which the physician provides judgment, technical guidance, and expertise and patients express their values and preferences.
- A broad array of scars and deformities exist, congenital and acquired, with a spectrum of perception of severity. Ethical issues relating to the treatment of scars may be specific to the circumstances of the scar.

In Nathaniel Hawthorne's story *The Birthmark*, an esteemed philosopher and scientist marries a beautiful woman who is aesthetically perfect save for a small red birthmark on her cheek.[1] He becomes progressively obsessed with this imperfection and seeks to develop a potion to rid his wife of the "frightful object." The potion succeeds in removing the birthmark but she dies as a side effect of the treatment. Renowned ethicist Leon Kass used this vignette to open the 2002 President's Council on Bioethics as a prelude to discussing the effects and consequences of biomedical innovations and intervention.[2] Hawthorne's story raises many issues that are relevant to the topic of deformities, one principal issue of which is the benefit–risk ratio of treating such deformities, either congenital ones as in *The Birthmark* or acquired ones, such as scars after a surgical procedure.

Scars exert far greater effect than simply their physiologic consequences. One need not venture past the popular literature to find examples of this sentiment. Nora Ephron writes in her book *I Feel Bad About My Neck:* "If you learn nothing else from reading this essay, dear reader, learn this: Never have an operation on any part of your body without asking a plastic surgeon to come stand by in the operating room and keep an eye out. Because even if you are being operated on for something serious or potentially serious, even if you honestly believe that your health is more important than vanity, even if you wake up in the hospital room thrilled beyond imagining that it wasn't cancer, even if you feel elated, grateful to be alive, full of blinding insight about what's important and what's not, even if you vow to be eternally joyful about being on the planet Earth and promise never to complain about anything ever again, I promise you that one day soon, sooner than you can imagine, you will look in the mirror and think, I hate this scar."[3]

Ethics underlies all medical practice and plays a fundamental role in decision-making in health care. Without ethics, medicine would be a "disembodied" discipline, one that would not consider the importance of the patient, his or her goals, and the broader meaning of the interventions that are performed.[4] This chapter will discuss ethical principles and tenets related to the management of scars, including congenital and iatrogenically acquired scars, with the goal of providing a framework for pertinent decision-making in the field of scar management.

Medicine and Ethics

Clinical Medical Ethics

The ethics of medicine and the interaction between physicians and patients has been of interest since the Hippocratic Oath in the 5th century BC. The "first do no harm" ethos is found in the Hippocratic writing *Epidemics, Book I*, and forms the historical impetus for contemporary medical ethics, based on the four principles of beneficence, nonmaleficence, respect for autonomy, and justice.[5] Beneficence means that practitioners should always work in the best interest of the patient. Nonmaleficence is a modern statement of the "first do no harm" principle. Respect for autonomy mandates that the patient has the right to choose or refuse treatment and holds primary responsibility in decision-making for medical treatment. In other words, autonomy recognizes the patient's right to self-determination. The principle of justice concerns itself with fairness and equality and the elimination of disparity in health care and health.

A well-regarded contemporary approach to assessing clinical ethical issues is Jonsen, Siegler, and Winslade's use of four different categories to analyze the issues: medical indications, patient preferences, quality of life, and contextual features.[6,7] Medical indications refer to the clinical facts of the medical situation and the goals of treatment. Patient preferences relate to the principle of respect for autonomy: has the patient been informed about the appropriate risks and benefits and have any choices or predilections been expressed? Quality of life explores the probable future of a patient, with or without treatment. Under this heading, the risks, benefits, and potential side effects are weighed in order to ascertain potential medical outcome. The contextual features category examines issues of justice, fairness, and disparities, for instance, whether there are entities outside of the physician and the patient that may be affected, including family members, the health care organization, or society at large (Fig. 4-1).

Surgical Ethics

Surgical ethics represents a subset of medical ethics specific to surgeons and other proceduralists.[8] One of the original goals of the American College of Surgeons upon its founding in 1913 was to eliminate unethical practices in surgery, particularly fee-splitting, itinerant surgical procedures, and the practice of performing surgery at a distance from one's local hospital and practice, which left the postoperative care to local physicians.

The practice of surgery and of other invasive procedures poses a direct challenge to the ancient doctrine of "do no harm" (i.e., nonmaleficence). Modern commentators have agreed that the "do no harm" rule is not an absolute prohibition. Rather, "do no harm" is a caution for physicians to balance the benefits of their interventions with the likelihood of bad effects or harms. The development of iatrogenic scars after surgical procedures is a prime example for the need for this benefit–harm balancing test.

On a daily basis, surgeons shoulder heavy responsibility. Because of the trust engendered in the surgeon–patient relationship, the surgeon feels a strong sense of personal responsibility for patient outcomes.[9] Frequently, they perform invasive procedures with high levels of associated risk, adding further complexity to the practice of surgery and surgical ethics.[10] In addition to invasive procedures, which may be performed when the patient is anesthetized and thus incapacitated, surgeons must adequately obtain informed consent, deliver bad news, and address end-of-life issues.[11] In the case of emergency surgeries, this relationship must be established quickly and under pressure, as the proceduralist must ascertain the patient's values in a brief time period and act upon those values while a patient is potentially incapacitated by anesthesia.

Further, the everyday, frequent potential for surgical innovation at the operating table distinguishes surgical ethics from the general field of clinical medical ethics.[12] For instance, in the early history of organ transplantation, patients were often harmed by the procedure. Laparoscopy and minimally invasive techniques in surgery were adopted widely in the absence of clinical trials because of patient demand after reports of decreased pain and shorter length of stay, even though early assessments on the novel techniques showed significantly increased complication rates.[13] Thus surgical ethics is a unique subset of clinical medical ethics, set apart by a distinct set of questions and by situations that distinguish them from the larger field of clinical ethics.

Medical Indications (Beneficence and nonmaleficence)	Patient Preferences (Autonomy)
Quality of Life	"External" Considerations (Resources/Money) ("The Law")

FIGURE 4-1 The four-box model, providing a structured approach to ethical and clinical decision-making. *(Adapted from Jonsen AR, Siegler M, Winslade WJ.* Clinical Ethics: A Practical Approach to Ethical Decisions in Clinical Medicine. *8th ed. New York, NY: McGraw Hill Medical; 2015.)*

Ethical Questions Specific to Scar Treatment

Medical Indications

What Is a Scar?

A scar generally forms as the body attempts to heal a wound. It is the natural endpoint of inflammation and subsequent fibrosis. Scars can result from trauma, infection, and certain diseases as well as from iatrogenic causes.

What Is Normal?

"As I contend that the desire for the normal is a powerful one, not easily swayed by a rational weighing of costs and benefits, I believe it is important to consider what means there are to satisfy that desire without necessarily acquiescing to the norm implied in the standard of normal."[14] It is also important to remember that the concept of "normalcy" is crucial to patients, especially ones with scars. This concept ought to be explicitly discussed and the possible outcomes explicitly conveyed. Thus we may consider that when a patient presents for consultation for improvement of an unsightly scar, the surgeon is generally thinking of how they may improve the scar or deformity. By contrast, the patient's goals are frequently to erase the scar and return to the preinjury state, and so, it is imperative that the surgeon's expectations be concordant with that of the patient's. We must recognize that what is "normal" or "acceptable" is often determined by the perception of the patient, a concept that conforms to the ethical principle of autonomy. For example, a military patient may wear a scar as a badge of honor or a reminder of bodily sacrifice. However, a victim of domestic abuse will likely have very negative feelings associated with his or her scars. A patient may consider any skin scarring "abnormal." Even a scar that is not visible may cause itching or pain and thus be considered "abnormal" by the patient. These differences contribute to the difficulty in managing scars as well as the difficulty in justifying compensation for these procedures from outside parties such as insurance companies.

What is "normal" can vary not only from person to person but geographically and culturally as well. For instance, in Nigeria, pediatric umbilical hernias are nearly ubiquitous. Anecdotal reports exist of Nigerian mothers bringing their children to medical centers because they did not have an umbilical hernia.[15] In some cultures, an umbilical hernia is seen as a sign of beauty.[16] Certain tribal cultures of eastern Africa have embraced and indeed celebrated their tendency to heal with hypertrophic scars and keloids by purposeful injury and scarification to produce decorative scarring, which has not only become the social norm but imparts social status.

Further, the implications of deviation from normal can be different culturally and geographically. Take Nora Ephron's example from this chapter's opening: a scar after a thyroidectomy is in a cosmetically sensitive anatomic location in the United States. However, in places such as Korea and Japan, this neck scar holds an even greater impact with a severe social stigma.[17] This has led Southeast Asian surgeons to develop innovative techniques for thyroidectomy, including using trans-axillary incisions to reach the neck. These techniques, however, are recognized to carry greater risk.

In describing the risk and benefits of altering the technique of a surgical procedure with the goal of a less noticeable scar, it is ethically imperative that surgeons present not only the benefit of reducing scars, but also the increased risk of scars from the procedure. Surgeons are well trained in assessing different risks for the same procedure based on ethnicity, skin type, incision location and direction, history, duration of symptoms, and comorbidities. However, physicians must also recognize that the same procedure may carry different benefits for individual patients. For instance, a fashion model may elect to have her gallbladder removed using natural orifice techniques to avoid the scars, even when informed that the novel technique is less well understood in terms of complications when compared with traditional gallbladder removal.

What Is the Nature of the Intervention to Repair the Scar?

Precise classification of the nature of the intervention is not only important for billing purposes but also provides a rationale for both the patient and the physician as to the necessity and goal of treatment. The majority of scar interventions are elective in nature, in that most are "unnecessary, or at least not immediately necessary."[18] However, the term "elective" may not adequately stratify procedures. "Elective" should be defined as any procedure that is not urgent or emergent. The term "elective" does not imply that the procedure is "not medically necessary," but only that there is more flexibility in its timing. For instance, repair of a myocardial laceration from a penetrating knife wound to the chest is not an elective procedure; it is urgent because the patient will die immediately if the surgery is not performed. However, a colectomy for colon cancer and a cholecystectomy for biliary colic are medically necessary procedures that may be done "semi-electively," whereas a cosmetic breast augmentation is generally not medically necessary and may be done electively. A breast reconstruction after mastectomy falls someplace in between these two examples; it is considered medically necessary to complete the treatment of breast cancer; however, its timing could be elective. Scar interventions may fall anywhere across this spectrum. Release of a scar that is limiting excursion of the eyelid, putting the patient at risk for an exposure keratopathy, would be a medically necessary procedure that should be done urgently. Alternatively, revision of an unsightly abdominal scar after surgery for a hysterectomy should be considered an elective operation. Release of a scar contracture of the elbow hampering a patient's ability to perform activities of daily living falls someplace in between these two examples: while it is considered medically necessary to improve the range of motion of the elbow, its timing could be elective. It is important to understand that the term "elective" does not adequately describe or classify an operation as anything other than "not currently a life- or limb-threatening emergency."

Although there may be an aesthetic component to revising a scar, and sometimes the improvement of the aesthetics of an unsightly scar is the primary goal, this still should be considered a reconstructive procedure. In general, the goal of a reconstructive procedure is to improve the abnormal—a specific pathology—and bring it closer toward normal, whereas the goal of a cosmetic procedure is to "improve" the normal—not necessarily a pathology but an undesired characteristic. This distinction is attributed to two pioneers of plastic surgery: Sir Harold Gillies and D. Ralph Millard.[19] Cosmetic procedures may be viewed as ethically different in that, though risk is assumed, there is not a specific physiological benefit for the patient. An interesting similarity arises in patients undergoing cosmetic procedures and living donors for organ transplantation. In both cases, it has been said that the patient does not "benefit" physiologically from the procedure. The living donor assumes great risk while not deriving any physiologic benefit from the medical intervention. The living donor does, however, often derive enormous psychological and social benefit from the act of donation. Similarly, for the patient having a "cosmetic" scar revision, there are direct personal, psychological, and often social benefits. In both instances, from an ethics perspective, the conclusion that the "benefits"—physiological, psychological, or social—outweigh the risks should be left in the hands of the donor or the patient with the scar.[20,21]

Patient Preferences

Should Any Intervention That a Patient Wants Be Performed by a Physician?

"Aesthetic surgery is the one area of medicine that makes widespread use of the term *client* rather than *patient*."[18] From a provider perspective, the decision to treat a patient is based on risks, benefits, and expectations. From a patient perspective, the assessment of potential benefit may outweigh other considerations.

For example, suppose a 70-year-old woman presents to your office for revision of her abdominal scar from a cesarean section 40 years prior. She states the scar is not only unsightly but brings her to tears every night as it reminds her of the pain of that day. It significantly reduces her quality of life and she would be willing to undergo any procedure for the possibility of improving the appearance of her abdomen. However, this patient has a long list of comorbidities, including hypertension, morbid obesity, uncontrolled type 2 diabetes, and chronic obstructive pulmonary disease, putting her at high risk for any type of anesthetic. The assessment of risks and benefits from the procedure may differ between the provider and the patient, who in this case may place a higher value on the intervention and thus be willing to undergo greater risk. The autonomy of the patient conflicts with the judgment of the physician, and this potentially limits the patient's autonomy.

Limiting patient autonomy may be more difficult in this era as contemporary patients may be more demanding. This is a function, at least in part, of the ease of availability of medical information via the Internet and other readily accessible resources, and the increase in direct-to-consumer advertising in which nonphysician health care entities (i.e., pharmaceutical companies, health care systems) encourage patients to ask physicians about specific diagnostics and treatments. When patient preferences and physician recommendations align, there is no conflict. However, a physician may feel morally obliged to refute a patient. In his 1987 essay, Siegler gives three criteria by which a clinician may refute a patient's demand: "1. General moral principles that apply to physicians and to all moral agents, 2. Uncertainty concerning the limits of one's role and responsibility as a physician, and 3. Responsibilities in one's role as a good physician."[22] In the first criterion, a physician may refute a patient's demand if it involves an immoral act. For instance, a clinician should not admit a patient to inpatient care under a false diagnosis to expedite what would be a lengthier (in terms of time) outpatient workup. Under the second criterion, a physician should not overstep his or her boundaries in care, for instance, admitting a patient overnight because of homelessness. In this case, homelessness is not defined as a medical problem under the purview of the physician's care. The third criterion states that a physician may refute a demanding patient based on one's role as a good physician. The physician is an educated provider of medical care and often functions as the "gatekeeper" to interventions. The decisions under which this "gatekeeper" role is executed are set forth by the physician's standards, the health care organization's standards, and society's standards.

Quality of Life

What Is the Goal of Scar Intervention?

This question is fundamental in the treatment of a scar: what is the goal of the intervention? Is the goal of intervention to return the patient to "normal"—either a societal understanding of normal in the case of a congenital blemish like a birthmark, or a prescar state in the case of a scar acquired through a disease process such as scleroderma, a trauma such as a burn, or iatrogenically from surgery? Is the goal an improvement of quality of life, either functional (as in the case of a burn contracture) or perceived (as in the case of cosmesis)? Even when the goal is for aesthetics, one needs to ask, what is the function of skin? In addition to the physiologic functions, a dominant function is to look normal or human. Improving the appearance of skin (especially on exposed areas like the face and hands) is important for social interactions and for the patient's ability to function in society without being self-conscious of their deformity.

Is a scar just a "cosmetic problem," such as a larger than average nose? Or does it qualify as pathology in its own right? The answers to questions such as these form the governing models of health care that guide our practices. Perhaps the prevailing contemporary model is the biopsychosocial model, expanding on the traditional biomedical model to include a framework for other patient-centered aspects of illness, including social, psychological, and behavioral facets.[23]

These models drive at the definition of "health" and thus what constitutes health care. To illustrate the importance of this understanding, Leon Kass has written: "Medicine, as well as the community which supports it, appears to be perplexed regarding its purpose. It is ironic, but not accidental, that medicine's great technical power should arrive in tandem with great confusion about the standards and goals for guiding its use... For without a clear view of its end, medicine is at risk of becoming merely a set of powerful means, and the doctor at risk of becoming merely a technician and engineer of the body, a scalpel for hire, selling his services upon demand."[24] Kass espoused a conservative view of health care and its goals, stating that patient happiness and other quality of life measures constituted false goals in health care. Implying a paternalistic view where physicians should guide the delivery and limits of health care, Kass rhetorically asks: "Who is the best judge of health, the doctor or the patient?"[24] Siegler and others have advocated a more liberal definition, stating that an issue becomes a health matter when the doctor and patient agree that it is one.[25] In Siegler's view, one of the central goals of medicine is to improve the patient's quality of life, and the determination of what is improved quality rests largely, albeit not exclusively, with the patient. This incorporates the patient perspective into the definition of health and health care, emphasizing autonomy and incorporating insights from the biopsychosocial model.

The difference in perspective between Kass and Siegler can act as a lens by which to view a fundamental question in scar treatment: should a scar be considered a medical problem? If so, should all scars and deformities—congenital ones, those acquired from trauma, those acquired iatrogenically, and others—be considered in the same manner?

Changes in the relationship of doctor and patient during the past 50 years, from a paternalistic model to one of autonomy, and now, to a shared decision-making model, suggest that Siegler's view on the ethical basis of decision-making may now be the dominant ethical paradigm. Further, Kass' proposal that medicine address only narrowly construed medical or physiological abnormalities seems to have been rejected in favor of an ever-expanding realm for medicine and medical interventions.

Contextual Features

Should Everyone Have Access to the Same Scar Interventions?

Issues of justice arise with scar intervention, as they do with every other health care issue. If scar interventions are deemed an important part of clinical care, should they not be distributed equally? What about iatrogenic scars: should a senior plastic surgeon close every incision in every hospital? Should they be on call for emergency procedures as well? Clearly, this is not feasible as that limited resource—a plastic surgeon—is not available in sufficient quantity to meet every request. Thus, is it ethically and clinically permissible to have a "reasonably" well-done skin closure? And for which patients should a skin closure be performed by a plastic surgeon and for whom should a skin closure be done in a "reasonable" manner? Consideration should be given to the fact that the ultimate quality of the resultant scar not only is determined by how each superficial stitch is placed, but actually begins with where, how, and in what direction incisions are made. Further the scar quality depends on whether or not complete hemostasis is obtained, how gently the tissue was handled, how "dead space" is dealt with, what tissue layers are closed, and what deep and superficial sutures are used. Also, the timing of when sutures are removed, subsequent treatment, compliance to postoperative instruction, and the individual genetic tendency either to scar or not all influence the ultimate quality of scars. In these issues, there is a need to also balance optimal medical treatment with available resources.

Special Categories

Pediatric Patients

Pediatric patients require special consideration because they are often too young to be informed and to participate in the consent process.[26] Infants are clearly unable to be informed, although the age of consent becomes debatable as children grow into teenagers. In the pediatric population, parents or guardians are the ones who consent; however, the physician must be wary that the intervention be in the child's best interest. Shame can be an important and hidden motivating factor for parents and guardians, as stated by Cassandra Aspinall, "This is where time needs to be spent carefully considering the motivations behind the surgical change. The relationship between external change and an internal state of mind is very important to assess. Shame is an important part of that relationship."[27]

Where does scar intervention fall on this spectrum as compared with other surgeries that children undergo without their own consent but with the consent of a parent or guardian? For instance, circumcision is performed routinely in the United States on newborns boys with parental consent; there is little discussion as to the child's future desire with respect to his foreskin. Similarly, repair of a cleft lip is considered "appropriate" given the societal attitude about this congenital problem. However, surgical intervention on gynecomastia in teenage boys is more controversial. And what of a parent that desires her teenage girl to undergo breast augmentation? Would one think differently if a parent of the same age girl desires unilateral breast augmentation for severe breast asymmetry? In all these cases, as with scar intervention, clinical and ethical standards mandate that the physician must ascertain the risks and benefits to the minor patient, despite the fact that the parent or guardian is the one consenting to, or requesting, the procedure. Assent of the child should always be obtained in children who are mature enough to understand, despite the standard that ultimate decision is that of the parents or guardians.

Precedent is common in other pediatric fields for understanding the role of parents and guardians as surrogate decision-makers. In regard to predictive genetic testing, a "best interest standard" is utilized. However, there is no specific standard as to which criteria count as the "best interest."[28] For instance, how does a parent weigh current interests against future interests? With cleft lip repair, a child must undergo a general anesthetic at a young age, which carries risk. However, repair at a young age can lead to an improved cosmetic outcome. Similarly, and perhaps more importantly, timely repair of a cleft palate will have a major effect on speech development, which may be irreparably compromised if repair is delayed. The situation is different for most conditions where predictive genetic testing is used. In those instances, early interventions and treatment do not improve the child's situation.

Keloids

Whereas any scar may be troubling to patients, keloids present an exceptionally difficult management issue given the limited efficacious interventions for the disease. Whereas we have strict definitions of hypertrophic scars and keloids, based on whether or not the scar falls inside or outside the boundary of the incision, this classification scheme pays little attention to the impact on the patients. Almost all keloids recur within 2 years of surgical excision alone, leading to the institution of additional treatment such as low-dose radiation. The data on using radiation or other adjuvant modalities are varied and there are very limited data looking at any potential secondary consequences of these modalities. Treatment protocols frequently require multiple interventions over many years. Given the propensity for these lesions to recur, physicians must heed the concept of beneficence in treatment and nonmaleficence and accurately communicate potential outcomes to the patient. Keloids and other unsightly scars may cause significant psychosocial burden. When evaluating these scars for treatment, it is important to attend to the psychological consequences on the patient when considering intervention.

Disfiguring Scars

How often do we see patients with major facial scars and deformities out and about in society? Rarely, because severely disfiguring scars can cause patients to live as hermits or in isolation except for close friends and families.

Although standard reconstructive techniques can improve most scars and deformities, there are some that are not reconstructable using conventional techniques. In the past two decades, vascularized composite allotransplantation of nonlife-saving body parts (e.g., face, hand transplants) has become a reality. Numerous ethical issues have been debated about this topic for many years. The most obvious question has been: Is it reasonable to put patients on life-long immunosuppressive medication for a nonlife-saving, quality of life operation? More than 20 face transplants have been successfully performed since the first successful partial face transplant in 2005 in France for Isabelle Diniore, a patient who had been mauled by her dog.[29] New ethical issues continue to arise including, Should we exhaust all conventional techniques attempting to repair irreparable defects before we consider whether the patient is a candidate for a face transplant, or do we save those "second-tier" conventional reconstructive techniques as a backup if the face transplant fails? Concern about leaving visible scars has changed how face transplants are done. Although the partial face transplant of Ms. Diniore was a spectacular advance in facial reconstruction, the seams (suture lines) and less than perfect skin tone and color match with partial face transplants has led most to move toward performing complete face transplants. This requires removing "normal" skin just to minimize the visibility of the scars. As more and more "normal" tissue is removed to optimize the aesthetics and function, the less likely the patient would survive if the face transplant were lost.

Physicians who treat disfiguring scars must be sensitive in balancing the risks and benefits of the treatment to the patient in the process of approaching their socially acceptable normalcy. A patient may take on considerable, potentially life-threatening physiological risk, as in the case of face transplant, in order for social benefit and reintegration into society.

Quantitative versus Qualitative Scars

Incisions are required for most surgical procedures and scars are the result of all incisions. Usually the length of a linear scar (quantity) is far less important than the quality of the scar. An incision placed in or parallel to a natural skin fold will usually result in a favorable scar. In contradistinction, an incision placed in the wrong direction or closed under tension will usually result in an unfavorable scar. The same incision made in the elderly will generally be more favorable than one made in a young person.

We have no control of the size, location, or direction of scars from traumatic origin. We do, however, have some control of the *quality* of the scar that forms as a result of traumatic injuries. Expeditious debridement of nonviable or severely traumatized tissue and closure of wounds in a timely fashion will limit the amount and duration of inflammation and thereby decrease the amount of scar formation.

One of the most important components of a consultation regarding scar revision is to determine what the patient's level of expectation is. Scars cannot be erased and scar revision has the potential of having one of four outcomes: (1) it is clearly improved and the patient is happy, (2) it is clearly improved but the patient is still bothered or embarrassed by it, (3) it is different but not significantly improved, or (4) it is made worse, which may happen if there is a wound healing complication. If it is clear that the patient will be just as unhappy with an improved (but still present) scar, it is best not to intervene. The surgeon should only commence with scar revision if it is more likely than not that the patient will not only have an improved scar but that the improvement will satisfy patient expectation and desires.

In the age of minimally invasive and robotic surgery, larger single scars are being traded for multiple small incisions. Specimen extraction sites, often the determining factor on the size of a scar, are being moved to cosmetically preferred areas. For instance, during a laparoscopic nephrectomy, the kidney can be removed via a Pfannenstiel incision, hiding the largest scar below the waistline. However, though these scar locations may be perceived as advantageous by physicians, it is important to respect patient autonomy in the planning process and provide the patient with adequate understanding of the number and location of scars.

Conclusion

There are many types of scars: congenital and acquired, physiologically limiting and aesthetically disfiguring. Ethical issues relating to scars are grounded in the context of the specific scar and the preferences of the particular patient. The clinical facts of the situation and the agreement between physician and patient that the scar is a medical/surgical issue is the first ethical requirement before scar treatment is considered. Ethical considerations in the management of scars also mandate respect of patient autonomy. The patient perspective determines whether they want the scar to be treated. The physician executes this request through the process of shared decision-making. The physician provides judgment, technical guidance, and expertise while patients express their values and preferences. It is imperative that the patient understands the limitations of what can be accomplished with scar revision and that their expectation of the final outcome is the same as those of the surgeon's.

In our view, one of the highest ethical considerations is the patient's perception of their own quality of life and whether, in the patient's view, surgical revision of a scar will improve their quality of life. Even though this decision is the patient's own, the surgeon is an independent moral agent and must agree that the scar procedure request is safe, likely to be effective, falls within the general category of "good medical care," and will contribute to improving the patient's quality of life.

Additionally, all medical care takes place in the context of limited individual and societal resources. Ethical approaches to scar management must acknowledge these limitations. Nevertheless, the old adage of never rationing at the bedside should hold for decisions about scar management. Those bedside decisions should be based on social, political, financial, and clinical agreements that antedate individual case decisions.

As an additional ethical point, we wish to discuss the doctrine of double effect and its application to surgery and specifically to iatrogenic scars.[30] The double effect doctrine states that (1) The action (in this case a needed surgical procedure) is ethically good and (2) the surgeon intends the good effect of the surgery and not the bad effect, that is, scar formation. And yet, in most instances, the scar is an inevitable result of the surgical procedure. The act of surgery is undertaken to achieve the good result while recognizing the likelihood that some scar formation will occur.

In this view, the performance of necessary surgery is entirely ethical and the surgeon's ethical obligation with regard to iatrogenic scars is to warn the patient of this necessary occurrence and to use all of his/her surgical/technical skill to reduce the extent of the scar formation. This leads to our final ethical conclusion: since surgery is often essential to benefit patients, it is equally essential as an ethical priority that we, as a society, support the kind of basic and translational research necessary to decrease scar formation and to treat unwanted scars efficaciously and cost-effectively when they do form.

REFERENCES

1. Hawthorne N. The birthmark. In: *Mosses from an Old Manse*. New York, NY: Wiley & Putnam; 1846.
2. O'Brien C. The US President's council on bioethics (2001–2009). *The Embryo Project Encyclopedia*. https://embryo.asu.edu/pages/us-presidents-council-bioethics-2001-2009. Accessed September 1, 2015.
3. Ephron N. *I Feel Bad About My Neck: And Other Thoughts on Being a Woman*. New York, NY: Knopf Doubleday Publishing Group, 2008.
4. Seldin DW. Donald Wayne Seldin, MD: a conversation with the editor. Interview by William Clifford Roberts. *Proc (Bayl Univ Med Cent)*. 2003;16(2):193–220.
5. Beauchamp TL, Childress JF. *Principles of Biomedical Ethics*. 6th ed., New York, NY: Oxford University Press, 2009.
6. Jonsen AR, Siegler M, Winslade WJ. *Clinical Ethics: A Practical Approach to Ethical Decisions in Clinical Medicine*. 1st ed. New York, NY: McGraw Hill Medical; 1982.
7. Jonsen AR, Siegler M, Winslade WJ. *Clinical Ethics: A Practical Approach to Ethical Decisions in Clinical Medicine*. 8th ed. New York, NY: McGraw Hill Medical, 2015.
8. Namm JP, Siegler M, Brander C, et al. History and evolution of surgical ethics: John Gregory to the twenty-first century. *World J Surg*. 2014;38(7):1568–1573.
9. Bosk CL. *Forgive and Remember*. 2nd ed. Chicago, IL: University of Chicago Press; 1979.
10. Wall A, Angelos P, Brown D, et al. Ethics in surgery. *Curr Probl Surg*. 2013;50(3):99–134.
11. Little M. The fivefold root of an ethics of surgery. *Bioethics*. 2002; 16(3):183–201.
12. Geiger JD, Hirschl RB. Innovation in surgical technology and techniques: Challenges and ethical issues. *Semin Pediatr Surg*. 2015;24(3):115–121.
13. The Southern Surgeons Club A prospective analysis of 1518 laparoscopic cholecystectomies. *N Engl J Med*. 1991;325:1517–1518.
14. Kittay EF. Thoughts of the desire for normality. In: Parens E, ed. *Surgically Shaping Children: Technology, Ethics, and the Pursuit of Normality*. Baltimore, MD: Johns Hopkins Press; 2008:90–112.
15. Meier DE, OlaOlorun DA, Omodele RA, et al. Incidence of umbilical hernia in African children: redefinition of "normal" and reevaluation of indications for repair. *World J Surg*. 2001;25(5):645–648.
16. Crump EP. Umbilical hernia. I. Occurrence of the infantile type in Negro infants and children. *J Pediatr*. 40:214, 1952.
17. Foley CS, Agcaoglu O, Siperstein AE, et al. Robotic transaxillary endocrine surgery: a comparison with conventional open technique. *Surg Endosc*. 2012;26(8):2259–2266.
18. Gilman SL. *Making the Body Beautiful*. Princeton, NJ: Princeton University Press; 1999.
19. Stanek J. *10 Years Younger Cosmetic Surgery Bible*. London: Transworld Publishers, 1997.
20. Testa G, Carlisle E, Simmerling M, et al. Living donation and cosmetic surgery: a double standard in medical ethics? *J Clin Ethics*. 2012;23(2):110–117.
21. Ross LF, Glannon W, Gottlieb LJ, et al. Different standards are not double standards: all elective surgical patients are not alike. *J Clin Ethics*. 2012;23(2):118–128.
22. Siegler M. Physicians' refusals of patient demands: an application of medical discernment. In: Bayer R, Caplan AL, Daniels N, eds. *In Search of Equity: Health Needs and the Health Care System*. New York, NY: Plenum Press, 1983:199–227.
23. Engel GL. The need for a new medical model: a challenge for biomedicine. *Science*. 1977;196(4286):129–136.
24. Kass L. Regarding the end of medicine and the pursuit of health. In: Caplan AL, Engelhardt Jr HT, McCartney JJ, eds. *Concepts of Health and Disease: Interdisciplinary Perspectives*. Reading, PA: Addison-Wesley Publishing Group, 1981:3–30.
25. Siegler M. The nature and limits of clinical medicine. In: Cassell EJ, Siegler M, eds. *Changing Values in Medicine*. Frederick, MD: University Publications of America, 1979:19–42.
26. Alderson P. *Children's Consent to Surgery*. Philadelphia, PA: Open University Press, 1993.
27. Aspinall C. Do I make you uncomfortable? In: Parens E, ed. *Surgically Shaping Children: Technology, Ethics, and the Pursuit of Normality*. Baltimore, MD: Johns Hopkins Press, 2008:13–28.
28. Ross LF. Predictive genetic testing of children and the role of the best interest standard. *J Law Med Ethics*. 2013;41(4):899–906.
29. Devauchelle B, Badet L, Lengelé B, et al. First human face allograft: early report. *Lancet*. 2006;368(9531):203–209.
30. Sulmasy DP, Pellegrino ED. The rule of double effect: clearing up the double talk. *Arch Intern Med*. 1999;159(6):545–550.

Formation

SECTION II

5

Scar Histopathology and Morphologic Classification

MOLLY POWERS, DAVID OZOG, and MARSHA CHAFFINS

KEY POINTS

- A more complete understanding of the relationship between clinical scar appearance and the corresponding histology over time may help guide management and the evaluation of the treatment response.
- Additional noninvasive technologies, such as reflectance confocal microscopy, may aid in the microscopic evaluation of scars.
- The morphology of a scar is classified into its physical characteristics, appearance, and symptoms.
- Scar assessment scales have been developed and implemented for the objective analysis of scars. Each scale differs from the next and may only be applicable to a unique set of scars.

The assessment and classification of scars in various conditions is essential for guiding therapy and advancing research. However, to our knowledge no consensus has been drawn on the best method to evaluate scar morphology. This chapter will help to review the basic histologic and morphologic characteristics of the various scar types and to discuss the classification of these lesions.

Scar Histology

There is limited research relating to scar histology. Hypertrophic and keloidal scars are better described, though to our knowledge there is no conclusive body of literature that examines the histology of each of the varying types of scars. The standard histologic description of a mature scar notes thicker collagen bundles with spindle cells that are arranged parallel to the epidermis, as compared with the basket weave appearance of the surrounding normal dermis as demonstrated in Figure 5-1.[1] The underlying vessels are typically oriented vertical (perpendicular) to the epidermis and are equal in number to the uninjured dermis after approximately 12 months of scar maturation.[1,2] In a mature scar there is often loss of elastic tissue with the effacement of the epidermis (Fig. 5-2).[3]

From the moment of injury to the skin and through the lifetime of the scar, there is a consistent change and remodeling, which is reflected in the corresponding histology. For example, in an early scar there are more inflammatory cells, but this usually normalizes after approximately 1 month absent any derangement in the scar maturation process.[1] Dermal vasculature also undergoes dynamic changes. One to three months after tissue injury, scars have a higher density of blood vessels in the dermis. However, as the scar continues to mature, the density decreases but blood vessel size increases in comparison to earlier scars.[1] Bond et al.[1] evaluated "poor" and "excellent" scar outliers based on their appearance in comparison to the representative group. Scars deemed "poor" were found to have higher density of blood vessels. "Excellent" scars had a lower blood vessel density and approached that of normal skin after a shorter duration of injury. These findings support the use of vascular lasers in younger scars (see Chapter 13). As a scar continues to mature, the vasculature of nonpathologic scars (excluding hypertrophic scars and keloids) approaches that of normal skin.[4] Clinically, this is associated with diminishing erythema. A maturing scar, however, does not fully recover its preinjury histology. There is complete loss of skin appendages, incomplete reformation of the rete ridges and papillary dermis, as well as alterations in the collagen fiber bundles.[1] This maturation process is further outlined in Table 5-1.

Hypertrophic (Fibroproliferative) Scars

There are important histopathologic distinctions among different scarring processes that may guide prognosis and management. However, distinguishing a hypertrophic scar from a keloid histopathologically is sometimes very difficult.[4] Keloids and hypertrophic scars both differ from normal skin as they have increased deposition of connective tissue as well as rich vasculature.[5] In the literature there is conflicting information regarding the vasculature of keloids and hypertrophic scars. Many theories suggest the role of hypoxia in the formation of pathologic scars. Kischer et al.[6] found an increased number of occluded or partially occluded

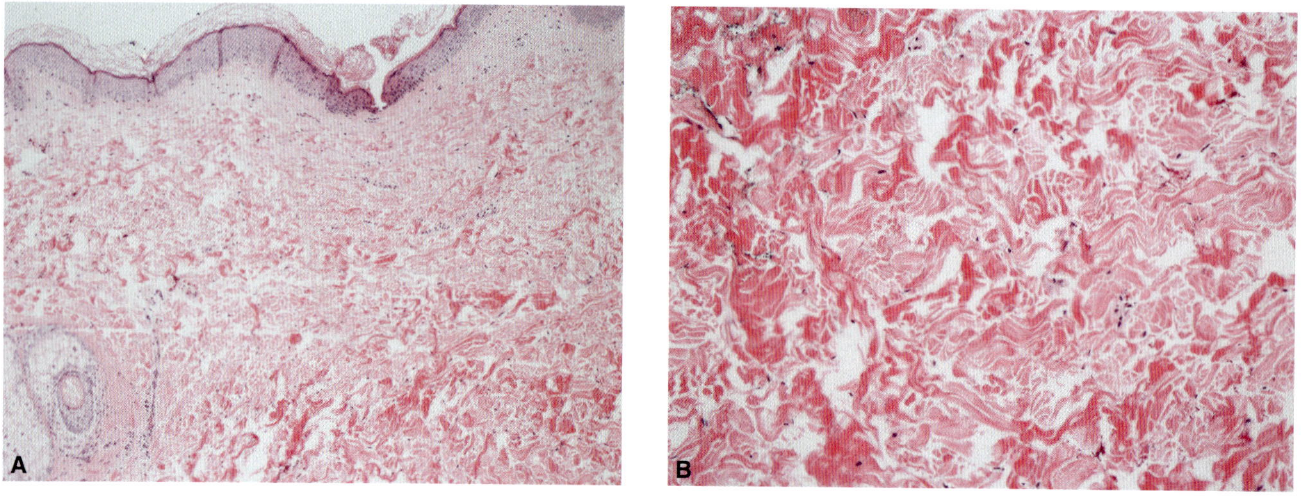

FIGURE 5-1 **Histology of normal skin**. **A:** Low-power image of normal skin with fine collagen and elastic fibers noted in the papillary dermis. **B:** Higher power image of normal reticular dermis with more compact collagen and thicker elastic fibers.

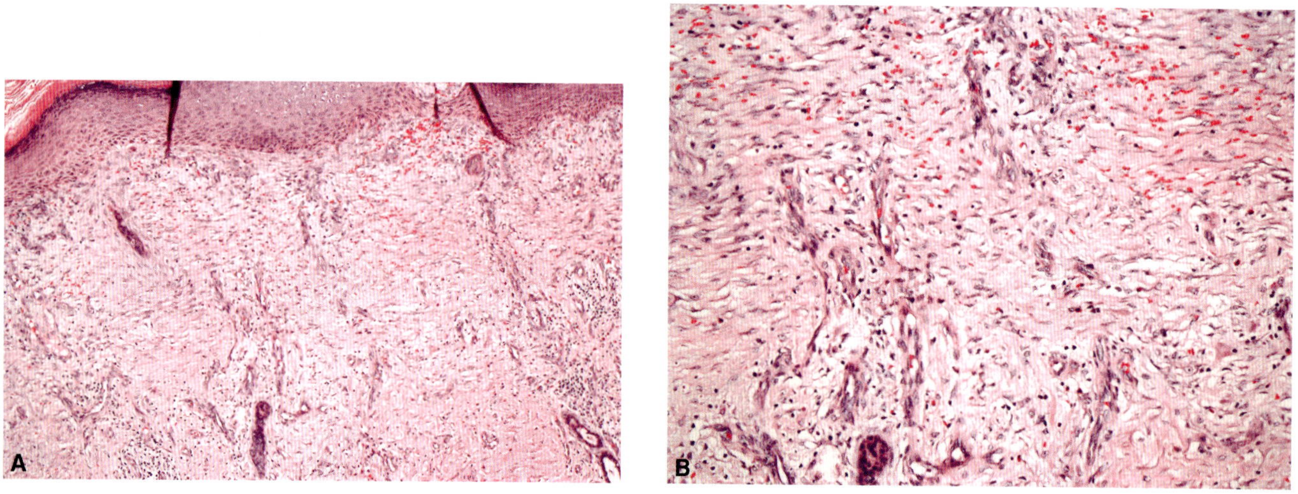

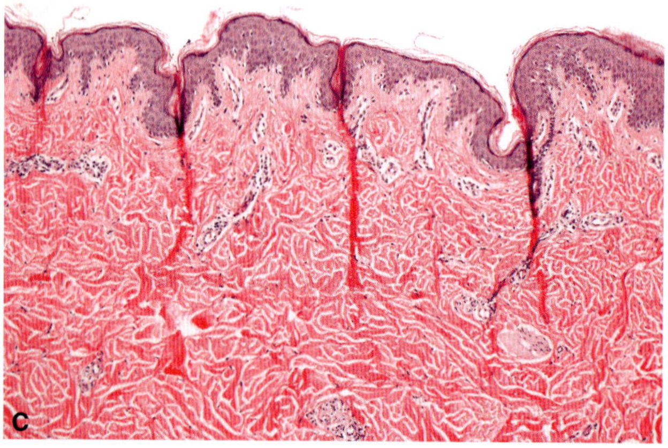

FIGURE 5-2 **The histologic comparison of an early and a late scar.** **A:** Low-power image of a newly forming scar demonstrating the cellular reticular dermis, increased vasculature, and absence of rete ridges and papillary dermis. **B:** Higher power image of a newly forming scar with fine, horizontally oriented collagen bundles and increased vasculature with vessels oriented vertically. **C:** An established scar with horizontally oriented thicker and more densely packed collagen bundles and loss of all skin appendages.

Table 5-1 Flowchart Describing the Histologic Maturation of a Scar Over Time

Months 1–3	Months 4–6	Months 7–9	Months 10–12
• Flat DEJ • Cellular reticular dermis • ECM immature with fine collagen bundles • Increased blood vessels and fibroblasts • No increased number of inflammatory cells seen after 1 mo	• Rete ridge and papillary dermis reformation minimal • Collagen fibers thicker and denser around month 4 • Scars highly vascular with larger vessels but still reduced from months 1 to 3	• Rete ridge reformation has begun • Collagen fibers becoming thicker and denser • Small reduction in blood vessel density	• Some scars with rete ridge and papillary dermal formation • Collagen fiber bundle maturity equal to the surrounding normal dermis • Fibers were dense and arranged horizontally • Blood vessel density higher than normal skin at 10 mo, but equaled that of normal skin at 12 mo

DEJ, dermoepidermal junction; ECM, extracellular matrix.

microvessels in hypertrophic and keloidal scars in comparison to normal scars and normal dermis because of endothelial cell swelling and increased endothelial cell density. Additionally the degree of vascular occlusion was higher in keloids with fewer and more flattened vessels, especially centrally within the lesion, suggesting less vascular supply in a keloid as compared with a hypertrophic scar. The growth of fibroblasts and increased collagen deposition may result in this occlusion.[7,8] On the contrary, other studies have demonstrated increased vasculature of keloids and hypertrophic scars in comparison with normal scars and normal skin.[1] Amadeu et al.[4] reported that the volume occupied by vessels in the papillary dermis was 79.7% higher in hypertrophic scars ($P < 0.01$) and 62.5% higher in keloids ($P < 0.05$) as compared with normal skin. Similar findings were noted in the reticular dermis, with hypertrophic scars having 62.9% higher vessel volume ($P < 0.025$) and keloids having 68.5% higher vessel volume than normal skin ($P < 0.001$). The benefit of pressure dressings and vascular lasers for the treatment of these pathologic scars contradicts our understating of the role of hypoxia in their pathogenesis. At this point, further research needs to be conducted to fully understand this interplay.

Aside from their vasculature, keloids and hypertrophic scars each have a high mesenchymal cell density and inflammatory cell infiltration, with an absence of subepidermal appendages including sebaceous glands and rete ridges.[1] Both lesions have a predominant active fibroblast cell type, but keloids tend to have more quiescent forms.[9] The dermis of a keloid comprises characteristic large, thick collagen bundles that are brightly eosinophilic and hyalinized with hematoxylin and eosin staining as demonstrated in Figure 5-3. These bundles are closely packed with thin fibrils and form the characteristic "keloidal collagen." Lee et al.[10] reported distinct keloidal collagen in approximately 55% of all keloids included in their study. They concluded that the histologic absence of keloidal collagen does not rule out the diagnosis of a keloid, but its presence is of high diagnostic value as it is only discovered in keloidal scars. Keloidal collagen is arranged in a nodular fashion in contrast to the parallel architecture of collagen in ordinary scars. In comparison, hypertrophic scars contain distinct smaller nodules present in the dermis (demonstrated in Fig. 5-4), aiding in the histologic distinction from keloids and normal scars, which often lack these nodules. The compaction of the collagen bundles in keloids has no effect on the overlying epidermis.[7,11] Additionally, hypertrophic scars have an accumulation of myofibroblasts expressing α-smooth muscle actin, whereas keloidal myofibroblasts often lack the expression of α-smooth muscle actin.[5]

Atrophic Scars

In contrast to keloids and hypertrophic scars, the histologic appearance of striae can be very subtle and may be difficult to distinguish from normal skin (Fig. 5-5). As with other scar types, the histologic appearance of striae depends on the stage of evolution. In earlier (younger) striae, there is often dermal edema with perivascular infiltrates. The epidermis can appear normal in earlier stages, but later may flatten and have blunting of the rete ridges (atrophy). Earlier striae may also demonstrate elastolysis and a relative lack of mast cells. There are structural changes seen in collagen bundles with prominent fibroblasts and reduced microfibrils. Earlier striae have been referred to as *striae rubra*, as they often appear erythematous in color.[12]

Well-established striae may be termed *striae alba*, owing to their hypopigmented (white) appearance over time. Striae alba demonstrate epidermal atrophy and decreased dermal thickness. Collagen fibers are generally found running parallel to the skin and transverse to the direction of the individual stria. There are variable alterations in the elastic fibers with reduced and fragmented dermal elastin on special stains. There is also loss of skin appendages including hair follicles and adnexal structures, as with all scars.[9]

Dyspigmentation

There are very few studies that examine the histologic findings associated with clinical dyspigmentation in scars. However, Travis et al.[13] evaluated the optical and histologic properties of wounds and their relationship with dyspigmentation in a porcine model. Hyperpigmented scars, hypopigmented scars, and uninjured tissue were evaluated by fixing and embedding these samples for histologic examination using Azure B stain and primary antibodies to

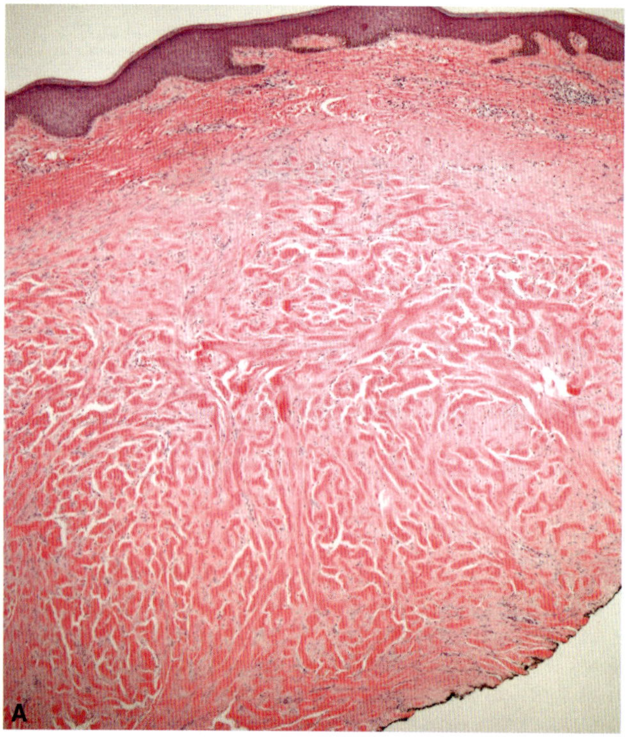

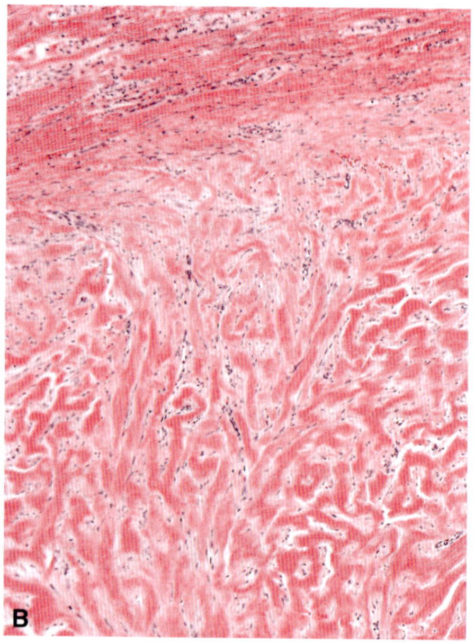

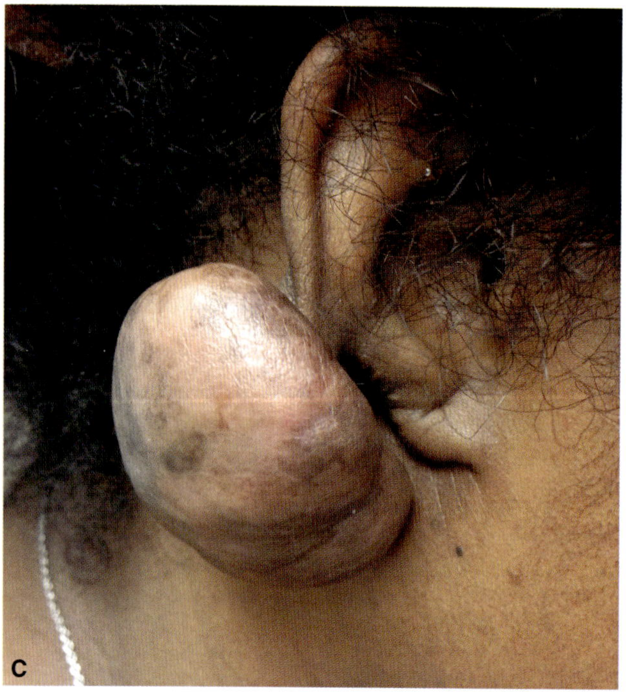

FIGURE 5-3 **Histology and clinical appearance of a keloid. A:** Low-power image demonstrating the large, thick collagen bundles that are closely packed with thin fibrils. **B:** Higher power image illustrating the unique thick nodular "keloidal collagen." **C:** Clinical picture of a keloid. Keloid on the right earlobe of this young African-American woman. The earlobe is a common site for keloid formation after ear piercing.

S100B, HMB45, and α-melanocyte-stimulating hormone (α-MSH) for comparison. They discovered no statistically significant difference in melanocyte number between hyperpigmented and hypopigmented scars and uninjured skin samples. There was, however, a statistically significant difference in the amount of melanin and α-MSH, and immunohistochemical evidence of stimulated melanocytes in hyperpigmented versus hypopigmented scars.

Histologic Effects of Fractional Laser Treatment

Whereas there has been extensive research conducted on certain scar types, elucidation of the relationship between clinical scar appearance and the corresponding histology may help guide treatment and evaluation of the response. For example, Ozog et al.[14] delineated the histologic changes

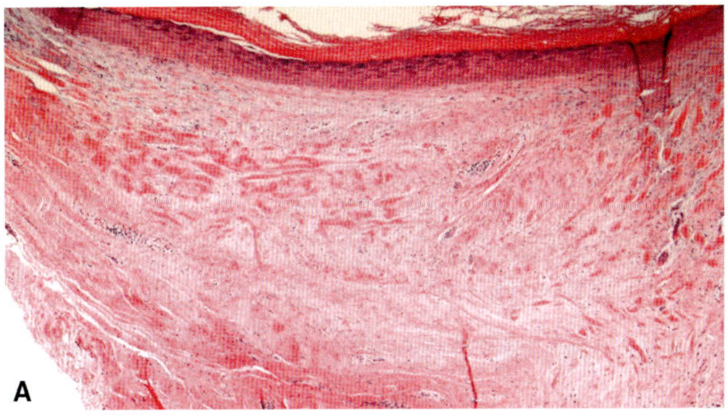

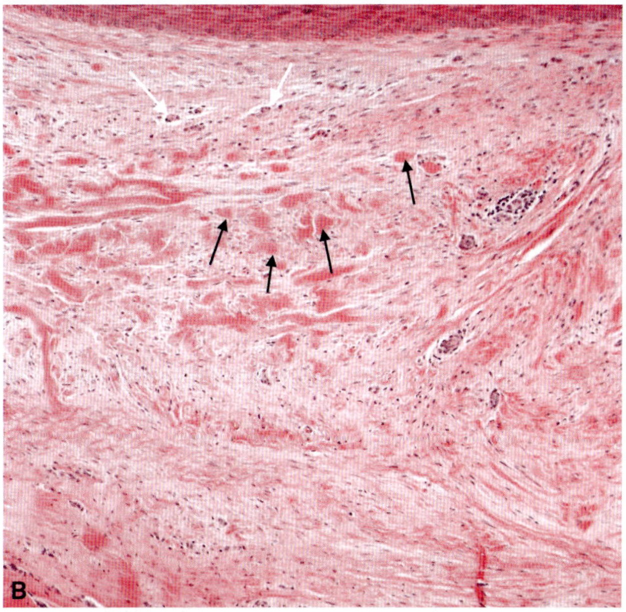

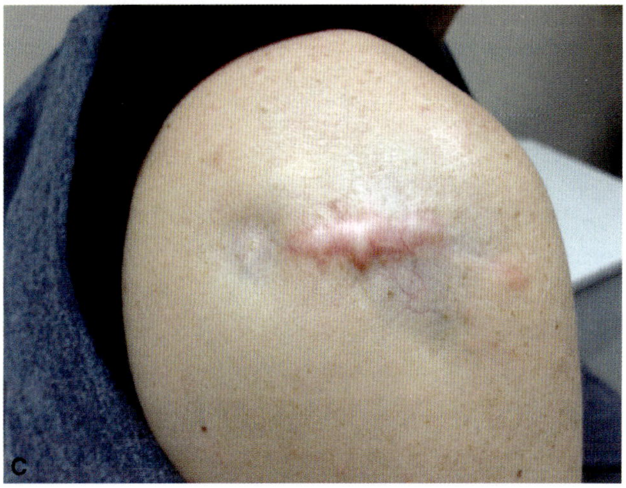

FIGURE 5-4 **Histology and clinical appearance of a hypertrophic scar**. **A:** Low-power view demonstrating the smaller nodules in the dermis. **B:** Higher power view illustrating again the smaller nodules as demonstrated by the black arrows and occluded microvessels superficially (*white arrows*) with increased deposition of connective tissue. **C:** Clinical picture of a scar with areas of atrophy and hypertrophy. Shoulder of a woman who underwent multiple intralesional steroid injections for a hypertrophic scar, resulting in steroid-induced atrophy.

in collagen typing between laser-treated and -untreated burn scars. It is well described that normal skin contains a combination of type I and type III collagen; fetal skin contains a higher proportion of type III collagen, and burn scars contain a higher proportion of type I to type III collagen. A course of three ablative fractionated CO_2 laser treatments to burn scars eventuated in a collagen profile approaching that of normal skin, with a posttreatment increase in type III collagen as demonstrated by the Herovici stain (Fig. 5-6). Additionally, Taudorf et al.[15] found statistically significant clinical improvement in various scar types (normal, hypertrophic, and atrophic) after three monthly nonablative fractional laser treatments ($P < 0.0001$ vs. untreated), with corresponding histology indicative of collagen remodeling. There is a predominance of thickened collagen within a scar as compared with the normal surrounding dermis. The healing process that follows fractionated photothermal injury ultimately leads to the remodeling and reorganization of collagen that begins to approach that of normal skin. A later study completed by Connolly et al.[16] discovered that, counterintuitively, treatment of erythematous burn scars with a fractionated CO_2 laser led to a statistically significant *increase* in vascular density as determined by anti-CD31 immunostaining, despite a *decrease* in clinically apparent erythema during the treatment course (Fig. 5-7). These histologic findings as illustrated above have both supported and challenged our understanding of the mechanisms leading to clinical improvement in scars. Perhaps we may use these predicted and unforeseen findings to further propel scientific discovery and improved management.

Reflectance Confocal Microscopy

To date, light microscopy of tissue has been the principal technique to evaluate the histology and microstructure of the skin. In vivo reflectance confocal microscopy (RCM) is a relatively new, noninvasive technology that has recently been utilized for the evaluation of various types of scars.[17–20] RCM provides real-time viewing with similar

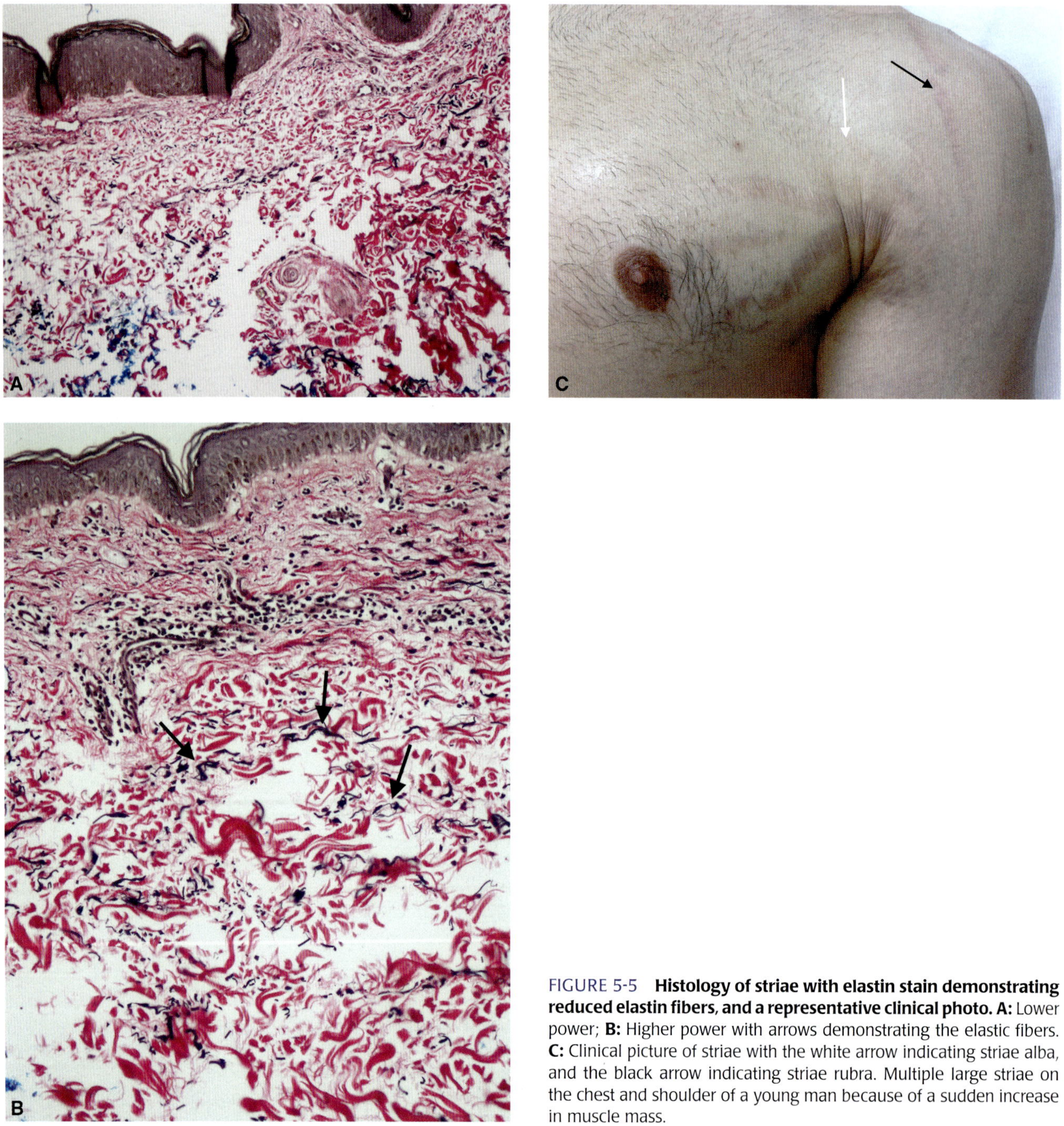

FIGURE 5-5 **Histology of striae with elastin stain demonstrating reduced elastin fibers, and a representative clinical photo. A:** Lower power; **B:** Higher power with arrows demonstrating the elastic fibers. **C:** Clinical picture of striae with the white arrow indicating striae alba, and the black arrow indicating striae rubra. Multiple large striae on the chest and shoulder of a young man because of a sudden increase in muscle mass.

resolution to classical histology, without tissue damage (Fig. 5-8). Additionally, it may be used to detect the dynamic microscopic changes of a particular skin lesion over time. RCM may provide promising in vivo evaluation and comparison of many scar types, and may also be used for the pre- and posttreatment analyses of scars, among other dermatologic conditions.

Figure 5-8 provides a clinical comparison of a hypertrophic scar with the associated confocal microscopic imaging. At a depth of 152.4 μm below stratum corneum, collagen fibers and bundles (red arrow) are present inside the lesion since it is raised compared with adjacent normal skin.

For this particular site, 152.4 μm was not deep enough to image collagen for adjacent normal skin.

Scar Assessment

There are multitudes of ways to assess a scar; as with any dermatologic condition, assessment begins with a history of the lesion. It is important to determine the mechanism,

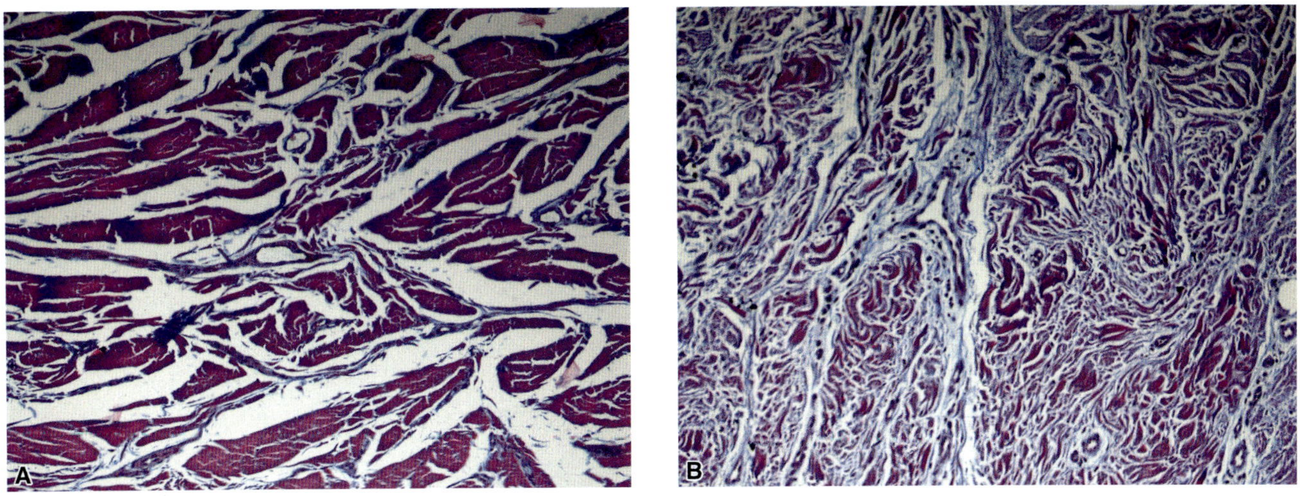

FIGURE 5-6 **A:** Pretreatment histologic image of burn scar utilizing the Herovici stain with diffuse red color indicating more type I collagen. **B:** Posttreatment of burn scar demonstrating a bluer color with Herovici stain consistent with more type III collagen.

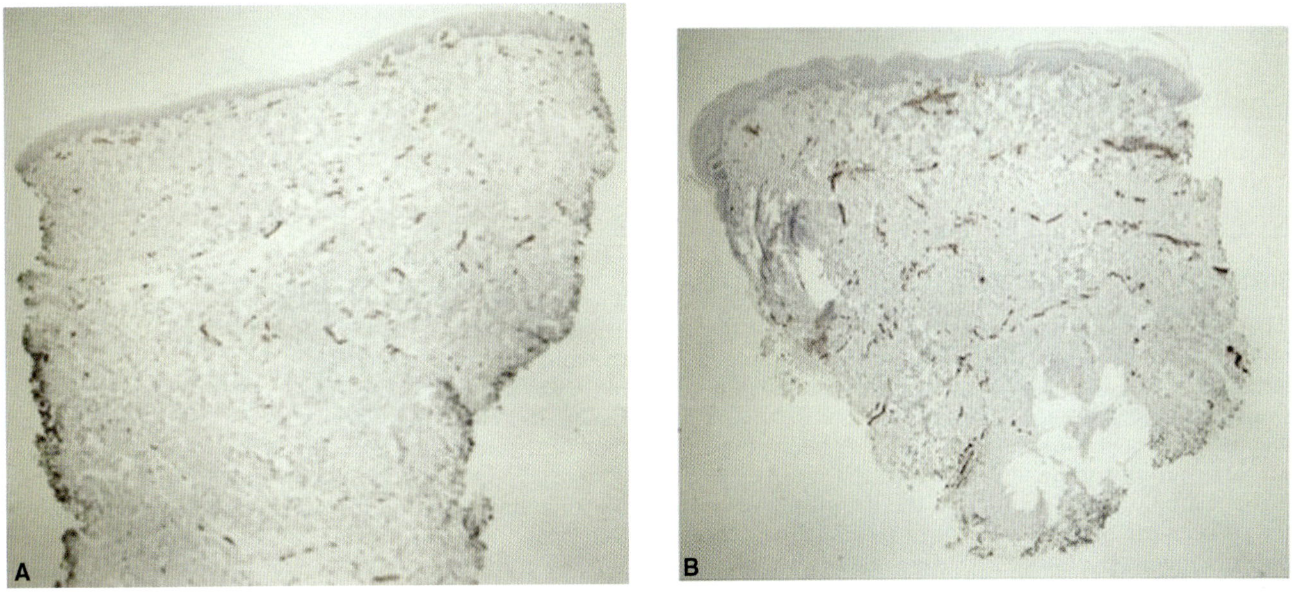

FIGURE 5-7 Pretreatment histologic image of a burn scar utilizing anti-CD31 immunostaining to highlight blood vessels demonstrated decreased blood vessels in the pretreatment scar (**A**) as compared with increased vasculature in the scar after three treatments with a fractionated CO_2 laser (**B**).

age, location, symptoms, and associated injuries. These factors are crucial to predict future behavior, and thus guide management.

The appearance of a scar is highly dependent on its stage of evolution. Granted each scar's assessment is primarily subjective, and interobserver biases will be present. There are instruments that can be utilized to more objectively analyze a scar, and these will be discussed later in this section (see also Chapter 28). The full comprehensive evaluation of a scar should include three primary measures: physical characteristics, appearance, and symptoms.[21]

Physical Characteristics

The physical characteristics of a scar are determinate of how that scar may function physiologically and mechanically. These characteristics as defined below offer vital clues to how the scar will serve in its role as repaired skin. For example, a lack of pliability will reduce the flexibility of the scar, and loss of tissue and scar contractures can lead to reduced range of motion. Assessing for these attributes may help to predict behavior and track the course of treatment (see Chapter 19).

Surface Texture (Profilometry[22])

The surface texture (relief) of a scar refers to irregularities and "lumpiness/bumpiness" when compared with normal skin.[23] For example, Figure 5-9 demonstrates the chest and shoulders of a woman after an extensive burn. The surfaces of these scars are highly variable and demonstrate many contour irregularities. Optical and mechanical profilometers

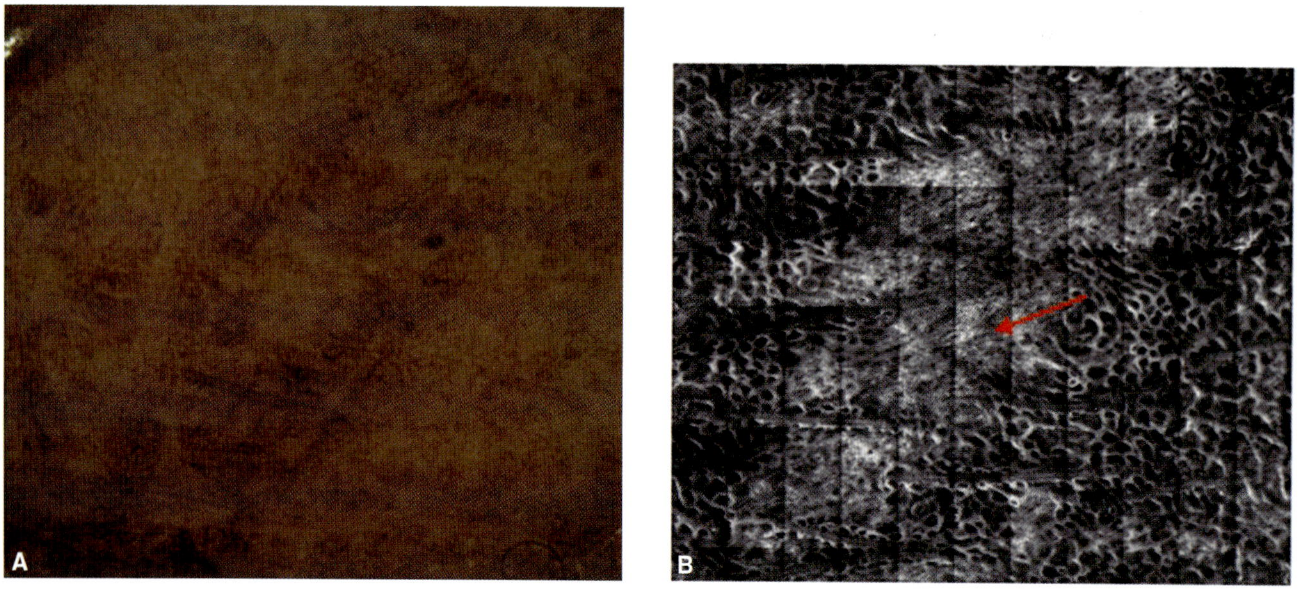

FIGURE 5-8 **A:** Clinical dermatoscopic image of a hypertrophic scar of the forearm. **B:** Confocal microscopy of the same hypertrophic scar on the forearm imaged at 152.40 μm below the stratum corneum. Collagen fibers and bundles (*red arrow*) are present within the hypertrophic scar; however, there is no collagen noted at that depth in the surrounding normal skin.

are available to provide objective measurements, but are used more commonly for cosmetic evaluations than for scar evaluations at this time.[22]

Surface Area (Planimetry[22])

This refers to the area the scar occupies in relation to the original wound size, and can be larger or smaller than the initial wound.[23] This can be assessed with simple dimensions to derive a surface area. However, more objective measures have been used in clinical studies because of the varying contours of the underlying normal and posttraumatic anatomy. More commonly, the margins have been traced on clear plastic film or grid paper, or have been photographed. For more extensive scars, such as burn scars, it may also be appropriate to quantify the scar as a percentage of total body surface area.

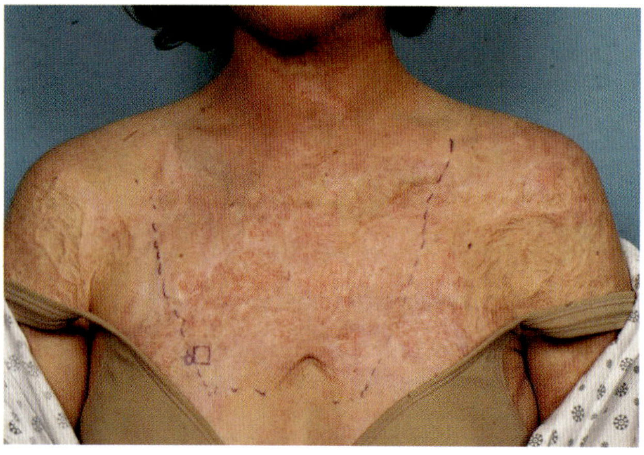

FIGURE 5-9 Clinical picture of a burn patient. Extensive burns on the chest, neck, and bilateral arms in this middle-age woman

Thickness/Height

The thickness and height of a scar is related to the scar's degree of hypertrophy. It is defined as the distance between the subcutaneous–dermal junction and epidermal surface of the scar.[23] One can measure the height of the scar from the epidermal surface of the surrounding normal skin to that of the scar; however, this will not account for the dermal component. Ultrasonography provides an accurate, reproducible, and objective method for measuring scar thickness. It also has the advantages of being noninvasive and relatively inexpensive.[24] It does have limitations, as do all imaging modalities. For example, it has limited specificity in evaluating thin lesions and lesions with surrounding inflammation. Fortunately, these limitations are not as applicable to the ultrasonographic evaluation of scars.[25] Scar thickness and height can vary tremendously based on genetic predispositions, medical conditions, and type and extent of injury.

Pliability

By definition, pliability refers to the quality of being easily bent or flexible. When pertaining to scars, it encompasses both morphologic and physiologic properties, and the pliability of a scar is crucial to its functional performance. Pliability can be evaluated grossly by assessing the range of motion over an affected joint, or by stretching the scar between two fingers.[26] A goniometer can be used to assess the maximum degree of extension or flexion prior to therapy. A relatively pliable scar will have a degree of stretch that is comparable to that of normal skin. Several tools have been developed to objectively assess this characteristic.

These include the pneumatonometer,[27] cutometer,[24] and the cicatronometer.[28] The pneumatonometer was derived from ocular tonometry. It uses similar principles to detect the pliability of a scar, measuring the flow and pressure of air in the instrument after applying pressure on the area of interest.[27] Fong et al.[24] used a cutometer to measure the pliability of burn scars. A cutometer uses gentle suction to measure the viscoelasticity of a scar. The cicatronometer is a form of a handheld tonometer. It has a loaded spring with an indicator rod attached. When applied vertically to the skin, the indicator rod is depressed to a certain degree; the further the depression, the firmer the scar.[28]

Color

The color of a scar comprises both its pigmentation and its vascularity. When assessing scars, it is important to make the distinction between the two components. As previously mentioned, the vascularity of a scar is highly associated with the age of the lesion. Earlier scars are more vascular, whereas mature nonpathologic scars eventually reach the vascularity of normal, uninjured skin. Therefore, the clinical appearance of erythema of a nonpathologic scar will subside as its vascularity normalizes over time.[1] Diascopy, or blanching of the vessels with a transparent device by applying gentle pressure, is a simple and effective way of assessing the vascularity of a scar. It also aids in eliminating the effects of vascularity when assessing the scar's pigmentation.[29] Colorimetry can also objectively assess measures of vascularity and pigmentation in the skin. A colorimeter is a device that analyzes color by measuring it in terms of a standard color, a color scale, or certain primary colors. Jones' review found high concurrent reliability, validity, and reproducibility of colorimeters in assessing vascularity; however, they fell short with pigmentation assessment as compared with the visual scoring systems.[30] Draijers et al. discovered that colorimeters produced much higher reliability in pigmentation assessment as compared with a single observer. Three observers were necessary to achieve adequate pigmentation assessment in comparison to the colorimeter. When assessing vascularity, a single observer could reliably assess the scar in comparison to the colorimeter.[31] Based on these studies, colorimeters may be particularly useful in evaluating pigmentation since this can be challenging (even for trained observers). On histologic examination, both vascularity and the pigmentation can be appreciated. For example, Travis et al.[13] discovered an increased amount of melanin, α-MSH, and stimulated melanocytes in hyperpigmented hypertrophic scars in comparison to hypopigmented hypertrophic scars, whereas there was no statistically significant difference in the number of melanocytes.

Appearance

A focus on individual characteristics such as color or elevation reveals little about the overall impact of a scar upon a patient's quality of life. A biopsychosocial approach is more informative, considering scar biology in the context of the patient's needs and expectations in their individual and social environment (see Chapter 24). For example, where is the scar located? Does it adhere to the cosmetic contours and relaxed skin tension lines? Does the scar cause any cosmetic disfigurement or loss of function? Is it located in a particularly relevant area for the patient and his/her background? Are there particularly negative associations surrounding the inciting trauma? These are all essential factors to consider with scar assessment, as cosmetically defective and functionally inhibitive scars can lead to significant psychological as well as physical distress.

Symptoms

Arguably, one of the most important aspects of a patient's scar is how it impacts him/her, if at all. The two most common symptoms related to scars are pruritus and pain. In a study by Van Loey et al.,[32] itch was rated to be one of the most important factors in a patient's assessment of his/her own scar. Other common symptoms to assess for include pain, pulling, heaviness, tightness, pinching, achiness, and tenderness. Underestimating the subjective symptoms in these patients may be detrimental to their psychological as well as physical health, and perhaps lead to undertreatment. It is well documented that the symptoms a patient may experience in their scars can lead to lasting and significant psychosocial impairments (see Chapter 11).[33,34]

Special Scar Assessment

Although there are morphologic characteristics and terms that are useful for the description and classification of all scar types regardless of origin, those resulting from acne and burns are worthy of special note because of their universality and demonstrative nature.

Acne Scar Assessment

As with any inflammatory condition of the skin, the lesions associated with acne can be both transient and persistent (see Chapter 17). Transient "scarring" of the skin in patients with acne includes postinflammatory changes such as dyspigmentation and erythematous to violaceous macules (Fig. 5-10). Postinflammatory changes may resolve with time with or without treatment, though contour changes can result. Persistent acne scars have primarily been categorized into three main subtypes: ice pick, rolling, and boxcar scars according to Jacob et al.[35] Ice pick scars are defined as narrow (<2 mm), deep scars that extend to the deeper dermis, and occasionally to the subcutaneous tissue. They are typically described as conical in shape (as if created with an ice pick), with the apex extending into the deeper dermis and a wider, well-demarcated opening at the epidermis. Boxcar scars are also sharply marginated, often oval to round in shape. As their name implies, they have vertical edges leading to the bottom portion, which can be classified as either shallow (<0.5 mm) or deep (≥0.5 mm). They are typically not as deep as ice pick scars, with the bottom-most portion of the depression remaining confined to the dermis. Many compare boxcar scars to those formed from varicella, each with the characteristic flat-bottomed, discrete depressions. Figure 5-11 illustrates a woman who had suffered from scarring acne resulting

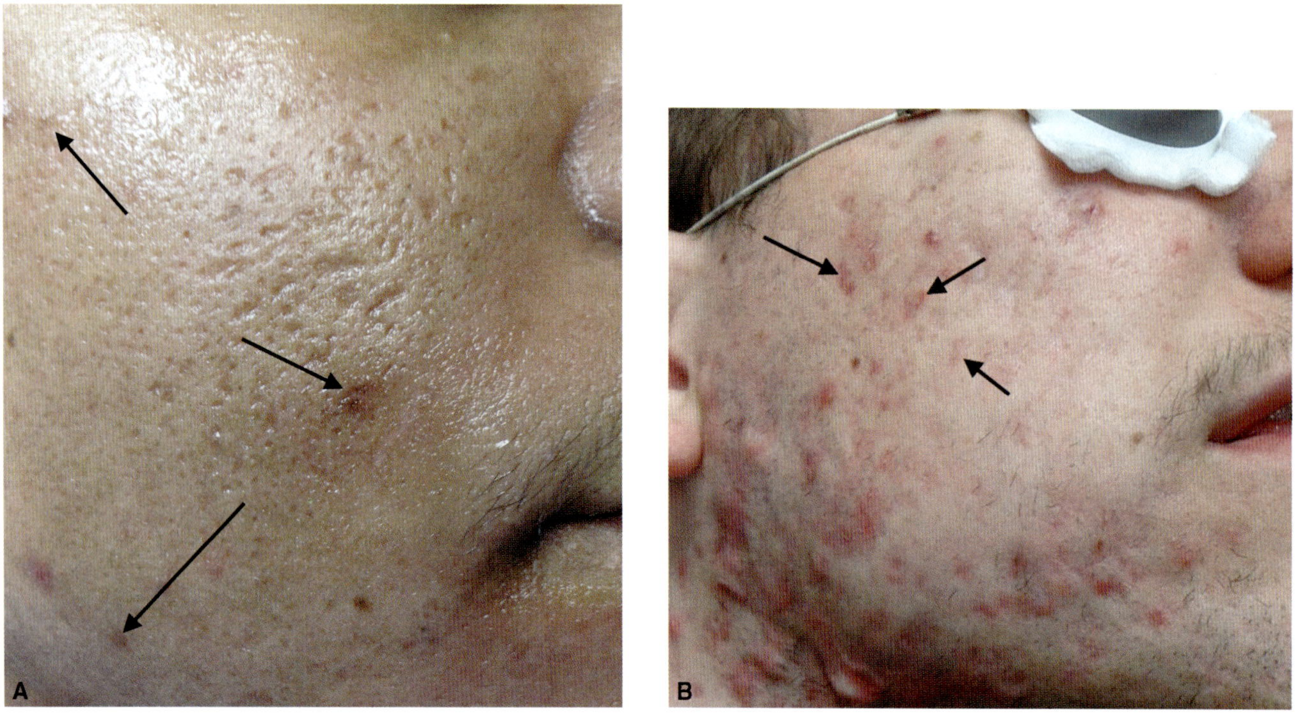

FIGURE 5-10 **A:** Hyperpigmented macules (*black arrows*) on the right cheek from previous inflammatory acne lesion. **B:** Erythematous to violaceous macules (*black arrows*) on the cheek of an adolescent man with a history of severe inflammatory acne.

in many ice pick and boxcar scars on the cheek. The third type of acne scar results from tethering of the dermis to the underlying superficial fascia, producing what we describe as rolling scars. Clinically, these scars are poorly demarcated and alter the contour of the skin to create an undulating appearance. Their appearance can be visualized best with tangential lighting to highlight these sometimes subtle depressions. Frontal flash photography will minimize or even eliminate the appearance because of lack of shadowing in the depressions, and should be avoided when used in clinical settings (Fig. 5-12).

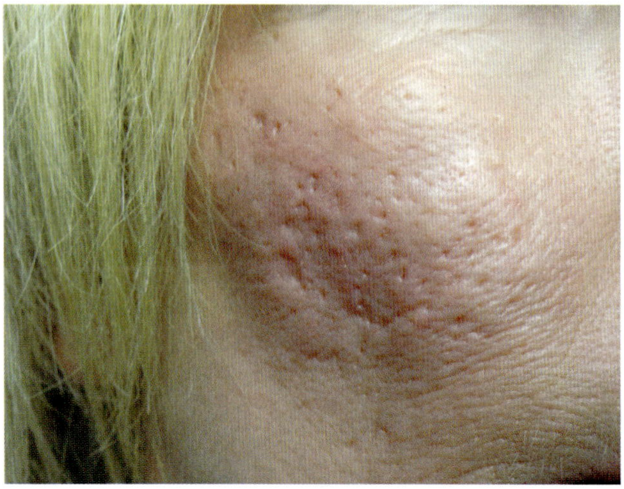

FIGURE 5-11 Ice pick and boxcar scarring associated with acne on the right cheek of an adult woman.

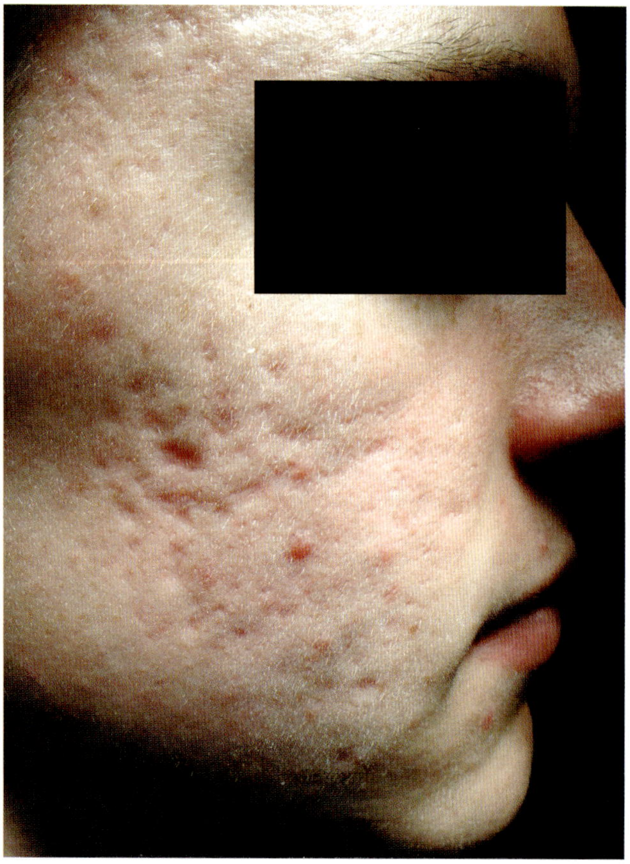

FIGURE 5-12 Picture of rolling scars in an individual with history of severe nodulocystic acne.

Burn Scar Assessment

Burn victims suffer from a distinctive set of scarring processes that can lead to significant cosmetic and functional disfigurement (see Chapter 6). Although the scars can be classified and described using the aforementioned criteria, the authors find it helpful to emphasize additional characteristics in this context. Describing the location and the surface area (sometimes given as a body surface area percentage) is of particular importance for two reasons: cosmetic appearance and functional impairment. For example, a small burn on the central face may be of more concern for one patient than a large burn scar covering the entire back. Similarly, a large burn scar with significant contraction over a joint may lead to a reduced range of motion and ultimately functional disability. Psychological assessment must also be taken into account given the multifactorial impact of burn scars on overall quality of life (see Chapter 24). Lastly, assessing the subjective components, especially pain and itch, is critical (see Chapter 11). It has been reported that the pain, tightness, and itch associated with burn scars may be more disturbing than the actual cosmetic appearance, and can have a larger negative impact on one's quality of life.[36,37]

Additionally, when assessing a burn scar, we propose to report the scar in terms of volume rather than surface area alone. As burn scars can have varying degrees of height and thickness, it is important to investigate the scar using a three-dimensional approach. This will allow for a more comprehensive understanding of the scar appearance as well as its effects on function. Determining the most effective and appropriate treatment for each scar hinges on the evaluator's ability to ultimately understand and visualize the scar volume. We propose standardized surface area measurements in conjunction with depth assessment utilizing high-frequency ultrasound to compose a volume analysis of a scar. This may be used to evaluate pre- and posttreatment scar volume.

Scar Assessment Scales

As additional advances in scar management are made, there is an increasing need to accurately assess scars in an objective manner to guide further research and management decisions (see Chapter 28). For this reason, a variety of scar assessment scales have been adapted to help determine the efficacy of therapeutic interventions over time.[38] Morphologic characteristics that are most commonly assessed with scar scales include the thickness, vascularity, and pigmentation in comparison to the subject's own uninvolved skin as a control. Further adaptations have incorporated the surface area and location of the scar as well as associated symptoms such as pain and pruritus. Additionally, the most comprehensive assessment scales have included the patient's perception of the scar's overall appearance, the observer's perceptions of the scar's overall appearance, psychosocial factors, functional impairment, and the reaction received from other individuals.

There is extensive literature to address the varying scar assessment scales. The goals of these scales are quite broad and differ depending on who is assessing the scar and for what purpose the scar necessitates an objective rating. In general, a scale should be relatively simple and reproducible to reduce inter-rater variability, allow for both quantitative and qualitative assessment, should be applicable across a wide variety of scar types in a diverse patient population, and incorporate additional factors such as psychosocial effects that may ultimately impact quality of life. The scar assessment scales chosen for review include the keystone scales and current scales that have been most recently utilized in the scar literature.

The first scar evaluation scale to enjoy widespread use was the Vancouver Scar Scale (VSS), introduced in 1990 to assess burn scars.[39] Although developed over 25 years ago, this scale is still widely used today and is the second most common scar assessment scale implemented.[40] It assesses scars based on four principal characteristics: vascularity, pigmentation, pliability, and height.[39] A modified VSS was adapted to improve the evaluation of pigmentation. The original scale assessed pigmentation categories as normal pigmentation, hypopigmentation, and hyperpigmented as 0, 1, and 2 points, respectively. This implies that a hypopigmented scar would have an overall lower VSS score than a hyperpigmented scar. The modified scale now uses an ordinal pigmentation scale ranging from normally pigmented skin to severely hypo- or hyperpigmented. Interestingly, this has not shown an increase in validity, reliability, and responsiveness.[38]

The VSS follows the Patient and Observer Scar Assessment Scale (POSAS) in frequency of use.[40] The POSAS was initially developed in 2004 and later modified in 2005.[41,42] The original POSAS evaluated surface area, thickness, vascularity, pigmentation, pain, pruritus, the patient's assessment of the overall appearance, and the observer's assessment of the overall appearance. The modified form published in 2005 added the category of functional impairment. In a recent study conducted by Bae and Bae, the POSAS was found to be the most frequently used scar assessment scale across all scar types.[40] The POSAS is one of the most comprehensive scales, and among the first to include both observer and patient assessments. This scale was compared against the VSS and found to have reduced variability and greater reliability for single observers.[41] In our own scar research, we have used both the VSS and POSAS and found them both to have considerable utility. We do believe that significantly more information is gathered from POSAS with minimal additional time and effort. Specifically in our work evaluating mature burn scars, patient subjective self-evaluation of improvement after fractional CO_2 laser treatment was much greater than physician observers. This led to an understanding that the overall "feel" of these scars is markedly improved from the patient perspective, correlating to histologic improvement but only moderately correlating with external physician observation.

The Visual Analog Scale (VAS) was introduced in 1995 as a means to assess a patient's subjective experience with pain. It was not specifically created for the evaluation of scar-related pain, but has been used in scar assessment as a simple and quick subjective evaluation of a patient's own scar. It does not evaluate the clinical morphology of scars. Patients are asked to select a point on a 100 mm line, ranging from no pain to the worst pain imaginable.[43] This scale has shown high observer reliability and internal

Table 5-2 Comparison of Components Included in the Most Commonly Used Scar Assessment Scale

	Vancouver Scar Scale–VSS (1990)	Modified VSS (1995)	Visual Analog Scale–VAS (1994)	Manchester Scar Scale–MSS (1998)	Patient and Observer Scar Assessment Scale–POSAS (2004)	Modified POSAS (2005)	Stony Brook Scar Evaluation Scale–SBSES (2007)
Surface area					✔	✔	✔
Thickness	✔	✔		✔	✔	✔	✔
Location							
Vascularity	✔	✔			✔	✔	
Pigmentation	✔	✔		✔	✔	✔	✔
Psychosocial factors							
Reaction from others							
Pain		✔	✔		✔	✔	
Pruritus		✔			✔	✔	
Dysesthesias							
Functional impairment						✔	
Patient's assessment of overall appearance					✔	✔	
Observer's assessment of overall appearance					✔	✔	✔

consistency in the expert panel, but shows only moderate reliability when used among the nonexperts.[44,45]

The Manchester Scar Scale (MSS) was introduced in 1998 by Beausang et al.[46]; it is unique as it includes an overall VAS that is added to the individual attribute scores, and a mismatch level between the scar and the surrounding normal skin. The mismatch comparison assesses seven parameters: *color* (perfect, slight, obvious, or gross mismatch to surrounding skin), *skin texture* (matte or shiny), *relationship to surrounding skin* (range from flush to keloid), *texture* (range from normal to hard), *margins* (distinct or indistinct), *size* (<1, 1 to 5, >5 cm), and *single or multiple*. It is excellent in the evaluation of linear and widespread scars, but does not account for patient symptoms. The MSS has also demonstrated statistically significant correlations with its score and the histology of the scar.[40] It does not, however, distinguish pigmentation from vascularity regarding the color mismatch assessment. The MSS has not been used significantly in research to date.[29]

The Stony Brook Scar Evaluation Scale described in 2007 sought to evaluate five principal characteristics of scars: *width*, *elevation/depression*, *color*, *suture/staple marks*, and the *overall appearance*. This scale lacks a subjective component.[47] It was designed to evaluate short-term, rather than long-term cosmetic outcomes at approximately 5 to 10 days after surgery.[29] Therefore, it has limited applicability in long-term pathologic scar assessment.

As with any subjective rating system, there are inherent strengths and weaknesses to each scale and it is important for all observers/raters to be familiar with them.[48] There is no single scale that will assess all scars reproducibly across all characteristics among different raters. Clinicians and researchers utilizing scar assessment scales must select the most appropriate scale based on the parameters of interest.

Table 5-2 illustrates the more commonly used scar assessment scales and reviews the components evaluated in each scale.

REFERENCES

1. Bond JS, Duncan JA, Sattar A, et al. Maturation of the human scar: an observational study. *Plast Reconstr Surg*. 2008;121:1650–1658.
2. Ko CJ, Barr RJ. *Dermatopathology: Diagnosis by First Impression*. 2nd ed. Wiley-Blackwell; 2008.
3. Elston DM, Ferringer T, Ko CJ, et al. *Dermatopathology*. China: Elsevier Limited; 2014.
4. Amadeu T, Braune A, Mandarim-de-Lacerda C, et al. Vascularization pattern in hypertrophic scars and keloids: a stereological analysis. *Pathol Res Pract*. 2003;199:469–473.
5. Ehrlich HP, Desmouliere A, Diegelmann RF, et al. Morphological and immunochemical differences between keloid and hypertrophic scar. *Am J Pathol*. 1994;145(1):105–113.

6. Kischer CW, Thies AC, Chvapil M. Perivascular myofibroblasts and microvascular occlusion in hypertrophic scars and keloids. *Hum Pathol.* 1982;13(9):819–824.
7. Kischer CW, Shetlar MR. Microvasculature in hypertrophic scars and the effects of pressure. *J Trauma.* 1979;19(10):757–764.
8. Kurokawa N, Ueda K, Tsuji M. Study of microvascular structure in keloid and hypertrophic scars: density of microvessels and the efficacy of three-dimensional vascular imaging. *J Plast Surg Hand Surg.* 2010;44:272–277.
9. Kischer CW. Comparative ultrastructure of hypertrophic scars and keloids. *Scan Electron Microsc.* 1984:423–431.
10. Lee JY, Yang CC, Chao SC, et al. Histopathological differential diagnosis of keloid and hypertrophic scar. *Am J Dermatopathol.* 2004;26:379–384.
11. Niessen FB, Spauwen PH, Schalkwijk J, et al. On the nature of hypertrophic scars and keloids: a review. *Plast Reconstr Surg.* 1999;104:1435–1458.
12. Arem AJ, Kischer CW. Analysis of striae. *Plast Reconstr Surg.* 1980;65(1):22–29.
13. Travis TE, Ghassemi P, Ramella-Roman JC, et al. A multimodal assessment of melanin and melanocyte activity in abnormally pigmented hypertrophic scar. *J Burn Care Res.* 2015;36:77–86.
14. Ozog DM, Liu A, Chaffins ML, et al. Evaluation of clinical results, histological architecture, and collagen expression following treatment of mature burn scars with a fractional carbon dioxide laser. *JAMA Dermatol.* 2013;149:50–57.
15. Taudorf EH, Danielsen PL, Paulsen IF, et al. Non-ablative fractional laser provides long-term improvement of mature burn scars—a randomized controlled trial with histological assessment. *Lasers Surg Med.* 2015; 47(2):141–147.
16. Connolly KL, Chaffins M, Ozog D. Vascular patterns in mature hypertrophic burn scars treated with fractional CO_2 laser. *Lasers Surg Med.* 2014;46:597–600.
17. Bencini PL, Tourlaki A, Galimberti M, et al. Nonablative fractional photothermolysis for acne scars: clinical and in vivo microscopic documentation of treatment efficacy. *Dermatol Ther.* 2012;25:463–467.
18. Rolfe H, Wurm E, Gilmore S. An investigation of striae distensae using reflectance confocal microscopy. *Australas J Dermatol.* 2012;53(3):181–185
19. Cameli N, Mariano M, Serio M, et al. Preliminary comparison of fractional laser with fractional laser plus radiofrequency for the treatment of acne scars and photoaging. *Dermatol Surg.* 2014;40:553–561.
20. Lo WC, Villiger M, Golberg A, et al. Longitudinal, 3D imaging of collagen remodeling in murine hypertrophic scars in vivo using polarization-sensitive optical frequency domain imaging. *J Invest Dermatol.* 2016;136(1):84–92.
21. Vercelli S, Ferriero G, Sartorio F, et al. How to assess postsurgical scars: a review of outcome measures. *Disabil Rehabil.* 2009;31(25):2055–2063.
22. van Zuijlen PP, Angeles AP, Kreis RW, et al. Scar assessment tools: implications for current research. *Plast Reconstr Surg.* 2002;109:1108–1122.
23. van de Kar AL, Corion LU, Smeulders MJ, et al. Reliable and feasible evaluation of linear scars by the Patient and Observer Scar Assessment Scale. *Plast Reconstr Surg.* 2005;116:514–522.
24. Fong SS, Hung LK, Cheng JC. The cutometer and ultrasonography in the assessment of postburn hypertrophic scar—a preliminary study. *Burns.* 1997;23(suppl 1):S12–S18.
25. Mandava A, Ravuri PR, Konathan R. High-resolution ultrasound imaging of cutaneous lesions. *Indian J Radiol Imag.* 2013;23:269–277.
26. Silverberg R, Johnson J, Moffat M. The effects of soft tissue mobilization on the immature burn scar: results of a pilot study. *J Burn Care Rehabil.* 1996;17:252–259.
27. Spann K, Mileski Wj, Atiles L, et al. The 1996 Clinical Research award. Use of a pneumatonometer in burn scar assessment. *J Burn Care Rehabil.* 1996;17(6 Pt 1):515–517
28. Katz SM, Frank DH, Leopold GR, et al. Objective measurement of hypertrophic burn scar: a preliminary study of tonometry and ultrasonography. *Ann Plast Surg.* 1985;14(2):121–127.
29. McOwan CG, MacDermid JC, Wilton J. Outcome measures for evaluation of scar: a literature review. *J Hand Ther.* 2001;14:77–85.
30. Jones HG. Clinimetrics of tristimulus colourimeters in scar assessment: a review of evidence. *J Wound Care.* 2012;21:30–35.
31. Draaijers LJ, Tempelman FR, Botman YA, et al. Colour evaluation in scars: tristimulus colorimeter, narrow-band simple reflectance meter or subjective evaluation? *Burns.* 2004;30:103–107.
32. Van Loey NE, Bremer M, Faber AW, et al. Itching following burns: epidemiology and predictors. *Br J Dermatol.* 2008;158:95–100.
33. Sidgwick GP, McGeorge D, Bayat A. A comprehensive evidence based review on the role of topicals and dressings in the management of skin scarring. *Arch Dermatol Res.* 2015;307:461–477.
34. Sobanko JF, Sarwer DB, Zvargulis Z, et al. Importance of physical appearance in patients with skin cancer. *Dermatol Surg.* 2015;41:183–188.
35. Jacob CI, Dover JS, Kaminer MS. Acne scarring: a classification system and review of treatment options. *J Am Acad Dermatol.* 2001;45:109–117.
36. Van Loey NE, Van Son MJ. Psychopathology and psychological problems in patients with burn scars: epidemiology and management. *Am J Clin Dermatol.* 2003;4:245–272.
37. Patterson DR, Everett JJ, Bombardier CH, et al. Psychological effects of severe burn injuries. *Psychol Bull.* 1993;113:362–378.
38. Tyack Z, Simons M, Spinks A, et al. A systematic review of the quality of burn scar rating scales for clinical and research use. *Burns.* 2012;38(1):6–18.
39. Sullivan T, Smith J, Kermode J, et al. Rating the burn scar. *J Burn Care Rehabil.* 1990;11:256–260.
40. Bae SH, Bae YC. Analysis of frequency of use of different scar assessment scales based on the scar condition and treatment method. *Arch Plast Surg.* 2014;41(2):111–115.
41. Draaijers LJ, Tempelman FR, Botman YA, et al. The patient and observer scar assessment scale: a reliable and feasible tool for scar evaluation. *Plast Reconstr Surg.* 2004;113:1960–1965; discussion 66–67.
42. Fearmonti R, Bond J, Erdmann D, et al. A review of scar scales and scar measuring devices. *Eplasty.* 2010;10:e43.
43. Scott J, Huskisson EC. Graphic representation of pain. *Pain.* 1976;2(2):175–184.
44. Micomonaco DC, Fung K, Mount G, et al. Development of a new visual analogue scale for the assessment of area scars. *J Otolaryngol Head Neck Surg.* 2009;38:77–89.
45. Duncan JA, Bond JS, Mason T, et al. Visual analogue scale scoring and ranking: a suitable and sensitive method for assessing scar quality? *Plast Reconstr Surg.* 2006;118:909–918.
46. Beausang E, Floyd H, Dunn KW, et al. A new quantitative scale for clinical scar assessment. *Plast Reconstr Surg.* 1998;102:1954–1961.
47. Singer AJ, Arora B, Dagum A, et al. Development and validation of a novel scar evaluation scale. *Plast Reconstr Surg.* 2007;120:1892–1897.
48. Nguyen TA, Feldstein SI, Shumaker PR, et al. A review of scar assessment scales. *Semin Cutan Med Surg.* 2015;34:28–36.

6

The Cellular and Molecular Basis of Scarring: The Paradigm of Hypertrophic Scarring After Thermal Injury

EDWARD E. TREDGET and JIE DING

KEY POINTS

- Hypertrophic scar(s) (HTS) are a common dermal form of fibroproliferative disorder.
- HTS commonly develop after thermal and other injuries to the deep layers of the dermis where prolonged inflammation occurs.
- Although HTS have a low mortality, they can result in functional limitations and cosmetic and psychological difficulties for burn survivors.
- Very few satisfactory treatment exists currently, which emphasizes the necessity of improving understanding of the mechanisms upon which novel therapy can be developed.

Clinical Significance of Fibroproliferative Disorders of the Skin

Fibroproliferative disorders (FPD) can involve many tissues throughout the body and constitute a leading cause of mortality in the United States, where they are involved as reported in 45% of annual deaths (see Chapter 3). Hypertrophic scars (HTS) and keloids are the dermal equivalent of FPD (Fig. 6-1).

HTS are a dermal form of FPD resulting from fibrotic wound healing after injuries to the deep dermis, because of burn injury, laceration, abrasions, surgery, and other trauma. HTS are red, raised, rigid and can cause pruritus, pain, and joint contractures. HTS formed in the facial area can cause cosmetic disfigurement, which predisposes to difficulties in psychological and social recovery after injury. HTS differ from keloids, which are characterized by frequent extension beyond the boundary of the original skin injury, occurrence even after very minor insults, and a higher incidence in darkly pigmented races. HTS occur commonly in all racial groups and are confined to the boundaries of the original wound.

HTS impose relatively low mortality but great morbidity, varying in incidence from 44% following surgical wounds to up to 91% following burn wounds, depending on the depth of injury.[1–3] In the United States, 1.25 million people are treated for burns annually, 50,000 of them requiring hospitalization.[4–6] In Canada, thermal injury necessitating hospitalization affects 26.4 patients per 100,000 people, amounting to greater than 7,000 significant thermal injuries annually; approximately 80% involve patients less than 45 years of age.[7,8] Although the mortality rate for thermal injury has improved, burn patients experience a prolonged period of hospitalization (mean 26.2 days) and prolonged rehabilitation,[9,10] requiring an average of 12.7 weeks off work for patients with thermal injuries greater than 30% of the total burn surface area (TBSA). Much of the rehabilitative phase is related to functional and cosmetic limitations imposed by HTS,[10] including a reduction in range of motion of the extremities and the intense pruritus and heat intolerance making early return to work prohibitive[6,7,10] (see Chapter 11).

Risk Factors for Hypertrophic Scars of the Skin

Risk factors such as young age, race/ethnicity, location of injury, and severity of injury (TBSA burn >20%) are well-recognized clinical features in the development of FPD of the skin.[3,8,11] Prospective randomized studies have revealed that high body mass index, non-Caucasian ethnic background, and scar discomfort including pain and itch are positively associated with HTS, especially in individuals <50 years of age. The presence of hypertension is positively associated with the development of HTS,

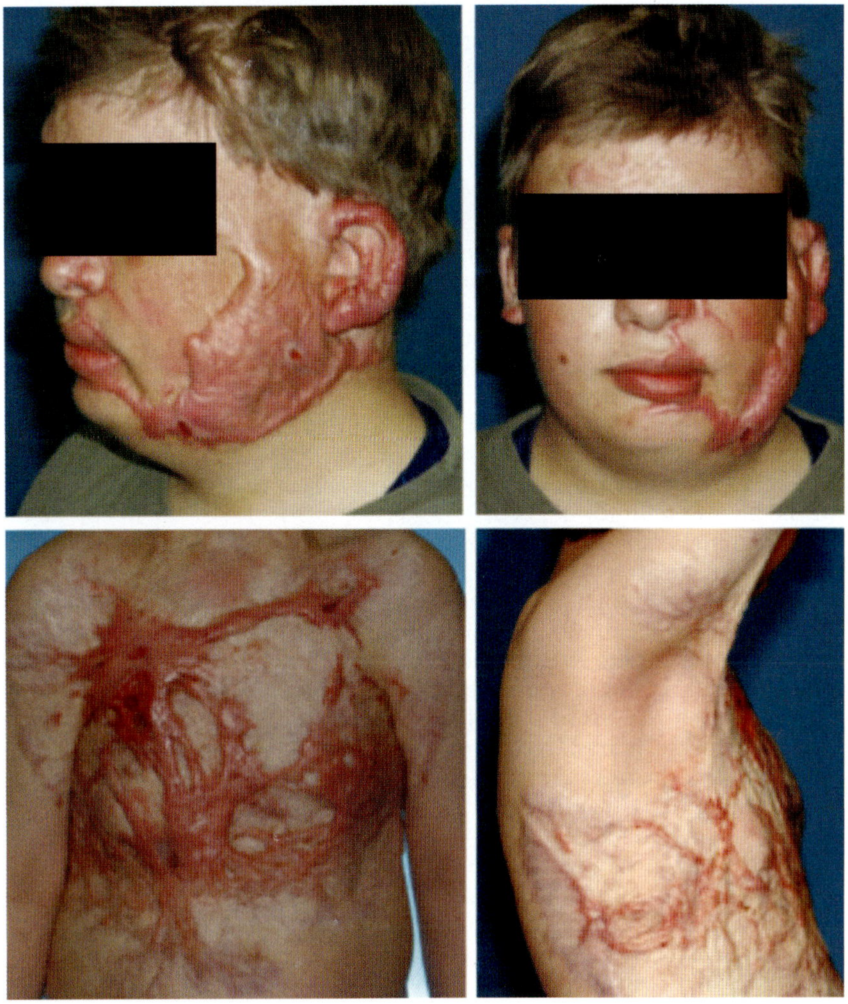

FIGURE 6-1 HTS in a 15-year-old boy 20 months after burn injury. (*From Ladak A, Tredget EE. Pathophysiology and management of the burn scar.* Clin Plast Surg. *2009;36(4):661–742.*)

and antihypertensive drugs and erythropoiesis-influencing agents appear to have antifibrotic affects.[11] HTS develop with very high frequency after prolonged inflammation of slowly healing deep dermal wounds independent of other factors,[12] with an incidence ranging up to 30% to 72% of burn patients as documented by Bombaro in injured military personnel.[13,14] Unfortunately, HTS and keloids are known to respond poorly to current forms of therapy including pressure garments, topically applied silicone, and intralesional steroids (see Chapter 10). Improvements usually accrue slowly over months or years, and often incompletely.[3,11,12,15–18] Genetic abnormalities associated with FPD, including single nucleotide polymorphisms (SNP), have been identified in some racial subpopulations such as the p27kip1 SNP in American Indian/Alaskan Natives.[19]

As burn mortality rates improve, the resulting severe sequelae lead to prolonged periods of hospitalization and extensive rehabilitation, much of which is related to functional and psychological limitations imposed by HTS. A degree of remodeling of their HTS is a prerequisite for returning to their preinjury duties.[20,21] Although most burn survivors recover, physical and psychiatric rehabilitation are significantly affected by the stigmatization, which occurs from their resulting scars[22,23] (see Chapters 19 and 24).

Morphology and Composition of the Matrix in Hypertrophic Scars

Highlights:

- HTS have thinner collagen fibrils with extensive regions of hyaline-appearing proteoglycans and glycoproteins in the interfibrillar spaces.
- Ultrastructural nodules or whorls are present in HTS.
- HTS contain higher proportions of types III and V collagens and low amounts of the small leucine-rich proteoglycan decorin, as compared with normal skin.

Collagen is the predominant extracellular matrix (ECM) protein in normal skin and HTS, where it functions to provide tensile strength of the tissue. However, collagen represents only about 30% of the dry weight of HTS because of other components including proteoglycans and glycoproteins, such as fibronectin and tenascin.[24] The major genetic form of collagen in skin is type I, assembled into thick fibrils, fibers, and fiber bundles. In HTS, thinner collagen fibrils averaging around 60 nm are present compared with 100 nm in normal dermis. This is in part because of higher proportions of thinner types III and V collagens in HTS, as much as 33% and 10%, respectively.[25] In light microscopy, much of the collagen in HTS is in whorls or nodules rather than thick fibers or fiber bundles that are normally oriented parallel to the surface in unaffected skin[26] (see Chapter 5). Extensive regions of hyaline-appearing material exist in HTS with little organization of the fine collagen fibrils, leading to an ovoid or irregular cross-section on electron microscopy. The interfibrillar space is occupied by proteoglycans and glycoproteins, which normally function to provide turgor, resilience, and resistance to compression as well as influencing cell adhesion and other functions, partly by modifying growth factor activity. Proteoglycans, which account for the water holding capacity of tissues, consist of one or more glycosaminoglycan chains as linear anionic polymers of disaccharides covalently attached to a protein core.[27] In HTS there is a 2.4-fold increase in glycosaminoglycan content and they are hyperhydrated relative to normal dermis and mature scars, accounting for the increased turgor in HTS.[24,27]

HTS contain only 2% of the normal amount of a small dermatan sulfate proteoglycan, decorin, which is the major proteoglycan found in normal dermis. Instead, there is a sixfold higher concentration of a large proteoglycan versican, which carries 12 to 30 chrondroitin sulfate chains. It is found normally in hyaline cartilage, and in small amounts in proliferating regions of the epidermis and associated with elastin in the dermis. Decorin regulates collagen fibril formation; decorin knockout animals display collagen fibrils that are variable in diameter and irregular in outline,[28] similar to that seen in HTS.[27]

As scars mature spontaneously, collagen fibers become coarser and better organized and there is a return of decorin (detected by immunohistochemistry) associated with a large increase in the number of decorin expressing cells.[27,29] Mature scars ultimately show contents of collagen, proteoglycans, and water that are indistinguishable from those in normal dermis.[24]

The Cellular Basis of Hypertrophic Scarring

Fibroblasts and Myofibroblasts

Highlights:

- Dermal fibroblasts are the predominant cell type in the dermis.
- HTS fibroblasts have many unique properties different from normal skin fibroblasts.
- Myofibroblasts are a contractile phenotype of fibroblasts.

Normal fibroblasts and HTS fibroblasts have been found to have significantly different features in vitro (Table 6-1). Many HTS strains synthesize fibronectin, pro-α2[I] collagen mRNA and protein, and transforming growth factor beta (TGF-β)[30] at higher levels than normal dermal fibroblasts. All strains of HTS fibroblasts consistently demonstrate reduced collagenase (matrix metalloproteinase—MMP-1),[31] nitric oxide,[32] and decorin production.[33]

Increased numbers of myofibroblasts constitute a prominent component of the hypercellular matrix in HTS; they contain microfilament bundles and alpha smooth muscle actin (α-SMA) important for wound contraction, a significant comorbid complication of HTS and other FPD.[34,35] The development of myofibroblasts appears to be induced by TGF-β[33,36] and strongly correlates with the severity of burn injury (TBSA). Myofibroblasts appear to differentiate not only from regional fibroblasts in the wounds under the influence of TGF-β,[36] but also from bone marrow–derived blood-borne sources.[37–39] Different from fibroblasts, myofibroblasts show highly modulated responses to TGF-β1 and interferon (IFN)-γ during wound healing, and in collagen synthesis and contractile capacity.[36] Myofibroblast formation can be induced by the application of tension in the

Table 6-1 Features of Normal, HTS, and Deep Dermal Fibroblasts

	Normal Fibroblasts	HTS Fibroblasts	Deep Dermal Fibroblasts
Cell size	+	++	+
Proliferation rate	++	+++	+
Collagen synthesis	+	++	++
Collagenase activity	++++	+	+
α-SMA expression	+	+++	+++
Collagen contraction	+	+++	+++
TGF-β	+	+	+
TGF-β T II receptor	+	+++	+++
CTGF	+	+++	+++
Osteopontin	+	+++	+++
Decorin	++++	+	+
Fibromodulin	++++	+	+
Biglycan	+	+++	+++
Versican	+	+++	+++
TLRs	+	+++	++

α-SMA, alpha smooth muscle actin; TGF-β, transforming growth factor beta; CTGF, connective tissue growth factor; TLRs, toll-like receptors.

absence of wounding[38] (see Chapter 7). As granulation tissue is converted to HTS and to mature scar tissue, a reduction in cellularity occurs through the induction of apoptosis, a process that is abrogated in myofibroblasts present in HTS by the expression of α-SMA in stress fibers.[39,40]

Fibroblast Heterogeneity and the Profibrotic Microenvironment

Highlights:

- The end result of scar formation (as opposed to regeneration) after a burn injury beyond a critical depth is presumed to be influenced by the heterogeneity in fibroblast populations at different levels (Fig. 6-2).[41]

Sorrell and Caplan have found that normal adult human skin contains at least three separate subpopulations of fibroblasts; these occupy unique niches depending on the depth in the dermis and exhibit distinctive differences when isolated by limited dilution cloning.[42,43] Fibroblasts associated with hair follicles show distinctive characteristics from cells in the papillary and reticular dermis.[44,45] Papillary dermal fibroblasts, which reside in the superficial dermis, are heterogeneous in terms of morphology and proliferation kinetics; reticular fibroblasts in the deep dermis possess myofibroblast-like characteristics associated with greater collagen lattice contraction and α-SMA expression.[46–49]

Fibroblasts that arise from the deeper layers proliferate at a slower rate,[48] are significantly larger morphologically,[49] and MMP-1 mRNA is significantly lower. Fibroblasts from the deeper layers produce more TGF-β, connective tissue growth factor (CTGF), and heat shock protein 47 (HSP47), a human chaperone protein for type I collagen. Fibroblasts from the deeper layer also produce more α-SMA protein and contract collagen gels more efficiently.[49] They also produce more collagen, more of the fibrocartilaginous proteoglycan versican, and less decorin.[48,49] As discussed earlier, decorin and other members of the small leucine-rich repeated protein (SLRP) family, fibromodulin and lumican, function to bind type I collagen in the ECM and regulate the kinetics of collagen fibrillogenesis and the diameter and distance between fibrils.[49] Decorin and fibromodulin can also bind to and inhibit TGF-β1 activity in vitro[50] and in vivo.[51,52] Low levels of growth factor production by fetal cells, especially TGF-β1, is a major factor in the absence of excess collagen deposition and scar formation[51,52] (see Chapter 27). In contrast, overexpression of TGF-β1 results in marked lung fibrosis, which is significantly reduced by concomitant increased expression of decorin.[52] Fibroblasts isolated from the deep dermis produce less decorin and more large cartilage-like proteoglycans, including versican and aggrecan, which can account for the ultrastructural abnormalities in HTS. Recently fibrocytes, a bone marrow–derived circulating monocyte, have also been described to produce less SLRPs and more versican, hyaluronan, perlecan, and biglycan in the ECM.[46,53] The profibrotic characteristics of deep dermal fibroblasts can be upregulated by bone marrow–derived mesenchymal stem cells.[54]

The Role of Toll-Like Receptor Signaling in Fibrosis

Highlights:

- Toll-like receptors (TLRs) are present on normal and HTS fibroblasts.
- They appear to mediate inflammation and the activation of dermal fibroblasts in HTS, and antagonism of this pathway may lead to novel therapeutic options.

TLRs are a group of highly conserved molecules that allow the innate immune system to sense molecules commonly present in bacteria and viruses, termed pathogen-associated molecular patterns (PAMPs), or endogenous molecules that are released from necrotic tissue, termed damage-associated molecular patterns (DAMPs).[55] They function as activators of the innate immune system, but have increasingly been implicated in the switch from normal wound healing responses to fibrosis in many different organs and tissues.[55,56] Ten different members that bind specific ligands exist; TLR2 recognizes gram-positive bacteria and TLR4 senses gram-negative bacteria by binding lipopolysaccharide (LPS).[57] The mechanism of fibrosis has not been established in the skin and many other tissues. However, in the liver TLR4-dependent fibrosis is stimulated by LPS directly, targeting fibroblast precursors which release chemokines to activate macrophage-like Kupffer cells. This results in unrestricted TGF-β-mediated activation of hepatic stellate cells, increased deposition of ECM, and the promotion of liver fibrosis.[58–62] TLRs are not just expressed in immune cells and monocytes, but are found in a range of tissues such as cardiac myocytes, vascular cells, cortical tubule cells, mesangial cells, podocytes, and dermal fibroblasts, which may contribute to the inflammation and resulting fibrosis of heart, kidney, lung, and skin.[63–69]

Recently, aberrant TLR activation by endogenous molecules released by necrotic or activated cells and ECM molecules upregulated upon injury or degraded following tissue damage (DAMPs) have been implicated in a number of diseases where inappropriate, pathogenic inflammation is at the basis of the fibrosis.[70,71] One such DAMP is the matrix proteoglycan biglycan, which has been found to be highly expressed in human HTS tissue and HTS fibroblasts in vitro; deep dermal fibroblasts have been shown to produce more biglycan (Table 6-1).[33,53] Although fibroblasts play an important structural role in wound healing, emerging evidence suggests that fibroblasts modify the healing microenvironment by inducing inflammation through activation of the TLRs and signaling through nuclear factor

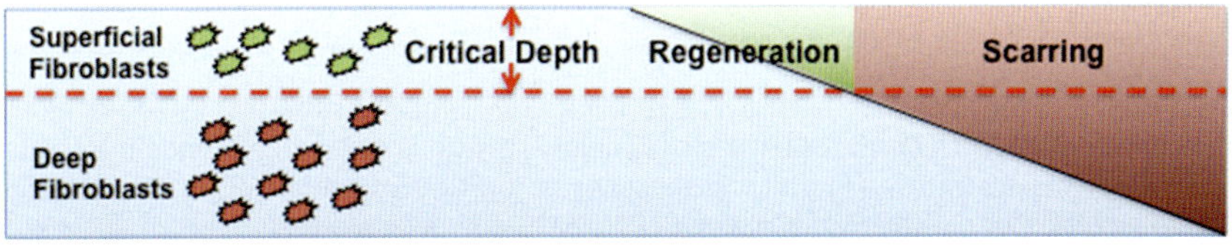

FIGURE 6-2 Regeneration occurs in superficial wounds while scarring occurs in deeper wounds. *(From Kwan P, Hori K, Ding J, et al. Scar and Contracture:* Hand Clin. *2009;25(4):511–528.)*

kappa B (NF-κB); this can lead to both the recruitment of monocytes and immune cells and subsequent production of inflammatory cytokines.[72,73]

Thus, fibroblasts appear capable of stimulating inflammation *via* TLR activation, likely *via* NF-κB and mitogen-activated protein kinase (MAPK), which upregulates the infiltration of inflammatory cells. In addition, activated deep dermal fibroblasts appear very important in the development of severe FDP of the skin. Future investigation of these profibrotic cells may improve the understanding of the role of TLRs in fibrosis and lead to novel therapeutic options to antagonize abnormal activation of fibroblasts by inflammation.

The Role of Blood-Borne Cells in Wound Healing and Fibrosis

Fibrocytes

Highlights:

- Circulating bone marrow–derived fibrocytes are recruited to the wound site after injury.
- They contribute to wound healing and fibrosis by producing ECM, secreting cytokines including TGF-β, and presenting antigen to T cells.
- They regulate fibroblasts and promote myofibroblast differentiation (Fig. 6-3).

Previously, Bucala has identified an adherent and proliferating population of cells with a fibroblast-like morphology that expresses a variety of biomarkers including some hematopoietic cell markers, mesenchymal cell markers, chemokine receptors, antigen-presenting cell markers, and others.[74–77] They make up 0.5% of peripheral blood leukocytes, but can constitute 10% of cells infiltrating acute wounds.[76] The chemokines CCL12 and CXCL12 and secondary lymphoid chemokines and their receptors CCR2, CXCR4, and CCR7 are involved in fibrocyte migration in vivo.[78] These migrating fibrocytes are capable of synthesizing ECM proteins, proteases including collagenase, and growth factors such as TGF-β1, tumor necrosis factor alpha (TNF-α), interleukin (IL)-6 and IL-10, but can also present antigens and thereby prime naïve T lymphocytes.[79,80] It has been demonstrated that fibrocytes differentiate into fibroblasts and myofibroblasts via in vivo and in vitro experiments.[81–82]

Fibrocytes have been identified in burn patients from the peripheral blood mononuclear cells (PBMCs), where the percentage of type I collagen–positive fibrocytes was significantly higher (up to 10% of PBMCs) than for control individuals (normal level <0.5%) and correlated with serum levels of TGF-β.[83,84] In vitro, fibrocytes can be cultured from $CD14^+$ PBMCs, but required TGF-β in the conditioned media from $CD14^-$ PBMCs for differentiation.[85] Leukocyte-specific protein 1 (LSP-1) is a unique marker for fibrocytes and is upregulated in burn patients, remaining stable through differentiation.[84,85] Double staining with antibodies to LSP-1 and the C-propeptide of type 1 collagen (COL-I) has identified a 300% increase in fibrocytes in HTS tissue, located primarily in deeper layers of the papillary dermis (Fig. 6-4).[84] Characteristic morphologic alterations in fibrocytes occur in vitro after exposure to endotoxin, which are corrected by treatment with IFN-α2b.[85–87]

From serial analysis of burn patients with HTS, increased numbers of fibrocytes are present in HTS tissues compared to mature scars and normal skin.[86–88] Quantitatively, fibrocytes produce less collagen than HTS fibroblasts; however, fibrocytes from burn patients differ from that of normal individuals because of their paracrine effects that include stimulating dermal fibroblasts to proliferate, production and contraction of the ECM, and producing TGF-β and its downstream effector, CTGF.[87,88] These findings resemble others,[89–92] where the principal source of collagen in other fibrosis models appears to be local fibroblasts. However, bone marrow–derived immune cells resembling fibrocytes

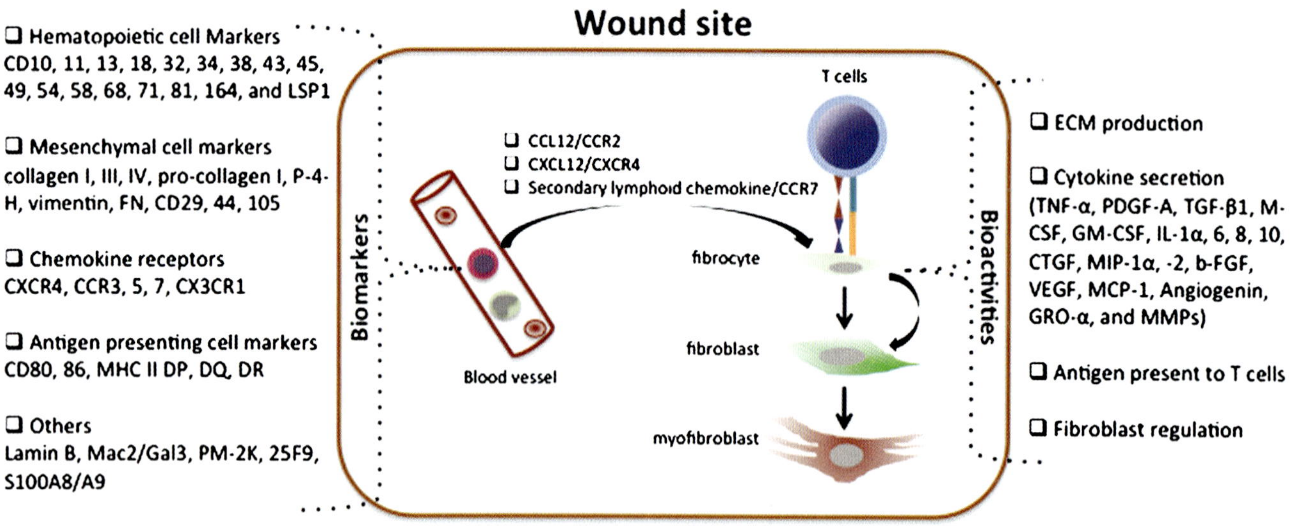

FIGURE 6-3 Biomarkers and bioactivities of fibrocytes. Fibrocytes express a variety of biomarkers including hemotopoietic cell markers, mesenchymal cell markers, chemokine receptors, antigen-presenting cell markers, and others. After injuries, circulating fibrocytes are recruited to the wound site and are involved in wound healing or scar formation by producing ECM, secreting cytokines, presenting antigen to T cells, regulating local fibroblasts, or directly differentiating to fibroblasts and myofibroblasts.

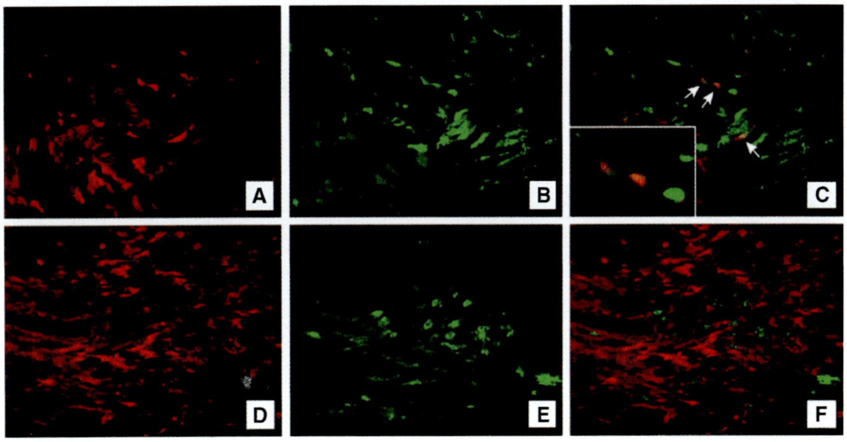

FIGURE 6-4 Dual immunofluorescent labeling of fibrocytes in scar tissue. Cryosections of (**A–C**) hypertrophic scar (**A–C**) and mature scar (**D–F**) were stained for type I collagen (A and D in red color) and leukocyte-specific protein 1 (LSP-1) (**B** and **E** in *green color*). The colocalization of the two molecules displayed a *yellow-colored* outline of the fibrocytes (**C** and **F**, *arrows*). Original magnifications ×100. *(From Yang L, Jiao H, Shankowsky HA, et al. Identification of fibrocytes in post-burn hypertrophic scar.* Wound Repair Regen. *2005;13(4):398–404.)*

persist in the matrix, suggesting an important paracrine role of fibrocytes in HTS and other FPD. It is possible to antagonize many of these fibrogenic effects of fibrocytes in vitro with IFN-α; significantly decreased numbers of fibrocytes were also found in the tissues of burn patients in response to systemic IFN treatment in vivo and were associated with a concomitant resolution of fibrosis and scar remodeling.[88] In addition, increased angiogenesis associated with increased vascular endothelial growth factor (VEGF) in HTS is reduced by IFN-α, in part because of suppression of endothelial cell proliferation and tubule formation through reduction in VEGF receptor expression in endothelial cells.[87] Coexpression of VEGF mRNA with the stromal cell–derived factor 1 (SDF-1) mRNA further implicates fibrocytes in the pathophysiology of idiopathic pulmonary fibrosis and other fibroses.[92]

Heterotopic ossification (HO) is a clinical condition where mature lamellar bone is formed in nondamaged tissues such as muscle, tendon, and fascia, particularly after burns and traumatic injuries.[93,94] HO can lead to skin breakdown, significant soft tissue deformity, joint ankylosis, and chronic pain that can prolong rehabilitation. In burn patients, the incidence of HO varies between 0.2% and 4%,[93] and is more frequent in patients with extensive burns (>20% TBSA). Although HO may occur in joints unrelated to burn injuries, lesions may develop under areas of deep burns complicated by HTS, especially in the elbow,[95,96] and it is associated with prolonged loss of consciousness, mechanical ventilation, long-term immobilization, burn wound infection and/or delayed closure, loss of skin grafts, and recurring local trauma including passive range of motion.[95–98] Therapeutic strategies for the prevention of HO are of limited success and include local radiation, but concerns of long-term side effects of radiation, including the development of secondary malignancies, stress the need for better animal models to develop and adequately test novel therapies before application to patients.[99]

Recently, a large population of fibrocytes (LSP-1$^+$ COL-I$^+$) have been identified within HO specimens as distinctive blood-borne cells that traffic to injured and apparently noninjured tissues and interact with resident cells.[100] Fibrocytes have the potential to differentiate into osteoblasts and chondrocytes[101] and can be reprogrammed into antifibrotic cells stimulating MMP-1 production in dermal fibroblasts, collagen breakdown, and scar remodeling.[102] Thus, HO and FPD such as HTS have common features and appear to be causally related. In this concept, after significant initial local tissue injury generates a systemic inflammatory response, unique PBMCs including fibrocytes contribute to the development of fibrosis and osteogenic matrix in injured and noninjured tissues in as yet unidentified mechanisms.

Type 1/Type 2 T-Helper Cells (T_H1/T_H2)

Highlights:

- After thermal injury, a polarized T_H2 environment favors the subsequent development of increased T_H3 cells (a different lineage from naturally arising CD25$^+$ CD4$^+$ Treg cells) and fibrocytes that can induce fibrosis in a paracrine fashion.
- Evidence suggests that monocytes and other inflammatory cells may also contribute to the development of dermal fibrosis.

In animal models of trauma and fibrosis as well as humans with acute burn injury, evidence for reduced IL-2 and IFN-γ production and increased T_H2 cytokines (IL-4, IL-5, IL-10, IL-13) is emerging.[103–105] In burn patients with HTS, a deficiency of circulating IFN-γ-producing lymphocytes exists very early after injury. Within 3 months postburn, increased numbers of IL-4-containing lymphocytes develop, which persist for up to 1 year after injury—consistent with a polarized T_H2 response.[104] Significant decreases in IL-10 within the first 2 months postinjury persist for 1 year, whereas IL-12 levels were significantly elevated and inversely related to IL-10.[103] IFN-γ mRNA was not detected in PBMCs and in HTS tissues until 6 months postinjury. IL-4 was undetected in normal controls, but was increased in HTS patients in PBMCs within 2 months postinjury, as well as in HTS tissues (Fig. 6-5).[103] CD4$^+$ TGF-β$^+$ lymphocytes are present in increased frequency in the circulating immune cells of burn patients as compared to normal control individuals.[105] These cells secrete increased levels of TGF-β, which promotes proliferation of dermal fibroblasts as well as α-SMA and wound contraction. The development of CD4$^+$ TGF-β$^+$ cells may contribute to the suppression of T_H1 immunity similar to trauma patients where increased T-regulatory CD4$^+$ CD25$^+$ cells, which produce TGF-β and other cytokines, have been found systemically.[106,107] Pilling et al. have

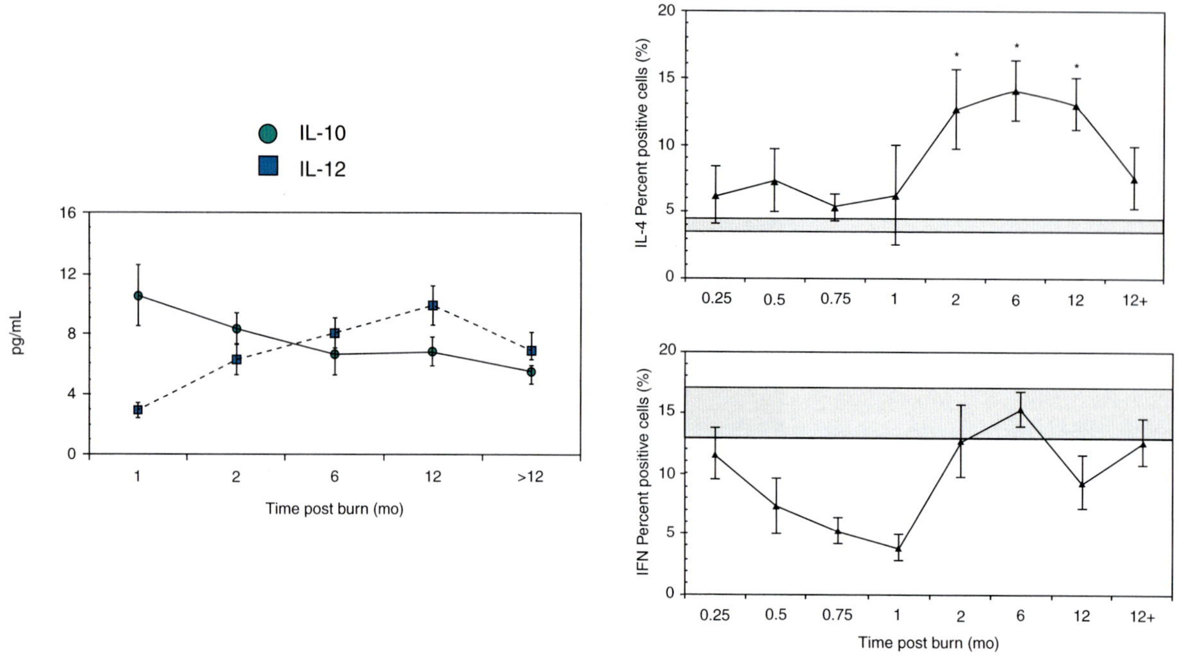

FIGURE 6-5 Time course of IL-10 and IL-12 from peripheral blood mononuclear cells (PBMCs) isolated from burn patients. The percentages of IL-4 or IFN-positive cells in burn patient PBMCs determined by flow cytometry. *(From Medina A, Ghahary A. Reprogrammed fibrocytes induce a mixed T_H1/T_H2 cytokine response of naïve CD4(+) T cells.* Mol Cell Biochem. *2011 346(1/2):89–94.)*

described that T_H2 cytokines (IL-4, IL-13) promote, whereas T_H1 cytokines (IFN-γ, IL-12) inhibit, fibrocyte differentiation in fibrosis.[107]

In liver and pulmonary fibrosis, macrophage subsets have been identified as key producers of TGF-β1 *via* TLR4 that promotes fibrosis. In addition to inducing fibrosis, TGF-β1 produced by regulatory T cells may suppress inflammation.[108,109] Like lymphocytes, macrophages respond to T_H2 cytokines where numerous studies have shown that macrophages exposed to IL-4 develop an alternate activation state termed "alternatively activated macrophages" or M2 macrophages, and their role may be equal to if not more important than the type of $CD4^+$ T-helper cell response in many different types of fibrosis.[109,110] Using an animal model of dermal fibrosis in human skin following transplantation into immunodeficient mice, animals which lack T cells, natural killer (NK) cells, and NK-T cells still develop significant fibrosis. This suggests that fibrosis can develop in the absence of lymphocytes and helps confirm an important role for other immune cells in the development of dermal fibrosis.[111] For this reason, emphasis has shifted to the importance of the role of monocytes/macrophages in HTS and other forms of FPD.

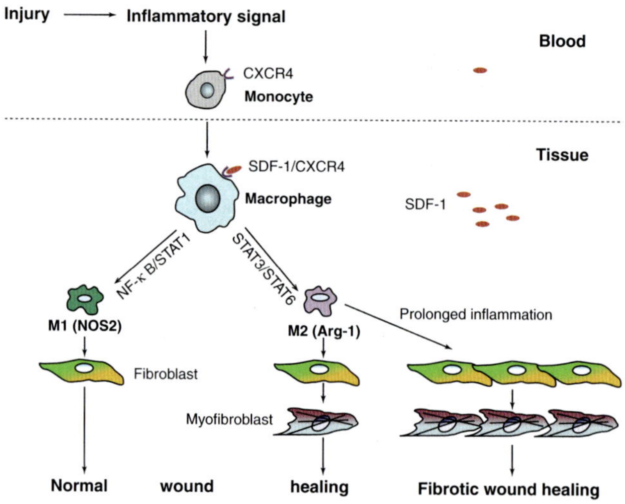

FIGURE 6-6 The roles of monocytes and polarized macrophages in HTS formation. It is hypothesized that blood monocytes are recruited into the injured site via the SDF-1/CXCR4 signaling pathway and differentiate into polarized macrophages. The polarized M1 and M2 macrophages then exert their functions via various signaling pathways involved in wound healing and HTS formation. *(From Zhu Z, Ding J, Ma Z, et al. The natural behavior of mononuclear phagocytes in HTS formation.* Wound Repair Regen. *2016. 24(1):14–25. doi:10.1111/wrr.12378.)*

M1/M2 Macrophages

Highlights:

- M1 macrophages are associated with normal wound healing and signal through the NF-κB/STAT1 pathway.
- M2 macrophages promote scar formation via the STAT3/STAT6 signaling pathway (Fig. 6-6).[112]

Since the initial discovery of macrophages by Metchnikoff in 1884, these mononuclear cells have been considered to play a vital role in the wound healing process. When they are ablated immunologically, studies have shown significant impairment in wound healing associated with a decreased number of macrophages at the injured site.[113,114] Conversely, increased numbers of activated polarized macrophages can lead to disordered wound healing, eventuating in dermal fibrosis.[115] Macrophages appear to differentiate into multiple phenotypes, but principally into classically activated macrophages (M1 macrophages) and alternatively activated macrophages (M2 macrophages) that appear to have distinct opposite functions in the wound healing process.[115] M1 macrophages induce nitric oxide synthase (NOS), which increases MMP-1 production and promotes ECM degradation, whereas M2 macrophages secrete large amounts of TGF-β1, which can stimulate myofibroblast differentiation and promote ECM deposition. It is also hypothesized that prolonged inflammation during wound healing attracts increased numbers of macrophages, which will initially be predominantly the proinflammatory M1 phenotype before a switch to the more profibrotic M2 phenotype occurs to counter the intense proinflammatory stimuli in the microenvironment.[116,117] With the shift from M1 macrophages, arginine is metabolized to nitric oxide and citrulline via NOS as a part of the inflammatory process in the healing wound. With the resolution of inflammation, arginine is metabolized by arginase I (Arg-1), leading to ornithine and polyamines modulated by M2 macrophages and leading to increased proline and collagen synthesis as well as other polyamines necessary for cell proliferation.[118] Growing evidence suggests that M2 macrophages are not a uniform population but can be further subdivided into M2a, M2b, and M2c subsets.[119] M2a macrophages are induced by IL-4 and IL-13, which are involved in an antiparasitic immune response and are considered to be profibrotic; M2b macrophages are induced by IL-1β, LPS, and immune complexes, whereas M2c macrophages are induced by IL-10, TGF-β, and glucocorticoids.[120] The fourth subtype of macrophages differentiates from an M1 phenotype into an angiogenic M2-like phenotype, which has been termed M2d by Leibovich et al.[121,122]

Using an animal model of human skin transplanted to immunodeficient mice, Zhu et al.[123] have demonstrated the development of contracted and thickened scars grossly. These resembled human HTS tissue histopathologically based on enhanced thickness, fibrotic orientation of collagen bundles, increased collagen level, and infiltration of myofibroblasts. Circulating monocytes decreased at 1 week after transplantation and returned to normal levels in the following 8 weeks. In the dermal tissues, F4/80$^+$NOS2$^+$ M1-like macrophages were found predominantly at 1 week after grafting, whereas F4/80$^+$Arg-1$^+$ M2-like macrophages were abundant at 3 weeks postgrafting (Fig. 6-7), coincident with the development of fibrosis in the human skin tissues. This understanding of the natural behavior of mononuclear phagocytes in vivo in the dermal mouse model of fibrosis provides evidence for the role of M2 macrophages in fibrosis of human skin, and suggests that macrophage depletion in the subacute phases of wound healing might reduce or prevent HTS formation.[124]

With the above discussion in mind, it is hypothesized that deep skin burn injury activates fibroblasts in the deep dermis via PAMPs like LPS and DAMPs like biglycan (and others) to stimulate the TLRs/NF-κB pathway in fibroblasts. This in turn releases chemokines and growth factors including TGF-β that recruit bone marrow–derived progenitor cells (such as M2 macrophages, fibrocytes, and T_H2 cells) to further activate fibroblasts to produce excessive ECM proteins and ultimately to the development of HTS (Fig. 6-8).[54]

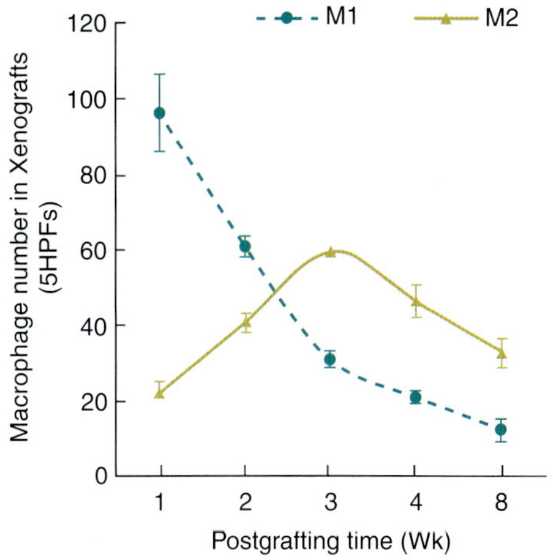

FIGURE 6-7 M1- and M2-like macrophages in xenografts. Human skin grafts were transplanted to the backs of nude mice. F4/80$^+$NOS2$^+$ M1-like macrophages were found predominantly at 1 week, whereas F4/80$^+$Arg-1$^+$ M2-like macrophages were abundant at 3 weeks postgrafting in the xenografts.

Newly Evolving Therapies Based on the Pathology of Hypertrophic Scars

IFN and Other Cytokine Therapy

Highlights:

- IFN-α treatment upregulates collagen degradation.
- IFN-α and -γ downregulate TGF-β production and mast cell function.

With greater understanding that three subtypes of helper T cells (T_H1, T_H2, and T_H3) are involved in scarring after thermal injury by regulating fibrocytes (Fig. 6-9),[8] newer therapeutics have emerged attempting to shift the systemic T_H2-polarized immune response toward a T_H1 response. IFN-α, a T_H1 cytokine, is reduced in HTS.[105] Type I IFNs in humans such as IFN-α, IFN-β, IFN-ε, IFN-κ, and IFN-ω are induced at a cellular level by viral infection, whereas type II IFN in humans (such as IFN-γ) is induced by mitogenic and antigenic stimulation of the immune system. Type I IFNs are produced by leukocytes and fibroblasts, whereas type II IFNs are synthesized only by certain immune cells including NK cells, CD4 T_H1 cells, and CD8 cytotoxic suppressor cells.[124,125] IFNs exert their effects through binding of high-affinity receptors associated with intracellular tyrosine kinases. In vitro, both IFN-α and IFN-γ are shown to decrease cell proliferation and collagen synthesis in fibroblasts from normal and HTS tissues.[3] Additionally, in HTS fibroblasts IFN-α2b increases MMP-1 mRNA levels and activity while decreasing the activity of tissue inhibitors of metalloproteinases (TIMPs),[31] features that would favor scar remodeling and that IFN-γ does not appear to possess.[30,31]

In a prospective clinical trial evaluating the effect of subcutaneous systemic treatment with IFN-α2b in nine burn patients with HTS,[126] seven of nine patients demonstrated significant improvement on scar assessment, and three of nine patients demonstrated significant reductions in scar volume compared to the control group. Prior to

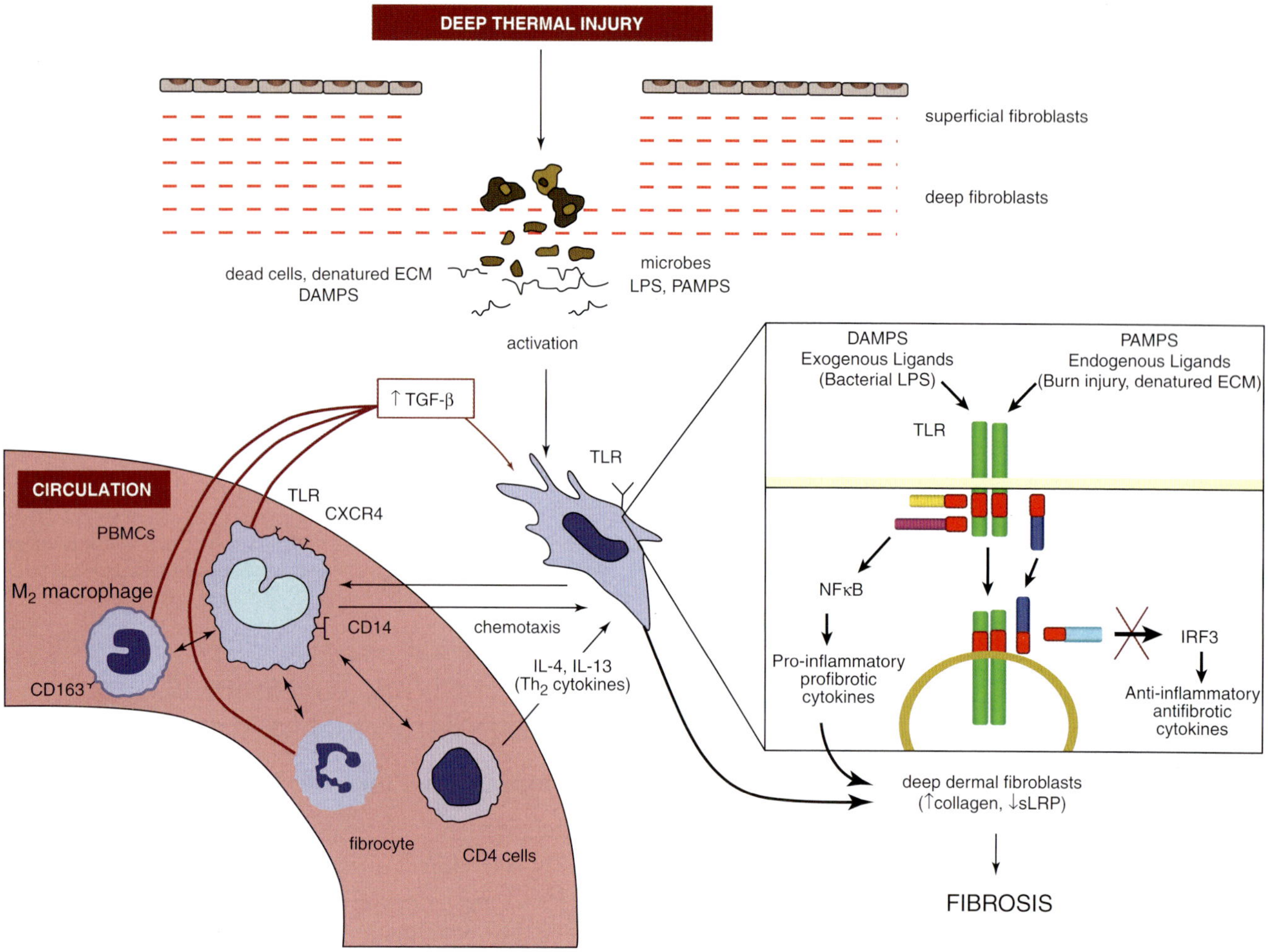

FIGURE 6-8 Proposed mechanism. Diagram illustrates that once a deep dermal burn injury occurs, the inflammatory signals derived from both infectious pathogens, such as lipopolysaccharide (LPS), and endogenous molecules released from necrotic tissue, such as biglycan, activate deep dermal fibroblasts through the toll-like receptors (TLRs)/nuclear factor kappa-light-chain-enhancer of activated B cells (NF-κB) pathway. Subsequently the activated fibroblasts in turn release chemokines, such as SDF-1, which lead to the recruitment of bone marrow–derived progenitor cells into wounds; there they contribute to hypertrophic scarring by further activating fibroblasts through many cytokines, most importantly TGF-β. *(From Ding J, Ma ZS, Shankowsky HA, et al. Deep dermal fibroblast profibrotic characteristics are enhanced by bone marrow-derived mesenchymal stem cells (BM-MSCs).* Wound Repair Regen. *2013;21(3):448–455.)*

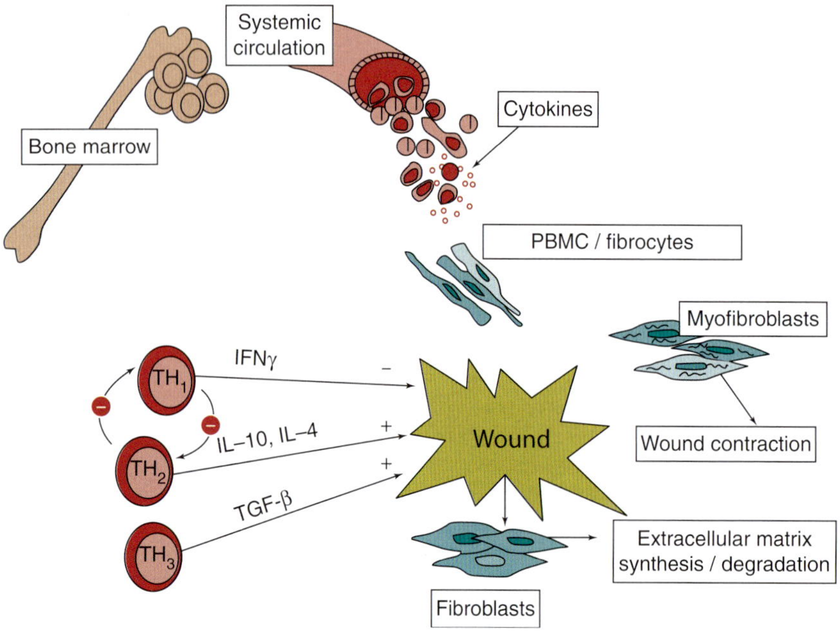

FIGURE 6-9 Hypothetical diagram of the role of $T_H1/T_H2/T_H3$ fibrogenic growth factors in the systemic circulation that may stimulate bone marrow stem cells to differentiate, migrate into wounds, and stimulate ECM synthesis and wound contraction in HTS. *(From Armour A, Scott PG, Tredget EE. Cellular and molecular pathology of HTS: basis for treatment.* Wound Repair Regen. *2007;15(suppl 1):S6–S17.)*

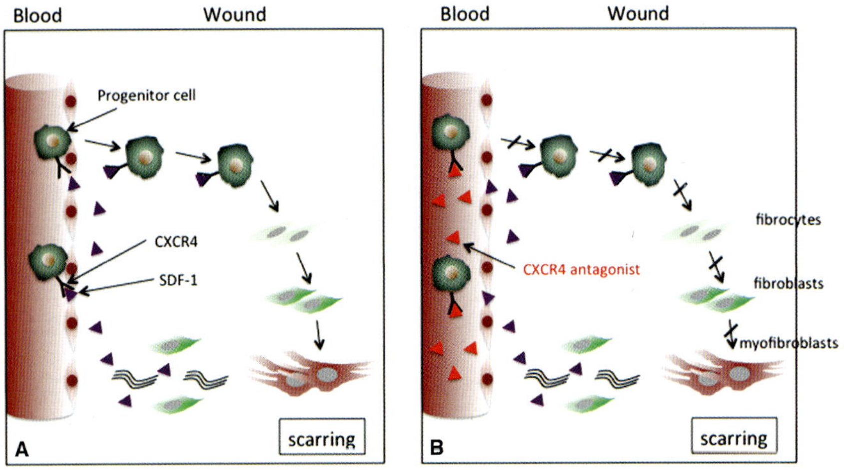

FIGURE 6-10 Schematic representation of the chemotaxis of circulating fibrocytes from blood to wound sites via the SDF-1/CXCR4 signaling pathway (**A**), and the blockade of excessive fibrocyte homing into wounds by CTCE-9908, a small peptide antagonist of CXCR4 (**B**).

IFN treatment, TGF-β levels were significantly higher in burn patients with HTS compared to a control group. With treatment, levels of TGF-β normalized to control levels with no increase following cessation of IFN treatment. The level of plasma Nτ-methylhistamine, which is an objective measure of mast cell mass and degranulation, was significantly elevated in HTS patients compared to controls, and a significant reduction in levels was achieved with treatment. These findings demonstrate an antagonistic relationship between IFN-α2b and TGF-β, and reinforce similar findings in vitro.[127–129]

Intralesional injection of IFN-α has been suggested for preventing recurrence of keloids and HTS after excision; however, our own experience and that of others have found minimal benefit in treating established proliferative scars intralesionally.[130] This suggests that TGF-β and other components of the T_H2 response may require systemic therapy to shift the inflammatory response toward a T_H1 cytokine profile. Systemic IFN-α2b, used in dosage regimes similar to the initial treatment of hepatitis C and B,[131,132] has been found effective in a double-blind placebo-controlled preliminary trial in 21 burn patients with HTS.[126] IFN-treated patients demonstrated significant improvements in overall scar assessment and color following treatment. Mild side effects of IFN treatment in this group of patients included myalgias, low-grade fever, and fatigue; however, significant depression with IFN therapy is a concern requiring careful observation of patients on systemic therapy.[131,132] Thus, despite early encouraging results, larger phase III trials are required to evaluate IFN treatment in patients with HTS and other FPD before routine off-label use can be advocated.

Chemokines and CXCR4 Inhibitors

Highlights:

- The SDF-1/CXCR4 signaling pathway is thought to be involved in the chemotaxis of circulating fibrocytes into wound sites.
- Excessive fibrocyte homing may lead to hypertrophic scarring via differentiation into fibroblasts and myofibroblasts.
- Blockade of this pathway has therapeutic potential for dermal fibrosis (Fig. 6-10).

Chemokines are small 8 to 10 kDa proteins that induce chemotaxis in cells surrounding the sites of injury. They can be divided into four subtypes depending on the spacing and location of two cysteine residues in the molecules, and include CC, CXC, C, and CX3C subfamilies.[133]

Increased expression of the chemokine monocyte chemotactic protein 1 (MCP-1) in fibroblasts from HTS compared to normal fibroblasts suggests a role for MCP-1 in fibrotic diseases.[133] SDF-1, also known as CXCL12, belongs to the CXC group. SDF-1 is similarly expressed in human, swine, and rat skin and is produced by pericytes, endothelial cells, and fibroblasts.[133,134] CXCR4 is a CXC chemokine receptor and it exclusively binds to SDF-1. This property is unique among receptors because most chemokines have more than one receptor, and most receptors have more than one ligand.[134,135] The SDF-1/CXCR4 signaling pathway mediates the migration of hematopoietic cells from fetal liver to bone marrow,[136] stimulates angiogenesis by recruiting progenitor cells,[137] regulates stem/progenitor cell trafficking,[136] and participates in the pathogenesis of lung fibrosis.[134] Increased expression of SDF-1 in human burn blister fluid has been found, with improved wound healing after blockade of the SDF-1/CXCR4 pathway.[137] Upregulation of SDF-1/CXCR4 signaling with increased SDF-1 levels in HTS and serum has been described in burn patients. SDF-1/CXCR4 signaling in burn wounds stimulates activated $CD14^+$ $CXCR4^+$ cells to migrate to the injured tissue where they appear to differentiate into fibrocytes, fibroblasts, and myofibroblasts, contributing to the pathogenesis of HTS.[37]

Using newly developed antagonists of CXCR4, a significant reduction in scar formation in a human skin on nude mice model in vivo has been found, in part by reducing the recruitment of macrophages and myofibroblasts and downregulating gene and protein expression of fibrotic factors in the engrafted human skin. Human skin tissues transplanted to mice treated with the vehicle control contained more compact collagen fibers and fibril bundles at each stage of wound healing, resembling the disoriented collagen fiber bundles typical of human HTS. In contrast, collagen fibers in the group treated with CTCE-9908 (CXCR4 antagonist) were thicker and more loosely arranged in the dermis, more closely resembling human normal skin (see Chapter 5). This strongly suggests that blockade of

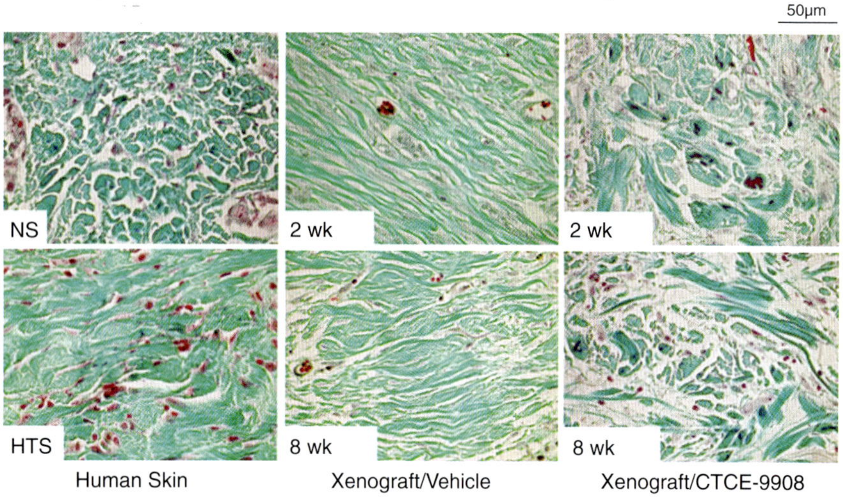

FIGURE 6-11 Masson's Trichrome staining for collagen fibers in the dermis of xenografts. Masson's Trichrome stain was performed in paraffin-embedded human normal skin (NS), human hypertrophic scar (HTS), and xenograft biopsies collected from mice treated with CXCR4 antagonist (CTCE-9908) or vehicle at 2 and 8 weeks after grafting, which stains keratin red, collagen green, cell cytoplasm pink, and cell nuclei dark brown. *(From Ding J, Ma Z, Liu H, et al. The therapeutic potential of a C-X-C chemokine receptor type 4 (CXCR4) antagonist on hypertrophic scarring in vivo.* Wound Repair Regen. *2014;22(5); 622–630.)*

the SDF-1/CXCR4 pathway enhances collagen remodeling in the murine dermal fibrotic model (Fig. 6-11).[138] In vitro, chemotaxis of fibrocyte precursor cells induced by recombinant human SDF-1 and fibroblast conditioned medium was inhibited by CXCR4 antagonists, suggesting a potential therapeutic value of this CXCR4 antagonist for the treatment of postburn HTS in the future.[138]

Other Potential Therapeutic Agents in the Future

Highlights:

- Specific targeting of the profibrotic factor TGF-β and antifibrotic factor decorin may have important therapeutic potential for the treatment of HTS.

Active research into TGF-β antagonists, including TGF-β antibodies and antisense oligonucleotides, suggests potential future roles for this approach in the management of HTS after burn injuries.[139] Similar strategies involve decorin (described earlier), a key proteoglycan deficient in HTS fibroblasts and tissues. Decorin binds TGF-β and has been demonstrated effective in renal fibrosis. A CAR–decorin fusion protein enhanced wound healing and suppressed scar formation in mice.[140] The development of target-seeking antifibrotic compounds may help establish the reduction of scar formation as a part of skin tissue engineering strategies for burn wounds.

Recently, microRNAs (miRs) that downregulate decorin in HTS as compared to normal skin have been identified, and in the deep as compared to superficial dermis.[141] Increased levels of miR-181b in deep dermal fibroblasts in vitro and in the HTS and deep dermal tissues in vivo were identified. TGF-β stimulation increased miR-181b in deep dermal fibroblasts; after blockade with an antagomir (a small synthetic RNA that is perfectly complementary to the specific miR-181b target and prevents other molecules from binding to a desired site on decorin mRNA molecule), reversal of TGF-β-induced decorin downregulation and myofibroblast differentiation occurred, suggesting a potential therapy for HTS.[141]

CURRENT PREVENTATIVE AND TREATMENT MODALITIES

Highlights:

- Treatment of postburn wounds has classically been thought of as surgical and nonsurgical, with surgical management reserved for wounds believed to be too deep to heal by secondary intention.[3,142]
- Traditional methods of nonsurgical management focus on attenuation of the ongoing fibrotic response and improvement/remodeling of the existing scar tissue (see Chapter 10).
- Current preventative strategies focus on inhibiting profibrotic responses before abnormal scarring and fibrosis occur.

Prevention of Scarring

A number of clinicians have demonstrated that HTS following burn injuries develops with high frequency in deep burns that require prolonged time to heal spontaneously.[142] In progressively deeper scratch wounds, the deep portions of the healed wound that developed HTS contained significantly more fibrocytes.[53] Activated fibroblasts from the deep regions of the skin very closely resemble HTS fibroblasts. Therefore, early recognition of deep dermal burn injuries allows prompt resurfacing and an improved quality of wound healing.[142] Using scanning laser Doppler, thermography, and other instruments, many investigators have demonstrated acceptable levels of accuracy in the prediction of deep burn wounds that can be targeted for early skin graft surgery to mitigate the development of HTS, which would likely occur if the wounds were allowed to heal spontaneously.[53,142,143–149] These instruments are common components of surgical decision-making in many burn centers, providing objective information in addition to wound observation and judgment, which has been demonstrated to be subjective and of limited accuracy.[143,149]

Pressure Garment Therapy

Compression therapy is believed to enhance ECM remodeling, although the exact mechanism through which it acts is not completely understood.[150,151] An in vitro study examining the effect of compression therapy on HTS tissue demonstrated increased MMP-9 activity in samples obtained from HTS tissue cultures following 24 hours of sustained compression.[150] Other proposed mechanisms of ECM remodeling stimulated by compression therapy include inhibition of α-SMA-expressing cells, and generalized induced tissue ischemia leading to cellular damage and reduced collagen synthesis.[151] A meta-analysis incorporating six clinical trials found that the clinical use of pressure garments postburn injury did not alter global scar scores.[152] The study did find a small but statistically significant decrease in scar height with pressure garment therapy, although the clinical relevance of this was undetermined. However, in a 12-year prospective study of moderate to severe HTS in burn patients with forearm injuries using objective outcome measurements, pressure garments led to significant improvements in hardness, color, and thickness of wounds with overall improvements in clinical appearance independent of patient ethnicity.[153] Pressure garment therapy is expensive and has recognized complications including skin breakdown, obstructive sleep apnea, dental alveolar deformation, bony deformity, and patient discomfort, making them difficult to wear for many patients such that compliance is often low[53] (see Chapter 19).

Silicone Therapy

Silicone gels are a commonly used treatment modality, even though its mechanism of action is poorly understood.[154] Silicone sheeting treatment is reported to soften, increase elasticity, and improve the appearance of HTS; conflicting results remain in the literature, which may be attributed to patient compliance.[155] The proposed mechanisms of action include increased oxygen delivery to the epidermis and dermis, hydration of the stratum corneum, increased surface skin temperature, and reduced tissue turgor.[156] In vitro evidence demonstrates decreased TGF-β2 levels and fibroblast-mediated lattice contraction with silicone treatment.[155] Evidence for the benefit of silicone therapy in HTS remains qualitative, where a review of the literature failed to reveal reliable quantitative evidence.[155]

Research Approaches to Fibroproliferative Disorders of the Skin

Highlights:

- Applicable dermal fibrotic human and animal models improve the understanding of the pathogenesis of HTS and approaches to its therapy.

In Vitro Models

Morry et al. exploited a dermal fibrotic model based on TGF-β-stimulated dermal fibroblasts, with which they evaluated the efficacy of nicotinamide adenine dinucleotide phosphate (NADPH) oxidase 4 (NOX4) and HSP47 as targets in a new strategy to treat dermal fibrosis.[157] Primary murine dermal fibroblast cells isolated from normal mouse skin and scleroderma-like fibroblasts harvested from the skin of a mouse receiving intradermal bleomycin injections were seeded on 96-well plates overnight in complete Dulbecco's modified Eagle's medium (DMEM). The cells were then serum-starved in the medium with 0.5% fetal bovine serum (FBS) prior to treatment with mesoporous silica nanoparticles, which delivered small interfering RNA (siRNA) targeting HSP47 or imparted an antioxidant property by scavenging reactive oxygen species (ROS) and subsequently reducing NOX4 levels. The nanoparticle effectively modulated the profibrotic markers α-SMA and COL-I.

Human HTS-derived fibroblasts were used as in vitro cell model to explore the role of multidrug resistance–associated protein 1 (MRP1) in HTS formation. They were found to have higher expression and colocalization of MRP1 and α-SMA than normal human fibroblasts. MRP1 knockdown by targeted siRNA successfully decreased protein expression of type III collagen (COL-III) and α-SMA in HTS fibroblasts.[158]

Methods to expand fibroblasts from human and mouse skin have been widely used to study basic aspects of fibrosis in vitro in medical research. These models involve scraping the subcutaneous tissue from the dermis and removing the epidermis with dispase for human skin (or trypsin for mouse, rat, and rabbit skin) before dermal samples are cut into 2 to 3 mm square pieces. Several pieces can be placed in tissue culture dishes with sterile glass coverslips gently over the skin specimens before culturing in complete growth medium placed into the space below the coverslip, or into the dish or well in a warmed, humidified, 5% CO_2 incubator. After 80% of the dish area is covered or confluent, the coverslips are removed and the cells harvested.[159]

In response to the limitation of available donor skin for skin grafts after major burns, and to avoid scarring in the donor site from harvesting split-thickness skin autografts, cultured skin substitutes (CSS) have been developed and used for permanent wound closure in patients with massive skin loss.[160] These forms of tissue-engineered skin have been used in another in vitro model to explore the biologic events surrounding wound healing and dermal fibrosis. In vitro manipulation of the cells, ECM, or their combination can be explored in the production of skin substitutes to investigate their fibrotic properties.[161]

By culturing dermal fibroblasts (isolated from either the superficial or deep dermis of normal skin obtained from patients who underwent abdominoplasty) in collagen-glycosaminoglycan (C-GAG) matrices, Varkey et al.[162] found C-GAG matrices with deep fibroblasts were significantly stiffer, contracted more, contained higher collagen, and had more α-SMA-expressing cells than the matrices composed of superficial fibroblasts. This suggests that differential remodeling of C-GAG matrices occurs by fibroblasts from different layers of the skin. Superficial dermal fibroblasts enhance basement membrane and epidermal barrier formation in CSS.[163] Keratinocytes appear to be beneficial to improve the mechanical and biologic characteristics of CSS cultured with deep dermal fibroblasts.[164,165] Gene therapy of fibroblasts and keratinocytes offers potential to control scarring, such as with skin substitutes seeded with indoleamine 2,3-dioxygenase-expressing cells, where improved healing outcomes have been achieved in full-thickness hypertrophic rabbit ear wounds.[166]

Ex Vivo Models

Human skin cultures used as an ex vivo organ model of fibrosis have several advantages including viability in culture for at least 2 weeks, therapeutic feasibility of deep and/or superficial injections, the capability of exerting their range of physiologic effects, and inclusion of all cell types resident in the skin. Using this model, the fibrotic effects of insulin-like growth factor–binding proteins (IGFBPs) were assessed, which supports the use of such ex vivo models to assess the effects of fibrosis-inducing factors.[167] Similarly, by culturing HTS tissue ex vivo, MRP1 knockdown achieved by transfecting the skin explants with MRP1 siRNA successfully reduced excessive fibrosis.[158]

Animal Models of Fibroproliferative Disorders

The Rabbit Ear Model

Based on their observation of scar formation after the healing of dermal ulcers created in the rabbit ear,[168] Mustoe et al. extended these observations in the rabbit ear scar model to allow quantitative assessment of scar tissue from the histologic sections obtained. In brief, under anesthesia, full-thickness excisional wounds to the cartilage surface were created over the ventral surface of each ear in female New Zealand white rabbits. Irregular elevated HTS developed from day 35 after wounding in this chronic scarring model. On histology, the scars were markedly thickened compared with surrounding unwounded tissue. Predominantly horizontally arranged collagen fibers, increased vascularity, and mild chronic inflammation were seen in the scar tissue.[169] This model has been used to study new therapeutic approaches such as manipulation of the indolamine dioxygenase pathway by activation of the MAPK/extracellular signal–regulated kinase (ERK) ERK1/2 MAPK, where kynurenine markedly improved scar formation via increasing the levels of MMP-1 and MMP-3 expression.[170] Intralesional injections of adipose-derived stem cells or conditioned medium from the cells in the rabbit ear model both reduced the formation of rabbit ear HTS by decreasing the α-SMA and COL-I gene expression and ameliorating collagen deposition.[171] However, this model is a small, full-thickness wound leading to scar formation because of perichondrial hypertrophy and cartilage thickening,[169] which is quite different from large, partial-thickness burn injuries in humans,[172] where no cartilaginous perichondrium is present.

Red Duroc Pig Model

Highlights:

- The red Duroc pig model has been considered a relevant model of human hypertrophic scarring.[173]
- However, the costs and the difficulty associated with evaluating burns or other deep dermal injuries in this species limits its widespread usage.

The recognition that red Duroc pigs healed with the development of HTS-like responses after skin injury[174–176] was popularized by Zhu et al.,[172] who illustrated that the scar features that developed resembled human hypertrophic scarring. After creating multiple variable depth excisional wounds on the back of each Duroc pig, they described increased scar thickness corresponding to the depth of wounds. Scar tissue from superficial wounds healed with the appearance of essentially normal skin. Deeper wounds healed with thickened scar tissue, which was devoid of decorin seemingly replaced by versican, and associated with the expression of TGF-β1 in the depths of the healed wounds and IGF-1 in the fibroblasts and endothelial cells.

Mouse Models of Fibroproliferative Disorders in Human Skin Research

Highlights:

- Compared to other dermal fibrotic animal models, the approaches to recreate HTS in human skin grafted onto nude and other immunodeficient mice offer the advantages of lower cost, easier manipulation, and shorter time frame for scar formation and remodeling.
- They possess greater similarities to human scar morphology and histology as compared to pig or rabbit dermal scarring.

Yamamoto et al.[177] described a mouse dermal fibrotic model created by injecting bleomycin in Balb/C mice, in which the induced skin fibrosis closely resembles human systemic sclerosis both histologically and biochemically. The dermal fibrotic model has also been created successfully in C3H/HeJ mice. To identify the effects of genetic background and gender on the severity of skin fibrosis, Ruzehaji et al.[178] used three common mouse strains and different gender mice to assess their susceptibility to bleomycin-induced fibrosis. The Balb/C mice are reported more susceptible to bleomycin-induced fibrosis compared to C57BL/6 and DBA/2, and male Balb/C mice developed the most severe fibrosis phenotype compared to male C57BL/6 and male DBA/2.

Following Yamamoto's original protocol, Serratrice et al.[179] made the same dermal fibrotic model in nude mice. They compared the long-term efficacy of human micro-fat "enriched" with other therapeutic products including the stromal vascular fraction of fat and platelet-rich plasma from human blood in this murine model of scleroderma. All substances were found effective in treating skin-induced lesions of scleroderma with different levels of fibrosis and vascular involvement. The micro-fat-derived products are more stable and the stromal vascular fraction demonstrated better proangiogenic effects. An antifibrotic effect was found in the model by intradermal injection of antagonists to lysophosphatidic acid receptors, LPA1 and LPA3.[180]

Human skin has been grafted onto athymic nude mice since 1984[181–186] as a tool to study the regeneration of human skin.[182] Keloids, HTS, and granulation tissue after skin injury have been implanted in the nude mice for basic investigation of dermal fibrotic disorders. Although earlier studies did not recognize the magnitude of scar formation when normal human skin was transplanted,[187,188] Robb et al.[189] described scar formation in normal human skin after burn injury a month after grafting on the mouse or after linear incisions in fetal skin 7 days after transplantation to full-thickness defects on the dorsum of the mouse.[190] Subsequently, Yang et al.[191] described persistent scars 6 months after transplantation of human skin onto FOXN1-difficient nude mice, which had morphologic and histologic properties similar to those of human HTS.

Using this model, our group has found that split-thickness human skin grafts develop more scar tissue in a shorter period of time after they have been transplanted to full-thickness excisional wounds on the dorsum of nude mice (Fig. 6-12).[192] In this model, the involvement of blood-borne cells such as fibrocytes, macrophages, and mast cells similar to human HTS formation was found.[192,193] Using a peptide molecule to block CXRC4 receptors to inhibit migration of blood-borne cells to wound sites via the SDF-1/CXCR4 chemokine pathway, a significant reduction in the accumulation of mouse macrophages occurred with attenuated scar formation and wound contraction.[37]

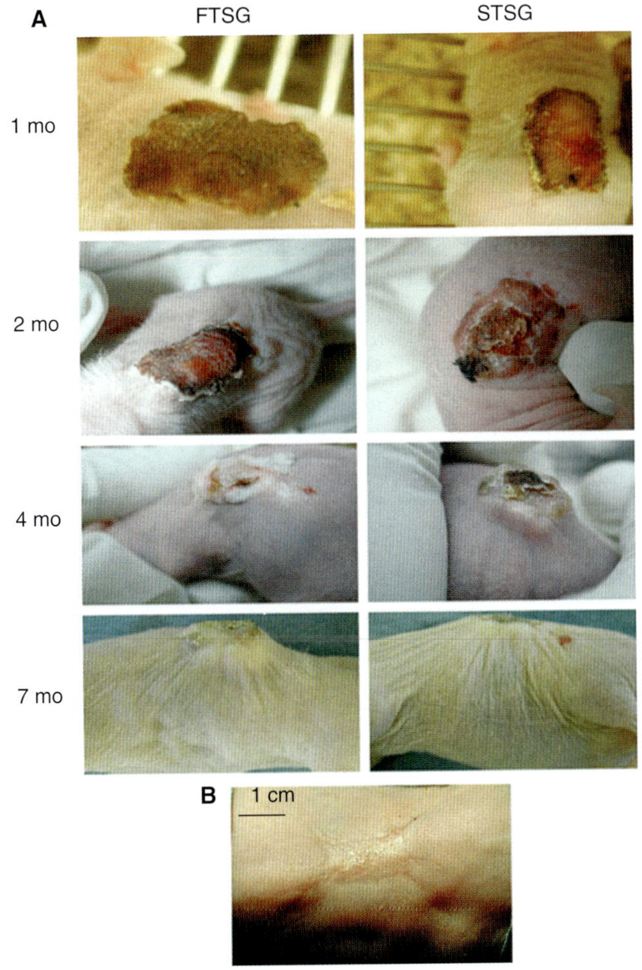

FIGURE 6-12 Photographs of scars after human skin grating. **A:** Macroscopic observation of scars developed in a full-thickness skin graft (FTSG) and a split-thickness skin graft (STSG). Scars were photographed using the same exposure and lighting settings, at the indicated time after transplantation. Representative results for the three animals in each group are shown. **B:** Macroscopic observation of rat skin transplantation. *(From Wang J, Ding J, Jiao H, et al. Human hypertrophic scar-like nude mouse model: characterization of the molecular and cellular biology of the scar process.* Wound Repair Regen. *2011;19(2):274–285.)*

Similar models of human skin transplantation have been performed in T-cell receptor α, β, γ, δ knockout mice, which lack genes for productive T-cell receptor rearrangement and are unable to produce functional T cells. These include RAG-1 knockout mice, which specifically are deficient in B and T cells, and RAG-2γc knockout mice, which lack NK cells. Significant amounts of dermal scarring still developed despite progressive ablation of increasing numbers of lymphocyte subsets, which suggests that macrophages, mast cells, or other nonspecific immune cells remain important in HTS formation in vivo.[194]

Using a deep dermal scratch injury in human skin either before or 1 week after transplantation to nude mice, significant amounts of additional scarring occurred in the wounded region of the transplanted tissue, which persisted beyond 12 months posttransplantation (Fig. 6-13). This suggests that human skin retains its profibrotic nature after transplantation. In dark African American skin samples transplanted in the same model, melanin-containing epidermal cells typical of the transplanted skin were retained in the raised elevated HTS-like tissues at 1 year after grafting (Fig. 6-14). This provides strong evidence for the persistent survival of human epidermal cells as well as dermal cells in the transplanted tissue and the developing hypertrophic-like scar.[195]

Gawronska-Kozak summarized an unusual model of scar-free skin healing in the African spiny mouse.[196] Different from the scar models mentioned above, full-thickness incisional wounds in the African spiny mouse heal in a scarless manner with tissue regeneration in the absence of human skin grafting. As such they are potentially an important animal model to explore the mechanisms of tissue regeneration.

Human Investigations of Dermal Fibrosis

Highlights:

- The dermal scratch model is an exciting representative, standardized, and acceptable traumatic wound model in humans.
- It is suitable for investigating the relationship of dermal injury depth to wound healing outcome and can be useful for the investigation of novel antifibrotic therapies.

Clinical experience with burns and other injuries to the skin suggests that scarring occurs after injury extends to a critical depth in dermis. Dunkin et al.[12] quantified the association between scarring and the depth of dermal injury in 113 human volunteers using a novel jig to create a scratch wound in a human dermal scratch model, eventuating in HTS and normotrophic scar within the same lesion. They found a threshold depth of dermal

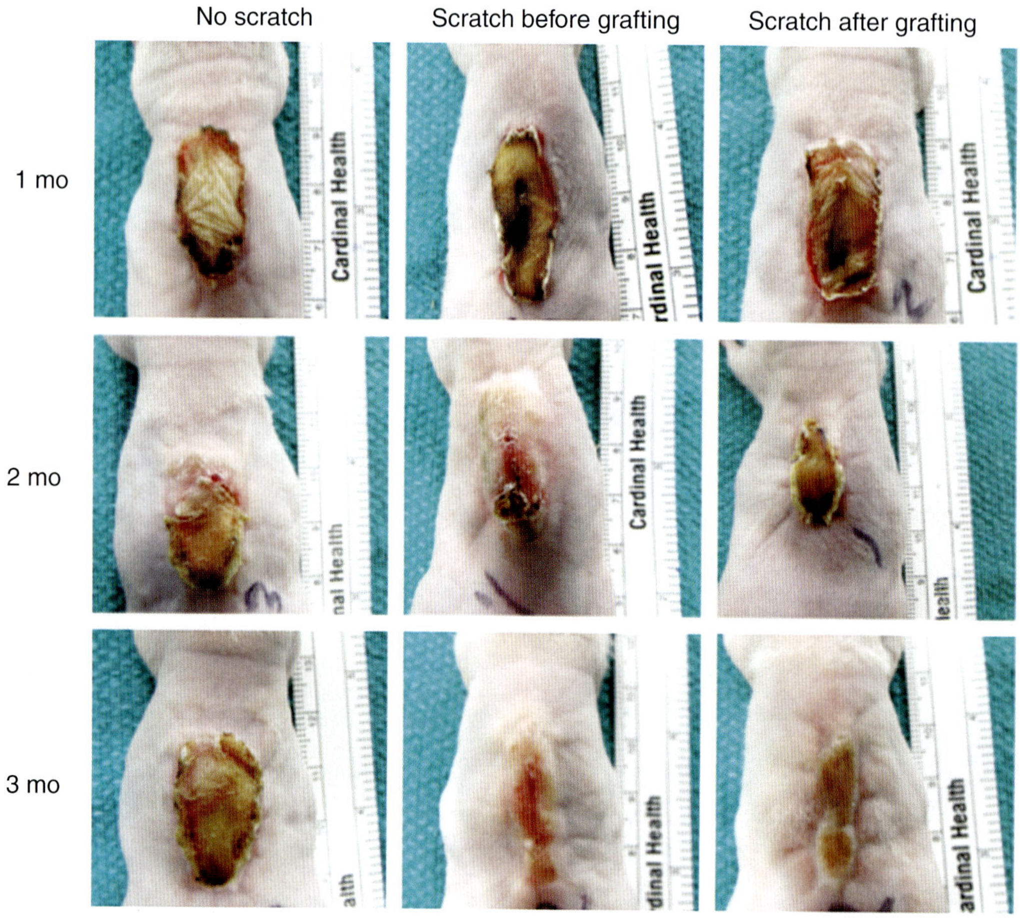

FIGURE 6-13 Morphologic observation of scar development over time after human skin grafting in nude mice. The scratch in the grafts before and after grafting made more contracted wounds than the ones without the scratch. *(From Alrobaiea SM, Ding J, Ma Z, Tredget EE. A novel nude mouse model of hypertrophic scarring using scratched full-thickness human skin grafts.* Adv Wound Care. *2016;5(7):299–313.)*

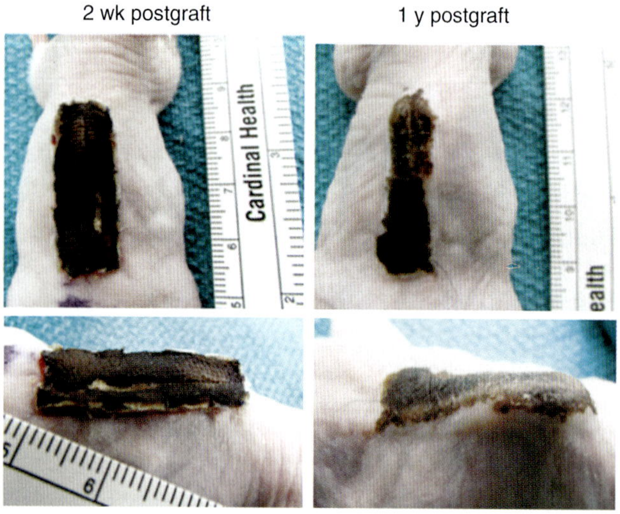

FIGURE 6-14 Survival of deep dermal injury in African American human skin in the athymic nude mouse model. The scratch wounds healed with significant scarring and preserved the color of African American human skin for 1 year after grafting, indicating the persistent viability of the human epidermal elements. *(From Alrobaiea SM, Ding J, Ma Z, Tredget EE. A novel nude mouse model of hypertrophic scarring using scratched full-thickness human skin grafts.* Adv Wound Care. *2016;5(7):299–313.)*

injury of 0.56 ± 0.03 mm (or 33% of the lateral hip thickness—high-frequency ultrasound showed skin thickness on the lateral hip to be 1.69 ± 0.1 mm), beyond which scarring develops. In each volunteer patient, two symmetrical wounds 6 cm long and 0 to 0.75 mm deep at one end and 0.76 to 3 mm deep at the other end were created on the skin of the anterior thigh. The superficial one-third of this scratch wound healed normally with minimal scar, whereas the deep dermal end region healed with a thickened scar typical of HTS and contained significantly greater numbers of fibrocytes.[46] Studies using this dermal scratch wound model in tissues from burn patients demonstrated a considerably lower expression of decorin, fibromodulin, and TGF-β3, higher expression of TGF-β1, and greater fibrocyte infiltration in deeper wound scars compared to superficial wounds, which ultimately healed with minimal thin flat smooth white scars (Fig. 6-15).[197] These data strongly demonstrate that fibroblasts from the deeper layers resemble HTS fibroblasts, and that activated deeper layer fibroblasts may play a critical role in the formation of HTS (Table 6-1).

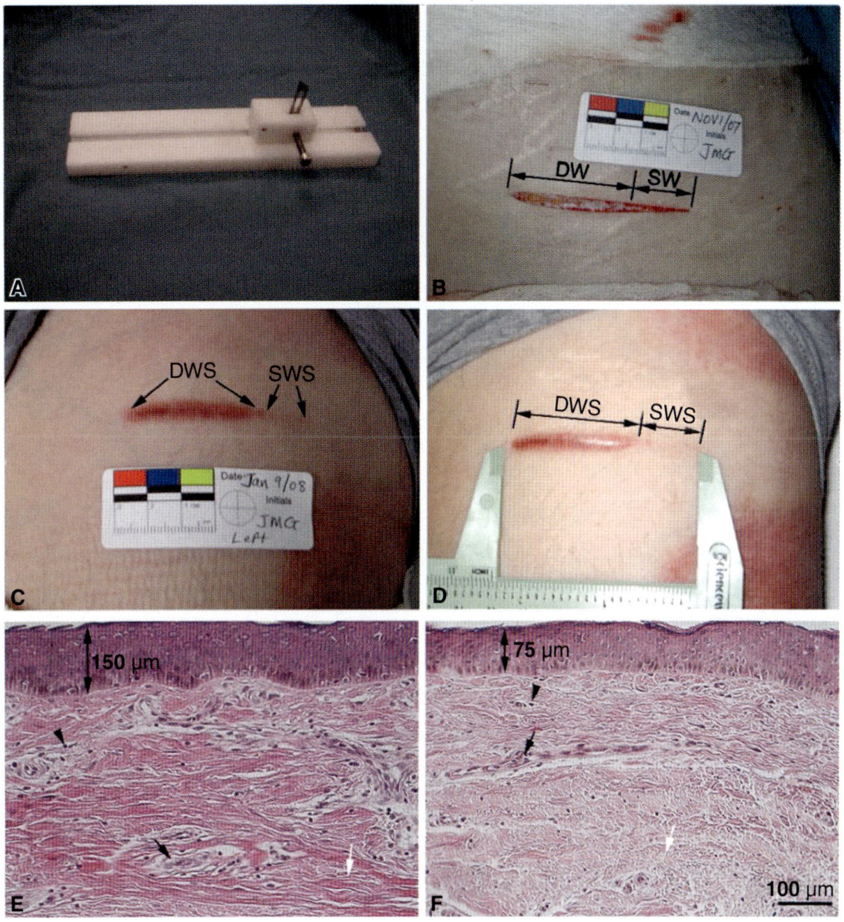

FIGURE 6-15 Creation of deep and superficial scratch wounds and histologic analysis of resulting scars. **A:** Jig used for the creation of scratch wound model. **B:** Wound created on the anterior thigh. **C:** Scratch wound 70 days postwounding. **D:** Deep and superficial wound scar. **E:** Deep wound scar tissue stained with hematoxylin and eosin staining (H&E). **F:** Superficial wound scar tissue stained with H&E. Double-headed arrows in (**E**) and (**F**) indicate average thickness of epithelium. Arrowheads point to cells. Black arrows point to blood vessels. White arrows point to collagen. DW, deep wound; SW, superficial wound; DWS, deep wound scar; SWS, superficial wound scar. *(From Honardoust D, Varkey M, Marcoux Y, et al. Reduced decorin, fibromodulin, and transforming growth factor-β3 in deep dermis leads to hypertrophic scarring.* J Burn Care Res. *2012;33(2):218–227.)*

Conclusions

Despite advancements in burn care, hypertrophic scarring remains a significant clinical problem after burn injury. Understanding of the pathophysiology of postburn scars and systemic responses to thermal injury have revealed potentially new therapeutic strategies including exogenous T_H1 cytokine administration, have specific antibody or antisense mRNA therapy toward fibrogenic cytokines including TGF-β and its downstream modulator CTGF, and hold significant promise in the prevention and treatment of hypertrophic scarring. In addition, methods of accurately assessing burn depth are improving, most recently with the advent of scanning laser Doppler imaging. As such, deep dermal wounds can be recognized at an early stage and appropriate interventions may potentially circumvent the complications of hypertrophic scarring, whereas superficial injuries can be allowed to heal without the development of HTS. Through continued investigation to enhance our understanding of the pathogenesis of dermal scar formation, advancements in the management of HTS and other FPD will occur to improve outcomes of patients with significant injury to the skin.

List of Abbreviations

FPD	Fibroproliferative disorders
HTS	Hypertrophic scar(s)
TBSA	Total burn surface area
SNP	Single-nucleotide polymorphisms
ECM	Extracellular matrix
TGF-β	Transforming growth factor beta
MMP	Matrix metalloproteinase
MMP-1	Matrix metalloproteinase 1 or collagenase
α-SMA	Alpha smooth muscle actin
CTGF	Connective tissue growth factor
HSP47	Heat shock protein 47
SLRP(s)	Small leucine-rich repeated proteoglycan(s)
TLRs	Toll-like receptors
PAMPs	Pathogen-associated molecular patterns

DAMPs	Damage-associated molecular patterns
LPS	Lipopolysaccharide
MyD88	Myeloid differentiation primary response gene 88
IL	Interleukin
IFN	Interferon
TRIF	Toll/interleukin (IL)-1R domain-containing adaptor inducing IFN-β factor
NF-κB	Nuclear factor kappa-light-chain-enhancer of activated B cells
MAPK	Mitogen-activated protein kinase
COL-I	Type I collagen
COL-III	Type III collagen
TNF-α	Tumor necrosis factor alpha
PBMCs	Peripheral blood mononuclear cells
LSP-1	Leukocyte-specific protein 1
VEGF	Vascular endothelial growth factor
SDF-1	Stromal cell–derived factor 1
HO	Heterotopic ossification
Th	T-helper cells
NK	Natural killer
M1	Classically activated macrophages
M2	Alternatively activated macrophages
NOS	Nitric oxide synthase
Arg-1	Arginase I
MCP-1	Monocyte chemotactic protein 1
NADPH	Nicotinamide adenine dinucleotide phosphate
NOX4	NADPH oxidase 4
ROS	Reactive oxygen species
DMEM	Dulbecco's modified Eagle's medium
MRP1	Multidrug resistance–associated protein 1
CSS	Cultured skin substitutes
C-GAG	Collagen-glycosaminoglycan
Ad	Adenoviral
IGF	Insulin-like growth factor
IGFBP	Insulin-like growth factor–binding protein
ERK	Extracellular signal–regulated kinase
LPA	Lysophosphatidic acid
PDGF	Platelet-derived growth factor
LDI	Laser Doppler imaging
si-RNA	Small inhibitory messenger ribonucleic acid

REFERENCES

1. Lee DE, Trowbridge RM, Ayoub NT, et al. Group box protein-1, matrix metalloproteinases, and vitamin D in keloids and hypertrophic scars. *Plast Reconstr Surg Glob Open*. 2015;3(6):e425.
2. Kozak L, Bacon W, Krzyzanowski M, et al. *Vital and Health Statistics*. Vol. 5 (ed. Office, GP); 2008.
3. Ladak A, Tredget EE. Pathophysiology and management of the burn scar. *Clin Plast Surg*. 2009;36(4):661–742.
4. Dissanaike S, Rahimi M. Epidemiology of burn injuries: highlighting cultural and socio-demographic aspects. *Int Rev Psychiatry*. 2009;21(6):505–119.
5. Ryan CM, Schoenfeld DA, Thorpe WP, et al. Objective estimates of the probability of death from burn injuries. *N Engl J Med*. 1998;338:362–366.
6. Tredget EE, Shankowsky HA, Taerum TV, et al. The role of inhalation injury in burn trauma. A Canadian experience. *Ann Surg*. 1990;212:720–727.
7. Snelling CF. Burn units' share of Canada's total burn care. *J Burn Care Rehabil*. 1995;16:519–524.
8. Armour A, Scott PG, Tredget EE. Cellular and molecular pathology of HTS: basis for treatment. *Wound Repair Regen*. 2007;15(suppl 1):S6–S17.
9. Engrav LH, Covey MH, Dutcher KD, et al. Impairment, time out of school, and time off from work after burns. *Plast Reconstr Surg*. 1987;79:927–934.
10. Helm P, Herndon DN, Delateur B. Restoration of function. *Burn Care Res*. 2007;28(4):611–614.
11. Butzelaar L, Soykam EA. Garre FG, et al. Going into surgery: risk factors for hypertrophic scarring. *Wound Rep Reg*. 2105;23:531–537.
12. Dunkin CS, Pleat JM, Gillespie PH, et al. Scarring occurs at a critical depth of skin injury: precise measurement in a graduated dermal scratch in human volunteers. *Plast Reconstr Surg*. 2007;119(6):1722–1733.
13. Jaskille AD, Shupp JW, Jordan MH, et al. Critical review of burn depth assessment techniques: Part I. Historical review. *J Burn Care Res*. 2009;30(6):937–947.
14. Bombaro KM, Engrav LH, Carrougher GJ, et al. What is the prevalence of hypertrophic scarring following burns? *Burns*. 2003;29:299–302.
15. Ripper S, Renneberg B, Landmann C, et al. Adherence to pressure garment therapy in adult burn patients. *Burns*. 2009;35(5):657–664.
16. Harte D, Gordon J, Shaw M, et al. The use of pressure and silicone in hypertrophic scar management in burns patients: a pilot randomized controlled trial. *J Burn Care Res*. 2009;30(4):632–642.
17. Brown JJ, Bayat A. Genetic susceptibility to raised dermal scarring. *Br J Dermatol*. 2009;161(1):8–18.
18. Ogawa R. The most current algorithms for the treatment and prevention of hypertrophic scars and keloids. *Plast Reconstr Surg*. 2010;125(2):557–568.
19. Thompson CM, Hocking AM, Honari S, et al. Genetic risk factors for hypertrophic scar development. *J Burn Care Res*. 2013;34(5):477–482.
20. Roeder RA, Schulman CI. An overview of war-related thermal injuries. *J Craniofac Surg*. 2010;21(4):971–975.
21. Kauvar DS, Wade CE, Baer DG. Burn hazards of the deployed environment in wartime: epidemiology of noncombat burns from ongoing United States military operations. *J Am Coll Surg*. 2009;209(4):453–460.
22. Esselman PC, Thombs BD, Magyar-Russell G, et al. Burn rehabilitation: state of the science. *Am J Phys Med Rehabil* 2006;85(4):383–413.
23. Stoddard FJ Jr, Ryan CM, Schneider JC. Physical and psychiatric recovery from burns. *Psychiatr Clin North Am* 2015;38(1):105–120.
24. Scott PG, Dodd CM, Tredget EE, et al. Chemical characterization and quantification of proteoglycans in human post-burn hypertrophic and mature scars. *Clin Sci*. 1996;90:417–425.
25. Lapiere CM, Nusgens B Pierard GE. Interaction between collagen type I and type III in conditioning bundles organization. *Connect Tissue Res*. 1977;5:21–29.
26. Linares HA, Kischer CW, Dorkovsky M, et al. The histiotypic organization of the hypertrophic scar in humans. *J Invest Dermatol*. 1972;59:323–331.
27. Scott PG, Dodd C, Tredget EE, et al. Immunohistochemical localization of the proteoglycans decorin, biglycan and versican and transforming growth factor-β in human post-burn hypertrophic and mature scars. *Histopathology*. 1995;26:423–431.
28. Danielson KG, Baribault, H, Holmes DF, et al. Targeted disruption of decorin leads to abnormal collagen fibril morphology and skin fragility. *J Cell Biol*. 1997;136:729–743.
29. Sayani K, Dodd CM, Nedelec B, et al. Delayed appearance of decorin in healing burn scars. *Histopathology*. 2000;36:262–272.
30. Tredget EE, Nedelec B, Scott PG, et al. Hypertrophic scars, keloids, and contractures. The cellular and molecular basis for therapy. *Surg Clin North Am*. 1997;77(3):701–730.

31. Ghahary A, Shen YJ, Nedelec B, et al. Collagenase production is lower in post-burn hypertrophic scar fibroblasts than in normal fibroblasts and is reduced by insulin-like growth factor-1. *J Invest Dermatol.* 1996;106(3):476–481.
32. Wang R, Ghahary A, Shen YJ, et al. Nitric oxide synthase expression and nitric oxide production are reduced in hypertropyic scar tissue and fibroablsts. *J Invest Dermatol.* 1997;108:438–444.
33. Scott PG, Dodd CM, Ghahary A, et al. Fibroblasts from post-burn hypertrophic scar tissue synthesize less decorin than normal dermal fibroblasts. *Clin Sci (Lond).* 1998;94:541–547.
34. Nedelec B, Shankowsky H, Scott PG, et al. Myofibroblasts and apoptosis in human hypertrophic scars: the effect of interferon-alpha2b. *Surgery.* 2001;130:798–808.
35. Nedelec B, Dodd CM, Scott PG, et al. Effect of interferon-alpha2b on guinea pig wound closure and the expression of cytoskeletal proteins in vivo. *Wound Repair Regen.* 1998;6:202–212.
36. Moulin V, Castilloux G, Auger FA, et al. Modulated response to cytokines of human wound healing myofibroblasts compared to dermal fibroblasts. *Exp Cell Res.* 1998;238:283–293.
37. Ding J, Hori K, Zhang R, et al. Stromal cell-derived factor 1 (SDF-1) and its receptor CXCR4 in the formation of postburn hypertrophic scar (HTS). *Wound Repair Regen.* 2011;19(5):568–578.
38. Squier CA. The effect of stretching on formation of myofibroblasts in mouse skin. *Cell Tiss Res.* 1981;220:325–335.
39. Desmouliere A, Badid C, Bochaton-Piallat ML, et al. Apoptosis during wound healing, fibrocontractive diseases and vascular wall injury. *Int J Biochem Cell Biol.* 1997;29:19–30.
40. Desmouliere A, Redard M, Darby I, et al. Apoptosis mediates the decrease in cellularity during the transition between granulation tissue and scar. *Am J Pathol.* 1995;146:56–66.
41. Kwan P, Hori K, Ding J, et al. Scar and contracture: *Hand Clin.* 2009;25(4):511–528.
42. Sorrell JM, Baber MA, Caplan AI. Clonal characterization of fibroblasts in the superficial layer of the adult human dermis. *Cell Tissue Res.* 2007;327:499–510.
43. Reynolds AJ, Jahoda CA. Inductive properties of hair follicle cells. *Ann N Y Acad Sci.* 1991;642:226–241.
44. Jahoda CA, Reynolds AJ. Dermal-epidermal interactions. Adult follicle-derived cell populations and hair growth. *Dermatol Clin.* 1996;14:573–583.
45. Ali-Bahar M, Bauer B, Tredget EE, et al. Dermal fibroblasts from different layers of human skin are heterogeneous in expression of collagenase and types I and III procollagen mRNA. *Wound Repair Regen.* 2004;12;175–182.
46. Honardoust D, Varkey M, Hori K, et al. Small Leucine-rich proteoglycans, decorin and fibromodulin, are reduced in post-burn hypertrophic scar. *Wound Healing Regen.* 2011;19(3):368–378.
47. Wang J, Dodd C, Shankowsky H, et al. Deep dermal fibroblast may dictate hypertrophic scarring. *Lab Invest* 2008;88(12):1278–1290.
48. Scott PG, Dodd CM, Tredget EE, et al. Immunohistochemical localization of the proteoglycans decorin, biglycan and versican and transforming growth factor-beta in human post-burn hypertrophic and mature scars. *Histopathology.* 1995;26:423–431.
49. Hildebrand A, Romarís M, Rasmussen LM, et al. Interaction of the small interstitial proteoglycans biglycan, decorin and fibromodulin with transforming growth factor beta. *Biochem J.* 1994;302(Pt 2):527–534.
50. Soo C, Hu FY, Zhang X, et al. Differential expression of fibromodulin, a transforming growth factor-beta modulator, in fetal skin development and scarless repair. *Am J Pathol.* 2000;157:423–433.
51. Kolb M, Margetts PJ, Sime PJ, et al. Proteoglycans decorin and biglycan differentially modulate TGF-beta-mediated fibrotic responses in the lung. *Am J Physiol Lung Cell Mol Physiol.* 2001;280:1327–1334.
52. Mattoli S, Bellini A, Schmidt M. The role of a human hematopoietic mesenchymal progenitor in wound healing and fibrotic diseases and implications for therapy. *Curr Stem Cell Res Ther.* 2009;4:266–280.
53. Honardoust D, Varkey M, Hori K, et al. Reduced decorin, fibromodullin and TGF-β3 in deep dermis lead to hypertrophic scar. *J Burn Care Res.* 2012;33(2):218–227.
54. Ding J, Ma ZS, Shankowsky HA, et al. Deep dermal fibroblast profibrotic characteristics are enhanced by bone marrow-derived mesenchymal stem cells (BM-MSCs). *Wound Repair Regen.* 2013;21(3):448–455.
55. Piccinini AM, Midwood KS. DAMPening inflammation by modulating TLR signaling. *Mediators Inflamm.* 2010. doi:10.1155/2010/672395.
56. Janeway CA Jr, Medzhitov R. Innate immune recognition. *Annu Rev Immunol.* 2002;20:197–216.
57. Kenny EF, O'Neill LAJ. Signaling adaptors used by toll-like receptors: an update. *Cytokine.* 2008;43(3):342–349.
58. Seki E, De Minicis S, Osterreicher CH, et al. TLR4 enhances TGF-beta signaling and hepatic fibrosis. *Nat Med.* 2007;13:1324–1332.
59. Isayama F, Hines IN, Kremer M, et al. LPS signaling enhances hepatic fibrogenesis caused by experimental cholestasis in mice. *Am J Physiol Gastrointest Liver Physiol.* 2006;290:1318–1328.
60. Huang H, Shiffman ML, Friedman S, et al. A 7 gene signature identifies the risk of developing cirrhosis in patients with chronic hepatitis C. *Hepatology.* 2007;46:297–306.
61. Watanabe A, Hashmi A, Gomes DA, et al. Apoptotic hepatocyte DNA inhibits hepatic stellate cell chemotaxis via toll-like receptor 9. *Hepatology.* 2007;46:1509–1518.
62. Seki E, Tsutsui H, Iimuro Y, et al. Contribution of Toll-like receptor/myeloid differentiation factor 88 signaling to murine liver regeneration. *Hepatology.* 2005;41:443–450.
63. Riad A, Jager S, Sobirey M, et al. Toll-like receptor-4 modulates survival by induction of left ventricular remodeling after myocardial infarction in mice. *J Immunol.* 2008;180:6954–6961.
64. Frantz S, Ertl G, Bauersachs J. Mechanisms of disease: toll-like receptors in cardiovascular disease. *Nat Clin Pract Cardiovasc Med.* 2007;4:444–454.
65. Wolf G, Bohlender J, Bondeva T, et al. Angiotensin II upregulates toll-like receptor 4 on mesangial cells. *J Am Soc Nephrol.* 2006;17:1585–1593.
66. Jiang D, Liang J, Fan J, et al. Regulation of lung injury and repair by toll-like receptors and hyaluronan. *Nat Med.* 2005;11:1173–1179.
67. Michelsen KS, Wong MH, Shah PK, et al. Lack of Toll-like receptor 4 or myeloid differentiation factor 88 reduces atherosclerosis and alters plaque phenotype in mice deficient in apolipoprotein E. *Proc Natl Acad Sci USA.* 2004;101:10679–10684.
68. Mullick AE, Tobias PS, Curtiss LK. Modulation of atherosclerosis in mice by toll-like receptor 2. *J Clin Invest.* 2005;115:3149–156.
69. Wang J, Hori K, Ding J, et al. Toll-like receptors expressed by dermal fibroblasts contribute to hypertrophic scarring. *J Cell Physiol.* 2011;226(5):1265–1273.
70. Babelova A, Moreth K, Tsalastra-Greul W, et al. Biglycan, a danger signal that activates the NLRP3 inflammasome via Toll-like and P2X receptors. *J Biol Chem.* 2009;284(36):24035–24048.
71. Schaefer L, Babelova A, Kiss E, et al. The matrix component biglycan is proinflammatory and signals through Toll-like receptors 4 and 2 in macrophages. *J Clin Invest.* 2005;115(8):2223–2233.
72. Shimazu R, Akashi S, Ogata H, et al. MD-2, a molecule that confers lipopolysaccharide responsiveness on Toll-like receptor 4. *J Exp Med.* 1999;189(11):1777–1782.
73. Jin MS, Lee J-O. Structures of the Toll-like receptor family and its ligand complexes. *Immunity.* 2008;29(2):182–191.
74. Bucala R, Spiegel LA, Chesney J, et al. Circulating fibrocytes define a new leukocyte subpopulation that mediates tissue repair. *Mol Med.* 1994; 1: 71–81.
75. Pilling D, Fan T, Huang D, et al. Identification of markers that distinguish monocyte-derived fibrocytes from monocytes, macrophages, and fibroblasts. *PLoS One.* 2009;4:e7475.
76. Quan TE, Cowper S, Wu SP, et al. Circulating fibrocytes: collagen-secreting cells of the peripheral blood. *Int J Biochem Cell Biol.* 2004;36:598–606.
77. Direkze NC, Hodivala-Dilke K, Jeffery R, et al. Bone marrow contribution to tumor-associated myofibroblasts and fibroblasts. *Cancer Res.* 2004;64:8492–8495.
78. Maharaj S, Shimbori C, Kolb M. Fibrocytes in pulmonary fibrosis: a brief synopsis. *Eur Respir Rev.* 2013;22(130):552–557.
79. Kuwana M, Okazaki Y, Kodama H, et al. Human circulating $CD14^+$ monocytes as a source of progenitors that exhibit mesenchymal cell differentiation. *J Leukoc Biol.* 2003;74:833–845.
80. Abe R, Donnelly SC, Peng T, et al. Peripheral blood fibrocytes: differentiation pathway and migration to wound sites. *J Immunol.* 2001;166:7556–7562.
81. Strieter RM, Keeley EC, Hughes MA, et al. The role of circulating mesenchymal progenitor cells (fibrocytes) in the pathogenesis of pulmonary fibrosis. *J Leukoc Biol.* 2009;86:1111–1118.
82. Quan TE, Cowper SE, Bucala R. The role of circulating fibrocytes in fibrosis. *Curr Rheumatol Rep.* 2006;8(2):145–150.
83. Yang L Shankowsky HA, Scott PG, et al. Peripheral blood fibrocytes from burn patients: identification and quantification of fibrocytes in adherent cells cultured from peripheral blood mononuclear cells. *Lab Invest.* 2002;82:1183–1192.
84. Yang L, Jiao H, Shankowsky HA, et al. Identification of fibrocytes in post-burn hypertrophic scar. *Wound Repair Regen.* 2005;13(4):398–404.
85. Wang J, Jiao H, Stewart TL, et al. Accelerated wound healing in leukocyte-specific, protein 1-deficient mouse is associated with

increased infiltration of leukocytes and fibrocytes. *J Leukoc Biol.* 2007;82:1554–1563.
86. Wang J, Stewart TL, Chen H, et al. Improved scar in post-burn patients following interferon alpha 2b treatment is associated with decreased angiogenesis mediated by vascular endothelial cell growth factor. *J Interferon Cytokine Res.* 2008;28(7):423–434.
87. Wang J, Jiao H, Stewart TL, et al. Improvement in postburn hypertrophic scar after treatment with IFN-alpha2b is associated with decreased fibrocytes. *J Interferon Cytokine Res.* 2007;27:921–930.
88. Wang JF, Jiao H, Stewart TL, et al. Fibrocytes from burn patients regulate the activities of fibroblasts. *Wound Repair Regen.* 2007;15(1):113–121.
89. Roufosse C, Bou-Gharios G, Prodromidi E, et al. Bone marrow-derived cells do not contribute significantly to collagen I synthesis in a murine model of renal fibrosis. *J Am Soc Nephrol.* 2006;17:775–782.
90. Barisic-Dujmovic T, Boban I, Clark SH. Fibroblasts/myofibroblasts that participate in cutaneous wound healing are not derived from circulating progenitor cells. *J Cell Physiol.* 2010;222(3):703–712.
91. Higashiyama R, Nakao S, Sibusawa Y, et al. Differential contribution of dermal resident and bone marrow-derived cells to collagen production during wound healing and fibrogenesis. *J Invest Dermatol.* 2011;131(2):529–536.
92. Antoniou KM, Soufla G, Lymbouridou R, et al. Expression analysis of angiogenic growth factors and biological axis CXCL12/CXCR4 axis in idiopathic pulmonary fibrosis. *Connect Tissue Res.* 2010;51:71–80.
93. Chen HC, Yang JY, Chuang SS, et al. Heterotopic ossification in burns: our experience and literature reviews. *Burns.* 2009;35(6):857–862.
94. Evans EB. Heterotopic bone formation in thermal burns. *Clin Orthop Relat Res.* 1991;(263):94–101.
95. Tsionos I, Leclercq C, Rochet JM. Heterotopic ossification of the elbow in patients with burns. Results after early excision. *J Bone Joint Surg Br.* 2004;86(3):396–403.
96. Gaur A, Sinclair M, Caruso E, et al. Heterotopic ossification around the elbow following burns in children: results after excision. *J Bone Joint Surg Am.* 2003;85A(8):1538–1543.
97. Michelsson JE, Rauschning W. Pathogenesis of experimental heterotopic bone formation following temporary forcible exercising of immobilized limbs. *Clin Orthop Relat Res.* 1983;176:265–272.
98. Medina A, Shankowsky HA, Savaryn B, et al. Characterization of heterotopic ossification in burn patients. *J Burn Care Res.* 2014;35(3):448–455.
99. Zuo KJ, Tredget EE. Multiple Marjolin's ulcers arising from irradiated post-bun hypertrophic scars: a case report. *Burns.* 2014;40(4): e21–e215.
100. Medina A, Ma Z, Varkey M, et al. Fibrocytes participate in the development of heterotopic ossification. *J Burn Care Res.* 2015;35(3):251–256.
101. Choi YH, Burdick MD, Strieter RM. Human circulating fibrocytes have the capacity to differentiate osteoblasts and chondrocytes. *Int J Biochem Cell Biol.* 2010;42(5):662–671.
102. Medina A, Ghahary A. Reprogrammed fibrocytes induce a mixed Th1/Th2 cytokine response of naïve CD4(+) T cells. *Mol Cell Biochem.* 2011;346(1/2):89–94.
103. Miller AC, Rashid RM, Elamin EM. The "T" in trauma: the helper T-cell response and the role of immunomodulation in trauma and burn patients. *J Trauma.* 2007;63(6):1407–1417.
104. Tredget EE, Yang L, Delehanty M, et al. Polarized T helper cells Th2 cytokine production in patients with hypertrophic scar following thermal injury. *J Interferon Cytokine Res.* 2006;26:179–189.
105. Wang J, Jiao H, Stewart TL, et al. Increased TGF-beta-producing $CD4^+$ T lymphocytes in postburn patients and their potential interaction with dermal fibroblasts in hypertrophic scarring. *Wound Repair Regen.* 2007;15(4):530–539.
106. MacConmara MP, Maung AA, Fujimi S, et al. Increased $CD4^+$ $CD25^+$ T regulatory cell activity in trauma patients depresses protective Th1 immunity. *Ann Surg.* 2006;244:514–523.
107. Shao DD, Suresh R, Vakil V, et al. Pivotal advance: Th-1 cytokines inhibit, and Th-2 cytokines promote fibrocyte differentiation. *J Leukoc Biol.* 2008;83:1323–1333.
108. Seki E, De Minicis S, Osterreicher CH, et al. TLR4 enhances TGF-beta signaling and hepatic fibrosis. *Nat Med.* 2007;13:1324–1332.
109. Wynn TA, Barron L. Macrophages: master regulators of inflammation and fibrosis. *Semin Liver Dis.* 2010;30(3):245–257.
110. Barron L, Wynn TA. Fibrosis is regulated by Th2 and Th17 responses and by dynamic interactions between fibroblasts and macrophages. *Am J Physiol Gastrointest Liver Physiol.* 2011;300(5):723–728.
111. Montazi M, Ding J, Kwan P, et al. Morphologic and histologic comparison of hypertrophic scar in nude mice, T-cell receptor and recombination activating gene knockout mice. *Plast Reconstr Surg.* 2015;136(6):1192–1204.
112. Zhu Z, Ding J, Tredget EE. The molecular basis of hypertrophic scars. *Burns Trauma.* 2016; 4:2.
113. Nagaoka T, Kaburagi Y, Hamaguchi Y, et al. Delayed wound healing in the absence of intercellular adhesion molecule-1 or L-selectin expression. *Am J Pathol.* 2000;157:237–247.
114. Eming SA, Werner S, Bugnon P, et al. Accelerated wound closure in mice deficient for interleukin-10. *Am J Pathol.* 2007;170:188–202.
115. Mahdavian Delavary B, van der Veer WM, van Egmond M, et al. Macrophages in skin injury and repair. *Immunobiology.* 2011;216:753–762.
116. Wynn TA. Fibrotic disease and the T(H)1/T(H)2 paradigm. *Nat Rev Immunol.* 2004;4:583–594.
117. Song E, Ouyang N, Horbelt M, et al. Influence of alternatively and classically activated macrophages on fibrogenic activities of human fibroblasts. *Cell Immunol.* 2000;204:19–28.
118. Mills CD, Kincaid K, Alt JM, et al. M1/M2 macrophages and the Th1/Th2 paradigm. *J Immunol.* 2000;164:6166–6173.
119. Mantovani A, Sica A, Sozzani S, et al. The chemokine system in diverse forms of macrophage activation and polarization. *Trends Immunol.* 2004;25:677–686.
120. Martinez FO, Sica A, Mantovani A, et al. Macrophage activation and polarization. *Front Biosci.* 2008;13:453–461.
121. Grinberg S, Hasko G, Wu D, et al. Suppression of PLC β2 by endotoxin plays a role in the adenosine A(2A) receptor-mediated switch of macrophages from an inflammatory to an angiogenic phenotype. *Am J Pathol.* 2009;175:2439–2453.
122. Sica A, Mantovani A. Macrophage plasticity and polarization: *in vivo* veritas. *J Clin Invest.* 2012;122:787–795.
123. Zhu Z, Ding J, Ma Z, et al. The natural behavior of mononuclear phagocytes in HTS formation. *Wound Repair Regen.* 2015. doi:10.1111/wrr.12378.
124. Stark GR, Kerr IM, Williams BR, et al. How cells respond to interferons. *Annu Rev Biochem* 1998;67:227–264.
125. Platanias LC. Interferons: laboratory to clinic investigations. *Curr Opin Oncol* 1995;7(6):560–565.
126. Tredget EE, Shankowsky HA, Pannu R, et al. Transforming growth factor-beta in thermally injured patients with hypertrophic scars: effects of interferon alpha-2a. *Plast Reconstr Surg.* 1998;102(5):1317–1328.
127. Ghahary A, Shen YJ, Scott PG, et al. Immunolocalization of TGF-beta 1 in human hypertrophic scar and normal dermal tissues. *Cytokine.* 1995;7:184–190.
128. Wang R, Ghahary A, Dodd, C, et al. Hypertrophic scar tissues and fibroblasts produce more transforming growth factor-beta1 mRNA and protein than normal skin and cells. *Wound Repair Regen.* 2009;8:128–137.
129. Berman B, Viera MH, Amini S, et al. Prevention and management of hypertrophic scars and keloids after burns in children. *J Craniofac Surg.* 2008;19(4):989–1006.
130. Wong TW, Chiu HC, Yip KM. Intralesional interferon alpha-2b has no effect in the treatment of keloids. *Br J Dermatol.* 1994;130(5):683–685.
131. Poynard T, Colombo M, Bruix J, et al. Peginterferon alfa-2b and ribavirin: effective in patients with hepatitis c who failed interferon-alfa/ribavirin therapy. *Gastroenterology.* 2009;136(5):1618–1628.
132. Yang YF, Zhao W, Zhong YD, et al. Interferon therapy in chronic hepatitis B reduces progression to cirrhosis and hepatocellular carcinoma: a meta-analysis. *J Viral Hepat.* 2009;16(4):265–271.
133. Rees PA, Greaves NS, Baguneid M, et al. Chemokines in wound healing and as potential therapeutic targets for reducing cutaneous scarring. *Adv Wound Care.* 2015;4(11):687–703.
134. Xu J, Mora A, Shim H, et al. Role of the SDF-1/CXCR4 axis in the pathogenesis of lung injury and fibrosis. *Am J Respir Cell Mol Biol.* 2007;37(3):291–299.
135. Zou YR, Kottmann AH, Kuroda M, et al. Function of the chemokine receptor CXCR4 in haematopoiesis and in cerebellar development. *Nature.* 1998;393(6685):595–599.
136. Nagasawa T. Role of chemokine SDF-1/PBSF and its receptor CXCR4 in blood vessel development. *Ann N Y Acad Sci.* 2001;947:112–115.
137. Avniel S, Arik Z, Maly A, et al. Involvement of the CXCL12/CXCR4 pathway in the recovery of skin following burns. *J Invest Dermatol.* 2006;126(2):468–476.
138. Ding J, Ma Z, Liu H, et al. The therapeutic potential of a C-X-C chemokine receptor type 4 (CXCR-4) antagonist on hypertrophic scarring in vivo. *Wound Repair Regen.* 2014;22(5);622–630.

139. Jarvinen TAH, Ruoshlahti E. Targeted antiscarring therapy for tissue injuries. *Adv Wound Care*. 2015;2(5):51–55.
140. Jarvinen TAH, Ruoshlahti E. Target seeking antifibrotic compound enhances wound healing and suppresses scar formation. *Proc Natl Acad Sci USA*. 2010;107:21671–21676.
141. Kwan P, Ding J, Tredget EE. MicroRNA 181b regulates decorin production by dermal fibroblasts and may be a potential therapy for hypertrophic scar. *PLoS One*. 205;10(4):e0123054.
142. Heimbach D, Engrav L, Grube B, et al. Burn depth: a review. *World J Surg*. 1992;16(1):10–15.
143. Mladick R, Georgiade N, Thorne F. A clinical evaluation of the use of thermography in determining degree of burn injury. *Plast Reconstr Surg*. 1966;38(6):512–518.
144. Cole RP, Jones SG, Shakespeare PG. Thermographic assessment of hand burns. *Burns*. 1990;16(1):60–63.
145. Droog EJ, Steenbergen W, Sjoberg F. Measurement of depth of burns by laser Doppler perfusion imaging. *Burns*. 2001;27(6):561–568.
146. Smits GJ, Roman RJ, Lombard JH. Evaluation of laser-doppler flowmetry as a measure of tissue blood flow. *J Appl Physiol*. 1986;61(2):666–672.
147. Bray R, Forrester K, Leonard C, et al. Laser Doppler imaging of burn scars: a comparison of wavelength and scanning methods. *Burns*. 2003;29(3):199–206.
148. Niazi ZB, Essex TJ, Papini R, et al. New laser Doppler scanner, a valuable adjunct in burn depth assessment. *Burns*. 1993;19(6):485–489.
149. Hoeksema H, Van de Sijpe K, Tondu T, et al. Accuracy of early burn depth assessment by laser Doppler imaging on different days post burn. *Burns*. 2009;35(1):36–45.
150. Reno F, Grazianetti P, Stella M, et al. Release and activation of matrix metalloproteinase-9 during in vitro mechanical compression in hypertrophic scars. *Arch Dermatol*. 2002;138(4):475–478.
151. Costa AM, Peyrol S, Porto LC, et al. Mechanical forces induce scar remodeling. Study in non-pressure-treated versus pressure-treated hypertrophic scars. *Am J Pathol*. 1999;155(5):1671–1679.
152. Anzarut A, Olson J, Singh P, et al. The effectiveness of pressure garment therapy for the prevention of abnormal scarring after burn injury: a meta-analysis. *J Plast Reconstr Aesthet Surg*. 2009;62(1):77–84.
153. Engrav LH, Heimbach DH, Rivara FP, et al. 12-year within-wound study of the effectiveness of pressure garment therapy. *Burns*. 2010;36:975–983.
154. Borgognoni L. Biological effects of silicone gel sheeting. *Wound Repair Regen*. 2002;10(2):118–121.
155. So K, Umraw N, Scott J, et al. Effects of enhanced patient education on compliance with silicone gel sheeting and burn scar outcome: a randomized prospective study. *J Burn Care Rehabil*. 2003;24(6): 411–417.
156. Gilman TH. Silicone sheet for treatment and prevention of hypertrophic scar: a new proposal for the mechanism of efficacy. *Wound Repair Regen*. 2003;11(3):235–236.
157. Morry J, Ngamcherdtrakul W, Gu S, et al. Dermal delivery of HSP47 siRNA with NOX4-modulating mesoporous silica-based nanoparticles for treating fibrosis. *Biomaterials*. 2015;66:41–52.
158. O'Brien L, Jones DJ. Silicone gel sheeting for preventing and treating hypertrophic and keloid scars. *Cochrane Database Syst Rev*. 2013;(9):CD003826.
159. Li Y, Yang L, Zheng Z, et al. Knockdown down-regulates the deposition of collagen and leads to a reduced hypertrophic scar fibrosis. *J Mol Histol*. 2015;46(4/5):357–364.
160. Boyce, Steven T. Kagan, et al. Cultured skin substitutes reduce donor skin harvesting for closure of excised, full-thickness burns. *Ann Surg*. 2002;235:269–79.
161. Kamel RA, Ong JF, Eriksson E, et al. Tissue engineering of skin. *J Am Coll Surg*. 2013;217(3):533–555.
162. Varkey M, Ding J, Tredget EE. Differential collagen-glycosaminoglycan matrix remodeling by superficial and deep dermal fibroblasts: potential therapeutic targets for hypertrophic scar. *Biomaterials*. 2011;32(30):7581–7891.
163. Varkey M, Ding J, Tredget EE. Superficial dermal fibroblasts enhance basement membrane and epidermal barrier formation in tissue-engineered skin: implications for treatment of skin basement membrane disorders. *Tissue Eng Part A*. 2014;20(3/4):540–552.
164. Varkey M, Ding J, Tredget EE. Fibrotic remodeling of tissue-engineered skin with deep dermal fibroblasts is reduced by keratinocytes. *Tissue Eng Part A*. 2014;20(3/4):716–727.
165. Varkey M, Ding J, Tredget EE; The effect of keratinocytes on the biomechanical characteristics and pore microstructure of tissue engineered skin using deep dermal fibroblasts. *Biomaterials*. 2014;35(36):9591–9598.
166. Hartwell R, Poormasjedi-Meibod MS, Chavez-Munoz C, et al. An in-situ forming skin substitute improves healing outcome in a hypertrophic scar model. *Tissue Eng Part A*. 2015;21(5/6):1085–1094.
167. Yasuoka H, Larregina AT, Yamaguchi Y, et al. Human skin culture as an ex vivo model for assessing the fibrotic effects of insulin-like growth factor binding proteins. *Open Rheumatol J*. 2008;2:17–22.
168. Mustoe TA, Pierce GF, Morishima C, et al. Growth factor-induced acceleration of tissue repair through direct and inductive activities in a rabbit dermal ulcer model. *J Clin Invest*. 1991;87(2): 694–703.
169. Morris DE, Wu L, Zhao LL, et al. Acute and chronic animal models for excessive dermal scarring: quantitative studies. *Plast Reconstr Surg*. 1997;100(3):674–681.
170. Li Y, Kilani RT, Rahmani-Neishaboor E, et al. Kynurenine increases matrix metalloproteinase-1 and -3 expression in cultured dermal fibroblasts and improves scarring in vivo. *J Invest Dermatol*. 2014;134(3):643–650.
171. Zhang Q, Liu LN, Yong Q, et al. Intralesional injection of adipose-derived stem cells reduces hypertrophic scarring in a rabbit ear model. *Stem Cell Res Ther*. 2015;18;6(1):145.
172. Zhu KQ, Engrav LH, Gibran NS, et al. The female, red Duroc pig as an animal model of hypertrophic scarring and the potential role of the cones of skin. *Burns*. 2003;29(7):649–664.
173. Domergue S, Jorgensen C, Noël D. Advances in research in animal models of burn-related hypertrophic scarring. *J Burn Care Res*. 2015;36(5):e259–e266.
174. Silverstein P, Goodwin M Jr, Raulston G. Hypertrophic scarring, etiology and control. In: *Ann Res Progress Report of the US Army Institute of Surgical Research* (Section 37); 1972.
175. Matsumura H, Engrav LH, Reichenbach D, et al. *Cones. Fat Domes and Hypertrophic Scarring in the Female, Red, Duroc Pig*. Loma Linda, CA: Plastic Surgery Council; 1998.
176. Gallant C, Wright J, Olson M, et al. *The Red Duroc Pig Model of Hypertrophic Wound Healing*. Albuquerque, NM: Wound Healing Society; 2001.
177. Yamamoto T, Takagawa S, Katayama I, et al. Animal model of sclerotic skin. I: local injections of bleomycin induce sclerotic skin mimicking scleroderma. *J Invest Dermatol*. 1999;112:456–462.
178. Ruzehaji N, Avouac J, Elhai M, et al. Combined effect of genetic background and gender in a mouse model of bleomycin-induced skin fibrosis. *Arthritis Res Ther*. 2015;17(1):145.
179. Serratrice N, Bruzzese L, Magalon J, et al. New fat-derived products for treating skin-induced lesions of scleroderma in nude mice. *Stem Cell Res Ther*. 2014;5(6):138.
180. Ohashi T, Yamamoto T. Antifibrotic effect of lysophosphatidic acid receptors LPA1 and LPA3 antagonist on experimental murine scleroderma induced by bleomycin. *Exp Dermatol*. 2015;24(9): 698–702.
181. Czernielewski J, Demarchez M, Prunieras M. Human Langerhans cells in epidermal cell culture, in vitro skin explants and skin grafts onto "nude" mice. *Arch Dermatol Res*. 1984;276(5):288–292.
182. Demarchez M, Desbas C, Prunieras M. Wound healing of human skin transplanted on to the nude mouse. *Br J Dermatol*. 1985;113(suppl 28):177–182.
183. Czernielewski JM, Demarchez M. Further evidence for the self-reproducing capacity of Langerhans cells in human skin. *J Invest Dermatol*. 1987;88(1):17–20.
184. Demarchez M, Hartmann DJ, Prunieras M. An immunohistological study of the revascularization process in human skin transplanted onto the nude mouse. *Transplantation*. 1987;43(6):896–903.
185. Démarchez M, Hartmann DJ, Herbage D, et al. Wound healing of human skin transplanted onto the nude mouse. II. An immunohistological and ultrastructural study of the epidermal basement membrane zone reconstruction and connective tissue reorganization. *Dev Biol*. 1987;121(1):119–129.
186. Rossio-Pasquier P, Casanova D, Jomard A, et al. Wound healing of human skin transplanted onto the nude mouse after a superficial excisional injury: human dermal reconstruction is achieved in several steps by two different fibroblast subpopulations. *Arch Dermatol Res*. 1999;291(11):591–599.
187. Shetlar MR, Shetlar CL, Hendricks L, et al. The use of athymic nude mice for the study of human keloids. *Proc Soc Exp Biol Med*. 1985;179(4):549–552.

188. Kischer CW, Pindur J, Krasovitch P, et al. Characteristics of granulation tissue which promote hypertrophic scarring. *Scanning Microsc.* 1990;4(4):877–887.
189. Robb EC, Waymack JP, Warden GD, et al. A new model for studying the development of human hypertrophic burn scar formation. *J Burn Care Rehabil.* 1987;8(5):371–375.
190. Lorenz HP, Longaker MT, Perkocha LA, et al. Scarless wound repair: a human fetal skin model. *Development.* 1992;114(1):253–259.
191. Yang DY, Li SR, Wu JL, et al. Establishment of a hypertrophic scar model by transplanting full-thickness human skin grafts onto the backs of nude mice. *Plast Reconstr Surg.* 2007;119(1):104–109.
192. Wang J, Ding J, Jiao H, et al. Human hypertrophic scar-like nude mouse model: characterization of the molecular and cellular biology of the scar process. *Wound Repair Regen.* 2011;19(2):274–285.
193. Momtazi M, Kwan P, Ding J, et al. A nude mouse model of hypertrophic scar shows morphologic and histologic characteristics of human hypertrophic scar. *Wound Repair Regen.* 2013;21(1):77–87.
194. Momtazi M, Ding J, Kwan P, et al. Morphologic and histologic comparison of hypertrophic scar in nude mice, T-cell receptor, and recombination activating gene knockout mice. *Plast Reconstr Surg.* 2015;136(6):1192–1204.
195. Alrobaiea SM, Ding J, Ma Z, et al. A novel nude mouse model of hypertrophic scarring using scratched full-thickness human skin grafts. *Adv Wound Care.* 2016;5(7):299–313.
196. Gawronska-Kozak B, Grabowska A, Kopcewicz M, et al. Animal models of skin regeneration. *Reprod Biol.* 2014;14(1):61–67.
197. Honardoust D, Varkey M, Marcoux Y, et al. Reduced decorin, fibromodulin, and transforming growth factor-β3 in deep dermis leads to hypertrophic scarring. *J Burn Care Res.* 2012;33(2):218–227.

7 The Biomechanics of Scar Formation

DOMINIK DUSCHER, MICHAEL T. LONGAKER, and GEOFFREY C. GURTNER

KEY POINTS

- All phases of wound healing are influenced by mechanical forces, and mechanotransduction, the mechanisms by which mechanical force is converted to biochemical stimuli, plays a pivotal role in cutaneous fibrosis.
- Extracellular biomechanical cues are transduced by the extracellular matrix (ECM), a dynamic structure with multiple functions. Mechanical stimuli can expose hidden domains and alter spatial concentration of growth factors within the ECM, resulting in changes of cellular behavior and phenotype. Additionally, stored factors within the ECM can be released based on the effects of mechanical force.
- Intracellular mechanotransduction, the mechanisms by which cells "feel" and interact with their environment, is mediated by mechanoresponsive ion channels (e.g., Ca^{2+}), growth factor, and cytokine receptors (e.g., for transforming growth factor (TGF)-β or stromal cell–derived factor (SDF)-1), integrin–matrix interactions (e.g., involving focal adhesion kinase (FAK)) and G protein–coupled receptors (GPCRs).
- Mechanomodulation can be utilized therapeutically. Randomized controlled clinical trials have demonstrated that mechanomodulation of the wound environment using an elastomeric silicone dressing significantly reduces scar development.

Scar formation is among the most complex biologic processes and represents a substantial source of morbidity worldwide. In humans, scarring is the typical response to tissue injuries. The process of fibrotic repair, prioritizing early restoration of tissue integrity rather than functional regeneration, offers a survival advantage and is therefore highly conserved in evolution.[1,2] Despite extensive research efforts dedicated to the expansion of our understanding of the mechanisms underlying scar formation, effective clinical therapies for scar mitigation are only beginning to be developed. A detailed understanding of the numerous signaling pathways involved is essential to develop remedies for fibrosis and scarring. During initial research efforts concentrated on elaborating the biochemical mechanisms involved in scar formation, however, evidence has emerged that mechanical forces play a previously underestimated role in the modulation of these pathways. The impact of mechanical forces on cutaneous scarring was first observed as early as the 19th century,[3] but only recently have the underlying signaling mechanisms begun to be elucidated. Mechanotransduction, which refers to the mechanisms by which mechanical forces are converted to biochemical stimuli, has been closely linked to inflammation and is believed to play a pivotal role in cutaneous fibrosis.[4] There is increasing evidence that all phases of wound healing are influenced by mechanical forces,[5] but the field of wound mechanobiology is still in its infancy. However, utilizing the recent insights into how mechanotransduction of environmental cues effects the behavior of cells and tissues will help us to formulate effective therapeutics and may lead to the achievement of the ultimate goal, to transform fibrotic healing into tissue regeneration.

Molecular Biomechanics of Scar Formation

The field of mechanobiology continues to advance rapidly. The application of innovative in vitro and in vivo models leads to a more thorough understanding of the effects of mechanical forces on biologic processes.[6] It has been demonstrated that cells are able to convert mechanical stimuli into biochemical or transcriptional changes via the process of mechanotransduction.[7] Signal transduction from the microenvironment involves numerous proteins and molecules of the extracellular matrix (ECM), the cytoplasmic membrane, the cytoskeleton, and the nuclear membrane, which transport mechanical cues down to the nuclear chromatin to alter cellular programs at the genetic and epigenetic level.[8]

Several attempts to define the role of mechanical influences in molecular biology have been made. The most widely accepted system linking the different levels of mechanotransduction is known as tensional integrity or "tensegrity."[9] First described as an architectural concept,[10] this principle, based on isolated components in compression inside a net of continuous tension, was adapted and developed by Ingber et al.[9] to explain how cellular structures and processes are influenced by mechanical force. However, a complete understanding of the complex mechanotransduction pathways in living organisms remains elusive. Nevertheless, the observations made in small and large animal studies implicate a significant involvement of mechanical influences in the development of cutaneous scarring. Translating these findings into clinical therapies must be our principal goal.

Extracellular Mechanotransduction

The ECM is much more than just an inert three-dimensional network passively offering structural support. It is a dynamic and living tissue responsible for numerous functions. The ECM governs cell adhesion, migration, differentiation, proliferation, and apoptosis and is highly involved in the complex processes of mechanotransduction[11,12] (Fig 7-1). Mechanical cues transported through the ECM to cells can directly affect gene expression because of a direct link between structural proteins of the ECM to nuclear chromatin.[13]

Additional evidence supporting the theories how ECM can alter cell functionality and phenotype is provided by the fact that tissue stiffness and rigidity can be linked to tumor growth and malignancy.[14] The extracellular environment can function in both ways, being pro-oncogenic in some circumstances,[15] but also may reverse malignant behavior if corrected.[16] Similarly, microenvironmental signals can influence scarring and fibrosis.[17–19] It has been demonstrated that scar progression results from a positive feedback loop connecting the accumulation of ECM and increased matrix stiffness to the enhancement of fibroblast proliferation and collagen production via mechanoresponsive mechanisms.[20,21]

In addition to direct effects on cell behavior via ECM–cell membrane/cytoskeletal interfaces, mechanical cues can also execute indirect effects. Specifically, alterations in ECM structure can expose normally hidden domains and binding sites that have regulatory capabilities.[22] The ECM can also alter the spatiotemporal composition of the microenvironment by changing the concentrations of soluble and matrix-bound effector molecules and growth factors, such as transforming growth factor beta (TGF-β), resulting in considerable impact on biologic functions.[23]

Intracellular Mechanotransduction

The mechanisms by which cells "feel" and interact with their environment are incompletely understood. However, recent efforts have led to the identification of key signaling pathways involved in intracellular mechanotransduction. The central mediators of mechanotransduction include mechanoresponsive ion channels (e.g., Ca^{2+}), growth factor and cytokine receptors (e.g., TGF-β and stromal cell–derived factor 1 [SDF-1]), integrin–matrix interactions, and G protein–coupled receptors (GPCRs)[24,25] (Fig. 7-2).

The fact that conformational alterations of ion channels govern numerous cellular functions is an established biologic concept. However, an understanding of how mechanoresponsive calcium channels influence fibrotic pathways has only recently begun to emerge.[26] Specifically, calcium-dependent ion channels have been demonstrated to be heavily involved in the arrangement of elements of the cytoskeleton, which are associated with mechanotransduction.[27] Additionally, Ca^{2+} influx caused by mechanical stimulation of the cell membrane activates mitogen-activated kinases (MAPKs), which enhance profibrotic gene expression.[28]

Growth factors and cytokines together with their receptors are implicated in all stages of wound healing and the development of cutaneous scarring. Recent work has shown

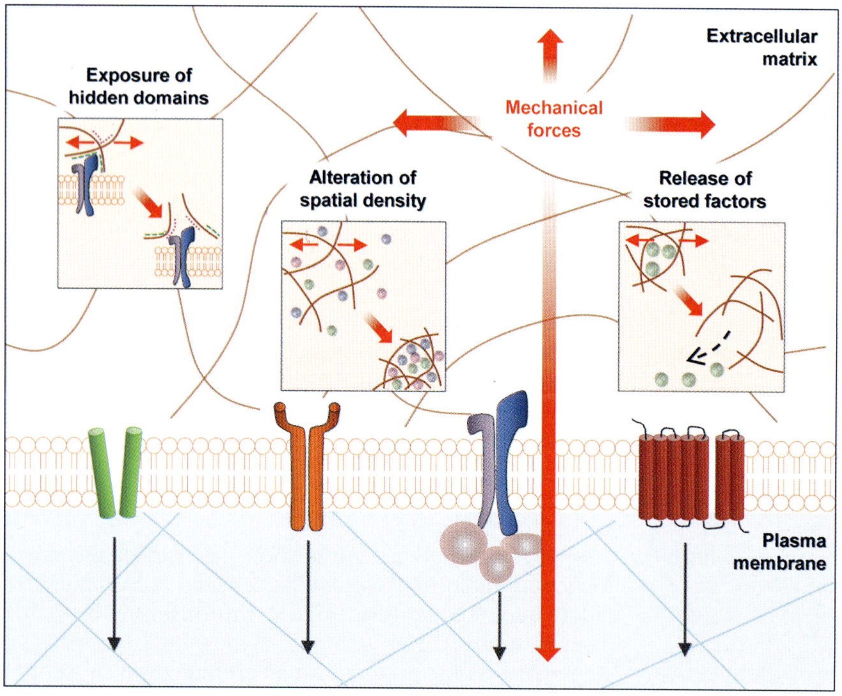

FIGURE 7-1 **Extracellular mechanotransduction.** Biomechanical cues directly affect the extracellular matrix (ECM), which is a dynamic structure with multiple functions. Mechanical stimuli can expose hidden domains and alter spatial concentration of growth factors within the ECM, resulting in changes of cellular behavior and phenotype. Additionally, stored factors within the ECM can be released based on the effects of mechanical force. *(Reproduced with permission from Wong VW, Akaishi S, Longaker MT, Gurtner GC. Pushing back: wound mechanotransduction in repair and regeneration.* J Invest Dermatol. *2011;131(11):2186–2196.)*

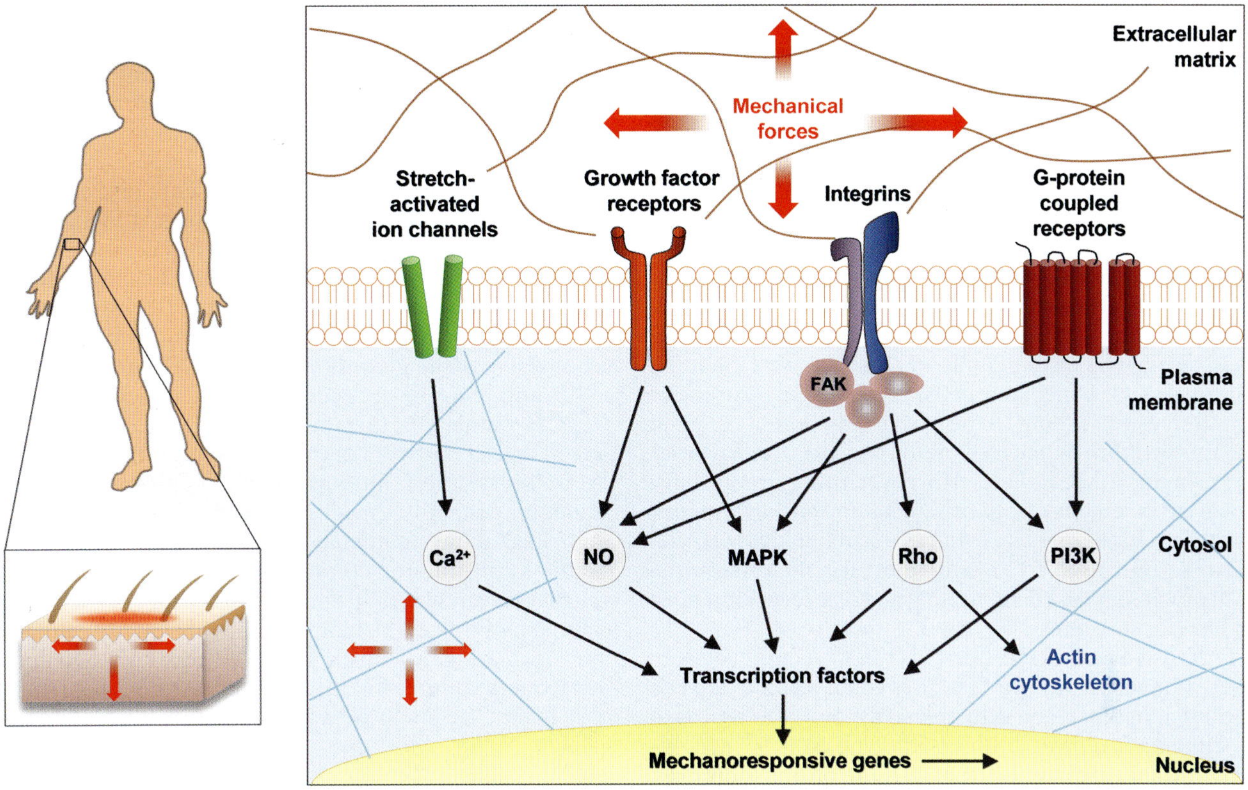

FIGURE 7-2 **Intracellular mechanotransduction.** Key players of mechnotransduction on the cellular level are mechanoresponsive ion channels (e.g., Ca^{2+}), growth factor and cytokine receptors (e.g., for TGF-β or SDF-1), integrin–matrix interactions, and G protein–coupled receptors (GPCRs). *(Reproduced with permission from Wong VW, Akaishi S, Longaker MT, Gurtner GC. Pushing back: wound mechanotransduction in repair and regeneration.* J Invest Dermatol. *2011;131(11):2186–2196.)*

promising results regarding scar formation and appearance when the cytokine system is manipulated.[29] Specifically, modulating the ratios of subsets of TGF-β in the wound microenvironment has received significant attention (see below). Mechanical stimuli result in a release of TGF-β from its reservoir in the extracellular latent complexes.[30–32] This growth factor is associated with numerous fibrotic diseases, and acts mainly via the TGF-β receptor 2 and its downstream effector proteins SMAD 2 and 3. The TGF-β signaling cascade controls numerous profibrotic mechanisms, such as collagen production and fibroblast to myofibroblast differentiation.[33,34] Another mechanoresponsive signaling molecule responsible for the regulation of cutaneous healing and fibrosis is SDF-1 or CXCL12. It has been demonstrated that mechanical stretching can upregulate SDF-1a in skin, which directly leads to the recruitment of circulating proregenerative mesenchymal stem cells through the SDF-1a/CXCR4 axis.[35] However, somewhat contradictory results regarding the influence of SDF-1 on wound healing and scar formation have been reported. Whereas hypertrophic burn scars could be associated with increased SDF-1a/CXCR4 signaling,[36] it could also be demonstrated that the therapeutic application of SDF-1 to cutaneous wounds of mice and pigs leads to enhanced healing with decreased fibrosis.[37,38] Additionally, a local increase of SDF-1 has been identified as the potential underlying mechanism of noncontact, low-frequency ultrasound therapy, which has been shown to have beneficial effects in the treatment of chronic wounds.[39] This further corroborates the pivotal role of cytokines at the intersection of mechanotransduction and tissue healing, and strongly merits further investigation.

Although ion channels and cytokines certainly play an important role in the mechanobiology of scar formation, the most extensively studied cellular elements in this context are integrins. The members of this family of heterodimeric transmembrane receptor proteins possess a cytoplasmic domain, which communicates with the actin cytoskeleton, and extracellular domain binding molecules of the ECM.[40] Integrins carry out both "outside-in" communication of environmental mechanical cues to the cell and "inside-out" interactions via forces produced by the cytoskeleton.[40] This two-way signaling process is influenced by intracellular proteins, which bind to integrins to form large macromolecular structures, the so-called focal adhesions.[41,42] The most prominent of these intracellular binding proteins is the focal adhesion kinase (FAK). Conformational changes in the complex macrostructure of the focal adhesions caused by mechanical stimuli lead to an activation of the nonreceptor protein tyrosine kinase FAK via autophosphorylation. Although integrins have no intrinsic enzymatic activity, they can affect downstream signaling pathways via FAK. Specifically, FAK signaling has been heavily linked to wound healing aberrations.[4,43] Although mechanical stimuli influence all cell types involved in wound healing,[44] the effects of FAK activation demonstrate how mechanical cues can change biologic mechanisms in different cell types in diametrically opposed directions. Our laboratory has previously demonstrated that FAK is a key regulator of mechanosensing in cutaneous fibroblasts and that a fibroblast-specific deletion of FAK leads to reduced fibrosis after injury in a mouse model of scar formation.[4] In stark contrast, the loss of FAK in cutaneous keratinocytes leads to a significant delay in wound healing and dermal proteolysis in mice,[43] suggesting a skin layer–specific effect of FAK signaling with a complex influence on ECM repair.

Further highlighting the important role that FAK plays in the mechanical regulation of tissue repair, our laboratory recently demonstrated how mechanically activated pathways link scar formation with extracellular-related kinase (Erk, part of the family of MAPKs). Erk could be identified as a key mediator in the FAK-related response to wound tension, leading to the overproduction of collagen and the profibrotic chemokine monocyte chemoattractant protein-1 (MCP-1).[4,45] Moreover, other groups have shown involvement of other MAPKs in tension-induced fibrotic reactions, namely c-Jun N-terminal kinase (JNK) and p38 isoforms.[46,47] However, their specific roles in the mechanobiology of wound healing and scar formation need further clarification.

FAK also executes its effects via the Rho family of GTPases. The activity of RhoGTPases could be linked to cell motility, adherence, and cytoskeletal dynamics, as well as to the stimulation of myofibroblast differentiation,[48,49] demonstrating their extensive mechanosensing utility. Moreover, evidence is accumulating that FAK-RhoGTPase signaling influences mechanobiology via two downstream effectors of the mammalian Hippo pathway. The Hippo pathway is an evolutionary highly conserved signaling pathway involved in cell proliferation, apoptosis, differentiation, stem cell function, and malignant transformation[50,51] (Fig. 7-3). Specifically, the mechanoresponsive Hippo-effectors YAP (Yes-associated protein) and TAZ (transcriptional coactivator with PDZ-binding motif, also known as WWTR1) have been identified as key factors of tissue regeneration,[52–54] and have pivotal roles in cutaneous wound healing.[55] Stimulated via biomechanical cues, YAP and TAZ are stabilized and trigger the transcription of profibrotic targets such as connective tissue growth factor (CTGF) and TGF-β.[54,56] YAP and TAZ have recently been characterized to be GPCR regulated. Specifically, G12/13 and Gs coupled receptors act upstream of these transcriptional coactivators to modulate the Hippo pathway.[57] Remarkably, GPCRs function generally as cell surface mechanoreceptors and have been shown to influence similar intracellular pathways as the focal adhesion complexes.[24,25] Despite the need for further research to fully understand the involvement of the Hippo pathway in the biomechanics of wound healing and scar formation, it is likely that YAP and TAZ signaling is an attractive target for antifibrotic treatment approaches.

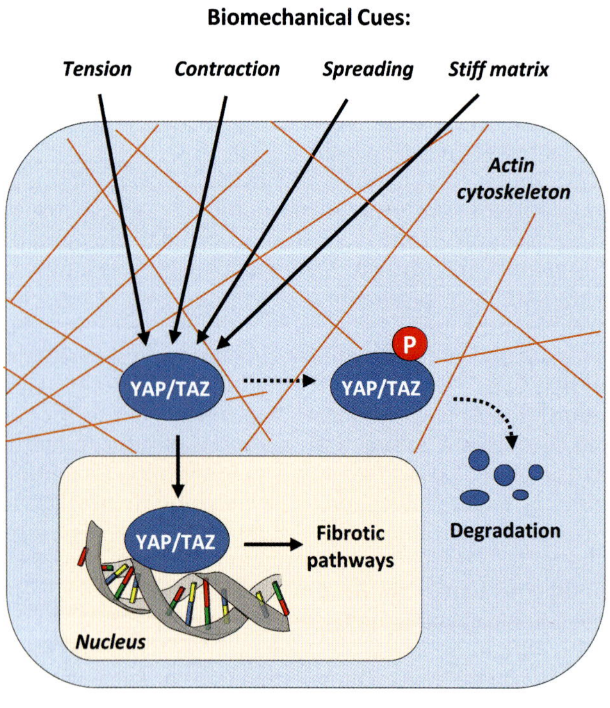

FIGURE 7-3 **The Hippo pathway in mechanotransduction**. The two main downstream Hippo-effectors,YAP and TAZ, have recently been identified to orchestrate biomechanical influences to alter cell behavior via the transcription of profibrotic signaling molecules such as connective tissue growth factor (CTGF) and TGF-β. This predisposes YAP and TAZ as potential targets for antifibrotic therapy. *(Reproduced with permission from Duscher D, Maan ZN, Wong VW, et al. Mechanotransduction and fibrosis.* J Biomech. *2014;47(9):1997–2005.)*

Modulation of Cutaneous Biomechanics to Reduce Scarring

Pharmacologic Approaches

Excessive scarring often results from aberrant signaling in response to injury. Deregulation of signaling pathways at the intersection of mechanotransduction and inflammation leads to a disruption of homeostasis between collagen production and collagen degradation. Therapies targeting fibrosis consequently seek to modulate these pathways for a shift from fibrosis toward regenerative healing.[58–61]

TGF-β controls collagen synthesis, and consequently fibrosis, which suggests its suitability as a target in antifibrotic therapy. TGF-β exists in at least three isoforms. Although TGF-β1 and TGF-β2 have profibrotic effects, TGF-β3 acts as an antifibrotic.[62] Based on the diverse effects of the TGF-β family on tissue fibrosis, strategies for therapeutic application include neutralizing antibodies to TGF-β1 and TGF-β2 or, alternatively, means to raise TGF-β3 levels. Surprisingly, the promising preclinical results of TGF-β antibodies have not been able to be translated from bench to bedside. Clinical trials evaluating anti-TGF-β antibodies for systemic sclerosis[63] and scleroderma[64] concluded with disappointing results. Similarly, TGF-β3 had no clinically significant antifibrotic effect despite promising results in experimental studies and failed in an international Phase III clinical trial.[65]

In addition to the TGF-β family, alternative therapeutic targets for the treatment of fibrosis are under current investigation. Promising areas of research include the hedgehog pathway,[66] extracellular cross-linking enzymes (transglutaminases, lysyl oxidases, and prolyl hydroxylases),[67–69] the transcriptional regulator early growth response gene-1 required for differentiation and mitogenesis,[58] canonical Wnt,[59] heat shock protein 90,[61] histone deacetylase,[60] and IL-10.[70–75]

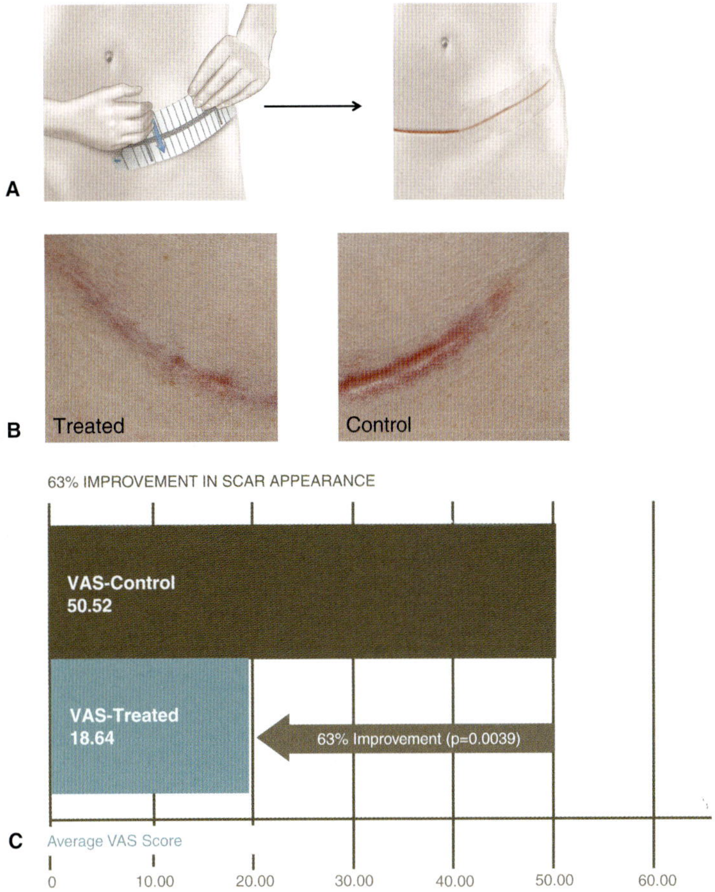

FIGURE 7-4 **Mechanomodulation therapy to reduce cutaneous scarring**. The embrace device is an elastomeric silicone dressing. The user applies the device using an applicator that prestrains the dressing. The dressing is applied directly over the center of the closed incision to mechanically offload the wound. Randomized controlled clinical trials have demonstrated that mechanomodulation of the wound environment using embrace significantly reduces scar development. *(Adapted with permission from Longaker MT, Rohrich RJ, Greenberg L, et al. A randomized controlled trial of the embrace advanced scar therapy device to reduce incisional scar formation.* Plast Reconstr Surg. *2014;134(3):536.)*

Despite remarkable results in preclinical models, translation of substances influencing mechanoresponsive profibrotic pathways has been lagging behind expectations and further innovation and refinement is needed before the clinical application of such therapies. The key to any mitigation of scar formation is the coordinated modulation of numerous cellular and molecular processes. Targeting a single element of a process as complex as scar formation is unlikely to yield clinically significant results and it is probable that only therapeutic approaches tackling multiple effectors in the aberrant physiology of problem wounds will be successful.

Mechanomodulatory Approaches

Evidence is accumulating that a mitigation of fibrosis in the setting of cutaneous injury can be achieved by modulating traction forces on wounds via mechanical offloading. In addition to the mode of injury[76] and genetic disposition,[77] environmental cues play a critical role in scar formation and development and studies suggest that mechanical tension is a driver of fibrosis.[4,78] Based on this theory it is not surprising that trials utilizing compression dressings,[79–83] chemoimmobilization via botolinum toxin,[84] or just paper tape for stable wound approximation[85] have revealed moderate efficacy in scar reduction.

Building upon these findings, approaches utilizing active mechanical offloading in contrast to passive approximation have recently been developed. Minimizing tension across healing wounds has proven effective in both preclinical and clinical studies, resulting in decreased scarring via influencing numerous mechanoresponsive signaling pathways.[4,86] Moving these insights from bench to bedside, a phase I clinical trial[86] as well as two multicenter randomized controlled trials[87,88] have demonstrated that stress-shielding of surgical incisions leads to a significant reduction of scar formation (Fig. 7-4). Lim et al.[87] showed that utilizing the principles of mechanomodulation significantly improves aesthetic outcomes following scar revision surgery. Similarly, Longaker et al.[88] observed a significant reduction of scarring following abdominoplasty surgery in a 12-month, prospective, open-label, randomized, multicenter clinical trial providing the first level I evidence for postoperative scar reduction. Collectively, these findings suggest that the complexity of the pathways involved in fibrosis and the limitations of our current understanding necessitate mechanomodulatory rather than pharmacologic approaches to mitigate fibrosis, at least in the cutaneous setting.

Conclusion and Future Perspectives

A profound understanding of the biomechanical principles influencing scarring and fibrosis is imperative to help alleviate a substantial health-care burden worldwide. Elucidating how mechanoresponsive signaling pathways affect scar development will help formulate effective strategies to mitigate fibrotic processes. Consequently, advances at the intersection of biology and material science have already led to novel therapeutics for hypertrophic scarring in the clinical realm. However, a complete understanding of the mechanobiology of scar formation has yet to be achieved. Future advances hold the promise to ultimately transform tissue fibrosis into regenerative healing.

Financial Disclosures/Conflicts of Interest

GCG and MTL are listed on the following patent assigned to Stanford University: inhibition of focal adhesion kinase for control of scar tissue formation (No: 2013/0165,463). GCG and MTL have equity positions in Neodyne Biosciences, Inc., a start-up company developing a device to shield wounds from tension to minimize postoperative scarring. DD has no potential conflicts of interest, affiliations, or financial involvement with any organization or entity with a financial interest in or financial conflict with the subject matter or materials discussed herein.

Acknowledgments

Funding for mechanobiology research conducted in our laboratory has been provided by the Hagey Family Endowed Fund in Stem Cell Research and Regenerative Medicine, the Armed Forces Institute of Regenerative Medicine (U.S. Department of Defense), and The Oak Foundation.

List of Abbreviations

ECM	Extracellular matrix
TGF-β	Transforming growth factor beta
SDF-1	Stromal cell–derived factor 1
GPCR	G protein–coupled receptors
Ca^{2+}	Calcium ions
NO	Nitric oxide
MAPK	Mitogen-activated kinases
PI3K	Phosphoinositide 3-kinase
CXCL	CXC chemokine ligand
CXCR	CXC chemokine receptor
FAK	Focal adhesion kinase
Erk	Extracellular-related kinase
MCP-1	Monocyte chemoattractant protein-1
JNK	c-Jun N-terminal kinase
YAP	Yes-associated protein
TAZ	Transcriptional coactivator with PDZ-binding motif
CTGF	Connective tissue growth factor
IL-10	Interleukin 10

REFERENCES

1. Gurtner GC, Werner S, Barrandon Y, et al. Wound repair and regeneration. *Nature*. 2008;453(7193):314–321.
2. Ting SB, Caddy J, Hislop N, et al. A homolog of Drosophila grainy head is essential for epidermal integrity in mice. *Science*. 2005;308(5720):411–413.
3. Langer K. Zur Anatomie und Physiologie der Haut. *Über die Spaltbarkeit der Cutis S. B. Acad Wiss Wein*. 1861;44.
4. Wong VW, Rustad KC, Akaishi S, et al. Focal adhesion kinase links mechanical force to skin fibrosis via inflammatory signaling. *Nat Med*. 2012;18(1):148–152.
5. Agha R, Ogawa R, Pietramaggiori G, et al. A review of the role of mechanical forces in cutaneous wound healing. *J Surg Res*. 2011;171(2):700–708.
6. Carver W, Goldsmith EC. Regulation of tissue fibrosis by the biomechanical environment. *Biomed Res Int*. 2013;2013:101979.
7. Alenghat FJ, Ingber DE. Mechanotransduction: all signals point to cytoskeleton, matrix, and integrins. *Sci STKE*. 2002;2002(119):pe6.
8. WangN, Tytell JD, Ingber DE. Mechanotransduction at a distance: mechanically coupling the extracellular matrix with the nucleus. *Nat Rev Mol Cell Biol*. 2009;10(1):75–82.
9. Ingber DE. The architecture of life. *Sci Am*. 1998;278(1):48–57.
10. Fuller B. Tensegrity. *Portfolio and Art News Annual*. 1961;4:112–127, 144, 148.
11. Huxley-Jones J, Pinney JW, Archer J, et al. Back to basics—how the evolution of the extracellular matrix underpinned vertebrate evolution. *Int J Exp Pathol*. 2009;90(2):95–100.
12. Oschman JL. Charge transfer in the living matrix. *J Bodyw Mov Ther*. 2009;13(3):215–228.
13. Gieni RS, Hendzel MJ. Mechanotransduction from the ECM to the genome: are the pieces now in place? *J Cell Biochem*. 2008;104(6):1964–1987.
14. Huang, S, Ingber DE. Cell tension, matrix mechanics, and cancer development. *Cancer Cell*. 2005;8(3):175–176.
15. Ingber DE. Tensegrity-based mechanosensing from macro to micro. *Prog Biophys Mol Biol*. 2008;97(2/3):163–179.
16. Kenny PA, Bissell MJ. Tumor reversion: correction of malignant behavior by microenvironmental cues. *Int J Cancer*. 2003;107(5):688–695.
17. Solon J, Levental I, Sengupta K, et al. Fibroblast adaptation and stiffness matching to soft elastic substrates. *Biophys J*. 2007;93(12):4453–4461.
18. Brown AC, Fiore VF, Sulchek TA, et al. Physical and chemical microenvironmental cues orthogonally control the degree and duration of fibrosis-associated epithelial-to-mesenchymal transitions. *J Pathol*. 2013;229(1):25–35.
19. Huang X, Yang N, Fiore VF, et al. Matrix stiffness-induced myofibroblast differentiation is mediated by intrinsic mechanotransduction. *Am J Respir Cell Mol Biol*. 2012;47(3):340–348.
20. Hinz B. Tissue stiffness, latent TGF-beta1 activation, and mechanical signal transduction: implications for the pathogenesis and treatment of fibrosis. *Curr Rheumatol Rep*. 2009;11(2):120–126.
21. Hadjipanayi E, Mudera V, Brown RA. Close dependence of fibroblast proliferation on collagen scaffold matrix stiffness. *J Tissue Eng Regen Med*. 2009;3(2):77–84.
22. Baneyx G, Baugh L, Vogel V. Fibronectin extension and unfolding within cell matrix fibrils controlled by cytoskeletal tension. *Proc Natl Acad Sci USA*. 2002;99(8):5139–5143.
23. Hynes RO. The extracellular matrix: not just pretty fibrils. *Science*. 2009;326(5957):1216–1219.
24. Jaalouk DE, Lammerding J. Mechanotransduction gone awry. *Nat Rev Mol Cell Biol*. 2009;10(1):63–73.
25. Wong VW, Longaker MT, Gurtner GC. Soft tissue mechanotransduction in wound healing and fibrosis. *Semin Cell Dev Biol*. 2012;23(9):981–986.
26. Goto M, Ikeyama K, Tsutsumi M, et al. Calcium ion propagation in cultured keratinocytes and other cells in skin in response to hydraulic pressure stimulation. *J Cell Physiol*. 2010;224(1):229–233.
27. Martinac B. The ion channels to cytoskeleton connection as potential mechanism of mechanosensitivity. *Biochim Biophys Acta*. 2014;1838(2):682–691.
28. Huang C, Akaishi S, Ogawa R. Mechanosignaling pathways in cutaneous scarring. *Arch Dermatol Res*. 2012;304(8):589–597.
29. Rees PA, Greaves NS, Baguneid M, et al. Chemokines in wound healing and as potential therapeutic targets for reducing cutaneous scarring. *Adv Wound Care*. 2015;4(11):687–703.
30. Margadant C, Sonnenberg A. Integrin-TGF-beta crosstalk in fibrosis, cancer and wound healing. *EMBO Rep*. 2010;11(2):97–105.
31. Buscemi L, Ramonet D, Klingberg F, et al. The single-molecule mechanics of the latent TGF-beta1 complex. *Curr Biol*. 2011;21(24):2046–2054.

32. Shi M, Zhu J, Wang R, et al. Latent TGF-beta structure and activation. *Nature*. 2011;474(7351):343–349.
33. Leask A, Abraham DJ. TGF-beta signaling and the fibrotic response. *FASEB J*. 2004;18(7):816–827.
34. LeBleu VS, Taduri G, O'Connell J, et al. Origin and function of myofibroblasts in kidney fibrosis. *Nat Med*. 2013;19(8):1047–1053.
35. Zhou SB, Wang J, Chiang CA, et al. Mechanical stretch upregulates SDF-1alpha in skin tissue and induces migration of circulating bone marrow-derived stem cells into the expanded skin. *Stem Cells*. 2013;31(12):2703–2713.
36. Ding J, Hori K, Zhang R, et al. Stromal cell-derived factor 1 (SDF-1) and its receptor CXCR4 in the formation of postburn hypertrophic scar (HTS). *Wound Repair Regen*. 2011;19(5):568–578.
37. Henderson PW, Singh SP, Krijgh DD, et al. Stromal-derived factor-1 delivered via hydrogel drug-delivery vehicle accelerates wound healing in vivo. *Wound Repair Regen*. 2011;19(3):420–425.
38. Rabbany SY, Pastore J, Yamamoto M, et al. Continuous delivery of stromal cell-derived factor-1 from alginate scaffolds accelerates wound healing. *Cell Transplant*. 2010;19(4):399–408.
39. Maan ZN, Januszyk M, Rennert RC, et al. Noncontact, low-frequency ultrasound therapy enhances neovascularization and wound healing in diabetic mice. *Plast Reconstr Surg*. 2014;134(3):402e–411e.
40. Schwarz US, Gardel ML. United we stand: integrating the actin cytoskeleton and cell-matrix adhesions in cellular mechanotransduction. *J Cell Sci*. 2012;125(Pt 13):3051–3060.
41. Wehrle-Haller B. Structure and function of focal adhesions. *Curr Opin Cell Biol*. 2012;24(1):116–124.
42. Zaidel-Bar R, Itzkovitz S, Ma'ayan A, et al. Functional atlas of the integrin adhesome. *Nat Cell Biol*. 2007;9(8):858–867.
43. Wong VW, Garg RK, Sorkin M, et al. Loss of keratinocyte focal adhesion kinase stimulates dermal proteolysis through upregulation of MMP9 in wound healing. *Ann Surg*. 2014;260(6):1138–1146.
44. Wong VW, Akaishi S, Longaker MT, et al. Pushing back: wound mechanotransduction in repair and regeneration. *J Invest Dermatol*. 2011;131(11):2186–2196.
45. Januszyk M, Wong VW, Bhatt KA, et al. Mechanical offloading of incisional wounds is associated with transcriptional downregulation of inflammatory pathways in a large animal model. *Organogenesis*. 2014;10(2):186–193.
46. Kook SH, Jang YS, Lee JC. Involvement of JNK-AP-1 and ERK-NF-kappaB signaling in tension-stimulated expression of type I collagen and MMP-1 in human periodontal ligament fibroblasts. *J Appl Physiol (1985)*. 2011;111(6):1575–1583.
47. Hofmann M, Zaper J, Bernd A, et al. Mechanical pressure-induced phosphorylation of p38 mitogen-activated protein kinase in epithelial cells via Src and protein kinase C. *Biochem Biophys Res Commun*. 2004;316(3):673–679.
48. Chiquet M, Tunc-Civelek V, Sarasa-Renedo A. Gene regulation by mechanotransduction in fibroblasts. *Appl Physiol Nutr Metab*. 2007;32(5):967–973.
49. Haudek SB, Gupta D, Dewald O, et al. Rho kinase-1 mediates cardiac fibrosis by regulating fibroblast precursor cell differentiation. *Cardiovasc Res*. 2009;83(3):511–518.
50. Tremblay AM, Camargo FD. Hippo signaling in mammalian stem cells. *Semin Cell Dev Biol*. 2012;23(7):818–826.
51. Zhao B, Tumaneng K, Guan KL. The Hippo pathway in organ size control, tissue regeneration and stem cell self-renewal. *Nat Cell Biol*. 2011;13(8):877–883.
52. Hiemer SE, Varelas X. Stem cell regulation by the Hippo pathway. *Biochim Biophys Acta*. 2013;1830(2):2323–2334.
53. Halder G, Dupont S, Piccolo S. Transduction of mechanical and cytoskeletal cues by YAP and TAZ. *Nat Rev Mol Cell Biol*. 2012;13(9):591–600.
54. Dupont S, Morsut L, Aragona M, et al. Role of YAP/TAZ in mechanotransduction. *Nature*. 2011;474(7350):179–183.
55. Lee MJ, Byun MR, Furutani-Seiki M, et al. YAP and TAZ regulate skin wound healing. *J Invest Dermatol*. 2013;134(2):518–525.
56. Varelas X, Samavarchi-Tehrani P, Narimatsu M, et al. The Crumbs complex couples cell density sensing to Hippo-dependent control of the TGF-beta-SMAD pathway. *Dev Cell*. 2010;19(6):831–844.
57. Yu FX, Zhao B, Panupinthu N, et al. Regulation of the Hippo-YAP pathway by G-protein-coupled receptor signaling. *Cell*. 2012;150(4):780–791.
58. Yamaguchi Y, Takihara T, Chambers RA, et al. A peptide derived from endostatin ameliorates organ fibrosis. *Sci Transl Med*. 2012;4(136):136ra71.
59. Beyer C, Reichert H, Akan H, et al. Blockade of canonical Wnt signalling ameliorates experimental dermal fibrosis. *Ann Rheum Dis*. 2013;72(7):1255–1258.
60. Diao JS, Xia WS, Yi CG, et al. Histone deacetylase inhibitor reduces hypertrophic scarring in a rabbit ear model. *Plast Reconstr Surg*. 2013;132(1):61e–69e.
61. Tomcik M, Zerr P, Pitkowski J, et al. Heat shock protein 90 (Hsp90) inhibition targets canonical TGF-beta signalling to prevent fibrosis. *Ann Rheum Dis*. 2013;73(6):1215–11215–1222.
62. Murata H, Zhou L, Ochoa S, et al. TGF-beta3 stimulates and regulates collagen synthesis through TGF-beta1-dependent and independent mechanisms. *J Invest Dermatol*. 1997;108(3):258–262.
63. Denton CP, Merkel PA, Furst DE, et al. Recombinant human anti-transforming growth factor beta1 antibody therapy in systemic sclerosis: a multicenter, randomized, placebo-controlled phase I/II trial of CAT-192. *Arthritis Rheum*. 2007;56(1):323–333.
64. Prey S, Ezzedine K, Doussau A, et al. Imatinib mesylate in scleroderma-associated diffuse skin fibrosis: a phase II multicentre randomized double-blinded controlled trial. *Br J Dermatol*. 2012;167(5):1138–1144.
65. Renovo, Juvista EU Phase 3 trial results. 2011. https://web.archive.org/web/20110903093511/http://www.renovo.com/en/news/juvista-eu-phase-3-trial-results. accessed 19.11.2016
66. Horn A, Kireva T, Palumbo-Zerr K, et al. Inhibition of hedgehog signalling prevents experimental fibrosis and induces regression of established fibrosis. *Ann Rheum Dis*. 2012;71(5):785–789.
67. Kolb MR Jr, Gauldie J. Idiopathic pulmonary fibrosis: the matrix is the message. *Am J Respir Crit Care Med*. 2011;184(6):627–629.
68. Barry-Hamilton V, Spangler R, Marshall D, et al. Allosteric inhibition of lysyl oxidase-like-2 impedes the development of a pathologic microenvironment. *Nat Med*. 2010;16(9):1009–1017.
69. Olsen KC, Sapinoro RE, Kottmann RM, et al. Transglutaminase 2 and its role in pulmonary fibrosis. *Am J Respir Crit Care Med*. 2011;184(6):699–707.
70. Shi JH, Guan H, Shi S, et al. Protection against TGF-beta1-induced fibrosis effects of IL-10 on dermal fibroblasts and its potential therapeutics for the reduction of skin scarring. *Arch Dermatol Res*. 2013;305(4):341–352.
71. Occleston NL, O'Kane S, Goldspink N, et al. New therapeutics for the prevention and reduction of scarring. *Drug Discov Today*. 2008;13(21/22):973–981.
72. Nakagome K, Dohi M, Okunishi K, et al. In vivo IL-10 gene delivery attenuates bleomycin induced pulmonary fibrosis by inhibiting the production and activation of TGF-beta in the lung. *Thorax*. 2006;61(10):886–894.
73. Yamamoto T, Eckes B, Krieg T. Effect of interleukin-10 on the gene expression of type I collagen, fibronectin, and decorin in human skin fibroblasts: differential regulation by transforming growth factor-beta and monocyte chemoattractant protein-1. *Biochem Biophys Res Commun*. 2001;281(1):200–205.
74. Reitamo S, Remitz A, Tamai K, et al. Interleukin-10 modulates type I collagen and matrix metalloprotease gene expression in cultured human skin fibroblasts. *J Clin Invest*. 1994;94(6):2489–2492.
75. Yuan W, Varga J. Transforming growth factor-beta repression of matrix metalloproteinase-1 in dermal fibroblasts involves Smad3. *J Biol Chem*. 2001;276(42):38502–38510.
76. Ruidiaz ME, Messmer D, Atmodjo DY, et al. Comparative healing of human cutaneous surgical incisions created by the PEAK PlasmaBlade, conventional electrosurgery, and a standard scalpel. *Plast Reconstr Surg*. 2011;128(1):104–111.
77. Sood RF, Hocking AM, Muffley LA, et al. Genome-wide association study of postburn scarring identifies a novel protective variant. *Ann Surg*. 2015;262(4):563–569.
78. Rustad KC, Wong VW, Gurtner GC. The role of focal adhesion complexes in fibroblast mechanotransduction during scar formation. *Differentiation*. 2013;86(3):87–91.
79. Engrav LH, Heimbach DM, Rivara FP, et al. 12-Year within-wound study of the effectiveness of custom pressure garment therapy. *Burns*. 2010;36(7):975–983.
80. Li-Tsang CW, Zheng YP, Lau JC. A randomized clinical trial to study the effect of silicone gel dressing and pressure therapy on post-traumatic hypertrophic scars. *J Burn Care Res*. 2010;31(3):448–457.
81. Steinstraesser L, Flak E, Witte B, et al., Pressure garment therapy alone and in combination with silicone for the prevention of hypertrophic scarring: randomized controlled trial with intraindividual comparison. *Plast Reconstr Surg*. 2011;128(4):306e–313e.
82. Ward RS. Pressure therapy for the control of hypertrophic scar formation after burn injury. A history and review. *J Burn Care Rehabil*. 1991;12(3):257–262.

83. Akaishi S, Akimoto M, Hyakusoku H, et al. The tensile reduction effects of silicone gel sheeting. *Plast Reconstr Surg*. 2010;126(2):109e–111e.
84. Kim YS, Lee HJ, Cho SH, et al. Early postoperative treatment of thyroidectomy scars using botulinum toxin: a split-scar, double-blind randomized controlled trial. *Wound Repair Regen*. 2014;22(5):605–612.
85. Atkinson JA, McKenna KT, Barnett AG, et al. A randomized, controlled trial to determine the efficacy of paper tape in preventing hypertrophic scar formation in surgical incisions that traverse Langer's skin tension lines. *Plast Reconstr Surg*. 2005;116(6):1648–1656; discussion 1657–1658.
86. Gurtner GC, Dauskardt RH, Wong VW, et al., Improving cutaneous scar formation by controlling the mechanical environment: large animal and phase I studies. *Ann Surg*. 2011;254(2):217–225.
87. Lim AF, Weintraub J, Kaplan EN, et al. The embrace device significantly decreases scarring following scar revision surgery in a randomized controlled trial. *Plast Reconstr Surg*. 2014;133(2):398–405.
88. Longaker MT, Rohrich RJ, Greenberg L, et al. A randomized controlled trial of the embrace advanced scar therapy device to reduce incisional scar formation. *Plast Reconstr Surg*. 2014;134(3):536.

SECTION III

Mitigation

8 An Approach to Scar Mitigation

FIONA WOOD

KEY POINTS

- The ultimate goal is skin regeneration, not repair that results in scar formation.
- Scar minimization begins at the time of the injury.
- Multiple interventions can impact the ultimate scar outcome.

Fibrosis is the repair mechanism in all human tissues when the capacity to heal by regeneration is overwhelmed.[1] The control of the process of fibrosis—the interplay between the cells and the extracellular matrix (ECM)—is key to retaining normal function of the organ.[2] In scar minimization the aim is to control the process to facilitate wound healing while avoiding excessive or abnormal ECM with the associated functional impact.[3]

The skin is a dynamic organ, responsive to the environment and replenishing its surface continuously. However, when injured it has a limited capacity for regeneration, and the resulting scarring leads to functional and aesthetic sequelae.[4] Cutaneous scarring may be classified related to its severity as normotrophic,[5,6] hypertrophic,[7,8] or keloid scarring.[9] The severity of the scar worn for life is influenced by a range of factors related to the following:

- Specific individual predispositions[10]
- The severity and type of injury[11]
- The interventions[12]
- Complications during the healing process[13]

The focus of this chapter is on the minimization of scarring postburn injury. The complexity of the process provides multiple therapeutic opportunities to limit scarring along the clinical journey. The scar continues to turnover throughout life as clearly seen in children as they grow, also providing an opportunity for intervention.[14]

It is well described that burn injury is associated with an aggressive scarring response related to the stimulation of a severe systemic inflammatory response (see Chapter 6).[15] However, there are many factors related to the pathophysiology and natural history of burn injury and recovery, which are common to all cutaneous injury repair responses (see Chapter 9).[16] The injury and individual's predisposition to scarring may not be amenable to direct influence at this time, but the knowledge of predisposition to poor outcome can guide timing and the type of intervention. The therapeutic opportunities to influence the scar outcome currently rely upon the understanding of the underlying mechanisms along the continuum of the total healing response.[17] Further, the goal can be extended by the knowledge of regenerative repair to achieve the ultimate aim of tissue restoration with scarless healing (see Chapter 27).[1,18]

The fundamental premise for this chapter is: **Every intervention from the point of injury will influence the scar worn for life**. It is with this in mind that the potential for incremental gains at every stage of the healing process will be considered. Key to minimizing scarring is a knowledge of the science of the healing response from hemostasis, inflammation, vascularization, and deposition of the ECM, through to the final remodeling of the scarred area.[19]

Understanding the mechanism of injury is the initial step in the scar risk assessment; a clean surgical procedure will clearly carry less risk of pathologic scarring than a contaminated blast wound or a burn injury. Factors affecting the speed of healing will have a profound impact on scar outcome; these may be classified as systemic or local. For example, a diabetic patient with a secondary infection will heal relatively more slowly with an increased risk of scarring.[13]

Attention to detail is essential at every stage of care in all circumstances, whether the intervention involves a clean excision and suture of a cutaneous lesion or excision and repair of a burn wound. The focus of clinical care is aimed at bringing together "the triangle of care," which is (1) the assessment of the patient's condition, (2) the experience and knowledge of the clinician, and (3) the environment of operation.[20]

The chapter will explore the opportunities related to scar minimization by reduction in the time to healing, with specific reference to burn wound injury and scarring. The basic understanding of essential topics will be introduced to link the concept of meticulous attention to detail in clinical care along the entire journey with the current scientific knowledge.

Skin Structure and Function

Scar minimization involves treatment of skin injury with the aim of maintaining function. Although a comprehensive review is beyond the scope of this chapter,[21] it is appropriate to spend a few moments considering the functionality of skin and the impact of the injury and repair process on the range of functions.

Skin consists of two main regions: (1) the outer epithelial tissue, the epidermis, which is a stratified squamous epithelium; (2) the dermis, which is the deeper thicker connective tissue layer. The tissue construct has cells derived from all three embryologic layers with specialized cell types and morphologic differences related to anatomical location.[22] The scar response to injury varies in relation to the body site of injury, with modulated responses linked to the cell phenotype.[23]

The skin's primary function is to act as a highly innervated and responsive protective barrier to the environment, restricting fluid losses and invasion of microorganisms. The secondary functions include vitamin D synthesis, thermoregulation, innate immune responses, as well as providing a range of homeostatic and sensory functions.[21]

As a complex multifunctional organ that is in a continuous state of regeneration, the epidermal layer is replaced every 6 to 8 weeks. The process of regeneration is stimulated in response to insult or injury, retaining a capacity of self-repair from the cells of the dermal–epidermal junction (DEJ) and skin adnexal structures.[24] The epidermis is responsive to both the external environment and to the systemic pathophysiology; optimal function is associated with retention of the epidermal integrity.

Epidermal damage is a frequent occurrence, and in the vast majority of instances the cells of the DEJ and those surrounding the skin adnexal structures are able to respond: proliferating, migrating, and differentiating to achieve a regenerative repair.[25] When the tissue damage is such that the capacity to regenerate is overwhelmed, the process of healing becomes associated with scarring. The time to achieve epidermal cover is directly related to the extent of injury.[26] The keratinocyte phenotype modified by the healing process has an influence on the underlying fibroblasts involved in scar formation.[27]

Although epidermal repair restores the essential barrier, the dermis provides the structural integrity and supports the skin adnexal structures and their functions, including the stem cell niche vital in regeneration and repair.

The balance of the turnover in the ECM is pivotal in the process of fibrosis and, hence, scar formation. An understanding of the processes of deposition and degradation of the matrix affords potential therapeutic opportunities.[19] However, the capacity of the dermal element of the skin to regenerate is severely limited and scar does not retain the architectural framework required for the maintenance of the adnexal structure environments, with the resulting loss of the specific functions (see Chapter 5).[28] Work to replace the dermis with a scaffold for cell migration and skin restoration has had some clinical success. Integra (Integra LifeSciences, Plainsboro, NJ) dermal template has been in clinical use for some decades and is a construct of bovine collagen and glycosaminoglycans with an average pore size of 80 μm.[29] When introduced into a full thickness skin defect, the cells migrate into the scaffold to establish a vascular network; the fibroblasts express a reticular dermal phenotype through a process of tissue-guided regeneration limited to the dermal ECM (Fig. 8-1). There is an impairment of neural ingrowth

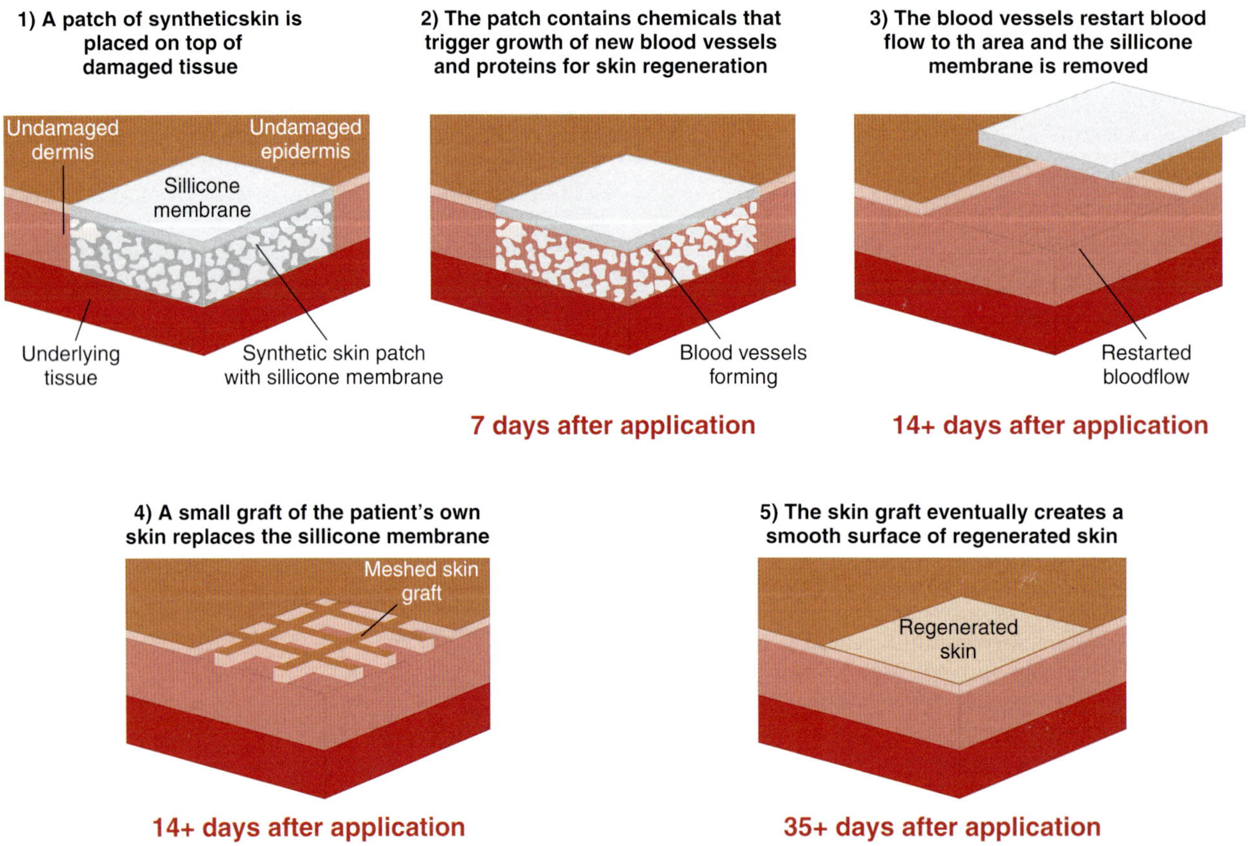

FIGURE 8-1 Integra dermal template introduced into a full thickness skin defect to facilitate dermal repair with a second-stage procedure to repair the epidermis. *(Courtesy of Integra Life Sciences.)*

into the construct and, at this stage of the technology, no restoration of hair follicles, sweat glands, or sebaceous units.[30]

Despite the restoration of the primary barrier functions, the scar will not function as normal skin, with significant differences seen in the architectural framework, chemistry of the ECM, and the cell phenotype. Clear differences are seen with the loss of skin and adnexal structures, and when investigating the impact on the peripheral nerve fields within the scar repair.[30] In some cases the extent of the skin loss is so great that it is life threatening (as in acute burn injury) with fluid loss and vulnerability to infection.[31]

In all cases the restoration of a full thickness skin construct specific for the functionality of the given body site is the ideal goal.[24] An understanding of the functions lost in the repair process directs us down a path of tissue salvage and guides the tissue engineering efforts to manufacture more than a two-layered structure of dermis and epidermis. It is clear that exploration of regenerative therapies for the restoration of the skin is the ultimate aim for full functional recovery.[25,32]

Basic Wound Healing

A breach in skin integrity results in the initiation of a complex series of overlapping processes driven locally and systemically.[33] The systemic optimization is a fundamental aspect of facilitating wound healing and is considered in the holistic approach to the assessment and treatment of the patient. The factors of influence are wide ranging, inclusive of pain, stress, nutrition, comorbidities, and cultural practices. Taking the time to consider all the factors and engagement in correction where possible will help in improving the clinical outcome.

The wound healing process is described as consisting of three phases—inflammation, tissue formation, and tissue remodeling (Fig. 8-2). An understanding of the underlying mechanisms provides therapeutic opportunities as highlighted in a review of the current literature.[34]

There are opportunities to improve clinical outcome by understanding the basic science behind our clinical observations. Initial hemostasis observed as clotting postinjury is associated with platelet degranulation and cytokine release that drives the inflammatory response. Endothelial cell changes allow cells and fluid to migrate from the circulation into the extracellular space.[35] The resulting edema is an essential aspect of the healing response, but can cause ongoing cellular and tissue damage if not controlled. The fluid shifts that increase proportionally with the percent of total body surface area (%TBSA) involved in burn injury may lead to significant pathology, possibly leading to compartment syndrome requiring targeted therapy.[36]

As the process of tissue formation progresses, manipulation of the cellular pathway can influence the balance of necrosis and apoptosis, with the potential for tissue salvage and limiting the ongoing inflammatory drive.[37] Tissue formation relies on the interaction of the cells and ECM, with the migration of fibroblasts to restore the dermal elements and keratinocytes to restore the epidermis. The processes are dynamic and a thorough knowledge of the applicable mechanisms provides opportunities for intervention over time, targeting the specific processes with an understanding of the triggers to phenotypic expression.[38] Investigation of the epigenetic processes in wound healing and scarring is important in understanding the potential for them to be returned to a regenerative state.[39] The methylation patterns seen in skin pathologies may also give insight into novel therapies.

Transforming growth factor (TGF)-β, a protein extensively investigated as a controller of cellular proliferation and differentiation in wound healing, is an example of how mechanistic understanding can drive therapeutic development.[40] It is a significant regulator of collagen deposition in the scarring process. Key to the feedback pathways for collagen buildup is the extracellular cross-linking forming the ECM framework, a process that maintains the aberrant collagen structure. The enzyme required for the cross-linking of collagen within the matrix is lysyl oxidase; its inhibition may provide an opportunity to manipulate the scar at the remodeling stage.[41]

The understanding of the basic science is an area of intense activity. From these brief examples it is clear that there is real potential for integrating the knowledge into clinical care and scar minimization.

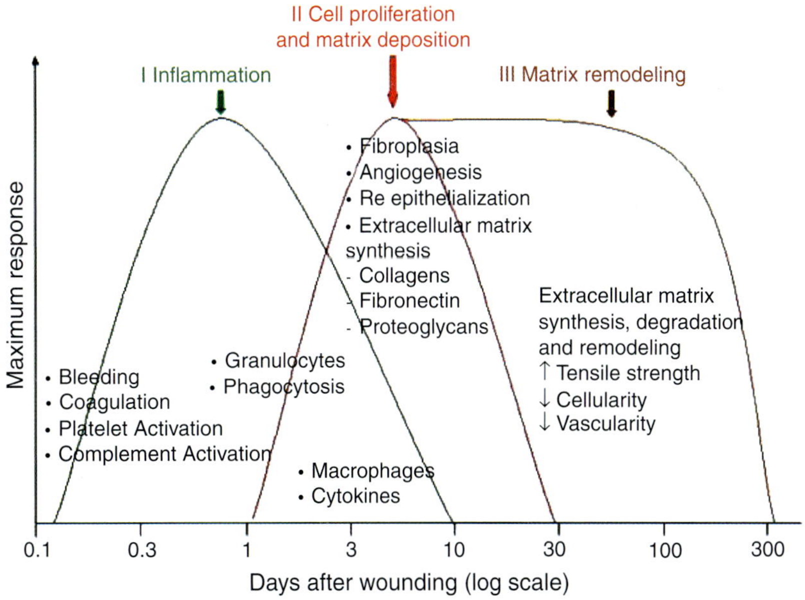

FIGURE 8-2 The phases of wound healing from injury to repair. *(Courtesy of www.worldwidewounds.com.)*

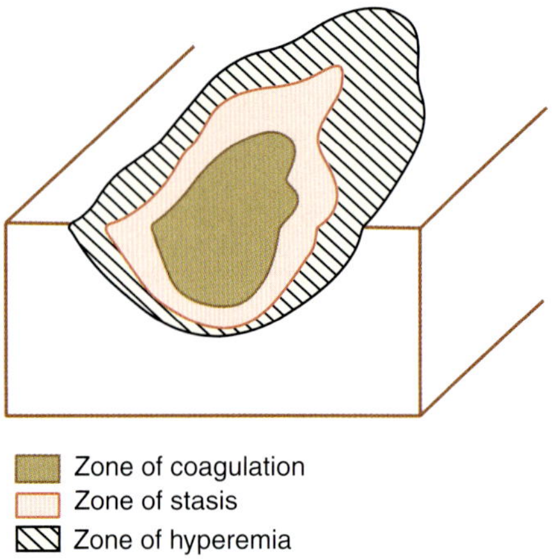

FIGURE 8-3 Jackson's burn wound model.

Burn Wound Pathophysiology

A basic understanding of burn injury responses is essential in linking the extent of the injury, the wound healing process, and the potential to improve clinical outcome by scar reduction.

In burn injury the tissue damage is well described by Jackson's burn wound model[42] (Fig. 8-3). The energy of the injury in contact with the skin results in an area of tissue destruction with associated cell death. The **zone of necrosis** is nonsalvageable and will be a significant driver of the overall scar outcome. In the future, mechanisms of repair might be found that could be applied to chemically repair denatured proteins.[43] Damage to ECM architecture and chemistry and cellular disruption are all triggers to inflammation.[37] The necrotic tissue interface is the driver of both the local and systemic inflammatory responses, which are essential for wound healing and also a driver of the pathologic scar when uncontrolled.[44]

The surrounding viable tissue rapidly becomes edematous as the loss of capillary integrity leads to the loss of fluid and small molecular weight proteins into the extracellular space along with cell migration. This **zone of stasis** is tissue that is potentially salvageable with appropriate intervention. Focusing therapy on salvage of this tissue will reduce the overall scarring.[45]

The surrounding **zone of hyperemia** is the primary vascular response to injury that facilitates the healing process. Much of the work to date has focused on the maintenance of the circulation to maintain vital organ function, specifically as the surface area of burn injury reaches 10 to 20 %TBSA and the associated fluid shifts compromise the circulation requiring fluid resuscitation.[46] The fluid resuscitation needs to be titrated to the patient's response in order to maintain the circulation, but also to limit the extent of the secondary edema and minimize the extension of the zone of stasis. As the zone of stasis extends, the relative hypoxia triggers apoptosis and necrosis, thereby extending the zone of necrosis. The resulting scar is directly related to the extent of the zone of necrosis. Therefore, limiting the zone of necrosis will have a direct effect on the scar outcome.[47]

The extent of the systemic responses postburn injury are such that as the %TBSA increases, the injury has a life-threatening impact systemically driven by the breach in barrier function of the skin. It is well known that the responses to burn injury are more severe than excisional injury, with a greater risk of severe pathologic scarring.[37] Reducing the time to healing is the key to scar minimization. The resulting fluid shifts and cellular responses, locally and systemically, are all opportunities to improve therapies by understanding the underlying mechanisms and targeted therapy.

Because the burned tissue drives the systemic responses, one solution would be burn wound excision. However, the excision of the wound must be undertaken in an appropriate environment based on a risk analysis of the patient, the assessment of the wound, and the environment of operation.

Assessment of the Individual's Risk of Scarring

There are well-documented factors that need consideration when assessing the individual's risk of scarring.[48] The age at the time of injury is known to influence not only survival, but the quality of survival and ultimate scar outcome. Therefore, this information needs acknowledgment in clinical decision making.[49] The elderly generally scar less but heal more slowly, and may have less tolerance of interventions such as surgery.[50] The young will scar more aggressively, and attention to reducing the time to healing requires special consideration.[51] The general condition of the patient in terms of nutrition, fitness, stress, in addition to smoking drugs and alcohol, has the potential to influence the healing trajectory and hence scarring (see Chapter 9). Further, there are a range of comorbidities such as diabetes, vascular disease, autoimmune disease, and medications such as steroids, all with the potential to influence healing and scarring. A clear understanding of the patient's condition is essential information in both clinical decision making and therapeutic interventions to improve the capacity to heal.[52]

Racial differences in scarring are well documented in the literature, with the genetic predisposition demonstrated to affect the level and quality of scar tissue formation in the wound.[53] With investigation of the genetic data, there appears to be a range of genes involved (e.g., African American differing from Han Chinese).[54] When investigating keloid disease, at the individual level the inheritance pattern is thought to be autosomal dominant with variable penetrance.[55]

Genetic screening studies have investigated some positive associations between polymorphisms in the major histocompatibility complex and scarring. The immunogenetic component to keloids and hypertrophic scars could potentially be explained as differing stages of the same disease, with different degrees of inflammation affected by genetic predisposition.[56] For example, investigation of known pathways has shown associations between a polymorphism in TGF-β associated with poor scar outcome after melanoma removal,[57] and between a polymorphism in the cell cycle regulator p27 and poor scar outcome after burn injury.[58]

Keloid formation is also described in some syndromes such as Rubinstein–Taybi syndrome,[59] Goeminne syndrome,[60] and Ehlers–Danlos syndrome,[61] with described genetic links. The investigation of the epigenetic pattern, which drives the cell phenotype, has shown differential regulation in a number of genes when comparing cells from scar and normal skin of the same individual. Further understanding of the underlying genetic links will provide the opportunity to better understand underlying mechanisms and investigate new therapeutic targets.

When planning intervention, a holistic assessment of the patient is essential to understanding scar risk and tailoring the interventions where possible. It is clear that further investigation of the differential scar risk at the genetic and epigenetic levels will provide opportunities for targeted care in the future.

Burn Wound Assessment

The capacity to heal by regeneration without scar is limited as the cells of the DEJ and the skin adnexal structures are damaged.[49] It is well known that the time to healing is a key driver of scar outcome.[26] The most significant factors driving the severity of the long-term scar postburn injury are the %TBSA of skin involved and the depth of the injury.[62] As the %TBSA increases, the systemic response and applicable interventions may also be associated with burn wound extension, increased tissue loss, and decreased capacity for healing.[63]

The use of clinical assessment and advancing technology along the clinical pathway is essential in guiding current interventions and measuring the impact of advancing therapies to reduce scarring. The %TBSA is based on a clinical assessment using the Lund and Browder chart and the rule of nines[64] (Fig. 8-4). The clinical assessment of the depth of injury based on appearance, blood supply, and sensation is complex and needs to be done with the understanding that the wound will change over time and repeated assessment is needed to guide treatment.[65] Laser Doppler imaging has been introduced to improve the accuracy of assessment by measuring the blood flow as an indicator of tissue viability; specifically, to guide the treatment in partial thickness wounds.[66] The application of other techniques based on color (e.g., spectroscopy) and in situ tissue imaging (e.g., optical coherence tomography)[67] provides opportunities to improve the understanding of the capacity of the injured skin to heal.

Therapeutic Interventions to Minimize Scarring from Injury to Full Rehabilitation

Having set the scene by briefly introducing an overview of patient factors and the process of healing, there is now some perspective of how to proceed in the manipulation of the healing trajectory to minimize the lifelong scar. The concept of bringing together the "triangle of care" (the assessment of the patient's condition, the experience and knowledge of the clinician, and the environment of operation) is essential at the time point of each intervention to optimize the outcome.

Lund and Browder Chart

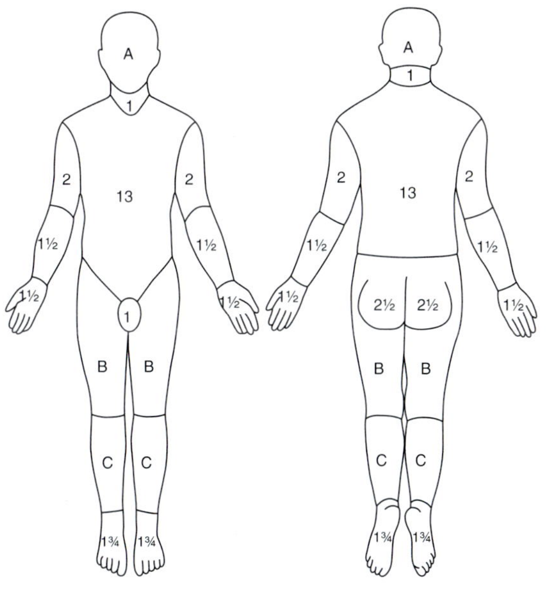

AREA /	AGE 0yr	1yr	5yrs	10yrs	15yrs	ADULT
A= ½ of HEAD	9½	8½	6½	5½	4½	3½
B= ½ of one THIGH	2¾	3¼	4	4½	4½	4¾
C = ½ of one LEG	2½	2½	2¾	3	3¼	3½

INSTRUCTIONS

1. Choose the figure most accurately resembling the child.
2. Shade the areas corresponding to the burn. DO NOT INCLUDE ERYTHEMA.
3. Use the charts to calculate the body surface area (BSA).
4. GUIDE: The patient's palm is equal to approx. 1% BSA.
5. See over the alternative charts.

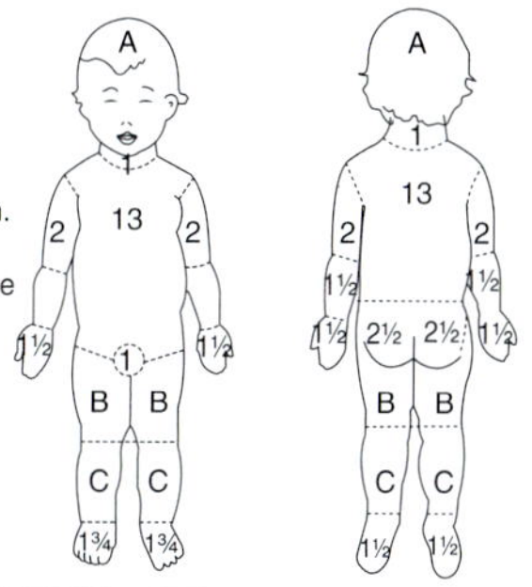

RELATIVE PERCENTAGE OF BODY SURFACE AREA AFFECTED BY GROWTH

AREA / AGE	0yr	1yr	5yrs	10yrs	15yrs	ADULT
A= ½ of head	9½	8½	6½	5½	4½	3½
B= ½ of one thigh	2¾	3¼	4	4½	4½	4¾
C = ½ of one leg	2½	2½	2¾	3	3¼	3½

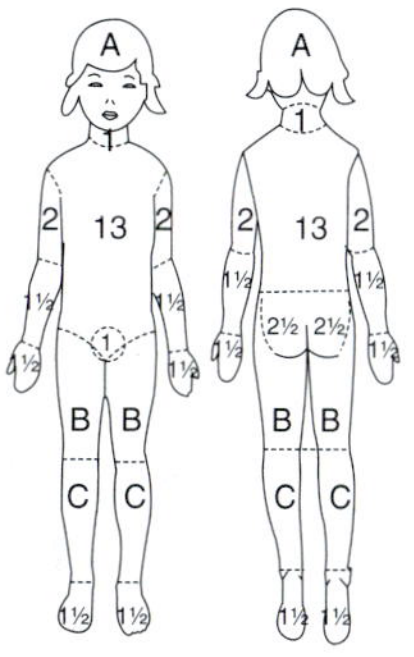

REGION	%
HEAD	
NECK	
ANT. TRUNK	
POST. TRUNK	
RIGHT ARM	
LEFT ARM	
BUTTOCKS	
GENITALIA	
RIGHT LEG	
LEFT LEG	
TOTAL BURN	

Name:..
Signature:..

FIGURE 8-4 The burn surface area assessment chart based on the Lund–Browder rule of nines. *(Courtesy of Burns Service of Western Australia.)*

First Aid Cooling and Cleaning

The first opportunity to limit scarring is at the time of injury, with good-quality first aid. Despite many alternatives the initial treatment of choice is clean, cool running water at 15°C to 18°C (59°F to 64°F) for 20 minutes. This is most effective in the first hour postinjury, but with some effect for at least 3 hours.[68]

The reduction of the destructive energy of the burn agent will of course reduce the injury. Community education programs include first steps such as to "stop, drop, and roll" to extinguish flames.[69] The impact of community education programs of cool water first aid has been analyzed to give insight into the potential reduction of injury. There is an associated reduction in a range of parameters that could be explained by limiting the secondary wound conversion.[70] The reported reduction in length of stay, infection rate, and incidence of surgical intervention indicates an effect on the rate of wound healing. Water irrigation may also have an effect on infection control by removing debris and reducing bacterial load.[71] There is evidence that the mechanism is more than simply reducing the energy in the wound; it also seems to have effects at the cellular level by changing pathways to limit cell death and escalation of the injury and inflammation.[72]

Edema Control

The response to injury involves essential changes in the endothelium of the small vessels, facilitating cytokine and cell migration into the area.[36] The resulting fluid shifts result in the expansion of the extracellular space as tissue edema. The volume of the edema can cause changes in tissue pressure, and may lead to tissue hypoxia and wound extension.[73] Persistent edema is associated with fibrosis within the tissue construct, further limiting functional recovery.[74]

In burn wound care edema control can be achieved by simple strategies such as elevation of the injured site.[75] Titration of the fluid resuscitation to the patient's urine output of 0.5 to 1 mL per kg body weight per hour has been shown to reduce the risk of compartment syndrome by restricting the extracellular fluid volume.[76] Maintaining mobilization will facilitate lymphatic drainage, which can be achieved by massage techniques.[77] Controlled compression therapy can also be used with the aim of tissue salvage and improved function.[78] Care must be taken in the acute stage with circumstances of increased tissue pressure requiring releasing escharotomy.[79] The use of negative pressure systems to control the local edema and salvage the underlying construct has been described both in the pre- and postsurgical phases with good effect.[80]

Wound salvage is core to the premise that every intervention from the time of injury influences the scar worn for life. The aim is to explore options to reduce tissue damage and salvage the tissue ECM construct. Manipulation of cell pathways has been explored in animal models and holds great promise, but is not yet in therapeutic use.[81]

Edema control can make an impact at every stage of the journey from injury to rehabilitation, with simple strategies being effective with low risk. With thoughtful care, the need for pharmacologic interventions for fluid management can be avoided to reduce the risk of such therapy on complex pathophysiology.[82]

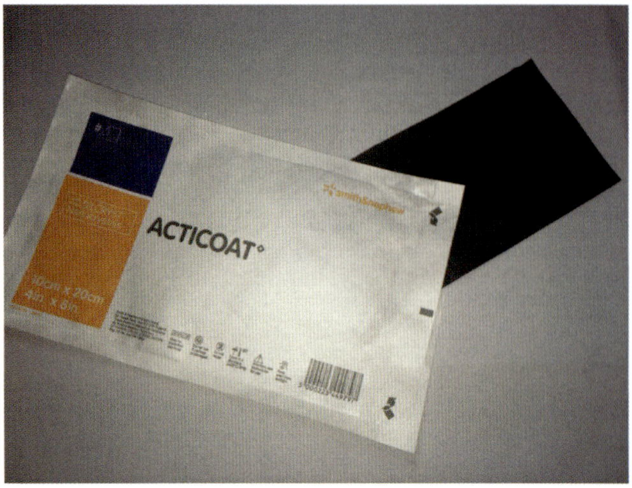

FIGURE 8-5 Acticoat nanocrystalline silver dressing. *(From Smith and Nephew.)*

Infection Control

Infection is well known to delay wound healing, and as such increases the scar risk. Meticulous attention to detail with a focus on infection control is essential.[83,84] In the initial phase cool water first aid can assist in cleaning, after which the wound can be treated to facilitate healing. Although in some environments an open wound care is advocated, in all but trivial wounds this requires a specific expertise. There has been much work on optimizing the wound healing environment with a range of dressings advocated to facilitate moist wound healing. In burn wounds the initial consideration is infection control, and for many decades silver in various forms has been the most commonly used topical antimicrobial agent. Nanocrystalline impregnated dressings have been shown to be effective and economical in our environment with reductions in infection rates and antibiotic use[85] (Fig. 8-5).

Infection control needs to be considered in the choice of primary covering for transfer to the burns center; consequently, the distance to travel is a key consideration. Once in the burn unit a specialized environment is advocated with air filtration and isolation capacity for major injuries.[86,87] The regular changing of dressings with appropriate barrier precautions is aimed at reducing the bacterial load and biofilm establishment.[88]

Microbial contamination of the wound surface has been shown to be associated with long-term wound infection at the time of secondary scar revision.[89] It is clear that a robust infection control bundle is a core element of the burn team strategy and must be integrated into clinical practice at every stage.[90]

Burn Wound Management

As noted above the time to healing is the main driver of scar outcome. The limited capacity to heal by regeneration and the sequelae of scarring have driven the exploration of techniques for expedient wound treatment to restore the cutaneous barrier. The patient and the wound are assessed clinically with respect to the capacity to heal within 10 to 14 days.[91] In instances where the wound is treated conservatively and reepithelializes within this time frame, the risk of scarring is low.[92] There is, therefore, a great deal of work ongoing to develop advanced dressing systems to facilitate rapid healing.

With the understanding that rapid epithelial repair is associated with an improved outcome, cellular responses have been well investigated. Topical applications of a wide range of molecules are in the development phase (e.g., manipulating heat shock proteins[93] and the application of erythropoietin gel,[94] focused on manipulating the rate of proliferation to improve the speed of healing). This is an expanding field, and a number of growth factors have been shown to increase the speed of healing in partial thickness wounds with associated scar reduction.[95] Enhancing the capacity to manipulate the wound may alter the threshold for surgical interventions in the future, and is driven by good outcome and good health economics. The manipulation of the inflammatory response may have a place using agents such as hemopexin, a glycoprotein scavenger of heme with a potential to reduce a specific driver of inflammation, and may also be useful in tissue salvage in more severe injuries, but requires careful analysis.[96]

If the extent of the injury is such that a prolonged healing time is predicted, despite efforts of tissue salvage, then surgical intervention is associated with the best outcome.[12]

Surgical intervention involves the removal of the damaged tissue in a safe environment to limit the blood loss and mitigate against hypothermia.[97] The technique of debridement relates to the extent and depth of tissue damage. A range of options are available including enzymatic techniques,[98] hydrosurgical debridement (VERSAJET™, Smith & Nephew, Fort Worth, TX), dermabrasion, diathermy, and sharp debridement (Fig. 8-6). The aim is to remove the necrotic tissue while leaving a viable clean wound bed for repair. The salvage of viable tissue is key in reducing the reconstructive needs and, hence, the scar.[99]

Technically full thickness restoration may not be possible if the area of cover exceeds available donor tissue. The use of split thickness skin grafting (STSG) techniques is effective in many instances but requires an adequate donor site and recipient wound bed. It should also be noted that despite widespread use of STSG, the result is always a scar.[100] The area the STSG can cover can be increased using meshing techniques, or even further using micrografting procedures.[101] The concept of laboratory-based tissue expansion and tissue-engineered solutions has been explored initially introduced as cultured epithelial autograft (CEA), or cell suspensions

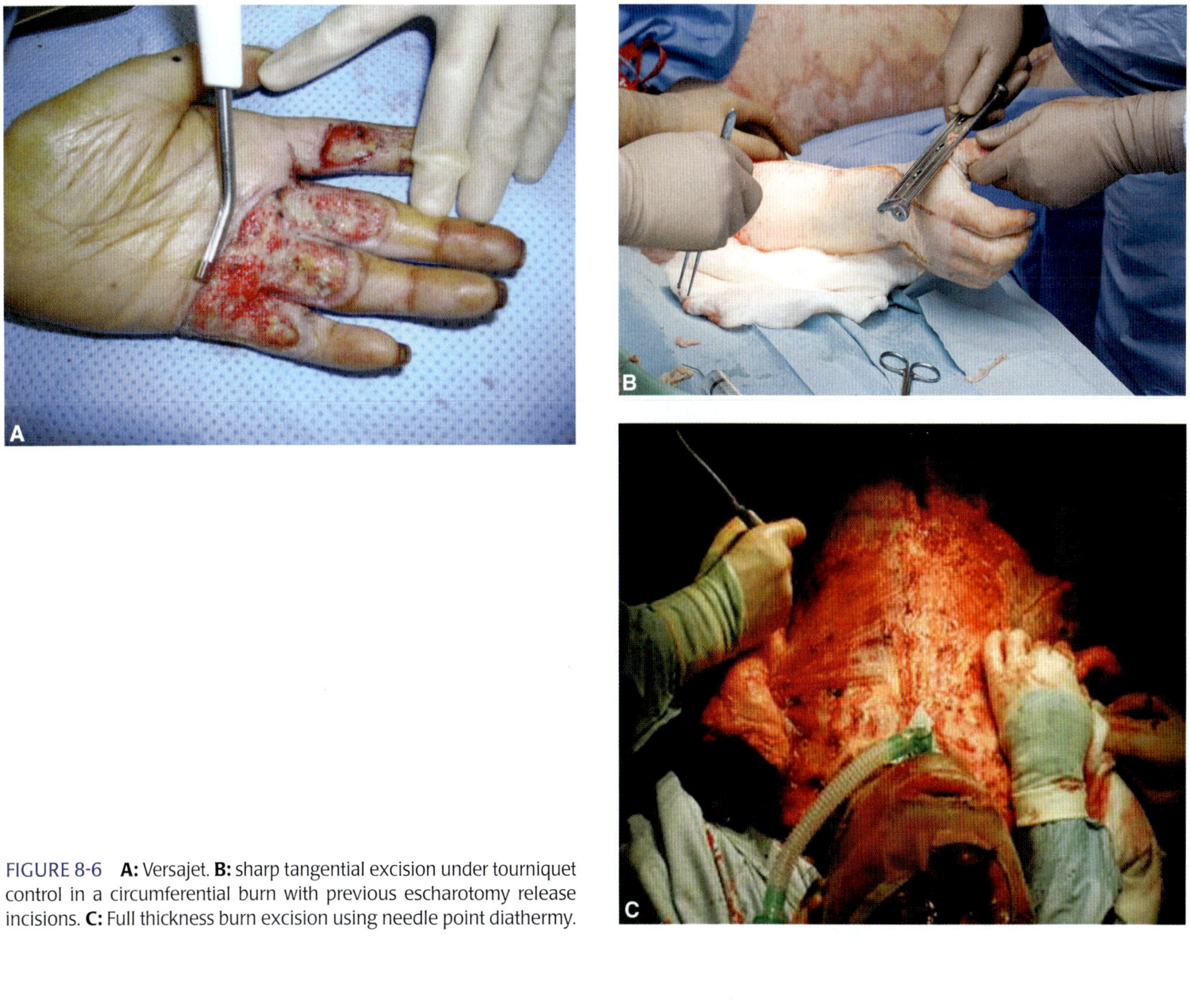

FIGURE 8-6 **A:** Versajet. **B:** sharp tangential excision under tourniquet control in a circumferential burn with previous escharotomy release incisions. **C:** Full thickness burn excision using needle point diathermy.

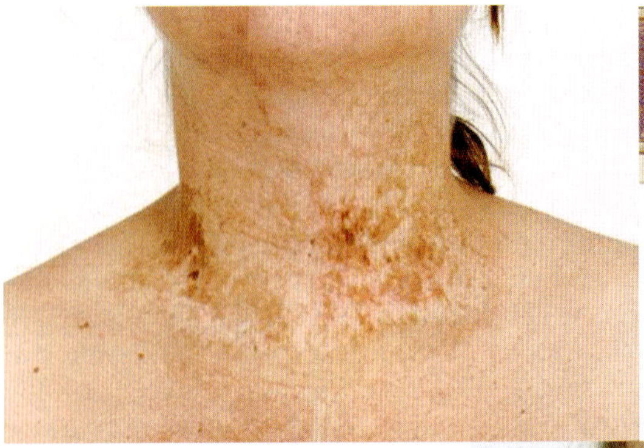

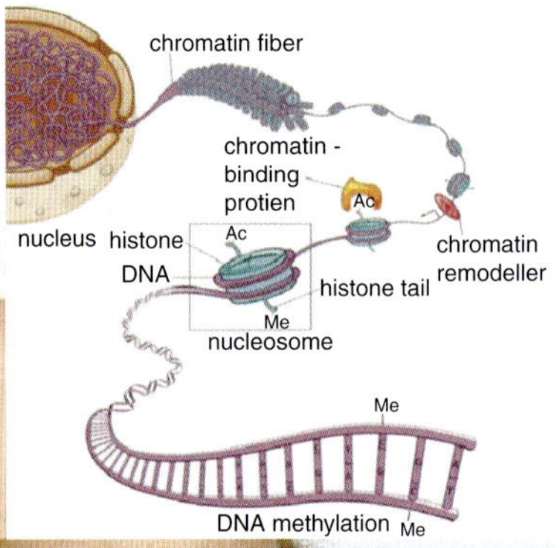

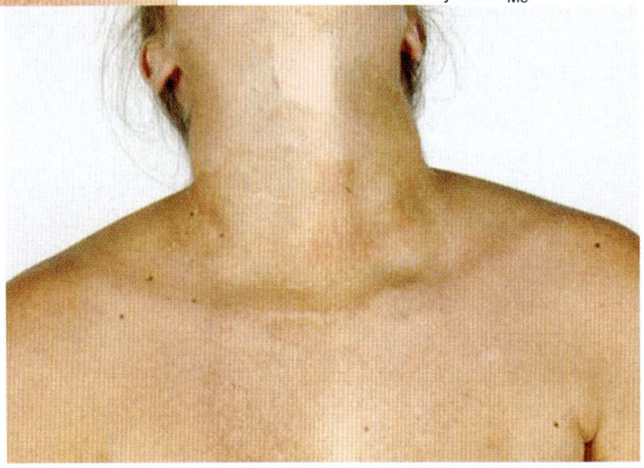

Scar postflame burn treated with dermabrasion and resurfacing using autologous cell suspension using a postauricular split thickness skin biopsy

harvested for immediate use.[102] Where the capacity for donor tissue is limited the potential solutions have been essentially:

- The use of dermal scaffolds with STSG.[103]
- Development of laboratory-based skin constructs with cultured cells seeded into ECM scaffolds (more recently exploring inkjet printing).[104]
- The harvest and transfer of cells for rapid use to facilitate dermal salvage in the wound bed, and in association with traditional skin grafting techniques and scaffold technologies.[105]

The cells of the DEJ are required to restore the normal physiology of the skin. The development of systems of cell isolation, proliferation, and delivery now provides a range of therapeutic options for cell-based therapies in clinical practice.

The use of cell-based therapies in acute burn wounds has been investigated over the last four decades. The clinical use of CEA (Fig. 8-7) confluent cell sheets was first reported in the early 1980s in a large surface area burn injury using the techniques described by Rhienwold and Green.[106] The drive to investigate laboratory-based tissue expansion was the need to provide skin repair in situations of severe injury with donor site limitation. Although potentially lifesaving, it has been clearly reported that CEA is limited to providing an epithelial repair without a consideration of the dermal elements, and resultant issues of long-term fragility.[107]

In a major burn injury the speed to healing influences both mortality and morbidity.[108] Therefore, the time taken to culture the CEA led to exploration of subconfluent cell use with specially designed carriers or using suspensions delivered via aerosol techniques[109] (Fig. 8-8). The capacity to use skin cell therapies earlier in the evolution of the burn wound enabled the exploration of its use in a range of circumstances such as with dermal substitutes, with traditional skin grafting techniques, and with dermal salvage.[110]

In the laboratory process of skin cell culture, cells harvested from the DEJ are seeded onto a layer of irradiated mouse fibroblasts (3T3 strain).[107] To improve the scope of the technology, the question asked was, can cells harvested from the DEJ be immediately delivered to a dermal wound bed using it as the "tissue culture environment?" Dermal salvage coupled with epithelialization to achieve rapid wound healing, with the reduction in scar risk, is the aim.[65] The ReCell device (Fig. 8-9) (Avita Medical, Perth Western Australia) was developed to provide a timely and convenient system for autologous cell harvest from a noninjured site with immediate delivery to the wound.[111]

Scald injuries in children are common, with a significant risk of hypertrophic scarring in instances of delayed healing (Fig. 8-10). The use of cells from the DEJ harvested for immediate use provides the opportunity to salvage dermis by facilitating rapid epidermal repair with minimal donor site morbidity, reducing the need for a prolonged period of dressing changes and the associated procedural pain.[112,113]

In areas where the dermis is more severely damaged, the introduction of a meshed STSG with DEJ cells delivered as an aerosolized suspension facilitates rapid healing of the interstices of the mesh and allows the extension of the area of wound covered and a reduction in the mesh pattern.[114] The combination of traditional and cell-based therapies has been reported using a range of cell techniques.

In major burn injuries the need for repeat harvesting of the donor site can lead to compromise of the donor's capacity to heal with resultant scarring.[115] The use of DEJ cells on the donor site as an adjunct can mitigate against this outcome. The use of dermal substitutes in full thickness injuries functions by providing an environment for tissue-guided regeneration. The cells from the base of the wound migrate into the scaffold and express a reticular dermal phenotype, predominantly fibroblasts and endothelial cells.[116] The scaffold is replaced by an autologous dermal construct. In an animal model, cells from the DEJ have been seeded into the dermal scaffold and have retained the ability to migrate and produce a functional epidermal layer.[117] The use of immediate cell seeding of dermal scaffolds holds promise for the future, driving in situ tissue-guided regeneration. The use of a range of stem cells as a source of cells to facilitate healing and rapid intervention is also under investigation.[118]

The time taken to prepare the patient for intervention is critical, but requires a consideration of the opportunities for repair.[69] In some cases where underlying vital structures are exposed there may be a need for free tissue transfer.[119] In cases where large areas are involved, tissue-engineered skin composites may be used to improve the quality of the repair despite the time taken to manufacture them in

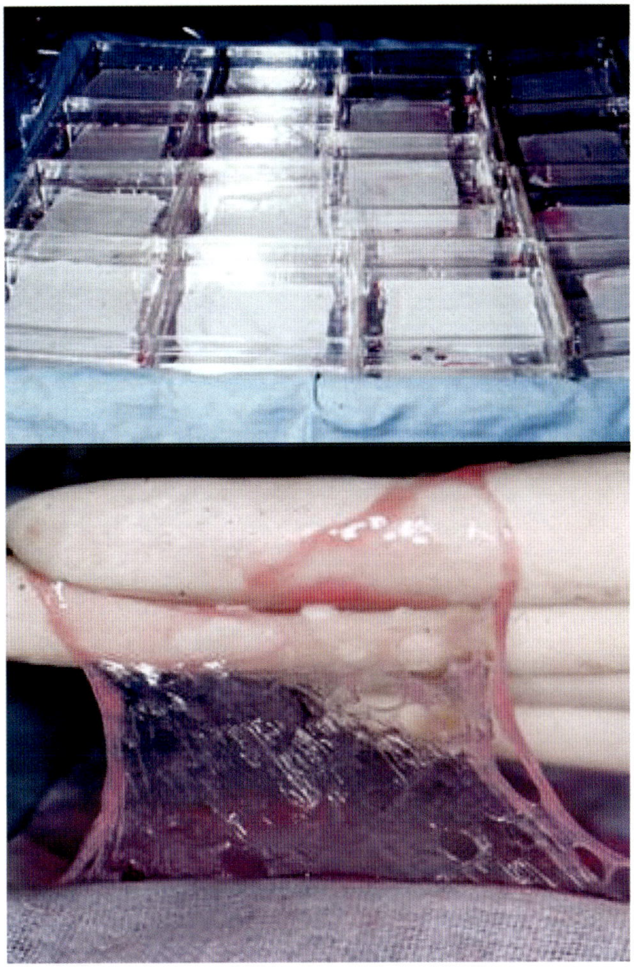

FIGURE 8-7 Laboratory-based tissue expansion, cultured epithelial autograft sheets for wound repair. *(Courtesy of Burns Service of Western Australia.)*

the laboratory.[120] Where the dermis can be salvaged, cell suspension provides a rapid wound repair technique for scar control.[121]

The clinical decision involves planning interventions based on the patient assessment at that particular point in time.

FIGURE 8-8 Autologous cell suspension delivered as an aerosol. *(Courtesy of AvitaMedical.)*

The timing of surgery is a complex decision involving the condition of the patient and the extent of the injury. Early intervention has been shown to be lifesaving in major burn situations.[122] When working with a complex network of interdependent factors that can influence the outcome, clear planning and communication are essential.[123] The surgical plan needs to factor in the timing, technique, and extent of debridement, and the technique of repair, all focused on reducing the time to healing and scar optimization.[124]

Scar Management

As the wound heals and the epidermis stabilizes, ongoing care is important to protect the fragile surface as secondary injury will prolong inflammation and increase scarring potential.[125] The functions of the skin take time to recover; ongoing protection is required, such as managing sun exposure until stabilization of pigmentation and moisturizing in the first 6 to 12 weeks until the sebaceous glands recover.[126]

Pressure garments have been used for decades to assist in scar maturation. Despite widespread use there is a lack of understanding with respect to the mechanism of action. Compression does have an element of edema control, and there is much discussion with respect to the timing, pressure, and wear pattern (see Chapter 19).[127] Commencing pressure early may reduce the extent of scar but can be associated with surface trauma. The use of advanced fabric technology introduces a range of opportunities, e.g., lighter, softer fabrics being easier to wear, impregnated fabrics for infection control, and advanced sensor technology to guide rehabilitation.[128]

Topical silicone contact media and gel preparations are also widely used to modulate the scar, with the aim of reducing hypertrophy and hastening scar maturation. Topical silicone can be applied as a sheet or in gel form.[129] Topical steroid preparations are advocated by some, and the use of steroid with tretinoin has been reported to be effective in scar modulation.[130] With increasing knowledge of the cellular mechanisms underlying the turnover of fibrosis, the targeting of relevant pathways may open up novel drug therapies.[131]

Massage of the scar area is widely practiced and can help with symptoms such as itch. Moisturizing the surface helps prevent drying with the associated risk of fissures and secondary infection. Hygiene is an important consideration as the skin recovers to reduce the bacterial load while the keratin layer matures.[132]

It is well described that scar matures over time, though the time frame is often measured in years with the need for continued therapy.[133] In children the situation is further complicated by growth over the subsequent years.[134] The scars can be associated with symptoms that are beyond the control of conservative scar therapies, with functional and psychological consequences requiring further intervention (see Chapter 24).[135]

Scar Revision

In situations where the symptoms of the scar are no longer tolerable there are a range of surgical options (see Chapter 12). Using the range of techniques of plastic surgery the outlook for the burn patient has improved considerably. The approach

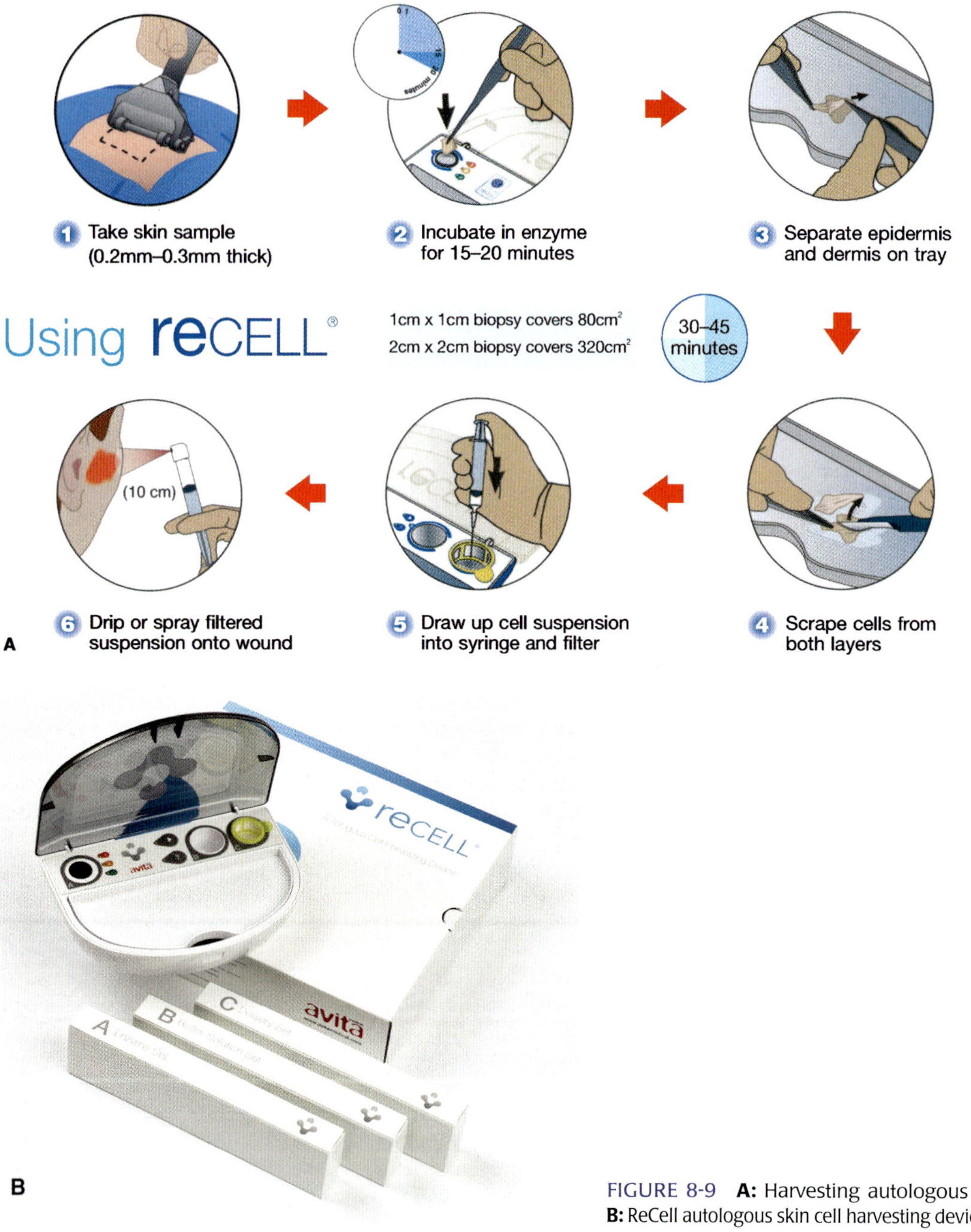

FIGURE 8-9 **A:** Harvesting autologous cells using ReCell device. **B:** ReCell autologous skin cell harvesting device. *(Courtesy of Avita Medical.)*

to burn scar reconstruction is also laid out comprehensively in the "Color Atlas of Burn Reconstructive Surgery."[115]

The decision-making matrix involves careful assessment of the patient, including potential donor sites, the techniques available, and the timing of the intervention. Traditional plastic surgical techniques may be used in combination with more recently developed therapies such as fractional laser resurfacing, tissue-engineered constructs, and cell-based therapies.

Laser therapy is covered more thoroughly in other sections of this book (see Chapter 13), but it should be noted that the recent use of the fractional laser approach has had a significant impact on burn scarring, especially in terms of pliability and tightness as well as aesthetic improvement.[136] The release of a contracture using a range of surgical techniques (e.g., Z-plasty), alone or in combination with laser treatment, can lead to a change in mechanosensing at the cellular level with a reduction in the hypertrophic scar response (see Chapter 7).[137]

Cell-based therapies can be used to resurface the scar to improve the overall color and texture following wound bed preparation using laser or mechanical dermabrasion. In large surface area scars the use of tissue-engineered composite skin constructs allows the excision of the scar and full thickness skin repair.[115] Understanding the interaction at the cellular level of the epidermis and dermis has led to the resurfacing of large areas with CEA[137] and autologous cell suspension harvested using the ReCell kit, with improved outcomes.[114]

The pharmacologic manipulation of the scar by intradermal delivery is also widely practiced, most frequently using steroid, either in isolation or in combination with other strategies driven by the patient's needs (see Chapter 14). The consistent delivery of drugs to influence the ECM remains a challenge to ensure the right dose is in the right place.[138]

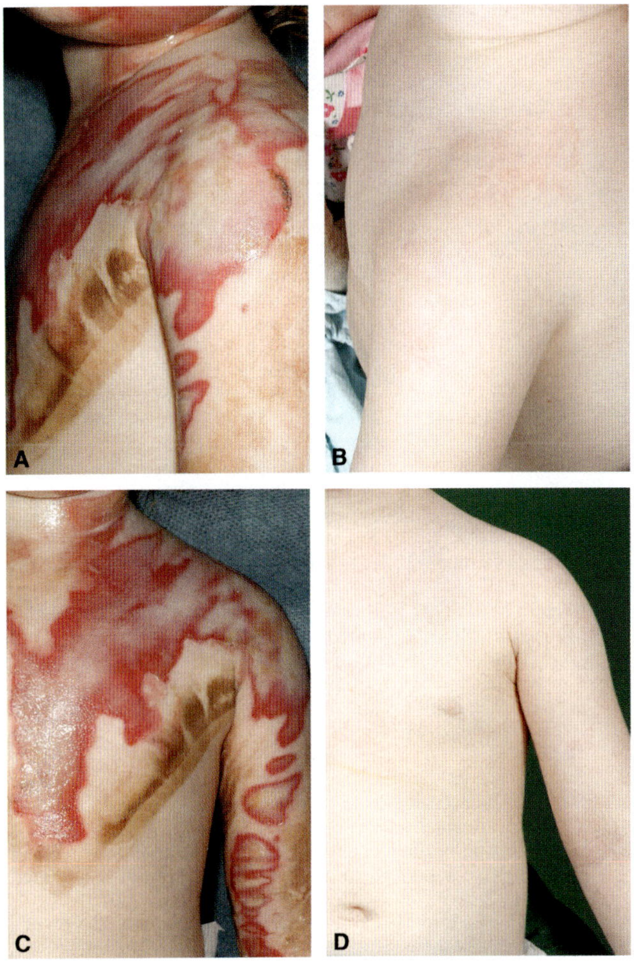

FIGURE 8-10 **A,C** Partial thickness scald injury treated at day 6 postinjury, dermabrasion, and autologous cell suspension harvested using a ReCell kit, with (**B, D**) follow-up at 6-months; the goal is scar minimization. *(Courtesy of Burns Service of Western Australia.)*

The key to scar revision is to assess the patient's needs linked to the range of options, with a clear risk–benefit analysis understanding the natural history of their scarring[139]

Conclusion

Scar minimization can be addressed along the whole healing journey, and there is no substitute for meticulous attention to detail at every stage to optimize the outcome. We are in a time with rapidly developing knowledge that is being translated into clinical practice: how to limit the scar response; how to control cell and ECM interactions; how to salvage damaged tissue; and how to drive toward tissue regeneration.

The implementation of innovative therapies needs to be on a background of using what we know well, then striving to continually improve without ignoring the basics: knowledge of first aid, infection control, edema management, tissue salvage, and tissue handling. The chapter has demonstrated the need to be aware of advancing knowledge in the science of wound healing and fibrosis and introduced some opportunities for clinical translation.

The clinical plan is driven by patient assessment and then bringing together all the appropriate therapeutic opportunities to achieve the best outcome. It involves a complex decision matrix with multiple factors, some of which may well be currently out of the control of the clinician.[140] However, the progress in knowledge toward regeneration makes scar minimization a reality and skin regeneration a possibility.

REFERENCES

1. Martinez-Hernandez A. Repair, regeneration, and fibrosis. In: Rubin E, Farber JL, eds. *Pathology*. Philadelphia, PA: JB Lippincott; 1988:66–95.
2. Nath N, Hyun J. Surface engineering strategies for control of protein and cell interactions. *Surf Sci*. 2004;570(1/2):98–110
3. Babu M, Wells A. Dermal-epidermal communication in wound healing. *Wounds*. 2008;13(5):183–189.
4. Fuchs E. Scratching the surface of skin development. *Nature*. 2007; 445(7130):834–842
5. Seifert O, Bayat A, Geffers R, et al. Identification of unique gene expression patterns within different lesional sites of keloids. *Wound Repair Regen*. 2008;16(2):254–265.
6. Uitto J, Olsen DR, Fazio MJ. Extracellular matrix of the skin: 50 years of progress. *J Invest Dermatol*. 1989;92(4, suppl):61S–77S.
7. Niessen F, Spauwen M, Schalkwijk J, et al. On the nature of hypertrophic scars and keloids: a review. *Plast Reconstr Surg*. 1999;104(5):1435–1458.
8. Gauglitz GG, Korting HC, Pavicic T, et al. Hypertrophic scarring and keloids: pathomechanisms and current and emerging treatment strategies. *Mol Med*. 2011;17(1/2):113–125.
9. Yang GP, Lim IL, Phan TT, et al. From scarless fetal wounds to keloids: molecular studies in wound healing. *Wound Repair Regen*. 2003;11(6):411–418.
10. Brown JJ, Bayat A. Genetic susceptibility to raised dermal scarring. *Br J Dermatol*. 2009:161(1):8–18.
11. Dunkin CS, Pleat JM, Gillespie PH, et al. Scarring occurs at a critical depth of skin injury: precise measurement in a graduated dermal scratch in human volunteers. *Plast Reconstr Surg*. 2007;119(6):1722–1732; discussion 1733–1744.
12. Munster AM, Smith-Meek M. The effect of early surgical intervention on mortality and cost effectiveness in burn care 1978–1991. *Burns*. 1994;20:61–64.
13. Basu S, Shukla V. Complications of wound healing. In: Mani R, Romanelli M, Shukla V, eds. *Measurement of Wound Healing*. New York: Springer; 2012:109–144.
14. Bayat A, McGrouther DA, Ferguson MW. Skin scarring. *BMJ*. 2003;326:88–92.
15. Hawkins HK, Pereira CT. Pathophysiology of the burn scar. In: Herndon DN, ed. *Total Burn Care*. 3rd ed. Philadelphia, PA: Saunders Elsevier; 2007:608–619.
16. Chavapil M, Koopmann C. Scar formation: physiology and pathological states. *Otolaryngol Clin North Am*. 1984;17:265–272.
17. Su CW, Alizadeh K, Boddie A, et al. The problem scar. *Clin Plast Surg*. 1998;25:451–465.
18. Fergurson MW, O'Kane S. Scar free healing from embryonic mechanisms to adult therapeutic intervention. *Trans R Soc Lond Biol Sci*. 2004;359:839–850.
19. Kemble J, Brown D. Enzyme activity in human scars, hypertrophic scars and keloids. *Br J Dermatol*.1976;94(3):301–305.
20. Wood F. Burn Injury Model of Care—Injury & Trauma Health Network. Department of Health; 2009. www.healthnetworks.health.wa.gov.au/modelsofcare/docs/Burn_Injury_Model_of_Care.pdf. Accessed November 2, 2016.
21. Saladin KS. *Anatomy and Physiology: The Unity of Form and Function*. New York, NY: McGraw-Hill; 2001.
22. Marieb E, Hoehn K. *Human Anatomy and Physiology*. 8th ed. San Francisco, CA: Pearson/Benjamin-Cummings; 2010.
23. Chipev CC, Simon M. Phenotypic differences between dermal fibroblasts from different body sites determine their responses to tension and tgfβ1. *BMC Dermatol*. 2002;2(1):1–13.
24. Wood FM. Tissue engineering of skin. *Clin Plast Surg*. 2012;39(1):21–32.
25. Martin P. Wound healing—aiming for perfect skin regeneration. *Science*. 1997;276;5309:75–81.
26. Deitch EA, Wheelahan TM, Paige Rose M, et al. Hypertrophic burn scars: analysis of variables. *J Trauma*. 1983;23(10):895–898.

27. Garner WL. Epidermal regulation of dermal fibroblast activity. *Plast Reconstr Surg*. 1998;102(1):135–139.
28. Diegelmann RF, Evans MC. Wound healing: an overview of acute, fibrotic and delayed healing. *Front Biosci*. 2001;9:283–289.
29. Yannas IV, Orgill DP, Burke JF. Template for skin regeneration. *Plast Reconstr Surg*. 2011;127:60s–70s.
30. Anderson JA, Fear MF, Phillips J, et al. A preliminary investigation of the reinnervation and return of sensory function in burn patients treated with Integra. *Burns*. 2011;37(7):1101–1108.
31. Marshall WG, Dimick AR. The natural history of major burns with multiple subsystem failure. *J Trauma—Injury Infect Crit Care*. 1983;23(2):230–245.
32. Robert MN. Tissue engineering: the hope, the hype, and the future. *Tissue Eng*. 2006;12(5):1143–1150.
33. Broughton GI, Janis JE, Attinger CE. The basic science of wound healing. *Plast Reconstr Surg*. 2008;117(7S):12S–34S.
34. Redd MJ. Wound healing and inflammation: embryos reveal the way to perfect repair. *Philos Trans R Soc Lond B Biol Sci*. 2004;359(1445):777–784.
35. Lund T, Onarheim HO, Reed RK. Pathogenesis of edema formation in burn injuries. *World J Surg*. 1992;16:2–9.
36. Lund T, Herndon DN. Pathophysiology of burn shock and burn edema. In: Herndon DN, ed. *Total Burn Care*. Saunders: London; 2002:78–85.
37. Valvis SM, Waithman J, Wood FM, et al. The immune response to skin trauma is dependent on the etiology of injury in a mouse model of burn and excision. *J Invest Dermatol*. 2015;135:2119–2128.
38. Robinson CM, Watson CJ, Baugh JA. Epigenetics within the matrix. *Epigenetics*. 2012;7(9):987–993.
39. Feinberg AP. Phenotypic plasticity and the epigenetics of human disease. *Nature*. 2007;447(7143):433–440.
40. Schiller MD, Javelaud H. TGF-β-induced SMAD signalling and gene regulation: consequences for extracellular matrix remodelling and wound healing. *J Dermatol Sci*. 2004;35(2):83–92.
41. Sazauter KM, Ordas A, Laxer RM. A novel fibrotic disorder associated with increased dermal fibroblast proliferation and downregulation of genes of the microfibrillar network. *Br Assoc Dermatol*. 2010;163:1102–1115.
42. Jackson DM. The diagnosis of the depth of burning. *Br J Surg*. 1953;40:588–596.
43. Bier M, Chen W, Gowrishankar TR, et al. Resealing dynamics of a cell membrane after electroporation. *Physics Rev E*. 2002;66(6 Pt 1):62905.
44. Rowan MP, Cancio LC, Elster EA, et al. Burn wound healing and treatment: review and advancements. *Crit Care*. 2015;19:243.
45. Farina JA Jr, Rosique MJ, Rosique RG. Curbing inflammation in burn patients. *Int J Inflamm*. 2013;2013:715645.
46. Shirani KZ, Vaughan GM, Mason AD Jr, et al. Update on current therapeutic approaches in burns. *Shock*. 1996;5:4–16.
47. Singh V, Devgan L, Bhat S, et al. The pathogenesis of burn wound conversion. *Ann Plast Surg*. 2007;59(1):109–115.
48. Gurtner GC, Werner S, Barrandon Y, et al. Wound repair and regeneration. *Nature*. 2008;453:314–321.
49. Guo S, DiPietro LA. Factors affecting wound healing. *J Dent Res*. 2010;89(3):219–229.
50. Du Noüy PL. Cicatrization of wounds. III. The relation between the age of the patient, the area of the wound, and the index of cicatrization. *J Exp Med*. 1916;24:461–470.
51. Ashcroft GS, Horan MA, Ferguson MW. Aging alters the inflammatory and endothelial cell adhesion molecule profiles during human cutaneous wound healing. *Lab Invest*. 1998;78:47–58.
52. Eming SA, Krieg T, Davidson JM. Inflammation in wound repair: molecular and cellular mechanisms. *J Invest Dermatol*. 2007;127:514–525.
53. Marneros A, Norris J, Olsen B, et al. Clinical genetics of familial keloids. *Arch Dermatol*. 2001;137(11): 1429–1434.
54. Zhu F, Wu B, Li J, et al. Association study confirmed susceptibility loci with keloid in the chinese han population. *PLos One*. 2013;8(5):e62377.
55. Bond JS, Duncan JA, Sattar A, et al. Maturation of the human scar: an observational study. *Plast Reconstr Surg*. 2008;121: 1650–1658.
56. Huang C, Murphy GF, Akaishi S, et al. Keloids and hypertrophic scars: update and future directions. *Plast Reconstr Surg Glob Open*. 2013;1(4):e25.
57. Ward S, CadbyG, Heyworth JS, et al. Association of TGFβ1 and clinical factors with scar outcome following melanoma excision. *Arch Dermatol Res*. 2012;304(5):343–351.
58. Thompson CM, Hocking AM, Honari S, et al. Genetic risk factors for hypertrophic scar development. *J Burn Care Res*. 2013;34(5):477–482.
59. Goodfellow A, Emmerson R, CalvertH. Rubinstein-taybi syndrome and spontaneous keloids. *Clin Exp Dermatol*. 1980;5(3):369–370.
60. Goeminne, L. A new probably x-linked inherited syndrome: congenital muscular torticollis, multiple keloids cryptorchidism and renal dysplasia. *Acta Genet Med Gemellol (Roma)*. 1968;17(3):439–467.
61. Heyen C, Delk P, Bull M, et al. A report of an apparent new genetic syndrome consisting of joint contractures, keloids, large optic cup-to-disc ratio and renal stones. *Am J Med Genet A*. 2008;146A(24):3120–3125.
62. Al-Mousawi AM, Mecott-Rivera GA, Jeschke MG, et al. Burn teams and burn centers: the importance of a comprehensive team approach to burn care. *Clin Plast Surg*. 2009;36:547–554.
63. Gibran NS, Boyce S, Greenhalgh DG. Cutaneous wound healing. *J Burn Care Res*. 2007;28(4):577–579.
64. Hettiaratchy S, Papini R. ABC of burns: initial management of a major burn: II—assessment and resuscitation. *BMJ*. 2004;329(7457):101–103.
65. Monstrey S, Hoeksema H, Verbelen J, et al. Assessment of burn depth and burn wound healing potential. *Burns*. 2008;34(6):761–769.
66. Pape S, Skouras CA, Byrne PO. An audit of the use of laser Doppler imaging (LDI) in the assessment of burns of intermediate depth. *Burns*. 2001;27(3):233–239.
67. Kim K, Pierce MC, Maguluri G, et al. In vivo imaging of human burn injuries with polarization-sensitive optical coherence tomography. *J Biomed Opt*. 2012;17(6):066012–066012.
68. Tiller G, Rea S, Silla R, et al. Burns first aid information on the Internet. *Burns*. 2007;32(7):897–901.
69. Kao CC, Garner WL. Acute burns. *Plast Reconstr Surg*. 2000;105(7): 2482–2493.
70. Wood FM, Phillips M, Jovic T, et al. Water first aid is beneficial in humans post-burn: evidence from a bi-national cohort study. *PLoS One*. 2016;11(1):e0147259.
71. Cuttle L, Kempfa M, Kravchuk O, et al. The efficacy of aloe vera, tea tree oil and saliva as first aid treatment for partial thickness burn injuries. *Burns*. 2008;34(8):1176–1182.
72. Bartlett N, Yuan J, Holland AJA, et al. Optimal duration of cooling for an acute scald contact burn injury in a porcine model. *J Burn Care Res*. 2008;29:828–834.
73. Detmar M, Brown LF, Berse B, et al. Hypoxia regulates the expression of vascular permeablilty factor/vascular endothelial growth factor (VPF/VEGF) and its receptors in human skin. *J Invest Dermatol*. 1997;108(3):263–268.
74. Boykin JV, Eriksson E, Pittman RN. In vivo microcirculation of a scald burn and the progression of the postburn dermal ischaemia. *Plast Reconstr Surg*. 1980;65(2):191–198.
75. Boland RA, Adams RD, The effects of arm elevation and overnight head-up tilt on forearm and hand volume. *J Hand Ther*. 1998;11:180–190.
76. Oda J, Yamashita K, Inoue T, et al. Resuscitation fluid volume and abdominal compartment syndrome in patients with major burns. *Burns*. 2006;32(2):151–154.
77. Infanger M, Schmidt O, Kossmehl P, et al. Vascular endothelial growth factor serum level is strongly enhanced after burn injury and correlated with local and general tissue edema. *Burns*. 2004;30(4):305–311.
78. Lowell M, Pirc P, Ward RS, et al. Effect of 3M™ Coban™ self-adherent wraps on edema and function of the burned hand: a case study. *J Burn Care Rehabil*. 2003;4(4):253–258.
79. Pegg SP. Escharotomy in burns. *Ann Acad Med Singapore*. 1992;21(5):682–684.
80. Wasiak J, Cleland H. Topical negative pressure (TNP) for partial thickness burns (Review). *Cochrane Database Syst Rev*. 2007;(3):CD006215.
81. Zielins ER, Brett EA, Luan A. Emerging drugs for the treatment of wound healing. *Expert Opin Emerg Drugs*. 2015;20(2):235–246.
82. Alvarado R, Chung KK, Cancio LC, et al. Burn resuscitation. *Burns*. 2009;35(1):4–14.
83. Allgower M, Schoenenberger GA, Sparkes BG. Burning the largest immune organ. *Burns*. 1995;21(suppl 1):S7–S47.
84. Backmann C, Marck PB, Krogman, et al. Barriers and bridges to infection prevention and control: results of a qualitative case study of a Netherlands surgical unit. *BMJ Open*. 2012;2:e000511.
85. Fong J, Wood F, Fowler B. A silver coated dressing reduces the incidence of early burn wound cellulitis and associated costs of inpatient treatment: Comparative patient care audits. *Burns*. 2005;31:562–567.
86. Sharma BR. Infection in patients with severe burns: causes and prevention thereof. *Infect Dis Clin N Am*. 2007;21:745–759.
87. Van Rijn, Kuiper EC, Kreis RW. Seven-year experience with a 'quarantine and isolation unit' for patients with burns. A retrospective audit. *Burns*. 1997;23:345–348.
88. Stoodley P, Sauer K, Davies DG, et al. Biofilms as complex differentiated communities. *Annu Rev Microbiol*. 2002;56:187–209.
89. Soleimani T, Evans TA, Sood R, et al. Predictors of reconstructive surgery among burn patients. *Plast Reconstr Surg*. 2015;136(4, suppl):126.

90. Borgert MJ, Goossens A, Dongelmans DA. What are effective strategies for the implementation of care bundles on ICUs: a systematic review. *Implement Sci*. 2015;10:119.
91. Cubison TC, Pape SA, Parkhouse N. Evidence for the link between healing time and the development of hypertrophic scars (HTS) in paediatric burns due to scald injury. *Burns*. 2006;32:992–999.
92. Wasiak J, Cleland H, Campbell F, et al. Dressings for superficial and partial thickness burns. *Cochrane Database Syst Rev*. 2013;(3):CD002106.
93. Wei L, Sahu D, Tsen F. Secreted heat shock protein-90 (Hsp90) in wound healing and cancer *Biochim Biophys Acta*. 2012;1823:730–741.
94. Giri P, Ebert S, Braumann UD. Skin regeneration in deep second-degree scald injuries either by infusion pumping or topical application of recombinant human erythropoietin gel. *Drug Des Devel Ther*. 2015:9 2565–2579.
95. Zhang Y, Wang T, Jinguang H. Growth factor therapy in patients with partial-thickness burns: a systematic review and meta-analysis. *Int Wound J*. 2016;13:354–366.
96. Lin T, Maita D, Thundivalappil SR, et al. Hemopexin in severe inflammation and infection:mouse models and human diseases. *Crit Care*. 2015;19:166.
97. Saaiq M, Zaib S, Ahmad S. Early excision and grafting versus delayed excision and grafting of deep thermal burns up to 40% total body surface area: a comparison of outcome. *Ann Burns Fire Disasters*. 2012;25:143–147.
98. Rosenberg L, Krieger Y, Bogdanov-Berezovski A, et al. A novel rapid and selective enzymatic debridement agent for burn wound management: a multi-center RCT. *Burns*. 2014;40(3):365–538.
99. Block L, King TW, Gosain A. Debridement techniques in pediatric trauma and burn-related wounds. *Adv Wound Care*. 2015;4(10):596–606.
100. Engrav LH, Heimbach DM, Reus JL, et al. Early excision and grafting vs. nonoperative treatment of burns of indeterminant depth: a randomized prospective study. *J Trauma*. 1983;23:1001–1004.
101. Zhang ML, Wang CY, Chang ZD, et al. Microskin grafting: clinical report. *J Burns*. 1986;12:544–548.
102. Hernon CA, Dawson RA, Freedlander E, et al. Clinical experience using cultured epithelial autografts leads to an alternative methodology for transferring skin cells from the laboratory to the patient. *Regen Med*. 2006;1(6):809–821.
103. Ryssel H, Gazykan E, Germann G, et al. The use of MatriDerm® in early excision and simultaneous autologous skin grafting in burns—a pilot study. *Burns*. 2008;34;1:93–97.
104. Boyce ST, Kagan RJ, Greenhalgh DG, et al. Cultured skin substitutes reduce requirements for harvesting of skin autograft for closure of excised, full-thickness burns. *J Trauma*. 2006;60(4):821–829.
105. Wood FM. Skin regeneration: the complexities of translation into clinical practise. *Int J Biochem Cell Biol*. 2014;56:133–140.
106. Rheinwald J, Green H. Serial cultivation of strains of human epidermal keratinocytes: The formation of keratinizing colonies from single-cells. *Cell*. 1975;6:331–344.
107. Wood FM, Kolybaba ML, Allen P. The use of cultured epithelial autograft in the treatment of major burn wounds: eleven years of clinical experience. *Burns*. 2006:32(5):538–544.
108. Burke JF, Bondoc CC, Quinby WC. Primary burn excision and immediate grafting: a method shortening illness. *J Trauma*. 1974;14: 389–395.
109. Worst PK, MacKenzie IC, Fusenig NE. Reformation of organised epidermal structure by transplantation of suspensions and cultures of epidermal and dermal cells. *Cell Tiss Res*. 1982:225:65–77.
110. MacNeil S, Progress and opportunities for tissue-engineered skin. *Nature*. 2007;445(7130):874–880.
111. Wood F, Martin L, Lewis D, et al. A prospective randomised clinical pilot study to compare the effectiveness of Biobrane® synthetic wound dressing, with or without autologous cell suspension, to the local standard treatment regimen in paediatric scald injuries. *Burns*. 2012:38(6):830–889.
112. Wood FM, Giles N, Stevenson A, et al. Characterisation of the cell suspension harvested from the dermal epidermal junction using a ReCell® kit. *Burns*. 2012;38(1):44–51.
113. Wood FM. Clinical potential of cellular autologous epithelial suspension. *Wounds*. 2002;15:16–22.
114. Navarro FA, Stoner ML, Park CS, et al. Sprayed keratinocyte suspensions accelerate epidermal coverage in a porcine microwound model. *J Burn Care Rehabil*. 2000;21(6):513–518.
115. Wood FM. ReCell. In: Hyakkusoku H, Orgill DP, Teot L, et al., eds. *Color Atlas of Burn Reconstructive Surgery*. Heidelberg, Germany: Springer-Verlag; 2010:26–37.
116. Kremer M, Lang E, Berger AC, Evaluation of dermal-epidermal skin equivalents ('composite-skin') of human keratinocytes in a collagen-glycosaminoglycan matrix(Integra artificial skin). *Br J Plast Surg*. 2000;53(6):459–465.
117. Wood FM, Stoner ML, Fowler BV, et al. The use of a non-cultured autologous cell suspension and Integra® dermal regeneration template to repair full-thickness skin wounds in a porcine model: A one-step process. *Burns*. 2007;33(6):693–700.
118. Wood FM. Advances in isolation and expansion of human cells for clinical application. In Albanna MZ, Holmes JH, eds. *Soft Tissue Engineering and Regenerative Medicine*. London: Elsevier; 2016.
119. Oni G, Saint-Cyr M, Mojallal A. Free tissue transfer in acute burns. *J Reconstr Microsurg*. 2012;28:77–84.
120. Supp DM, Boyce ST. Engineered skin substitutes: practices and Potentials. *Clin Dermatol*. 2005;23(4):403–412.
121. Wood F. Clinical potential of autologous epithelial suspension. *Wounds*. 2003;15(1):16–22.
122. Talbot SG, Pribaz JJ. Sophisticated surgical solutions for complex wound problems. *Clin Plastic Surg*. 2012;39:325–340.
123. Herndon DN, Barrow RE, Rutan RL, et al. A comparison of conservative versus early excision. Therapies in severely burned patients. *Ann Surg*. 1989;209(5):547–552.
124. Breederveld S, Kreis RW. Damage control in burn surgery. *Br J Surg*. 2009;96:1227–1228.
125. Van der Wal MBA, Offringa T, Derriks F, et al. Outcome after burns: a clinical observational study on the maturation of scar characteristics. *Burns*. 2009;35:S21.
126. Falder S, Browne A, Edgar D, et al. Core outcomes for adult burn survivors: a clinical overview. *Burns*. 2009;35(5):618–641.
127. Atiyeh BS, El Khatib AM, Dibo SA. Pressure garment therapy (PGT) of burn scars: evidence-based efficacy. *Ann Burns Fire Disasters*. 2013;26(4):205–212.
128. Qin Y. Smart wound care materials. In: Van Langenhove L, ed. *Smart Textiles for Medicine and Healthcare*. Cambridge: Woodhead Publishing; 2007.
129. Friedstat JS, Hultman CS. Hypertrophic burn scar management: what does the evidence show? A systematic review of randomized controlled trials. *Ann Plast Surg*. 2014;72(6):S198–S201.
130. Taheri A, Tuchayi S, Alinia H, et al. Topical clobetasol in conjunction with topical tretinoin is effective in preventing scar formation after superficial partial-thickness burn ulcers of the skin: a retrospective study. *J Dermatol Treat*. 2015;26(4):361–364.
131. Block L, Gosain A, King TW. Emerging therapies for scar prevention. *Adv Wound Care*. 2015;4(10):607–617.
132. Mustoe TA, Cooter RD, Gold MH, et al. International clinical recommendations on scar management. *Plast Reconstr Surg*. 2002;110:560–571.
133. Xue M. Jackson CJ. Extracellular matrix reorganization during wound healing and its impact on abnormal scarring. *Adv Wound Care*. 2013;4(3):119–136.
134. Argirova M, Hadjiski O, Victorova A. Non-operative treatment of hypertrophic scars and keloids after burns in children. *Ann Burns Fire Disasters*. 2006;19(2):80–87.
135. Gürol AP, Polat S, Akçay MN. Itching, pain, and anxiety levels are reduced with massage therapy in burned adolescents. *J Burn Care Res*. 2010;31(3):429–432.
136. Hultman CS, Friedstat JS, Edkins RE, et al. Laser resurfacing and remodeling of hypertrophic burn scars: the results of a large, prospective, before-after cohort study, with long-term follow-up. *Ann Surg*. 2014;260(3):519–529; discussion 529–532.
137. Humphrey JD, Dufresne ER, Schwartz MA. Mechanotransduction and extracellular matrix homeostasis. *Nat Rev Mol Cell Biol*. 2014;15;802–811.
138. Kadoya K, Amano S, Nishiyama T, et al. Changes in the expression of epidermal differentiation markers at sites where cultured epithelial autografts were transplanted onto wounds from burn scar excision. *Int Wound J*. 2014;13(3):412–417.
139. Korrapati PS, Karthikeyan K, Satish A, et al. Recent advancements in nanotechnological strategies in selection, design and delivery of biomolecules for skin regeneration. *Mater Sci Eng C Mater Biol Appl*. 2016;67:747–765.
140. Rea SM, Goodwin-Walters A, Wood FM. Surgeons and scars: differences between patients and surgeons in the perceived requirement for reconstructive surgery following burn injury. *Burns*. 2006;32(3):276–283.

9 Optimizing Wound Healing and Scar Formation

REINHARD DOLP, SAEID AMINI NIK, and MARC G. JESCHKE

KEY POINTS

- Absorbable staples combine the good cosmetic results of sutures with the fast wound closure time of conventional staples.
- Adhesive tape and tissue glue are reasonable alternatives for the closure of small wounds.
- Laser-assisted wound closure shows great results but is too expensive for routine clinical practice.
- Wnt/β-catenin, TGF-β, Hedgehog, and Notch pathways are key mechanisms for wound healing and scar formation.
- Intralesional steroid injection and silicone gel sheeting are the most recommended therapies for hypertrophic scars and keloids.
- Nutrition plays a key role in wound healing, and special recommendations have to be considered.
- Negative pressure dressings and hydrocolloid/hydrogel dressings are excellent in the treatment of complex wounds.
- Acellular skin substitutes are a life-saving component in the treatment of severe skin loss.
- Cellular skin substitutes are limited by the availability of cells and their high costs.
- Cytotherapy is the future in the treatment of wounds and scars.

With claimed annual health care costs for the treatment of chronic wounds of 25 billion dollars (in the United States alone) and a 15 billion dollar market for wound care products,[1] the optimization of wound healing and scar formation is essential in times of escalating health care costs.[2] Two to three percent of the American population is affected by wound healing disorders that require therapy.[1,3] This is not limited to insufficient or absent wound healing, but also includes excessive skin proliferation that can lead to keloids and hypertrophic scars.[4] The psychological and physical effects of skin diseases on patients can be devastating, and improving the treatment modalities can drastically improve a patient's quality of life (see Chapter 24).

Wounds are commonly classified as acute (<3 months) or chronic (>3 months). Recently, it was proposed to change this classification into acute and complex wounds.[5] A wound is considered complex if it displays one of the following characteristics: absence of healing within 3 months, infection, compromised viability of superficial tissues, necrosis, circulation impairment, or associated with systemic pathologies. Excessive skin proliferation after dermal injury can be divided into keloids and hypertrophic scars. Keloids are characterized by an abnormally increased deposition of collagen in the dermis that extends beyond the margin of the initial injury, whereas collagen deposition in hypertrophic scars is limited to the initial wound area.

Scar Formation and Wound Healing

In contrast to antenatal skin, postnatal skin usually heals by scar formation; scar tissue is inherently weaker and contains an extracellular matrix (ECM) that is more disorganized.[6,7] Posttraumatic inflammation plays a key role in this process (see Chapter 6). Although an inflammatory response is vital to prevent or contain wound site infections, the inflammatory cytokines and growth factors released during this process promote fibrosis and scar formation.[7–10] In addition to this inflammation (that can only take place in a fully developed immune system), the expression profile, concentration of growth factors and cytokines, as well as some ECM components (hyaluronic acid, fibronectin, elastin) differ in adult scar-forming wound healing as compared with embryonic scarless wound healing (see Chapter 27).[7,8,11–13] Understanding the molecular basis for scar formation and wound healing is essential for developing and applying novel medical therapies.[2] This chapter will explain the most important mechanisms together with the corresponding ways to enhance the process.

Measuring Scars

Despite obvious macroscopic criteria such as wound and scar size and time to wound closure, no consistent methodology exists to precisely determine the effects of therapy upon scar formation and wound healing (see Chapter 28).[14] In contrast to intact skin (with its loose, random, basket-weave-like organization of collagen bundles), scar tissue is composed of more parallel and tightly packed collagen bundles (see Chapter 5).[15] A total of 85% of the dermis consists of collagen and it dictates dermal elasticity and strength. This makes collagen one of the main targets in the evaluation of wound healing.[16,17]

Khorasani et al.[14] suggested a new method for analyzing scar tissue using fractal dimension (FD) and lacunarity (L) analysis. FD measures the degree to which an object fills a space, with a minimum value of 1 being a straight line and a maximum value of 2 occupying the whole space (=structural density). L determines the degree of structural variance within an object, with a minimal value of 0 representing complete homogeneity and a maximum value of 1 representing absolute heterogeneity (structural heterogeneity).[18] This method has already proved itself to be reliable and reproducible in the evaluation of complex biologic structures such as neurons[19] and capillary beds.[20,21] However, studies of Khorasani et al. were performed on a murine model, and the clinical usefulness of this more precise method of scar tissue determination is yet to be investigated in humans.

Procedural Optimization

Surgical Optimization

Surgical optimization of scar and wound healing starts with choosing a way of opening the skin with the least trauma possible, followed by closing the wound or by preparing it for healing by secondary intention with a technique that achieves the best cosmetic and functional results. It also includes the surgical treatment of aberrant/excessive scar formation after wound closure (see Chapter 12).

Incision Method: Electrocautery/ Diathermy

Since the first use of an electrosurgical device in 1926, diathermy has become ubiquitous because of its efficacy, convenience, advantages in hemostasis, and safety as compared with scalpels.[22,23] Recent meta-analyses and reviews show no significant difference in the wound infection rate,[24–26] but suggest a decrease in patient-perceived postoperative pain with the use of diathermy.[24] The use of diathermy to cut the epidermis and dermis remains controversial because of the believed inferior scar cosmesis owing to thermal damage. A recent Canadian double-blind randomized trial assessing 66 patients having received abdominal surgery (laparoscopic and open) could not detect any significant difference (on either subjective or objective measures) between epidermal incision with diathermy or with a scalpel, 6 months postoperatively.[22] This supports existing data on smaller patient cohorts that also failed to detect an inferior cosmetic result when using diathermy for skin incisions.[27,28] Further investigation is needed to elucidate if using diathermy for skin incisions is also legitimate in cosmetically sensitive areas like the head, neck, and breast.[22]

Wound Closure

The principal aim of skin/wound closure is to minimize tissue damage and inflammation, to promote a rapid acquisition of tissue strength, and good cosmesis. Accurate coaptation of the dermal margins is a key factor in this, and inappropriate eversion or inversion can lead to suboptimal healing.[29,30] There are different techniques available for skin/wound closure including sutures, staples, adhesive tape, and liquid adhesives. Sutures and staples are the most commonly used wound closure materials because they provide the often needed mechanical support.[31]

Absorbable versus Nonabsorbable Sutures

Luck et al.[32] could not detect significant differences in cosmesis or infection rate for absorbable vs. nonabsorbable suture materials after 3 months in facial lacerations. Also, no differences regarding the cosmetic outcome could be found in pediatric lacerations after 4 to 5 months.[33] However, nonabsorbable monofilament nylon sutures seemed to diminish the risk of hypertrophic scarring in comparison to absorbable sutures in a randomized clinical trial that looked at 60 patients who underwent midline sternotomy for cardiac surgery.[34] Skin was closed in a subcuticular continuous fashion either with a 4-0 braided polyglycolic acid suture or with a 4-0 nonabsorbable monofilamentous polypropylene suture that was removed 8 to 10 days after the surgery. Patients were evaluated 6 months after sternotomy. Interestingly, the benefit of the nonabsorbable monofilament suture was only apparent in the upper half of the sternum. The lower half did not show any difference. The authors concluded that increased tension and mobility of the skin in the lower half of the sternotomy led to the inferior scar appearance independently of the suture material. In terms of cost-effectiveness, it has to be considered that nonabsorbable sutures have a higher cost and require an additional physician visit for removal.[35]

Sutures versus Staples

Compared with sutures, stapling with metal staples is five to seven times faster and produces equivalent cosmetic results when used in an emergency setting.[36,37] A 2014 study evaluating 130 women that underwent an emergency cesarean section found skin closure with staples to have a better cosmesis and shorter duration of surgery, with comparable postoperative pain and wound complications.[38] Even in cosmetic surgery on more sensitive areas like the neck, no difference between stapling and suturing could be detected.[30] Two out of five randomized controlled trials evaluating chest and leg wounds after cardiovascular surgery found sutures to be superior cosmetically and were associated with fewer complications.[39] However, there are no large trials comparing sutures with staples in elective surgeries in cosmetically critical body regions. Staples puncture the epidermis and therefore carry a potential risk of scarring and wound contamination in comparison to absorbable sutures.[40] The use of staples has also been associated with increased tension along the incision line, precluding their use for reconstructive flap surgery.[41] Stapling has been found to be safer and easier to use.[37] Whether the removal of staples or nonabsorbable sutures is more or equally painful for the patient is not clear.[36,42] There are also controversial reports about which method is cheaper.[37,43]

Absorbable staples (tissue half-life of 10 weeks; Insorb) that are placed in the subcuticular tissue without puncturing the epidermis[40,44] are designed to combine the good cosmesis of absorbable sutures with the increased wound closure times of a stapler.[40] A randomized controlled trial comparing absorbable staples versus absorbable sutures conducted in patients receiving bilateral breast reconstruction found that the wound could be closed faster with staples, while showing a comparable cosmesis.[45] Absorbable staples also seem to be an adequate wound closure material in sensitive areas like the face and neck,[40] as well as in immunocompromised patients.[46] Nevertheless, there are no long-term data regarding absorbable staples and they are a relatively expensive alternative to other wound closure techniques.[47]

Adhesive Tape

Adhesive tapes contain an adhesive material consisting of iso-octo-acrylate and n-vinyl-pyrrolidone.[48] Microporous strips enable the passage of gas and water from the skin surface, reducing the suitable environment for bacterial growth and wound site infections.[49,50] In clean contaminated wounds (wounds that are clean, but carry a high risk of contamination in locations such the gastrointestinal, respiratory, or genitourinary tract), a lower rate of infection has been reported in wounds closed with adhesive tape in comparison to sutures.[51] The difficulty in approximating the wound edges accurately[49] and achieving sufficient adhesiveness, which in turn is dependent on correct usage and the presence of a dry wound site, limits the use of adhesive tape.[49,52]

Tissue Glue

A liquid adhesive (*n*-alkyl-alpha-cyanoacrylate tissue adhesives, e.g., Dermabond) polymerizes once applied on the wound, bridging the edges of the wound together.[53] The film is water resistant and sloughs off about 9 days after application.[53,54] It is supposed to be used in small lacerations replacing sutures that are 5-0 or smaller.[54] For the closure of surgical or traumatic wounds, Dermabond was considered to be faster,[55,56] less painful,[55] and with a similar,[57,58] equal,[56] or improved[59,60] cosmesis compared with standard wound closure methods. No higher rates of dehiscence have been detected.[56,59] Whereas the experience of the surgeon is a key factor for a good cosmesis using suturing,[61] it seems to be negligible for the outcome with tissue glue.[62] Another positive side effect is that liquid tissue adhesive seems to inhibit bacterial growth and wound site infection to a certain degree.[60,63,64] Tissue adhesives are now being commonly and successfully used for facial wounds, groin wounds, hand surgery, blepharoplasty, laparoscopic wounds, hair transplantation, and lacrimal punctum closure.[63,65] In addition, it can be a good method for wound closure in patients who are at risk for keloid or hypertrophic scar formation.[66] Tissue glue is not suitable for patients at risk for delayed wound healing (diabetics or patients with collagen vascular diseases),[59] in wounds that are in difficult areas (moist, hairy), or wounds that are complicated by edema, infection, high tension, or bleeding.[67,68] Depending on the situation (size of wound, experience of the doctor with different wound closure techniques), liquid tissue adhesives can be more costly than conventional wound closure techniques.[52]

Laser Therapy

Laser-Assisted Tissue Bonding

Laser techniques to optimize wound healing and scar formation are a promising and highly investigated alternative to currently established procedures.[69] In laser tissue welding (LTW), the laser energy is directed to opposed wound margins, causing their partial liquefaction (conversion of photonic energy into heat energy), which is followed by their fusion.[52] In this process, collagen fibers from both sides of the wound are intertwined,[70] leading to an immediate wound seal, thereby promoting a faster reepithelialization without the need for a large formation of granulation tissue.[52,69]

In laser tissue soldering (LTS), a solder (a protective proteinaceous barrier such as a semisolid/solid serum albumin) is added to enhance the fusion of opposed wound margins.[71] Data suggest that the use of wavelength-specific dye absorbers such as indocyanine green and adhesive proteins such as albumin to LTW may lead to an increased strength and speed of wound closure than that achieved with traditional suture techniques.[71–73]

Laser-assisted tissue bonding is expected to be a fast and efficient technique for wound closure, potentially decreasing scar formation and complications associated with standard surgical alternatives.[52] LTS has shown very promising results in various tissues (e.g., skin, vessels) in animal models regarding strength and tissue quality.[73–75] Temperature-controlled LTS in rats showed comparable histologic and cosmetic results to those of standard sutures.[70] In a porcine model, the scars after LTS were almost undetectable 7 days following surgical skin incision.[75] A 2001 study compared the results of LTS with conventional suturing for hypospadias repair in 183 boys. The authors reported fewer complications (fistulas and stenosis) in the LTS group and concluded that LTS is an acceptable and faster method of tissue closure in hypospadias repair.[76] Furthermore, the reduced need for suture materials appeared to decrease local inflammation.[76] However, only a few studies regarding LTW and LTS have been conducted in humans.[52] The concerns of low tensile strength, the potential for excessive thermal damage to the skin, and the high costs of the equipment will likely exclude this technology from use in routine clinical practice.[52]

Laser-Assisted Scar Treatment

In addition to their applications in connecting wounded tissues, lasers are a promising treatment option for existing keloids and hypertrophic scars (see Chapter 13), though the mechanism of action of laser treatment is still not fully understood. Suggested mechanisms include the thermo-induced breakdown of collagen fibers as well as the mediation of growth factor expression.[77–81] In comparison with other treatment options such as intralesional 5-fluorouracil (5-FU) and corticosteroids for keloidal and hypertrophic scars, pulsed dye laser therapy has shown comparable results without side effects (see Chapter 10).[77,78] Argon lasers, the first lasers used in the treatment of keloids, were dismissed in favor of carbon dioxide, neodymium-doped yttrium aluminum garnet (Nd:YAG), and pulsed dye lasers because of unsatisfying results.[82] As a monotherapy for keloids and hypertrophic scars, nonfractionated carbon dioxide laser ablation was associated with recurrence rates of 90% and higher,[83,84] whereas the nonablative Nd:YAG laser showed recurrence rates of 17%.[85] Laser-assisted scar treatment also seems to be effective in treating associated symptoms like itching, redness, and pain.[77,86] A review article on the treatment of keloids and hypertrophic scars published in the *Journal of the American Medical Association* stated that pulsed dye lasers are an emerging therapeutic option owing to their high efficacy, yielding fewer adverse effects.[82]

Recently, using a picosecond pulse width infrared (IR) laser that targets tissue water, Amini-Nik et al.[87] demonstrated a significant reduction of thermal damage and scar formation compared with conventional lasers and scalpels.[87] In principle, the shorter pulse duration mitigates the destructive photochemical and photothermal effects associated with conventional devices with longer pulse widths.[87] This highlights the role that novel surgical modalities might have in minimizing scar formation. However, this study was performed in a rodent model, whose skin and wound healing properties differ from those of humans.[88]

Pharmacologic Optimization

To understand the pharmacologic targets involved in wound healing and hypertrophic/keloid scar treatment, it is important to have a basic knowledge of important molecular pathways and regulators involved. Those pathways are not isolated entities, instead more and more data reveal an extensive cross-link between them.[89]

Molecular Pathways Involved in Wound Healing and Scar Formation

Wnt/β-Catenin

Wnts are glycoproteins that are important in embryonic and adult tissue maintenance.[90–93] Depending on the context, Wnt ligands signal through either the canonical (mediated through β-catenin) or the noncanonical (independently of β-catenin) Wnt signaling pathway.[92,94] The focus here will be on the canonical Wnt pathway because it plays an important role in skin development and in various aspects of cutaneous wound repair.[2,89,95–97] Various Wnt glycoproteins (Wnt 1, 3, 4, 5a, and 10b) can be found in cutaneous wounds in the early phase of healing and are present up to 7 days after injury.[98,99]

In this signaling pathway, Wnt binds to the membrane receptor Frizzled and the coreceptor low-density lipoprotein receptor–related protein 5/6 (LRP5/6). Once bound, the protein Dishevelled is activated. Dishevelled inhibits a protein complex—consisting of glycogen synthase kinase 3β (GSK-3β), adenomatous polyposis coli protein (APC), casein kinase I, and axin 1—that is responsible for the ubiquitin-mediated degradation of β-catenin. Ultimately Wnt leads to an intracellular accumulation of β-catenin.[91–93] β-catenin itself is a transcriptional coactivator (bound to T-cell factors; Tcfs) for genes that encode important proteins for wound healing such as fibronectin,[90] but it also functions as a structural protein in the adherens junction that mediates cell–cell contacts[91,100] (see Fig. 9-1).

The Wnt pathway participates in the dermal accumulation of β-catenin, but it does not seem to be a key mechanism of maintaining it during wound healing.[101,102] β-catenin levels can be elevated independently of the Wnt pathway by TGF-β1, a growth factor excreted during early wound healing,[103–105] as well as by fibronectin, an ECM component, through a β1-integrin-mediated GSK-3β-dependent pathway.[101] β-catenin and its target genes are elevated in dermal fibroblasts during the proliferation phase of wound healing, and return to baseline levels during the remodeling phase.[106,107] In humans the duration and level of β-catenin activity correlate with wound size[108,109] and the number of macrophage cells present in the wound.[110] In an uncharacterized process, the Wnt pathway can reprogram or endow other epidermal cells. Ito et al.[97] showed that in large wounds the Wnt pathway pushes epithelial cells toward de novo folliculogenesis.

β-catenin is essential for adequate wound repair, though excessive expression is found in human hypertrophic scars and keloids.[107,108] A high amount and activity of β-catenin leads to an enlarged and hypercellular dermal compartment with an increased dermal collagen deposition, scarring, and myofibroblast formation.[103,111,112] Genetic mutations that cause an unphysiologic stabilization of β-catenin lead to aggressive fibromatosis (desmoid tumor).[113] Interestingly the Wnt/β-catenin pathway also seems to have an inhibitory effect: it decreases the reepithelialization after wounding. A nuclear accumulation of β-catenin has been found in the edge of chronic ulcers, and in vitro pharmacologic stabilization of β-catenin inhibited the migration of keratinocytes.[114]

β-catenin plays a significant role in various cells during the process of wound healing, but its role in macrophages seems to be essential.[110] In mice, it has been shown that β-catenin promotes motility and adhesion of macrophages[110] by upregulating the expression of cadherins, catenins, ADAMs (a disintegrin and metalloproteinase), and integrins.[110] Macrophages are believed to be an essential mediator of granulation tissue formation after skin trauma.[115–121] These cells express multiple receptors for Wnts,[110] and deficient macrophage migration and adhesion has been

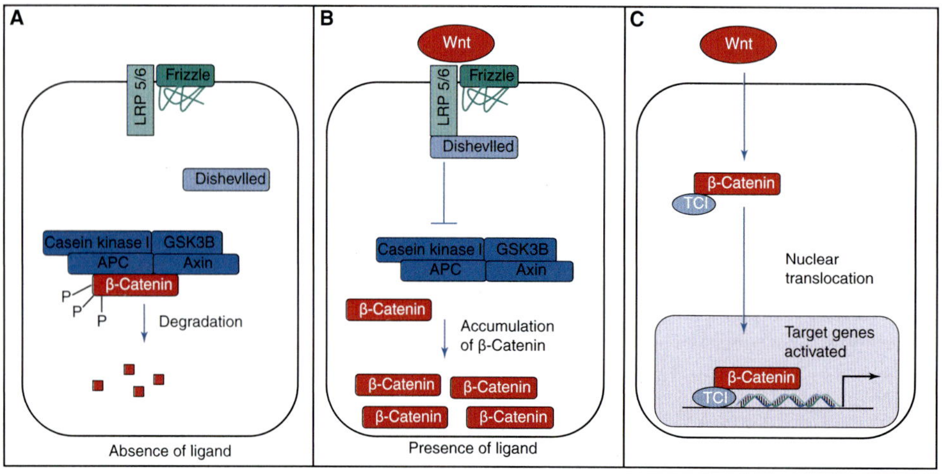

FIGURE 9-1 Wnt/β-catenin pathway. **A:** Without Wnt a protein complex (casein kinase1, GSK-3β, APC, and Axin) binds β-catenin and induces its degradation. **B:** Wnt binds to the receptor Frizzled and the coreceptor LRP5/6 which activates Dishevelled. Dishevelled inhibits the protein complex (casein kinase1, GSK-3β, APC, and Axin) and subsequently β-catenin accumulates in the cell. **C:** β-catenin, bound to Tcf, is translocated into the nucleus and activates the transcription of its target genes. LRP, low-density lipoprotein receptor–related protein; GSK, glycogen synthase kinase; APC, adenomatous polyposis coli; Tcf, T-cell factor.

associated with poor wound healing.[122] If macrophages lacked β-catenin, they also showed less TGF-β1 (a cytokine essential for wound healing; see below).[110] Furthermore, in the absence of β-catenin, macrophages were not able to achieve a fibroblast-like phenotype.[110] Scarless embryonic wound healing takes place in the absence of a fully developed monocyte lineage[118] and a less active Wnt signaling pathway.[123]

Manipulation of the Wnt/β-catenin signaling pathway and β-catenin activity could be a promising therapeutic approach in the treatment of deficient wound healing. Nefopam (5-methyl-1-phenyl-1,3,4,6-tetrahydro-2,5-benzoxazocine), a centrally acting nonopioid analgesic, reduced β-catenin levels to baseline even if the cells were highly stimulated with a Wnt ligand.[124] These cells showed a decrease in cell proliferation and viability in cell cultures derived from aggressive fibromatosis or hypertrophic wounds without affecting normal fibroblasts.[124] When this was used daily for 14 days in a murine model, there was a 50% reduction in scar diameter as compared with the control group. However, the exact mechanism of decreasing β-catenin levels and inhibiting fibroblast cell proliferation is unclear.[124] In a murine model a new laser—the picosecond IR laser—showed the ability to ablate tissue at a monocellular level, which causes less tissue trauma and less activation of the Wnt/β-catenin and TGF-β pathways.[87] It will be a future challenge to fully understand under which circumstances and in what amount Wnt/β-catenin regulation is beneficial in wound healing.

Growth Factors

In addition to the above-described Wnt/β-catenin pathway, various growth factors and cytokines such as fibroblast growth factors (FGFs), vascular endothelium growth factors (VEGFs), and interleukins (IL) have been linked to the process of wound healing; TGF-β is one of the crucial mediators.[2,125,126]

The TGF-β proteins consist of three isoforms—TGF-β1, TGF-β2, and TGF-β3—that are secreted by various cell types such as macrophages and fibroblasts.[126,127] Released as inactive precursors and adjacent to TGF-β binding protein, they require activation either through proteases or through conformational changes which are in part caused by cell traction forces of integrins.[9,127] Once activated, they are bound to TGF-β receptors. This initiates the formation of a SMAD complex (intracellular proteins that form a trimer of two receptor-regulated SMADs and one co-SMAD when they are activated by an extracellular stimulus) that acts as a transcription factor for various genes that encode important proteins for wound healing such as collagen (see Fig. 9-2).[9,10,127–129] TGF-β can also act through non-SMAD-dependent mechanisms including TGF-β-associated kinase I, mitogen-activated protein kinase, and GTPases, but the exact function of this pathway and its effect on wound healing are yet to be elucidated.[130,131]

The different isomers of the TGF-β superfamily have different effects on wound healing and scar formation (see Table 9-1). TGF-β1 promotes the proliferation of fibroblasts, their synthesis of collagen I and fibronectin as well as wound contraction, but inhibits keratinocyte migration and therefore wound reepithelialization[132–137,138]. TGF-β3 seems to have antiscarring effects, whereas TGF-β2 is required for hair follicle development.[11,139,140] Deficiencies in the TGF-β pathway lead to poor wound healing including a thin disorganized dermis, fewer fibroblasts, fibroblasts with cytoskeletal abnormalities, and a reduction of granulation tissue through reduced ECM deposition.[136,141–143] Interestingly, a deficiency in the TGF-β pathway also leads to smaller wound areas and less inflammation.[141,142]

The expression of TGF-β proteins by fibroblasts does not only affect keratinocytes in a unidirectional manner; rather, keratinocytes also have the ability to downregulate TGF-β1 secretion.[138,144] Excessive amounts of TGF-β1 lead to hypertrophic scars mediated either through the above-described β-catenin pathway or through connective tissue growth factor (CTGF; CCN2).[103,104,145–150] Topical

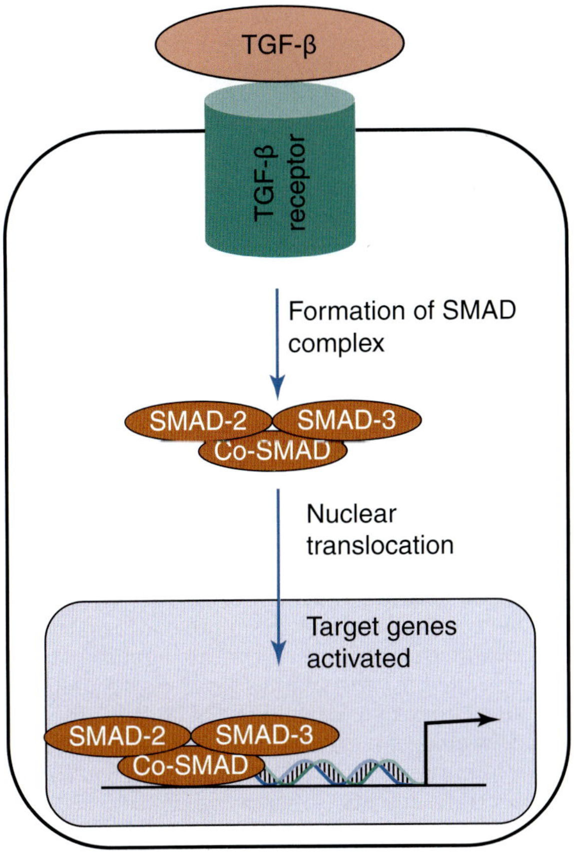

FIGURE 9-2 TGF-β pathway. Activated TGF-β binds to its receptor and leads to the formation of the SMAD complex (SMAD-2, SMAD-3, and Co-Smad). The SMAD complex is translocated into the nucleus and activates the transcription of its target gene.

TGF-β1 application on murine wounds causes accelerated healing and reepithelialization.[132] Interestingly, antagonizing TGF-β can also result in accelerated wound closure and increased keratinocyte proliferation and migration.[140,151,152] It seems to be of great importance at which exact point the TGF-β pathway is altered, suggesting a complex system of networks in this pathway that are yet to be elucidated.[2] In scarless embryonic wound healing, the ratio of TGF-β1 to TGF-β3 is lower as compared with what has been found in adults.[8,11,153] Applying TGF-β1 to embryonic wounds (in animal models) promotes scar formation, whereas TGF-β3 reduced it.[139,153] The promising results of wound treatment with tissue growth factor in animal models has led to various clinical trials. Despite positive preliminary data,[154] all of the clinical studies failed to establish a clinical benefit for TGF therapy in wound healing.[2,155–159] Additionally, TGF also contributes to the formation of hypertrophic scars.[105,160,161]

Table 9-1 Effects of TGF in Wound Healing and Scar Formation

TGF	Effect
β1	Proliferation of fibroblasts
	Production of collagen and fibronectin
	Wound contraction
	Inhibition of keratinocyte migration
β2	Hair follicle development
β3	Antiscarring

Today, only a few growth factors are approved for clinical treatment and their indications are very limited. Human recombinant platelet-derived growth factor-BB (PDGF-BB; becaplermin) is used for the treatment of chronic diabetic ulcers on the limbs. It led to a 15% increase in healing compared with standard wound care alone in those patients.[162–164] Health Quality Ontario stated that the efficacy of growth factors and granulocyte colony-stimulating factor (G-CSF) in enhancing the healing of chronic pressure ulcers has not been established yet.[165] PDGF (Regranex; approved by Health Canada for the treatment of diabetic ulcers on the lower extremities) was associated with an increased rate of deaths from cancer.[165] In Japan, FGF-2 is used postoperatively to reduce hypertrophy and widening of scars.[2] Next to its antiscarring effects,[166] FGF-2 showed promising results in the treatment of life-threatening, large disruptions of the skin integrity as in severe burns.[167]. More sophisticated, well-designed clinical trials will be necessary to evaluate the efficiency of growth factors in the treatment of wounds and scars.[125,168]

Hedgehog

The Hedgehog pathway plays important roles in embryonic skin development, angiogenesis, the regulation of epidermal stem cells, and the development of skin appendices in adults.[169–175] Among the three existing Hedgehog proteins—Indian Hedgehog (Ihh), Sonic Hedgehog (Shh), and Desert Hedgehog (Dhh)—Shh seems to be the main contributor to wound healing and scar formation.[169,176] Shh binds to Protein patched homolog (PTCH)—a transmembrane protein. PTCH is a tumor suppressor that prevents the activation of Gli transcription factors (see Fig. 9-3). Shh removes the inhibition of PTCH and activates Gli transcription factors that promote the encoding of a multitude of different proteins such as cyclin D2, a key regulator of the cell cycle.[169,176] The exact role of the Hedgehog pathway in wound healing and scar formation is relatively unknown.

Shh can be found in regenerated hair follicles after wounding, but not in the epidermis or keratinocytes.[177] Nevertheless, if diabetic mice are treated topically with Shh they show better reepithelialization and wound healing. The dermis is thicker, more collagen-rich, and better vascularized.[178] Shh stimulates the proliferation of fibroblasts and promotes the recruitment of bone marrow–derived endothelial progenitor cells and the excretion of VEGF.[178] If the Shh pathway is blocked, mice showed delayed wound healing, reduced granulation tissue formation, and decreased vascularization.[179]

Notch

The Notch pathway in mammals is activated by the binding of a transmembrane ligand (members of the Delta-like and Jagged families) to one of the four Notch receptors of an adjacent cell.[180–182] This binding causes the liberation of the Notch intracellular domain (NCID) by sequential

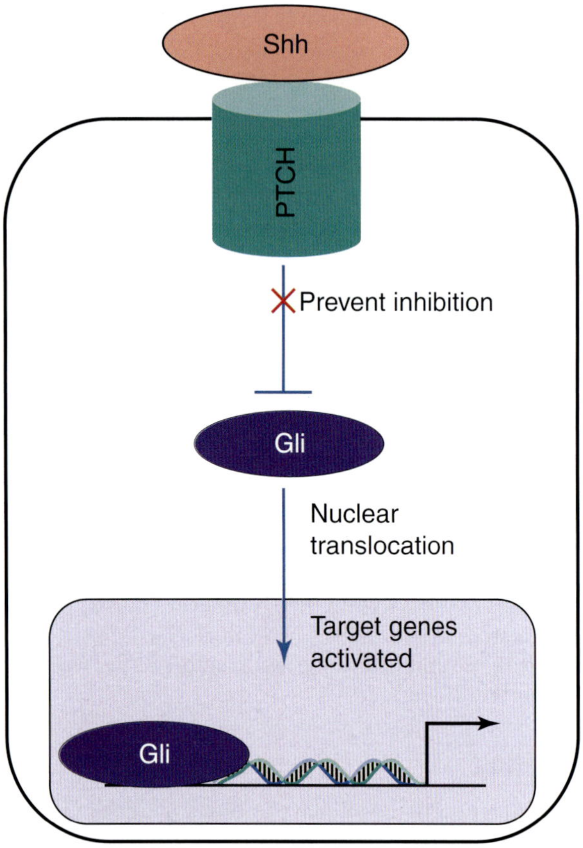

FIGURE 9-3 Sonic Hedgehog pathway. Shh binds to the tumor suppressor PTCH. By binding, Shh removes the inhibition of Gli and enables its translocation into the nucleus where it activates the transcription of target genes. Shh, Sonic Hedgehog; PTCH, Protein patched homolog; Gli, glioblastoma.

proteolytic cleavage. The NCID then translocates to the nucleus where it regulates gene expression (see Fig. 9-4).[180–182]

Notch plays a role in the development and maintenance of the epidermis and blood vessels.[180–183] It ensures the correct skin stratification during skin development.[183–185]

Downregulation of the Notch pathway leads to delayed wound healing, and stimulates increased wound closure in mice.[186] This might be because of an activating effect on the endothelial cells and the fibroblasts, increasing vascularization and collagen deposition.[186–188] In addition, recent data suggest that the Notch pathway promotes inflammatory activity by enhancing the recruitment of macrophages and the secretion of inflammatory cytokines.[187] However, the role of the Notch pathway in wound healing and scar formation is relatively unknown, as well as its impact on the different cell types contributing to this process (like macrophages, keratinocytes, and fibroblasts).[2]

Nonsteroidal Anti-inflammatory Drugs

Nonsteroidal anti-inflammatory drugs (NSAIDs) are the most widely used oral drugs to suppress inflammation.[189] They inhibit the activity of cyclooxygenase (COX), which is needed for the synthesis of prostaglandins and proinflammatory cytokines like IL-1β.[190,191] NSAIDs minimize swelling and pain by reducing the inflammatory response after skin injury.[192] Diclofenac also has a moderate antibacterial activity (in vitro and in vivo) because of its ability to inhibit DNA synthesis in bacteria.[193] Despite those positive aspects of NSAIDs, aspirin administration is associated with impaired wound healing.[194] Postoperative diclofenac treatment significantly inhibited collagen deposition in murine subcutaneous granulation tissue.[190] It has been postulated that NSAIDs decrease the degradation

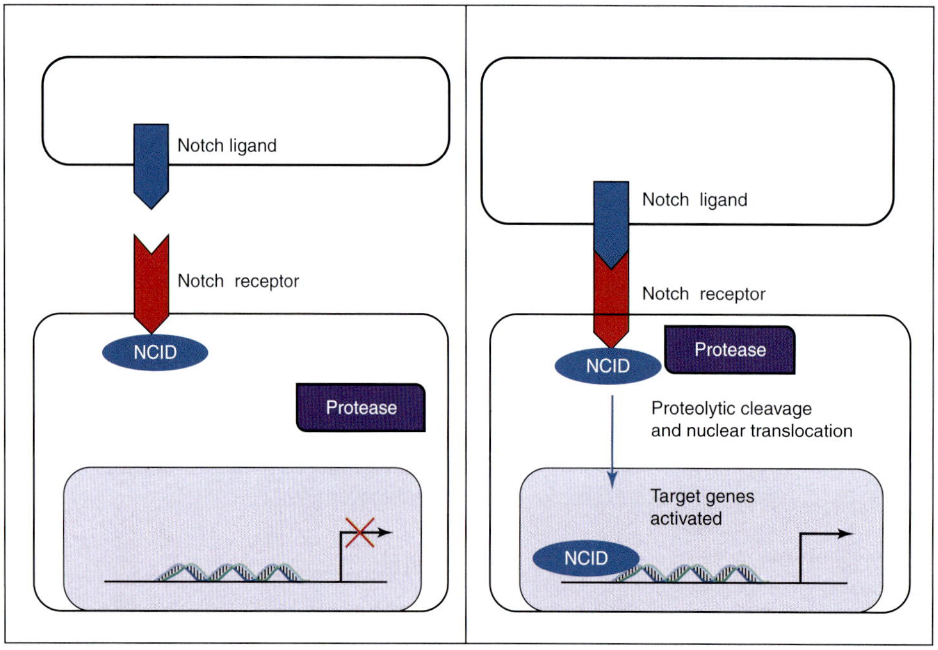

FIGURE 9-4 Notch pathway. Activation of the Notch receptor enables the translocation of NCID into the nucleus where it activates the transcription of its target genes. The left image shows a cell where the Notch receptor is not activated, the right one shows the intracellular process after binding of a Notch ligand. NCID, notch intracellular domain.

of collagen in the early phase of wound healing because of their anti-inflammatory properties and inhibition of matrix metalloproteinases (MMPs),[195–197] whereas they inhibit collagen synthesis in later stages.[196]

Antihistamines

Histamine is an important mediator of inflammatory skin reactions.[198–200] It is mainly released by basophils and mast cells.[200–202] The complex influence of histamine on the cellular and humoral immune system is not fully understood,[203] but studies suggest that it plays an important role in restoring the mechanical integrity of the skin barrier and in pathogen clearance at multiple levels.[204] Histamine-induced wound closure is mediated by all classic histamine receptors (HRs), with HR1 being the main one.[204]

If exposed to histamine, keratinocytes have shown an altered expression profile of multiple genes[204] including an upregulation of genes involved in the migration of epithelial cells like β5-integrin,[205] and a downregulation of the tumor suppressor gene p53.[204] This leads to a dose-dependent acceleration of reepithelialization in histamine-exposed keratinocytes.[204] Antagonizing HR1 results in delayed skin healing and reduces the breaking strength of collagen.[206] The antiproliferative and anti-inflammatory properties of HR1 antagonists[207,208] are promising for the potential treatment of keloidal and hypertrophic scars. Pheniramine, an antihistamine, reduced the proliferation and DNA and collagen synthesis rate in fibroblasts from abnormal scars, but also affected, to a lesser extent, fibroblasts from regular skin.[209] Tranilast, a histamine antagonist, reduced the synthesis of collagen in keloidal fibroblasts through suppression of the release of TGF-β1, but does not affect normal fibroblasts.[210] This drug is approved and has been used in Korea and Japan for the treatment of hypertrophic scars since 1993.[211]

Immune Suppressants and Modulators

Intralesional Steroid Injection

Intralesional steroid injection (triamcinolone acetonide suspension) has been considered a mainstay in the prophylaxis and treatment of hypertrophic and keloid scars for decades (see Chapter 10).[82] It leads to the degeneration of collagen bundles as well as to the inhibition of fibroblast growth.[212] In a 10-year follow-up study of keloid and hypertrophic scar patients, intralesional triamcinolone acetonide caused a 64% reduction in scar size and a 72% reduction in symptoms. Keloidectomy in combination with β-radiation showed a similar effect on the reduction of scar size (75%), whereas β-radiation alone was inferior to steroid injection and surgery (11% scar size reduction, 55% symptom control).[213]

Interferons

Interferons (INFs) are potent inhibitors of human fibroblast collagen production, with INF-γ being more potent than INF-α.[214] Intralesional injection of INF-γ used as a monotherapy led to a reduction in keloid size in 75% of patients.[215] As an adjunct to scar excision, INF-α reduced the recurrence rate of keloids from 58% to 19%.[216] Disadvantages of INF include adverse effects such as flu-like symptoms and high cost.[82]

Imidazoquinolines

Imidazoquinolines (imiquimod and resiquimod) are toll-like receptor (TLR) 7 and 8 agonists that induce key cytokines for wound healing like INF-α.[214,217] Data on the utility of topical application of imiquimod for the prevention of keloid recurrence after excision have been conflicting. The application of 5% imiquimod cream after[218] or before[219] surgical removal of keloids resulted in a good cosmesis and no recurrences at 4 and 12 months. However, less successful imiquimod treatment has also been reported. A study evaluating postsurgical administration of 5% imiquimod after surgical therapy of keloids of the trunk had a recurrence rate of 80% (8 out of 10).[220] In addition, pigmentary alteration is a common side effect.[218]

Fluorouracil

Fluorouracil inhibits fibroblast proliferation by blocking DNA synthesis through competitive inhibition of thymidylate synthase.[221] Intralesional injection of 5-FU has been reported to achieve a reduction of scar size of at least 50% in more than 75% of the treated patients.[222,223] A combination therapy of intralesional injection of 5-FU and triamcinolone acetonide paired with a pulsed laser dye treatment showed the highest success rate in a comparison of those three individual treatment modalities.[221] The most common adverse effects are pain, hyperpigmentation, and tissue sloughing.[82]

Bleomycin

Bleomycin as an intralesional injection is a common treatment for keloids and hypertrophic scars. The exact mechanism of this drug on fibroblasts is not fully understood. It directly inhibits collagen synthesis in skin fibroblasts in vitro, even under stimulation with TGF-β1.[224] Bleomycin induces apoptosis and reduces lysyl oxidase, an enzyme that is essential for collagen maturation.[225,226] When administered intralesionally to hypertrophic/keloidal scars that were unresponsive to steroid treatment, 73% of the treated patients (11 out of 15) showed complete regression of scar size with a significant reduction in associated symptoms.[227] Systemic adverse effects are uncommon with intralesional use.[82] Local side effects include hypo- and hyperpigmentation as well as moderate skin atrophy.[228]

Methotrexate

Methotrexate inhibits the enzyme dihydrofolate reductase that is essential for DNA synthesis.[229] Topical methotrexate has been reported for the prophylaxis of keloid formation after syndactyly release, and for suppression of recurrence during revision surgery for keloids.[230] No significant adverse effects after topical application were noted in a follow-up period of 10 years.[230]

Mitomycin C

Mitomycin C causes alkylation and cross-linkage of the DNA strands, inhibiting their replication.[231] As a topical treatment, mitomycin C shows very promising results in vitro and in clinical trials. In an in vitro study, human keloid fibroblasts showed decreased density and DNA synthesis in the first 3 weeks following mitomycin C exposure.[232] After surgical excision of head and neck keloids in 10 patients, only 1 recurrence was noted after topical mitomycin C was applied.[231] In another study evaluating subjective patient satisfaction, only 1 out of 10 patients was disappointed by the cosmetic outcome after surgical excision plus mitomycin C.[233] Despite those good results, other studies failed to achieve a reliable reduction of hypertrophic scars and keloids. In a study including eight patients evaluating combined surgical therapy followed by topical mitomycin C application, a complete recurrence could only be seen in two cases.[234] Interestingly, all patients were satisfied with the results. In another study including 15 patients, mitomycin C had no beneficial effect on recurrence when applied after surgical excision.[235] These contradictory results may be in part because of the limited number of patients, short follow-up periods, and great variance in dosing and application interval of mitomycin C.[236]

Studies on a large patient collective systematically comparing immune-modulatory and immune-suppressive drugs for the treatment of keloids and hypertrophic scars are lacking. In addition, treatment benefits of each drug are not clear. More studies need to be conducted until a definitive statement about the efficacy or a possible superiority of these drugs can be made.

Other Drugs and Topical Agents

The need to improve wound healing and ultimately scar formation has nourished vast research for new pharmaceuticals and bioactive agents.[236,237] The following focuses only on a few specific reagents.

Silver Sulfadiazine

A meta-analysis from 2012 published in the *British Journal of Medicine*[238] concludes that the use of silver sulfadiazine cream for burn wounds should be avoided because of wound healing delays (because of toxic effects on regenerating keratinocytes), increased infection rates, and increased pain[239–241]

Growth- and Colony-Stimulating Factors

G-CSF, administered subcutaneously or intravenously,[242] along with hyaluronic acid derivative[243] showed a clear benefit in the treatment of complex surgical wounds. However, a systematic review published in 2009 by Health Quality Ontario found that the efficacy of growth factors and G-CSF in enhancing the healing of chronic pressure ulcers has not yet been established.[165]

Honey

Honey applied topically onto wounds was strongly associated with a reduction in wound healing time compared with film or gauze-based dressings for burns.[244] However, the use of honey-containing dressings in contaminated wounds led to an increase in the local bacterial burden, in comparison to iodine- or silver-containing dressings.[245]

Tamoxifen

Tamoxifen citrate, a selective estrogen receptor modulator used in the treatment of breast cancer, has shown promising results in the treatment of keloids and hypertrophic scars.[246,247] The effect is thought to be because of a down-regulation in TGF-β, though the exact mechanism of action remains to be discovered.[248,249]

Several other agents have been investigated for the treatment of keloids and hypertrophic scars including IL-10, calcium channel blockers, mannose-6-phosphate, calcineurin inhibitors, and retinoids. However, none can be definitively advocated because results are either inconclusive, contradictory, or nonapplicable for clinical use because they lack sufficient power.[236] Additional studies are needed to extensively evaluate these agents in regard to their efficacy, practicability, side effects, and cost-effectiveness.[236,237]

Nutrition and Additives

A key factor to achieve optimal wound healing is adequate nutrition.[250–256] Malnourished patients are at a higher risk of pressure ulcers, delayed wound healing, and wound site infections.[251] The proliferation of fibroblasts, collagen formation, complement and antibody levels, T-cell function, and angiogenesis can all be impaired in a malnourished state.[250,256]

Updated information and current guidelines on correct nutrition and dosing of additives can be found at the webpage of The American Society for Parenteral and Enteral Nutrition: *https://www.nutritioncare.org*. The following section highlights the most important nutrients and additives for optimal wound healing. Table 9-2 gives an overview.

Caloric Intake

The American Society for Parenteral and Enteral Nutrition and the Wound Healing Society recommend a caloric intake of 30 to 35 kcal/kg/d for optimal wound healing.[251,257] If underweight, an increase of caloric intake up to 35 to 40 kcal/kg/d is suggested.[251,257,258] Geriatric or obese patients need an individualized nutrition plan.[259] Stratton et al.[252] have shown in their 2005 published meta-analysis that oral nutrition supplements (250 to 500 kcal per serving) given over 2 to 26 weeks were associated with a 25% reduction in the incidence of pressure ulcer development in at-risk patients (elderly, postsurgical, long-term care patients) when compared with standard care.

Vitamins

Multivitamin **preparations** with minerals are recommended for patients with large wounds, and if deficiencies are confirmed or suspected.[251,259,260] In particular, vitamins A and C play a key role in wound healing. **Vitamin A** improves wound healing by increasing collagen deposition and promoting epithelialization, along with its important

Table 9-2 Special Recommendations for Patients with Chronic Wounds According to the American Society for Parenteral and Enteral Nutrition; http://www.nutritioncare.org

Calories	30–35 kcal/kg/d	Adjustment for under/overweight and geriatric patients
Proteins	1.25–1.5 g/kg/d	Adjustment according to the protein loss over the wound
Fluids	30 mL/kg/d or 1–1.5 mL/kcal consumed	Adjustment according to the fluid loss over the wound
Vitamins	Standard multivitamin preparations with trace elements and minerals • **Vitamin C:** 100–200 mg/d PO (moderate wounds); 1,000–2,000 mg/d PO (severe wounds) • **Vitamin A:** 10,000–50,000 International Units/d PO or 10,000 International Units IM for 10 d	
Amino acids **Fatty acids**	Individual decision, no general recommendations	

role in stimulation of the local immune system.[250,253,259] Supplementation is recommended in patients with comorbidities including diabetes, tumors, radiation and in acute or chronic wounds.[250,259] Common dosages range from 10,000 to 50,000 International Units per day orally or 10,000 International Units intramuscularly for 10 days.[250,260–262] Interestingly, vitamin A has the potential to reverse the delayed wound healing in patients taking steroids by modifying the immune system.[250] For patients receiving corticosteroids, oral administration of 10,000 to 15,000 International Units per day of vitamin A is recommended to enhance wound healing.[259]

Vitamin C plays a key role in the synthesis of collagen.[259,260] If the patient suffers from vitamin C deficiency or has moderate chronic wounds such as stage 1 and 2 pressure ulcers, supplementation with 100 to 200 mg per day orally is recommended.[259,261] If wounds are more severe as in stage 3 and 4 pressure ulcers and severe trauma, 1,000 to 2,000 mg per day orally has been suggested until healing occurs.[259,261] High doses of vitamin C may cause the formation of kidney stones.[251]

Proteins

Adequate protein intake is vital for wound healing because it is required for the proliferation of cells and collagen, for the formation of connective tissue, and for the synthesis of enzymes involved in wound healing.[250,252,258,260,263–269] The requirement for exogenous protein in healthy adults is 0.8 and 1 g/kg/d in older people.[253,256,259] The recommended protein intake in the healing of chronic wounds is 1.25 to 1.5 g/kg/d.[256,259] In severely catabolic patients with more than one chronic wound, the protein requirements may even be higher.[256,259] A protein intake of 2 g/kg/d or higher may be associated with dehydration and should be monitored carefully.[250,259]

Amino and Fatty Acids

There are no evidence-based guidelines addressing the safe use and dosage of amino acids, especially arginine and glutamine for improved healing of wounds.[257,259,270,271] Arginine is contained in standard tube-feeding formulas,[259,272] and additional supplementation is only recommended if a depletion of body stores is suspected.[250] It is a substrate for protein synthesis and collagen deposition.[250] Glutamine is essential for gluconeogenesis, synthesis of other amino acids, and synthesis of nucleotides needed for optimal functioning of fibroblasts and epithelial cells.[250,259] The influence of different fatty acids on wound healing has not been elucidated sufficiently to give any recommendations.[250,258,259,273]

Micronutrients

Trace elements and micronutrients (e.g., copper, zinc, magnesium) are critical to cell metabolism, especially during wound healing.[250,259,260] A dose of 5 to 10 times the recommended daily allowance is usually suggested until protein–energy malnutrition is resolved.[256,259,260]

Physical Optimization

Ultrasound Therapy

Noncontact low-frequency ultrasound (NLFU) at 20 to 40 kHz has been shown in preclinical studies to reduce bacteria and pseudomonas biofilm on the wound, to upregulate VEGF, and downregulate proinflammatory cytokines such as IL-1β, IL-8, and MMPs.[274,275] NLFU has been shown to be a useful adjunctive in the treatment of chronic[276–278] and acute[279] wounds.

NLFU treatment on skin graft donor sites resulted in a better quality of healing, an accelerated healing time, reduced pain and itching as well as less wound site infections.[279] In diabetic leg/foot ulcers NLFU was found to be more effective than standard treatment alone.[276] However, a 2015 single-center, assessor-blinded, and randomized controlled trial conducted in 36 patients with venous leg ulcers could not detect a statistically significant advantage for the addition of NLFU to standard wound care.[280] The authors concluded that this might be because of the small patient collective and the short follow-up time of only 90 days.

Cryotherapy

In the treatment of hypertrophic/keloid scars, cryotherapy is less favored than other treatment modalities because of its association with postinterventional hypopigmentation and pain.[82] Despite its side effects, cryotherapy has shown variable efficacy in reducing scar size. One study using a liquid nitrogen spray has found a 73% success rate (48 out of 65 patients) in terms of scar size reduction,[281] whereas another study evaluating 93 patients found a response rate of only 32%.[282]

Scar Massage

Scar massage has two main effects: *reflex effects* (muscle relaxation, decrease in pain, and an overall sense of well-being because of stimulation of the afferent peripheral nerves) and *mechanical effects* (improvement in venous return, lymphatic drainage, and movement between muscle fibers).[283] There is growing evidence that scar massage leads to a clinically relevant improvement not only of pain, itching, and pliability of scars, but also of mood and anxiety of patients.[283–286] It is shown that massage therapy in postburn hypertrophic scars improves depression, pruritus, and appearance (measured by the Vancouver Scar Scale).[287] After operative therapy of bilateral cleft lip, scar massage therapy showed beneficial results in terms of oral range of motion, muscle strength, and adhesions.[288] Moreover, a patient's subjective perception of the scar improved.[288] Possible adverse effects include irritation from friction and irritant or contact dermatitis from the lubricant used for massage.[289] On a molecular level, in vitro studies suggest that mechanical strain has antifibrotic properties by reducing CTGF expression in fibroblasts,[290] as well as tumor necrosis factor (TNF)-α,[291] along with an increase in apoptosis.[291] However, there are no clear guidelines on which massage technique to use, when to start, and on the duration of the treatment.[283,292,293]

Electromagnetic Therapy

Pulsed electromagnetic field therapy (PEMFT) uses low-frequency magnetic waves such as sine waves with a frequency of 50 or 60 Hz to stimulate a tissue or area of interest.[294] It can promote wound healing by increasing angiogenesis promoting factors (angiopoietin-2 and VEGF) as well as fibroblast promoting factors (FGF-2). Furthermore, it can reduce inflammation via downregulation of proinflammatory cytokines such as TNF, IL-1β, and nuclear factor κB.[295–301] Ferroni et al.[302] described an increase in fibroblastic activity and keratinocyte differentiation in an in vitro model of 3D artificial skin.

PEMFT has shown to accelerate wound healing and improve microcirculation in patients with chronic diabetic foot[303] and venous leg ulcers.[304] The depth of the venous ulcers and their recurrence rates could be significantly reduced with this therapy.[305,306] However, a Cochrane database review published in 2010 could not find strong evidence supporting PEMFT in the treatment of pressure ulcers and called for more and higher powered studies.[307] Various clinical studies are currently evaluating PEMFT in regard to fracture[308,309] and skin wound[307,310] healing.

Pressure Therapy

The mechanism of pressure or occlusive dressings is not fully understood, but it is suggested that scar hydration and pressure promote collagen breakdown by decreasing α-macroglobulin (inhibitor of collagenase) and by causing apoptosis via vasoconstriction-induced hypoxia.[311,312] Pressure therapy is widely used in the treatment of hypertrophic and keloidal scars (see Chapter 19).[313] In hypertrophic scars of burn patients, pressure therapy led to an apoptotic decrease in myofibroblasts responsible for wound contracture, and to a partial restoration of the disorganized ECM to the phenotype of a regular, nonhypertrophic scar (e.g., elastin formed patch deposits in untreated hypertrophic scars, whereas under pressure therapy it was organized in fibers).[312] A 2005 published study compared silicone cushions (pressure therapy) with silicone gel (occlusive dressing) and found that pressure therapy alone reduced symptoms in 74% of the patient collective while achieving a complete reduction of the hypertrophic/keloid scar in 26% over an 8-month period. Occlusive dressings have shown a reduction of symptoms in 52% and a resolution of excessive scar tissue in 22%.[313] Four-layer bandages,[314,315] multilayer stockings,[314] compression bandages,[289,316] and elastic high compression[289] were found to be more effective in treating complex wounds (venous ulcers) than standard wound care. Four-layer bandages consisting of orthopedic wool, cotton crepe, elastic bandage, and cohesive bandage have shown to be more effective in treating mixed venous and arterial ulcers than other compression systems.[314]

It is recommended to use pressure therapy/dressings to reduce scar height and erythema for 23 hours per day for 12 months at a pressure of 20 to 30 mm Hg, with dressing changes every 2 to 3 months.[317] Despite the low costs and the few side effects, pressure dressings may cause a restriction in movement leading to a reduction in patient compliance.[82]

Radiation Therapy

The use of radiation to treat hypertrophic scars and keloids is very controversial because of two factors: (1) radiation is a potential carcinogen, especially in sensitive regions like breast and thyroid,[82] (2) the efficacy of this treatment varies greatly among the published studies.[213] Based on literature, no definitive conclusion can be made regarding the safety and the efficacy of this treatment.

A 10-year follow-up study found that the use of β-radiation, which involves high-energy and high-speed electrons that are emitted during the radioactive decay of a nucleus, showed an improvement of 55% in symptoms, but only a 11% success rate in the reduction of scar size. If β-radiation was applied within 48 hours after surgical excision of the hypertrophic/keloid scar, a success rate of 75% in the reduction of the initial size could be achieved.[213]

Hyperbaric Oxygen

In hyperbaric oxygen therapy (HBOT), the patient is placed in a sealed chamber where 100% oxygen is pressurized to 1.5 to 3 atm for 60 to 120 minutes.[318] HBOT increases the arterial oxygen pressure, which leads to an arterial vasoconstriction and subsequently to a reduction of capillary pressure.[318] Fluid absorption into the venous system is increased, and therefore HBOT reduces wound edema in addition to hyper-oxygenating the blood.[318] This additional oxygenation is believed to promote tissue repair in the wound where perfusion is impaired.[318] More recent studies also suggest a positive role of HBOT in neovascularization by increasing the number of first-endothelial progenitor cells.[319,320] The main adverse effects of this therapy include discomfort, claustrophobia, and neurologic oxygen toxicity.[318]

HBOT is used mainly as a supplementary method for treating complex wounds.[321] It significantly improves healing rates and decreases wound size in diabetic foot and venous ulcers compared with standard wound care.[322,323,324] A 2004 published Cochrane analysis including 147 patients with diabetic foot ulcers showed a significant reduction in the rates of major amputations, as well as an increase in the number of wounds that remained healed 1 year after treatment with HBOT in comparison to standard care.[322] The same analysis also showed the beneficial effect of HBOT in the treatment of venous ulcers in 16 patients regarding the reduction of wound size. HBOT also seems to be superior in the treatment of lower-extremity wounds compared with standard treatment.[322] Two additional studies in patients with diabetic foot ulcers also confirmed the superiority of HBOT therapy in comparison to standard wound care.[323,324] However, the exact mechanism of action of HBOT still remains unclear and therefore more studies are needed.[318]

The role of HBOT in the treatment of keloids and hypertrophic scars is less clear. In vitro HBOT decreased collagen production and fibroblast proliferation—one of the main problems in pathologic scar formation.[325] TGF-β and insulin-like growth factor type 1, the main mitogens during wound healing believed to contribute to hypertrophic scarring and keloid formation, were reduced through HBOT.[321] In vivo experiments could replicate those positive in vitro results. In rabbits HBOT was able to significantly inhibit hyperplastic scarring of the ear when exposed to hyperbaric oxygen for 1 hour daily until wound closure took place.[326] However, to date there is not enough evidence in literature to support the standard usage of HBOT in the treatment of hypertrophic scars and keloids.

Dressings

Improvements in technology and in the understanding of wound healing have led to an enormous expansion of commercially available wound dressing products.[240] The overall purpose of dressings, especially for larger wounds, is to prevent the loss of fluids and proteins from the wound site, to create an environment that favors granulation tissue formation and reepithelialization, and thus reduce the risk of subsequent bacterial infection and tissue damage.[327,328]

Table 9-3 gives an overview of the most commonly used dressings in the treatment of wounds and scars.

Table 9-3 Overview of Wound Dressings Used to Optimize Wound Healing and Scar Formation; Product Brand Names Are Only Exemplary

Dressing	Brand Name (Exemplary)	Key Characteristics	Picture
Negative pressure dressing	• **PICO**, Renasys (Smith & Nephew) • Invia Motion (Medela)	• Reduces wound edema and seroma • Promotes granulation tissue formulation and neovascularization • Removes wound secretions	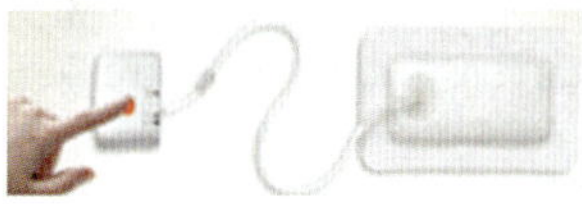
Hydrocolloid dressing	• **Comfeel** (Coloplast) • DuoDerrn (ConvaTec)	• Creates moist environment • Absorbs wound secretions • Promotes autolytic debridement	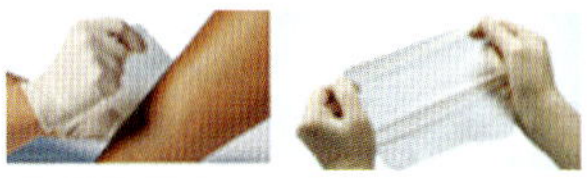
Hydrogel dressing	• **NuGel** (Systagenix) • Intrasite Gel (Smith & Nephew)		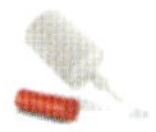
Silicone gel dressings (Silicone gel sheeting)	• **Cica-Care** (Smith & Nephew) • Epi-Derm (Biodermis)	• Reduces excessive collagen production	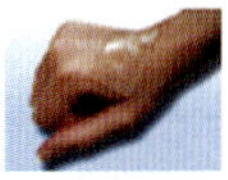
Polyurethane film dressing	• **Opsite** (Smith & Nephew) • Tegaderm (3M)	• Permeable for oxygen and vapor but not for liquids • Creates moist environment • Promotes autolytic debridement	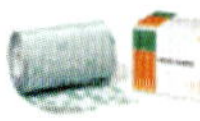
Silicone-coated nylon dressing	• **Mepithel** (Mölnlycke Health Care) • Jelonet (Smith & Nephew)	• Nonadherent dressing layer to enable frequent dressing changes	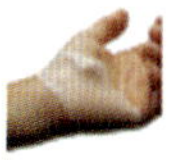
Antimicrobial dressing (silver or iodine)	• **Mepilex Ag** (Mölnlycke Health Care) • Inadine (Systagenix)	• Minimize wound infections	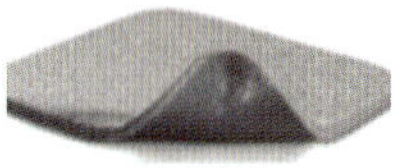

Negative-Pressure Dressings

Negative pressure is used in the treatment of chronic and complex wounds worldwide, with various studies confirming its efficacy.[329–332] Negative-pressure wound therapy (NPWT) has been shown to reduce wound edema[333,334] and the prevalence of postsurgical seromas[335] and to enhance the formation of granulation tissue along with neovascularization.[333,336–339] In the treatment of complex wounds, NPWT is superior to standard wound care.[329,340] A case report has shown beneficial effects of NPWT in a preterm neonate subjected to emergency abdominal surgery, underscoring the advantages of this technique with respect to wound closure and decreased need for dressing changes.[341]

Granulation tissue synthesis is believed to be caused by an upregulation of FGF-2,[342,343] TGF-β, and PDGF.[341,344,345] NPWT applies a mechanical strain to the underlying cells.[346] This physical force activates mechanoreceptors,[347,348] which results in ECM synthesis.[349] A key mediator of the mechanoreceptor pathway and NPWT efficacy is the transcription factor early growth response (EGR)-1, which increases the expression of VEGF, PDGF, TGF-β, and FGF-2.[350–354] However, in some studies NPWT did not show any effect on those factors.[344,355] Negative pressure on the wound bed reduces the underlying blood flow.[356] Hypoxic fibroblasts are believed to upregulate hypoxia-inducible factor (HIF)-1.[357,358] This promotes the encoding of proteins that increase collagen deposition and its alignment,[359] in addition to upregulating VEGF and FGF expression.[359] The role of HIF-1 is controversial because it was also shown that it also can be downregulated by NPWT.[360]

Neovascularization under NPWT seems to be facilitated by a significant elevation in VEGF.[355,362] However, a 2005 published study could not detect any effect of NPWT on VEGF expression.[364] Following NPWT in human traumatic wounds, an increase in local IL-8 was detected.[362] This chemokine is known to play an important role in regulating macrophage and neutrophil migration in addition to being a proangiogenetic factor.[364,365] NPWT also has anti-inflammatory properties: It reduces the expression of TNF[366,367] and proinflammatory cytokines such as IL-1β and IL-10.[344,361,366,367] No conclusive results exist for IL-6, a major proinflammatory cytokine.[344,355,362]

The latest Cochrane meta-analysis concluded that there is no rigorous evidence regarding the clinical effectiveness of NPWT in surgical wound healing by secondary intention.[368,369] The role of NPWT in treating burn wounds also remains unclear because of insufficient evidence.[371] Despite the positive effects of NPWT on wound healing, excessive formation of granulation tissue can result in thick and poorly compliant scar tissue.[334,371] Foam-based NPWT seems to result in thicker scar formation than gauze-based NPWT, but the underlying mechanism is yet to be discovered.[371] In terms of the treatment of hypertrophic scars and keloids, only little data of poor quality are available for NPWT such as a clinical study involving two patients that showed a better scar appearance and thickness after 1 month of NPWT treatment.[373] More studies will be needed to establish the use of this therapy for the treatment of hypertrophic scars and keloids.

Hydrocolloid and Hydrogel Dressings

The term hydrocolloid dressing is commonly used for two different products. The first are fibrous dressings, the true hydrocolloid dressings (e.g., Comfeel, DuoDerm), that have a hydrogel-forming component such as sodium carboxymethyl cellulose. Absorption of wound secretions causes the gel formation.[240,373] Some formulations contain alginate to increase absorption capabilities (e.g., Algosteril, Comfeel Alginate Dressing). The exchange of calcium ions from the dressing with sodium ions from the wound causes gel formation in these materials.[240] The second products are dressings that use an existing amorphous hydrogel (e.g., IntraSite, Nu-Gel) consisting of insoluble polymers such as modified carboxymethyl cellulose or pectin.[240] Both groups of dressings enable the absorption of wound fluids and promote autolytic debridement of the wound.

A systematic review published in 2009 by Health Quality Ontario found hydrocolloid dressings in the treatment of pressure ulcers to be associated with nearly a three-fold increase in complete wound healing, as compared with saline gauze (=standard wound care).[165] However, the same review found that hydrogel and hydropolymer are more efficacious than hydrocolloid dressings in the treatment of pressure ulcers.[165] A 2015 meta-analysis concluded that it is unclear if the treatment of pressure ulcers with hydrogel dressings is more or less effective than other treatments.[374] For diabetic foot/leg ulcers, hydrogel dressings were an effective alternative to standard care.[375] In a meta-analysis comparing hydrocolloid dressings with standard care for the treatment of complex wounds, hydrocolloid dressings were more effective.[376]

In superficial and partial thickness burns, hydrocolloids did not show any advantage in healing time, pain, or wound site infections in comparison to chlorhexidine-impregnated paraffin gauze dressing with[377] or without[378,379] the additional use of silver sulfadiazine. However, patients and doctors favored the subjective appearance of the wound after the use of hydrocolloid dressings.[379] In comparison to the use of silver sulfadiazine alone, hydrocolloids resulted in less pain for the patient and a shorter healing time.[380] Recent data suggest that hydrocolloid dressings may be superior to the commonly used paraffin-based gauze (Jelonet; see below), resulting in a decreased need for debridement and grafting.[381] Moreover, they seem to accelerate the healing of partial thickness burns.[240] In two studies hydrogel dressings, compared with standard wound care (basic wound contact dressings), showed either a statistically significant shorter healing time[382] or a trend that supports this assertion.[383] In addition, less pain was reported in the hydrogel group.[382]

The relative similarity of alginate dressings to the ECM makes them an ideal material for wound dressings, and for the delivery of bioactive agents (e.g., G-CSF[384] or silver sulfadiazine[385]) and cell transplantation.[384] A 2015 Cochrane analysis concluded that the effects of alginate dressings in the treatment of pressure ulcers as compared with alternative treatments are unclear, and that they should be used after considering their costs and their wound management properties.[386] A systematic review published in 2009 by Health Quality Ontario found that in deeper ulcers (stage III and IV), the use of alginate with hydrocolloid resulted in significantly greater reduction in the size of the ulcers as compared with hydrocolloid alone.[165]

Occlusive Dressings

The creation of a moist environment via occlusive or hydrocolloid dressings has been employed for almost 30 years to treat and prevent hypertrophic scars and keloids.[387] Although the mechanism of action is not fully understood, the clinical efficacy has been shown in various studies.[388,389] However, those studies vary in the extent of the efficacy of this treatment. During wound healing the newly forming tissue is more permeable to water until the reepithelialization is complete. This leads to a dehydration of the wound site. Keratinocytes in the dehydrated area stimulate collagen production in the surrounding fibroblasts, promoting scar formation. By maintaining sufficient hydration of the wound via hydrocolloid and occlusive dressings, excessive collagen production can be (partially) prevented.[388,389]

Silicone dressings (silicone gel sheeting; e.g., CicaCare, Epi-Derm) are recommended as the first-line treatment for scar management, followed by intralesional corticosteroid injection.[390] They have been shown to affect basic scar parameters such as size and texture, and scar-related discomfort such as itching and pain; several studies also reported favorable effects regarding scar color.[389,391–394] However, not all of those effects could be detected reliably at the same time. For example, a randomized controlled trial involving 20 patients compared a 2-month treatment period of occlusive silicone dressings (silicone sheet dressing) versus over-the-counter moisturizer (Eucerin). Silicone dressings were found to be superior in reducing scar itching and erythema. However, there was no difference noted in pain or physical features such as thickness.[395] The main limitations of those dressings is patient compliance, because they have to be worn over a longer period of time and can lead to discomfort, especially in warmer climates.[390,396]

See also section "Pressure therapy" in this chapter.

Polyurethane Film Dressings

Polyurethane film dressings (e.g., OpSite, Tegaderm) are transparent wound dressings that are permeable to water vapor, oxygen, and carbon dioxide, but not to liquid water or bacteria.[240] By keeping the wound moist, these products aid wound debridement and promote a favorable wound healing environment.[240] Surgical wounds covered with polyurethane film dressings have a lower risk for infection, blistering, and erythema compared with standard wound care with gauze and tape.[397] The slightly higher costs were outweighed by the reduction in the treatment cost of possible complications occurring in standard care.[397] In partial thickness burns they showed a faster healing time and caused less pain for the patient, though no effects on wound site infection were observed; the available evidence is of poor quality.[240,398] Compared with paraffin gauze dressing, polyurethane film dressings were not superior in terms of wound healing, patient satisfaction, wound site infection, and pain in partial thickness burns.[399]

Polyurethane dressings, similar to hydrocolloid and occlusive dressings, create a moist environment that reduces excessive collagen deposition (see previous section about hydrocolloid and hydrogel dressings). Few studies are available that compare polyurethane dressings with hydrocolloid/occlusive dressings or that look at their effects on hypertrophic scars and keloids. A 12-week clinical trial evaluating the effects of polyurethane versus silicone dressings on hypertrophic scars found that both were highly effective in reducing scar thickness and associated discomfort.[400] Polyurethane dressings, however, were statistically more effective and better tolerated by the patients. Dressings worn only overnight (12 hours) showed the same results as when used continuously for 24 hours for an 8-week period.[401]

Silicone-Coated Nylon Dressings

Silicone-coated nylon dressings (e.g., Mepitel, Jelonet) consist of a flexible polyamide net coated with soft silicone.[240] If applied to an open wound, it allows for the drainage of wound secretions and acts as a nonadherent dressing layer—enabling frequent dressing changes without causing damage to the wound.[240]

Compared with hydrocolloid dressings, silicone-coated dressings seem to be inferior with respect to the need for debridement and grafting.[381] In the treatment of complex wounds such as venous leg ulcers, Jelonet did not provide a significant advantage in comparison with hydrocolloid dressings.[402] Moreover hydrocolloid dressings showed a trend of increased healing rates, whereas silicone-coated dressings did not.[402] In a clinical phase III study including 167 patients, Jelonet alone was inferior to Jelonet combined with Repithel, a povidone–iodine-containing liposomal hydrogel, in the treatment of split-thickness skin grafts.[403] Jelonet is the most commonly used burn dressing worldwide.[381] Silicone-coated nylon dressings were superior to silver sulfadiazine dressings regarding the healing time of partial thickness burn wounds, along with an improvement in pain during and in between dressing changes.[240,404,405] It has to be mentioned that overall cost was almost twice that of standard wound care.[404]

Antimicrobial Dressings

Antimicrobial dressings most commonly contain silver (e.g., Contreet, Mepilex) or iodine (Inadine, Iodoflex) materials that are thought to minimize the risk of invasive wound site infections by reducing microbial wound colonization.[240]

Iodine- and silver-containing dressings have been shown to significantly reduce the local bacteria burden in heavily contaminated wounds.[245] Silver dressings improved wound healing and reduced odor, pain-related symptoms, and wound exudates as compared with standard wound care in a meta-analysis including 1,399 patients.[406] In a multicenter clinical evaluation of 126 patients with various wounds (acute and complex/chronic), the use of silver dressings led to an improvement in the condition of wound tissue and the surrounding skin, with a significant reduction in wound site infections and wound exudates.[407]

However, there was no clear superiority of antimicrobial dressings compared with standard wound care in terms of overall complete healing.[245] Healing time, on the other hand, seems to be improved by these dressings.[408] There is doubt concerning the long-term cost-effectiveness of antimicrobial dressings[409] and they cause more unpleasant local side effects when compared with standard care.[410,411] Further research is required before definitive conclusions can be made about the effectiveness of topical antimicrobial agents/dressings.[165,245]

Skin Substitutes

Skin substitutes provide mechanical coverage and bacterial protection and allow gas and fluid exchange while reepithelialization takes place.[240,318] Skin substitutes are either acellular or contain incorporated cells to further facilitate wound closure and reepithelialization. The range of cells used can include allogeneic and autologous differentiated cells such as fibroblasts and keratinocytes, as well as stem cells from different sources such as the bone marrow or umbilical cord. Depending on the material, they can be used as a temporary or permanent wound coverage.[412] Most of the skin substitutes are used to cover the wounds temporarily until definitive grafting can occur.

To date, there is no ideal substitute for human skin. Limitations of skin substitutes include immune rejection in allogeneic skin grafts, pain, scarring, slow healing and infection, and massive costs.[413,414] The need for improving wound care (especially of larger wounds) has stimulated intensive research in this area and led to multiple skin substitutes—both cellular and acellular.[412] The following focuses on the most commonly used skin substitutes to highlight their function and benefits.

Acellular Skin Substitutes

Some of the most commonly used acellular skin substitutes include Biobrane, Integra, and Alloderm. Biobrane consists of a silicone membrane and a nylon mesh, both embedded in porcine collagen. Integra is made of bovine collagen, shark chondroitin-6-sulfate glycosaminoglycan, and silicone. Alloderm is a cadaveric acellular matrix. Burn wounds are the major indication for the use of skin substitutes.[318] Wound coverage and the early excision of severely damaged tissue are recognized as fundamental aspects of burn management.[415–417] The goal of skin substitutes is to temporize the excised burn wound until autografting is possible.[418] In 45 burn patients with upper extremity burns, Biobrane was superior to cadaveric allografts in terms of procedure times and overall costs, with the added benefit of a lower complication rate.[419] Both acellular skin substitute and allograft skin coverage were previously found to be safe and effective in burn patients.[420,421] Two potential additional advantages of biosynthetic skin grafts are the possibility of initiating physical therapy in the immediate postoperative period, and a lesser tendency toward the formation of excessive granulation tissue. Overall this leads to a softer and smoother autograft appearance postoperatively.[419]

Available data show their promising role in the treatment of complex wounds.[165] Three meta-analyses revealed a clear benefit for the use of artificial skin grafts in comparison to standard care in the treatment of complex wounds.[422,423] Integra is used in complex soft tissue reconstruction after trauma over tendons, joints, and bone, as well as in vascular and pressure ulcers.[318,424] A 10-year follow-up study showed excellent results regarding cosmesis.[425] If placed over a joint, the resulting mobility has shown to be excellent, and it even has shown efficacy in pediatric patients.[425] The ability to cover up large (skin) defects may also reduce the rate of amputations.[426] However, a 2008 meta-analysis including 708 patients with venous leg ulcers and 1,201 patients with diabetic foot ulcers found inconclusive results regarding the efficacy of skin substitutes and advocated better designed trials with longer follow-up periods.[427] A systematic review published in 2009 by Health Quality Ontario concluded that because of limited, low-quality evidence on skin matrix and engineered skin equivalent efficacy in the treatment of pressure ulcers, no definitive conclusion regarding their usage could be drawn.[165] Next to the above-described indications, acellular skin substitutes can also be used in the treatment of epidermolysis bullosa and hidradenitis suppurativa.[428–430]

Cellular Skin Substitutes

Transcyte or Dermagraft contain only human fibroblasts, whereas Apligraf resembles human skin the closest as it not only contains a dermal component with fibroblasts, but also an epidermal layer with keratinocytes. Nevertheless, it still lacks important elements of human skin such as hair follicles, sweat glands, and macrophages.[412] Apligraf is approved for noninfected venous ulcers that have not responded to conventional treatment for at least 1 month, or for neuropathic diabetic ulcers that have failed to respond to conservative treatment for 3 weeks.[413,431,432] When compared with compression therapy alone, patients with venous leg ulcers additionally treated with Apligraf were twice as likely to achieve wound closure within half a year.[433] A higher rate in complete wound closure and a reduced healing time were seen in the treatment of diabetic foot ulcers with cellular skin substitutes.[434,435] It is also used for burn wounds, wounds in epidermolysis bullosa, donor sites, and skin cancer.[413,431] Cellular skin substitutes seem to be suitable for reconstructing keloids, but Integra also showed excellent clinical results and high patient satisfaction for this indication.[436,437]

One of the main obstacles in using cellular skin substitutes on a larger scale is their high cost. Apligraf, for example, sold as a circular disc of approximately 7.5 cm in diameter costs 1,000 to 1,200 USD.[438] For the treatment of a venous ulcer 1.41 applications were needed.[439] The high regeneration potential of stem cells combined with the favorable immune properties, especially of umbilical cord mesenchymal stem cells, makes them a promising future component to improve skin substitutes.[440]

Cytotherapy

Cytotherapy is an emerging field of medical research and describes the application of cells to wounds in order to promote accelerated healing.[441] The history of this type of therapy dates back to the early 1980s when cultured autologous keratinocytes were first applied to a burn patient.[442] The field of cytotherapy in wound healing has many facets, mostly relying on the differentiation of stem cells into the key players (keratinocytes and fibroblasts) whose interactions regulate skin homeostasis and promote the wound healing process.[441,443] Transplanted pluripotent adult-type stem cells are not necessarily responsible for enhanced wound healing, as evidence indicates that the benefits may be found in the soluble growth factors produced by these cells, especially in allogeneic transplants.[441] A focus of recent research in this area is upon the application of cultured cells, including but not limited to keratinocytes, fibroblasts, and adipose-derived stem cells, to wounds, and their further applications in this field.[442]

There is a large diversity in the nature of wounds, and the potential applications of cytotherapy. One study has reported a potentially viable matrix for a full-thickness wound using human adipose–derived stem cells; it takes advantage of their ability to self-renew and differentiate in cell-sheet technology transplanted onto mice.[444] Other models in mice have used bone marrow–derived mesenchymal stem cells to assess the delivery methods used to treat cutaneous wounds with cytotherapy; interestingly, there is enhanced healing and sweat gland formation with certain methods of cell transplantation.[445] Lymphatic endothelial cells derived from human pluripotent stem cells have recently been implicated as promoters of wound healing in both in vitro and in vivo murine models.[446] These developments in animal models are promising, especially in a field as new as cytotherapy. Recent explorations have identified human chorion–derived stem cells as another source of cells with comparable efficacy to adipose-derived stem cells.[447]

Optimal application techniques and standardization have yet to be determined in the field of cytotherapy in wound healing, though there are an increasing number of commercially available products derived from human cells. For example, in Korea, Haloderm is an autologous skin graft produced from biopsied cells that can reach the surface area of a human in 17 days.[442] The potential applications of these types of products in the context of burns and chronic wounds are vast.

A 2014 retrospective analysis of data collected and reported in randomized controlled trials, physician product prescribing information, and premarket approval summary documents from the U.S. Food and Drug Administration compared existing skin allografts (EpiFix, Apligraf, and Dermagraft). It showed that EpiFix, a human amnion/chorion membrane–derived allograft consisting of multiple layers of epithelial cells, a basement membrane, and an avascular connective tissue matrix, was associated with the most rapid improvement and resolution of diabetic foot ulcers in comparison to the other products.[448] A meta-analysis had already showed promising results for allograft skin substitutes versus standard care in the treatment of diabetic ulcers.[422]

There is much additional research required in the area of scar formation and cytotherapy. One study has implicated the delivery method (by microspheres) as key in maintaining mesenchymal stromal cell potency—which has been found to inhibit fibrotic tissue formation in mice. These actions are a result of the paracrine actions of these mesenchymal stromal cells, and microspheres may hold promise in the future of scar formation control utilizing cytotherapy.[449]

List of Abbreviations

APC	Adenomatous polyposis coli protein
CCN2	Connected tissue growth factor 2
CGRP	Calcitonin gene–related peptide
CTGF	Connective tissue growth factor
Dhh	Desert Hedgehog
ECM	Extracellular matrix
EDA	Extra-Domain-A
EGR	Transcription factor early growth response
FD	Fractal dimension
FGF	Fibroblast growth factor
G-CSF	Granulocyte colony–stimulating factor
GSK	Glycogen synthase kinase
GSK-3β	Glycogen synthase kinase 3β
HBOT	Hyperbaric oxygen therapy
HR	Histamine receptor
Ihh	Indian Hedgehog
IL	Interleukin
INF	Interferon
L	Lacunarity
LRP	Low-density lipoprotein receptor–related protein 5/6
LTS	Laser tissue soldering
LTW	Laser tissue welding
MMP	Matrix metalloproteinase
NCID	NOTCH intracellular domain
NLFU	Noncontact low-frequency ultrasound
NPWT	Negative-pressure wound therapy
NSAIDs	Nonsteroidal anti-inflammatory drugs
PDGF	Platelet-derived growth factor
PEMFT	Pulsed electromagnetic field therapy
Shh	Sonic Hedgehog
SSD	Silver sulfadiazine
Tcfs	T-cell factors
TGF	Tissue growth factor
TGF	Transforming growth factor
V(E)GF	Vascular (endothelial) growth factors

REFERENCES

1. Sen CK, Gordillo GM, Roy S, et al. Human skin wounds: a major and snowballing threat to public health and the economy. *Wound Repair Regen*. 2009;17:763–771.
2. Bielefeld KA, Amini-Nik S, Alman BA. Cutaneous wound healing: recruiting developmental pathways for regeneration. *Cell Mol Life Sci*. 2013;70:2059–2081.
3. Gottrup F. A specialized wound-healing center concept: importance of a multidisciplinary department structure and surgical treatment facilities in the treatment of chronic wounds. *Am J Surg*. 2004;187:38S–43S.
4. Gurtner GC, Werner S, Barrandon Y, et al. Wound repair and regeneration. *Nature*. 2008;453:314–321.
5. Ferreira MC, Tuma P Jr, Carvalho VF, et al. Complex wounds. *Clinics*. 2006;61:571–578.
6. Yamada KM, Clark RAF. *The Molecular and Cellular Biology of Wound Repair*. New York: Plenum Press; 1996.
7. Larson BJ, Longaker MT, Lorenz HP. Scarless fetal wound healing: a basic science review. *Plast Reconstr Surg*. 2010;126:1172–1180.
8. McCallion RL, Ferguson MWJ. *The Molecular and Cellular Biology of Wound Repair*. New York: Plenum Press; 1996.
9. Verrecchia F, Mauviel A. Control of connective tissue gene expression by TGF beta: role of Smad proteins in fibrosis. *Curr Rheumatol Rep*. 2002;4:143–149.
10. Leask A, Abraham DJ. TGF-beta signaling and the fibrotic response. *FASEB J*. 2004;18:816–827.
11. Soo C, Beanes SR, Hu FY, et al. Ontogenetic transition in fetal wound transforming growth factor-beta regulation correlates with collagen organization. *Am J Pathol*. 2003;163:2459–2476.
12. Li-Korotky HS, Hebda PA, Lo CY, et al. Age-dependent differential expression of fibronectin variants in skin and airway mucosal wounds. *Arch Otolaryngol—Head Neck Surg*. 2007;133:919–924.
13. Coolen NA, Schouten KC, Middelkoop E, et al. Comparison between human fetal and adult skin. *Arch Dermatol Res*. 2010;302:47–55.
14. Khorasani H, Zheng Z, Nguyen C, et al. A quantitative approach to scar analysis. *Am J Pathol*. 2011;178:621–628.
15. van Zuijlen PP, Ruurda JJ, van Veen HA, et al. Collagen morphology in human skin and scar tissue: no adaptations in response to mechanical loading at joints. *Burns*. 2003;29:423–431.
16. van Zuijlen PPM, de Vries HJC, Lamme EN, et al. Morphometry of dermal collagen orientation by Fourier analysis is superior to multi-observer assessment. *J Pathol*. 2002;198:284–291.
17. Peacock E. Contraction. In: Peacock E., editor. WB Saunders; Philadelphia: 1984. pp. 38–90.
18. Smith TG Jr, Lange GD, Marks WB. Fractal methods and results in cellular morphology–dimensions, lacunarity and multifractals. *J Neurosci Methods*. 1996;69:123–136.
19. Eblen-Zajjur A, Salas R, Vanegas H. Fractal analysis of spinal dorsal horn neuron discharges by means of sequential fractal dimension D. *Comput Biol Med*. 1996;26:87–95.
20. Guidolin D, Vacca A, Nussdorfer GG, et al. A new image analysis method based on topological and fractal parameters to evaluate the angiostatic activity of docetaxel by using the Matrigel assay in vitro. *Microvasc Res*. 2004;67:117–124.
21. Tinajero JP, Robledo RF, Lantz RC, et al. Fractal analysis of lung alveoli during the acute phase vs. repair phase of an adenoviral infection in canines. *Res Comm Mol Pathol Pharmacol*. 1997;95:275–285.
22. Aird LN, Bristol SG, Phang PT, et al. Randomized double-blind trial comparing the cosmetic outcome of cutting diathermy versus scalpel for skin incisions. *Br J Surg*. 2015;102:489–494.
23. Watt AM, Patkin M, Sinnott MJ, et al. Scalpel safety in the operative setting: a systematic review. *Surgery*. 2010;147:98–106.
24. Aird LNF, Brown CJ. Systematic review and meta-analysis of electrocautery versus scalpel for surgical skin incisions. *Am J Surg*. 2012;204:216–221.
25. Ly J, Mittal A, Windsor J. Systematic review and meta-analysis of cutting diathermy versus scalpel for skin incision. *Br J Surg*. 2012;99:613–620.
26. Ahmad NZ, Ahmed A. Meta-analysis of the effectiveness of surgical scalpel or diathermy in making abdominal skin incisions. *Ann Surg*. 2011;253:8–13.
27. Chau JK, Dzigielewski P, Mlynarek A, et al. Steel scalpel versus electrocautery blade: comparison of cosmetic and patient satisfaction outcomes of different incision methods. *J Otolaryngol—Head Neck Surg*. 2009;38:427–433.
28. Stupart DA, Sim FW, Chan ZH, et al. Cautery versus scalpel for abdominal skin incisions: a double blind, randomized crossover trial of scar cosmesis. *ANZ J Surg*. 2013;86(4):303–306.
29. Gatt D, Quick CR, Owen-Smith MS. Staples for wound closure: a controlled trial. *Ann R Coll Surg Engl*. 1985;67:318–320.
30. Ghosh A, Nanjappa M, Nagaraj V, et al. Comparison between stainless steel staples and silk sutures for primary closure of skin in patients undergoing neck dissection: a comparative clinical study. *Contemp Clin Dent*. 2015;6:51–55.
31. Bastian PJ, Haferkamp A, Albers P, et al. A new form of noninvasive wound closure with a surgical zipper. *J Urol*. 2003;169: 1785–1786.
32. Luck RP, Flood R, Eyal D, et al. Cosmetic outcomes of absorbable versus nonabsorbable sutures in pediatric facial lacerations. *Pediatr Emerg Care*. 2008;24:137–142.
33. Karounis H, Gouin S, Eisman H, et al. A randomized, controlled trial comparing long-term cosmetic outcomes of traumatic pediatric lacerations repaired with absorbable plain gut versus nonabsorbable nylon sutures. *Acad Emerg Med*. 2004;11:730–735.
34. Durkaya S, Kaptanoglu M, Nadir A, et al. Do absorbable sutures exacerbate presternal scarring? *Tex Heart Inst J*. 2005;32:544–548.
35. LaBagnara J Jr. A review of absorbable suture materials in head & neck surgery and introduction of monocryl: a new absorbable suture. *Ear Nose Throat J*. 1995;74:409–415.
36. George TK, Simpson DC. Skin wound closure with staples in the Accident and Emergency Department. *J R Coll Surg Edinb*. 1985;30:54–56.
37. MacGregor FB, McCombe AW, King PM, et al. Skin stapling of wounds in the accident department. *Injury*. 1989;20:347–348.
38. Sharma C, Verma A, Soni A, et al. A randomized controlled trial comparing cosmetic outcome after skin closure with 'staples' or 'subcuticular sutures' in emergency Cesarean section. *Arch Gynecol Obstet*. 2014;290:655–659.
39. Sanni A, Dunning J. Staples or sutures for chest and leg wounds following cardiovascular surgery. *Interact Cardiovasc Thorac Surg*. 2007;6:243–246.
40. Parell GJ, Becker GD. Comparison of absorbable with nonabsorbable sutures in closure of facial skin wounds. *Arch Fac Plast Surg*. 2003;5:488–490.
41. Coupland RM. Sutures versus staples in skin flap operations. *Ann R Coll Surg Engl*. 1986;68:2–4.
42. McClelland H, Nellis G. Surgical staple trial in accident and emergency. Accident and emergency nursing 1997;5:62–64.
43. Kanegaye JT, Vance CW, Chan L, et al. Comparison of skin stapling devices and standard sutures for pediatric scalp lacerations: a randomized study of cost and time benefits. *J Pediatr*. 1997;130:808–813.
44. Roolker W, Kraaneveld E, Been HD, et al. Results of a prospective randomised study comparing a non-invasive surgical zipper versus intracutaneous sutures for wound closure. *Arch Orthop Trauma Surg*. 2002;122:2–4.
45. Cross KJ, Teo EH, Wong SL, et al. The absorbable dermal staple device: a faster, more cost-effective method for incisional closure. *Plast Reconstr Surg*. 2009;124:156–162.
46. Tellis VA. Renal transplant incision closure using new absorbable subcuticular staple device. *Clin Transplant*. 2007;21:410–412.
47. Greenberg JA. INSORB® | 25 subcuticular skin stapler. Reviews in Obstetrics and Gynecology. 2008;1(3):141–142.
48. Katz KH, Desciak EB, Maloney ME. The optimal application of surgical adhesive tape strips. *Dermatol Surg*. 1999;25:686–688.
49. Kolt JD. Use of adhesive surgical tape with the absorbable continuous subcuticular suture. *ANZ J Surg*. 2003;73:626–629.
50. Marples RR, Kligman AM. Growth of bacteria under adhesive tapes. *Arch Dermatol*. 1969;99:107–110.
51. Conolly WB, Hunt TK, Zederfeldt B, et al. Clinical comparison of surgical wounds closed by suture and adhesive tapes. *Am J Surg*. 1969;117:318–322.
52. Al-Mubarak L, Al-Haddab M. Cutaneous wound closure materials: an overview and update. *J Cutan Aesthet Surg*. 2013;6:178–188.
53. Hollander JE, Singer AJ. Laceration management. *Ann Emerg Med*. 1999;34:356–367.
54. Bruns TB, Worthington JM. Using tissue adhesive for wound repair: a practical guide to Dermabond. *Am Fam Phys*. 2000;61:1383–1388.
55. Quinn J, Wells G, Sutcliffe T, et al. A randomized trial comparing octylcyanoacrylate tissue adhesive and sutures in the management of lacerations. *JAMA*. 1997;277:1527–1530.

56. Singer AJ, Quinn JV, Clark RE, et al. Closure of lacerations and incisions with octylcyanoacrylate: a multicenter randomized controlled trial. *Surgery*. 2002;131:270–276.
57. Quinn J, Wells G, Sutcliffe T, et al. Tissue adhesive versus suture wound repair at 1 year: randomized clinical trial correlating early, 3-month, and 1-year cosmetic outcome. *Ann Emerg Med*. 1998:645–649.
58. Zempsky WT, Parrotti D, Grem C, et al. Randomized controlled comparison of cosmetic outcomes of simple facial lacerations closed with Steri Strip Skin Closures or Dermabond tissue adhesive. *Pediatr Emerg Care*. 2004;20:519–524.
59. Toriumi DM, O'Grady K, Desai D, et al. Use of octyl-2-cyanoacrylate for skin closure in facial plastic surgery. *Plast Reconstr Surg*. 1998: 2209–2219.
60. Maartense S, Bemelman WA, Dunker MS, et al. Randomized study of the effectiveness of closing laparoscopic trocar wounds with octylcyanoacrylate, adhesive papertape or poliglecaprone. *Br J Surg*. 2002;89:1370–1375.
61. Singer AJ, Hollander JE, Valentine SM, et al. Association of training level and short-term cosmetic appearance of repaired lacerations. *Acad Emerg Med*. 1996;3:378–383.
62. Quinn JV, Drzewiecki A, Li MM, et al. A randomized, controlled trial comparing a tissue adhesive with suturing in the repair of pediatric facial lacerations. *Ann Emerg Med*. 1993;22:1130–1135.
63. Sterling JB, Skouge JW. Surgical glue to secure small split-thickness skin grafts: a cost-effective and time-saving technique. *Dermatol Surg*. 2008;34:246–247; discussion 7–8.
64. Grimaldi L, Cuomo R, Brandi C, et al. Octyl-2-cyanoacrylate adhesive for skin closure: eight years experience. *In Vivo*. 2015;29:145–148.
65. Dowson CC, Gilliam AD, Speake WJ, et al. A prospective, randomized controlled trial comparing n-butyl cyanoacrylate tissue adhesive (LiquiBand) with sutures for skin closure after laparoscopic general surgical procedures. *Surg Laparosc Endosc Percutan Techn*. 2006;16:146–150.
66. Lin M, Coates WC, Lewis RJ. Tissue adhesive skills study: the physician learning curve. *Pediatr Emerg Care*. 2004;20:219–223.
67. Scott GR, Carson CL, Borah GL. Dermabond skin closures for bilateral reduction mammaplasties: a review of 255 consecutive cases. *Plast Reconstr Surg*. 2007;120:1460–1465.
68. Beam JW. Tissue adhesives for simple traumatic lacerations. *J Athl Train*. 2008;43:222–224.
69. Bass LS, Treat MR. Laser tissue welding: a comprehensive review of current and future clinical applications. *Lasers Surg Med*. 1995;17:315–349.
70. Simhon D, Ravid A, Halpern M, et al. Laser soldering of rat skin, using fiberoptic temperature controlled system. *Lasers Surg Med*. 2001;29:265–273.
71. McNally KM, Sorg BS, Chan EK, et al. Optimal parameters for laser tissue soldering. Part II: Premixed versus separate dye-solder techniques. *Lasers Surg Med*. 2000;26:346–356.
72. Bleustein CB, Walker CN, Felsen D, et al. Semi-solid albumin solder improved mechanical properties for laser tissue welding. *Lasers Surg Med*. 2000;27:140–146.
73. McNally KM, Sorg BS, Chan EK, et al. Optimal parameters for laser tissue soldering. Part I: tensile strength and scanning electron microscopy analysis. *Lasers Surg Med*. 1999;24:319–331.
74. Oz MC, Johnson JP, Parangi S, et al. Tissue soldering by use of indocyanine green dye-enhanced fibrinogen with the near infrared diode laser. *J Vasc Surg*. 1990;11:718–725.
75. Simhon D, Halpern M, Brosh T, et al. Immediate tight sealing of skin incisions using an innovative temperature-controlled laser soldering device: in vivo study in porcine skin. *Ann Surg*. 2007; 245:206–213.
76. Kirsch AJ, Cooper CS, Gatti J, et al. Laser tissue soldering for hypospadias repair: results of a controlled prospective clinical trial. *J Urol*. 2001;165:574–577.
77. Manuskiatti W, Fitzpatrick RE. Treatment response of keloidal and hypertrophic sternotomy scars: comparison among intralesional corticosteroid, 5-fluorouracil, and 585-nm flashlamp-pumped pulsed-dye laser treatments. *Arch Dermatol*. 2002;138(9):1149–1155.
78. Alster T. Laser scar revision: comparison study of 585-nm pulsed dye laser with and without intralesional corticosteroids. *Dermatol Surg*. 2003;29:25–29.
79. Dierickx C, Goldman MP, Fitzpatrick RE. Laser treatment of erythematous/hypertrophic and pigmented scars in 26 patients. *Plast Reconstr Surg*. 1995;95(1):84–90.
80. Zhu R, Yue B, Yang Q, et al. The effect of 595 nm pulsed dye laser on connective tissue growth factor (CTGF) expression in cultured keloid fibroblasts. *Lasers Surg Med*. 2015;47:203–209.
81. Yang Q, Ma Y, Zhu R, et al. The effect of flashlamp pulsed dye laser on the expression of connective tissue growth factor in keloids. *Lasers Surg Med*. 2012;44:377–383.
82. Leventhal D, Furr M, Reiter D. Treatment of keloids and hypertrophic scars: a meta-analysis and review of the literature. *Arch Facial Plast Surg*. 2006;8:362–368.
83. Apfelberg DB, Maser MR, White DN, et al. Failure of carbon dioxide laser excision of keloids. *Lasers Surg Med*. 1989;9:382–388.
84. Norris JE. The effect of carbon dioxide laser surgery on the recurrence of keloids. *Plast Reconstr Surg*. 1991;87:44–49; discussion 50–53.
85. Kumar K, Kapoor BS, Rai P, et al. In-situ irradiation of keloid scars with Nd:YAG laser. *J Wound Care*. 2000;9:213–215.
86. Murray JC. Keloids and hypertrophic scars. *Clin Dermatol*. 1994;12:27–37.
87. Amini-Nik S, Kraemer D, Cowan ML, et al. Ultrafast mid-IR laser scalpel: protein signals of the fundamental limits to minimally invasive surgery. *PLoS One*. 2010;5(9):e13053.
88. van den Broek LJ, Limandjaja GC, Niessen FB, et al. Human hypertrophic and keloid scar models: principles, limitations and future challenges from a tissue engineering perspective. *Exp Dermatol*. 2014;23:382–386.
89. Yamaguchi Y, Hearing VJ, Itami S, et al. Mesenchymal-epithelial interactions in the skin: aiming for site-specific tissue regeneration. *J Dermatol Sci*. 2005;40:1–9.
90. Logan CY, Nusse R. The Wnt signaling pathway in development and disease. *Annu Rev Cell Dev Biol*. 2004;20:781–810.
91. Nelson WJ, Nusse R. Convergence of Wnt, beta-catenin, and cadherin pathways. *Science*. 2004;303:1483–1487.
92. Angers S, Moon RT. Proximal events in Wnt signal transduction. *Nat Rev Mol Cell Biol*. 2009;10:468–477.
93. Cadigan KM, Peifer M. Wnt signaling from development to disease: insights from model systems. *Cold Spring Harbor Perspect Biol*. 2009;1:a002881.
94. Gao C, Chen YG. Dishevelled: the hub of Wnt signaling. *Cell Signal*. 2010;22:717–727.
95. Widelitz RB. Wnt signaling in skin organogenesis. *Organogenesis*. 2008;4:123–133.
96. Ohtola J, Myers J, Akhtar-Zaidi B, et al. β-catenin has sequential roles in the survival and specification of ventral dermis. *Development*. 2008;135:2321–2329.
97. Ito M, Yang Z, Andl T, et al. Wnt-dependent de novo hair follicle regeneration in adult mouse skin after wounding. *Nature*. 2007;447:316–320.
98. Okuse T, Chiba T, Katsuumi I, et al. Differential expression and localization of WNTs in an animal model of skin wound healing. *Wound Repair Regen*. 2005;13:491–497.
99. Labus MB, Stirk CM, Thompson WD, et al. Expression of Wnt genes in early wound healing. *Wound Repair Regen*. 1998;6:58–64.
100. Lilien J, Balsamo J. The regulation of cadherin-mediated adhesion by tyrosine phosphorylation/dephosphorylation of beta-catenin. *Curr Opin Cell Biol*. 2005;17:459–465.
101. Bielefeld KA, Amini-Nik S, Whetstone H, et al. Fibronectin and beta-catenin act in a regulatory loop in dermal fibroblasts to modulate cutaneous healing. *J Biol Chem*. 2011;286:27687–27697.
102. Bafico A, Liu G, Yaniv A, et al. Novel mechanism of Wnt signalling inhibition mediated by Dickkopf-1 interaction with LRP6/Arrow. *Nat Cell Biol*. 2001;3:683–686.
103. Cheon SS, Wei Q, Gurung A, et al. Beta-catenin regulates wound size and mediates the effect of TGF-beta in cutaneous healing. *FASEB J*. 2006;20:692–701.
104. Cheon SS, Nadesan P, Poon R, et al. Growth factors regulate beta-catenin-mediated TCF-dependent transcriptional activation in fibroblasts during the proliferative phase of wound healing. *Exp Cell Res*. 2004;293:267–274.
105. Amini Nik S, Ebrahim RP, Van Dam K, et al. TGF-beta modulates beta-Catenin stability and signaling in mesenchymal proliferations. *Exp Cell Res*. 2007;313:2887–2895.
106. Cheon SS, Cheah AY, Turley S, et al. beta-Catenin stabilization dysregulates mesenchymal cell proliferation, motility, and invasiveness and causes aggressive fibromatosis and hyperplastic cutaneous wounds. *Proc Natl Acad Sci USA*. 2002;99:6973–6978.
107. Cheon S, Poon R, Yu C, et al. Prolonged beta-catenin stabilization and tcf-dependent transcriptional activation in hyperplastic cutaneous wounds. *Lab Invest*. 2005;85:416–425.

108. Sato M. Upregulation of the Wnt/beta-catenin pathway induced by transforming growth factor-beta in hypertrophic scars and keloids. *Acta Derm Venereol*. 2006;86:300–307.
109. Yu H, Bock O, Bayat A, et al. Decreased expression of inhibitory SMAD6 and SMAD7 in keloid scarring. *J Plast Reconstr Aesthet Surg*. 2006;59:221–229.
110. Amini-Nik S, Cambridge E, Yu W, et al. beta-Catenin-regulated myeloid cell adhesion and migration determine wound healing. *J Clin Invest*. 2014;124:2599–2610.
111. Kapoor M, Liu S, Shi-wen X, et al. GSK-3beta in mouse fibroblasts controls wound healing and fibrosis through an endothelin-1-dependent mechanism. *J Clin Invest*. 2008;118:3279–3290.
112. Poon R, Nik SA, Ahn J, et al. Beta-catenin and transforming growth factor beta have distinct roles regulating fibroblast cell motility and the induction of collagen lattice contraction. *BMC Cell Biol*. 2009;10.
113. Alman BA, Li C, Pajerski ME, et al. Increased beta-catenin protein and somatic APC mutations in sporadic aggressive fibromatoses (desmoid tumors). *Am J Pathol*. 1997;151:329–334.
114. Stojadinovic O, Brem H, Vouthounis C, et al. Molecular pathogenesis of chronic wounds: the role of beta-catenin and c-myc in the inhibition of epithelialization and wound healing. *Am J Pathol*. 2005;167:59–69.
115. Mirza R, DiPietro LA, Koh TJ. Selective and specific macrophage ablation is detrimental to wound healing in mice. *Am J Pathol*. 2009;175:2454–2462.
116. Geissmann F, Manz MG, Jung S, et al. Development of monocytes, macrophages, and dendritic cells. *Science*. 2010;327:656–661.
117. Goren I, Allmann N, Yogev N, et al. A transgenic mouse model of inducible macrophage depletion: effects of diphtheria toxin-driven lysozyme M-specific cell lineage ablation on wound inflammatory, angiogenic, and contractive processes. *Am J Pathol*. 2009;175:132–147.
118. Hopkinson-Woolley J, Hughes D, Gordon S, et al. Macrophage recruitment during limb development and wound healing in the embryonic and foetal mouse. *J Cell Sci*. 1994;107 (Pt 5):1159–1167.
119. Leibovich SJ, Ross R. The role of the macrophage in wound repair. A study with hydrocortisone and antimacrophage serum. *Am J Pathol*. 1975;78:71–100.
120. Simpson DM, Ross R. The neutrophilic leukocyte in wound repair a study with antineutrophil serum. *J Clin Invest*. 1972;51:2009–2023.
121. Werner S, Grose R. Regulation of wound healing by growth factors and cytokines. *Physiol Rev*. 2003;83:835–870.
122. Peters T, Sindrilaru A, Hinz B, et al. Wound-healing defect of CD18(–/–) mice due to a decrease in TGF-β(1) and myofibroblast differentiation. *EMBO J*. 2005;24:3400–3410.
123. Carre AL, James AW, MacLeod L, et al. Interaction of wingless protein (Wnt), transforming growth factor-beta1, and hyaluronan production in fetal and postnatal fibroblasts. *Plast Reconstr Surg*. 2010;125:74–88.
124. Poon R, Hong H, Wei X, et al. A high throughput screen identifies nefopam as targeting cell proliferation in β-catenin driven neoplastic and reactive fibroproliferative disorders. *PloS One*. 2012;7:e37940.
125. Barrientos S, Stojadinovic O, Golinko MS, et al. Growth factors and cytokines in wound healing. *Wound Repair Regen*. 2008;16:585–601.
126. Schultz GS, WysockiA. Interactions between extracellular matrix and growth factors in wound healing. *Wound Rep Regen*. 2009;17:153–162.
127. Margadant C, Sonnenberg A. Integrin-TGF-beta crosstalk in fibrosis, cancer and wound healing. *EMBO Rep*. 2010;11:97–105.
128. Owens P, Han G, Li AG, et al. The role of Smads in skin development. *J Invest Dermatol*. 2008;128:783–790.
129. Biernacka A, Dobaczewski M, Frangogiannis NG. TGF-beta signaling in fibrosis. *Growth Factors*. 2011;29:196–202.
130. Mu Y, Gudey SK, Landstrom M. Non-Smad signaling pathways. *Cell Tissue Res*. 2012;347:11–20.
131. Landstrom M. The TAK1-TRAF6 signalling pathway. *Int J Biochem Cell Biol*. 2010;42:585–589.
132. Puolakkainen PA, Reed MJ, Gombotz WR, et al. Acceleration of wound healing in aged rats by topical application of transforming growth factor-beta(1). *Wound Repair Regen*. 1995;3:330–339.
133. Schreier T, Degen E, Baschong W. Fibroblast migration and proliferation during in vitro wound healing. A quantitative comparison between various growth factors and a low molecular weight blood dialysate used in the clinic to normalize impaired wound healing. *Res Exp Med*. 1993;193:195–205.
134. Varga J, Rosenbloom J, Jimenez SA. Transforming growth factor beta (TGF beta) causes a persistent increase in steady-state amounts of type I and type III collagen and fibronectin mRNAs in normal human dermal fibroblasts. *Biochem J*. 1987;247:597–604.
135. Hocevar BA, Brown TL, Howe PH. TGF-beta induces fibronectin synthesis through a c-Jun N-terminal kinase-dependent, Smad4-independent pathway. *EMBO J*. 1999;18:1345–1356.
136. Martinez-Ferrer M, Afshar-Sherif AR, Uwamariya C, et al. Dermal transforming growth factor-beta responsiveness mediates wound contraction and epithelial closure. *Am J Pathol*. 2010;176:98–107.
137. Yang CC, Lin SD, Yu HS. Effect of growth factors on dermal fibroblast contraction in normal skin and hypertrophic scar. *J Dermatol Sci*. 1997;14:162–169.
138. Pietenpol JA, Holt JT, Stein RW, et al. Transforming growth factor beta 1 suppression of c-myc gene transcription: role in inhibition of keratinocyte proliferation. *Proc Natl Acad Sci USA*. 1990;87:3758–3762.
139. Shah M, Foreman DM, Ferguson MW. Neutralisation of TGF-beta 1 and TGF-beta 2 or exogenous addition of TGF-beta 3 to cutaneous rat wounds reduces scarring. *J Cell Sci*. 1995;108 (Pt 3):985–1002.
140. Foitzik K, Paus R, Doetschman T, et al. The TGF-β2 isoform is both a required and sufficient inducer of murine hair follicle morphogenesis. *Dev Biol*. 1999;212:278–289.
141. Ashcroft GS, Yang X, Glick AB, et al. Mice lacking Smad3 show accelerated wound healing and an impaired local inflammatory response. *Nat Cell Biol*. 1999;1:260–266.
142. Crowe MJ, Doetschman T, Greenhalgh DG. Delayed wound healing in immunodeficient TGF-beta 1 knockout mice. *J Invest Dermatol*. 2000;115:3–11.
143. Denton CP, Khan K, Hoyles RK, et al. Inducible lineage-specific deletion of TbetaRII in fibroblasts defines a pivotal regulatory role during adult skin wound healing. *J Invest Dermatol*. 2009;129:194–204.
144. Le Poole IC, Boyce ST. Keratinocytes suppress transforming growth factor-beta1 expression by fibroblasts in cultured skin substitutes. *Br J Dermatol*. 1999;140:409–416.
145. Leask A. CCN2: a bona fide target for anti-fibrotic drug intervention. *J Cell Comm Signal*. 2011;5:131–133.
146. Trojanowska M. Noncanonical transforming growth factor beta signaling in scleroderma fibrosis. *Curr Opin Rheumatol*. 2009;21:623–629.
147. Cicha I, Goppelt-Struebe M. Connective tissue growth factor: context-dependent functions and mechanisms of regulation. *BioFactors*. 2009;35:200–208.
148. Leask A, Parapuram SK, Shi-Wen X, et al. Connective tissue growth factor (CTGF, CCN2) gene regulation: a potent clinical bio-marker of fibroproliferative disease? *J Cell Comm Signal*. 2009;3:89–94.
149. Lee CH, Shah B, Moioli EK, et al. CTGF directs fibroblast differentiation from human mesenchymal stem/stromal cells and defines connective tissue healing in a rodent injury model. *J Clin Invest*. 2010;120:3340–3349.
150. Sisco M, Kryger ZB, O'Shaughnessy KD, et al. Antisense inhibition of connective tissue growth factor (CTGF/CCN2) mRNA limits hypertrophic scarring without affecting wound healing in vivo. *Wound Repair Regen*. 2008;16:661–673.
151. Singer AJ, Huang SS, Huang JS, et al. A novel TGF-beta antagonist speeds reepithelialization and reduces scarring of partial thickness porcine burns. *J Burn Care Res*. 2009;30:329–334.
152. Han G, Li F, Ten Dijke P, et al. Temporal smad7 transgene induction in mouse epidermis accelerates skin wound healing. *Am J Pathol*. 2011;179:1768–1779.
153. Lin RY, Adzick NS. The role of the fetal fibroblast and transforming growth factor-beta in a model of human fetal wound repair. *Semin Pediatr Surg*. 1996;5:165–174.
154. So K, McGrouther DA, Bush JA, et al. Avotermin for scar improvement following scar revision surgery: a randomized, double-blind, within-patient, placebo-controlled, phase II clinical trial. *Plast Reconstr Surg*. 2011;128:163–172.
155. Grose R, Werner S. Wound healing studies in transgenic and knockout mice. A review. *Methods Mol Med*. 2003;78:191–216.
156. Singer AJ, Clark RA. Cutaneous wound healing. *N Engl J Med*. 1999;341:738–746.
157. Fu X, Shen Z, Chen Y, et al. Randomised placebo-controlled trial of use of topical recombinant bovine basic fibroblast growth factor for second-degree burns. *Lancet*. 1998;352:1661–1664.
158. Brown GL, Nanney LB, Griffen J, et al. Enhancement of wound healing by topical treatment with epidermal growth factor. *N Engl J Med*. 1989;321:76–79.
159. Mohan VK. Recombinant human epidermal growth factor (REGEN-D 150): effect on healing of diabetic foot ulcers. *Diabetes Res Clin Pract*. 2007;78:405–411.

160. Lin RY, Sullivan KM, Argenta PA, et al. Exogenous transforming growth factor-beta amplifies its own expression and induces scar formation in a model of human fetal skin repair. *Ann Surg*. 1995;222:146–154.
161. Ghahary A, Shen YJ, Scott PG, et al. Enhanced expression of mRNA for transforming growth factor-beta, type I and type III procollagen in human post-burn hypertrophic scar tissues. *J Lab Clin Med*. 1993;122:465–473.
162. LeGrand EK. Preclinical promise of becaplermin (rhPDGF-BB) in wound healing. *Am J Surg*. 1998;176:48S–54S.
163. Mandracchia VJ, Sanders SM, Frerichs JA. The use of becaplermin (rhPDGF-BB) gel for chronic nonhealing ulcers. A retrospective analysis. *Clin Podiatr Med Surg*. 2001;18:189–209.
164. Smiell JM, Wieman TJ, Steed DL, et al. Efficacy and safety of becaplermin (recombinant human platelet-derived growth factor-BB) in patients with nonhealing, lower extremity diabetic ulcers: a combined analysis of four randomized studies. *Wound Repair Regen*. 1999;7:335–346.
165. Health Quality Ontario. Management of chronic pressure ulcers: an evidence-based analysis. *Ontario Health Technol Assess Ser*. 2009;9:1–203.
166. Ono I, Akasaka Y, Kikuchi R, et al. Basic fibroblast growth factor reduces scar formation in acute incisional wounds. *Wound Repair Regen*. 2007;15:617–623.
167. Berlanga-Acosta J, Gavilondo-Cowley J, Lopez-Saura P, et al. Epidermal growth factor in clinical practice—a review of its biological actions, clinical indications and safety implications. *Int Wound J*. 2009;6:331–346.
168. Barrientos S, Brem H, Stojadinovic O, et al. Clinical application of growth factors and cytokines in wound healing. *Wound Repair Regen*. 2014;22:569–578.
169. Athar M, Tang X, Lee JL, et al. Hedgehog signalling in skin development and cancer. *Exp Dermatol*. 2006;15:667–677.
170. Lavine KJ, White AC, Park C, et al. Fibroblast growth factor signals regulate a wave of Hedgehog activation that is essential for coronary vascular development. *Genes Dev*. 2006;20:1651–1666.
171. St-Jacques B, Dassule HR, Karavanova I, et al. Sonic hedgehog signaling is essential for hair development. *Curr Biol*. 1998;8:1058–1069.
172. Karlsson L, Bondjers C, Betsholtz C. Roles for PDGF-A and sonic hedgehog in development of mesenchymal components of the hair follicle. *Development*. 1999;126:2611–2621.
173. Niemann C, Unden AB, Lyle S, et al. Indian hedgehog and beta-catenin signaling: role in the sebaceous lineage of normal and neoplastic mammalian epidermis. *Proc Natl Acad Sci USA*. 2003;100(suppl 1):11873–11880.
174. Brownell I, Guevara E, Bai CB, et al. Nerve-derived sonic hedgehog defines a niche for hair follicle stem cells capable of becoming epidermal stem cells. *Cell Stem Cell*. 2011;8:552–565.
175. Chiang C, Swan RZ, Grachtchouk M, et al. Essential role for Sonic hedgehog during hair follicle morphogenesis. *Dev Biol*. 1999;205:1–9.
176. Tasouri E, Tucker K. Primary cilia and organogenesis: is Hedgehog the only sculptor? *Cell Tissue Res*. 2011;345:21–40.
177. Levy V, Lindon C, Zheng Y, et al. Epidermal stem cells arise from the hair follicle after wounding. *FASEB J*. 2007;21:1358–1366.
178. Asai J, Takenaka H, Kusano KF, et al. Topical sonic hedgehog gene therapy accelerates wound healing in diabetes by enhancing endothelial progenitor cell-mediated microvascular remodeling. *Circulation*. 2006;113:2413–2424.
179. Le H, Kleinerman R, Lerman OZ, et al. Hedgehog signaling is essential for normal wound healing. *Wound Repair Regen*. 2008;16:768–773.
180. Okuyama R, Tagami H, Aiba S. Notch signaling: its role in epidermal homeostasis and in the pathogenesis of skin diseases. *J Dermatol Sci*. 2008;49:187–194.
181. Watt FM, Estrach S, Ambler CA. Epidermal Notch signalling: differentiation, cancer and adhesion. *Curr Opin Cell Biol*. 2008;20:171–179.
182. Gridley T. Notch signaling in the vasculature. *Curr Top Dev Biol*. 2010;92:277–309.
183. Blanpain C, Fuchs E. Epidermal homeostasis: a balancing act of stem cells in the skin. *Nat Rev Mol Cell Biol*. 2009;10:207–217.
184. Moriyama M, Durham AD, Moriyama H, et al. Multiple roles of notch signaling in the regulation of epidermal development. *Dev Cell*. 2008;14:594–604.
185. Blanpain C, Lowry WE, Pasolli HA, et al. Canonical notch signaling functions as a commitment switch in the epidermal lineage. *Genes Dev*. 2006;20:3022–3035.
186. Chigurupati S, Arumugam TV, Son TG, et al. Involvement of notch signaling in wound healing. *PLoS One*. 2007;2:e1167.
187. Outtz HH, Wu JK, Wang X, et al. Notch1 deficiency results in decreased inflammation during wound healing and regulates vascular endothelial growth factor receptor-1 and inflammatory cytokine expression in macrophages. *J Immunol*. 2010;185:4363–4373.
188. Caiado F, Real C, Carvalho T, et al. Notch pathway modulation on bone marrow-derived vascular precursor cells regulates their angiogenic and wound healing potential. *PLoS One*. 2008;3:e3752.
189. Chang YC, Wang JD, Hahn RA, et al. Therapeutic potential of a non-steroidal bifunctional anti-inflammatory and anti-cholinergic agent against skin injury induced by sulfur mustard. *Toxicol Appl Pharmacol*. 2014;280:236–244.
190. Klein M, Krarup PM, Kongsbak MB, et al. Effect of postoperative diclofenac on anastomotic healing, skin wounds and subcutaneous collagen accumulation: a randomized, blinded, placebo-controlled, experimental study. *Eur Surg Res*. 2012;48:73–78.
191. Ku EC, Wasvary JM, Cash WD. Diclofenac sodium (GP 45840, Voltaren), a potent inhibitor of prostaglandin synthetase. *Biochem Pharmacol*. 1975;24:641–643.
192. Pawar HV, Tetteh J, Boateng JS. Preparation, optimisation and characterisation of novel wound healing film dressings loaded with streptomycin and diclofenac. *Colloids Surf B, Biointerfaces*. 2013;102:102–110.
193. Mazumdar K, Dastidar SG, Park JH, et al. The anti-inflammatory non-antibiotic helper compound diclofenac: an antibacterial drug target. *Eur J Clin Microbiol Infect Dis*. 2009;28:881–91.
194. de Santos JS, Monte-Alto-Costa A. Female, but not male, mice show delayed cutaneous wound healing following aspirin administration. *Clin Exp Pharmacol Physiol*. 2013;40:90–96.
195. Inan A, Koca C, Sen M. Effects of diclofenac sodium on bursting pressures of anastomoses and hydroxyproline contents of perianastomotic tissues in a laboratory study. *Int J Surg*. 2006;4:222–227.
196. Mastboom WJ, Hendriks T, van Elteren P, et al. The influence of NSAIDs on experimental intestinal anastomoses. *Dis Colon Rectum*. 1991;34:236–243.
197. Syk I, Agren MS, Adawi D, et al. Inhibition of matrix metalloproteinases enhances breaking strength of colonic anastomoses in an experimental model. *Br J Surg*. 2001;88:228–234.
198. Johnson HH Jr, Deoreo GA, Lascheid WP, et al. Skin histamine levels in chronic atopic dermatitis. *J Invest Dermatol*. 1960;34:237–238.
199. Ruzicka T, Gluck S. Cutaneous histamine levels and histamine releasability from the skin in atopic dermatitis and hyper-IgE-syndrome. *Arch Dermatol Res*. 1983;275:41–44.
200. Marone G, Casolaro V, Paganelli R, et al. IgG anti-IgE from atopic dermatitis induces mediator release from basophils and mast cells. *J Invest Dermat*. 1989;93:246–252.
201. Macfarlane AJ, Kon OM, Smith SJ, et al. Basophils, eosinophils, and mast cells in atopic and nonatopic asthma and in late-phase allergic reactions in the lung and skin. *J Allergy Clin Immunol*. 2000;105:99–107.
202. Ito Y, Satoh T, Takayama K, et al. Basophil recruitment and activation in inflammatory skin diseases. *Allergy*. 2011;66:1107–1113.
203. O'Mahony L, Akdis M, Akdis CA. Regulation of the immune response and inflammation by histamine and histamine receptors. *J Allergy Clin Immunol*. 2011;128:1153–1162.
204. Gutowska-Owsiak D, Selvakumar TA, Salimi M, et al. Histamine enhances keratinocyte-mediated resolution of inflammation by promoting wound healing and response to infection. *Clin Exp Dermatol*. 2014;39:187–195.
205. Goh YY, Pal M, Chong HC, et al. Angiopoietin-like 4 interacts with integrins beta1 and beta5 to modulate keratinocyte migration. *Am J Pathol*. 2010;177:2791–2803.
206. Bairy KL, Rao CM, Ramesh KV, et al. Effects of antihistamines on wound healing. *Indian J Exp Biol*. 1991;29:398–399.
207. Tanaka K, Honda M, Kuramochi T, et al. Prominent inhibitory effects of tranilast on migration and proliferation of and collagen synthesis by vascular smooth muscle cells. *Atherosclerosis*. 1994;107:179–185.
208. Miyazawa K, Hamano S, Ujiie A. Antiproliferative and c-myc mRNA suppressive effect of tranilast on newborn human vascular smooth muscle cells in culture. *Br J Pharmacol*. 1996;118:915–922.
209. Venugopal J, Ramakrishnan M, Habibullah CM, et al. The effect of the anti-allergic agent avil on abnormal scar fibroblasts. *Burns*. 1999;25:223–228.
210. Suzawa H, Kikuchi S, Arai N, et al. The mechanism involved in the inhibitory action of tranilast on collagen biosynthesis of keloid fibroblasts. *Jpn J Pharmacol*. 1992;60:91–96.
211. Occleston NL, O'Kane S, Goldspink N, et al. New therapeutics for the prevention and reduction of scarring. *Drug Discov Today*. 2008;13:973–981.

212. McCoy BJ, Diegelmann RF, Cohen IK. In vitro inhibition of cell growth, collagen synthesis, and prolyl hydroxylase activity by triamcinolone acetonide. *Proc Soc Exp Biol Med Soc Exp Biol Med.* 1980;163:216–222.
213. Darzi MA CN, Kaul SK, Khan M. Evaluation of various methods of treating keloids and hypertrophic scars: a 10-year follow-up study. *Br J Plast Surg.* 1992;45:374–379.
214. Jimenez SA, Freundlich B, Rosenbloom J. Selective inhibition of human diploid fibroblast collagen synthesis by interferons. *J Clin Invest.* 1984;74:1112–1116.
215. Granstein RD, Rook A, Flotte TJ, et al. A controlled trial of intralesional recombinant interferon-gamma in the treatment of keloidal scarring. *Arch Dermatol.* 1990;126:1295–1302.
216. Berman B, Flores F. Recurrence rates of excised keloids treated with postoperative triamcinolone acetonide injections or interferon alfa-2b injections. *J Am Acad Dermatol.* 1997;37:755–757.
217. Sauder DN, Smith MH, Senta-McMillian T, et al. Randomized, single-blind, placebo-controlled study of topical application of the immune response modulator resiquimod in healthy adults. *Antimicrob Agents Chemother.* 2003;47:3846–3852.
218. Berman B, Kaufman J. Pilot study of the effect of postoperative imiquimod 5% cream on the recurrence rate of excised keloids. *J Am Acad Dermatol.* 2002;47:S209–S211.
219. Stashower ME. Successful treatment of earlobe keloids with imiquimod after tangential shave excision. *Dermatol Surg.* 2006;32:380–386.
220. Cacao FM, Tanaka V, Messina MC. Failure of imiquimod 5% cream to prevent recurrence of surgically excised trunk keloids. *Dermatol Surg.* 2009;35:629–633.
221. Fitzpatrick RE. Treatment of inflamed hypertrophic scars using intralesional 5-FU. *Dermatol Surg.* 1999;25:224–232.
222. Kontochristopoulos G, Stefanaki C, Panagiotopoulos A, et al. Intralesional 5-fluorouracil in the treatment of keloids: an open clinical and histopathologic study. *J Am Acad Dermatol.* 2005;52:474–479.
223. Nanda S RB. Intralesional 5-fluorouracil as a treatment modality of keloids. *Dermatol Surg.* 2004;30:54–56.
224. Hendricks T, Martens MF, Huyben CM, et al. Inhibition of basal and TGF beta-induced fibroblast collagen synthesis by antineoplastic agents. Implications for wound healing. *Br J Cancer.* 1993;67:545–550.
225. Yeowell HN, Marshall MK, Walker LC, et al. Regulation of lysyl oxidase mRNA in dermal fibroblasts from normal donors and patients with inherited connective tissue disorders. *Arch Biochem Biophys.* 1994;308(1):299–305.
226. James MP, Collier PM, Aherne W, et al. Histologic, pharmacologic, and immunocytochemical effects of injection of bleomycin into viral warts. *J Am Acad Dermatol.* 1993;28(6):933–937.
227. Saray Y, Gulec AT. Treatment of keloids and hypertrophic scars with dermojet injections of bleomycin: a preliminary study. *Int J Dermatol.* 2005;44:777–784.
228. Derderian CA, Bastidas N, Lerman OZ, et al. Mechanical strain alters gene expression in an in vitro model of hypertrophic scarring. *Ann Plast Surg.* 2005;55:69–75; discussion 75.
229. Wallace CA. The use of methotrexate in childhood rheumatic diseases. *Arthritis Rheum.* 1998;41:381–391.
230. Tolerton SK, Tonkin MA. Keloid formation after syndactyly release in patients with associated macrodactyly: management with methotrexate therapy. *J Hand Surg.* 2011;36:490–497.
231. Stewart CE, Kim JY. Application of mitomycin-C for head and neck keloids. *Otolaryngol—Head Neck Surg.* 2006;135:946–950.
232. Simman R, Alani H, Williams F. Effect of mitomycin C on keloid fibroblasts: an in vitro study. *Ann Plast Surg.* 2003;50:71–76.
233. Bailey JNR, Waite AE, Clayton WJ, et al. Application of topical mitomycin C to the base of shave-removed keloid scars to prevent their recurrence. *Br J Dermatol.* 2007;156:682–686.
234. Talmi YP, Orenstein A, Wolf M, et al. Use of mitomycin C for treatment of keloid: a preliminary report. *Otolaryngol—Head Neck Surg.* 2005;132:598–601.
235. Sanders KW, Gage-White L, Stucker FJ. Topical mitomycin C in the prevention of keloid scar recurrence. *Arch Fac Plast Surg.* 2005;7:172–175.
236. Viera MH, Amini S, Valins W, et al. Innovative therapies in the treatment of keloids and hypertrophic scars. *J Clin Aesthet Dermatol.* 2010;3:20–26.
237. Rhett JM, Ghatnekar GS, Palatinus JA, et al. Novel therapies for scar reduction and regenerative healing of skin wounds. *Trends Biotechnol.* 2008;26:173–180.
238. Brolmann FE, Ubbink DT, Nelson EA, et al. Evidence-based decisions for local and systemic wound care. *Br J Surg.* 2012;99:1172–1183.
239. Storm-Versloot MN, Vos CG, Ubbink DT, et al. Topical silver for preventing wound infection. *Cochrane Database Syst Rev.* 2010;(3):CD006478.
240. Wasiak J, Cleland H, Campbell F, et al. Dressings for superficial and partial thickness burns. *Cochrane Database Syst Rev.* 2013;3:CD002106.
241. Wasiak J, Cleland H. Burns (minor thermal). *Clin Evid.* 2005;14: 2388–2396.
242. Cruciani M, Lipsky BA, Mengoli C. Granulocyte-colony stimulating factors as adjunctive therapy for diabetic foot infections. *Cochrane Database Syst Rev.* 2009;(3):CD006810.
243. Voigt J, Driver VR. Hyaluronic acid derivatives and their healing effect on burns, epithelial surgical wounds, and chronic wounds: a systematic review and meta-analysis of randomized controlled trials. *Wound Repair Regen.* 2012;20:317–331.
244. Jull AB, Rodgers A, Walker N. Honey as a topical treatment for wounds. Cochrane Database of Systematic Reviews, 2008. *Cochrane Database Syst Rev.* 20088;(4):CD005083.
245. Guthrie HC, Martin KR, Taylor C, et al. A pre-clinical evaluation of silver, iodine and Manuka honey based dressings in a model of traumatic extremity wounds contaminated with Staphylococcus aureus. *Injury.* 2014;45:1171–1178.
246. Gragnani A, Warde M, Furtado F, et al. Topical tamoxifen therapy in hypertrophic scars or keloids in burns. *Arch Dermatol Res.* 2010;302:1–4.
247. Hu D, Hughes MA, Cherry GW. Topical tamoxifen--a potential therapeutic regime in treating excessive dermal scarring? *Br J Plast Surg.* 1998;51:462–469.
248. Mikulec AA, Hanasono MM, Lum J, et al. Effect of tamoxifen on transforming growth factor beta1 production by keloid and fetal fibroblasts. *Arch Fac Plast Surg.* 2001;3:111–114.
249. Chau D, Mancoll JS, Lee S, et al. Tamoxifen downregulates TGF-beta production in keloid fibroblasts. *Ann Plast Surg.* 1998;40:490–493.
250. Arnold M, Barbul A. Nutrition and wound healing. *Plast Reconstr Surg.* 2006;117:42S–58S.
251. Stechmiller JK. Understanding the role of nutrition and wound healing. *Nutr Clin Pract.* 2010;25:61–68.
252. Stratton RJ, Ek AC, Engfer M, et al. Enteral nutritional support in prevention and treatment of pressure ulcers: a systematic review and meta-analysis. *Ageing Res Rev.* 2005;4:422–450.
253. Langemo D, Anderson J, Hanson D, et al. Nutritional considerations in wound care. *Adv Skin Wound Care.* 2006;19:297–298, 300, 3.
254. Posthauer ME. The role of nutrition in wound care. *Adv Skin Wound Care.* 2012;25:62–63.
255. Posthauer ME. The role of nutrition in wound care. *Adv Skin Wound Care.* 2006;19:43–52; quiz 3–4.
256. Campos AC, Groth AK, Branco AB. Assessment and nutritional aspects of wound healing. *Curr Opin Clin Nutr Metab Care.* 2008;11:281–288.
257. Stechmiller JK, Cowan L, Whitney JD, et al. Guidelines for the prevention of pressure ulcers. *Wound Repair Regen.* 2008;16:151–68.
258. Dorner B, Posthauer ME, Thomas D, et al. The role of nutrition in pressure ulcer prevention and treatment: National Pressure Ulcer Advisory Panel white paper. *Adv Skin Wound Care.* 2009;22:212–221.
259. Stechmiller JK, Cowan L, Logan K. Nutrition support for wound healing. *Supp Line.* 2009;31:2–8.
260. Ross V. Micronutrient recommendations for wound healing. *Supp Line.* 2002;24:3–9.
261. Standing Committee on the Scientific Evaluation of Dietary Reference Intakes FaNB. *Dietary Reference Intakes for Vitamin A, Vitamin K, Arsenic, Boron, Chromium, Copper, Iodine, Iron, Manganese, Molybdenum, Nickel, Silicon, Vanadium, and Zinc.* Washington, DC: National Academy Press; 2001.
262. American Dietetic Association and Morrison Health Care IPusI-Imntp. *Medical Nutrition Therapy Across the Continuum of Care.* Chicago, IL: American Dietetic Association; 1997.
263. Menke M, MenkeN, Boardman CH, et al. Biologic therapeutics and molecular profiling to optimize wound healing. *Clin Dermatol.* 2007;25:19–25.
264. Chernoff R. Policy: nutrition standards for treatment of pressure ulcers. *Nutr Rev.* 1996;54:43–4.
265. Gordon MD, Gottschlich M, Helvig EI. Review of evidence-based practice for the prevention of pressure sores in burn patients. *J Burn Care Rehabil.* 2004;25:388–410.
266. Chernoff R. Normal aging, nutritional assessment, and clinical practice. *Nutr Clin Pract.* 2003;18:12–20.

267. Williams JZ, Barbul A. Nutrition and wound healing. *Surg Clin N Am*. 2003;83:571–596.
268. Mathus-Vliegen EM. Old age, malnutrition, and pressure sores: an ill-fated alliance. *J Gerontol Ser A, Biol Sci Med Sci*. 2004;59:355–360.
269. Langer G, Schloemer G, Knerr A, et al. Nutritional interventions for preventing and treating pressure ulcers. *Cochrane Database Syst Rev*. 2003;(4):CD003216.
270. Whitney J, Phillips L, Aslam R, et al. Guidelines for the treatment of pressure ulcers. *Wound Repair Regen*. 2006;14:663–679.
271. Stechmiller JK, Childress B, Cowan L. Arginine supplementation and wound healing. *Nutr Clin Pract*. 2005;20:52–61.
272. Thompson C, Fuhrman MP. Nutrients and wound healing: still searching for the magic bullet. *Nutr Clin Pract*. 2005;20: 331–347.
273. Casaer MP, Van den Berghe G. Nutrition in the acute phase of critical illness. *N Engl J Med*. 2014;370:1227–1236.
274. Seth AK, Nguyen KT, Geringer MR, et al. Noncontact, low-frequency ultrasound as an effective therapy against Pseudomonas aeruginosa–infected biofilm wounds. *Wound Repair Regen*. 2013;21:266–274.
275. Maan ZN, Januszyk M, Rennert RC, et al. Noncontact, low-frequency ultrasound therapy enhances neovascularization and wound healing in diabetic mice. *Plast Reconstr Surg*. 2014;134.
276. Voigt J, Wendelken M, Driver V, et al. Low-frequency ultrasound (20-40 kHz) as an adjunctive therapy for chronic wound healing: a systematic review of the literature and meta-analysis of eight randomized controlled trials. *Int J Lower Extrem Wounds*. 2011;10:190–199.
277. Serena T, Lee SK, Lam K, et al. The impact of noncontact, nonthermal, low-frequency ultrasound on bacterial counts in experimental and chronic wounds. *Ostomy/Wound Manag*. 2009;55:22–30.
278. Escandon J, Vivas AC, Perez R, et al. A prospective pilot study of ultrasound therapy effectiveness in refractory venous leg ulcers. *Int Wound J*. 2012;9:570–578.
279. Prather JL, Tummel EK, Patel AB, et al. Prospective randomized controlled trial comparing the effects of noncontact low-frequency ultrasound with standard care in healing split-thickness donor sites. *J Am Coll Surg*. 2015;221(2):309–318.
280. White J, Ivins N, Wilkes A, et al. Non-contact low-frequency ultrasound therapy compared with UK standard of care for venous leg ulcers: a single-centre, assessor-blinded, randomised controlled trial. *Int Wound J*. 2015;13(5):588–842.
281. Rusciani L, Rossi G, Bono R. Use of cryotherapy in the treatment of keloids. *J Dermatol Surg Oncol*. 1993;19:529–534.
282. Zouboulis CC, Blume U, Buttner P, et al. Outcomes of cryosurgery in keloids and hypertrophic scars. A prospective consecutive trial of case series. *Arch Dermatol*. 1993;129:1146–1151.
283. Cho YS, Jeon JH, Hong A, et al. The effect of burn rehabilitation massage therapy on hypertrophic scar after burn: a randomized controlled trial. *Burns*. 2014;40:1513–1520.
284. Morien A, Garrison D, Smith NK. Range of motion improves after massage in children with burns: a pilot study. *J Bodyw Mov Ther*. 2008;12:67–71.
285. Hernandez-Reif M, Field T, Largie S, et al. Childrens' distress during burn treatment is reduced by massage therapy. *J Burn Care Res*. 2001;22.
286. Field T, Peck M, Scd, et al. Postburn itching, pain, and psychological symptoms are reduced with massage therapy. *J Burn Care Rehabil*. 2000;21:189–193.
287. Roh YS, Cho H, Oh JO, et al. Effects of skin rehabilitation massage therapy on pruritus, skin status, and depression inburn survivors. *Taehan Kanho Hakhoe Chi*. 2007;37:221–226.
288. Knott PD, Zins JE, Banbury J, et al. A comparison of dermabond tissue adhesive and sutures in the primary repair of the congenital cleft lip. *Ann Plast Surg*. 2007;58:121 125.
289. Cullum N, Nelson EA, Flemming K, et al. Systematic reviews of wound care management: (5) beds; (6) compression; (7) laser therapy, therapeutic ultrasound, electrotherapy and electromagnetic therapy. *Health Technol Assess*. 2001;5:1–221.
290. Kanazawa Y, Nomura J, Yoshimoto S, et al. Cyclical cell stretching of skin-derived fibroblasts downregulates connective tissue growth factor (CTGF) production. *Connect Tissue Res*. 2009;50:323–329.
291. Reno F, Sabbatini M, Lombardi F, et al. In vitro mechanical compression induces apoptosis and regulates cytokines release in hypertrophic scars. *Wound Repair Regen*. 2003;11:331–336.
292. Roques C. Massage applied to scars. *Wound Repair Regen*. 2002;10: 126–128.
293. Liuzzi F, Chadwick S, Shah M. Paediatric post-burn scar management in the UK: a national survey. *Burns*. 2015;41:252–256.
294. Markov MS. Expanding use of pulsed electromagnetic field therapies. *Electromagn Biol Med*. 2007;26(3):257–274
295. Goto T, Fujioka M, Ishida M, et al. Noninvasive up-regulation of angiopoietin-2 and fibroblast growth factor-2 in bone marrow by pulsed electromagnetic field therapy. *J Orthop Sci*. 2010;15:661–665.
296. de Girolamo L, Stanco D, Galliera E, et al. Low frequency pulsed electromagnetic field affects proliferation, tissue-specific gene expression, and cytokines release of human tendon cells. *Cell Biochem Biophys*. 2013;66:697–708.
297. Lei T, Jing D, Xie K, et al. Therapeutic effects of 15 Hz pulsed electromagnetic field on diabetic peripheral neuropathy in streptozotocin-treated rats. *PLoS One*. 2013;8:e61414.
298. Hao CN, Huang JJ, Shi YQ, et al. Pulsed electromagnetic field improves cardiac function in response to myocardial infarction. *Am J Transl Res*. 2014;6:281–290.
299. Ross CL, Harrison BS. Effect of pulsed electromagnetic field on inflammatory pathway markers in RAW 264.7 murine macrophages. *J Inflamm Res*. 2013;6:45–51.
300. Gomez-Ochoa I, Gomez-Ochoa P, Gomez-Casal F, et al. Pulsed electromagnetic fields decrease proinflammatory cytokine secretion (IL-1beta and TNF-alpha) on human fibroblast-like cell culture. *Rheumatol Int*. 2011;31:1283–1289.
301. Rohde CH, Taylor EM, Alonso A, et al. Pulsed electromagnetic fields reduce postoperative interleukin-1beta, pain, and inflammation: a double-blind, placebo-controlled study in TRAM flap breast reconstruction patients. *Plast Reconstr Surg*. 2015;135:808e–817e.
302. Ferroni L, Bellin G, Emer V, et al. Treatment by Therapeutic Magnetic Resonance (TMR) increases fibroblastic activity and keratinocyte differentiation in an in vitro model of 3D artificial skin. *J Tissue Eng Regen Med*. 2015. doi:10.1002/term.2031
303. Kwan RL, Wong WC, Yip SL, et al. Pulsed electromagnetic field therapy promotes healing and microcirculation of chronic diabetic foot ulcers: a pilot study. *Adv Skin Wound Care*. 2015;28:212–219.
304. Callaghan MJ, Chang EI, Seiser N, et al. Pulsed electromagnetic fields accelerate normal and diabetic wound healing by increasing endogenous FGF-2 release. *Plast Reconstr Surg*. 2008;121:130–141.
305. Cañedo-Dorantes L, García-Cantú R, Barrera R, et al. Healing of chronic arterial and venous leg ulcers with systemic electromagnetic fields. *Arch Med Res*. 2002;33:281–289.
306. Mulder G, Tenenhaus M, D'Souza GF. Reduction of diabetic foot ulcer healing times through use of advanced treatment modalities. *Int J Lower Extrem Wounds*. 2014;13:335–346.
307. Aziz Z, Flemming K. Electromagnetic therapy for treating pressure ulcers. *Cochrane Database Syst Rev*. 2012;(12):CD002930.
308. Li S, Yu B, Zhou D, et al. Electromagnetic fields for treating osteoarthritis. *Cochrane Database Syst Rev*. 2013;(12):CD003523.
309. Hannemann PF, Mommers EH, Schots JP, et al. The effects of low-intensity pulsed ultrasound and pulsed electromagnetic fields bone growth stimulation in acute fractures: a systematic review and meta-analysis of randomized controlled trials. *Arch Orthop Trauma Surg*. 2014;134:1093–1106.
310. Zhao M. Electrical fields in wound healing-An overriding signal that directs cell migration. *Semin Cell Dev Biol*. 2009;20:674–682.
311. Kelly AP. Medical and surgical therapies for keloids. *Dermatol Ther*. 2004;17:212–218.
312. Costa AM, Peyrol S, Porto LC, et al. Mechanical forces induce scar remodeling. Study in non-pressure-treated versus pressure-treated hypertrophic scars. *Am J Pathol*. 1999;155:1671–1679.
313. Amicucci G, Schietroma M, Rossi M, et al. Silicone occlusive sheeting vs silicone cushion for the treatment of hypertrophic and keloid scars. A prospective-randomized study [in Italian]. *Ann Ital Chir*. 2005;76:79–83.
314. O'Meara S, Cullum N, Nelson EA, et al. Compression for venous leg ulcers. *Cochrane Database Syst Rev*. 2012;(11):CD000265.
315. O'Meara S, Tierney J, Cullum N, et al. Four layer bandage compared with short stretch bandage for venous leg ulcers: systematic review and meta-analysis of randomised controlled trials with data from individual patients. *BMJ*. 2009;338:b1344.
316. Fletcher A, Cullum N, Sheldon TA. A systematic review of compression treatment for venous leg ulcers. *BMJ*. 1997;315:576–580.
317. Sharp PA, Pan B, Yakuboff KP, et al. Development of a best evidence statement for the use of pressure therapy for management of hypertrophic scarring. *J Burn Care Res*. 2016;37(4):255–264.

318. Murphy PS, Evans GR. Advances in wound healing: a review of current wound healing products. *Plast Surg Int*. 2012;2012:190436.
319. Thom SR, Bhopale VM, Velazquez OC, et al. Stem cell mobilization by hyperbaric oxygen. *Am J Physiol Heart Circ Physiol*. 2006;290:H1378–H1386.
320. Gallagher KA, Goldstein LJ, Thom SR, et al. Hyperbaric oxygen and bone marrow-derived endothelial progenitor cells in diabetic wound healing. *Vascular*. 2006;14:328–337.
321. Romero-Valdovinos M, Cardenas-Mejia A, Gutierrez-Gomez C, et al. Keloid skin scars: the influence of hyperbaric oxygenation on fibroblast growth and on the expression of messenger RNA for insulin like growth factor and for transforming growth factor. *In Vitro Cell Dev Biol Anim*. 2011;47:421–424.
322. Kranke P, Bennett M, Roeckl-Wiedmann I, et al. Hyperbaric oxygen therapy for chronic wounds. *Cochrane Database Syst Rev*. 2004;(2):CD004123.
323. Londahl M, Katzman P, Nilsson A, et al. Hyperbaric oxygen therapy facilitates healing of chronic foot ulcers in patients with diabetes. *Diabetes Care*. 2010;33:998–1003.
324. Abidia A, Laden G, Kuhan G, et al. The role of hyperbaric oxygen therapy in ischaemic diabetic lower extremity ulcers: a double-blind randomised-controlled trial. *Eur J Vasc Endovasc Surg*. 2003; 25:513–18.
325. Dimitrijevich SD, Paranjape S, Wilson JR, et al. Effect of hyperbaric oxygen on human skin cells in culture and in human dermal and skin equivalents. *Wound Repair Regen*. 1999;7(1):53–64.
326. Zhang Q, Shao Js, Yue Yg, et al. Effect of hyperbaric oxygen on the scar formation at the rabbit ears at an early stage [in Chinese]. *Zhonghua Zheng Xing Wai Ke Za Zhi*. 2013;29(1):55–58.
327. Chang CH, Lie HW, Huang CC. Designed drug-release systems having various breathable polyurethane film-backed hydrocolloid acrylated adhesive layers for moisture healing. *Bio-Med Mater Eng*. 2014;24:2081–2088.
328. Quinn KJ, Courtney JM, Evans JH, et al. Principles of burn dressings. *Biomaterials*. 1985;6:369–377.
329. Suissa D, Danino A, Nikolis A. negative-pressure therapy versus standard wound care: a meta-analysis of randomized trials. *Plast Reconstr Surg*. 2011;128:498e–503e.
330. Blume PA, Walters J, Payne W, et al. Comparison of negative pressure wound therapy using vacuum-assisted closure with advanced moist wound therapy in the treatment of diabetic foot ulcers: a multicenter randomized controlled trial. *Diabetes Care*. 2008;31:631–636.
331. Argenta LC, Morykwas MJ, Marks MW, et al. Vacuum-assisted closure: state of clinic art. *Plast Reconstr Surg*. 2006;117:127S–42S.
332. Campbell PE. Surgical wound case studies with the versatile 1 wound vacuum system for negative pressure wound therapy. *J Wound Ostomy Continence Nurs*. 2006;33:176–185; discussion 85–90.
333. Miller MS, McDaniel C. Postsurgical post-hysterectomy abdominal wound dehiscence treated with negative pressure wound therapy. *Int J Gynaecol Obstet*. 2006;93:264–266.
334. Morykwas MJ, Argenta LC, Shelton-Brown EI, et al. Vacuum-assisted closure: a new method for wound control and treatment: animal studies and basic foundation. *Ann Plast Surg*. 1997;38:553–562.
335. Nordmeyer M, Pauser J, Biber R, et al. Negative pressure wound therapy for seroma prevention and surgical incision treatment in spinal fracture care. *Int Wound J*. 2015. doi:10.1111/iwj.12436.
336. Shweiki D, Itin A, Soffer D, et al. Vascular endothelial growth factor induced by hypoxia may mediate hypoxia-initiated angiogenesis. *Nature*. 1992;359:843–845.
337. Saxena V, Hwang CW, Huang S, et al. Vacuum-assisted closure: microdeformations of wounds and cell proliferation. *Plast Reconstr Surg*. 2004;114:1086–96; discussion 97–8.
338. Pietramaggiori G, Liu P, Scherer SS, et al. Tensile forces stimulate vascular remodeling and epidermal cell proliferation in living skin. *Ann Surg*. 2007;246:896–902.
339. Erba P, Ogawa R, Ackermann M, et al. Angiogenesis in wounds treated by microdeformational wound therapy. *Ann Surg*. 2011;253: 402–409.
340. Sadat U, Chang G, Noorani A, et al. Efficacy of TNP on lower limb wounds: a meta-analysis. *J Wound Care*. 2008;17:45–48.
341. Mcgarrah B. Using negative pressure therapy for wound healing in the extremely low-birth-weight infant (Micropreemie). *J Wound Ostomy Continence Nurs*. 2015;42:409–412.
342. Lu F, Ogawa R, Nguyen DT, et al. Microdeformation of three-dimensional cultured fibroblasts induces gene expression and morphological changes. *Ann Plast Surg*. 2011;66:296–300.
343. Jacobs S, Simhaee DA, Marsano A, et al. Efficacy and mechanisms of vacuum-assisted closure (VAC) therapy in promoting wound healing: a rodent model. *J Plast Reconstr Aesthet Surg*. 2009;62:1331–1338.
344. Kilpadi DV, Bower CE, Reade CC, et al. Effect of vacuum assisted closure therapy on early systemic cytokine levels in a swine model. *Wound Repair Regen*. 2006;14:210–215.
345. McNulty AK, Schmidt M, Feeley T, et al. Effects of negative pressure wound therapy on cellular energetics in fibroblasts grown in a provisional wound (fibrin) matrix. *Wound Repair Regen*. 2009;17:192–199.
346. Wilkes R, Zhao Y, Kieswetter K, et al. Effects of dressing type on 3D tissue microdeformations during negative pressure wound therapy: a computational study. *J Biomech Eng*. 2009;131:031012.
347. Galbraith CG, Sheetz MP. Forces on adhesive contacts affect cell function. *Curr Opin Cell Biol*. 1998;10:566–571.
348. Shyy JY, Chien S. Role of integrins in cellular responses to mechanical stress and adhesion. *Curr Opin Cell Biol*. 1997;9:707–713.
349. Kessler D, Dethlefsen S, Haase I, et al. Fibroblasts in mechanically stressed collagen lattices assume a "synthetic" phenotype. *J Biol Chem*. 2001;276:36575–36585.
350. Schwachtgen JL, Houston P, Campbell C, et al. Fluid shear stress activation of Egr-1 transcription in cultured human endothelial and epithelial cells is mediated via the extracellular signal-related kinase 1/2 mitogen-activated protein kinase pathway. *J Clin Invest*. 1998;101:2540–2549.
351. Biesiada E, Razandi M, Levin ER. Egr-1 activates basic fibroblast growth factor transcription. Mechanistic implications for astrocyte proliferation. *J Biol Chem*. 1996;271:18576–18581.
352. Khachigian LM, Lindner V, Williams AJ, et al. Egr-1-induced endothelial gene expression: a common theme in vascular injury. *Science*. 1996;271:1427–1431.
353. Kim SJ, Jeang KT, Glick AB, et al. Promoter sequences of the human transforming growth factor-beta 1 gene responsive to transforming growth factor-beta 1 autoinduction. *J Biol Chem*. 1989;264:7041–7045.
354. Yan SF, Fujita T, Lu J, et al. Egr-1, a master switch coordinating upregulation of divergent gene families underlying ischemic stress. *Nat Med*. 2000;6:1355–1361.
355. Labler L, Mica L, Harter L, et al. Influence of V.A.C.—therapy on cytokines and growth factors in traumatic wounds [in German]. *Zentralbl Chir*. 2006;131(suppl 1):S62–S67.
356. Glass GE, Nanchahal J. The methodology of negative pressure wound therapy: separating fact from fiction. *J Plast Reconstr Aesthet Surg*. 2012;65:989–1001.
357. Dastouri P, Helm DL, Scherer SS, et al. Waveform modulation of negative-pressure wound therapy in the murine model. *Plast Reconstr Surg*. 2011;127:1460–1466.
358. Yang F, Hu D, Bai XJ, et al. The influence of oxygen partial pressure change and vascularization of rabbit wound through negative pressure wound therapy [in Chinese]. *Zhonghua Wai Ke Za Zhi*. 2012:650–654.
359. Gilkes DM, Bajpai S, Chaturvedi P, et al. Hypoxia-inducible factor 1 (HIF-1) promotes extracellular matrix remodeling under hypoxic conditions by inducing P4HA1, P4HA2, and PLOD2 expression in fibroblasts. *J Biol Chem*. 2013;288:10819–10829.
360. Liu L, Gao J, Yuan Y, et al. Hypoxia preconditioned human adipose derived mesenchymal stem cells enhance angiogenic potential via secretion of increased VEGF and bFGF. *Cell Biol Int*. 2013;37:551–560.
361. Glass GE, Murphy GF, Esmaeili A, et al. Systematic review of molecular mechanism of action of negative-pressure wound therapy. *Br J Surg*. 2014;101:1627–1636.
362. Labler L, Rancan M, Mica L, et al. Vacuum-assisted closure therapy increases local interleukin-8 and vascular endothelial growth factor levels in traumatic wounds. *J Trauma*. 2009;66:749–757.
363. Tang SY, Xu H, Qi LJ, et al. Effect of vacuum-assisted closure on angiogenesis during denervation of wound healing. *Zhongguo Linchuang Kangfu*. 2005;46:91–93.
364. Mukaida N, Harada A, Matsushima K. Interleukin-8 (IL-8) and monocyte chemotactic and activating factor (MCAF/MCP-1), chemokines essentially involved in inflammatory and immune reactions. *Cytokine Growth Factor Rev*. 1998;9:9–23.
365. Koch AE, Polverni P, Kunkel SL, et al. Interleukin-8 as a macrophage-derived mediator of angiogenesis. *Science*. 1992:1798–1801.
366. Stechmiller JK, Kilpadi DV, Childress B, et al. Effect of vacuum-assisted closure therapy on the expression of cytokines and proteases in wound fluid of adults with pressure ulcers. *Wound Repair Regen*. 2006;14:371–374.
367. Eisenhardt SU, Schmidt Y, Thiele JR, et al. Negative pressure wound therapy reduces the ischaemia/reperfusion-associated

inflammatory response in free muscle flaps. *J Plast Reconstr Aesthet Surg*. 2012;65:640–649.
368. Dumville JC, Owens GL, Crosbie EJ, et al. Negative pressure wound therapy for treating surgical wounds healing by secondary intention. *Cochrane Database Syst Rev*. 2015;(6):CD011278.
369. Dumville JC, Webster J, Evans D, et al. Negative pressure wound therapy for treating pressure ulcers. *Cochrane Database Syst Rev*. 2015;(5):CD011334.
370. Wasiak J, Cleland H. Topical negative pressure (TNP) for partial thickness burns. *Cochrane Database Syst Rev*. 2007;(3):CD006215.
371. Fraccalvieri M, Zingarelli E, Ruka E, et al. Negative pressure wound therapy using gauze and foam: histological, immunohistochemical and ultrasonography morphological analysis of the granulation tissue and scar tissue. Preliminary report of a clinical study. *Int Wound J*. 2011;8:355–364.
372. Fraccalvieri M, Sarno A, Gasperini S, et al. Can single use negative pressure wound therapy be an alternative method to manage keloid scarring? A preliminary report of a clinical and ultrasound/colour-power-doppler study. *Int Wound J*. 2013;10(3):340–344.
373. Phipps AR, Lawrence JC. Use of a hydrocolloid dressing in the ambulatory treatment of burns [in French]. *Rev Infirm*. 1989;39:7–9.
374. Dumville JC, Stubbs N, Keogh SJ, et al. Hydrogel dressings for treating pressure ulcers. *Cochrane Database Syst Rev*. 2015;(2):CD011226.
375. Dumville JC, Deshpande S, O'Meara S, et al. Hydrocolloid dressings for healing diabetic foot ulcers. *Cochrane Database Syst Rev*. 2012;(2):CD009099.
376. Singh A, Halder S, Menon GR, et al. Meta-analysis of randomized controlled trials on hydrocolloid occlusive dressing versus conventional gauze dressing in the healing of chronic wounds. *Asian J Surg*. 2004;27:326–332.
377. Afilalo M, Dankoff J, Guttman A, et al. DuoDERM hydroactive dressing vs silver sulphadiazine/Bactigras in the emergency treatment of partial skin thickness burns. *Burns*. 1992;18:313–316.
378. Thomas SS, Lawrence JC, Thomas A. Evaluation of hydrocolloids and topical medication in minor burns. *J Wound Care*. 1995;4:218–220.
379. Wright A, MacKechnie D, Paskins JR. Management of partial thickness burns with Granuflex 'E' dressings. *Burns*. 1993:128–130.
380. Wyatt D, McGowan DN, Najarian MP. Comparison of a hydrocolloid dressing and silver sulfadiazine cream in the outpatient management of second-degree burns. *J Trauma*. 1990;30:857–865.
381. Martin FT, O'Sullivan JB, Regan PJ, et al. Hydrocolloid dressing in pediatric burns may decrease operative intervention rates. *J Pediatr Surg*. 2010;45:600–605.
382. Guilbaud J. European comparative clinical study of Inerpan: a new wound dressing in treatment of partial skin thickness burns. *Burns*. 1992;18:419–422.
383. Guilbaud J, Honde C. Multicentre comparative clinical study of a new wound dressing: PA286 (Inerpan). *Eur J Plast Surg*. 1993;16:73–76.
384. Huang G, Sun T, Zhang L, et al. Combined application of alginate dressing and human granulocyte-macrophage colony stimulating factor promotes healing in refractory chronic skin ulcers. *Exp Therap Med*. 2014;7:1772–1776.
385. Boateng J, Burgos-Amador R, Okeke O, et al. Composite alginate and gelatin based bio-polymeric wafers containing silver sulfadiazine for wound healing. *Int J Biol Macromol*. 2015;79:63–71.
386. Dumville JC, Keogh SJ, Liu Z, et al. Alginate dressings for treating pressure ulcers. *Cochrane Database Syst Rev*. 2015;(5):CD011277.
387. Perkins K, Davey RB, Wallis KA. Silicone gel: a new treatment for burn scars and contractures. *Burns*. 1983;9:201–204.
388. Bleasdale B, Finnegan S, Murray K, et al. The use of silicone adhesives for scar reduction. *Adv Wound Care (New Rochelle)*. 2015;4(7):422–430.
389. Mustoe TA. Evolution of silicone therapy and mechanism of action in scar management. *Aesthet Plast Surg*. 2008;32:82–92.
390. Mustoe TA, Cooter RD, Gold MH, et al. International clinical recommendations on scar management. *Plast Reconstr Surg*. 2002;110:560–571.
391. Eishi K, Bae SJ, Ogawa F, et al. Silicone gel sheets relieve pain and pruritus with clinical improvement of keloid: possible target of mast cells. *J Dermatolog Treat*. 2003;14:248–252.
392. Li-Tsang CW, Lau JC, Choi J, et al. A prospective randomized clinical trial to investigate the effect of silicone gel sheeting (Cica-Care) on post-traumatic hypertrophic scar among the Chinese population. *Burns*. 2006;32:678–683.
393. O'Brien L, Jones DJ. Silicone gel sheeting for preventing and treating hypertrophic and keloid scars. *Cochrane Database Syst Rev*. 2013;(9):CD003826.
394. Mercer NS. Silicone gel in the treatment of keloid scars. *Br J Plast Surg*. 1989;42:83–87.
395. Phillips TJ, Gerstein AD, Lordan V. A randomized controlled trial of hydrocolloid dressing in the treatment of hypertrophic scars and keloids. *Dermatol Surg*. 1996;22:775–778.
396. Puri N, Talwar A. The efficacy of silicone gel for the treatment of hypertrophic scars and keloids. *J Cutan Aesthet Surg*. 2009;2:104–106.
397. Arroyo AA, Casanova PL, Soriano JV, et al. Open-label clinical trial comparing the clinical and economic effectiveness of using a polyurethane film surgical dressing with gauze surgical dressings in the care of post-operative surgical wounds. *Int Wound J*. 2015;12:285–292.
398. Neal D, Whalley P, Flowers M, et al. The effects of an adherent polyurethane film and conventional absorbent dressing in patients with small partial thickness burns. *Br J Clin Pract*. 1981;35:254–257.
399. Poulsen TD, Freund KG, Arendrup K, et al. Polyurethane film (Opsite) vs. impregnated gauze (Jelonet) in the treatment of outpatient burns: a prospective, randomized study. *Burns*. 1991;17:59–61.
400. Wigger-Albert W, Kuhlmann M, Wilhelm D, et al. Efficacy of a polyurethane dressing versus a soft silicone sheet on hypertrophic scars. *J Wound Care*. 2009;18:208, 210–214.
401. Schmidt A, Gassmueller J, Hughes-Formella B, et al. Treating hypertrophic scars for 12 or 24 hours with a self-adhesive hydroactive polyurethane dressing. *J Wound Care*. 2001;10:149–153.
402. Handfield-Jones SE, Grattan CE, Simpson RA, et al. Comparison of a hydrocolloid dressing and paraffin gauze in the treatment of venous ulcers. *Br J Dermatol*. 1988;118:425–427.
403. Hauser J, Rossbach O, Vogt PM, et al. Efficacy of treatment with Repithel and Jelonet in comparison to treatment with Jelonet alone—a randomized clinical trial in patients receiving meshed skin grafts [in German]. *Zentralbl Chir*. 2006;131:315–321.
404. Bugmann P, Taylor S, Gyger D, et al. A silicone-coated nylon dressing reduces healing time in burned paediatric patients in comparison with standard sulfadiazine treatment: a prospective randomized trial. *Burns*. 1998;24:609–612.
405. Gotschall CS, Morrison MIS, Eichelberger MR. Prospective, randomized study of the efficacy of Mepitel* on children with partial-thickness scalds. *J Burn Care Res*. 1998;19(4):279–283.
406. Lo SF, Chang CJ, Hu WY, et al. The effectiveness of silver-releasing dressings in the management of non-healing chronic wounds: a meta-analysis. *J Clin Nurs*. 2009;18:716–728.
407. Kotz P, Fisher J, McCluskey P, et al. Use of a new silver barrier dressing, ALLEVYN(◊) Ag in exuding chronic wounds. *Int Wound J*. 2009;6:186–194.
408. O'Meara S, Al-Kurdi D, Ologun Y, et al. Antibiotics and antiseptics for venous leg ulcers. *Cochrane Database Syst Rev*. 2014;(1):CD003557.
409. Michaels JA, Campbell B, King B, et al. Randomized controlled trial and cost-effectiveness analysis of silver-donating antimicrobial dressings for venous leg ulcers (VULCAN trial). *Br J Surg*. 2009;96:1147–1156.
410. Holloway GA Jr, Johansen KH, Barnes RW, et al. Multicenter trial of cadexomer iodine to treat venous stasis ulcer. *West J Med*. 1989;151:35–38.
411. Ormiston MC, Seymour MT, Venn GE, et al. Controlled trial of Iodosorb in chronic venous ulcers. *Br Med J*. 1985;291:308–310.
412. Daugherty S, Spear M. Skin and skin substitutes—an overview. *Plast Surg Nurs*. 2015;35:92–97.
413. Horch RE, Jeschke MG, Spilker G, et al. Treatment of second degree facial burns with allografts—preliminary results. *Burns*. 2005;31:597–602.
414. Lee KH. Tissue-engineered human living skin substitutes: development and clinical application. *Yonsei Med J*. 2000;41:774–779.
415. Cope O, Langohr JL, Moore FD, et al. Expeditious care of full-thickness burn wounds by surgical excision and grafting. *Ann Surg*. 1947;125:1–22.
416. Hart DW, Wolf SE, Chinkes DL, et al. Effects of early excision and aggressive enteral feeding on hypermetabolism, catabolism, and sepsis after severe burn. *J Trauma*. 2003;54:755–761; discussion 61–64.
417. Janzekovic Z. A new concept in the early excision and immediate grafting of burns. *J Trauma*. 1970;10:1103–1108.
418. Shores JT, Gabriel A, Gupta S. Skin substitutes and alternatives: a review. *Adv Skin Wound Care*. 2007;20:493–508; quiz 9–10.
419. Austin RE, Merchant N, Shahrokhi S, et al. A comparison of Biobrane and cadaveric allograft for temporizing the acute burn wound: cost and procedural time. *Burns*. 2015;41:749–753.
420. Purdue GF, Hunt JL, Gillespie RW, et al. Biosynthetic skin substitute versus frozen human cadaver allograft for temporary coverage of excised burn wounds. *J Trauma*. 1987;27:155–157.

421. Whitaker IS, Prowse S, Potokar TS. A critical evaluation of the use of biobrane as a biologic skin substitute: a versatile tool for the plastic and reconstructive surgeon. *Ann Plast Surg*. 2008;60:333–337.
422. Ho C, Tran K, Hux M, et al. *Artificial Skin Grafts in Chronic Wound Care: A Meta-Analysis of Clinical Efficacy and a Review of Cost-Effectiveness*. Ottawa, Canada: Canadian Coordinating Office for Health Technology Assessment; 2005.
423. Tricco AC, Antony J, Vafaei A, et al. Seeking effective interventions to treat complex wounds: an overview of systematic reviews. *BMC Med*. 2015;13:89.
424. Lineen E, Namias N. Biologic dressing in burns. *J Craniofac Surg*. 2008;19:923–928.
425. Jones I, Currie L, Martin R. A guide to biological skin substitutes. *Br J Plast Surg*. 2002;55:185–193.
426. Jeng JC, Fidler PE, Sokolich JC, et al. Seven years' experience with integra as a reconstructive tool. *J Burn Care Res*. 2007;28:120–126.
427. Barber C, Watt A, Pham C, et al. Influence of bioengineered skin substitutes on diabetic foot ulcer and venous leg ulcer outcomes. *J Wound Care*. 2008;17:517–527.
428. Melkun ET, Few JW. The use of biosynthetic skin substitute (Biobrane) for axillary reconstruction after surgical excision for hidradenitis suppurativa. *Plast Reconstr Surg*. 2005;115(5):1385–1388.
429. Shakespeare P, Shakespeare V. Survey: use of skin substitute materials in UK burn treatment centres. *Burns*. 2002;28(4):295–297.
430. Shakespeare PG. The role of skin substitutes in the treatment of burn injuries. *Clin Dermatol*. 2005;23:413–418.
431. Supp DM, Boyce ST. Engineered skin substitutes: practices and potentials. *Clin Dermatol*. 2005;23:403–412.
432. Ho W-S. Skin substitutes: an overview. *Ann Coll Surg Hong Kong*. 2002;6:102–108.
433. Falanga V, Sabolinski M. A bilayered living skin construct (APLIGRAF) accelerates complete closure of hard-to-heal venous ulcers. *Wound Repair Regen*. 1999;7:201–207.
434. Marston WA, Hanft J, Norwood P, et al. The efficacy and safety of Dermagraft in improving the healing of chronic diabetic foot ulcers: results of a prospective randomized trial. *Diabetes Care*. 2003;26:1701–1705.
435. Veves A, Falanga V, Armstrong DG, et al. Graftskin, a human skin equivalent, is effective in the management of noninfected neuropathic diabetic foot ulcers: a prospective randomized multicenter clinical trial. *Diabetes Care*. 2001;24(2):290–295.
436. Clayman MA, Clayman SM, Mozingo DW. The use of collagen-glycosaminoglycan copolymer (Integra) for the repair of hypertrophic scars and keloids. *J Burn Care Res*. 2006;27:404–409.
437. Osswald SS, Elston DM, Vogel PS. Giant right plantar keloid treated with excision and tissue-engineered allograft. *J Am Acad Dermatol*. 2003;48:131–134.
438. Hanft JR. Are tissue replacements cost effective? *Podiat Today*. 2003;16.
439. Atillasoy E. The safety and efficacy of Graftskin (Apligraf) in the treatment of venous leg ulcers: a multicenter, randomized, controlled clinical trial. *Wounds*. 2000;12(5, suppl A):20A–26A.
440. Chen M, Przyborowski M, Berthiaume F. Stem cells for skin tissue engineering and wound healing. *Crit Rev Biomed Eng*. 2009;37:399–421.
441. Kwon SH, Bhang SH, Jang HK, et al. Conditioned medium of adipose-derived stromal cell culture in three-dimensional bioreactors for enhanced wound healing. *J Surg Res*. 2015;194:8–17.
442. You HJ, Han SK. Cell therapy for wound healing. *J Korean Med Sci*. 2014;29:311–319.
443. Martin P, Parkhurst SM. Parallels between tissue repair and embryo morphogenesis. *Development*. 2004;131:3021–3034.
444. Lin YC, Grahovac T, Oh SJ, et al. Evaluation of a multi-layer adipose-derived stem cell sheet in a full-thickness wound healing model. *Acta Biomater*. 2013;9:5243–5250.
445. Huang S, Lu G, Wu Y, et al. Mesenchymal stem cells delivered in a microsphere-based engineered skin contribute to cutaneous wound healing and sweat gland repair. *J Dermatol Sci*. 2012;66:29–36.
446. Lee S-J, Park C, Lee JY, et al. Generation of pure lymphatic endothelial cells from human pluripotent stem cells and their therapeutic effects on wound repair. *Sci Rep*. 2015;5:11019.
447. Kim MK, Seo BF, Kim KJ, et al. Secretory factors of human chorion-derived stem cells enhance activation of human fibroblasts. *Cytotherapy*. 2015;17:301–309.
448. Fetterolf DE, Istawan N, Stanziano GJ. An evaluation of healing metrics associated with commonly used advanced wound care products for the treatment of chronic diabetic foot ulcers. *Manag Care*. 2014;23:31–38.
449. Huang S, Wu Y, Gao D, et al. Paracrine action of mesenchymal stromal cells delivered by microspheres contributes to cutaneous wound healing and prevents scar formation in mice. *Cytotherapy*. 2015;17:922–931.

Rehabilitation

SECTION IV

10 Medical Management of Scars

JULIAN POETSCHKE, MARKUS REINHOLZ, and GERD G. GAUGLITZ

KEY POINTS

- Excessive scarring represents a frequently observed medical problem around the world.
- In addition to their bothersome appearance, hypertrophic scars and keloids are commonly associated with significant pain, pruritus, and functional impairment.
- Despite a variety of currently available therapeutic approaches, treatment remains challenging.
- Injection of 5-Fluorouracil for therapy-refractory keloids and the introduction of fractional laser therapy for the improvement of hypertrophic scars have significantly contributed to recent advances in this area.

Scars are common and can be cosmetically, physically, and psychologically debilitating. As recently described by our group,[1] keloids, atrophic acne scars, self-harm scars, and burn scars may significantly affect patients in their daily well-being. Thus, adequate assessment of associated symptoms and appropriate treatment remains crucial to improve the overall quality of life of these patients. Although many studies have been published on the pathophysiology of excessive scarring, the complex alterations underlying hypertrophic and keloid scar formation remain relatively poorly understood (see Chapter 6). The lack of appropriate animal models in this area may significantly contribute to this fact.

Pathophysiology Underlying Physiological and Excessive Scar Formation

In order to understand the altered wound healing response underlying excessive scarring, it may be best compared to physiological wound healing.[2]

Scars regularly occur after trauma of the deeper dermis following a complex physiological wound healing cascade. This cascade can be subdivided into three phases: inflammation, proliferation, and remodeling. Traumatic injuries are immediately followed by the onset of hemostasis. As a fibrin-rich blood clot develops, it serves as a scaffold for the ensuing wound repair and the degranulation of activated thrombocytes sets free a variety of chemotactic and proinflammatory agents. Macrophages and neutrophil granulocytes are attracted and dissolve necrotic tissue. Released cytokines like epidermal growth factor, platelet-derived growth factor, insulin-like growth factor I, and transforming growth factor (TGF)-β mediate the stimulation of fibroblasts and keratinocytes and mark the transition into the proliferative phase.[2,3] During this phase, a scaffold of extracellular matrix (ECM), consisting of immature type III collagen, elastin, proteoglycans, and hyaluronic acid, is constructed by the activated fibroblasts. Mediated by vascular endothelial growth factor, vascular ingrowth is induced. As myofibroblasts facilitate wound contraction and closure, the remodeling phase begins. During this final phase, abundant ECM is degraded and immature matrix components are converted into their mature form. This is most notably achieved through the transformation of procollagen type III into mature type I collagen.[2–5]

Typically, immature scars (Fig. 10-1) have a reddish appearance. Sometimes they cause itching and are slightly elevated. Within months, they regularly turn into a flat, frequently depigmented scar without any further symptoms (Fig. 10-2).[6] Based on a published study observing the natural history of scar redness and maturation after incisional and excisional wounds, scars commonly fade within approximately 7 months.[7]

The successful conversion of a wound clot into granulation tissue necessitates a balance between degradation and deposition of ECM proteins.[2] Alteration of this process can lead to abnormalities in scarring. Several risk factors have shown to increase abnormal (pathological) scarring such as specific anatomic locations, infection, genetic susceptibility, and delayed epithelialization (Table 10-1). The occurrence of keloids has been reported after negligible surgical or laser procedures, and even without apparent trauma—primarily in predisposed individuals.[2]

Both keloids (Fig. 10-3) and hypertrophic scars (Fig. 10-4) reveal fundamental aberrations in the wound healing cascade, which may be best characterized by an imbalance between the anabolic and catabolic phases.[8] A scar is densely infiltrated with inflammatory cells that secrete fibrogenic factors, such as TGF-β1 and TGF-β2. Increased

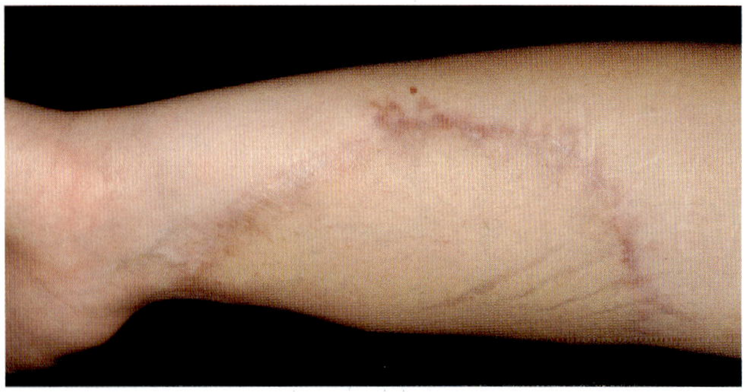

FIGURE 10-1 Immature scar with raised edges and erythema.

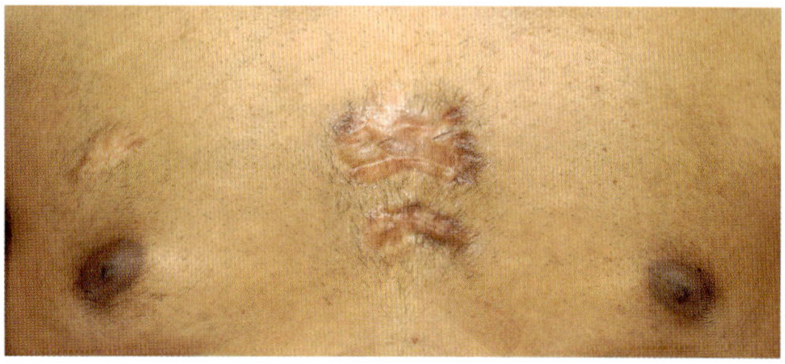

FIGURE 10-3 Spontaneous presternal keloid.

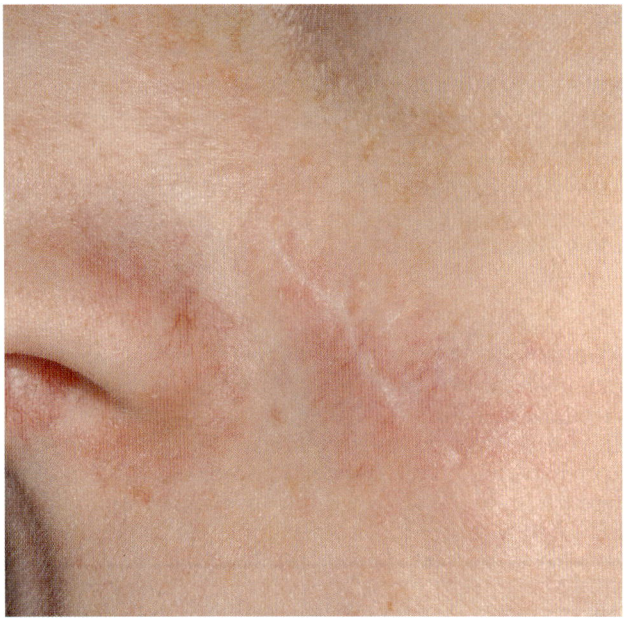

FIGURE 10-2 Physiological scar healing after surgery. *(From Reinholz M, Poetschke J, Schwaiger H, et al. The dermatology life quality index as a means to assess life quality in patients with different scar types.* J Eur Acad Dermatol Venereol. *2015;29(11):2112–2119.)*

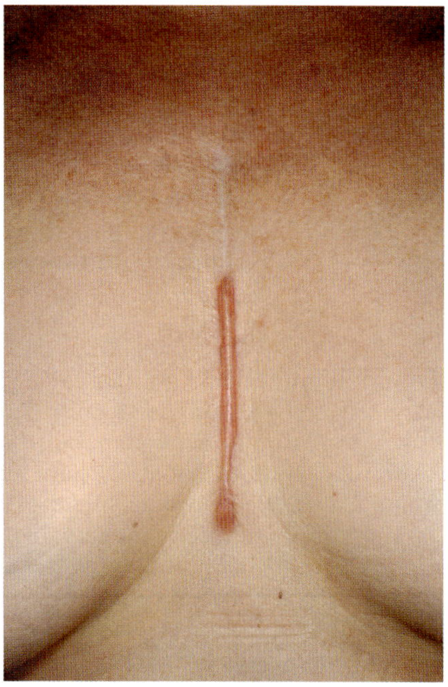

FIGURE 10-4 Hypertrophic scar after open heart surgery; the scar remains within the confines of the original injury. *(From Reinholz M, Poetschke J, Schwaiger H, et al. The dermatology life quality index as a means to assess life quality in patients with different scar types.* J Eur Acad Dermatol Venereol. *2015;29(11):2112–2119.)*

Table 10-1 Main Risk Factors for Hypertrophic Scars and Keloids

Hormones (higher incidence during puberty and pregnancy)
Genetic predisposition
Topography
Chronic inflammation (e.g., acne)
Tension on wound margins
Delayed epithelialization (>21 d)

PEARL 10-1 *Based on clinical experience, keloids seem to represent the more aggressive and persistent fibrotic disorder compared to hypertrophic scars.*[8]

levels of TGF-β1 and TGF-β2 promote an accumulation of ECM, whereas their degradation through decreased levels of TGF-β3 and matrix metalloproteinases (MMPs) is impaired. Both the severity of inflammation and the type of immune response predispose to excess scar formation.[9] An increased T_H2 response stimulates fibrogenesis, whereas a T_H1 preponderance reduces tissue fibrosis.[10,11]

There is evidence that a more prolonged inflammatory period with increased infiltrates of immune cells present in the scar tissue of keloids may contribute to increases in fibroblast activity with greater deposition of ECM proteins.[9] This may help explain why keloids continue expanding beyond the margins of the initial injury, whereas hypertrophic scars (in which the immune cell infiltrate decreases over time) remain restricted to the initial wound bed and commonly show involution over time.[9]

Therapeutic Approaches for the Treatment of Hypertrophic Scars and Keloids

Various studies elaborating on the formation of excessive scarring have resulted in a multitude of therapeutic strategies (Table 10-2). A vast number of articles on the prevention or improvement of keloid and hypertrophic scars have been published. Despite the rapidly increasing options in this area, some considerations are worth being highlighted in this context:

- Many of the therapeutic approaches available to date are being used for both prevention and treatment of excessive scarring.
- Only a limited number of these strategies have been supported by controlled and well-designed prospective studies.
- Differentiating between keloids and hypertrophic scars is crucial prior to any therapeutic manipulation because of augmented recurrence rates with keloids (Table 10-3).
- Lasers continue to play an increasingly important role and are being marketed accordingly.

But:

- By utilizing basic options such as silicone sheeting/gel, intralesional triamcinolone acetonide (TAC), cryotherapy, or pressure, improvement can frequently be observed without any extensive cost for the respective patients.

The following paragraph will provide a summary of the currently available options for the prevention and treatment of scarring, starting with the most common.

Surgical Approaches for the Prevention and Therapy of Hypertrophic Scars and Keloids

Five main principles should be taken into consideration when considering any surgical approach for the prevention or treatment of excessive scarring[2]:

1. Common prophylactic approaches in order to reduce the possibility of postoperative pathological scarring:
   - Delayed epithelialization beyond 10 to 14 days is well known to increase the incidence of hypertrophic scarring[12]; fostering rapid epithelialization is crucial to avoid excessive scar growth.
   - Wounds subjected to high tension due to motion, body location, or tissue loss are at increased risk of excessive scarring and spreading of scars (see Chapter 7). Patients undergoing surgery in these body areas should be aware of this significant risk prior to any surgery.[13]
   - The modern understanding of wound healing is based on the knowledge of restoring skin anatomy and function, and a thoughtful selection of suture materials and closure techniques. Surgical approaches should precisely coapt the tissue layers and margins. This is necessary to minimize new tissue formation within the wound. Suitable surgical closing techniques will also eliminate a potential cavity by approximating the subcutaneous tissue. If misalignment and dead space is minimized adjacent to the opposed wound edges, new tissue has limited room to grow. Atraumatic handling of tissue in combination with avoiding tight closures result in better aesthetic outcomes. Additionally, reduced tension on the wound margins facilitated by cautious undermining and loosening of the surrounding tissue contributes to better results. As an example, a combination of polydioxanone (PDS II, Ethicon Inc.) monofilament synthetic absorbable subcutaneous sutures (which provide extended wound support for up to 6 months) with absorbable sutures or Steri-Strip (3M) for optimal epidermal wound closure might be used. It has been shown that subcutaneous fascial tensile reduction sutures in a predisposed patient population, where the tension is placed on the layer of deep fascia and superficial fascia, revealed good clinical results. Here 2-0 or 3-0 PDS II sutures were preferred for subcutaneous/fascial sutures, and 4-0 or 5-0 PDS II sutures for dermal sutures.[14]
2. If hypertrophic scarring occurs, determining the optimal timing for procedural intervention (including surgical excision/revision) is key. Hypertrophic scars have the potential to mature over a year or more after injury and significantly flatten and soften without any medical intervention, potentially obviating the need for surgical excision.[15] Nevertheless postexcisional relapse rates of the original hypertrophic scar are commonly negligible.[16,17] On the other hand, if scar (joint) contractures occur, then invasive approaches that release contractures should be performed earlier (see Chapter 12).[14]
3. The development of hypertrophy is facilitated when there is an increased tension on wound margins. Consequently, employing surgical techniques such as Z- or W-plasty, grafts, or local skin flaps to interrupt the vicious circle between scar tension and scar thickening due to permanently stimulated ECM production may help mitigate pathological scar formation.[18]
4. Delayed would healing (e.g., after deep dermal burn or wound infection) may increase the risk of hypertrophic scars and keloids. Transforming selected lesions by surgery (excision with suture or graft) into a wound with appropriate healing time may reduce the risk of new excessive scar formation.[18]
5. If excessive scar tissue is surgically removed, a situation similar to a fresh wound is created. In this new setting disproportionate scarring might be reduced by adjuvant conservative therapy straight from the beginning.[18] Nonetheless, the excision of keloids without any further conservative therapy (e.g., corticosteroid or 5-Fluorouracil [5-FU] injections, intrainterventional cryotherapy, pressure, or radiation) should be rigorously avoided because of a strongly elevated risk of recurrence (45% to 100%). The postexcision scar may even grow larger than the initial one in this new area of trauma.[19,20] Remarkably good cosmetic results were obtained after a surgical repair approach (core excision with low-tension wound closure or shave excision) of earlobe keloids with postinterventional

Table 10-2 Hypertrophic Scars and Keloids: Current Therapeutic Strategies

Treatment	Use	Mechanisms of Action	Indications, Efficiency, and Comments
Prophylaxis			
Pressure therapy	Continuous pressure (15–40 mm Hg) for at least 23 h/d ≥6 mo of scar healing	Collagen synthesis↓, Apoptosis↑ via limiting the supply of blood and oxygen to scar tissue	• Prophylaxis of hypertrophic burn scars, ear keloids (postexcision) • Controversial success • Reduced compliance due to frequent patient discomfort
Silicone gel sheeting	≥12 h/d for ≥2 mo beginning 2 wk after wound healing	Pressure↑; hydration of the stratum corneum; temperature ↑→ collagenase activity↑	• Prophylaxis of hypertrophic scars and keloids • Controversial benefit • No effects on mature keloids and hypertrophic scars
Flavonoids	e.g., Contractubex gel (Merz Pharma, Frankfurt, Germany), Mederma Skin Care Gel (Merz, Pharmaceuticals, Greensboro, NC, USA). Twice daily for 4 to 6 mo	Antiproliferative, anti-inflammatory, reduction in TGF-β expression	• Limited to management and prophylaxis of hypertrophic scars and keloids
Current Therapies			
Corticosteroids	Intralesional injections of triamcinolone acetonide (10–40 mg/mL), several treatments once or twice a month	Anti-inflammatory effects. Vasoconstriction↑→ oxygen and nutrients↓ Anti-mitotic effects on keratinocytes and fibroblasts α2-macroglobulin↓→ collagenase↑ Production of TGF-β1and 2↓	• First-line therapy for the treatment of keloids and second-line therapy for the treatment of hypertrophic scars • Combination with surgery, PDL, and cryotherapy • Beware: skin and subcutaneous fat atrophy, telangiectasias
Cryotherapy	Contact/spray freezing with liquid nitrogen using 10–20 s freeze–thaw cycles	Induction of vascular damage → anoxia and tissue necrosis. Collagen synthesis↓	• Overall effective for hypertrophic scars, for keloids in combination with triamcinolone acetonide injections recommended • Limited to management of smaller scars • Beware: blistering and pain
Scar revision	Excision with linear, tension-free closure, split- or full-thickness skin grafting, Z-plasty, W-plasty	Surgical removal of excessive scarring	• Efficacious for treatment of hypertrophic scarring • Recurrence rates of 45%–100% after keloid excision
Radiotherapy	Superficial X-rays, dosages15–20 Gy, overall limit 40 Gy. Over 5–6 sessions in the early postoperative period	Inhibition and apoptosis of proliferating fibroblasts	• Overall good efficiency rates of adjuvant radiotherapy after keloid excision • Beware: potential risk of malignant change/carcinogenesis
Laser therapy	Pulsed dye laser (585-nm PDL) with doses ranging from 6.0 to 7.5 J/cm^2 (7-mm spot) or from 4.5 to 5.5 J/cm^2 (10-mm spot), 2–6 treatments every 2–6 wk	Local ischemia via destroying blood vessels → tissue hypoxia↑	• Excellent therapeutic option for the treatment of younger keloids and hypertrophic scars • High recurrence rates with other (ablative) laser techniques for the treatment of keloids
Emerging Therapies			
Interferon	Intralesional injection of INF-α2b (1.5–2 million International Units) twice daily over 4 d	Antiproliferative properties	• Clinical studies report overall effectiveness • Beware: flu-like symptoms on injection
5-FU	Intralesional injection of 5-FU 50 mg/mL	Increased fibroblast apoptosis via inhibiting DNA synthesis	• Overall effective for the treatment of keloids and hypertrophic scars • Beware: blood count monitoring (anemia, leukopenia, thrombocytopenia). No therapy in pregnant women or patients with bone marrow suppression

From Gauglitz GG, Korting HC, Pavicic T, et al. Hypertrophic scarring and keloids: pathomechanisms and current and emerging treatment strategies. *Mol Med*. 2011;17(1/2):113–125.

Table 10-3 Hypertrophic Scars and Keloids: Epidemiological, Clinical, and Histological Differences

	Hypertrophic Scarring	Keloids
Incidence	40%–70% following surgery, up to 91% following burn injury.[150–152]	6%–16% in African populations.[153,154]
	Equal in sex distribution with highest incidence in the second to third decade.[155,156]	
Predilection sites	Shoulders, neck, presternum, knees, and ankles.[17,157,158]	Anterior chest, shoulders, earlobes, upper arms, and cheeks.[154,159,160]
	Less affected: Eyelids, cornea, palms, mucous membranes, genitalia, and soles.[154]	
Time course	Within 4–8 wk following wounding,[161] rapid growth phase for up to 6 mo, then regression over a period of a few years.[158,162,163]	Within years after minor injuries or spontaneous formation on the mid-chest in the absence of any known injury. Persistence for long periods of time. No spontaneous regression.[41]
	Low recurrence rates after excision of the original hypertrophic scar.[16,17]	High recurrence rates following excision.
Appearance	Do not extend beyond the initial site of injury.[164]	Project beyond the original wound margins.[164,165]
	Both lesions are commonly pruritic, but keloids may even be the source of significant pain or hyperesthesia.[158,161]	
Histological characteristics	Primarily fine, well-organized, wavy type III collagen bundles oriented parallel to the epidermis surface with abundant nodules containing myofibroblasts and plentiful acidic mucopolysaccharide.[3]	Disorganized, large, thick, type I and III hypocellular collagen bundles with no nodules or excess myofibroblasts.[3,166] Poor vascularization with widely scattered dilated blood vessels.[167]
	PCNA/p53-level/ATP expression low.[168]	PCNA/p53-level/ATP expression high.[168]

From Gauglitz GG, Korting HC, Pavicic T, et al. Hypertrophic scarring and keloids: pathomechanisms and current and emerging treatment strategies. *Mol Med.* 2011;17(1/2):113–125.

corticosteroid or 5-FU injections, postoperative pressure (e.g., pressure earrings), application of imiquimod 5% cream or intraoperative cryotherapy on the incision site.[21]

Silicone-Based Products

Silicone-based products are currently mostly available as gels, patches, and sheets. Silicone is also frequently being combined with pressure, and a multitude of ready-to-use products are available to date. Silicone gel sheeting has been incorporated frequently into scar management paradigms since its introduction in the early 1980s.[22–26] The mechanism of action appears to involve a normalization of transepidermal water loss, among other possible pathways, rather than any inherent antiscarring property of silicone.[15,27] Silicone-based products should usually be employed for 12 to 24 hours per day over a period of 12 to 24 weeks, beginning approximately 2 weeks after wounding after complete reepithelialization has been achieved.[18] Although published studies generally support the use of silicone-based therapy, a recent Cochrane review analyzing effectiveness of silicone gel sheeting determined that the efficacy remains unclear because of the poor quality of most studies.[28] Nevertheless, for many years silicone gel sheeting has been considered a first-line therapy for linear hypertrophic, widespread hypertrophic burn scars, and minor keloids as stated in the international guidelines on scar management published in 2002.[12] In the last decade, more and more studies have endorsed the use of silicone gels as prophylaxis for excessive scarring, particularly in areas where movement or other factors preclude the consistent use of silicone sheets.[29–33] According to updated guidelines,[34,35] silicone gels and sheets can be recommended as first-line therapy for various scar types including hypertrophic scars, minor keloids, and the prevention of pathological scarring.

PEARL 10-2 Treatment Pearl: Silicone Products *The authors recommend silicone-based gels merely as preventative tools for patients with an increased risk of excessive scar formation or for those who are significantly concerned about unpleasant scarring. We also combine silicone-based products with injectables or nonablative lasers in order to increase efficacy in between treatment sessions.*

Intralesional Corticosteroid Injections and Cryotherapy

Since the mid-1960s intralesional steroid injections have been used for the treatment of excessive scarring.[36] Even after its long history of use, intralesional TAC remains a standard therapy for hypertrophic scars as well as early keloids.[12,18] Additionally, TAC injections effectively relieve common symptoms such as pain and pruritus. The clinical response to corticosteroid treatment is mainly achieved by reducing the inflammatory response in the wound,[15] inhibiting collagen and glycosaminoglycan synthesis by reducing fibroblast proliferation,[37] and enhancing collagen and fibroblast degeneration.[38] The common therapeutic scheme would consist of three to four injections of TAC 10 to 40 mg per mL every 3 to 4 weeks. This number of injections may be generally sufficient, although sometimes injections continue for 6 months and even longer.[36] Based on current literature, response rates vary from 50% to

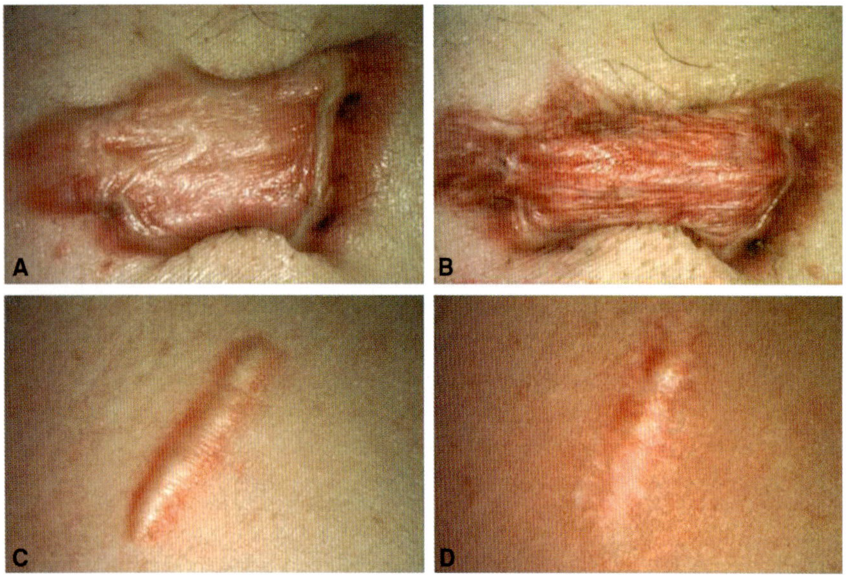

FIGURE 10-5 Keloids and hypertrophic scars after cryotherapy and triamcinolone acetonide (TAC) injections. **A,C:** Before treatment. **B,D:** After four sessions of cryotherapy and intralesional TAC injections (40 mg per mL).

100%, and recurrence rates vary from 9% to 50%.[20] Side effects of corticosteroid injection include dermal atrophy, telangiectasia, and pain at the injection site. To improve the pain, topical anesthesia and/or regional injections of local anesthetics around the scars may be employed.[5]

Although systemic side effects of intralesional corticosteroid injections are rarely observed, cases of Cushing's syndrome following TAC injections for keloid and hypertrophic scar treatment in children have been reported in the literature. A review by Fredman and Tenenhaus recommends a maximum dose of 30 mg of intralesional corticosteroids per month in children, while acknowledging that close observation of young patients is required after treatment.[39] In adults, very few cases of iatrogenic Cushing's syndrome after intralesional TAC injections have been reported; generally among these, extremely large doses (up to 1,200 mg) were applied within 1 month to treat multiple keloids.[40] Although the possibility of adrenal complications in adults exists, it is highly unlikely in most patients after intralesional injection of the corticosteroid alone. In patients with multiple or larger lesions, alternating treatment of the different scars or scar segments can be taken into consideration as a precaution.

For older hypertrophic scars and larger keloids, the combination with cryotherapy represents a popular practical approach in daily routine and seems to be highly effective (Fig. 10-5).[41,42] Marked improvement of hypertrophic scars and keloids after application of cryotherapy in combination with intralesional TAC injections has been reported.[43–45] The exact mechanism of action of cryotherapy is not yet understood; aside from physical destruction of fibrotic tissue, it is believed to induce vascular damage, hypoxia, and ultimately tissue necrosis.[2] An interval of at least 3 to 4 weeks between each treatment (approximately three to six sessions are needed) is commonly required to allow for postinterventional healing. Common side effects include permanent hypo- and hyperpigmentation, blistering, and postoperative pain.[46–48] Based on communications among experts, cryotherapy performed directly prior to the injection of TAC appears to increase the therapeutic success rate. Though the mechanism is uncertain, this might be due to the edema formation caused by the preceding cryotherapy facilitating the injection and enabling the deposition of larger amounts of the drug.

PEARL 10-3 Treatment Pearl: Intralesional Corticosteroid *The use of TAC remains our most frequently used approach for both hypertrophic scars and keloids. Used in combination with cryotherapy, the scar tissue is softened facilitating the injection of TAC. In patients with very small keloids or hypertrophic scars we may use TAC 40 mg per mL as a monotherapy and inject small droplets of highly concentrated solution by employing an insulin syringe (0.3 mL, 30G needle). We usually perform three sessions around 4 weeks apart, before we either switch to 5-FU (in case of nonresponse) or continue with a vascular laser in order to improve erythema or newly formed telangiectasia.*

Pressure Therapy

Since the 1970s pressure therapy has been a mainstay for the management of hypertrophic scars and keloids. Pressure garments remain a common choice for the prevention of excessive scar formation after burn injury, although the mechanism of action and efficacy remain vague. Decreased collagen production through reduced capillary perfusion, tissue hypoxia,[49–51] and an increased rate of fibroblast apoptosis[52] are presumed.

Special methods are frequently used to apply pressure in various anatomical areas including suits or bandages, transparent plastic masks, or buttons of padding in specific locations. The recommendations for the amount of applied pressure are based on mainly empirical observation, because research on the topic has been inconsistent. A continuous pressure of 15 to 40 mm Hg for at least 23 hours per day for more than 6 months is the norm.[50,53]

Recent research has revealed that a slightly higher pressure of 20 to 25 mm Hg was significantly superior to lower pressure (10 to 15 mm Hg) in the treatment of hypertrophic scars.[54] However, another recent systematic meta-analysis on the use of compression garments revealed no significant benefit.[55] Because pressure therapy is mainly dependent on the compliance of the patient and the body location, adequate counseling on the importance of regular use and proper fitting to the wound area has to be assured (see Chapter 19). Side effects such as maceration, eczema, and odor emanating from the garment may decrease the adherence to the therapy. Nevertheless, when adequately employed postoperative pressure (e.g., pressure earrings after surgical repair of earlobe keloids) may significantly reduce the recurrence rates after surgery.[56,57] Moreover, pressure garments may possibly represent a promising alternative to intralesional TAC or cryotherapy, particularly in children because of fewer side effects and decreased potential for painful procedures.

PEARL 10-4 Treatment Pearl: Pressure Therapy *The authors have good experience with pressure for multiple applications: the prevention of recurrence after surgical removal of ear keloids (pressure earrings); pressure gowns for patients suffering from multiple acne keloids, which helps soften the scar tissue and eases the injections of TAC or 5-FU; and convincing results in younger children suffering from minor hypertrophic scars or keloids on the extremities.*

Laser Therapy

A variety of different lasers have been applied and evaluated in the past decades for the treatment of hypertrophic scars and keloids (see Chapter 13).[58] However, studies comparing different wavelengths and laser settings are generally lacking. In the early 1990s the 585-nm pulsed dye laser (PDL) was described as a promising new tool in the treatment of younger hypertrophic scars and keloids.[59] The mechanism of action is not yet fully understood, but it is thought that the PDL improves keloids or hypertrophic scars by inducing capillary injury or destruction, with favorable resultant alterations in collagen synthesis and breakdown.[60–62] Increased production of MMPs (e.g., collagenase) has been described following PDL treatment.[63] The current recommendation comprises nonoverlapping laser pulses at lower fluences ranging from 6.0 to 7.5 J per cm^2 (7 mm spot) or from 4.5 to 5.5 J per cm^2 (10 mm spot) for the treatment of hypertrophic scars and keloids.[64] According to Alster and coworkers,[59] two to six laser treatments are necessary to successfully improve scar color, height, pliability, and texture. However, these findings could not be reproduced in several subsequent studies.[65] Also, later case–control studies revealed no significant differences from the untreated control group after longer follow-up observation periods.[66,67] Frequent weaknesses of these kinds of studies include a lack of control group or a small number of study participants. Also, hypertrophic scars and keloids are often not differentiated, or there is a lack of information on the age and activity of the scars. These are all contributing factors to potentially explain why the level of evidence in regard to laser treatment for hypertrophic scarring and keloids is currently low.[68]

Mild side effects may be observed with PDL treatment, including purpura persisting for 7 to 14 days. Depending on the applied energy density, vesicles and crusts may also occur. Persistent hyperpigmentation may be observed in darker skin types, but is less frequent with use of the 595-nm wavelength than with that of 585 nm.[18] The authors and others have occasionally observed reactivation of younger keloids following PDL treatment.[69] For this reason, the authors often initiate keloid treatment using a combination of cryotherapy and TAC in addition to the PDL.

Recently, a 1,064-nm neodymium-doped yttrium aluminum garnet (Nd:YAG) laser has been suggested as a promising treatment for the improvement of keloids and hypertrophic scars.[63] The underlying mechanism of action may be similar to that of PDL therapy, though the Nd:YAG laser has a greater penetration depth than PDL and should be better tolerated by darker skin types because of more modest absorption by melanin (see Chapter 13). The utility of nonablative lasers may be limited in thicker keloids, however, since efficacy appears to decrease with the thickness of the scar.[63] Another study showed improvements of pigmentation, vascularity, pliability, and scar height in keloids and hypertrophic scars after 5 to 10 treatments (at 1- to 2-week intervals) using low fluences. The observed side effects were mild and included a prickling sensation during intervention and posttreatment erythema.[70] However, additional studies are necessary to clarify the use of Nd:YAG nonablative laser treatment for excessive scarring. Recently published German guidelines for the therapy of excessive scarring primarily recommend PDL for the reduction of erythema, particularly in fresh, highly vascularized scars and those associated with pruritus.[18] According to these guidelines, additional laser platforms including full-field (nonfractionated) ablative carbon dioxide (CO_2) or erbium (Er):YAG lasers may be recommended for the ablation of inactive hypertrophic scars. However, their use for removal of keloids without additional anticipatory management should be avoided because of recurrence rates similar to those after excision.[18]

The concept of fractional photothermolysis (FP) dramatically changed the spectrum of laser applications. The favorable reaction to pixelated coagulative and ablative injury in the deeper layers of the dermis represents a revolution in laser therapy. This new application mode promises to decrease the risk of worsening scarring as well as the downtime associated with traditional ablative resurfacing. FP consistently leads to the stimulation of collagen remodeling and rapid wound healing.[71,72] The rationale behind FP is the creation of relatively narrow and deep microscopic thermal wounds while relatively large surrounding areas of skin remain untreated. In practice this appears to minimize side effects while maintaining good clinical efficacy.[71,72] Ablative as well as nonablative fractional laser systems have been well studied for different indications such as the improvement of photoaging, periorbital wrinkles, and atrophic scars.

Based on a vigorous collagen remodeling response mediated by various inflammatory immunoactive molecules like heat shock proteins, MMP-1, TGF-β2, β-fibroblast growth factor, and TGF-β3, fractional lasers have also been suggested for the management of postsurgical and hypertrophic (burn) scars.[73–75] Interestingly two different randomized controlled trials comparing FP with PDL therapy in the treatment of surgical scars have shown that clinical outcomes were better after fractional laser therapy, both ablative and nonablative.[76,77]

Another study compared fractional CO_2 laser treatment with dermabrasion for severe posttraumatic and surgical scars. Again, the outcomes favored fractional ablative treatment.[78] Remarkable clinical improvements with corresponding histological/structural improvements have recently been reported after fractional laser therapy.[79–81] Based on current understanding, ablative fractional lasers may be preferred over nonablative ones because ablative fractional devices usually require fewer treatment sessions and can achieve greater depths of penetration for the treatment of symptomatic contractures.[34,35,81]

PEARL 10-5 Treatment Pearl: Laser Therapy
Depending on the type of scar and associated symptoms, the choice of the respective laser may vary. Although erythematous elevated scars may benefit from PDL or Nd:YAG laser treatment, the limited penetration depth should be taken into consideration before initiating any therapy. Thus, the initiation of an anti-inflammatory treatment such as intralesional TAC may be useful before starting laser therapy, particularly with inflamed keloids. Next to the anti-inflammatory effect, the main goal is to reduce the scar height, which may be more effectively achieved when combined with cryotherapy. Multiple treatments are generally necessary in order to achieve satisfying results. With older linear or widespread hypertrophic scars, frequently an improvement of scar texture, pliability, and softening of the scar tissue is desired. Here, fractional lasers play an increasingly important role. Although both ablative and nonablative devices may be employed, current guidelines favor of the fractional CO_2 because of its penetration depth (up to 4 mm) and the ability to ablate excessive scar tissue. As with most modalities, multiple sessions are needed and final results are only seen months after the last procedure because of gradual collagen remodeling.

5-Fluorouracil

5-FU has been successfully employed in the treatment of hypertrophic scars and keloids for decades (Fig. 10-6).[82] 5-FU, a pyrimidine analog, inhibits fibroblast proliferation and collagen deposition. Studies show that about half of the treated keloids respond positively to therapy in both "high-dose" (40 to 50 mg per mL)[83] and "low-dose" (1.4 to 3.5 mg per mL) regimens.[84–86] Other studies have evaluated the combination of intralesional 5-FU and TAC. One prospective study including 69 patients revealed that the combination of TAC (40 mg per mL):5-FU (50 mg per mL) (1:9) injected intralesionally once weekly for 2 months combined with PDL resulted in greater improvements than intralesional TAC 40 mg per mL alone.[87] Another double-blind, prospective study including 40 patients with keloids and hypertrophic scars demonstrated that the combination of intralesional TAC (40 mg per mL):5-FU (50 mg per mL) (1:9) was more effective than TAC 40 mg per mL in reducing scar size and redness.[88] Another study demonstrated that the combination of intralesional 5-FU/TAC and excision was superior to intralesional TAC alone and excision for overall scar reduction.[89] According to the presently available study data, intralesional 5-FU represents a safe and effective approach to the treatment of hypertrophic scars and keloids. Typical adverse events include pain at the injection side, hyperpigmentation, skin irritation, and ulceration. Ulceration is mostly seen in dark-skinned individuals and commonly resolves within weeks. Contraindications to 5-FU therapy include anemia, leukopenia, thrombocytopenia, pregnancy, bone marrow depression, and infection. To date no systemic side effects have been observed. According to the updated German and international guidelines for the therapy of pathological scarring, treatment of therapy-refractory keloids with 5-FU can be considered.[18,34,35,90]

PEARL 10-6 Treatment Pearl: 5-Fluorouracil *Over the past years, the authors have used 5-FU more and more frequently for the treatment of keloids and the prevention of recurrence of ear keloids after surgical excision. For keloids without prior treatment, we inject them with TAC (+ cryotherapy) for three sessions at 4-week intervals. If no significant improvement is noted, we switch to 5-FU (50 mg per mL) and TAC (40 mg per mL) in a ratio of 3:1. In case patients are being referred to our center and TAC, cryotherapy, or silicone has been employed for longer than 3 months, we immediately start with the combination of 5-FU and TAC if no contraindications exist. For prevention of recurrence of ear keloids after surgery, we inject small amounts of 5-FU (50 mg per mL) directly into the fresh scar tissue, usually beginning around 2 weeks after surgery at 2-month intervals.*

Onion Extract (Extractum Cepae)

Onion extract appears to have anti-inflammatory as well as bactericidal properties. The potential positive effects of onion extract in scar management, including the inhibition of fibroblast proliferation and collagen synthesis, have been attributed speculatively to flavonoids including quercetin. Recently it has been suggested that these inhibitory effects may be mediated through inhibition of the TGF-β1, TGF-β2, and SMAD signaling pathways.[91,92] Nevertheless, the effects of onion extract–containing creams on excessive scarring remain to be fully elucidated.[93–97] Based on the latest studies, however, onion extract–containing scar creams have been reported to significantly improve scar height and associated symptoms compared to vehicle.[94] Furthermore, they appear to be effective for the prevention of pathological scars in patients having laser removal of tattoos[98] as well as in combined approaches with intralesional TAC.[99] According to the recently published German and

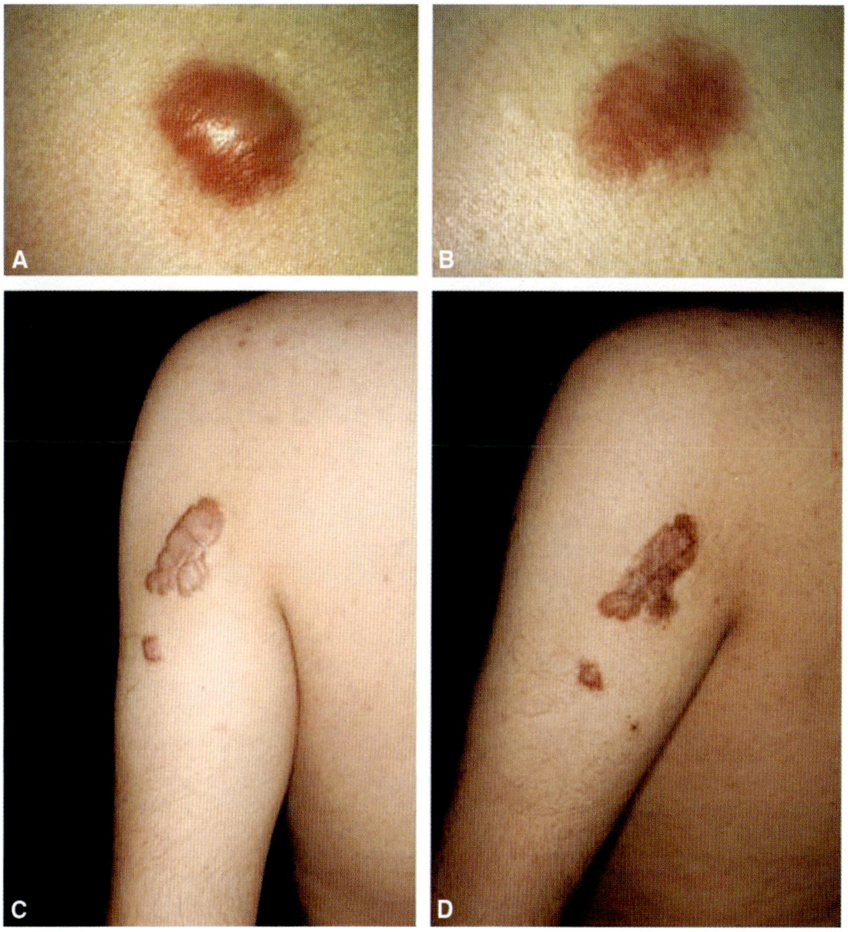

FIGURE 10-6 Keloids after intralesional 5-FU injection. **A, C:** Scars were refractory to triamcinolone acetonide and cryotherapy. **B, D:** After four 5-FU intralesional injections at 4-week intervals. 5-FU, 5-Fluorouracil.

international guidelines on scars, the application of onion extract–containing scar creams can be considered in the treatment of active hypertrophic scars and for postsurgical prevention of excessive scarring.[18,34,35,90]

PEARL 10-7 Treatment Pearl: Onion Extract *Onion extract represents an attractive alternative to the use of silicone gels, because it is frequently less expensive and study data are improving. Recently, onion extract has been brought onto the market as a patch, which may be of potential interest, even though study data on this application form is widely missing.*

Intralesional Cryotherapy

Recently, the novel approach of intralesional cryosurgery for hypertrophic and keloid scars has been introduced (Figs. 10-7 and 10-8).[100–102] The cryoneedle (CryoShape, Etgar Group Ltd, Kfar Saba) is connected to a reservoir with liquid nitrogen and inserted into the hypertrophic scar, freezing the scar tissue from the inside out. One study demonstrated up to 70% of volume reduction for ear keloids and 60% reduction for keloids on the upper back, shoulder, and chest following a single cryo-session. In addition to volume reduction, clinical symptoms were also decreased. Treatments appear to be well tolerated, with only discrete hypopigmentation and no obvious tendency toward worsening scars or infection.

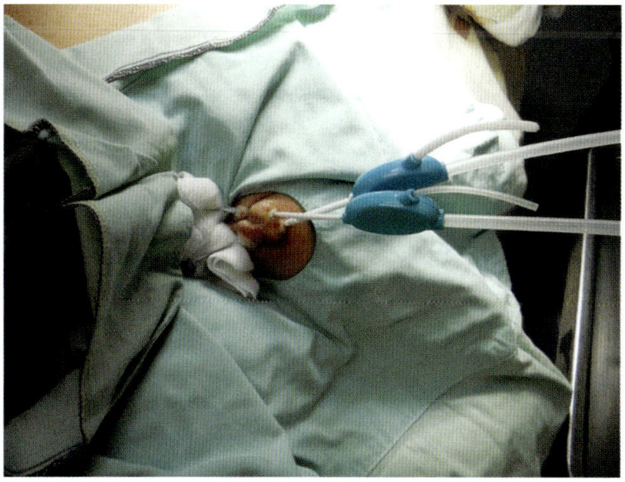

FIGURE 10-7 Cryoneedle after insertion (following translesional local anesthesia) into keloid. *(From Gauglitz GG. Management of keloids and hypertrophic scars: current and emerging options.* Clin Cosmet Invest Dermatol. 2013;6*(10):103–114.)*

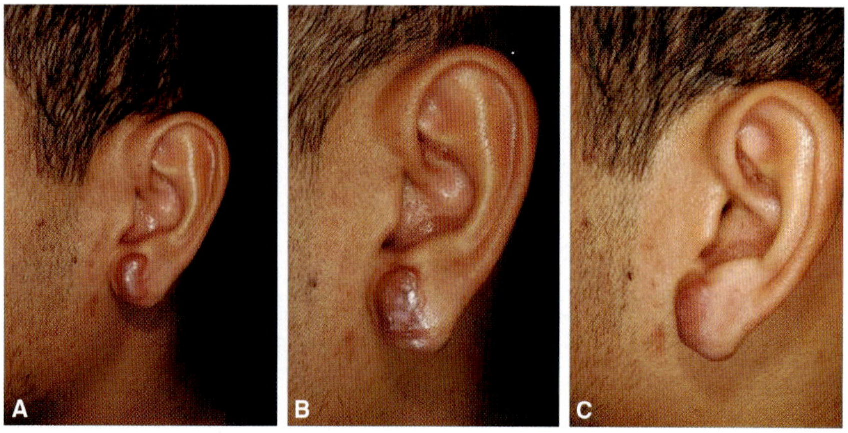

FIGURE 10-8 Results of intralesional cryotherapy of an ear keloid. **A:** Before intralesional cryotherapy. **B:** 4 weeks after intralesional cryotherapy. **C:** 12 weeks after intralesional cryotherapy.

PEARL 10-8 Treatment Pearl: Intralesional Cryotherapy *With favorable early reports of safety and efficacy in comparison to contact/spray probes, intralesional cryotherapy may represent a promising alternative scar reduction strategy.[103] Unfortunately, the costs of this treatment are relatively high because of the price of the cryoneedle.*

Imiquimod

Imiquimod is a toll-like receptor 7 ligand, which activates innate immune pathways and thereby acts as an immune response modifier. Imiquimod 5% cream has been approved for the treatment of actinic keratosis, superficial basal cell carcinoma, and genital warts.[87] Imiquimod promotes the release of interferon (IFN), a proinflammatory cytokine, and collagen breakdown. Moreover, imiquimod modulates the expression of genes inducing programmed cell death.[104] Efficacy in keloid management after surgical intervention has been reported in several trials, observational studies, and case reports. Varying successful treatment regimens (starting on the night of surgery with daily treatments or 2 weeks after the operation every other night for 8 weeks) have been proposed.[105–107] In contrast, a prospective, double-blind, placebo-controlled pilot study including 20 patients undergoing keloid excision with a subsequent treatment with imiquimod 5% cream or placebo revealed no significant differences in 6-month keloid recurrence rates.[108] Another study revealed a keloid recurrence rate of 80% in a total of 10 treated patients with imiquimod.[109] Consequently, additional studies are necessary to elaborate on the efficacy and the side-effect profile (persistent inflammation, erosions, depigmentation, etc.) of this immunomodulatory approach in regard to the reduction of recurrence rates after keloid excision.

PEARL 10-9 Treatment Pearl: Imiquimod *Study data unfortunately are too contradictory for this rather expensive approach. Therefore, the panel of the recently updated international guidelines did not include it in their recommendations.*

Bleomycin

Bleomycin sulfate is a glycopeptide that is typically used as a systemic chemotherapeutic agent, but has been employed for intralesional use in the treatment of excessive scarring. It is thought to inhibit collagen synthesis by decreasing stimulation by TGF-β1.[110] Several previous studies have revealed a significant improvement in height, pliability, and erythema, as well as subjective symptoms such as pruritus and pain of hypertrophic scars and keloids after three to five injections using the serial needle puncture or jet injection technique.[110–112] In rare cases long-term depigmentation and dermal atrophy may occur after intralesional bleomycin. As bleomycin is a chemotherapeutic with high toxicity, systemic administration is associated with serious side effects in the pulmonary, renal, hepatic, and other organ systems. Despite the cytotoxic potential, systemic side effects after intralesional bleomycin appear to be rare.[16] Still, further investigation and trials on the efficacy on bleomycin are necessary in order to establish the proper role for this agent in future treatment protocols.

PEARL 10-10 Treatment Pearl: Bleomycin *The approach is in general similar to the use of 5-FU. Although 5-FU currently appears somewhat better studied, the efficacy of injected bleomycin has been proven scientifically and through extensive clinical use. One advantage of bleomycin is that it is less frequently associated with ulcerations (which may be observed with 5-FU) leading to a higher popularity in darker skinned patient populations.*

Radiotherapy

Radiotherapeutic approaches such as superficial X-rays, electron beam, and low- or high-dose-rate brachytherapy have been employed primarily as an adjunct to the surgical removal of keloids. This combinational therapeutic approach has generally revealed good results in terms of reduced recurrence,[113–116] except for one report.[117] Radiotherapy acts through inhibition of vascular budding and fibroblast proliferation, resulting in decreased collagen synthesis.[15] Early initiation of electron beam irradiation after keloid excision (within 24 to 48 hours) appears to be favorable for enhanced results. A cumulative dose of up to 12 Gy in 6 or 10 fractions of 2 Gy applied daily or every other day is currently recommended by dermatologists.[18] Common side effects of radiotherapy include hypo- and hyperpigmentation, erythema, telangiectasia, and atrophy.[118] As ionizing irradiation has carcinogenic side effects, it should be handled with caution in younger patients and in sensitive areas such as the breast or thyroid.[16,46]

PEARL 10-11 Treatment Pearl: Radiotherapy *We only utilize radiotherapy as an additional approach to prevent recurrence after excision of keloids. Nevertheless, in patient populations such as Asians who may suffer from a completely different magnitude of keloids, radiotherapy may be considered, even as monotherapy.*

Interferon

IFN is a potent inhibitor of collagen I and III synthesis, and as such it has been considered for the treatment of excessive scarring.[16,119] IFN-α2b may exert antiproliferative effects, and may improve the pathologic features of dermal fibrosis directly or by antagonizing the effects of TGF-β and histamine.[120] In one report intralesional injection of IFN-α2b (1.5 million International Units, given twice daily over 4 days) reduced keloid size by 50% within only 9 days, and was determined to be more effective than intralesional corticosteroids.[120] Keloids injected three times weekly with IFN-α2b showed significant improvement and reduced serum TGF-β levels.[121] However, side effects after IFN administration are common, including flu-like symptoms and pain at the injection site.[16]

PEARL 10-12 Treatment Pearl: Interferon *Despite being an expensive therapeutic approach for excessive scarring, IFN may be of benefit in patients with scars resistant to other treatments.*

Botulinum Toxin A

Botulinum toxin A (BTA) has been previously reported as a successful treatment and prevention method for pathological scars, although its mechanism of action has yet to be fully elucidated. BTA is well known for its potential to immobilize facial muscles to reduce skin tension caused by muscle pull. By decreasing microtrauma and subsequent inflammation in the vicinity of the wound, the ultimate scar appearance may also improve.[122,123] This hypothesis was tested in a clinical trial by Gassner et al.[124] wherein 15 units of BTA (Botox, Allergan, Irvine, CA) per 2 cm of intraoperative length was injected into the musculature adjacent to the wound within 24 hours after wound closure. The authors noted enhanced wound healing and less noticeable scars compared to the control group.

A prospective, uncontrolled study involving 12 patients documented excellent efficacy following a course of intralesional BTA for keloids of varying sizes and durations.[125] BTA was injected at intervals of 3 months at a concentration of 35 units per mL, with a total dose ranging from 70 to 140 units per session. At 1 year follow-up, 25% (3 of 12 patients) demonstrated excellent results, 5 patients good, and 4 patients fair results without any therapeutic failures. As this study illustrates, in addition to reducing tension BTA likely also exerts direct effects on scar formation at the molecular and cellular level through mechanisms including the inhibition of fibroblast proliferation, TGF-β1 expression, and fibroblast-to-myofibroblast differentiation.[126,127] Despite these findings, a recently published study could not verify previously described results using intralesional BTA for existing keloid management; no differences were detected after BTA therapy compared to baseline using optical profilometry.[128] Additionally, no in vitro effect of BTA on TGF-β subtypes or fibroblast proliferation could be confirmed. Although results using intralesional BTA for existing keloids have been somewhat contradictory, a recent split-scar, double-blind randomized controlled trial demonstrated that a single BTA injection directly into the surgical site within 10 days of surgery was safe and effective for modulating thyroidectomy scars.[129] Thus, cutaneous BTA injection is a promising option for scar mitigation, and its various proposed inhibitory effects are consistent with its use in the early postoperative period.

PEARL 10-13 Treatment Pearl: Botulinum Toxin *Additional larger clinical studies are certainly required to further elucidate the role of BTA in scar treatment and prevention.*

Photodynamic therapy

Topical photodynamic therapy (PDT), the application of a photosensitizing medication such as aminolevulinic acid followed by light activation after an incubation period, is a well-accepted therapy for actinic keratosis, superficial basal cell carcinoma, and Bowen's disease (superficial squamous cell carcinoma). In recent years the treatment of keloids with PDT has also been proposed. It is known that PDT induces the production of reactive oxygen species (ROS), which are thought to contribute to the therapeutic effects through membrane and mitochondrial damage and cell apoptosis. Additionally ROS activate various signaling molecules such as TNF-α. PDT was shown to reduce the type I collagen synthesis and fibroblast proliferation in vitro, and these effects may be responsible for the improvement seen clinically.[130] Another group demonstrated in a small study population of 20 patients that three treatments of PDT (37 J per cm^2) at weekly intervals were effective in reducing pruritus and pain, as well as in increasing pliability of symptomatic keloids.[131]

PEARL 10-14 Treatment Pearl: Photodynamic Therapy *PDT is a promising and noninvasive approach in the treatment of scars. However, additional studies are needed to further evaluate the efficacy and optimal PDT treatment regime for this indication.*

Recombinant TGF-β3

In the first trimester of human fetal development, cutaneous tissue is able to heal scarlessly (see Chapter 27). Later in gestation there is a transition so that injuries result in scar formation similar to that of adult skin. Among the key differences observed between scar-free and scar-forming skin is the ratio of TGF-β isoform expression. Early fetal tissue is characterized by a high ratio of TGF-β3 to TGF-β1 and TGF-β2, whereas the reverse is true in adult skin. Furthermore, TGF-β1 and TGF-β2 are known to promote fibrosis.[132] Recombinant human TGF-β3 (avotermin) was thus identified as a promising potential therapeutic agent for scar treatment based in part on these observations. Ferguson and colleagues summarized the results of three double-blind, placebo-controlled trials in a landmark study published in 2009 in the *Lancet*.[133] Intradermal avotermin (recombinant human TGF-β3) administered in healthy subjects to the wound margins was judged to be effective in improving scar appearance by both lay observers and clinicians. However, in a 2011 study avotermin failed to hit its primary and secondary endpoints in a pivotal phase III trial.[134]

PEARL 10-15 Treatment Pearl: TGF-β3 *Although the clinical future and potential of recombinant TGF-β3 in scar management remain uncertain, work continues to identify methods to replicate the wound healing environment of early fetal tissue.*

Clinical Approach

The request for appropriate scar therapy is continuously increasing for both functional/symptomatic and cosmetic improvement. With many options available, it may help to follow a certain treatment regime based on scientific data as well as on clinical practicability.

Differentiation of Scar Types

Based on the updated international guidelines published in 2014, excessive scarring is differentiated into minor and major keloids, as well as immature, linear, and widespread (burn) hypertrophic scars.[35] In our own clinical routine, we mainly differentiate between mature and immature scars, linear hypertrophic scars, and widespread (burn) scars, as well as keloids (Fig. 10-9) (see Chapter 5). We further differentiate scars (of any type) into those that have never been treated and those that have been pretreated elsewhere with minimal or no response (as mentioned above). For the latter ones, we currently utilize noninvasive objective measurements in order to monitor progress of the scar therapy more closely.

Objective Measurements and Evaluation of Treatment Progress

Although many different scar assessment scales such as the Vancouver Scar Scale (VSS) and the Patient and Observer Scar Assessment Scale (POSAS) have been described over the last two decades, the POSAS has rapidly become one of the most frequently employed method for scar documentation and evaluation after its initial introduction in 2004 (see Chapter 28). It consists of two six-item scores, one based on the observer's assessment and the other based on the patient's assessment, and additionally provides an overall opinion for both sides. Patients rate pain, pruritus, color, stiffness, thickness, and irregularity of the scar, whereas observers rate vascularity, pigmentation, thickness, relief, pliability, and surface area.[135] Every item and the overall opinion can be scored from 1 to 10 points, resulting in scores between 12 and 120 points and overall opinion scores between 2 and 20 points.[136] Although the first publication of the POSAS focused on the rating of burn scars, it has subsequently been utilized to successfully analyze, document, and monitor a variety of different scar types such as keloids, hypertrophic scars, and fresh postsurgical scars.[29,137–141] In recent years, the POSAS has been demonstrated to produce reliable and valid documentation and appears to provide more consistent and reliable results than the VSS.[136,142,143]

In specific cases, combination with a noninvasive imaging method may be warranted, especially when minor differences in scar size and height may influence decisions with regard to more invasive treatment options. Here, the PRIMOS (Phaseshift Rapid In-vivo Measurement

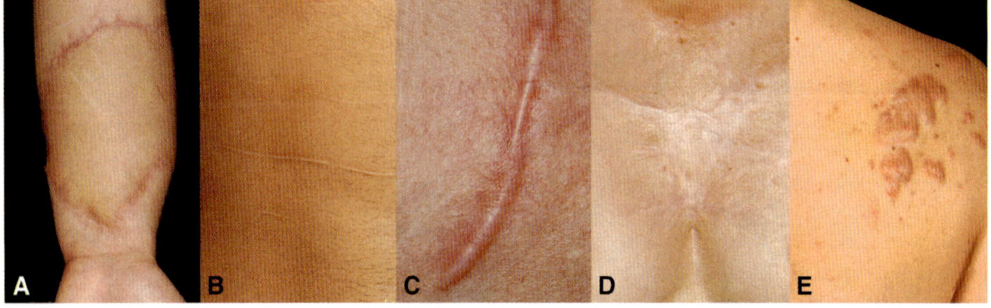

FIGURE 10-9 Classification of scar types in the authors' clinical practice. **A:** immature scar, **B:** mature scar, **C:** linear hypertrophic scar, **D:** widespread hypertrophic scar (burn), **E:** keloid. *(From Poetschke J, Gauglitz GG. Aktuelle Therapieoptionen zur Behandlung von überschießenderNarbenheilung.* J Dtsch Dermatol Ges. *2016 May;14(5):467-78.)*

Of Skin; GFMesstechnik, Teltow, Germany) represents a valuable tool that is able to render three-dimensional (3D) high-resolution images of skin surfaces in vivo. The device uses micro-mirrors to project a stripe pattern with a sinusoidal light intensity onto the surface of the measured object, which is then captured by a charge-coupled device camera. The information about the displacement of the stripe pattern and its gray levels is then utilized to construct a detailed height map that can subsequently be used for a variety of analyses.[135]

The PRIMOS system was primarily designed for the measurement and documentation of wrinkles and skin roughness.[144,145] Based on its abilities to provide high-resolution 3D models of the measured surfaces that ascertain information such as height, width, elevation, and volume of the captured lesions, the PRIMOS system has found its use in a variety of studies on the treatment of acneiform scars, keloids, and hypertrophic scars, where it proved to produce valid and reliable results.[128,146–149] Other 3D imaging options include the VISIA system by Canfield Scientific, the Minolta Vivid 910, the Polhemus FastSCAN, or the Steinbichler Comet.[135] Alternatively, diagnostic ultrasound can also be employed to evaluate the extent and the density of the intracutaneous scar tissue as well as the superficial dimensions of the respective scars.

Treatment Paradigm

See Figure 10-10.

Prevention

Next to appropriate surgical techniques, we recommend silicone-based products for patients at increased risk for pathological scarring or patients with increased concerns about scar outcome. In case of scarring in visible areas we prefer gels to patches and highlight the importance of sun protection in order to prevent potential postinflammatory hyperpigmentation. Alternatively, an onion extract–containing gel can be considered. In patients with pressing aesthetic concerns, a fractional (nonablative) laser may be employed early after wounding every 2 to 4 weeks. Even though settings do vary with every device, moderate energies and densities are usually sufficient.

Treatment

Keloids (Body)

If not pretreated elsewhere, we usually start with combination of cryotherapy (two cycles of 10 seconds each) directly followed by injection of TAC (20 to 40 mg per mL) every 4 weeks. If no significant improvement is noted, we switch to 5-FU (50 mg per mL) and TAC (40 mg per mL) in a ratio of 3:1. In case patients are being referred to our center and TAC, cryotherapy, or silicone has been employed for longer than 3 months, we immediately start with the combination of 5-FU and TAC if no contraindications exist. As soon as signs of maturation or a stable steady state is achieved and the scar has significantly flattened, we may continue with a vascular laser in order to improve erythema or newly formed

Keloids (body):
- apply cryotherapy twice for 10 seconds at a time
- afterwards lesions are injected with TAC (20 mg/mL) until a blanching effect (visible deposition of crystalline glucocorticoid) shows

This approach is repeated every 4 weeks
If no significant improvement after 3–4 treatment sessions is apparent:
- commence intralesional injections of 5-FU (50 mg/mL) and TAC (40 mg/mL) in a ratio of 3:1

In case of prior treatment with cryotherapy, TAC or silicone for over 3 months:
- immediately start with combination of 5-FU and TAC

After achieving significant scar flattening or a steady state, consider vascular laser therapy for the improvement of erythema and telangiectasia

Keloids (earlobe):
- surgical removal indicated as primary therapy

For prevention of recurrence, further means are necessary:
- apply cryotherapy twice for 10 seconds at a time, directly after surgery
- pressure earrings should be worn for at least 3 months
- small amounts of 5-FU (50 mg/mL) can be injected into the fresh scar tissue, starting 2 weeks after surgery, every 2 months

Hypertrophic scars (immature):
- primary means of therapy similar to scar prevention (silicone products, onion extract, pressure therapy)
- current developments include the early use of fractional lasers and intralesional TAC injections (10 mg/mL)

Hypertrophic scars (linear):
- combination of cryotherapy and TAC usually yields quick and satisfying results
- use of vascular lasers can be included after scar flattening to alleviate residual erythema and telangiectasia
- in case of remaining surface irregularities, fractional lasers can be considered

In case of mature hypertrophic scarring, conventional CO_2 laser therapy may be used to ablate scar tissue. After reepithelialization, silicone based products can help optimize the healing process

Hypertrophic scars (widespread/burn):
- fractional CO_2 laser therapy can be used to alleviate the scarring
- steps include deep fractional application of the laser to induce the collagen remodeling process in the dermis and afterwards the targeted ablation of individual scar strands and the general superficial scar ablation for further scar surface flattening

FIGURE 10-10 Treatment paradigm for scars. TAC, triamcinolone acetonide, 5-FU, 5-Fluorouracil.

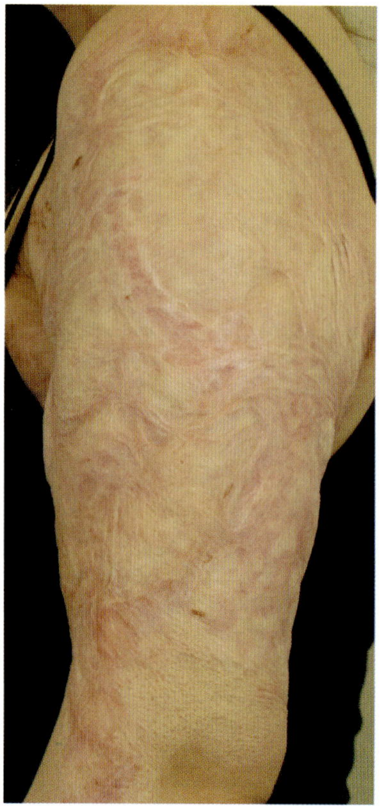

FIGURE 10-11 Hypertrophic burn scar on the upper arm.

telangiectases. Here, multiple sessions are necessary in order to significantly reduce erythema, especially in keloids.

In very rare cases, if 5-FU treatment has not been successful we may consider a surgical approach, which then is always combined with postsurgical radiotherapy, pressure, or other preventative measures.

Keloids (Earlobes)

Surgery remains our first choice. For prevention of recurrence of ear keloids after surgery, we perform cryotherapy directly after the surgery (two cycles of 10 seconds each), prescribe pressure earrings (to be worn for at least 3 months), and inject small amounts of 5-FU (50 mg per mL) directly into the fresh scar tissue, usually beginning around 2 weeks postsurgery at 2-month intervals.

Hypertrophic Scars (Immature)

See prevention, similar regime; trend to use fractional lasers in combination with intralesional TAC (10 mg per mL) more often.

Linear Hypertrophic Scars

We usually start with the combination of cryotherapy and TAC. Because hypertrophic scars usually respond well, we often do not need alternative treatment regimens besides vascular lasers for the improvement of erythema or fractional lasers for the improvement of scar texture. In case of older mature hypertrophic scars, we may even ablate the scar tissue with a conventional (nonfractionated) CO_2 laser and use silicone-based products for amelioration of the scar healing process as soon as the wound has closed.

Hypertrophic Burn Scars

Usually patients are being referred to our department from burn centers; thus, any reconstructive surgical procedures have already been undertaken (Fig. 10-11). Frequently pressure garments and silicone-based products have already been used extensively and patients worry about persistent uneven scar texture, pliability, and tension. After the scars have matured (usually about 1.5 years after the injury), we frequently utilize a fractional CO_2 laser in three distinct steps. First, in order to initiate the scar remodeling process,

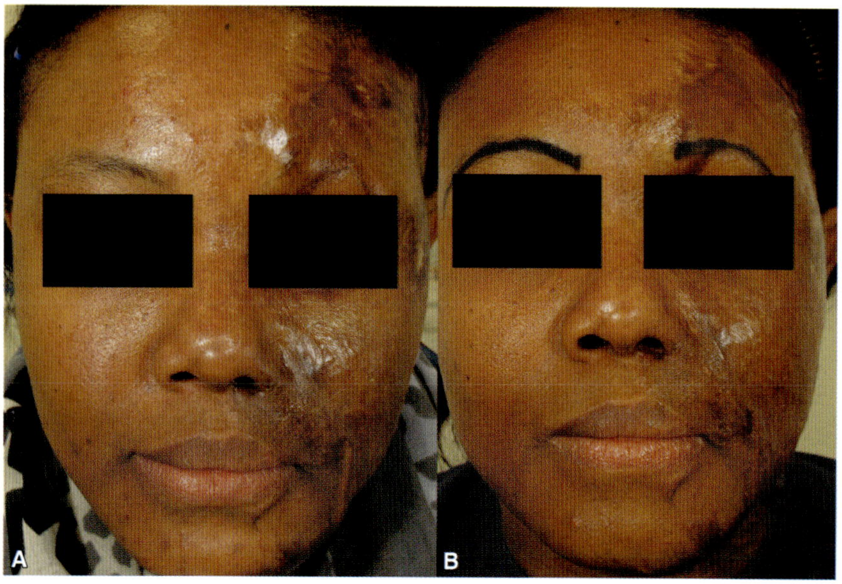

FIGURE 10-12 Burn scar before and after fractional CO_2 laser therapy. **A:** Before. **B:** After two fractional CO_2 laser treatment sessions. (Lumenis Ultrapulse SCAAR FX 70 to 110 mJ, 250 Hz, density setting 1; Active FX 1st pass: 60 to 100 mJ, 200 Hz, CPG 1-4-7, for ablation of individual scar strands; 2nd pass: 100 to 125 mJ, 125 Hz, CPG 2-7-3, for general superficial scar ablation.)

a fractionated CO_2 modality is often employed (Lumenis Ultrapulse, SCAAR FX, Yokneam, Israel) with pulse energies ranging from 70 to 110 mJ and a microcolumn density of 1%. Next, the elevated scar areas are ablated to the desired level in a nonfractionated full-field mode (Active FX) with a small spot size, pulse energy from 60 to 100 mJ, and high density (setting 9). Last the overall area is treated with another pass in a macrofractionated mode using pulse energies of 100 to 125 mJ and a moderate density (setting 3) to smoothen the respective area (Fig. 10-12). The whole procedure is performed after applying a topical anesthetic cream for 1 hour (Piaglis, Galderma) and 1 g of oral paracetamol, and is repeated every 3 months until the desired results are achieved. Although objective data on the optimum number of treatment sessions are still lacking, we usually inform patients about the necessity of at least three treatment sessions for sufficiently satisfying results. Postoperatively, we cover the treated area with a fusidic acid–containing crème, paraffin gauze, and a sterile wound dressing. After 24 hours, the dressings are changed for the first time. In case of weeping, further dressing of the wound is recommended. A dry wound, however, can be left undressed, if its location and patient comfort allow it. For the prevention of wound infections, we recommend continued wound care with a fusidic acid–containing crème three times a day for a total of 5 days postoperatively. After the removal of the dressings, patients can carefully clean the wounds with sterile water. To help with postoperative swelling and pain, local cooling can be considered. After ablative laser treatment, special care should be taken in regard to minimizing exposure to sunlight and the use of strong sunscreen is highly recommended.

Conclusions

Pathological scarring following a surgical intervention or trauma remains difficult to predict and treat. Current standard prophylactic and therapeutic strategies comprise pressure therapy, silicone, intralesional TAC, cryotherapy, radiation, lasers, surgical excision, and various combinations of these methods (see Chapter 16). Most of these are merely supported by clinical experience, whereas only few have been supported by well-designed prospective studies with adequate control groups. Emerging techniques such as the intralesional injection of 5-FU, fractional lasers, and intralesional cryotherapy extend the spectrum of treatment for excessive scarring. Innovative therapeutic approaches such as PDT and BTA and novel compounds such as avotermin may have therapeutic potential but also require additional investigation.

REFERENCES

1. Reinholz M, Poetschke J, Schwaiger H, et al. The dermatology life quality index as a means to assess life quality in patients with different scar types. *J Eur Acad Dermatol Venereol*. 2015;29(11):2112–2119.
2. Gauglitz GG. Management of keloids and hypertrophic scars: current and emerging options. *Clin Cosmet Investig Dermatol*. 2013;6:103–114.
3. Slemp AE, Kirschner RE. Keloids and scars: a review of keloids and scars, their pathogenesis, risk factors, and management. *Curr Opin Pediatr*. 2006;18(4):396–402.
4. Reinke JM, Sorg H. Wound repair and regeneration. *Eur Surg Res*. 2012;49(1):35–43.
5. Tredget EE, Nedelec B, Scott PG, et al. Hypertrophic scars, keloids, and contractures. The cellular and molecular basis for therapy. *Surg Clin North Am*. 1997;77(3):701–730.
6. Gauglitz GG, Pavicic T. Emerging strategies for the prevention and therapy of excessive scars [in German]. *MMW Fortschr Med*. 2012;154(15):55–58.
7. Bond JS, Duncan JA, Mason T, et al. Scar redness in humans: how long does it persist after incisional and excisional wounding? *Plast Reconstr Surg*. 2008;121(2):487–496.
8. Gauglitz GG, Korting HC, Pavicic T, et al. Hypertrophic scarring and keloids: pathomechanisms and current and emerging treatment strategies. *Mol Med*. 2011;17(1–2):113–125.
9. Brown JJ, Bayat A. Genetic susceptibility to raised dermal scarring. *Br J Dermatol*. 2009;161(1):8–18.
10. Wynn TA. Fibrotic disease and the T(H)1/T(H)2 paradigm. *Nat Rev Immunol*. 2004;4(8):583–594.
11. Doucet C, Brouty-Boyé D, Pottin-Clémenceau C, et al. Interleukin (IL) 4 and IL-13 act on human lung fibroblasts. Implication in asthma. *J Clin Invest*. 1998;101(10):2129–2139.
12. Mustoe TA, Cooter RD, Gold MH, et al; International Advisory Panel on Scar Management. International clinical recommendations on scar management. *Plast Reconstr Surg*. 2002;110(2):560–571.
13. Mutalik S. Treatment of keloids and hypertrophic scars. *Indian J Dermatol Venereol Leprol*. 2005;71(1):3–8.
14. Ogawa R, Akaishi S, Huang C, et al. Clinical applications of basic research that shows reducing skin tension could prevent and treat abnormal scarring: the importance of fascial/subcutaneous tensile reduction sutures and flap surgery for keloid and hypertrophic scar reconstruction. *J Nippon Med Sch*. 2011;78(2):68–76.
15. Reish RG, Eriksson E. Scar treatments: preclinical and clinical studies. *J Am Coll Surg*. 2008;206(4):719–730.
16. Leventhal D, Furr M, Reiter D. Treatment of keloids and hypertrophic scars: a meta-analysis and review of the literature. *Arch Facial Plast Surg*. 2006;8(6):362–368.
17. Muir IF. On the nature of keloid and hypertrophic scars. *Br J Plast Surg*. 1990;43(1):61–69.
18. Nast A, Eming S, Fluhr J, et al; German Society of Dermatology. German S2k guidelines for the therapy of pathological scars (hypertrophic scars and keloids). *J Dtsch Dermatol Ges*. 2012;10(10):747–762.
19. Poochareon VN, Berman B. New therapies for the management of keloids. *J Craniofac Surg*. 2003;14(5):654–657.
20. Robles DT, Berg D. Abnormal wound healing: keloids. *Clin Dermatol*. 2007;25(1):26–32.
21. Zuber TJ, DeWitt DE. Earlobe keloids. *Am Fam Physician*. 1994;49(8):1835–1841.
22. Sawada Y, Sone K. Hydration and occlusion treatment for hypertrophic scars and keloids. *Br J Plast Surg*. 1992;45(8):599–603.
23. Fulton JE Jr. Silicone gel sheeting for the prevention and management of evolving hypertrophic and keloid scars. *Dermatol Surg*. 1995;21(11):947–951.
24. Ahn ST, Monafo WW, Mustoe TA. Topical silicone gel: a new treatment for hypertrophic scars. *Surgery*. 1989;106(4):781–786; discussion 786-7.
25. Carney SA, Cason CG, Gowar JP, et al. Cica-Care gel sheeting in the management of hypertrophic scarring. *Burns*. 1994;20(2):163–167.
26. Lee SM, Ngim CK, Chan YY, et al. A comparison of Sil-K and Epiderm in scar management. *Burns*. 1996;22(6):483–487.
27. Mustoe TA. Evolution of silicone therapy and mechanism of action in scar management. *Aesthetic Plast Surg*. 2008;32(1):82–92.
28. O'Brien L, Pandit A. Silicon gel sheeting for preventing and treating hypertrophic and keloid scars. *Cochrane Database Syst Rev*. 2006;(1):CD003826.
29. Bianchi FA, Roccia F, Fiorini P, et al. Use of Patient and Observer Scar Assessment Scale for evaluation of facial scars treated with self-drying silicone gel. *J Craniofac Surg*. 2010;21(3):719–723.
30. van der Wal MB, van Zuijlen PP, van de Ven P, et al. Topical silicone gel versus placebo in promoting the maturation of burn scars: a randomized controlled trial. *Plast Reconstr Surg*. 2010;126(2):524–531.
31. Steinstraesser L, Flak E, Witte B, et al. Pressure garment therapy alone and in combination with silicone for the prevention of hypertrophic scarring: randomized controlled trial with intraindividual comparison. *Plast Reconstr Surg*. 2011;128(4):306e–313e.

32. Chernoff WG, Cramer H, Su-Huang S. The efficacy of topical silicone gel elastomers in the treatment of hypertrophic scars, keloid scars, and post-laser exfoliation erythema. *Aesthetic Plast Surg*. 2007;31(5):495–500.
33. Stoffels I, Wolter TP, Sailer AM, et al. The impact of silicone spray on scar formation. A single-center placebo-controlled double-blind trial [in German]. *Hautarzt*. 2010;61(4):332–338.
34. Gold MH, Berman B, Clementoni MT, et al. Updated international clinical recommendations on scar management. Part 1: evaluating the evidence. *Dermatol Surg*. 2014;40(8):817–824.
35. Gold MH, McGuire M, Mustoe TA, et al; International Advisory Panel on Scar Management. Updated international clinical recommendations on scar management. Part 2: algorithms for scar prevention and treatment. *Dermatol Surg*. 2014;40(8):825–831.
36. Jalali M, Bayat A. Current use of steroids in management of abnormal raised skin scars. *Surgeon*. 2007;5(3):175–180.
37. Cruz NI, Korchin L. Inhibition of human keloid fibroblast growth by isotretinoin and triamcinolone acetonide in vitro. *Ann Plast Surg*. 1994;33(4):401–405.
38. Boyadjiev C, Popchristova E, Mazgalova J. Histomorphologic changes in keloids treated with Kenacort. *J Trauma*. 1995;38(2):299–302.
39. Fredman R, Tenenhaus M. Cushing's syndrome after intralesional triamcinolone acetonide: a systematic review of the literature and multinational survey. *Burns*. 2013;39(4):549–557.
40. Liu MF, Yencha M. Cushing's syndrome secondary to intralesional steroid injections of multiple keloid scars. *Otolaryngol Head Neck Surg*. 2006;135(6):960–961.
41. Murray JC. Keloids and hypertrophic scars. *Clin Dermatol*. 1994; 12(1):27–37.
42. Lawrence WT. In search of the optimal treatment of keloids: report of a series and a review of the literature. *Ann Plast Surg*. 1991;27(2):164–178.
43. Boutli-Kasapidou F, Tsakiri A, Anagnostou E, et al. Hypertrophic and keloidal scars: an approach to polytherapy. *Int J Dermatol*. 2005;44(4):324–327.
44. Jaros E, Priborsky J, Klein L. Treatment of keloids and hypertrophic scars with cryotherapy [in Czech]. *Acta Medica (Hradec Kralove) Suppl*. 1999;42(2):61–63.
45. Yosipovitch G, Widijanti Sugeng M, Goon A, et al. A comparison of the combined effect of cryotherapy and corticosteroid injections versus corticosteroids and cryotherapy alone on keloids: a controlled study. *J Dermatolog Treat*. 2001;12(2):87–90.
46. Atiyeh BS. Nonsurgical management of hypertrophic scars: evidence-based therapies, standard practices, and emerging methods. *Aesthetic Plast Surg*. 2007;31(5):468–494.
47. Zouboulis CC, Blume U, Büttner P, et al. Outcomes of cryosurgery in keloids and hypertrophic scars. A prospective consecutive trial of case series. *Arch Dermatol*. 1993;129(9):1146–1151.
48. Barara M, Mendiratta V, Chander R. Cryotherapy in treatment of keloids: evaluation of factors affecting treatment outcome. *J Cutan Aesthet Surg*. 2012;5(3):185–189.
49. Baur PS, Larson DL, Stacey TR, et al. Ultrastructural analysis of pressure-treated human hypertrophic scars. *J Trauma*. 1976;16(12):958–967.
50. Macintyre L, Baird M. Pressure garments for use in the treatment of hypertrophic scars--a review of the problems associated with their use. *Burns*. 2006;32(1):10–15.
51. Kelly AP. Medical and surgical therapies for keloids. *Dermatol Ther*. 2004;17(2):212–218.
52. Reno F, Sabbatini M, Lombardi F, et al. In vitro mechanical compression induces apoptosis and regulates cytokines release in hypertrophic scars. *Wound Repair Regen*. 2003;11(5):331–336.
53. Van den Kerckhove E, Stappaerts K, Fieuws S, et al. The assessment of erythema and thickness on burn related scars during pressure garment therapy as a preventive measure for hypertrophic scarring. *Burns*. 2005;31(6):696–702.
54. Candy LH, Cecilia LT, Ping ZY. Effect of different pressure magnitudes on hypertrophic scar in a Chinese population. *Burns*. 2010;36(8):1234–1241.
55. Anzarut A, Olson J, Singh P, et al. The effectiveness of pressure garment therapy for the prevention of abnormal scarring after burn injury: a meta-analysis. *J Plast Reconstr Aesthet Surg*. 2009;62(1):77–84.
56. Bran GM, Brom J, Hörmann K, et al. Auricular keloids: combined therapy with a new pressure device. *Arch Facial Plast Surg*. 2012;14(1):20–26.
57. Kadouch DJ, van der Veer WM, Mahdavian Delavary B, et al. Therapeutic hotline: an alternative adjuvant treatment after ear keloid excision using a custom-made methyl methacrylate stent. *Dermatol Ther*. 2010;23(6):686–692.
58. Apfelberg DB, Maser MR, Lash H, et al. Preliminary results of argon and carbon dioxide laser treatment of keloid scars. *Lasers Surg Med*. 1984;4(3):283–290.
59. Alster TS, Handrick C. Laser treatment of hypertrophic scars, keloids, and striae. *Semin Cutan Med Surg*. 2000;19(4):287–292.
60. Alster T. Laser scar revision: comparison study of 585-nm pulsed dye laser with and without intralesional corticosteroids. *Dermatol Surg*. 2003;29(1):25–29.
61. Alster TS, Williams CM. Treatment of keloid sternotomy scars with 585 nm flashlamp-pumped pulsed-dye laser. *Lancet*. 1995;345(8959):1198–1200.
62. Dierickx C, Goldman MP, Fitzpatrick RE. Laser treatment of erythematous/hypertrophic and pigmented scars in 26 patients. *Plast Reconstr Surg*. 1995;95(1):84–92.
63. Akaishi S, Koike S, Dohi T, et al. Nd:YAG laser treatment of keloids and hypertrophic scars. *Eplasty*. 2012;12:e1.
64. Tanzi EL, Alster TS. Laser treatment of scars. *Skin Therapy Lett*. 2004;9(1):4–7.
65. Paquet P, Hermanns JF, Pierard GE. Effect of the 585 nm flashlamp-pumped pulsed dye laser for the treatment of keloids. *Dermatol Surg*. 2001;27(2):171–174.
66. Allison KP, Kiernan MN, Waters RA, et al. Pulsed dye laser treatment of burn scars. Alleviation or irritation? *Burns*. 2003;29(3):207–213.
67. Wittenberg GP, Fabian BG, Bogomilsky JL, et al. Prospective, single-blind, randomized, controlled study to assess the efficacy of the 585-nm flashlamp-pumped pulsed-dye laser and silicone gel sheeting in hypertrophic scar treatment. *Arch Dermatol*. 1999;135(9):1049–1055.
68. Durani P, Bayat A. Levels of evidence for the treatment of keloid disease. *J Plast Reconstr Aesthet Surg*. 2008;61(1):4–17.
69. Shih PY, Chen HH, Chen CH, et al. Rapid recurrence of keloid after pulse dye laser treatment. *Dermatol Surg*. 2008;34(8):1124–1127.
70. Cho SB, Lee JH, Lee SH, et al. Efficacy and safety of 1064-nm Q-switched Nd:YAG laser with low fluence for keloids and hypertrophic scars. *J Eur Acad Dermatol Venereol*. 2010;24(9):1070–1074.
71. Manstein D, Herron GS, Sink RK, et al. Fractional photothermolysis: a new concept for cutaneous remodeling using microscopic patterns of thermal injury. *Lasers Surg Med*. 2004;34(5):426–438.
72. Laubach HJ, Tannous Z, Anderson RR, et al. Skin responses to fractional photothermolysis. *Lasers Surg Med*. 2006;38(2):142–149.
73. Dams SD, de Liefde-van Beest M, Nuijs AM, et al. Pulsed heat shocks enhance procollagen type I and procollagen type III expression in human dermal fibroblasts. *Skin Res Technol*. 2010;16(3):354–364.
74. Kwan JM, Wyatt M, Uebelhoer NS, et al. Functional improvement after ablative fractional laser treatment of a scar contracture. *PM R*. 2011;3(10):986–987.
75. Helbig D, Paasch U. Molecular changes during skin aging and wound healing after fractional ablative photothermolysis. *Skin Res Technol*. 2011;17(1):119–128.
76. Tierney E, Mahmoud BH, Srivastava D, et al. Treatment of surgical scars with nonablative fractional laser versus pulsed dye laser: a randomized controlled trial. *Dermatol Surg*. 2009;35(8):1172–1180.
77. Oh G, Ahn HH, Choi JE, et al. Postoperative treatment of surgical scars with ablative fractional laser versus pulsed dye laser: a randomized controlled trial. *J Am Acad Dermatol*. 2012;66(4 suppl 1):AB12.
78. Cervelli V, Gentile P, Spallone D, et al. Ultrapulsed fractional CO_2 laser for the treatment of post-traumatic and pathological scars. *J Drugs Dermatol*. 2010;9(11):1328–1331.
79. Qu L, Liu A, Zhou L, et al. Clinical and molecular effects on mature burn scars after treatment with a fractional CO(2) laser. *Lasers Surg Med*. 2012;44(7):517–524.
80. Ozog DM, Liu A, Chaffins ML, et al. Evaluation of clinical results, histological architecture, and collagen expression following treatment of mature burn scars with a fractional carbon dioxide laser. *JAMA Dermatol*. 2013;149:50–57.
81. Suh D-H, Chang, KY, Song KY, et al. Revision of burn scars using ablative fractional CO_2 laser. *J Am Acad Dermatol*. 2012;66(4, suppl 1):AB216.
82. Fitzpatrick RE. Treatment of inflamed hypertrophic scars using intralesional 5-FU. *Dermatol Surg*. 1999;25(3):224–232.
83. Nanda S, Reddy BS. Intralesional 5-fluorouracil as a treatment modality of keloids. *Dermatol Surg*. 2004;30(1):54–56; discussion 56–57.

84. Liu W, Wu X, Gao Z, et al. Remodelling of keloid tissue into normal-looking skin. *J Plast Reconstr Aesthet Surg*. 2008;61(12): 1553–1554.
85. Wu XL, Liu W, Cao YL. Clinical study on keloid treatment with intralesional injection of low concentration 5-fluorouracil [in Chinese]. *Zhonghua Zheng Xing Wai Ke Za Zhi*. 2006;22(1):44–46.
86. Wu XL, Gao Z, Song N, et al. Clinical study of auricular keloid treatment with both surgical excision and intralesional injection of low-dose 5-fluorouracil and corticosteroids [in Chinese]. *Zhonghua Zheng Xing Wai Ke Za Zhi*. 2009;28(89):1102–1105.
87. Asilian A, Darougheh A, Shariati F. New combination of triamcinolone, 5-fluorouracil, and pulsed-dye laser for treatment of keloid and hypertrophic scars. *Dermatol Surg*. 2006;32(7):907–915.
88. Darougheh A, Asilian A, Shariati F. Intralesional triamcinolone alone or in combination with 5-fluorouracil for the treatment of keloid and hypertrophic scars. *Clin Exp Dermatol*. 2009;34(2):219–223.
89. Davison SP, Dayan JH, Clemens MW, et al. Efficacy of intralesional 5-fluorouracil and triamcinolone in the treatment of keloids. *Aesthet Surg J*. 2009;29(1):40–46.
90. Monstrey S, Middelkoop E, Vranckx JJ, et al. Updated scar management practical guidelines: non-invasive and invasive measures. *J Plast Reconstr Aesthet Surg*. 2014;67(8):1017–1025.
91. Phan TT, Lim IJ, Sun L, et al. Quercetin inhibits fibronectin production by keloid-derived fibroblasts. Implication for the treatment of excessive scars. *J Dermatol Sci*. 2003;33(3):192–194.
92. Phan TT, Lim IJ, Chan SY, et al. Suppression of transforming growth factor beta/smad signaling in keloid-derived fibroblasts by quercetin: implications for the treatment of excessive scars. *J Trauma*. 2004;57(5):1032–1037.
93. Maragakis M, Willital GH, Michel G, et al. Possibilities of scar treatment after thoracic surgery. *Drugs Exp Clin Res*. 1995;21(5):199–206.
94. Chanprapaph K, Tanrattanakorn S, Wattanakrai P, et al. Effectiveness of onion extract gel on surgical scars in asians. *Dermatol Res Pract*. 2012;2012:212945.
95. Jackson BA, Shelton AJ. Pilot study evaluating topical onion extract as treatment for postsurgical scars. *Dermatol Surg*. 1999;25(4):267–269.
96. Chung VQ, Kelley L, Marra D, et al. Onion extract gel versus petrolatum emollient on new surgical scars: prospective double-blinded study. *Dermatol Surg*. 2006;32(2):193–197.
97. Beuth J, Hunzelmann N, Van Leendert R, et al. Safety and efficacy of local administration of contractubex to hypertrophic scars in comparison to corticosteroid treatment. Results of a multicenter, comparative epidemiological cohort study in Germany. *In Vivo*. 2006;20(2):277–283.
98. Ho WS, Ying SY, Chan PC, et al. Use of onion extract, heparin, allantoin gel in prevention of scarring in chinese patients having laser removal of tattoos: a prospective randomized controlled trial. *Dermatol Surg*. 2006;32(7):891–896.
99. Koc E, Arca E, Surucu B, et al. An open, randomized, controlled, comparative study of the combined effect of intralesional triamcinolone acetonide and onion extract gel and intralesional triamcinolone acetonide alone in the treatment of hypertrophic scars and keloids. *Dermatol Surg*. 2008;34(11):1507–1514.
100. Har-Shai Y, Sabo E, Rohde E, et al. Intralesional cryosurgery enhances the involution of recalcitrant auricular keloids: a new clinical approach supported by experimental studies. *Wound Repair Regen*. 2006;14(1):18–27.
101. Har-Shai Y, Amar M, Sabo E. Intralesional cryotherapy for enhancing the involution of hypertrophic scars and keloids. *Plast Reconstr Surg*. 2003;111(6):1841–1852.
102. Har-Shai Y, Brown W, Labbé D, et al. Intralesional cryosurgery for the treatment of hypertrophic scars and keloids following aesthetic surgery: the results of a prospective observational study. *Int J Low Extrem Wounds*. 2008;7(3):169–175.
103. Tziotzios C, Profyris C, Sterling J. Cutaneous scarring: pathophysiology, molecular mechanisms, and scar reduction therapeutics. Part II: strategies to reduce scar formation after dermatologic procedures. *J Am Acad Dermatol*. 2012;66(1):13–24; quiz 25-6.
104. Zurada JM, Kriegel D, Davis IC. Topical treatments for hypertrophic scars. *J Am Acad Dermatol*. 2006;55(6):1024–1031.
105. Berman B, Kaufman J. Pilot study of the effect of postoperative imiquimod 5% cream on the recurrence rate of excised keloids. *J Am Acad Dermatol*. 2002;47(4, suppl):S209–S211.
106. Chuangsuwanich A, Gunjittisomram S. The efficacy of 5% imiquimod cream in the prevention of recurrence of excised keloids. *J Med Assoc Thai*. 2007;90(7):1363–1367.
107. Stashower ME. Successful treatment of earlobe keloids with imiquimod after tangential shave excision. *Dermatol Surg*. 2006;32(3):380–386.
108. Berman B, Harrison-Balestra C, Perez OA, et al. Treatment of keloid scars post-shave excision with imiquimod 5% cream: a prospective, double-blind, placebo-controlled pilot study. *J Drugs Dermatol*. 2009;8(5):455–458.
109. Cacao FM, Tanaka V, Messina MC. Failure of imiquimod 5% cream to prevent recurrence of surgically excised trunk keloids. *Dermatol Surg*. 2009;35(4):629–633.
110. Espana A, Solano T, Quintanilla E. Bleomycin in the treatment of keloids and hypertrophic scars by multiple needle punctures. *Dermatol Surg*. 2001;27(1):23–27.
111. Naeini FF, Najafian J, Ahmadpour K. Bleomycin tattooing as a promising therapeutic modality in large keloids and hypertrophic scars. *Dermatol Surg*. 2006;32(8):1023–1030.
112. Saray Y, Gulec AT. Treatment of keloids and hypertrophic scars with dermojet injections of bleomycin: a preliminary study. *Int J Dermatol*. 2005;44(9):777–784.
113. Ragoowansi R, Cornes PG, Moss AL, et al. Treatment of keloids by surgical excision and immediate postoperative single-fraction radiotherapy. *Plast Reconstr Surg*. 2003;111(6):1853–1859.
114. Guix B, Henríquez I, Andrés A, et al. Treatment of keloids by high-dose-rate brachytherapy: a seven-year study. *Int J Radiat Oncol Biol Phys*. 2001;50(1):167–172.
115. Escarmant P, Zimmermann S, Amar A, et al. The treatment of 783 keloid scars by iridium 192 interstitial irradiation after surgical excision. *Int J Radiat Oncol Biol Phys*. 1993;26(2):245–251.
116. Sallstrom KO, Larson O, Hedén P, et al. Treatment of keloids with surgical excision and postoperative X-ray radiation. *Scand J Plast Reconstr Surg Hand Surg*. 1989;23(3):211–215.
117. van de Kar AL, Kreulen M, van Zuijlen PP, et al. The results of surgical excision and adjuvant irradiation for therapy-resistant keloids: a prospective clinical outcome study. *Plast Reconstr Surg*. 2007;119(7):2248–2254.
118. Ogawa R, Mitsuhashi K, Hyakusoku H, et al. Postoperative electron-beam irradiation therapy for keloids and hypertrophic scars: retrospective study of 147 cases followed for more than 18 months. *Plast Reconstr Surg*. 2003;111(2):547–555.
119. Jimenez SA, Freundlich B, Rosenbloom J. Selective inhibition of human diploid fibroblast collagen synthesis by interferons. *J Clin Invest*. 1984;74(3):1112–1116.
120. Berman B, Duncan MR. Short-term keloid treatment in vivo with human interferon alfa-2b results in a selective and persistent normalization of keloidal fibroblast collagen, glycosaminoglycan, and collagenase production in vitro. *J Am Acad Dermatol*. 1989;21(4, Pt 1):694–702.
121. Tredget EE, Shankowsky HA, Pannu R, et al. Transforming growth factor-beta in thermally injured patients with hypertrophic scars: effects of interferon alpha-2b. *Plast Reconstr Surg*. 1998;102(5):1317–1328; discussion 1329-30.
122. Viera MH, Amini S, Valins W, et al. Innovative therapies in the treatment of keloids and hypertrophic scars. *J Clin Aesthet Dermatol*. 2010;3(5):20–26.
123. Lee BJ, Jeong JH, Wang SG, et al. Effect of botulinum toxin type a on a rat surgical wound model. *Clin Exp Otorhinolaryngol*. 2009;2(1):20–27.
124. Gassner HG, Brissett AE, Otley CC, et al. Botulinum toxin to improve facial wound healing: a prospective, blinded, placebo-controlled study. *Mayo Clin Proc*. 2006;81(8):1023–1028.
125. Zhibo X, Miaobo Z. Intralesional botulinum toxin type A injection as a new treatment measure for keloids. *Plast Reconstr Surg*. 2009;124(5):275e–277e.
126. Xiao Z, Zhang F, Lin W, et al. Effect of botulinum toxin type A on transforming growth factor beta1 in fibroblasts derived from hypertrophic scar: a preliminary report. *Aesthetic Plast Surg*. 2010;34(4):424–427.
127. Jeong HS, Lee BH, Sung HM, et al. Effect of botulinum toxin type A on differentiation of fibroblasts derived from scar tissue. *Plast Reconstr Surg*. 2015;136(2):171e–178e.
128. Gauglitz GG, Bureik D, Dombrowski Y, et al. Botulinum toxin A for the treatment of keloids. *Skin Pharmacol Physiol*. 2012;25(6):313–318.
129. Kim YS, Lee HJ, Cho SH, et al. Early postoperative treatment of thyroidectomy scars using botulinum toxin: a split-scar, double-blind randomized controlled trial. *Wound Repair Regen*. 2014;22(5): 605–612.
130. Mendoza-Garcia J, Sebastian A, Alonso-Rasgado T, et al. Ex vivo evaluation of the effect of photodynamic therapy on skin scars and

striae distensae. *Photodermatol Photoimmunol Photomed*. 2015;31(5): 239–251.
131. Ud-Din S, Thomas G, Morris J, et al. Photodynamic therapy: an innovative approach to the treatment of keloid disease evaluated using subjective and objective non-invasive tools. *Arch Dermatol Res*. 2013;305(3):205–214.
132. Occleston NL, O'Kane S, Laverty HG, et al. Discovery and development of avotermin (recombinant human transforming growth factor beta 3): a new class of prophylactic therapeutic for the improvement of scarring. *Wound Repair Regen*. 2011;19(suppl 1):s38–s48.
133. Ferguson MW, Duncan J, Bond J, et al. Prophylactic administration of avotermin for improvement of skin scarring: three double-blind, placebo-controlled, phase I/II studies. *Lancet*. 2009;373(9671):1264–1274.
134. McKee S. Renovo stock demolished by Justiva trial failure. http://www.pharmatimes.com/Article/11-02-15/Renovo_stock_demolished_by_Justiva_trial_failure.aspx. Accessed November 11, 2016.
135. Poetschke J, Schwaiger H, Gauglitz GG. Current and emerging options for documenting scars and evaluating therapeutic progress. *Dermatol Surg*. 2016. doi:10.1097/DSS.0000000000000698 (in press).
136. Draaijers LJ, Tempelman FR, Botman YA, et al. The patient and observer scar assessment scale: a reliable and feasible tool for scar evaluation. *Plast Reconstr Surg*. 2004;113(7):1960–1965; discussion 1966–1967.
137. Cromi A, Ghezzi F, Gottardi A, et al. Cosmetic outcomes of various skin closure methods following cesarean delivery: a randomized trial. *Am J Obstet Gynecol*. 2010;203(1):36.e1–36.e8.
138. Jina H, Simcock J. Median sternotomy scar assessment. *N Z Med J*. 2011;124(1346):57–62.
139. Khoo TL, Halim AS, Zakaria Z, et al. A prospective, randomised, double-blinded trial to study the efficacy of topical tocotrienol in the prevention of hypertrophic scars. *J Plast Reconstr Aesthet Surg*. 2011;64(6):e137–e145.
140. Maher SF, Dorko L, Saliga S. Linear scar reduction using silicone gel sheets in individuals with normal healing. *J Wound Care*. 2012;21(12):602, 604–606, 608–609.
141. Nicholas RS, Falvey H, Lemonas P, et al. Patient-related keloid scar assessment and outcome measures. *Plast Reconstr Surg*. 2012;129(3):648–656.
142. van de Kar AL, Corion LU, Smeulders MJ, et al. Reliable and feasible evaluation of linear scars by the Patient and Observer Scar Assessment Scale. *Plast Reconstr Surg*. 2005;116(2):514–522.
143. van der Wal MB, Tuinebreijer WE, Bloemen MC, et al. Rasch analysis of the Patient and Observer Scar Assessment Scale (POSAS) in burn scars. *Qual Life Res*. 2012;21(1):13–23.
144. Luebberding S, Krueger N, Kerscher M. Comparison of Validated Assessment Scales and 3D digital fringe projection method to assess lifetime development of wrinkles in men. *Skin Res Technol*. 2014;20(1):30–36.
145. Prager W, Steinkraus V. A prospective, rater-blind, randomized comparison of the effectiveness and tolerability of Belotero (R) Basic versus Restylane (R) for correction of nasolabial folds. *Eur J Dermatol*. 2010;20(6):748–752.
146. Barolet D, Boucher A. Prophylactic low-level light therapy for the treatment of hypertrophic scars and keloids: a case series. *Lasers Surg Med*. 2010;42(6):597–601.
147. Bloemen MC, van Gerven MS, van der Wal MB, et al. An objective device for measuring surface roughness of skin and scars. *J Am Acad Dermatol*. 2011;64(4):706–715.
148. Chapas AM, Brightman L, Sukal S, et al. Successful treatment of acneiform scarring with CO_2 ablative fractional resurfacing. *Lasers Surg Med*. 2008;40(6):381–386.
149. Friedman PM, Skover GR, Payonk G, et al. Quantitative evaluation of nonablative laser technology. *Semin Cutan Med Surg*. 2002;21(4):266–273.
150. Deitch EA, Wheelahan TM, Rose MP, et al. Hypertrophic burn scars: analysis of variables. *J Trauma*. 1983;23(10):895–898.
151. Elliot D, Cory-Pearce R, Rees GM. The behaviour of presternal scars in a fair-skinned population. *Ann R Coll Surg Engl*. 1985;67(4):238–240.
152. Lewis WH, Sun KK. Hypertrophic scar: a genetic hypothesis. *Burns*. 1990;16(3):176–178.
153. Murray CJ, Pinnel SR. Keloids and excessive dermal scarring. In: Cohen IK, Diegelmann RF, Lindblad WJ, eds. *Woundhealing, Biochemical and Clinical Aspects*. Philadelphia,PA: Saunders Elsevier; 1992:500–509.
154. Niessen FB, Spauwen PH, Schalkwijk J, et al. On the nature of hypertrophic scars and keloids: a review. *Plast Reconstr Surg*. 1999;104(5):1435–1458.
155. Moustafa MF, Abdel-Fattah MA, Abdel-Fattah DC. Presumptive evidence of the effect of pregnancy estrogens on keloid growth. Case report. *Plast Reconstr Surg*. 1975;56(4):450–453.
156. Oluwasanmi JO. Keloids in the African. *Clin Plast Surg*. 1974;1(1): 179–195.
157. From L, Assad D. Neoplasms, pseudoneoplasms, and hyperplasia of supporting tissue origin. In: Jeffers JD, Englis MR, eds. *Dermatology in General Medicine*. New York, NY: McGraw-Hill; 1993:1198–1199.
158. Hawkins HK. Pathophysiology of the burn scar. In: Herndon DN, ed. *Total Burn Care*. Philadelphia, PA: Saunders Elsevier; 2007:608–119.
159. Buchwald C, Nielsen LH, Rosborg J. Keloids of the external ear. *ORL J Otorhinolaryngol Relat Spec*. 1992;54(2):108–112.
160. Ketchum LD. Hypertrophic scars and keloids. *Clin Plast Surg*. 1977;4(2):301–310.
161. Wheeland RG. Keloids and hypertrophic scars. In: Arndt KA, et al, eds. *Cutaneous Medicine and Surgery*. Philadelphia, PA: Saunders Elsevier; 1996:900–905.
162. Gold MH. Topical silicone gel sheeting in the treatment of hypertrophic scars and keloids. A dermatologic experience. *J Dermatol Surg Oncol*. 1993;19(10):912–916.
163. Alster TS, West TB. Treatment of scars: a review. *Ann Plast Surg*. 1997;39(4):418–432.
164. Mancini RE, Quaife JV. Histogenesis of experimentally produced keloids. *J Invest Dermatol*. 1962;38:143–181.
165. Peacock EE Jr, Madden JW, Trier WC. Biologic basis for the treatment of keloids and hypertrophic scars. *South Med J*. 1970;63(7):755–760.
166. Sephel GC, Woodward SC. Repair, regeneration, and fibrosis. In: Rubin E, ed. *Rubin's Pathology*. Baltimore, MD: Lippincott, Williams & Wilkins; 2001:84–117.
167. Wenig BM. Modern surgical pathology. In: Weidner N, ed. Vol 1. Philadelphia, PA: Saunders; 2003.
168. Kose O, Waseem A. Keloids and hypertrophic scars: are they two different sides of the same coin? *Dermatol Surg*. 2008;34(3)336–346.

11 Neurobiology of Scars: Managing Pain and Itch

KENDRA GRIM and MICHAEL E. NEMERGUT

KEY POINTS

- Optimal management of scar-related pain and itch often requires multimodal therapy.
- Children with scars commonly acquire them in the setting of trauma; assessment for and treatment of comorbid psychological disease may incur significant treatment benefit.
- Although the focus of this text is on scars in general, much of the pediatric data are based on adult studies as data from children are limited.
- Given limitations of current data, a general understanding of pain and itch perception is warranted to optimize scar treatment, develop future treatment strategems, and conduct future studies that are needed in the pediatric and adult populations.

The history of procedural sedation and anesthesia for children has been a story of extremes.[1] Although experience in adult patients dictated the importance of providing analgesia, hypnosis, and amnesia to all such patients undergoing invasive diagnostic and therapeutic procedures, the importance of providing these goals for infants and children has historically been less clear. Indeed, in the past many have questioned the ability of neonates to sense pain, develop memories (explicit and/or implicit), as well as possess the higher order cognition necessary for consciousness.[2,3] These abilities were more than just academic—they had profound implications on therapeutic decision making. Indeed, because modulating nociception, memory formation, and/or consciousness confers overt risk (e.g., hypotension, apnea, airway obstruction, etc.), one might argue it illogical to provide analgesia to a person insensate, amnesia to a person without memory formation, and/or hypnosis to an unconscious person. In its extreme, such a point of view led to the practice of allowing infants to undergo major surgical procedures (such as an exploratory laparotomy) in the presence of paralysis but absence of sedative or analgesic medications.[4,5]

Today, it would be at variance with care standards to have a pediatric patient undergo a significant invasive procedure in the absence of analgesia as there are incontrovertible data that newborns not only feel pain, but that failure to provide adequate analgesia may result in both short- and long-term adverse consequences.[6–9] In this chapter, we will review the basic pathways involved in the transmission of pain and itch, as well as review pharmacologic methods for their assessment and for controlling these unpleasant sensations. It should be noted that although much is known about the nuances of these pathways, comparatively little is known with regard to how these pathways interact specifically with scars; furthermore, data with regard to stimulus mitigation are limited. When able, we will expound upon extant data with regard to scars and we will indicate when inferring from more generalized data. Surgical methods are discussed in a separate chapter (see Chapter 12).

Physiology

Pain

Pain Transmission

The sensation, delivery, and interpretation of pain sensation are complex. The discussion below will highlight the mechanisms involved, which have clinical implications of how patients sense/describe pain as well as provide a basis for pharmacologic treatment.

In its most simplified form, nociception signals begin in primary afferent neurons, which are subsequently transmitted through the dorsal horn of the spinal cord and along ascending pathways to the thalamus and somatosensory cortex. Primary afferents are the principal sensory neurons for nociception. The cell bodies of these sensory neurons are located in the dorsal root ganglia (DRG) or in the corresponding ganglion of specific cranial nerves (Fig. 11-1).[10] As sensory neurons can be very diverse, they are categorized in the Erlanger–Gasser classification according to the size of the axon and presence or absence of myelin. The three major categories are, in order from largest diameter to

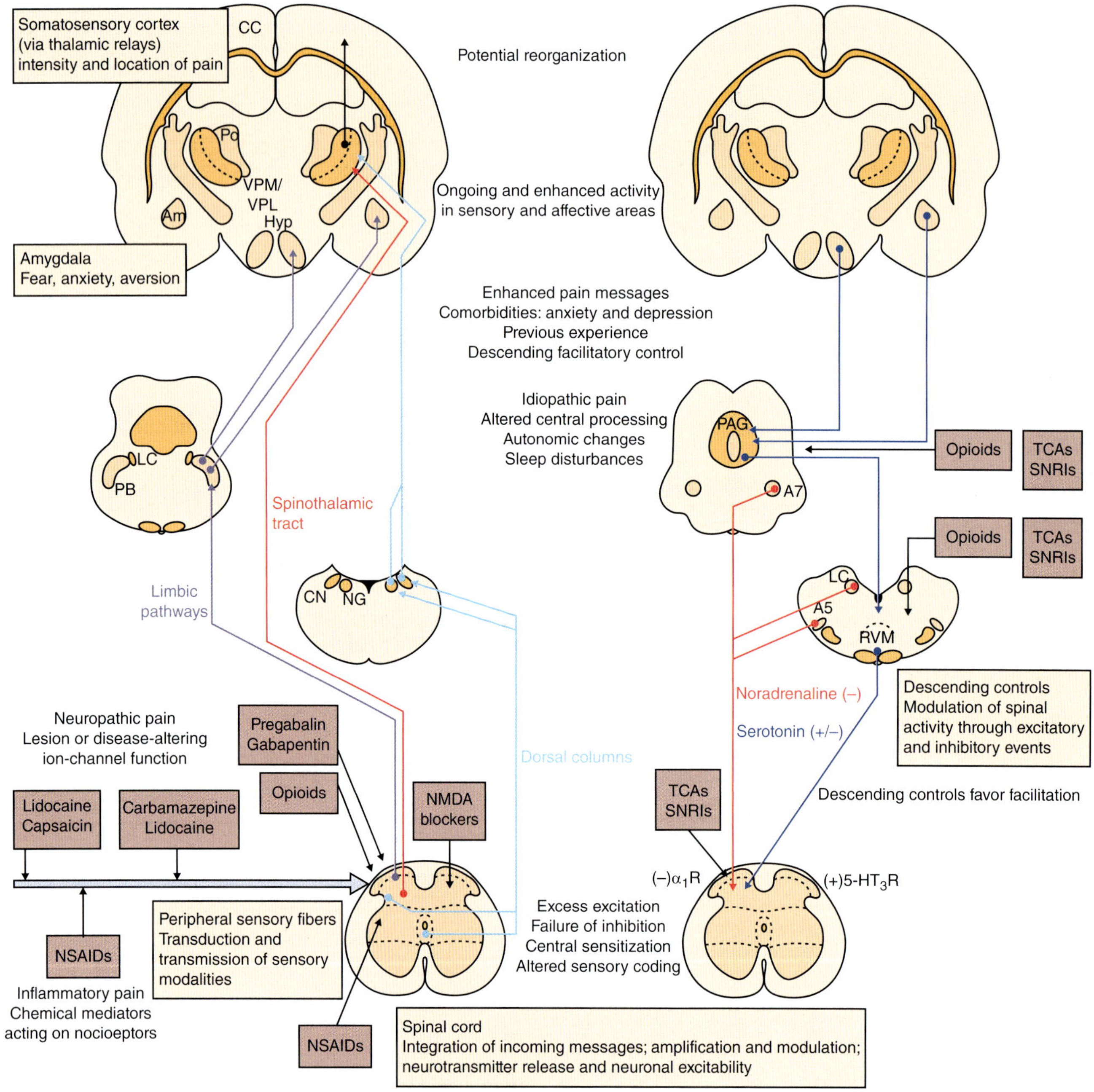

FIGURE 11-1 **Pain pathway transmission and modulation**. The ascending sensory and affective components are shown on the left. Processes by which higher centers can alter spinal function are shown on the right. The major functional roles of different neural components in these pathways are summarized in boxes. Changes that occur after tissue or nerve damage are listed, and pharmacologic agents are shown at their sites of action. Peripheral inputs are indicated by arrows. (–)α_2R=inhibition of neuronal activity. (+) 5-HT3R, stimulation of neuronal activity; Am, amygdala; A5 and A7, brainstem nuclei containing noradrenergic neurons; CC, cerebral cortex; CN, cuneate nucleus; Hyp, hypothalamus; LC, locus coeruleus; NG, nucleus gracilis; NMDA, N-methyl-D-aspartate; NSAID, nonsteroidal anti-inflammatory drug; PAG, periaqueductal gray matter; PB, parabrachial nucleus; Po, posterior nuclei of the thalamus; RVM, rostroventral medial medulla; SNRI, serotonin–norepinephrine reuptake inhibitor; TCA, tricyclic antidepressant; VPM and VPL, ventrobasal thalamus, medial and lateral components. *(Gilron I, Baron R, Jensen T. Neuropathic pain: principles of diagnosis and treatment. Mayo Clin Proc. 2015(Apr);90(4):532–545.)*

smallest, A, B, and C (Table 11-1).[10] Neurons of Groups A and B are coated with myelin, which enhances nerve conduction speed. Group A is further subdivided into four subgroups, of which Aβ and Aδ are important to pain sensation and signaling. Aβ provide cutaneous touch and pressure afferents, whereas Aδ are mechanoreceptors, nociceptors, thermoreceptors, and sympathetic postganglionic fibers.[10] Group B are sympathetic preganglionic fibers.[10] Group C are small, unmyelinated mechanoreceptors, nociceptors, thermoreceptors, and sympathetic postganglionic fibers.[10]

The primary afferents that contribute to pain sensation are Aδ and C fibers, and each transmits different types of pain sensation. As Aδ are myelinated, they transmit acute pain rapidly, typically sensed as "sharp" by a patient. C fibers are small and unmyelinated, and thereby transmit pain in a more delayed fashion, often described as "burning" in

Table 11-1 Peripheral Nerve Fiber Classifications

Fiber	Innervation	Conduction Velocity (mm/s)
Aα	Primary muscle spindle, motor to skeletal muscle	100
Aβ	Cutaneous touch and pressure afferents	50
Aγ	Motor to muscle spindles	20
Aδ	Mechanoreceptors and nociceptors, sympathetic postganglionic	15
B	Sympathetic preganglionic	7
C	Mechanoreceptors, nociceptors, thermoreceptors, and sympathetic postganglionic fibers	1

Adapted from Davis PJ, Cladis FP, Motoyama EK. *Smith's Anesthesia for Infants and Children*. New York, NY: Elsevier Health Sciences; 2011. Chapter 15, Table 15-4.

quality. Free nerve endings of both Aδ and C fibers respond to varied stimuli intensity including tissue injury, possible tissue injury, and even threatened injury.[10] This graded response may be intended to prevent injury, although it may also contribute a mechanism to development of chronic pain states.

Cell bodies for both Aδ and C fibers are located in the DRG of the spinal cord or respective cranial nerves they serve. Most of the sensory neurons terminate in the ipsilateral dorsal horn. However, the spinal neurons bifurcate into ascending and descending branches to innervate several spinal segments. The dorsal horn is divided anatomically into locations known as Rexed laminae. Aδ and C fibers converge on lamina I (marginal zone), lamina II (substantia gelatinosa), and lamina X (central canal). Lamina V comprises wide dynamic range neurons. In lamina V, Aβ, Aδ, and C fibers converge, which leads to the phenomenon of "referred pain." An example of referred pain is how visceral pain from myocardial infarction can be felt as pain in the left arm.

In the dorsal horn, the sensory nerves connect with the second-order neurons of the spinothalamic and spinoreticulothalamic tracts. Sensory nerves to the spinothalamic tract cross the contralateral ventrolateral tract and ascend the ventral horn to the thalamus. Sensory nerves to the spinoreticulothalamic tract ascend ipsilaterally in the ventrolateral tract, have medullary projections, and finally ascend to the thalamus.

From the thalamus, a nociceptive signal is transmitted to the somatosensory cortex for discriminative sensation, or to the anterior cingulate gyrus or inferior insula for sensation of the affective–motivational sensation of pain. These pathways are responsible for the affective phenomenon of how pain is experienced physically and emotionally.

Anatomically, the vascular supply of the spinal cord has important clinical implications. Although the posterior spinal cord is supplied by two posterior spinal arteries, the anterior spinal cord is supplied by a solitary anterior spinal artery. The largest anterior spinal artery, the artery of Adamkiewicz, has variable anatomic locations and is vulnerable to injury or spasm. Infarction of the anterior spinal cord is a devastating complication that leads to paraplegia with intact proprioception.

Table 11-2 Neuropathic Pain Taxonomy

Type	Definition
Allodynia	Pain generated by a typically non-noxious stimulus (light touch)
Hyperalgesia	Increased pain from a typically noxious stimulus
Hyperpathia	Abnormally painful reaction to a stimulus, especially repetitive stimulus (raised threshold, painful response)
Dysesthesia	Unpleasant abnormal sensation, spontaneous or evoked
Paresthesia	Abnormal sensation, spontaneous or evoked (with or without pain)
Hyperesthesia	Increased sensitivity to stimulation (with or without pain)
Hypoalgesia	Diminished response to normally noxious stimulus (raised threshold, decreased response)
Hypoesthesia	Decreased sensitivity to stimulation, excluding special senses

From International Society of Pain Taxonomy 2012. http://www.iasp-pain.org/Taxonomy. Accessed November 12, 2016.

Mechanisms of Neuropathic Pain

Understanding the mechanisms of pain is important, as the sensation described by the patient can identify the type of injury/aberrancy that governs treatment. Mechanisms involved in neuropathic pain are multiple and overlapping. As such, a single patient may report multiple mechanisms of pain with one nidus or injury. This understanding supports the clinical importance of multimodal analgesia for treatment of pain.

As the description of pain is important to understanding its mechanism, the International Society of Pain developed a taxonomy of pain descriptors (Table 11-2; http://www.iasp-pain.org/Taxonomy). These descriptors can be divided into positive and negative symptoms, based on the response of the patient to stimuli. Positive painful symptoms include allodynia (pain generated by a nonpainful stimulus, such as light touch), hyperalgesia (increased pain from a painful stimulus), and hyperpathia (raised threshold or heightened pain response). Positive symptoms that may or may not be associated with pain include dysesthesia (unpleasant abnormal sensation, spontaneous, or evoked), paresthesia (abnormal sensation, may not be unpleasant, spontaneous, or evoked), and hyperesthesia (increased sensitivity to stimulation, but may not be painful). Negative symptoms include hypoalgesia (decreased sensitivity to painful stimulus) and hypoesthesia (decreased sensitivity to stimulus, not necessarily painful stimulus).

There are at least five accepted mechanisms for neuropathic pain that explain the sensations described above. These mechanisms include ectopic activity, peripheral sensitization, central sensitization, impaired inhibitory modulation, and activation of microglia (Table 11-3).[11] Ectopic activity is thought to be secondary to hyperexcitability

Table 11-3 Neuropathic Pain Mechanisms

Type	Mechanism	Associated Symptomatology
Ectopic	Spontaneous, sodium and potassium channel changes	Neuroma, demyelination, trigeminal neuralgia
Peripheral sensitization	Hyperexcitability of sensory neurons, TRPV1 channel changes	Hyperalgesia, allodynia
Central sensitization	Change in Aβ fibers. Increase CGRP, substance P, and NMDA	Fibromyalgia, IBS, chronic fatigue syndrome
Impaired sensory modulation (inhibition)	Apoptosis of GABAergic spinal inhibitory neurons	Postinjury pain, postherpetic neuralgia, entrapment neuropathy
Activation of microglia	Upregulation of chemokine receptors, release of glial cytokines	Central sensitization, hyperalgesia, allodynia, anticipation

and spontaneous firing of neurons occurring after an insult, thereby explaining spontaneous symptoms such as paresthesia and dysesthesia; such neuropathic pain can be constant, intermittent, or paroxysmal. Ectopic activity has been attributed to changes in voltage-gated sodium and potassium channels, and hyperpolarization of cyclic nucleotide-gated channels.[11]

Peripheral sensitization results from hyperexcitability and reduced activation threshold of primary afferent neurons, described by the patient as hyperalgesia or allodynia.[11] Peripheral sensitization may be thought of as inflammatory pain, and may be due to changes in the transient receptor potential cation channel subfamily V member 1 (TRPV1) ion channel.[12]

Central sensitization is classified as central neuroplastic changes involving spinal or supraspinal nerves. The patient may describe exaggerated response to painful stimulus, hyperalgesia, allodynia, and/or anticipation. Aβ touch fibers develop phenotypic changes including increased neuropeptide expression of substance P and increased excitatory amino acid transmission via *N*-methyl-D-aspartate (NMDA) receptors.[11] These changes may explain some of the purported analgesic benefit of NMDA modulating agents such as ketamine (see below). Microglial activation occurs following injury by upregulation of chemokine receptors and release of glial cytokines and growth factors.[11] These changes are believed to contribute to central sensitization and increased pain sensation reported by the patient.

Inhibitory neurons project from the central nervous system (CNS) and serve to modify painful stimuli. Apoptosis of spinal inhibitory interneurons has been reported as a consequence of some injuries, which may explain abnormalities in inhibitory neuron signaling.[13] Without modulation from inhibitory neurons, a peripheral painful stimulus may be interpreted by the CNS as pain of significantly increased severity.

Itch

Centuries ago, Samuel Haffenreffer defined itch as an unpleasant sensation that causes the urge to scratch, the act of which is subsequently rewarded by a pleasant sensation and/or itch relief. Itch is primarily carried by C-fibers, then transmitted by the spinothalamic tract to the brain.[14] In research, itch is induced by histamine, extracts from cowhage (a tropical legume), or electrical stimulation. Importantly, cowhage-induced itch cannot be inhibited by antihistamines and suggests different mechanisms are involved in pruritus. Indeed, the transmission between histamine and cowhage appears to be different in the peripheral nervous system as well as the spinal cord and brain[15]; nevertheless, both involve regions that are also involved in pain transmission. The mechanism for electrically evoked itch, while preliminary, does appear to involve C-fibers.[15] Centrally, multiple areas of the brain respond to both histamine and cowhage-induced pruritus, including the prefrontal cortex, supplementary motor area, premotor cortex, primary motor cortex, primary somatosensory cortex, parietal cortex, cingulate cortex, precuneus, opercular cortex (secondary somatosensory cortex and insular cortex), claustrum, and basal ganglia.[15] Of particular interest, the precuneus is thought to participate in pain modulation and has been shown to activate on functional magnetic resonance imaging to itch stimuli.[16] The primary somatosensory cortex and secondary somatosensory cortex are thought to be the primary regions for sensory interpretation, in addition to their roles in the perception of pain intensity.[15] The cingulate cortex has also been shown to activate in response to itch.

Once transmitted, the sensation of itch is modulated centrally. Similar to nociception, both spinal cord and supraspinal areas participate in stimulus modulation. Inhibitory neurons attenuate signals from ascending the spinal cord. Supraspinal inhibition has been shown to contribute to itch suppression; however, the exact mechanism is not known.[15] Periaqueductal gray area and rostral medulla are well documented to be involved with descending inhibitory control for pain transmission, and modulation of itch is hypothesized to involve the same or a similar pathway.[15]

The pleasure induced by scratching an itch is hypothesized to involve the reward system of the CNS, including the midbrain, striatum, medial prefrontal cortex, and anterior cingulate cortex.[15] Dopamine release has been purported to be central to the pleasure sensation associated with scratching, and the midbrain has a particularly high density of dopaminergic receptors.[15]

Chronic pruritus can be agonizing for patients, as compulsive scratching may lead to a cycle of further tissue damage, further histamine release, and further pruritus (i.e., the so-called "itch–scratch–itch" cycle). Scratching can also become a maladaptive habit. A central mechanism for perpetuation of itch has also been hypothesized, as patients with atopic dermatitis have shown higher activity in the basal ganglia,[17] and patients with pruritus secondary to end-stage renal disease have higher density of gray matter with enhanced baseline activity in the basal ganglia.[18] Further research is required to understand the central mechanisms that contribute to chronic itch.

Assessment

Clinical

Pain is defined as an unpleasant sensory and emotional experience caused by a noxious or perceived noxious stimulus. No two individuals experience the same pain in an identical manner, and the ability to communicate pain does not correlate with the pain experienced.[19] Nociception describes how neurons respond to noxious stimuli including autonomic and behavioral changes, such as elevated heart rate and withdrawal reflex, respectively. Nociception, however, does not always induce pain. Neuropathic pain includes spontaneous positive and negative symptoms as described above, and it is imperative to understand the patient's particular pain experience to formulate an appropriate treatment plan.[19,20]

Itch is also an unpleasant sensory experience, and patients "self-treat" by scratching or applying a painful stimulus. Scratching causes a sensation of pleasure and relief. However, prolonged scratching can lead to excoriation, skin disruption, secondary infection, and poor wound healing and/or scarring.

Psychosocial Impact

It is difficult to overstate the impact of pain on psychosocial function. Pain is often associated with significant negative emotional changes and maladaptive behavior problems; in response, emotion and mental health can change how pain signals are interpreted centrally.[21] It is recommended that patients with severe acute or chronic pain be evaluated for concurrent mental health illness as comorbid conditions such as anxiety and depression are common (see Chapter 24).[22] In addition, preexisting anxiety and depression are commonly worsened by pain, even if previously well controlled. Mental health changes associated with chronic pain or itch can have impact on the patients' overall health, quality of life, and productivity.

Treatment

Topical Agents

Topical analgesics for skin and scar-related pain logically target stimuli at their site of origin. As the noxious stimulus is often instigated in the skin and first sensed by primary afferent neurons, treatment at this site may inhibit excitation of the peripheral neurons, prevent transmission centrally, and may prevent central sensitization.[23] The pharmacokinetics and pharmacodynamics of topical analgesics also have many appealing characteristics. Topical medications provide nearly constant therapeutic levels of drug at the site of action, unlike systemic medications that may undergo significant first-pass metabolism as well as having peak and trough concentrations associated with unwanted side effects and decreased efficacy, respectively. These features, combined with limited systemic absorption, allow systemic toxicity to be avoided. Indeed, several systemic medications that are commonly avoided in certain populations (e.g., nonsteroidal anti-inflammatory agents [NSAIDs] in the elderly population) can be used topically with relative safety. Topical medications can be customized for the patient (e.g., type of drug, concentration, etc.) and are relatively easy to use.[24] Finally, adding a topical medication in combination with an oral medication can act synergistically to improve pain relief.[25]

Topical medications are most commonly studied under conditions where they are placed over intact and nonmucosal skin. As mucosal membranes have increased absorption, a reduction in concentration is recommended. Data on particular dosage reduction for medications are very limited, however. In general, emulsions are typically employed as vehicles; Zur[23] and colleagues recommended a ~10-fold reduction in concentration for application to mucosal tissue.

Topical Local Anesthetics

Local anesthetics reversibly bind the α subunit of neuronal sodium channels, inhibiting channel activation and the sodium influx required for membrane depolarization, thereby inhibiting conduction and propagation of nerve impulses. Local anesthetics have an attractive mechanism of action for treatment of neuropathic pain as they have been shown to preferentially block hyperexcitable cells.[26] Sodium channel blockade may not entirely account for the topical local anesthetic mechanism of action, however, as the clinical response to lidocaine therapy has been shown to be independent of epidermal nerve fiber density. In addition, topical lidocaine paste has been effective in nociceptor-deprived skin, suggesting that sodium channel blockade made not be required for analgesia.[20] Lidocaine also activates transient receptor potential cation channel families TRPV1 and TRPA1, which may account for some of its analgesic benefits.[27]

When given systemically, lidocaine has less cardiotoxicity than other local anesthetics (such as bupivacaine), a reasonably well-defined dose–response curve, as well as readily available laboratory tests to determine serum lidocaine levels (Table 11-4). As such, lidocaine is commonly used for chronic pain management. Although intravenous lidocaine has been used via infusion for pain management, the beneficial effect typically does not extend beyond the duration of the infusion.[10] Pain specialists commonly transition lidocaine infusions to oral mexiletine to avoid complications inherent with constant intravenous infusions;

Table 11-4 Phases of Local Anesthetic Toxicity

1. Lethargy
2. Perioral paresthesias
3. Tinnitus
4. Seizures
5. Respiratory arrest
6. Cardiac arrest

however, doses must be escalated slowly to avoid side effects such as nausea, vomiting, diplopia, and tremor. Mexiletine cannot be used in patients with second- or third-degree heart block as atrioventricular conduction time can be increased.

Lidocaine is available, however, as a topical analgesic in multiple forms, including gel, lotion, and patch, and can be of significant benefit for patients that have pain and/or itching from scars. Lidocaine 5% patch (Lidoderm) has a gentle adhesive, which is easy to apply without the mess associated with topical gel or cream. The patch can be cut to fit the affected area without changing the pharmacokinetics of the drug, according to the Lidoderm product label. Each patch contains 700 mg of lidocaine released slowly as a deposition, and it is worn for 12 hours of a 24-hour period. Patients with allodynia or itch may have discomfort while placing the patch and may prefer to wear the patch during the day so that it also helps protect the area from touch and clothing. Other patients may prefer to wear the patch for 12 hours at night to avoid the inconvenience of wearing the patch during the day. For best therapeutic effect, the patch should be worn daily for at least 2 weeks before ascertaining treatment efficacy. If the lidocaine patch is only used sporadically, the subdermal lidocaine deposition may not be sufficient in concentration or depth to provide therapeutic benefit.

Lidoderm 5% is considered first-line therapy for localized neuropathic pain,[28] and it is effective in treating sensory polyneuropathy, postoperative or posttraumatic neuropathic cutaneous pain, and chemotherapy-related peripheral neuropathy.[23] Currently Lidoderm 5% is approved only for postherpetic neuralgia and diabetic peripheral neuropathy by the Food and Drug Administration (FDA), and some insurance providers may require prior authorization. The manufacturer recommends the patch be placed on intact skin only because placement on open skin (such as denuded, burned, eroded, or eczematous) or mucus membranes will increase absorption. Drug absorption over scars has not been reported, although one would predict similar absorption to normal skin as long as the scar is intact. The lidocaine patch can be placed alongside open wounds, however, and may help with pain while maintaining safety.

Lidocaine is also available in cream and gel form, in 4% or 5% concentrations; these can be applied two to three times daily over intact skin. Lidocaine is also frequently mixed with other medications as part of compounded cream. As local anesthetic toxicity can be life-threatening and numerous local anesthetic formulations are extant, we refer the reader to individual manufacturers with regard to the maximum surface area of intact skin that may be used, as highlighted by a recent review.[29]

Ketamine

Ketamine is commonly used as a dissociative anesthetic, but it also has significant acute/chronic pain management properties secondary to its effect on glutamate signaling. Glutamate is released by stimuli at sensory nerve endings in response to noxious stimuli, inflammation, or tissue damage. Glutamate NMDA receptors are present on primary afferent nerve endings as well as keratinocytes, the stimulation of which activates sensory nerves. Ketamine is a potent antagonist of glutamate NMDA receptor function. Ketamine also binds multiple opioid receptors, monoamine transporters, muscarinic and nicotinic cholinergic receptors, dopamine and serotonin receptors.[20] Peripheral pain relief from ketamine may also be due to effects on nitric oxide/cyclic guanosine monophosphate and adenosine triphosphate–sensitive potassium channels.[20]

Topical ketamine has been studied for treatment of complex regional pain syndrome, postherpetic neuralgia, diabetic neuropathy, and other neuropathic pain syndromes. Case reports and case series found that patients with complex regional pain syndrome responded to ketamine 0.25% to 1.5%.[30] Another study of patients with postherpetic neuralgia showed response to topical 0.5% ketamine[31]; however, a study by Barros et al. of 12 patients with ketamine 1% treatment did not show any difference from placebo. Ketamine 0.5%, combined with amitriptyline 1% or 2%, showed benefit for neuropathic itching[32] as well as localized pruritus in one study.[33] Importantly, a single application of topical ketamine 0.5% to 10% did not produce systemic plasma blood levels of ketamine nor its metabolite norketamine; however, analyses of repeat doses of higher concentrations (5% to 10%) have not been reported.[20]

Topical Amitriptyline–Ketamine Combination

Modulation of itch by topical amitriptyline may occur by inhibiting nerve transmission of sensitized A and C fibers.[33] A study by Poterucha et al.[33] showed that the majority (62%) of patients (n = 16) with recalcitrant localized pruritus experienced some relief of itching with topical amitriptyline and ketamine. The combination of amitriptyline and ketamine was also effective in the treatment of brachioradial pruritus, a syndrome of intense itching between the wrist and elbow without known cause.[32]

Amitriptyline 5% and 10% creams have been used to treat diabetic peripheral neuropathy. However, amitriptyline 10% was associated with somnolence, suggesting significant systemic absorption.[34] Amitriptyline 1% and amitriptyline 1%–ketamine 0.5% in combination did not produce analgesia for neuropathic pain with treatment over 2 to 7 days.[35] However, amitriptyline 2% with ketamine 1% treated neuropathic pain when treatment was continued over 6 to 12 months.[36]

Amitriptyline may be less efficacious alone than in combination with other topicals. Amitriptyline 5% cream has been reported to be an effective treatment for posttraumatic neuropathic pain without systemic side effects.[37] However, a new meta-analysis concluded topical amitriptyline is not effective for treatment of neuropathic pain,[38] and randomized placebo-controlled trial for amitriptyline treatment of neuropathic pain also concluded topical amitriptyline was ineffective.[39] Data for combination agents, however, appear more promising and suggest an additive effect.

The cause of the pain contributes to the expected benefit of amitriptyline combination creams. For instance, amitriptyline and ketamine cream did not significantly improve neuropathic pain in patients with chemotherapy-induced neuropathy; however,[40] it did treat the majority of patients (75%) with pain from erythromelalgia.[41] Pelvic pain has also been effectively treated with topical amitriptyline–ketamine.[42] An amitriptyline–ketamine–lidocaine combination was also effective in the treatment of radiation-induced dermatitis.[43]

Topical Gabapentin

Data on topical gabapentin are limited. Its theoretical utility stems from the observation that gabapentin-compounded creams produced local antinociception against formalin as pain control.[44] Topical gabapentin 5% produced a response similar to systemic gabapentin (100 mg per kg).[44] Gabapentin 6% has also been reported to be effective at reducing pain for postherpetic neuralgia with negligible systemic absorption.[45]

Topical NSAIDs

NSAIDs are potent analgesics that decrease prostaglandin synthesis. Systemic NSAID use is associated with potentially serious adverse events including gastrointestinal bleeding, renal failure, myocardial infarction, and cerebrovascular accident. The FDA has issued a black box warning for NSAIDs because of these adverse events, particularly in the elderly. Thus, systemic NSAID use should be of limited duration and with extreme caution in the elderly.

Topical diclofenac has been reported safe in patients, even those at high risk for systemic NSAID side effects (renal dysfunction, diabetes mellitus type II, cardiovascular disease, bleeding tendency/coagulopathy).[46–48] Gastrointestinal side effects are rare.[49] Although systemic absorption is thought to be minimal, case-reported bleeding complications in ill patients (especially those already taking anticoagulants) have been reported.[50]

Although the gel formulation of diclofenac had a faster rate of onset, the transdermal patch delivers more constant and concentrated drug release.[51] The majority of diclofenac appears to remain in the subcutaneous tissue in animal studies, although some systemic absorption was detected.[52] Many studies regarding efficacy of diclofenac are for treatment of osteoarthritis, which show benefit, minimal side effects, and the presence of the drug in the synovium of the joint treated.[53–55] Topical diclofenac has not been studied for scar pain, per se, but has been shown to be an effective treatment for neuropathic pain from tissue injury.[56–58] Topical diclofenac also effectively treated back strain,[59] postherpetic neuralgia,[60] and complex regional pain syndrome.[60] Diclofenac's analgesic activity was found to be additive to the analgesic effect of topical capsaicin treatment.[61] Side effects including skin irritation and photosensitivity[62] have been reported.

Topical Doxepin

Doxepin is a dibenzoxepin tricyclic antidepressant with competitive antihistaminergic (H1 and H2) activity. Because of H1 receptor blockade, systemic absorption can lead to significant drowsiness, and multiple studies warn of clinically significant drowsiness or toxicity with topical doxepin.[63–66] Topical doxepin should therefore be used cautiously in consideration of these reports. Doxepin has been used to treat neuropathic pain from complex regional pain syndrome.[67] Doxepin 3.3% is often combined with capsaicin 0.075%. Doxepin 3.3%, both with and without capsaicin, has reported efficacy in the treatment of neuropathic pain versus placebo,[26] although doxepin combined with capsaicin produced analgesia more quickly.[68] Topical doxepin also has reported efficacy for the treatment of pruritus,[63,69] with the antipruritic benefit persisting for 2 weeks after doxepin is stopped.[66]

Capsaicin

Although capsaicin is primarily used for postherpetic neuralgia, it can be used for cutaneous neuropathic pain of other etiologies. Capsaicin is thought to be particularly efficacious on allodynia.[68] Capsaicin is thought to work by decreasing TRPV1 expression and decreasing the density of epidermal nerve fibers.[23] This effect has been termed "defunctionalization" of nociceptive nerve fibers.[70] This defunctionalization renders the nociceptor unable to transmit nerve signals.

Capsaicin is available in over-the-counter strength in various topical forms, including lotion, cream, gel (0.1% to 1% capsaicin), patch (0.025%), and stick "roll on" (0.03%) forms. Capsaicin 8% patch is available for prescription use. Previous high-concentration capsaicin creams required adequate ventilation and respirators for the treating medical personnel out of concern for inhalation injury. The capsaicin 8% patch, however, requires only gloves. The patch should be administered by experienced medical personnel. Treatment can be extremely painful, with pain lasting for up to a week. The area to be treated should first be treated with topical anesthetic (typically provided in the "administration kit" by the manufacturer). The patient may also require systemic analgesics, including opioids, after the treatment for up to 1 week. Other adverse effects include application site erythema, which also resolves within 1 week.

Topical Clonidine

Clonidine is an α_2-adrenergic agonist. Topical clonidine 0.1% has been reported to reduce signaling from hyperactive cutaneous nociceptors in peripheral diabetic neuropathy. Systemic absorption is minimal, with studies showing undetectable plasma levels. The neuropathic stimulus must be within superficial skin layers, however, as the effect is superficial and local.[23]

Topical Opioid Antagonists

Pruritus is a common side effect of opioid therapy, and opioid antagonism has been used to treat pruritus in a wide variety of settings in both the presence and absence of systemic opioids.[10] Small studies found benefit with the application of 1% topical naltrexone; however, a larger study with the long-acting opioid antagonist nalmefene did not show benefit over placebo.[11,71] Use of topical opioid antagonists is thus of unclear efficacy based upon the available literature.

Systemic Medications

Systemic medications can be considered if topical analgesics are contraindicated, if patients continue to have significant pain after topical agents, or if the pain and dysfunction are severe enough that a synergistic effect with topical and systemic medication is desired. Systemic medications are more likely to have associated side effects, however, and the patient should be selected carefully and educated regarding use.

α_2-δ Ligands

Systemic α_2-δ ligands (gabapentin, pregabalin) are frequently used and well-tolerated medications for treatment of pain

Table 11-5 Gabapentin Titration Calendar Example

	Capsule or Tablet Size (mg)	Time of Dose			Total Daily Dose (mg)
		Morning	Noon	Evening	
Week 1	300	0	0	1	300
Week 2	300	1	0	1	600
Week 3	300	1	1	1	900
Week 4	300	1	1	2	1,200
Week 5	300	2	1	2	1,500
Week 6	300	2	2	2	1,800
Ongoing	600	1	1	1	1,800

and itch. Neuropathic pain reduction from this class of medication is well studied. Pruritus relief from multiple causes continues to be of interest, although uremia is one of the most studied causes. In one study, 85% of 71 chronic kidney disease patients with uremic pruritus experienced relief of itching with either gabapentin or pregabalin.[72] In this study, pregabalin was started in patients who did not tolerate gabapentin due to side effects. Overall, multiple studies show improvement in uremic pruritus with gabapentin[72–79] or pregabalin.[72,75,80–83] Gabapentin has been shown to treat pruritus from notalgia paresthetica,[84] brachioradial pruritus,[85,86] and postburn itch.[87]

Gabapentin

Gabapentin was initially marketed for seizure management but was found to have analgesic properties. Gabapentin primarily works by binding to the α_2-δ site of voltage-gated calcium channels. FDA-approved indications include seizure management and postherpetic neuralgia. Non-FDA approved uses include hemodialysis-associated pruritus, perioperative pain, diabetic peripheral neuropathy, and fibromyalgia. Gabapentin is renally cleared and must be dose adjusted for renal insufficiency, but it may be used with a stable hemodialysis regimen after dose adjustment. Gabapentin is rated class C for pregnancy and lactation, with limited data on risk to the developing fetus. Common side effects include drowsiness, difficulty with concentration, and mood changes. Other common side effects include peripheral edema, nausea, and fatigue. Serious side effects that have been reported include Stevens–Johnson syndrome, drug hypersensitivity, dizziness, drowsiness, and severe mood disturbance including hostile behavior and suicidal thoughts (particularly in adolescents).

Multiple dosing strategies have been outlined with gabapentin; however, slow titration seems to be best tolerated. A common dosing strategy (for healthy adults and adolescents more than 50 kg) is: start 300 mg at bedtime; after 1 week, add 300 mg in the morning; after one additional week, add 300 mg in the afternoon (for a total of 300 mg three times daily). Titration may be continued by increasing by 300 mg per day every week until a goal therapeutic effect has been achieved or until dose-limiting side effects or a maximal dose has been obtained (Table 11-5). A calendar is a good tool to share with patients to help clarify dosing escalation. Maximum gabapentin dosing for healthy adults and adolescents is typically 1,800 to 3,600 mg per day. Gabapentin should not be stopped abruptly as it can precipitate a withdrawal seizure. The dose can be decreased by 300 mg every 3 days when titrating off gabapentin for side effects or if the medication is not effective.

Pregabalin

Pregabalin is in the same drug class as gabapentin and is thought to work by the same mechanism of action. FDA indications are similar to gabapentin, with the addition of neuropathic pain after spinal cord injury. Pregabalin has also reported efficacy for the treatment of pruritus.[72]

Some patients who experience intolerable side effects with gabapentin may tolerate pregabalin. Side effects of pregabalin include drowsiness, dizziness, mood change, and peripheral edema (similar to gabapentin), but pregabalin is more likely than gabapentin to cause increased appetite and weight gain. Serious side effects include angioedema, increased creatinine kinase, jaundice, hypersensitivity, and suicidal thoughts. Pregabalin is also renally cleared and must be dose adjusted for patients with renal insufficiency. Pregabalin is also category C for pregnancy and lactation.

Like gabapentin, pregabalin is titrated slowly to minimize side effects and promote tolerability. Healthy adults and adolescents >50 kg can be started on pregabalin 75 mg twice daily and, subsequently, increased by 75 mg twice daily on a weekly basis (Table 11-6). The maximum daily dose for pregabalin is 300 mg twice daily. Pregabalin should also be titrated off instead of being stopped abruptly.

Tricyclic Antidepressants

Tricyclic antidepressants have multiple mechanisms of action including the blockade of serotonin and noradrenaline reuptake, interacting with sodium and calcium channels, and blocking acetylcholine and histamine signaling.[10] Tricyclic antidepressants are well studied in the treatment of neuropathic pain.

Tricyclic antidepressants may prolong the QT interval, and routine electrocardiogram screening to identify patients with congenital prolonged QT syndrome is recommended (especially in children, adolescents, and young adults). The most prominent side effect of tricyclic antidepressants is somnolence; therefore, the one-time daily dose can be given 2 hours before desired bedtime to facilitate sleep onset. If patients have difficulty arousing in the morning, then the dose can be taken with the evening meal. Other side effects include dry mouth, constipation, and weight gain. Tricyclic antidepressants have a black box warning for suicidal thoughts, ideation, or action, particularly in young adults and adolescents. This risk should be discussed

Table 11-6 Pregabalin Titration Calendar Example

	Capsule Size (mg)	Time of Dose		Total Daily Dose (mg)
		Morning	Evening	
Week 1	75	1	1	150
Week 2	75	2	2	300
Week 3	75	2	2	300
Week 4	75	3	3	450
Week 5	75	4	4	600
Ongoing	300	1	1	600

with patients and family members, if appropriate. Of note, tricyclic antidepressant overdose can be fatal.

Amitriptyline and nortriptyline are the most commonly used tricyclic antidepressants. Amitriptyline is a prodrug that is metabolized to nortriptyline, and it has more anticholinergic side effects than nortriptyline. Therefore, patients that have dose-limiting side effects with amitriptyline may find nortriptyline more tolerable. Nortriptyline is also the only tricyclic drug available in a liquid formulation, which may facilitate enteral administration in pediatric patients. Tricyclic antidepressants are hepatically metabolized via the cytochrome P450 pathway CYP2D6. Approximately 25% of patients are poor metabolizers of tricyclic antidepressants, which may result in increased plasma concentrations. An amitriptyline level should be measured by a simple trough blood test once a total daily dose of 1 mg per kg has been obtained to rule out the possibility that the patient is a slow metabolizer; the dose can then be titrated to patient symptomatology. Importantly, many patients experience analgesic benefit at doses (and drug levels) substantially less than that which was defined for clinical depression. As such, subtherapeutic plasma levels are common in patients with reported analgesic efficacy. If pain control is adequate, the dose should not be reflexively increased to the defined "therapeutic" plasma range, which was defined for clinical depression rather than analgesia.

Typical dosing for amitriptyline or nortriptyline in adult patients is 10 mg 2 hours before bedtime, escalating by 10 mg per week to a goal dose of 50 mg per day. After confirming nontoxic blood level, the dose can further be increased to approximately 1 mg per kg (ideal body weight) per day. The therapeutic dose is typically between 50 and 100 mg per day. As with other agents, these medications should not be abruptly discontinued.

Opioids

Chronic opioid management for the treatment of scar pain or pruritus is rarely indicated as the mu receptor agonist activity of opioids is well known to precipitate pruritus, especially when administered centrally (intrathecal, epidural). Opioids are most effective at treating nociceptive pain (such as postsurgical pain) and less effective at treating the neuropathic pain commonly associated with scars. Chronic opioid therapy results in decreased efficacy over time as tolerance develops. At high doses, opioids can actually increase pain by a phenomenon known as opioid-induced hyperalgesia; opioid taper results in improved pain control for these affected patients. Opioid misuse, including addiction, abuse, and diversion, is a disastrous consequence of prescription drug use, and overdose can be fatal. Patients with known abuse or diversion should be tapered off prescription opioids. Unfortunately, some patients in that situation can revert to use of illegal opioids such as heroin. A single prescription for opioids has been linked with chronic opioid use.[88] Therefore, starting a patient on a plan for long-term opioid therapy carries significant risk and should be done only for end of life management or after all treatment has been exhausted *and* opioid therapy improves the patient's function. An opioid contract with routine urine drug screen should be in place.

Interventional Procedures

Interventional procedures can be considered for patients that do not have pain, itch, or functional improvement with topical or systemic medications; furthermore, localized injections may be first-line therapy for specific lesions (such as corticosteroid injections for localized hypertrophic scar). As the severity and area of lesions increase, patients should be carefully chosen and informed of perceived risk and benefit of the procedure so that realistic expectations may be established. For patients with severe scarring, interventional therapy may be most efficacious when performed as a part of multidisciplinary therapy, especially with physical therapy and desensitization (see Chapters 10, 13, and 19). Invasive procedures always carry risk of bleeding and infection, as the skin's integrity is compromised. Scar tissue may have impaired would healing because of altered blood supply. Other risk depends on the specific procedure performed. Injections typically consist of local anesthetic with corticosteroid. Subcutaneous corticosteroid risks atrophy of skin or subcutaneous tissue (resulting in "skin dimple"), which may be a detrimental cosmetic outcome for the patient even if pain and disability improve.

Scar Injections

Although a formal study of scar injections for pain relief has not been performed, clinical practice may utilize scar injection to decrease pain, decrease keloid formation, or be coupled with physical therapy to improve patient function. The injectate typically consists of corticosteroid with or without local anesthetic. Particulate corticosteroids (methylprednisolone, triamcinolone) are often used as they theoretically deliver the steroid as a depot, which may remain in the scar for a period of time. Corticosteroid injections may cause asymmetric atrophy of the scar[89] or skin dimpling because of degradation of subcutaneous adipose tissue by the steroid. These cosmetic changes may be undesirable, and thus physicians and patients should carefully consider this specific risk of injection.

Peripheral Nerve Block

Peripheral nerve block may be used for large scars. A single injection of local anesthetic or placement of an indwelling catheter for delivery of local anesthetic for a few hours per day can be performed. Outpatient drug delivery systems for infusion of local anesthetics into peripheral nerve catheters have been developed. With these devices, patients may not require hospitalization for peripheral nerve catheter infusion. The primary goal of the peripheral nerve block is to improve pain (especially medically refractory neuropathic symptoms) so the patient is able to tolerate physical therapy, including stretching, range of motion, and desensitization.

Spinal Cord Stimulation

Spinal cord stimulation involves neuromodulation of the dorsal columns by percutaneous placement of epidural electrodes. Spinal cord stimulation could be considered for pain refractory to medical management, especially pain with neuropathic features. Spinal cord stimulation has not been studied to treat chronic itch; however, as itch involves the same pathways for transmission it would be an area open to study.

Intrathecal Drug Delivery

Intrathecal drug delivery systems are placed for medically refractory pain. A catheter is placed into the intrathecal sac and then tunneled to the reservoir device, which is usually placed subcutaneously over the abdomen. Medications that can be infused include opioids, local anesthetics, clonidine, and baclofen. Long-term therapy with intrathecal drug delivery can be fraught with complications. Mechanical complications include kinking of the catheter, migration, and granuloma formation. Tolerance to medications (particularly opioids) develops, leading to decreased efficacy.

Physical

Rehabilitation

Physical rehabilitation is important for patients suffering from debilitating chronic pain or itch from scars. Graduated return to cardiovascular exercise has been shown to improve pain and quality of life.[90] Pain itself should not prohibit activity. Patients should be educated to start with a daily attainable goal for cardiovascular activity, with gradual escalation. For patients with severe disability, or limitations from scarring, evaluation by a physiatrist or physical therapist can help determine appropriate physical activity and set goals for improvement (see Chapter 19).

Massage

The evidence to support use of massage for the treatment of scar pain is poor; however, small studies have shown efficacy.[91] Massage with a medicated topical agent versus simple lubricant alone showed similar improvement, suggesting massage may be beneficial as an independent mechanism.[92] The caveat is that methods of massage therapy for scar pain are varied and not standardized; therefore, there may be significant interprovider results due to technique. One meta-analysis reported 45.7% of patients had clinical improvement in range of motion, pruritus, pain, mood, depression, or anxiety.[91] Of the subset of patients with surgical scars, however, 90% experienced improvement; the authors concluded massage efficacy may be better for postsurgical scars than traumatic or burn scars.[91] Subsequent to that meta-analysis, massage was shown to be helpful specifically for the treatment of burn patients, with a report by Cho et al.[93] demonstrating a decrease in scar thickness, melanin, erythema, pain, and pruritus in burn patients. Skin distensibility (immediate and delayed retraction) also improved.

Transcutaneous electrical nerve stimulation is a method of peripheral neuromodulation. The unit includes a pulse generator, amplifier, and two to four electrodes. The conventional settings are a waveform of 40 to 70 Hz frequency and 0.1 to 0.5 ms pulse width. Current is constant. The stimulus feels like vibrations or tingling to the patient and can be placed over the area of pain or along the nerve innervating the pain. The mechanism is thought to include modulation of central pain perception[94] and has also been shown to activate descending inhibitory pathways,[95] thus decreasing pain perception.

Psychological

Patients with disfiguring scars are at risk for developing psychopathology, including depression and anxiety. As patients with chronic pain often have concurrent mental health disease that may impact treatment and ability to cope with any stressor, they should be screened for underlying psychological illness as a part of their pain management (see Chapter 24).[96] Beck Depression Inventory, Psychological Adjustment to Illness Scale, and Impact of Event Scale (for posttraumatic stress disorder) have been used to assess psychological comorbidity. Patients may require counseling for anxiety, depression, posttraumatic stress disorder, and return to social situations (prevention of social anxiety).

Biobehavioral strategies for pain and itch are also important therapeutic tools. Itch in particular can be treated with a biopsychological model, as itch can be provoked by audiovisual stimuli, and can have significant input from personality traits and psychological stress/emotions.[97] Habit reversal training and relaxation techniques can treat itch, interrupt further skin damage that can propagate the sensation of itch, and also improve psychological health.[97] A meta-analysis by Lavda et al.[98] found large improvements in itch with psychological therapy, as well as medium improvement in overall skin condition and psychological comorbidity. Progressive muscle relaxation has also been helpful for pruritic symptoms of atopic dermatitis.[99,100]

Multidisciplinary

Multidisciplinary assessment and management of chronic pain and itch may be beneficial to some patients, particularly those refractory to medical therapy or who present initially with significant disability from their symptoms. The multidisciplinary team can be tailored to the patient's needs for management of scar pain or itch and may consist of a dermatologist, plastic surgeon, pain physician, physical medicine and rehabilitation physician, physical therapist, psychologist, and psychiatrist.

When patients have significant pain or disability, medication and/or interventional procedures combined with physical therapy and reintroduction into physical activity improves pain. A graduated cardiovascular exercise program promotes endorphin and enkephalin release that helps to improve pain, neuromodulate, and interrupt the central sensitization phenomenon of chronic pain and itch.[21] The patient should be educated to perform exercise daily with a goal that is attainable. For instance, severely debilitated patients can start with walking for 5 minutes daily. It can be increased by 5 minutes every week to a goal of 30 minutes per day. After this goal is achieved, the patient can start 5 minutes of strenuous cardiovascular activity (running, elliptical) and 25 minutes of walking. The daily goal should be advanced slowly with active patient encouragement. A support system is important for patients to complete this goal, given by family members, if available, and/or a physical therapist. If motivation or a mood disorder is prohibitive, a counselor or psychologist can help with goal setting, maintenance, and positive reinforcement.

Sleep hygiene is also very important. Sleep is often disrupted because of pain or itch, and pain is typically worse at night. Sleep time (bed time and morning wakening) should be scheduled and consistent to facilitate adequate sleep quality. Sleep onset may be facilitated by encouraging quiet activities ("wind down") and avoidance of artificial light (including cell phones, tablets, and television) 2 hours prior to the desired bedtime. If sleep onset remains disrupted, supplemental melatonin can be given 2 hours prior to desired sleep. Dosing of melatonin is variable; however, 1 to 3 mg of melatonin is sufficient. Avoidance of daytime naps and physical activity during the day will also facilitate sleep onset and quality of sleep at night. If patients have signs of sleep disorder, such as sleep apnea, referral to a sleep specialist may help improve sleep and, consequently, pain.

Reintegration into life activities that provide pleasure for the patient is important, and although it may seem counterintuitive and daunting to the patient, doing so successfully actually improves pain and quality of life significantly. Encourage patients to choose activities, hobbies, or social avenues that are likely to be successful and provide pleasure. Return to work is also important for patients, who may benefit from accommodations initially to facilitate compliance and productivity at work. An occupational health physician typically manages this process, and accommodations can be decreased as the patient improves.

Treatment of underlying mood disorders is crucial, as both anxiety and depression are prevalent in patients with chronic pain and itch. Inadequate treatment of an underlying mood disorder often leads to persistence of somatic symptoms. In addition, biobehavioral strategies for pain and itch are well documented to decrease pain and improve quality of life and function. Biobehavioral strategies include biofeedback, mindfulness, deep relaxation, diaphragmatic breathing, and hypnosis.

Conclusion

Overall, mitigating pain and itch associated with scars requires an understanding of the pathophysiology to provide management for affected patients. The mechanisms described in this chapter also highlight why multimodal therapy is often required for successful treatment and a possible flowchart is included (Fig. 11-2). In addition to topical and pharmacologic methods, physical therapy, exercise, sleep counseling, and recognition of mood disturbance is important as part of pain and itch management.

For all patients:

1. Consider scar-reduction therapy as indicated
2. Assess severity of underlying pain/pruritus as well as functional impairment
   a. If symptoms are mild–moderate and without functional impairment, no specific treatment may be indicated; reassurance may be helpful.
   b. If symptoms are moderate–severe with/without functional impairment, consider referral to pain specialist

Pain

A. Localized Scar

1. Consider topical therapy
   a. Topical local anesthetics
   b. Topical NSAIDs
   c. Topical doxepin
2. Consider systemic therapy
   a. Acetaminophen
   b. NSAIDs
   c. If refractive to the above, refer to pain specialist for consideration of gabapentin, TCA, as well as other systemic analgesics. Opioids typically are not indicated for chronic scar pain; refer to pain specialist if considering opioid therapy
3. Injections—local anesthetic and steroid trigger point, focal peripheral nerve block.

B. Generalized Scar

1. Assess for comorbid psychological disorders and refer for treatment as indicated
2. Physical therapy
3. Acetaminophen
4. NSAIDs
5. If refractive to the above, refer to pain specialist for consideration of gabapentin, TCA, as well as other systemic analgesics. Opioids are typically not indicated for chronic scar pain; refer to pain specialist if considering opioid therapy.
6. Injections, or other advanced interventional pain procedures, including spinal cord stimulation may be considered for large and debilitating scars. Refer to pain specialist.

Pruritus

A. Localized Scar

1. Consider topical therapy
   a. Doxepin
   b. Amitriplyline/ketamine

B. Generalized Scar

1. Assess for comorbid psychological disorders and refer for treatment as indicated
2. Consider topical therapy
   a. Doxepin
   b. Amitriptyline/ketamine
3. Physical therapy, possible desensitization
4. Systemic medications
5. Injections, or other advanced interventional pain procedures, including spinal cord stimulation may be considered for large and debilitating scars. Refer to pain specialist.

FIGURE 11-2 Suggested flowchart for the management of scar-related pain and itch.

REFERENCES

1. Nemergut ME, Aganga D, Flick RP. Anesthetic neurotoxicity: what to tell the parents? *Paediatr Anaesth*. 2014;24:120–126.
2. Nemergut ME, Yaster M, Colby CE. Sedation and analgesia to facilitate mechanical ventilation. *Clin Perinatol*. 2013;40:539–558.
3. Davidson AJ. Neurotoxicity and the need for anesthesia in the newborn: does the emperor have no clothes? *Anesthesiology*. 2012;116:507–509.
4. Williamson PS, Williamson ML. Physiologic stress reduction by a local anesthetic during newborn circumcision. *Pediatrics*. 1983;71:36–40.
5. Weber F. Evidence for the need for anaesthesia in the neonate. *Best Pract Res Clin Anaesthesiol*. 2010;24:475–484.
6. Taddio A, Katz J, Ilersich AL, et al. Effect of neonatal circumcision on pain response during subsequent routine vaccination. *Lancet*. 1997;349:599–603.
7. Anand KJ, Hickey PR. Halothane-morphine compared with high-dose sufentanil for anesthesia and postoperative analgesia in neonatal cardiac surgery. *N Engl J Med*. 1992;326:1–9.
8. Whitfield MF, Grunau RE. Behavior, pain perception, and the extremely low-birth weight survivor. *Clin Perinatol*. 2000;27:363–379.
9. Anand KJ, Sippell WG, Aynsley-Green A. Randomised trial of fentanyl anaesthesia in preterm babies undergoing surgery: effects on the stress response. *Lancet*. 1987;1:62–66.
10. Pongcharoen P, Fleischer AB Jr. An evidence-based review of systemic treatments for itch. *Eur J Pain*. 2016;20:24–31.
11. Herzog JL, Solomon JA, Draelos Z, et al. A randomized, double-blind, vehicle-controlled crossover study to determine the anti-pruritic efficacy, safety and local dermal tolerability of a topical formulation (srd174 cream) of the long-acting opiod antagonist nalmefene in subjects with atopic dermatitis. *J Drugs Dermatol*. 2011;10:853–860.
12. Kim YH, Park CK, Back SK, et al. Membrane-delimited coupling of TRPV1 and mGluR5 on presynaptic terminals of nociceptive neurons. *J Neurosci*. 2009;29:10000–10009.
13. Scholz J, Broom DC, Youn DH, et al. Blocking caspase activity prevents transsynaptic neuronal apoptosis and the loss of inhibition in lamina II of the dorsal horn after peripheral nerve injury. *J Neurosci*. 2005;25:7317–7323.
14. Andrew D, Craig AD. Spinothalamic lamina I neurons selectively sensitive to histamine: a central neural pathway for itch. *Nat Neurosci*. 2001;4:72–77.
15. Mochizuki H, Papoiu ADP, Yosipovitch G. Brain processing of itch and scratching. In: Carstens E, Akiyama T, eds. *Itch: Mechanisms and Treatment*. Boca Raton (FL): CRC Press; 2014:494.
16. Herde L, Forster C, Strupf M, et al. Itch induced by a novel method leads to limbic deactivations a functional MRI study. *J Neurophysiol*. 2007;98:2347–2356.
17. Schneider G, Stander S, Burgmer M, et al. Significant differences in central imaging of histamine-induced itch between atopic dermatitis and healthy subjects. *Eur J Pain*. 2008;12:834–841.
18. Papoiu AD, Emerson NM, Patel TS, et al. Voxel-based morphometry and arterial spin labeling fMRI reveal neuropathic and neuroplastic features of brain processing of itch in end-stage renal disease. *J Neurophysiol*. 2014;112:1729–1738.
19. Baron R, Binder A, Wasner G. Neuropathic pain: diagnosis, pathophysiological mechanisms, and treatment. *Lancet Neurol*. 2010;9:807–819.
20. Sawynok J. Topical analgesics for neuropathic pain: preclinical exploration, clinical validation, future development. *Eur J Pain*. 2014;18:465–481.
21. Boomershine CS. Fibromyalgia: the prototypical central sensitivity syndrome. *Curr Rheumatol Rev*. 2015;11:131–145.
22. Adams MH, Lovejoy TI, Turk DC, et al. Pain-related anxiety mediates the relationship between depressive symptoms and pain interference in veterans with hepatitis C. *Gen Hosp Psychiatry*. 2015;37:533–537.
23. Zur E. Topical treatment of neuropathic pain using compounded medications. *Clin J Pain*. 2014;30:73–91.
24. Lynch ME, Craig KD, Peng PWH. *Clinical Pain Management: A Practical Guide*. Hoboken, NJ: Blackwell Publishing Ltd; 2011:xii, 371.
25. Mao J, Gold MS, Backonja MM. Combination drug therapy for chronic pain: a call for more clinical studies. *J Pain*. 2011;12:157–166.
26. Peppin JF, Albrecht PJ, Argoff C, et al. Skin matters: a review of topical treatments for chronic pain. Part two: treatments and applications. *Pain Ther*. 2015;4:33–50.
27. Leffler A, Fischer MJ, Rehner D, et al. The vanilloid receptor TRPV1 is activated and sensitized by local anesthetics in rodent sensory neurons. *J Clin Invest*. 2008;118:763–776.
28. Dworkin RH, O'Connor AB, Audette J, et al. Recommendations for the pharmacological management of neuropathic pain: an overview and literature update. *Mayo Clin Proc*. 2010;85:S3–S14.
29. Sobanko JF, Miller CJ, Alster TS. Topical anesthetics for dermatologic procedures: a review. *Dermatol Surg*. 2012;38:709–721.
30. Ushida T, Tani T, Kanbara T, et al. Analgesic effects of ketamine ointment in patients with complex regional pain syndrome type 1. *Reg Anesth Pain Med*. 2002;27:524–528.
31. Quan D, Wellish M, Gilden DH. Topical ketamine treatment of postherpetic neuralgia. *Neurology*. 2003;60:1391–1392.
32. Poterucha TJ, Murphy SL, Davis MD, et al. Topical amitriptyline-ketamine for the treatment of brachioradial pruritus. *JAMA Dermatol*. 2013;149:148–150.
33. Poterucha TJ, Murphy SL, Sandroni P, et al. Topical amitriptyline combined with topical ketamine for the management of recalcitrant localized pruritus: a retrospective pilot study. *J Am Acad Dermatol*. 2013;69:320–321.
34. Kopsky DJ, Hesselink JM. High doses of topical amitriptyline in neuropathic pain: two cases and literature review. *Pain Pract*. 2012;12:148–153.
35. Lynch ME, Clark AJ, Sawynok J. A pilot study examining topical amitriptyline, ketamine, and a combination of both in the treatment of neuropathic pain. *Clin J Pain*. 2003;19:323–328.
36. Lynch ME, Clark AJ, Sawynok J, et al. Topical amitriptyline and ketamine in neuropathic pain syndromes: an open-label study. *J Pain*. 2005;6:644–649.
37. Liebregts R, Kopsky DJ, Hesselink JM. Topical amitriptyline in post-traumatic neuropathic pain. *J Pain Symptom Manag*. 2011;41:e6–e7.
38. Thompson DF, Brooks KG. Systematic review of topical amitriptyline for the treatment of neuropathic pain. *J Clin Pharm Ther*. 2015. doi:10.1111/jcpt.12297.
39. Ho KY, Huh BK, White WD, et al. Topical amitriptyline versus lidocaine in the treatment of neuropathic pain. *Clin J Pain*. 2008;24:51–55.
40. Gewandter JS, Mohile SG, Heckler CE, et al. A phase III randomized, placebo-controlled study of topical amitriptyline and ketamine for chemotherapy-induced peripheral neuropathy (CIPN): a University of Rochester CCOP study of 462 cancer survivors. *Support Care Cancer*. 2014;22:1807–1814.
41. Poterucha TJ, Weiss WT, Warndahl RA, et al. Topical amitriptyline combined with ketamine for the treatment of erythromelalgia: a retrospective study of 36 patients at Mayo Clinic. *J Drugs Dermatol*. 2013;12:308–310.
42. Poterucha TJ, Murphy SL, Rho RH, et al. Topical amitriptyline-ketamine for treatment of rectal, genital, and perineal pain and discomfort. *Pain Physician*. 2012;15:485–488.
43. Uzaraga I, Gerbis B, Holwerda E, et al. Topical amitriptyline, ketamine, and lidocaine in neuropathic pain caused by radiation skin reaction: a pilot study. *Support Care Cancer*. 2012;20:1515–1524.
44. Bryson E, Asbill S, Sweitzer S. Skin permeation and antinociception of topical gabapentin formulations. *Int J Pharm Compd*. 2014;18:504–511.
45. Hiom S, Patel GK, Newcombe RG, et al. Severe postherpetic neuralgia and other neuropathic pain syndromes alleviated by topical gabapentin. *Br J Dermatol*. 2014;173:300–302.
46. Peniston JH, Gold MS, Wieman MS, et al. Long-term tolerability of topical diclofenac sodium 1% gel for osteoarthritis in seniors and patients with comorbidities. *Clin Interv Aging*. 2012;7:517–523.
47. Baraf HS, Gold MS, Petruschke RA, et al. Tolerability of topical diclofenac sodium 1% gel for osteoarthritis in seniors and patients with comorbidities. *Am J Geriatr Pharmacother*. 2012;10:47–60.
48. Taylor RS, Fotopoulos G, Maibach H. Safety profile of topical diclofenac: a meta-analysis of blinded, randomized, controlled trials in musculoskeletal conditions. *Curr Med Res Opin*. 2011;27:605–622.
49. Brewer AR, Pierchala LA, Yanchick JK, et al. Gastrointestinal tolerability of diclofenac epolamine topical patch 1.3%: a pooled analysis of 14 clinical studies. *Postgrad Med*. 2011;123:168–176.
50. Lee J, Burke DT. Lower gastrointestinal bleeding associated with diclofenac topical patch in a patient with colonic mass and on antiplatelet therapy for atrial fibrillation. *Am J Phys Med Rehabil*. 2014;93:1014–1017.
51. Folzer E, Gonzalez D, Singh R, et al. Comparison of skin permeability for three diclofenac topical formulations: an in vitro study. *Pharmazie*. 2014;69:27–31.
52. Wible JH Jr, Barrett T, Devarakonda K, et al. Biodistribution of diclofenac following repeated topical applications of two diclofenac sodium formulations to minipigs. *Biopharm Drug Dispos*. 2014;35:87–96.

53. Roth SH, Fuller P. Diclofenac topical solution compared with oral diclofenac: a pooled safety analysis. *J Pain Res*. 2011;4:159–167.
54. Roth SH, Fuller P. Diclofenac sodium topical solution 1.5% w/w with dimethyl sulfoxide compared with placebo for the treatment of osteoarthritis: pooled safety results. *Postgrad Med*. 2011;123:180–188.
55. Baraf HS, Gloth FM, Barthel HR, et al. Safety and efficacy of topical diclofenac sodium gel for knee osteoarthritis in elderly and younger patients: pooled data from three randomized, double-blind, parallel-group, placebo-controlled, multicentre trials. *Drugs Aging*. 2011;28:27–40.
56. Kuehl K, Carr W, Yanchick J, et al. Analgesic efficacy and safety of the diclofenac epolamine topical patch 1.3% (DETP) in minor soft tissue injury. *Int J Sports Med*. 2011;32:635–643.
57. Mueller EA, Kirch W, Reiter S. Extent and time course of pain intensity upon treatment with a topical diclofenac sodium patch versus placebo in acute traumatic injury based on a validated end point: post hoc analysis of a randomized placebo-controlled trial. *Expert Opin Pharmacother*. 2010;11:493–498.
58. McCarberg BH, Argoff CE. Topical diclofenac epolamine patch 1.3% for treatment of acute pain caused by soft tissue injury. *Int J Clin Pract*. 2010;64:1546–1553.
59. Gimbel J, Jacobs D, Pixton G, et al. Effectiveness and safety of diclofenac epolamine topical patch 1.3% for the treatment of acute pain due to back strain: an open-label, uncontrolled study. *Phys Sportsmed*. 2011;39:11–18.
60. Ahmed SU, Zhang Y, Chen L, et al. Effect of 1.5% topical diclofenac on clinical neuropathic pain. *Anesthesiology*. 2015;123:191–198.
61. Ercan N, Uludag MO, Agis ER, et al. The anti-inflammatory effect of diclofenac is considerably augmented by topical capsaicinoids-containing patch in carrageenan-induced paw oedema of rat. *Inflammopharmacology*. 2013;21:413–419.
62. Akat PB. Severe photosensitivity reaction induced by topical diclofenac. *Indian J Pharmacol*. 2013;45:408–409.
63. Sabroe RA, Kennedy CT, Archer CB. The effects of topical doxepin on responses to histamine, substance P and prostaglandin E2 in human skin. *Br J Dermatol*. 1997;137:386–390.
64. Zell-Kanter M, Toerne TS, Spiegel K, et al. Doxepin toxicity in a child following topical administration. *Ann Pharmacother*. 2000;34:328–329.
65. Jones ME, Skaufle ML. Systemic adverse effects from topical doxepin cream. *Ann Pharmacother*. 2001;35:505–506.
66. Karaz SS, Moeckli JK, Davis W, et al. Effect of topical doxepin cream on skin testing. *J Allergy Clin Immunol*. 1995;96:997–998.
67. McCleane G. Topical application of doxepin hydrochloride can reduce the symptoms of complex regional pain syndrome: a case report. *Injury*. 2002;33:88–89.
68. McCleane G. Topical application of doxepin hydrochloride, capsaicin and a combination of both produces analgesia in chronic human neuropathic pain: a randomized, double-blind, placebo-controlled study. *Br J Clin Pharmacol*. 2000;49:574–579.
69. Drake LA, Fallon JD, Sober A. Relief of pruritus in patients with atopic dermatitis after treatment with topical doxepin cream. The Doxepin Study Group. *J Am Acad Dermatol*. 1994;31:613–616.
70. Anand P, Bley K. Topical capsaicin for pain management: therapeutic potential and mechanisms of action of the new high-concentration capsaicin 8% patch. *Br J Anaesth*. 2011;107:490–502.
71. Bigliardi PL, Stammer H, Jost G, et al. Treatment of pruritus with topically applied opiate receptor antagonist. *J Am Acad Dermatol*. 2007;56:979–988.
72. Rayner H, Baharani J, Smith S, et al. Uraemic pruritus: relief of itching by gabapentin and pregabalin. *Nephron Clin Pract*. 2012;122: 75–79.
73. Cheikh Hassan HI, Brennan F, Collett G, et al. Efficacy and safety of gabapentin for uremic pruritus and restless legs syndrome in conservatively managed patients with chronic kidney disease. *J Pain Symptom Manag*. 2015;49:782–789.
74. Yong AS, Lee KY. Uremic pruritus is improved by gabapentin. *Int J Dermatol*. 2014;53:e404–e405.
75. Solak Y, Biyik Z, Atalay II, et al. Pregabalin versus gabapentin in the treatment of neuropathic pruritus in maintenance haemodialysis patients: a prospective, crossover study. *Nephrology (Carlton)*. 2012;17: 710–717.
76. Razeghi E, Eskandari D, Ganji MR, et al. Gabapentin and uremic pruritus in hemodialysis patients. *Ren Fail*. 2009;31:85–90.
77. Vila T, Gommer J, Scates AC. Role of gabapentin in the treatment of uremic pruritus. *Ann Pharmacother*. 2008;42:1080–1084.
78. Naini AE, Harandi AA, Khanbabapour S, et al. Gabapentin: a promising drug for the treatment of uremic pruritus. *Saudi J Kidney Dis Transpl*. 2007;18:378–381.
79. Gunal AI, Ozalp G, Yoldas TK, et al. Gabapentin therapy for pruritus in haemodialysis patients: a randomized, placebo-controlled, double-blind trial. *Nephrol Dial Transplant*. 2004;19:3137–3139.
80. Yue J, Jiao S, Xiao Y, et al. Comparison of pregabalin with ondansetron in treatment of uraemic pruritus in dialysis patients: a prospective, randomized, double-blind study. *Int Urol Nephrol*. 2015;47:161–167.
81. Ahuja RB, Gupta GK. A four arm, double blind, randomized and placebo controlled study of pregabalin in the management of post-burn pruritus. *Burns*. 2013;39:24–29.
82. Shavit L, Grenader T, Lifschitz M, et al. Use of pregabalin in the management of chronic uremic pruritus. *J Pain Symptom Manag*. 2013;45:776–781.
83. Aperis G, Paliouras C, Zervos A, et al. The use of pregabalin in the treatment of uraemic pruritus in haemodialysis patients. *J Ren Care*. 2010;36:180–185.
84. Maciel AA, Cunha PR, Laraia IO, et al. Efficacy of gabapentin in the improvement of pruritus and quality of life of patients with notalgia paresthetica. *An Bras Dermatol*. 2014;89:570–575.
85. Uldall Pallesen KA, Bygum A. Brachioradial pruritus effectively treated with gabapentin [in Danish]. *Ugeskr Laeger*. 2012;174:1830–1831.
86. Yilmaz S, Ceyhan AM, Baysal Akkaya V. Brachioradial pruritus successfully treated with gabapentin. *J Dermatol*. 2010;37:662–665.
87. Ahuja RB, Gupta R, Gupta G, et al. A comparative analysis of cetirizine, gabapentin and their combination in the relief of post-burn pruritus. *Burns*. 2011;37:203–207.
88. Hooten WM, St Sauver JL, McGree ME, et al. Incidence and risk factors for progression from short-term to episodic or long-term opioid prescribing: a population-based study. *Mayo Clin Proc*. 2015;90:850–856.
89. Ashley FL. Atrophy following cortisone injection for hypertrophic scar. *Calif Med*. 1973;119:65–66.
90. Sabharwal R, Rasmussen L, Sluka KA, et al. Exercise prevents development of autonomic dysregulation and hyperalgesia in a mouse model of chronic muscle pain. *Pain*. 2016;157:387–398.
91. Shin TM, Bordeaux JS. The role of massage in scar management: a literature review. *Dermatol Surg*. 2012;38:414–423.
92. Ko WJ, Na YC, Suh BS, et al. The effects of topical agent (kelo-cote or contractubex) massage on the thickness of post-burn scar tissue formed in rats. *Arch Plast Surg*. 2013;40:697–704.
93. Cho YS, Jeon JH, Hong A, et al. The effect of burn rehabilitation massage therapy on hypertrophic scar after burn: a randomized controlled trial. *Burns*. 2014;40:1513–1520.
94. Kocyigit F, Akalin E, Gezer NS, et al. Functional magnetic resonance imaging of the effects of low-frequency transcutaneous electrical nerve stimulation on central pain modulation: a double-blind, placebo-controlled trial. *Clin J Pain*. 2012;28:581–588.
95. Choi JC, Kim J, Kang E, et al. Brain mechanisms of pain relief by transcutaneous electrical nerve stimulation: a functional magnetic resonance imaging study. *Eur J Pain*. 2016;20:92–105.
96. Twillman RK. Mental disorders in chronic pain patients. *J Pain Palliat Care Pharmacother*. 2007;21:13–19.
97. Schut C, Kupfer J. Itch and psyche [in German]. *Hautarzt*. 2013;64:414–419.
98. Lavda AC, Webb TL, Thompson AR. A meta-analysis of the effectiveness of psychological interventions for adults with skin conditions. *Br J Dermatol*. 2012;167:970–979.
99. Bae BG, Oh SH, Park CO, et al. Progressive muscle relaxation therapy for atopic dermatitis: objective assessment of efficacy. *Acta Derm Venereol*. 2012;92:57–61.
100. Ehlers A, Stangier U, Gieler U. Treatment of atopic dermatitis: a comparison of psychological and dermatological approaches to relapse prevention. *J Consult Clin Psychol*. 1995;63:624–635.

12 Surgical Scar Revision

MATTHIAS B. DONELAN, BENJAMIN LEVI, and CURTIS GABALL

KEY POINTS

- All injuries to the skin that significantly damage the papillary dermis result in scars.
- Scars are not inherently bad, they are an essential part of life.
- Scar revision improves scars by favorably altering their characteristics, not necessarily by excising them.
- Scar revision has been greatly improved by a more thorough understanding of scar maturation and novel technologies.

Scar revision requires analysis, diagnosis, treatment selection, surgical technique, and total patient care. That makes it an infinitely challenging and rewarding part of plastic surgery.

A long-term view of how scars have been managed over the course of medical history is informative and gives perspective (see Chapter 1). The management of scars can be divided into five different eras:

1. Prior to the development of anesthesia there was primarily acceptance and disguise, except for totally life-altering deformities (e.g., nasal reconstruction for punitive amputation).
2. After the emergence of anesthesia (both general and local) in the late 19th century, there was a burgeoning interest, and an extensive literature, in scar revision techniques. Among these the Z-plasty is most notable.
3. After World War I, scar excision and resurfacing gained popularity following Sir Harold Gillies' monumental work on soldiers using flaps to restore facial appearance.
4. During the mid- to late 20th century, scar excision and ever more complex replacement with the patient's other undamaged body parts has dominated thinking, particularly for large scars.
5. In the 21st century, scar rehabilitation—preserving original tissue—and regeneration have the potential to revolutionize how we "revise" scars.

Without scars there would be no wound healing, so scars are an essential part of life. The goal of this chapter on surgical scar revision is to demonstrate how understanding scar etiology and pathogenesis enables us to enhance normal wound healing during surgical scar revision therapy. We have now reached a point where scar excision is often not the best option for improving scars; there is nothing like original equipment in its original location. Understanding how and why scars heal well or unsatisfactorily is a fascinating and evolving process. Careful analysis of an individual scar's qualities is the most essential part of planning a successful scar revision procedure.

The term "scar" originates from the Greek word "eskara," meaning the scab (eschar), or wound caused by burning. It has come to mean any visible mark remaining after the healing of a wound or other pathological process. "Scar" is therefore a term applied to a wide range of visible skin abnormalities that can be composed of very different kinds of pathologic tissue, with or without pigmentary abnormalities. These include such varied presentations as linear surgical scars, hypertrophic burn scars, atrophic scars (such as those that follow severe acne), and skin grafts placed during reconstruction; each presents different clinical problems.

All scars are unique, but from a strategic thinking standpoint they can be roughly divided into four fundamentally different categories.

Category I: Linear scars from an incision or laceration through the full thickness of the dermis without "significant" associated tissue loss. Their most important attribute is their relationship to relaxed skin tension lines (RSTLs)[1,2] (Figs. 12-1 and 12-2).

Category II: Scars following injury to the mid- to deep dermis from burns or trauma that have not completely transected the dermis, but are conspicuous and have associated hypertrophy and contractures (Fig. 12-3).

Category III: Scars associated with full-thickness loss of the integument and deeper tissues from trauma, surgical resection, or extensive third-degree burn injury (Fig. 12-4).

Category IV: Keloid scars, a benign proliferative disease process that behaves differently from other physiologic scarring processes (Fig. 12-5).

Appreciating the environment within which an individual scar lives is an essential factor in planning scar revision, particularly the presence of tension and an awareness of absolute tissue loss (see Chapter 7). Each of the above four categories presents different challenges and opportunities

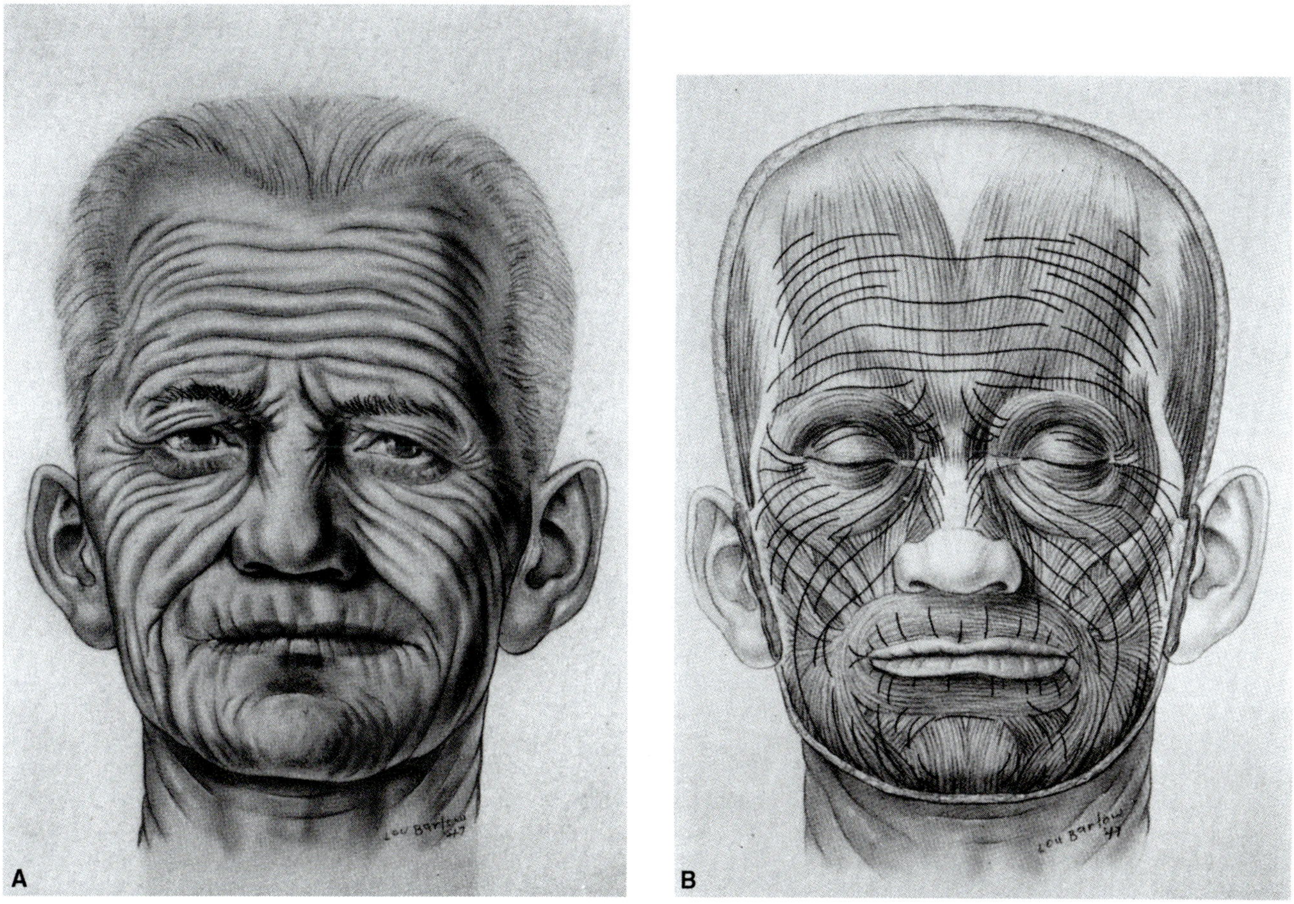

FIGURE 12-1 **A:** Relaxed skin tension lines (RSTLs) differ from Langer's lines and most closely follow the natural wrinkle lines, as demonstrated in this facial schematic. **B:** RSTLs are usually perpendicular to the orientation of the muscles beneath. *(Kraisel CJ. The selection of appropriate lines for elective surgical incisions.* Plast Reconstr Surg. *1951;8:1–28.)*

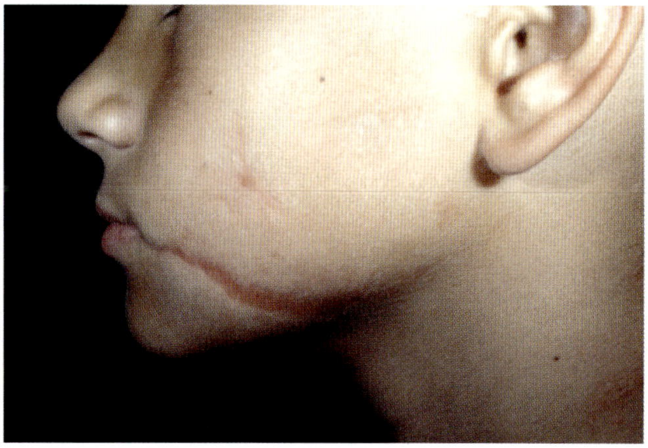

FIGURE 12-2 Traumatic lacerations which do not follow relaxed skin tension lines, particularly if they are perpendicular to them as in this example, heal unfavorably. *(From Krakowski AC, Totri CR, Donelan MB, Shumaker PR. Scar management in the pediatric and adolescent populations.* Pediatrics. *2016;137(2):e20142065.)*

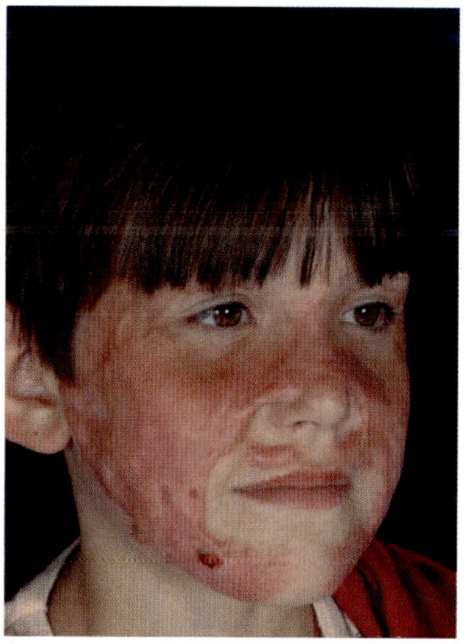

FIGURE 12-3 A 11-year-old girl who sustained mixed second- and third-degree facial burns. One year after the injury they have healed with contraction, hypertrophy, and ulceration.

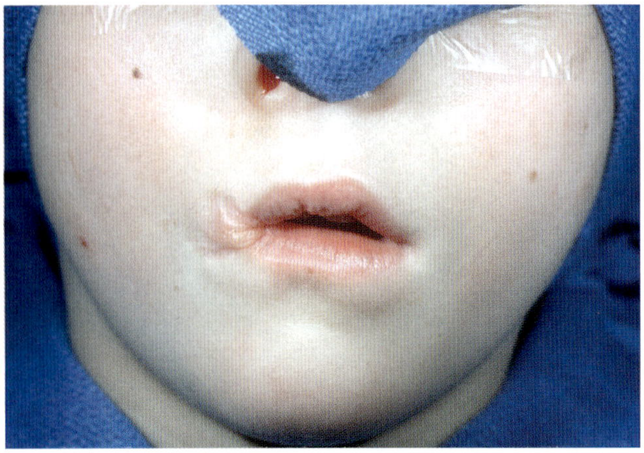

FIGURE 12-4 A 5-year-old child who sustained an electrical burn injury to the right oral commissure with full-thickness loss of vermilion, muscle, mucosa, and skin. His deformity has extensive contractures with displacement of the philtrum and the midpoint of the lower lip.

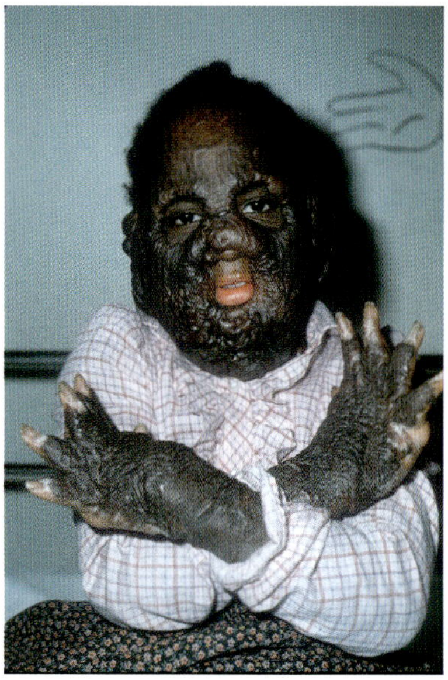

FIGURE 12-5 A 10-year-old girl following a second- and third-degree burn injury with massive keloid scar formation in all areas, including donor sites.

for surgical scar revision. It is of critical importance to understand these differences in order to determine the most appropriate treatment plan. Scar orientation is of profound importance and plays a role in all categories except IV.[1] RSTLs differ from Langer's lines and most closely follow natural wrinkle lines, particularly in the head and neck (Fig. 12-1A). These lines are usually perpendicular to the orientation of the muscles beneath (Fig. 12-1B). They also can be identified by gentle compression of the skin.[1,3] Elective incisions should be made as much as possible along these lines in order to obtain the best healing (Fig. 12-6A, B).

The decision of whether to treat or not to treat an "unsatisfactory" scar is extremely important (see Chapter 4). Some scars are unsatisfactory because they restrict range of motion or distort facial features; others, despite being very subtle, are objectionable because they evoke unpleasant memories. The perspectives of the patient and the evaluating surgeon are often very different. The patient frequently desires that the scar be "removed," as

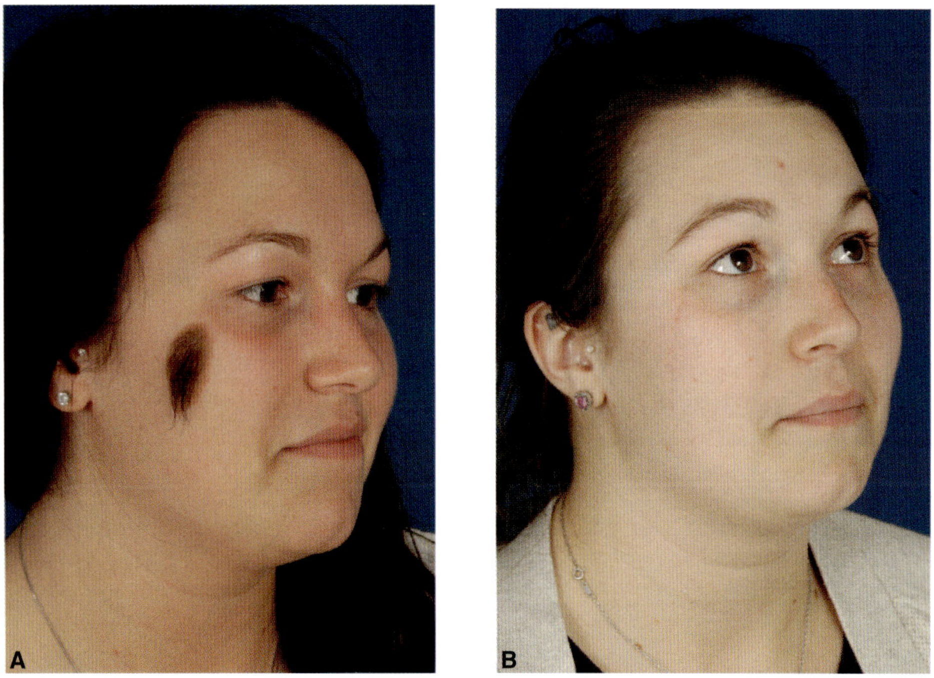

FIGURE 12-6 **A:** A 20-year-old woman who had always been reluctant to have her congenital nevus excised because of concerns about a scar. **B:** Scars parallel to RSTLs result in the best possible healing for both elective incisions and traumatic lacerations. Fusiform scar revision should always adhere as much as possible to this principle.

in eliminated completely. This is clearly not possible. The surgeon must determine which scars are possible to improve and whether the improvement will be adequate to make an individual patient pleased with the outcome. Arriving at a satisfactory meeting of the minds is an essential first step in creating reasonable patient expectations. Creating that joint understanding is a subtle but important learned skill that is an integral part of successful scar revision surgery. In some cases the decision is easy to make. For example, a linear scar on the face that is unfavorably oriented to RSTLs, and has an unsatisfactory appearance because of either hypertrophy or widening with atrophy, almost always can be improved by a correctly performed surgical scar revision (Fig. 12-7).

Goals of Scar Revision

The overriding goal is to unequivocally improve the appearance of the scar. Simply creating a new deformity to modify an old one is not a successful outcome. Surgery should only be undertaken when the surgeon feels confident that the scar will be made clearly better to both patient and surgeon. There should be minimal to no additional iatrogenic deformity caused by the scar revision procedure. When possible, favorably altering the environment in which the scar will heal is very beneficial. Decreasing or eliminating tension is of the utmost importance. Using lasers for drug delivery, to obscure scar margins, and to initiate scar remodeling/regeneration are new game-changing advances, discussed in detail in other chapters (see Chapters 13 and 14).

Category I: Scars parallel to RSTLs in general are favorable and usually cannot be improved by revisional surgery.[2] Antitension line (ATL) scars, which are unfavorably oriented to RSTLs, frequently result in hypertrophy, atrophy, "trapdooring," and widening and can frequently be improved by scar revision. With experience, and taking these simple factors into consideration, it is a rare unsatisfactory linear scar that cannot be improved.

Category II: Scars require an accurate diagnosis of what has caused their unsatisfactory characteristics, followed by a rehabilitative approach that eliminates tension and facilitates scar remodeling.

Category III: Scars require the provision of adequate tissue to enable the best possible restoration of satisfactory appearance.

Category IV: Keloid scars are unsolved clinical and surgical problems, often requiring multimodal therapies geared toward palliation and symptomatic improvement.

Surgical Technique

It goes without saying that scar revision surgery must be performed well. The plan must make sense, and the execution

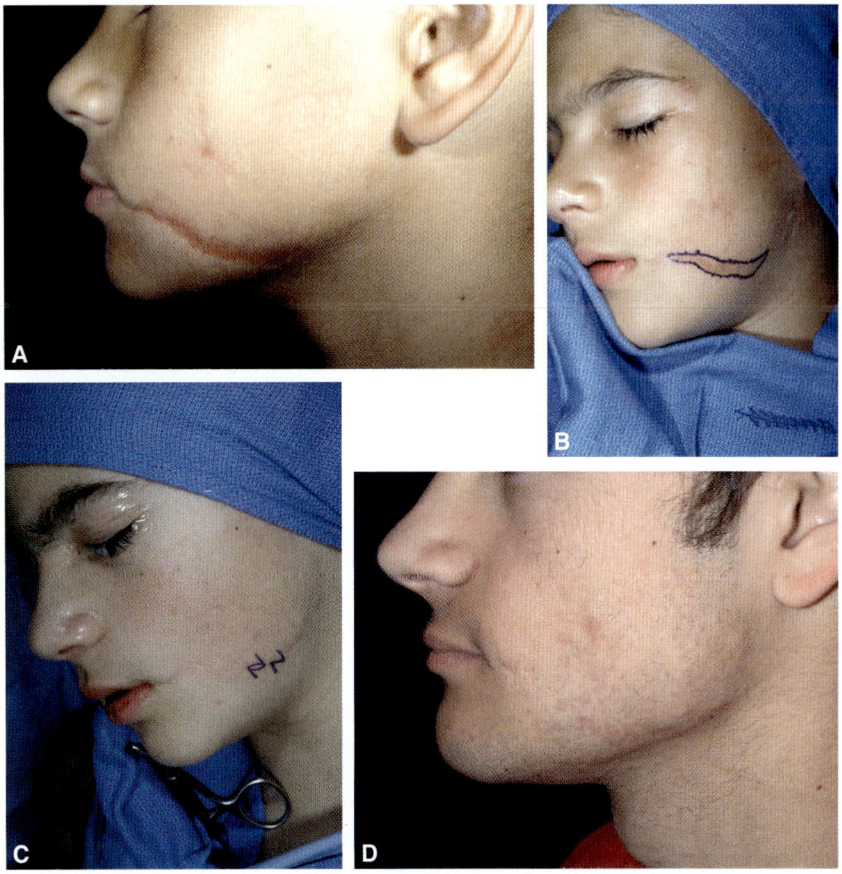

FIGURE 12-7 **A:** Transverse facial laceration perpendicular to relaxed skin tension lines with widening and atrophy. **B:** The atrophic depressed scar was excised and the defect closed incorporating four Z-plasties with the lateral limbs oriented parallel to relaxed skin tension lines. **C:** The most posterior extent of the excision was not closed with Z-plasties. That area widened again and 2 years later it was revised with two Z-plasties similarly oriented to the original excision. **D:** Six years following the last scar revision the deformity is not noticeable. *(From Krakowski AC, Totri CR, Donelan MB, Shumaker PR. Scar management in the pediatric and adolescent populations.* Pediatrics. *2016;137(2):e20142065.)*

must be meticulous. Basic surgical techniques are described in detail in many excellent texts,[4–6] and only a few relevant caveats will be highlighted here. Incisions must be made exactly perpendicular to the skin's surface unless specific local conditions, such as hair follicle angulation, dictate a different approach. When dealing with tissue that includes a combination of indurated scar and uninjured skin, scalpel control is extremely important. The different resistance of the tissues can easily result in inaccurate incisions. Preserving the minimally injured skin at the margin of a scar can be helpful in masking the transition from normal skin into the reconstructed area, and helps with camouflage. Surgical incisions made in normal skin always heal with the appearance of a surgical scar and this looks unnatural in most circumstances.

Scar Analysis

Everyone can treat, but few can diagnose.
—Dr. Samuel Moschella

Many factors play a role in whether a scar has healed in a satisfactory or unsatisfactory fashion. It is mandatory to take a complete history to understand the etiology and pathogenesis of an individual scar. If previous attempts at revision have occurred, details of treatment should be obtained to avoid a repeat disappointment. Important physical findings to note include anatomical location, orientation to RSTLs, shape, hypertrophy or atrophy, presence of tension, pigmentation, step-off deformities, presence of extrinsic contractures, patient age, scar maturity, and the presence of foreign bodies.

Anatomic Region

Scars on the face tend to heal more favorably than scars in other areas of the body. Favorably oriented scars on the face can end up looking much like normal skin lines. Neck skin is notorious for poor healing, perhaps because it is thin and has fewer skin appendages. Linear scars in other areas, such as the deltoid region, the presternal area, and around the knee, frequently result in widening, hypertrophy, and an unsightly appearance. Scars on the trunk have much more of a propensity to widen than do scars in the region of the head and neck, even if they approximate RSTLs.

Orientation

As noted, this is probably the most important component for linear scars. "Practically speaking few tension lines (TL) scars are unaesthetic, but most, if not all, anti-tension lines (ATL) scars are unsatisfactory."[2]

Hypertrophic Scars

Hypertrophic scars are a normal physiologic response of the skin to trauma, influenced by multiple factors which cause them to hypertrophy (see Chapter 6). Keloid scars, on the other hand, are a benign proliferative diathesis leading to hypertrophy that is not in response to normal physiologic stimuli (see Chapter 5). Hypertrophic scars can be improved by correct diagnosis and appropriate scar revision. Keloid scars are a completely separate entity and will be discussed separately in Category IV.

It is essential to diagnose the etiology of the hypertrophic scar. Is it hypertrophied because of an unfavorable orientation to RSTL? Is it hypertrophic because it was a partial-thickness burn injury which has contracted and is now under tension? Is it the result of tension and relaxation across a flexion joint, or because it bridges a concavity? Is it the result of healing complicated by infection or foreign bodies? Before embarking on the correction of a hypertrophic scar, the etiology must be diagnosed and there must be a plan to favorably alter the factors that resulted in the hypertrophy.

Depressed Scars

Depressed scars can result from unfavorable orientation, fat atrophy following a contusion or laceration, loss of tissue, or adhesions between the surface of the scar and the underlying deep structures such as fascia. Depressed scars are frequently seen as a result of overly aggressive steroid injection for hypertrophic scars (Fig. 12-8). When atrophy is present, regardless of etiology (with the frequent exception of steroid-induced atrophy), it is often necessary to remove all or part of the atrophic tissue (Fig. 12-7). Fat grafting can be helpful in selected cases (see Chapter 15). Because the transposed limbs of Z-plasties originate from the level surface of the normal skin on either side of a depression they can be very effective in elevating depressed scars.

Shape

Curvilinear scars create a trapdoor effect because of the tightening of the margin of the scar like a "purse string." Lengthening the scar by multiple Z-plasties, with the limbs of the Z-plasties paralleling RSTLs as one moves along the curvilinear scar, is a uniformly successful technique in the authors' experience.

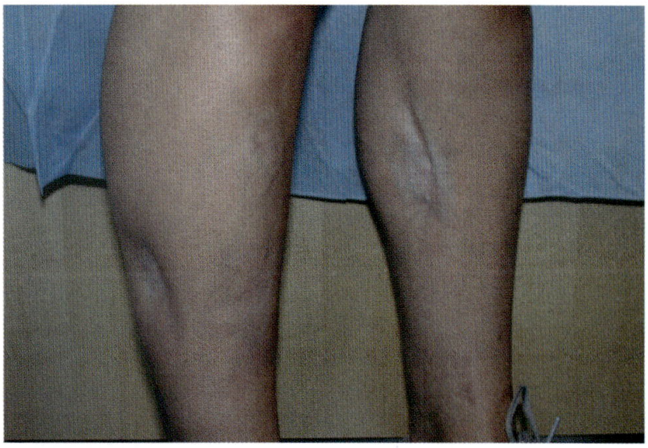

FIGURE 12-8 A 20-year-old woman athlete who underwent elective orthopedic fasciotomies for compartment syndrome. Following multiple steroid injections for hypertrophic scarring she developed severe atrophy of both the skin and subcutaneous fat.

Step-off Deformities

These are usually the result of an inadequate, or absent, closure of a laceration. This type of deformity, once clearly diagnosed, requires reopening of the scar and then appropriate, meticulous, closure. If the scar is unfavorably oriented, such that unfavorable future healing is likely, appropriate revisional techniques should be considered at the same time. Otherwise, a careful simple closure is adequate.

Patient Age

The very young and the very old heal with the best scars. Adolescents are the healthiest patients and make the most exuberant scars.

Scar Maturity

As mentioned under hypertrophic scars, the timing of the scar analysis is pivotal as scars go through a normal maturation phase that lasts for years. A hypertrophic scar in a fair-skinned blue-eyed patient which is extremely erythematous, even though favorably oriented, is likely to mature well if given enough time. Experience is very important, as well as patient patience, in determining when and how to intervene after a scar has become unsatisfactory.

Pigmentary Abnormalities

Scars can be either hyperpigmented, hypopigmented, or both (i.e., mottled). They also can have pigmentary abnormalities as a result of foreign bodies from the time of the original trauma.

Foreign Bodies

Traumatic tattooing diffusely interspersed through a wound can be treated by excision of the involved area. Lasers now offer greater flexibility in posttraumatic tattoo treatment and excision is less frequently indicated (see Chapters 13 and 23).

Genetic Background

Genetic background is well known to affect the ways scars evolve. Despite the complexity of the human genome, there are racial patterns to the wound healing process that can be helpful to discuss in generalities. Fair-skinned, blue-eyed, Northern European, and Celtic patients (that are Fitzpatrick type I or II) tend to make hypertrophic scars early on in their postinjury or post-op course. As time goes by these scars tend to mature favorably and often end up flat and hypopigmented. Fitzpatrick type III through VI show varying tendencies toward postinflammatory hyperpigmentation and are particularly prone to developing hyperpigmentation in both grafts and skin flaps (Fig. 12-9A,B). Careful examination of the patient's prior injuries or operative sites is paramount in determining, as much as possible, whether a reconstructive operation could result in a more harmful pigmentary abnormality. Fitzpatrick type V and VI patients can be so dark that hyperpigmentation following surgical intervention is nearly irrelevant. These groups of patients, however, have a greater tendency to develop hypertrophic or keloid scars (Figs. 12-5 and 12-9). Once again, clinical judgment and caution are of extreme importance.

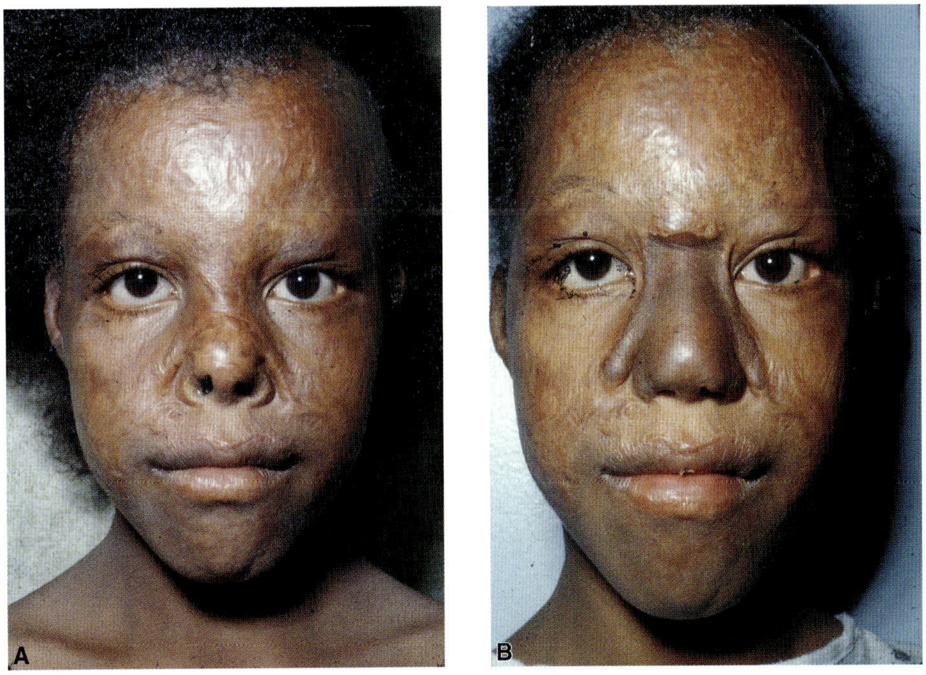

FIGURE 12-9 **A:** An 8-year-old girl with contracted hypertrophic scars following a mixed second- and third-degree burn. Color match of scars on the face was acceptable. **B:** Following scar excision and replacement with a full-thickness skin graft, the hyperpigmented graft is her most conspicuous deformity. This mistake required removal of the entire graft and resurfacing with a median forehead flap. The scars could potentially be improved today with local tissue rearrangement and laser therapy.

Category I: Linear Scars

As noted previously, orientation relative to TLs is the principal determinant of whether a linear scar without tissue loss develops into a satisfactory or unsatisfactory scar.[2] If scars are not correctly oriented to RSTLs, they may hypertrophy or atrophy.[7] Alternatively, as they mature linear scars may also form contractures that distort surrounding tissues and even cause functional impairments. Relieving tension surgically is crucial in this situation, and can be performed in several ways. The goal of scar revision surgery is to make a scar less abnormal and, as a result, make it less noticeable. For linear scars this is accomplished by improving orientation to RSTL, leveling the surface, relieving and avoiding unfavorable tension, eliminating trapdoor deformities, and obscuring the transition from normal skin into the area of scarring.

There are four basic techniques to accomplish these goals for linear scars:

1. Fusiform scar revision (FSR)
2. Z-plasty
3. W-plasty[2,8]
4. Geometric broken line closure (GBLC)[2,7,9,10]

A combination of these techniques may be employed in long and irregularly shaped scars depending on the specific position, shape, and local environment.

1. *Fusiform scar revision*
   The simplest technique to accomplish improvement in linear scars is the FSR. FSR consists of excising the existing scar in a lenticular fashion, sometimes including small amounts of adjacent normal tissue in order to more closely approximate RSTL, and then meticulously closing the defect in layers to create a level surface. If the scar is depressed or there is a concern that the scar may become depressed, leaving the old deepithelializing scar and advancing normal tissue over it can help prevent this by giving the new scar a bed of support (Fig. 12-10). This can be employed with any excisional technique, including fusiform, W-pasty, and GBLC (described below). For short scars, particularly in the facial region, this technique can be quite successful and is a mainstay of simple scar revision. Surgical technique is important for successful outcome, as is the absence of excessive tension perpendicular to the line of the scar. The presence of perpendicular tension will always tend to widen scars, even if they are well oriented, and preoperative judgment regarding this factor is paramount in choosing FSR as a technique.

   Curvilinear scars are problematic because they obviously do not follow RSTL. When the scar completes the majority of a circle, a "trapdoor" effect is often created.[4,11] The contracting band of scar causes a "purse string" effect, bulging the central tissue and possibly interrupting lymphatic drainage, which further contributes to the perceived fullness. If a trapdoor scar is small, and a fusiform excision can be carried out along RSTL, that can be a satisfactory solution. The most effective correction in our experience has been to eliminate the purse string effect by carrying out Z-plasties to lengthen the scar. At the same time, this type of revision recruits tissue from the central redundant area into the lateral normal tissue, both leveling and stretching the contour abnormality. The Z-plasties should be designed so that the limbs most closely follow RSTL in the different regions of the trapdoor scar. In our hands, this has been a uniformly effective trapdoor scar revision technique.

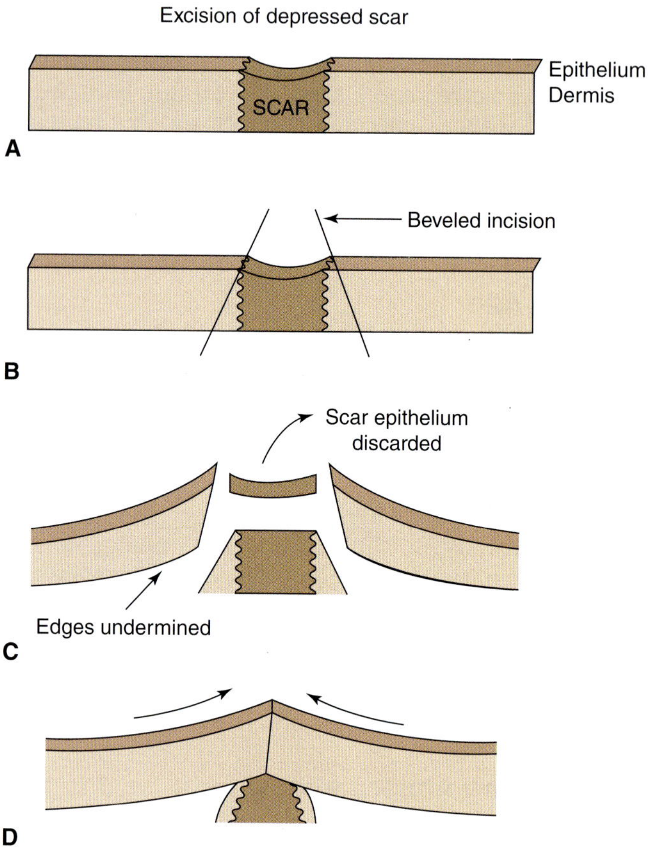

FIGURE 12-10 Excision of a depressed scar. **A:** Depressed scar through dermis. **B:** Beveling incisions out around scar facilitates eversion for closure. **C:** Undermine adjacent skin in the subcutaneous plane and deepithelialize the scar, leaving the scar base in place. **D:** Normal skin is advanced over old scar base to help maintain contour.

2. *Z-plasty*
   The history of "zigzag" linear scar revision is an integral part of the history of plastic surgery and makes for fascinating reading.[9] The most important of these techniques, by far, is the Z-plasty. The evolution of the Z-plasty parallels the increasing sophistication of plastic surgery during the late 19th and early 20th centuries. This technique involves creating an incision along the length of the scar to be released, then creating equilateral incisions that extend from the ends of the original incision to opposite sides and at equal angles, creating a Z-shaped incision. Increasing the angle at which these limbs are designed increases the length gained by the Z-plasty. The incisions create two opposing flaps in the shape of isosceles triangles, which are then elevated (including release

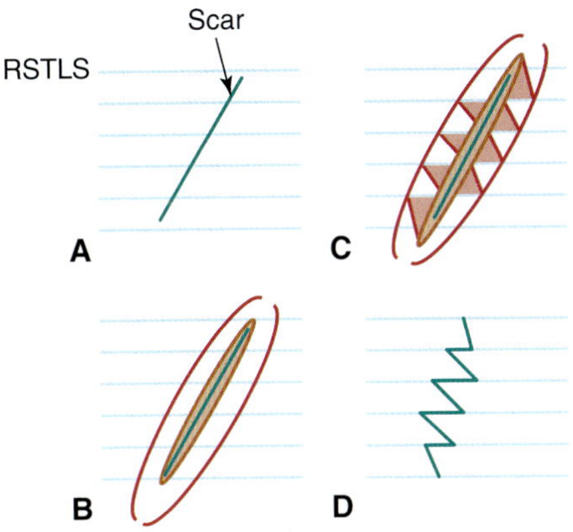

FIGURE 12-11 W-plasty. **A:** Linear scar with unfavorable orientation to RSTLs. **B:** Parallel lines are drawn 3 to 6 mm from the edge of the planned scar excision. **C:** Triangles are drawn (shaded areas ultimately discarded) with one limb parallel to RSTLs. Triangles are drawn (shaded areas ultimately discarded) with one limb parallel to RSTLs. The angles at the ends of the excision must be 30 degrees or less to avoid prominent standing cones. **D:** Final result breaks linearity, has short limbs (3 to 6 mm), and runs maximally in RSTLs.

of any deeper fibrous scar) and transposed relative to one another, before being reinset with their apices now positioned at the opposite base of the opposing triangle. The flaps are then sutured in place.

3. *W-plasty*
The W-plasty was first proposed in 1959 and has had many advocates and practitioners since then.[8] The W-plasty can be thought of as an extension of the fusiform scar excision, with the goal of making a linear scar irregular. It requires the excision of both the scar and some of the surrounding normal tissue (Fig. 12-11). The normal tissue is excised as a series of repetitive, triangular advancement flaps. These flaps are designed such that they are equilateral and interdigitate with the flaps from the opposite side of the defect. On the face or neck, each limb should be approximately 3 to 6 mm in length so that they are of adequate size with which to work, yet not too visually obvious. Because a significant amount of skin is removed, this technique should only be applied where there is a reservoir of recruitable skin that will not distort surrounding mobile structures when advanced. The angles of the flaps should be designed such that they are maximally oriented along RSTLs.

4. *Geometric broken line closure*
Another technique that has been described is the so-called GBLC.[10] The alleged advantage of this technique is that it is less noticeable than the regular repetitive pattern of a W-plasty. The purpose of "breaking up a scar" is that it breaks up the visual line of the scar into smaller segments and confuses the visual cortex, the purpose of camouflage. GBLC is an extension of the W-plasty concept and is designed to create a scar that is not only irregular, but also random (Fig. 12-12). Classically, GBLC also consists of excising the existing scar and adjacent normal tissue to create a mixture of interdigitating triangular, rectangular, or semicircular flaps in alternating patterns. Eliminating semicircular flaps is recommended by the authors to eliminate their tendency to "pin cushion." As with W-plasty, acute angles at the end of the closure should be designed in order to minimize raised cutaneous deformities. Every effort should be made to orient incisions maximally along RSTLs.[7]

In the view of the authors, the advantages of the classic Z-plasty over these other two irregularization techniques are significant and deserve discussion.[12] Both W-plasty and GBLC create an irregular scar line and a level surface by excising both the scar and adjacent normal tissue, and then carrying out a meticulous primary closure. Both of these techniques consist of excision of scar and normal tissue, creating shorter and more favorably oriented segments, and then a primary closure which changes the geometric shape of the scar. The closure is therefore carried out completely in normal tissue, creating a brand new scar without any gradual transitions. The classic Z-plasty, in contrast, accomplishes both of those goals and maximally preserves tissue. In addition, the well-planned Z-plasty is dynamic and physiologic, improving scar appearance in

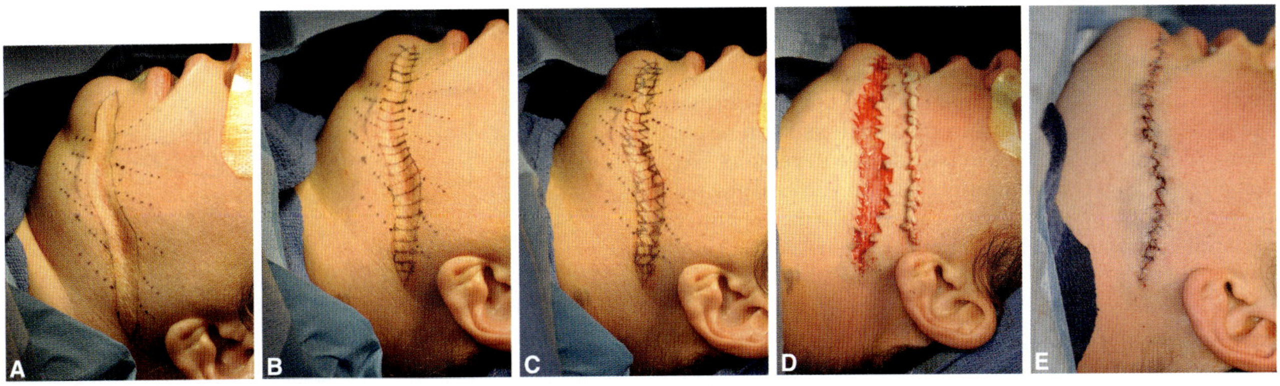

FIGURE 12-12 Geometric broken line closure. **A:** A 5 mm border is marked outside the scar to be excised and RSTLs are identified. **B:** 5 mm lines perpendicular to the scar are drawn, effectively making 5 mm squares on each side of the scar. **C:** Pseudorandom combinations of triangles and squares are designed to interdigitate, with as many limbs as possible aligning with RSTLs. **D:** After excision with acute corners, the wound "springs open" because of normal skin elasticity. Consider leaving the deepithelialized scar base in place to help maintain contour (Fig. 12-10). **E:** Undermine surrounding skin and advance edges together, interdigitating shapes with their directly apposed counterparts to close.

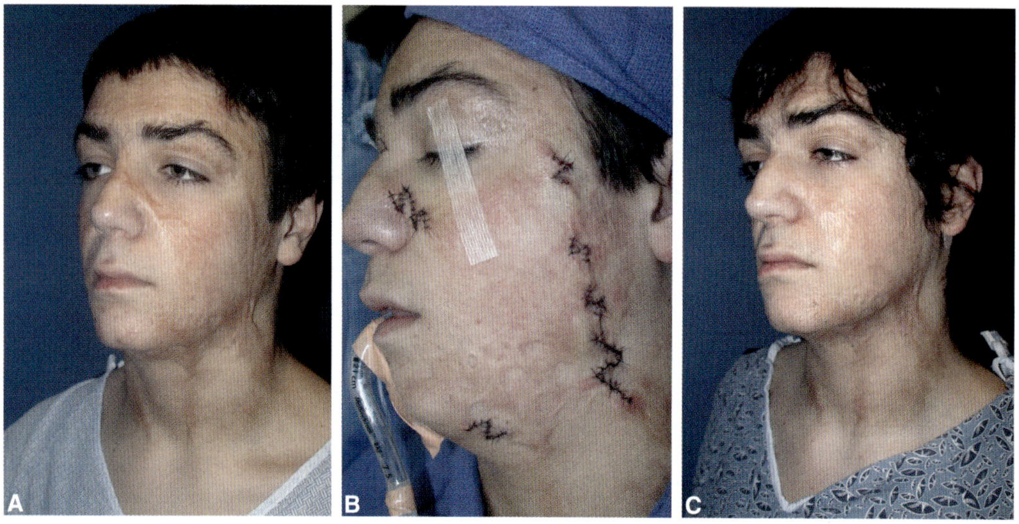

FIGURE 12-13 **A:** A 14-year-old boy with diffuse, linear, contracted, hypertrophic scars going from the bridge of the nose onto the cheek and from the cheek onto the neck. **B:** The scars were lengthened with Z-plasties, decreasing tension, and the limbs of the Z-plasties were oriented along RSTLs. **C:** Two years following scar revision, the geometric shape of the Z-plasties is inconspicuous. Note particularly the transition from the dorsum of the nose onto the cheek.

four dimensions, as time results in continuing improvement. Z-plasty also allows for the preservation of minimally damaged tissue, which helps to make the transition from normal skin into scar less conspicuous. Z-plasties in scar tissue are almost undetectable unless one knows they have been performed. This is a fact well known to experienced scar revision surgeons (Fig. 12-13).[13]

The W-plasty and GBLC are both static, and only change appearance in two dimensions. Both anatomically rearrange the scar to better follow RSTL at the expense of excising normal tissue. Z-plasty, however, in addition to breaking up the linear scar, relieves tension by recruiting lateral tissue and creates new transverse tension in a favorable direction that will improve with time—a form of tissue expansion in reverse. The goals of central scar lengthening and linear tension relief are accomplished on the day of the operation at the expense of creating elective lateral tension. The new, more favorably oriented, lateral tension can then proceed to rearrange itself in a beneficial way. Z-plasties also lower hypertrophic scars and elevate depressed scars without removing any normal tissue.[14] All of this is accomplished while preserving all of the normal skin elements. This is particularly important in the revision of scars which have resulted from partial-thickness dermal injuries with resulting hypertrophy, such as burn scars. Preservation of the dermis is important whenever possible. There is no reason to gratuitously excise and discard normal skin and dermis by converting a partial-thickness injury into a full-thickness iatrogenic injury by surgical excision.

Z-Plasty Fundamentals

Z-plasty is without doubt the most useful and valuable tool in surgical scar revision procedures. The first reported example of the Z-plasty—as we know and use it today—was described by Berger in 1904 for correction of an axillary burn contracture.[9] As noted before, the procedure consists of lengthening a central linear scar by transposing two lateral flaps centrally, providing additional tissue that allows the scar to be lengthened (Fig. 12-14).[15] In order for a Z-plasty to work, there must be a relative excess of tissue in the lateral location, allowing the flaps to move centrally without undue tension or unacceptable distortion of the adjacent lateral tissues. The concept is simple, brilliant, and actually capable of many more accomplishments than solely the lengthening of the central limb. In addition to lengthening the central linear contracture, Z-plasty can also be used to camouflage scars by making them more closely parallel skin TLs (Fig. 12-7).[7] As noted previously, it can lower hypertrophic scars, it can elevate depressed scars, and it can also be used to separate broad areas of scarring under tension, allowing them to mature in a much more favorable fashion.

FIGURE 12-14 Z-plasty. Lateral tissue is recruited centrally by transposing the two triangular flaps. This results in a lengthening of the scar as well as narrowing of the scar. The borders are made much more irregular which creates camouflage. *(Donelan MB. Principles of burn reconstruction. In: Thorne CH, ed.* Grabb & Smith's Plastic Surgery. *6th ed, Philadelphia, PA: Lippincott Williams & Wilkins; 2007.)*

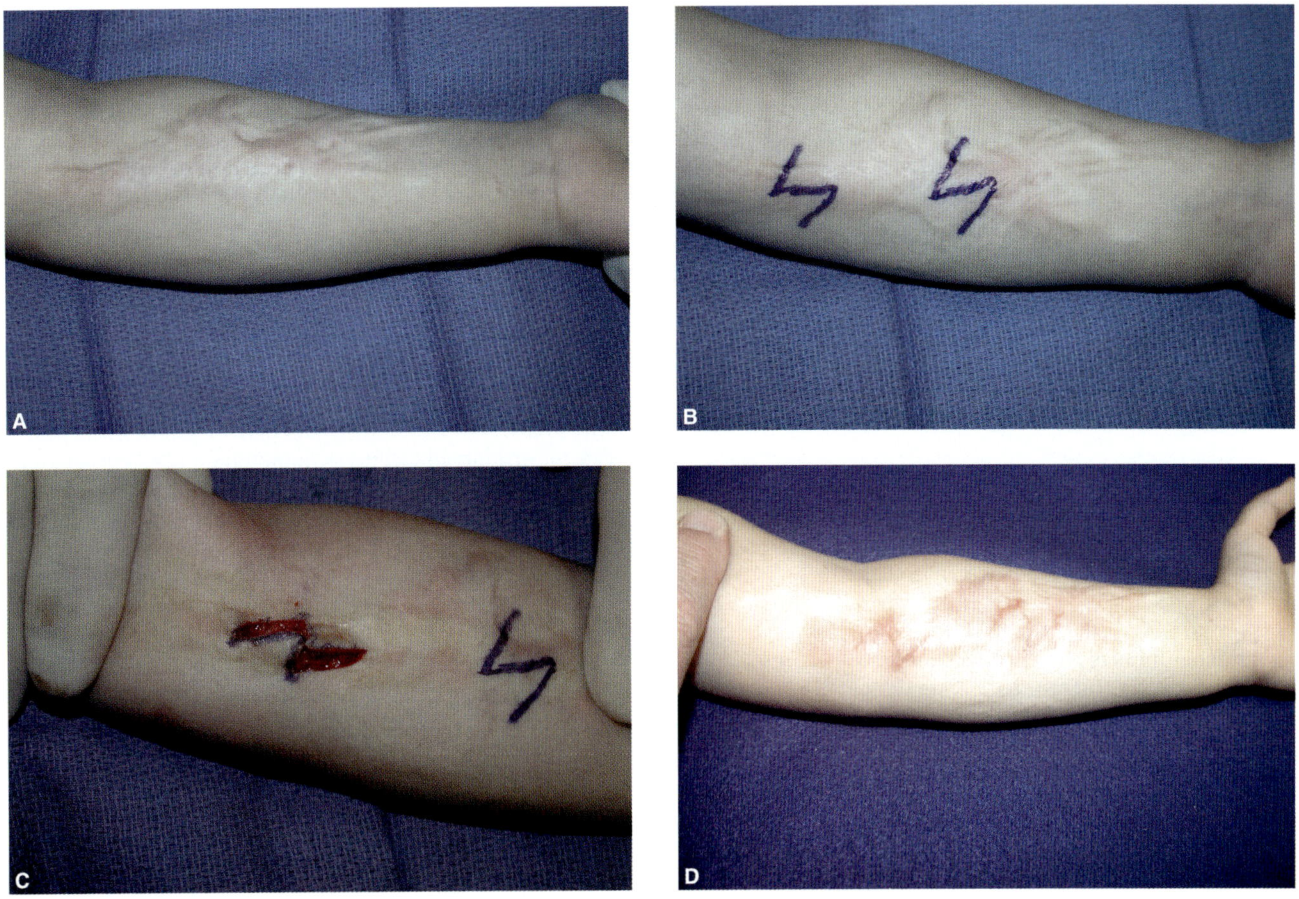

FIGURE 12-15 **A:** The beneficial effect of tension relief on scars with Z-plasty is profound. This patient had diffuse, hypertrophic, contracted scars of the forearm with narrow connecting segments. **B:** Two Z-plasties were designed to lengthen, narrow, and flatten the scars, as well as obscure the margins. **C:** Intraoperatively the Z-plasty almost transposes itself because of the favorable redistribution of tension. **D:** Six weeks later the remarkable effect of tension relief on scar maturation is dramatically illustrated by this case.

The design principles and effectiveness of the Z-plasty are well illustrated by the case shown in Figure 12-15. The narrow areas of the scars are identified. The central limb of each Z-plasty is drawn along the main line of longitudinal tension. The transverse limbs are designed parallel to the RSTLs as much as possible, and extended into normal tissue on either side of the hypertrophic scars.

In Figure 12-15C longitudinal tension is placed on the scar after the Z-plasty has been incised. It can be seen that the lateral tissue moves comfortably into the central location, decreases the longitudinal tension, and is easily recruited from its elastic base. The elasticity of the lateral tissue is essential for successful Z-plasty. The hypertrophic scars are flattened immediately in the operating room because the bases are located in the normal skin.

Figure 12-15D illustrates the powerful way the Z-plasty favorably alters the local environment of the scar, with dramatic improvement in maturation and appearance occurring after only 6 weeks. These same design concepts apply when using the Z-plasty technique in every type of scar revision situation. Z-plasty principles, and the technique itself, are simple and can be easily understood and performed. The endless number of different clinical situations is what makes it an art form. It is analogous to surgical jazz. The melody is simple but the variations are infinite and dependent only on the skill of the practitioner. Scar excision should be carried out only when the scar is unacceptable because of atrophy, hyperpigmentation, or other negative qualities.

The Z-plasty is typically described as dealing best with linear scars. The narrowing of wide scars by Z-plasty revision, however, can be very effective. A 60 degree Z-plasty lengthens the scar by 75%, while narrowing it by approximately 30%.[15] It is essential to note, however, that skin tension, flap thickness, location, and other individual factors can alter the theoretical changes in length and width of a Z-plasty.[16] As the shortest distance between two points is a straight line, as the lateral flaps are transposed with their base in normal tissue, a leveling effect is accomplished by the transverse limb (Fig. 12-15).

Because Z-plasty flaps are largely performed within scarred or previously grafted tissues, meticulous attention to technique is essential in order to prevent flap necrosis. Incisions must be made exactly perpendicular to the surface and every effort made to create flaps to look like "cheesecake" as opposed to "apple pie" (Fig. 12-16).

Accomplishing this technical goal prevents the deeper tissues from falling away from the surface, creating a dead space under the tip of the flap. This can lead to hematoma and ischemia, which cause flap tip necrosis. Attention to

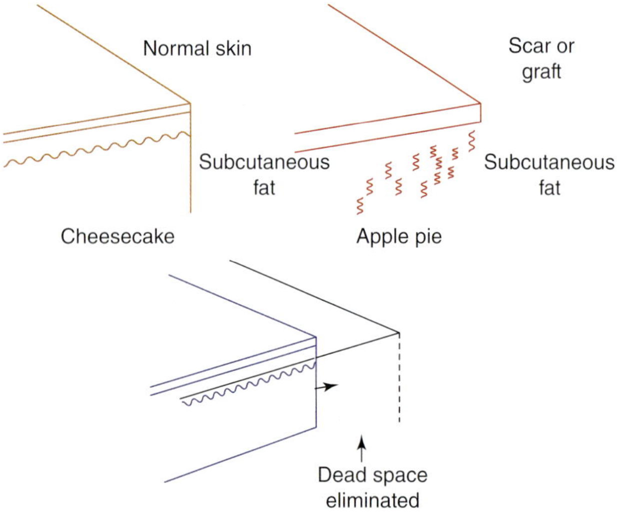

FIGURE 12-16 Attention to detail in the execution of the Z-plasty in scarred and grafted tissue is extremely important.

technique minimizes this problem and enables the Z-plasty to be a very powerful tool in dealing with contractures and scar irregularities in all types of tissues.

Category II: Scars After Injury to the Mid- to Deep Dermis from Burns or Trauma

This category of scars presents very different clinical challenges, and opportunities than linear scars from lacerations or full-thickness injuries. Scar revision surgery for this category involves all the principles previously discussed, while providing the opportunity to incorporate new scar rehabilitation principles currently transforming scar management. For over 50 years a great deal of emphasis has been placed on the improvement of posttraumatic deformities, in particular those stemming from burns, based on the concept of aesthetic units.[17] The rationale is that if an aesthetically important area is marred by scarring, then removing the scarred area in an aesthetic unit (even including normal tissue) and replacing it with either a graft or a flap from an uninjured part of the patient's body will result in a more natural appearance than improving the scars themselves. This was an innovative and intriguing concept in 1956 that has come to dominate modern plastic surgery thinking in many areas. It most likely has its true origin in the seminal work of Sir Harold Gillies as depicted in *The Principles and Art of Plastic Surgery*.[18] His outcomes in restoring facial appearance with tubed pedicle flaps were transformational and implied that flap replacement of scars was the best way to recreate normal appearance. Unfortunately, although that may have been true 100 years ago, today nothing could be further from the truth (Fig. 12-17).

At the present time it is necessary to rethink the concept of scar excision and resurfacing in aesthetic units. Patients' hypertrophic and contracted scars may well be their most valuable anatomy for reconstructive surgery. When scars can be effectively rehabilitated using local plastic surgery techniques and regenerative stimulation with photomedicine and pharmaceuticals, it provides great benefits to both the patient and the reconstructive surgeon.[19] Using the local scar tissue effectively to achieve your reconstructive goals is advantageous for multiple obvious reasons including those listed below:

- It is autologous tissue.
- It is in the right location.

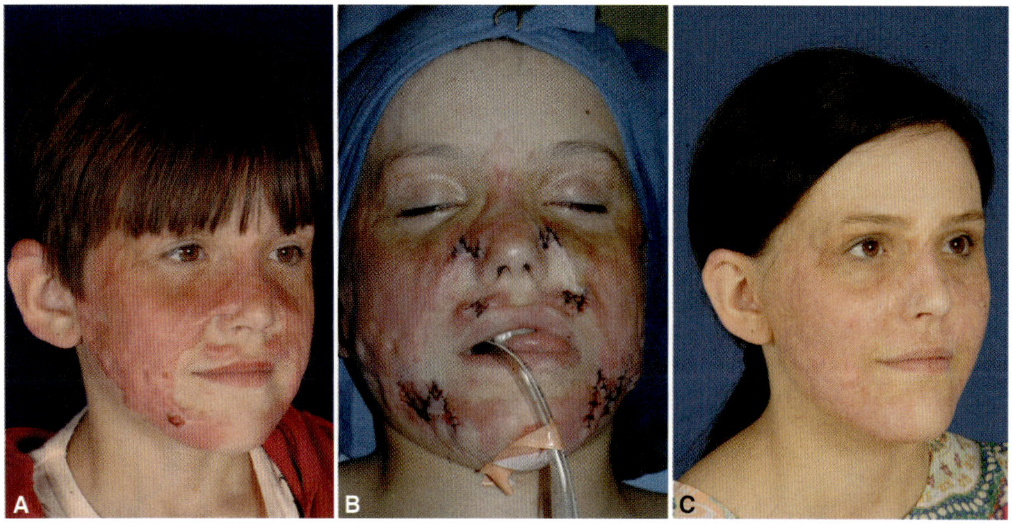

FIGURE 12-17 **A:** A 10-year-old girl 1 year following second- and third-degree burns to the face with contracture, hypertrophy, and ulceration. **B:** Contracted, hypertrophic scars are lengthened and narrowed in multiple areas where scars cross concavities, relieving tension on all the scars, and eliminating "bow-stringing." Z-plasties were also performed on the upper lip scars to flatten and relieve tension. **C:** Six years later following three small Z-plasty procedures and 12 laser treatments, her appearance is markedly improved with only mild dyspigmentation.

- It is original equipment.
- There is no additional deformity from elective donor sites.
- It allows for minimally morbid interventions.
- It is less complicated surgery with fewer risks of bad complications.

Futile and misguided efforts to "eliminate scars" by excising areas in aesthetic units have been a potential "fool's gold" since first proposed and have become far more dangerous for patients since the advent of tissue expansion and microsurgical capabilities. It is remarkable how much iatrogenic damage can be done by excisional scar therapy in Category II patients (Fig. 12-18). Equally remarkable, however, is how much "real gold" can be found within patients' hypertrophic and contracted scars, particularly patients who have sustained extensive burn injuries. As noted above, their scars are perfect reconstructive material, autologous, and in the right location. It is the responsibility of the reconstructive surgeon to be able to visualize the ways in which unfavorably acting and appearing scar tissue can be "rehabilitated" and turned into an asset for the patient. The patient shown in Figure 12-19 is an excellent example of what is possible through a combination of very minor, minimally morbid, surgical revisions to relieve tension combined with treatment using the pulsed-dye laser and fractional CO_2 laser with laser-assisted topical corticosteroid delivery (see Chapters 13 and 14). Excellent results can now be consistently obtained with minimal morbidity and tremendous patient satisfaction. We are truly at the dawn of a new era of revisional scar management that will likely result in less, and less extensive, scar excisions and fewer complex flap or graft reconstructions, which irreversibly harm other areas of the body with their donor site morbidity. We must strive to get better and better at rehabilitating scars, and at helping scars do the best possible job at regenerating themselves.

Category III: Full-Thickness Loss of Extensive Soft Tissue with Scarring

Category III scarring is important to include in this chapter because the absence of significant amounts of soft tissue clearly changes the prospects of improving a patient with a scar revision procedure. When there is absolute tissue loss and the scarring is already under significant tension, directing one's attention only to the revision of the objectionable scar itself can lead to very unfavorable outcomes for the patient. As noted before, the decision of whether to treat or not to treat an unsatisfactory scar is extremely important. When the underlying deformity that includes scarring is also predominantly the result of significant tissue loss, the tissue loss must be addressed. There is nothing worse than performing a procedure, or series of procedures, to improve the appearance of a scar and be left with a patient who has been devastated by the process. Before embarking on a scar revision sequence, it is essential that the treating physician/surgeon make the correct diagnosis, perform an accurate scar analysis, and be certain that the patient has realistic expectations. The patient shown in Figure 12-20 sustained significant tissue loss of the skin, vermilion, muscle, and mucosa from an electrical burn injury. Directing surgery at the thickened oral commissure scar would likely have worsened his condition. After adding new tissue from his tongue, and removing no scar, his appearance was significantly improved. Adequate tissue replacement was the most important part of this scar revision.[20]

Category IV: Keloid Scars

The distinction between hypertrophic and keloid scars is crucial (see Chapter 5). Keloids are fibroproliferative

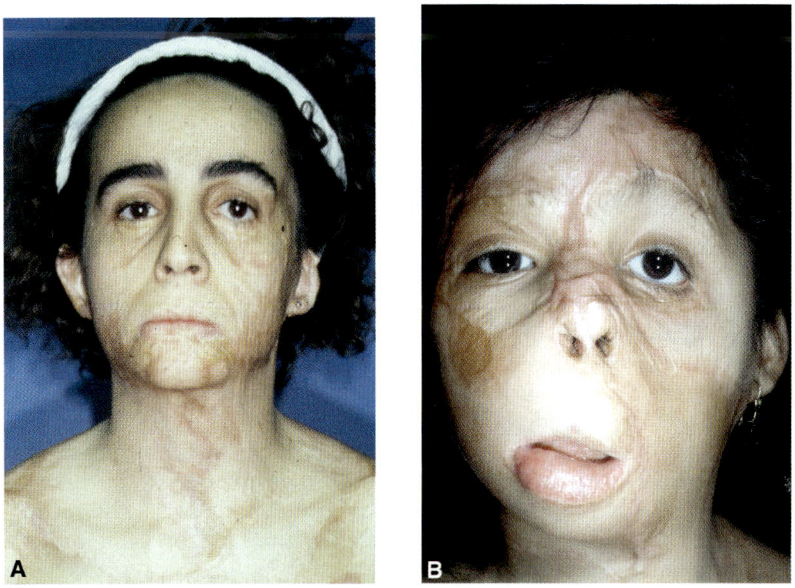

FIGURE 12-18 Both of these patients underwent more than 20 reconstructive operations consisting of extensive scar excision and replacement with flaps including tissue expansion and free tissue transfers.

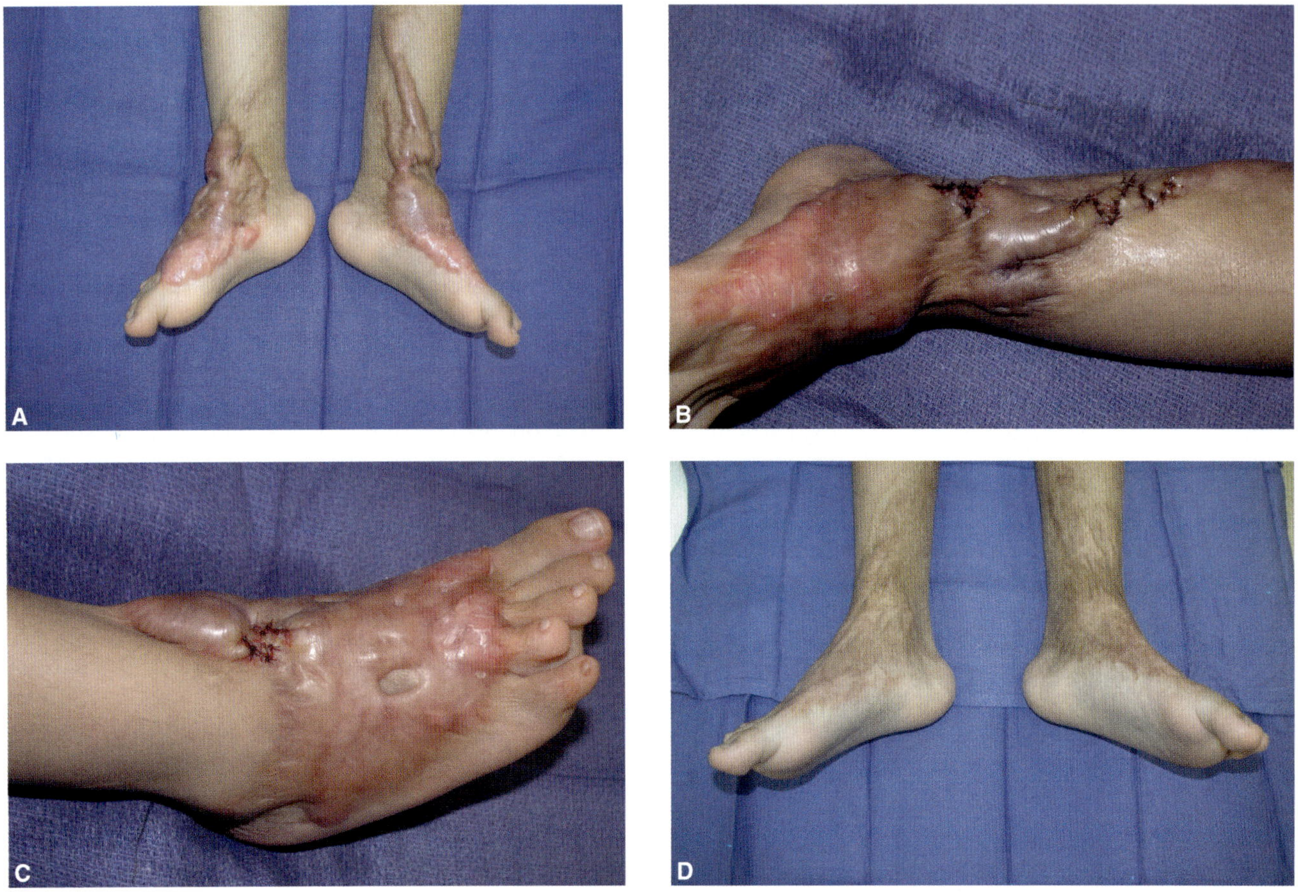

FIGURE 12-19 **A:** A 3-year-old child with bilateral scald burn injuries to the dorsum of the foot and ankle with massive hypertrophic scarring. **B, C:** Tension-relieving Z-plasties were carried out on both feet on two separate occasions. Multiple treatments were performed with the pulsed dye laser and fractionated CO_2 laser with laser-assisted topical corticosteroid delivery. **D:** Four years later the patient is asymptomatic with minor contractures.

dermal tumors with effusive accumulation of extracellular matrix components, particularly collagen, and result from excessive expression of growth factors and cytokines resulting in continual growth and rare regression. Keloids, unlike hypertrophic scars, traditionally do not appear to enter a quiescent/regenerative phase, and continue to infiltrate surrounding tissues growing beyond the original scar borders.[21] Additionally, keloid patients have a genetic predisposition consistent with an autosomal dominant condition. Keloids are thought to form in areas of high skin tension; however, they can occur in areas of low tension such as the earlobe. Keloids are very likely to recur after surgical excision and closure alone; current literature suggests a recurrence rate of 45% to 100% in these circumstances.[22] Therefore, the excision of keloids should only be performed in conjunction with adjuvant therapies such as steroids or radiation.[23] Steroids reduce the recurrence of excised keloids to less than 50%, whereas radiation reduces recurrence to less than 10%.[7] In the particular instance of earlobe keloids, button compression after excision reduces recurrence rates.[24] Given the unpredictable response of keloids to any tissue injury, case series demonstrating the failure of full-field (nonfractionated) CO_2 laser intervention to prevent recurrence, and the paucity of data on the efficacy of fractionated CO_2 laser interventions, ablative laser procedures should be used with caution even in the hands of experienced scar surgeons.[21,25] Similarly, a Z-plasty or a local tissue rearrangement which decreases tension may further exacerbate keloid formation and should also be embarked upon with similar caution.

Conclusion

History, science, technology, and a better understanding of wound healing and scar maturation have ushered in the greatest era ever for performing scar revision. Local tissue rearrangement to relieve scar tension, in combination with photomedicine and pharmacology, has created a new paradigm for surgical scar revision. Accurate scar analysis and these powerful tools allow us to maximize the benefit of the patient's own wound healing and scar remodeling abilities. This is a remarkable improvement in the way we think of scars. One thing is certain—in the future it should become less and less common that the first step in a scar revision procedure is the excision of the scar.

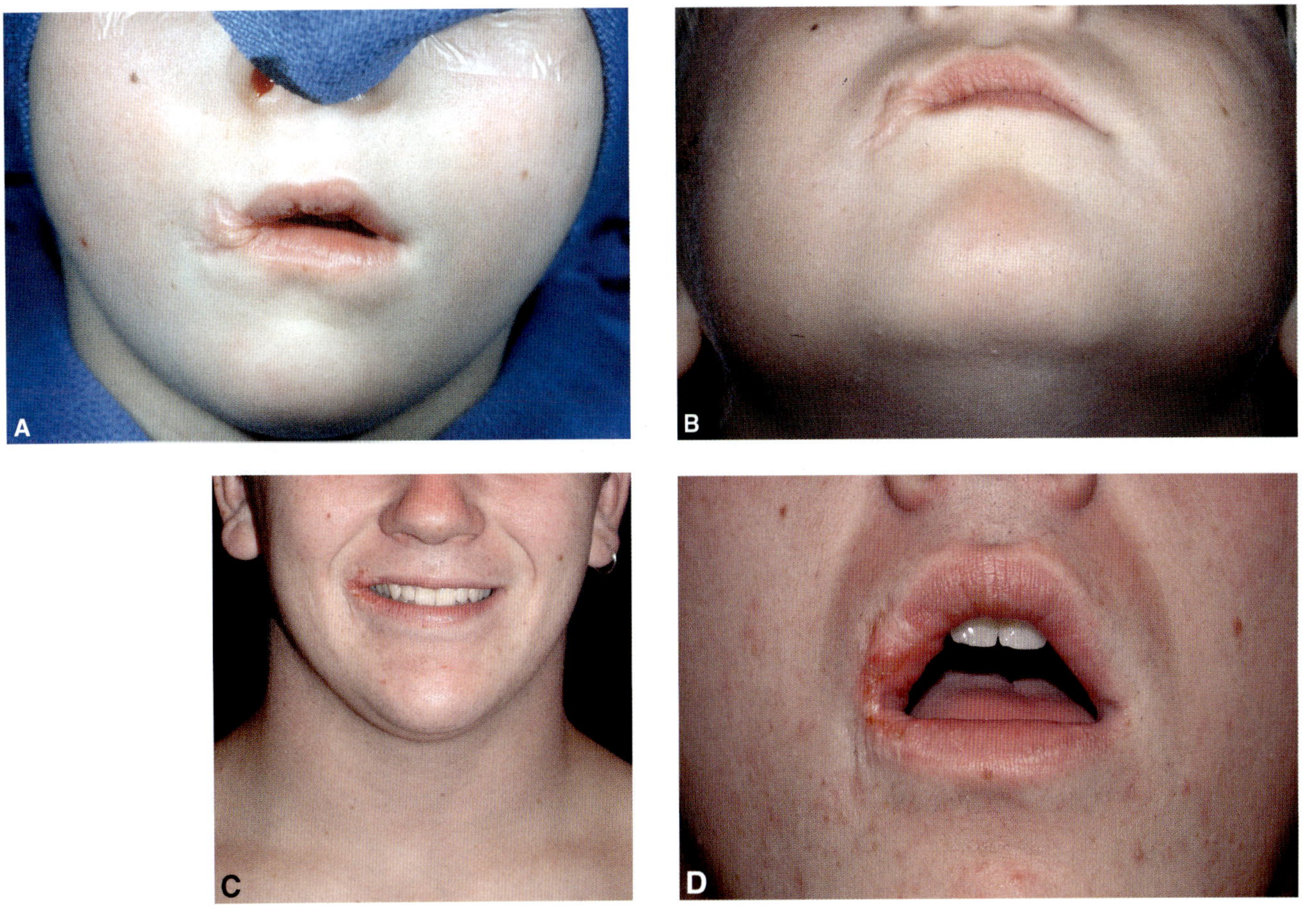

FIGURE 12-20 **A, B:** A 5-year-old boy 3 years after an electrical burn of the right oral commissure. There was extensive loss of skin, vermilion, mucosa, and muscle. Contraction during the wound healing process caused obvious displacement of the upper and lower lips, as well as a thick, prominent scar. **C, D:** Following the provision of additional tissue from the ventral surface of his tongue including muscle and mucosa, the oral commissure scar has become inconspicuous even though no scar tissue was removed.

Disclaimer

The views expressed in this chapter are those of the authors and do not necessarily reflect the official policy or position of the Department of Defense or the United States Government. Dr. Gaball is a military service member. This work was prepared as part of his official duties. Title 17, USC, § 105 provides that 'Copyright protection under this title is not available for any work of the United States Government.' Title 17, USC, § 101 defines a U.S. Government work as a work prepared by a military service member or employee of the U.S. Government as part of that person's official duties.

REFERENCES

1. Kraisel CJ. The selection of appropriate lines for elective surgical incisions. *Plast Reconstr Surg*. 1951;8:1–28.
2. Borges AF. Scar analysis and objectives of revision procedures. *Clin Plast Surg*. 1977;4:223–227.
3. Courtiss E, Longacre JJ, Destefano GA, et al. The placement of elective skin incisions. *Plast Reconstr Surg*. 1963;31:31–44.
4. McGregor IA. *Fundamental Techniques of Plastic Surgery and Their Surgical Applications*. Edinburgh, Sweden: Churchill Livingstone; 1962.
5. McCarthy J. *Plastic Surgery General Principles*. Philadelphia, PA: Saunders; 1990.
6. Thorne I. *Grabb & Smith's Plastic Surgery*. 7th ed. Philadelphia, PA: Lippincott Williams and Wilkins; 2014.
7. Shockley WW. Scar revision techniques: z-plasty, w-plasty, and geometric broken line closure. *Facial Plast Surg Clin North Am*. 2011;19(3):455–463.
8. Borges AF. Improvement of anti-tension line scars by the W-plastic operation. *Br J Plast Surg*. 1959;12:27.
9. Borges AF. Historical review of Z-plastic techniques. *Clin Plast Surg*. 1977;4:207–215.
10. Wessberg GA, Hill SC. Revision of facial scars with geometric broken line closure. *J Oral Maxillofac Surg*. 1982;40:492–496.
11. Ausin A. The "trap door" scar deformity. *Clin Plast Surg*. 1977;4: 255–261.
12. MacGregor IA. The Z-plasty. *Br J Plast Surg*. 1966;9:82–87.
13. Davis JS. Relaxation of scar contractures by means of the Z-, or reversed Z-type incision; stressing the use of scar infiltrated tissues. *Ann Surg*. 1931;94:871.
14. Marino H. The levelling effect of Z-plasties on lineal scars of the face. *Br J Plast Surg*. 1959;12:34–42.

15. Donelan MB. Principles of burn reconstruction. In: Thorne CH, ed. *Grabb & Smith's Plastic Surgery*. 6th ed, Philadelphia, PA: Lippincott Williams & Wilkins; 2007.
16. Rohrich RJ, Zbar RI. A simplified algorithm for the use of Z-plasty. *Plast Reconstr Surg*. 1999;103(5):1513–1518.
17. Gonzalez-Ulloa M. Restoration of the face covering by means of selected skin in regional aesthetic units. *Br J Plast Surg*. 1956;9:212–221.
18. Gilles H, Millard R. *The Principles and Art of Plastic Surgery*. London: Butterworth; 1957:463.
19. Donelan MB, Parrett BM, Sheridan RL. Pulsed dye laser therapy and z-plasty for facial burn scars: the alternative to excision. *Ann Plast Surg*. 2008;60:480–486.
20. Donelan MB. Reconstruction of electrical burns of the oral commissure with a ventral tongue flap. *Plast Reconstr Surg*. 1995;95:1155–1164.
21. Norris JE. The effect of carbon dioxide laser surgery on the recurrence of keloids. *Plast Reconstr Surg*. 1991;87(1):44–49.
22. Mustoe TA, Cooter RD, Gold MH, et al. International clinical recommendations on scar management. *Plast Reconstr Surg*. 2002;110(2):560–571.
23. Gauglitz GG, Korting HC, Pavicic T, et al. Hypertrophic scarring and keloids: pathomechanisms and current and emerging treatment strategies. *Mol Med*. 2011;17(1–2):113.
24. Berman B, Bieley HC. Adjunct therapies to surgical management of keloids. *Dermatol Surg*. 1996;22(2):126–130.
25. Apfelberg DB, Maser MR, White DN, et al. Failure of carbon dioxide laser excision of keloids. *Lasers Surg Med*. 1989;9(4):382–388.

13

Lasers and Light Devices in Scar Management

EDWARD VICTOR ROSS and JAMES DANIEL JENSEN

KEY POINTS

- Scar treatment with lasers should be guided by the features of the scar and the respective mechanisms of action of available technologies.
- Typical scar reduction requires multiple treatments, potentially with multiple modalities; slow incremental improvement is the rule.
- Laser treatment is often combined with injectable antimetabolites or corticosteroids to optimize outcomes.

Almost everyone has a scar, and although the prevalence of scars remains relatively unchanged, lasers and light sources have advanced their treatment. The foundation of the proper management of scars with lasers is an understanding of laser–tissue interactions. The outcome of these interventions depends both on the immediate laser–tissue interaction and on the cascade of wound healing events that follow.

The pathogenesis and wound healing aspects of scars are examined in other sections of the book (see Chapters 6, 9, and 10). In brief, at least in the case of a scar that begins as an open wound, early reepithelialization is the best predictor of the behavior of the scar over the next 6 months. Longer reepithelialization times, typically associated with deeper injures or those located on "underprivileged" skin (i.e., neck, upper chest, legs—almost any region off the face), are associated with a greater risk of hypertrophic or atrophic scarring.

In this chapter, we will concentrate on "open wound" scars as opposed to wounds that are closed primarily. However, the same principles may be applied to suboptimal scars resulting from surgical procedures. Once the skin has reepithelialized, typically occurring over a period of 1 to 4 weeks, a role for laser technology is most commonly considered. Not every scar requires an intervention, and the treating physician must consider which scars would benefit from laser treatment versus those that will benefit from tincture of time alone. Most studies of the role of lasers in scar reduction rely on nonobjective findings, and a healthy amount of skepticism should be directed toward publications or other observations that rely solely on visual improvements. The natural tendency for most scars is typically one of progressive gradual improvement. Therefore, the role of lasers is potentially twofold: (1) accelerate the spontaneous improvement in color, tone, and texture and (2) improve the ultimate form and function of scars that would otherwise not be observed in the natural course of healing. Another role for devices in scar management is "prevention." Some studies have reported that laser procedures performed at the time of surgery or just before surgery can modulate the wound healing process.[1,2] In some scenarios, this intervention can reduce the potential for adverse scarring.

Introduction to Lasers

Laser is an acronym for Light Amplification by Stimulated Emission of Radiation.[3] Initially postulated by Albert Einstein in 1917 when he first introduced the concept of stimulated emission, the idea was enabled by the work of several scientists over the next four decades. The first viable laser device was demonstrated in 1960. Since that time, lasers have become available for numerous medical applications. In the early days of lasers, physicians feared that lasers, like ionizing radiation, might have some potential long-term effects on the skin such as mutagenicity and cancer. Fifty-five years later, these concerns have been largely dismissed.

Principles of Laser–Tissue Interactions

The laser operator should appreciate the fundamental principles of laser–tissue interactions. An understanding of how laser light interacts with the skin from a macroscopic and microscopic perspective allows the treating physician to optimize treatment results. Scar enhancement with lasers relies on a normalization of histology and a reduction in the contrast between scar tissue and adjacent unscarred skin.

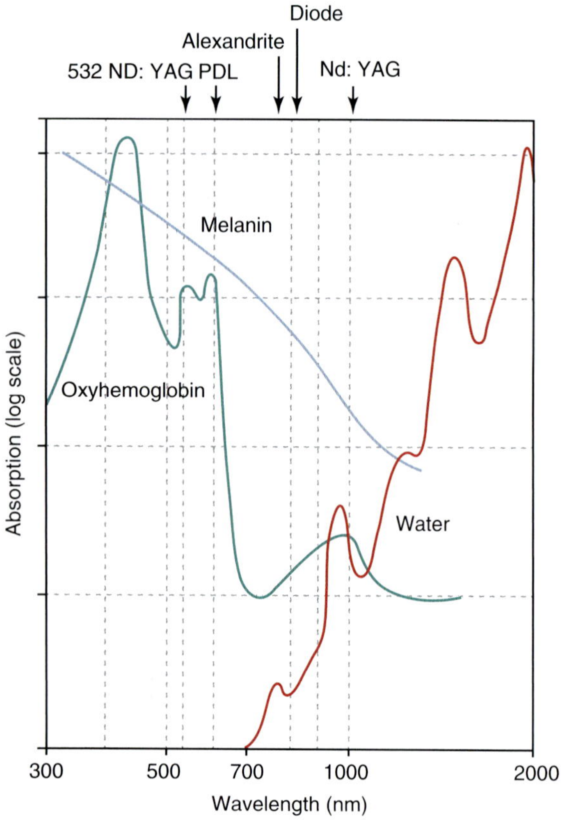

FIGURE 13-1 Absorption spectra for three major skin chromophores. *(From Figure 1.15 in Goldman MP, Fitzpatrick RE, Ross EV, et al., eds., 2013.* Lasers and Energy Devices for the Skin. *Boca Raton, FL: CRC Press.)*

Any light-based technology that modulates the behavior of a scar must take into account all of the potential opportunities to exploit the "contrast agents," or chromophores, that differentiate the scar from normal skin.[4–7] These contrast agents allow for selective heating of various components of the skin and, thus, selective modulation of the histology, appearance, and function of the scar.[8] For example, when selectively targeting the red color in a scar, one applies wavelengths that selectively heat the blood vessels associated with the scar and avoids damaging the innocent bystander—in this case, the normal skin (Fig. 13-1).

Likewise, for treating a pigmented scar with a nonfractional technology, one might apply a wavelength that takes advantage of any pigment difference between the scar and surrounding skin.

There are several ways to limit heating with lasers to specific targets. In one scenario, using ubiquitous tissue water as the chromophore, laser "beams" are spatially confined by either using a microbeam with scanners or simply by having the operator, with the aid of magnifying loupes, use a small beam (0.2 to 2 mm) to precisely target a scar. An example is an exophytic scar related to acne, where the physician can precisely "whittle" the scar down, as one would knock down a stack of coins one by one. The other scenario is where the laser targets the scar based on the theory of selective photothermolysis (SPT), where wavelength and pulse duration direct heating only to areas with excess melanin or blood.[5,9,10] According to this theory, through appropriate selection of pulse duration and wavelength, one can confine heat to a particular chromophore (i.e., pigment, hemoglobin [HgB], or water) within the scar. Shorter pulses generally are more likely to confine heat to the target, whereas longer pulses are less selective in heating. On the other hand, extremely short pulses can result in a very "violent" heating of the target (particularly in the case of Q-switched nanosecond or picosecond range lasers) where the subsequent inflammatory reaction can result in postinflammatory hyperpigmentation (PIH). This is of particular concern in darker skinned patients (see Chapter 18).[11,12] Moreover, in the case of vascular scars, very short pulses can result in purpura; although purpura is sometimes a desirable reaction, in the setting of facial scar treatment purpura might limit social or work obligations.

The other primary determinant of selective heating is wavelength. In the absence of absorption—that is, in the absence of significant water, blood, or melanin absorption—longer wavelengths over the range of 400 to 2,000 nm penetrate deeper than shorter wavelengths. However, as wavelengths increase beyond 2,000 nm, the relative absorption of water increases, thereby limiting the depth of penetration (Fig. 13-2A,B). This phenomenon should be a consideration in proper selection of parameters for optimal scar management.

One can think of light interacting with the skin in a similar manner as with other optical phenomena, where there is a loss of a fraction of incident light from reflection and scattering upon contact with the skin surface. In short, upon initial impact of light on the surface, a portion of the incident light is reflected (about 5%), and the remainder enters into the skin just below the stratum corneum.[7,13] Once the light has penetrated the skin surface, the skin's optical properties determine the propagation of light.

In general, three effects guide the propagation of light in the skin (Fig. 13-3):

1. Reflection and refraction
2. Absorption
3. Scattering

For purposes of the skin, where the medium is opaque, refraction is hard to measure within the context of absorption and scattering. If we consider a slice of skin in cross section, only a portion of photons will be transmitted to the base of the slice. These are the nonreflected, nonabsorbed, and forward-scattered photons. When a surface is smooth, the reflection is said to be "specular," and when it is rough, the reflection is said to be "diffuse." As most tissue is rough, save for some wet surfaces, diffuse reflection typically exceeds specular reflection (Fig. 13-4). Refraction occurs when two media show different light velocities in their respective regions. This causes bending of the light at the interface (Fig. 13-5). Reflectance is the ratio of the intensities of reflected light to the intensity of the light propagating to the next layer. Reflectance depends on the angle of incidence, the polarization of the radiation, and indices of refraction of the two media at the boundary.

Generally, as the angle of incidence (the angle between the light ray and the direction perpendicular to the skin

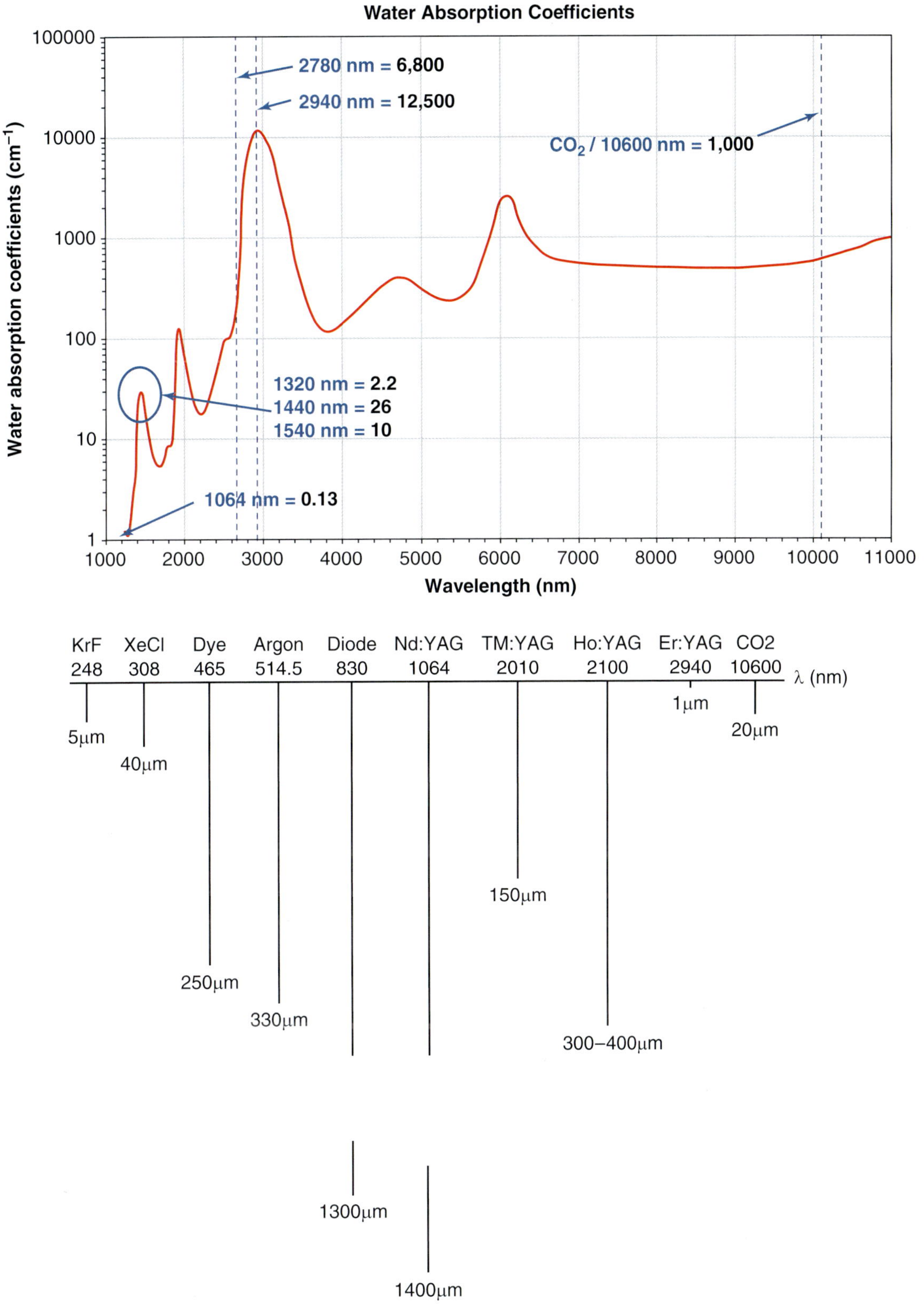

FIGURE 13-2 **A:** Water absorption spectrum. **B:** Relative depths of penetration for various wavelengths. *(B from Figure 2.11 in Welch AJ, Van Gemert MJ, eds.* Optical-Thermal Response of Laser-Irradiated Tissue. *New York, NY: Plenum Press; 1995.)*

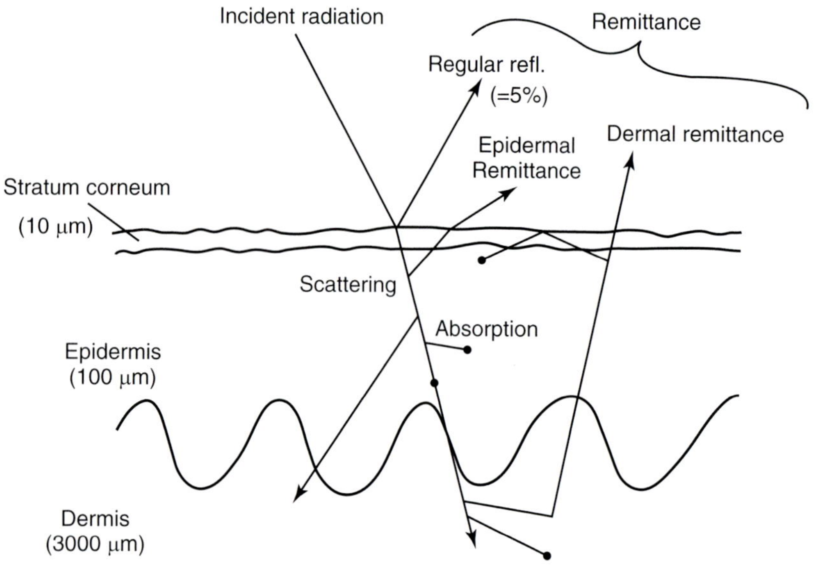

FIGURE 13-3 Figure showing the behavior of light at the skin interface. *(From Figure 1 in Anderson RR, Parrish JA. The optics of human skin.* J Investig Dermatol. *1981;77(1):13–19.)*

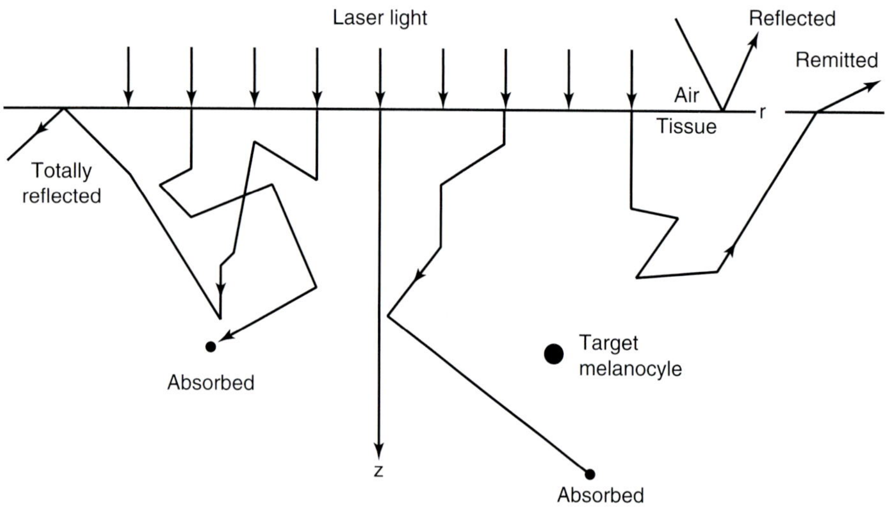

FIGURE 13-4 Random path of photons in skin. *(From Figure 2.3 in Welch AJ, Van Gemert MJ, eds.* Optical-Thermal Response of Laser-Irradiated Tissue. *New York, NY: Plenum Press; 1995.)*

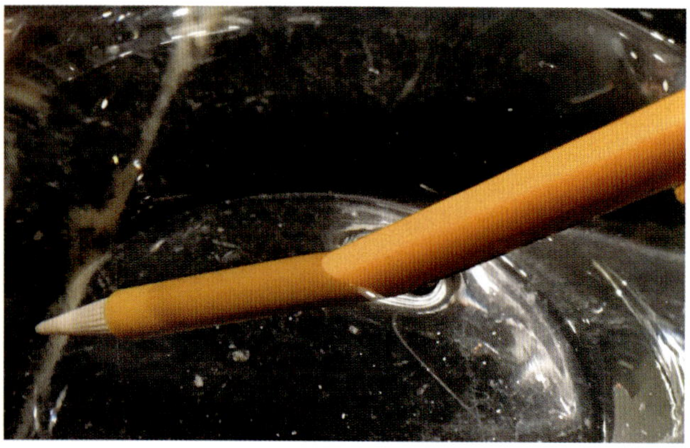

FIGURE 13-5 Effect of refraction as light moves from materials of different indices of refraction.

surface) approaches 90 degrees, reflectance increases. The absorbance of a medium is defined as the ratio of the absorbed and incident intensities. Selective absorption is the absorption of certain wavelengths over others.

Attenuation of the laser beam due to absorption is directed by Beer–Lambert law.

This law states that the absorption "length" in the tissue is given by

$$Z = \frac{1}{\propto}\ln\left(\frac{I_0}{I_z}\right), \qquad \text{(Eq. 1)}$$

where Z is the distance over which the intensity diminishes to $1/e$ of its incident "strength," I_z is the intensity at the depth z, I_o is the incident intensity, and α is the absorption coefficient.

The inverse of this coefficient is the absorption length, or

$$L = 1/\propto . \qquad \text{(Eq. 2)}$$

In the infrared (IR) region, water is the main absorber, whereas in the visual and ultraviolet (UV) portions of the spectrum, proteins and pigment are the primary absorbers. The two primary discrete absorbers in skin are HgB and melanin. Melanin is the main chromophore in the epidermis, and its absorption decreases almost linearly as a function of wavelength over 400 to 1,000 nm. HgB has relative peaks at 280, 420, 540, and 580 nm, with a much smaller peak at 940 nm (Fig. 13-1). As neither water nor HgB absorbs strongly between 600 and 1,200 nm, there is a so-called therapeutic window in this range where light penetrates more deeply.[7,13]

Absorption is related to specific wavelength-dependent bonds, where particles are set into motion by electromagnetic (EM) fields; the frequency of the wave makes for transitional (electron transition level changes in the shell chemical model) or vibrational changes in the target. With scattering, the frequencies do not match but rather result in forced vibration, causing photons to slow down in a denser medium.

Usually we consider a turbid medium (like the skin) as showing both absorption and scattering, and we can define two coefficients that characterize the attenuation of light in the skin (scattering and absorption coefficients). A good "phantom" for the dermis is milk, a turbid material that scatters light much like the skin. If one, for example, takes a laser pointer and applies it to the surface of a glass of milk, one will observe the linear beam spread just beneath the surface. There are many methods to analyze the nature of scattering in the skin, among them Monte Carlo models (where statistical models of chance characterize the migration of photons in the skin).[14,15] One should note that the skin is heterogeneous and fragile, and many of the predicted behaviors of light and the skin are not reliably observed. Ultimately, the immediate end response is the best predictor of the therapeutic outcome for any laser tissue interaction,[16,17] and this concept is especially true in scar management and rehabilitation.

The nonpigmented portion of the epidermis and the dermis serves as a scattering medium, whereas blood, melanin, and water contained in these layers act as the most significant chromophores (absorbers) within the skin. If one examines the absorbance of blood, melanin, and water along the EM spectrum shown in Figure 13-1, blood and melanin absorption is most prominent along the 400 to 800 nm portion of the EM spectrum, whereas water has little absorbance within this range. The absorbance of water, however, increases significantly in the IR portion of the EM spectrum, with an absorption peak at 2,940 nm (Fig. 13-2A).

In any laser–tissue interaction, the local peak elevation in temperature is characterized by the following equation:

$$\Delta T = \frac{F_z \mu_a}{\rho c}\left(\frac{\tau_r}{\tau_r + \tau_p}\right)^{g/2}, \qquad \text{(Eq. 3)}$$

where F_z is the local subsurface fluence, ρ is the density, c is the specific heat, g is a geometric factor ("1" for planes, "2" for cylinders, and "3" for spheres), τ_p is the laser pulse duration, and τ_r is the thermal relaxation time of the target (time for target to cool to 37% of peak temperature), defined by:

$$\tau_r = \frac{D^2}{gK}, \qquad \text{(Eq. 4)}$$

where D is the thickness or diameter of the target, g is the geometric factor referenced earlier, and K is the thermal diffusivity (a measure that includes the heat capacity and thermal conductivity of the material). For example, a potato would show a relatively low thermal diffusivity because of its low thermal conductivity and high specific heat, whereas a small metal tattoo particle would show a high thermal diffusivity.

F_z is determined largely by the attenuation by scattering and absorption. The probabilities of absorption or scattering (designated μ_a and μ_s, respectively) are determined by experiment. For example, for a μ_a of 0.3 per cm, the mean free path before absorption is $1/\mu_a$, or 3.3 cm. Generally, light is attenuated as it propagates through tissue. In turbid tissue (i.e., the dermis, where collagen acts as the major scatterer), the fluence attenuation can be described by:

$$F(z) = F_o k^{e(-z/\delta)}, \qquad \text{(Eq. 5)}$$

where F_o is the incident fluence, $F(z)$ is the local subsurface fluence at some depth z, k is a constant that accounts for backscattered light, and δ is the wavelength-dependent optical penetration depth of light, or the depth at which there is attenuation to 37% of the surface value (37% = $1/e$, where $e = 2.7$, the base of the natural logarithm). This depth is determined by absorption and scattering coefficients, as related by the simple equation below:

$$\delta = \frac{1}{\sqrt{3\mu_a(\mu_a + \mu_s(1-g))}}. \qquad \text{(Eq. 6)}$$

Blood

The greatest practical absorption peaks for blood are in the green and yellow spectral regions. Most of the blood in the skin is in the form of oxygenated HgB; however, approximately 30% is in the deoxygenated state, and a still smaller fraction is in the methemoglobin state.[18]

Recent work has highlighted the optimal wavelengths for targeting venous versus arterial blood (primarily mirroring the relative fractions of oxygenated and deoxygenated HgB). However, the optimal wavelengths for targeting venous versus arterial blood also have overall lower associated blood absorption coefficients. For example, a much lower fluence would be required to generate reduction of erythema using green-yellow light wavelengths (e.g., 532 and 595 nm) than, for example, the alexandrite laser (755 nm, near-IR spectrum, preferentially targeting deoxygenated HgB), where very large fluences must be delivered to achieve a similar effect.[19]

Melanin

Melanin has a broad absorption spectrum. This broad absorption helps to protect the skin from harmful radiation from the sun. In patients with a lighter skin phenotype (i.e., Fitzpatrick type I, II), pigment lying within a scar is easily targeted because of the relative lack of pigment in the surrounding, normal skin. In darker skin types, however, the laser operator should take care not to overtreat pigment within a scar and cause further dyspigmentation (i.e., hypopigmentation). The broad absorption spectrum of melanin is a double-edged sword. On one hand, the broad absorption allows many types of lasers to target pigment within the skin, thus giving the laser operator many choices for treating unwanted melanin deposition. On the other hand, many lasers that are intended to target other chromophores (i.e., blood) can also unintentionally be absorbed

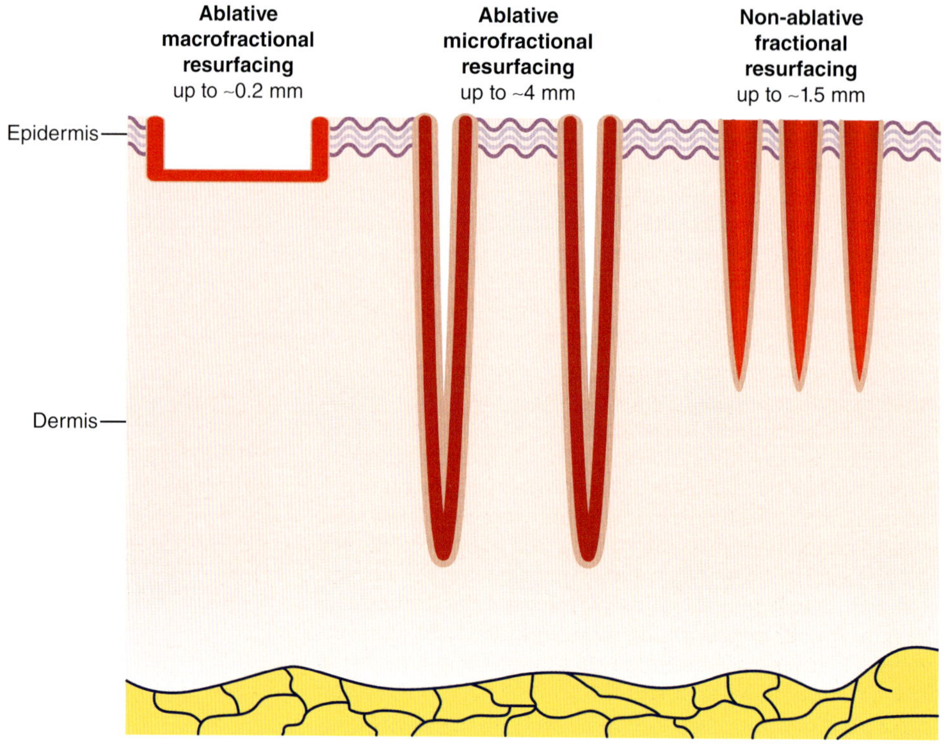

FIGURE 13-6 Cross section of the fractional pattern of injury associated with CO_2 ablative fractional laser resurfacing. Each ablative column is surrounded by a narrow rim of coagulation, and ample areas of untreated intervening tissue allow for depths of penetration up to several millimeters and rapid healing.

by melanin.[20] Usually, melanin is found in the epidermis superficial to the excess blood (with the exception of some scars with excess dermal melanin—usually long-standing scars or acne scars associated with medication-induced dyspigmentation, such as from the drug minocycline). It follows that treating a red scar in dark skin is a challenge. This is because melanin has a broad and relatively nonspecific spectrum of absorption, and will absorb the energy from a laser directed toward blood. Consequently, if a patient with Fitzpatrick type IV skin were to present for treatment of hyperemia associated with a thyroid scar, the operator must reduce settings to avoid overtreatment of the epidermis. Fortunately, however, the same melanin that poses such a concern for the laser operator also tends to mask underlying hyperemia.[21–23]

Water

Water is ubiquitous in the skin, and wavelength ranges from 1,200 to 2,000 nm show intermediate absorption, whereas 2,940 nm (erbium:yttrium–aluminum–garnet—Er:YAG laser output) and 10,600 nm (carbon dioxide—CO_2 laser output) show very strong absorption. It follows that the former wavelengths are associated with nonablative or semi-ablative treatments, and the latter with purely ablative treatments. Both ablative and nonablative wavelengths are applied with scanners that can deliver the energy in a fractional manner, meaning that a grid-like pattern of columns of controlled tissue damage may be reliably produced (Fig. 13-6).[24–27] Through proper selection of wavelength, pulse duration, and microspot diameter (normally between 100 and 430 μm), a particular cross-sectional density and depth of wounds can be created. The typical geometry of the wounds is cylindrical craters. However, other manufacturers have designed lasers that create a cross-hatched grid pattern of microinjuries. Radiofrequency (RF) needle devices can also create controlled thermal injuries in a fractionated pattern; deeper injuries with relative epidermal sparing can be achieved through the use of insulated needles.[28]

Interaction Types

Most laser–tissue interactions are thermal in nature. Other potential mechanisms are photochemical (e.g., photodynamic therapy, PDT) and plasma-induced ablation (termed photoablation or photodisruption) (Fig. 13-7). Photodisruption is a form of minimally invasive surgery used in ophthalmology; IR neodymium (Nd):YAG lasers form a plasma ("lightning bolt"), which then causes acoustic shock waves (like a "thunderclap"), which in turn affects tissue.

Photochemical

PDT has been used in the management of some scars. In one study Chang et al.[29] examined aminolevulinic acid (ALA) PDT in scars and the mechanism of action. They found that for fibroblast cell cultures from hypertrophic scars, apoptosis was observed through a p53-associated signaling pathway. Challenges in PDT include (a) achieving sufficient accumulation of ALA in fibroblasts versus the epidermis and (b) pain management. Another obstacle is penetration of the light, as the presumed fibroblast targets reside up to several millimeters deep in the dermis for thicker scars.[29,30]

Another type of intervention is *biostimulation* (aka low-level light therapy, LLLT), where presumably certain frequencies of light can modify mitochondrial behavior through the cytochrome system. For example, Freitas et al.[31] showed that LLLT works by interacting with the cytochrome system in cells, such that changes in adenosine triphosphate and

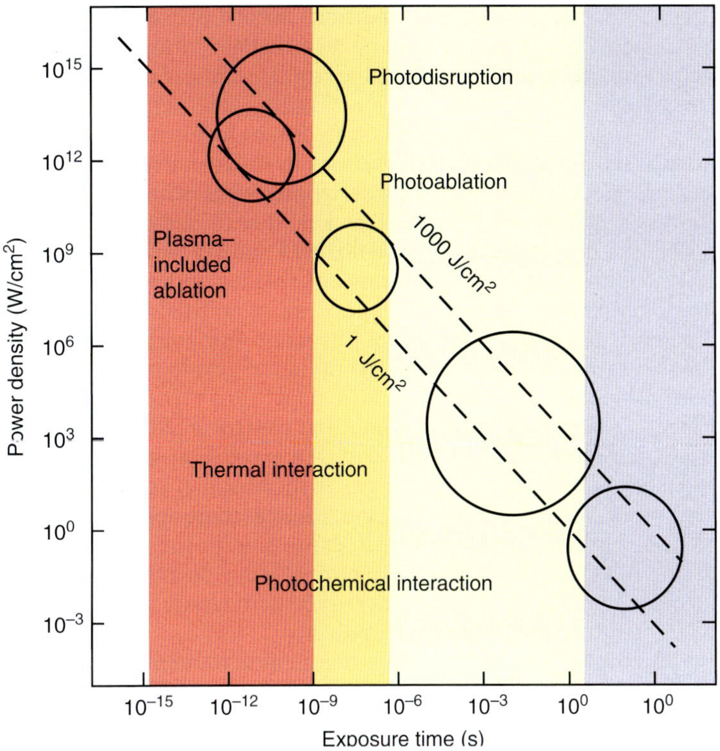

FIGURE 13-7 Range of tissue interactions as a function of power density. *(From Boulnois JL. Photophysical processes in recent medical laser developments: a review.* Lasers Med Sci. *1986;1(1):47–66.)*

interleukin 6 expression have been noted. LLLT usually involves wavelengths between 600 and 1,100 nm so that adequate penetration depth is achieved. In one study 800 nm light at 500 mW was applied at 1 W per cm^2 for a total of 4 J per cm^2, three times per week for 5 weeks. Overall, they found no significant differences between placebo and experimental groups evaluated using the Vancouver Scar Scale (VSS). However, tendencies toward greater improvement in the treatment group were found.[31]

In scar management, very short–pulsed lasers (picosecond and nanosecond 1,064-nm lasers) have been applied as well (outside of pigment-specific Q-switched lasers and ruby lasers).[32] These lasers, even though their pulse widths are very short, work primarily through photothermal rather than photomechanical mechanisms. Acne scars in particular have been treated with Q-switched lasers (1,064 nm), where presumably there is some focal heating of blood vessels and possibly even tissue water, leading to scar improvement via a wound healing and remodeling response. Tian[33] recently reported the use of a rapid-fire pulse-stacking technique for remediation of blepharoplasty scarring using a low-fluence (2 J per cm^2) Q-switched 1,064-nm Nd:YAG laser.

Role of Pulse Duration

Selectivity and the theory of SPT rely on

1. Preferential ablation of the targets based on wavelength (see spectra)
2. Sufficient energy to affect the target
3. Optimal pulse duration range that achieves preferential target heating, rather than nonspecific bulk heating through diffusion

An understanding of item #3 is often the greatest challenge for the novice laser practitioner. If one examines the thermal relaxation time equation (Eq. 4), that value is related to the time it takes for the target to cool to about 37% of its peak temperature. Larger targets cool more slowly than smaller targets (e.g., a small cupful of water will cool much faster than a bathtub full of water). Likewise, a minute traumatic tattoo particle will cool much faster than a much larger hair bulb. These findings are important in designing optimal laser parameters in scar reduction; the smaller the target, the shorter the associated pulse duration to help minimize thermal diffusion.

More recently, a focused lens array has been applied to acne scars using a 700-ps, 755-nm laser. In this approach, small "fractional" intraepidermal zones of laser-induced optical breakdown (caused by plasma-induced photodisruption) are noted; the resulting pressure wave is thought to be operative in the improvement in scar pigment as well as tone and texture. At present the 755-nm laser has been used, though newer 1,064-nm lasers are now available that also tout these short-pulsed microbeams to enhance scars.[34]

Potential Mechanisms of Action for Device-Based Scar Treatments

Dermal fibroblasts, which form the majority of the dermal cellular architecture and produce and maintain the extracellular matrix (i.e., collagen and elastic fibers), can be divided into two subpopulations: superficial and deep. Fibroblasts in the superficial (papillary) dermis help regulate hair growth and assist in the development of the arrector pili muscle. Fibroblasts of the deep (reticular) dermis synthesize the bulk of the extracellular matrix and compose the progenitors of the preadipocytes and adipocytes of the subcutis.[35] Initial healing of wounded adult skin is mediated by the reticular dermal fibroblasts, whereas superficial dermal fibroblasts participate only in the process of reepithelialization; this helps explain the lack of mature hair follicles in scar tissue (see Chapter 6).

The microarchitecture of a scar differs from that of normal skin. Furthermore, alterations in collagen expression are specific to scar type. Hypertrophic scars primarily express type III collagen, whereas keloid scars are composed of a disordered array of collagen I and III bundles. Histologically, collagen bundles are thicker and more homogeneous in scars when compared to normal skin. They are arranged in a parallel formation horizontal to the skin surface, whereas collagen bundles of histologically normal skin are arranged in a more haphazard manner.[36] Elastin expression in scars is somewhat controversial; one study demonstrated a decreased elastin expression in the superficial dermis for all scar types (hypertrophic, keloid, etc.) when compared to normal skin, whereas there appears to be a relative increase in elastin expression in the deep dermis of keloidal scars relative to normal skin.[37] In a recent keloid scar study by Tong et al., a reduction of elastic fibers was noted by multiphoton spectroscopy.[38]

The overall aim of laser scar treatment is to help normalize the histologic architecture and composition of the abnormal components of injured skin, and ultimately to enhance function and appearance. Both ablative and nonablative modalities have been shown to stimulate collagen remodeling. Ablative lasers, which may be categorized as fully or fractionally ablative, promote vigorous dermal remodeling and stimulate collagen expression.[39] They have been shown to stimulate procollagen I and III mRNA expression by up to 700% to 800% above baseline.[40–42] Ablative lasers have also been shown to induce thinner, better-organized collagen bundles histologically, and to modify expression of collagens I and III to more closely mimic that of normal skin.[43] Nonablative laser treatment has similar, albeit more attenuated effects; a 47% and 84% increase in type I procollagen mRNA expression has been demonstrated in scars treated with the 585 nm pulsed dye laser (PDL) and nonfractional 1,320 nm laser, respectively, 1 week following treatment in one study.[44]

The loss of elastic tissue in scars contributes to their cosmetic and functional deficits. Scar behavior has been studied with respect to stress and strain (see Chapter 7). The ideal scar should show a normalized elasticity, where the stress/strain relationship is improved by restoration of elastic fiber microarchitecture. A recent paper by Ozog et al.[43] showed no effect on elastic tissue staining after a course of fractional CO_2 laser therapy. On the other hand, Hantash et al.[45] showed that after RF needling, neoelastogenesis was observed. Botulinum toxin has been applied in the same session as PDL in one report; the neuromodulator was injected to decrease the hypermobility of the chin during recovery after trauma.[46]

Treatment Approach Based on Clinical Setting

Treatment algorithms for laser and other energy-based devices in scar management are based on a synthesis of history, symptoms, and clinical findings for a specific area, in an individual patient, at a particular time point (Table 13-1). A basic algorithm driven by scar features appears in Figures 13-8 and 13-9; these should serve as a starting point as opposed to a firm set of rules. All scars require individualized treatment based on the experience of the operator to obtain optimal results. A range of devices may be used in any given patient or area on a concurrent or alternating basis. Although multiple modalities may often be safely combined in a single session, cumulative injury through excessive settings and/or overly aggressive combinations can result in worsening scarring.

Table 13-1 Diagnostic Points of Scar Treatment

Period after injury	⇨	Fresh and acute/residual and chronic
Depth	⇨	Epidermis/dermis/subcutaneous tissue
Color	⇨	Red (inflammation/white/brown [pigmentation])
Aspect	⇨	Raised/flat/depressed/rough/smooth
Property	⇨	Planate/linear
Symptoms	⇨	Painful (achy)/itchy (pruritus)/dysesthesia, etc.
Others	⇨	Skin phototype, medicine use, prior treatments, etc.

Red Scars

Almost every scar begins with redness, such that a logical first approach to the rehabilitation of early scars frequently includes a vascular-specific device such as the 532-nm potassium titanyl phosphate (KTP) or frequency-doubled

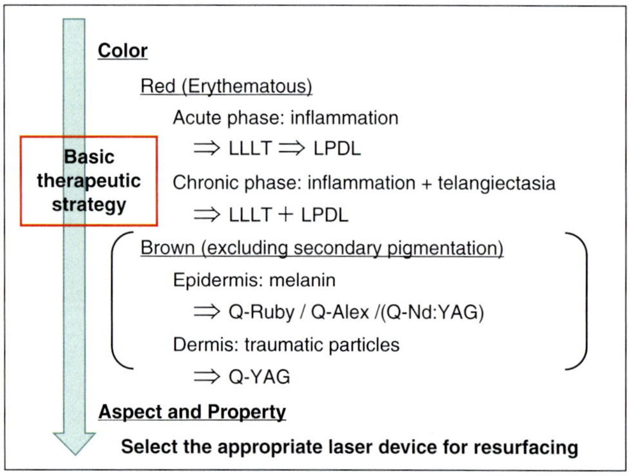

FIGURE 13-8 Therapeutic planning and procedures. LLLT = Low level light therapy; LPDL = Long pulsed dye laser; Q = Q-switched (short-pulsed). *(Adapted from Ohshiro T, Ohshiro T, Sasaki K. Laser scar management technique.* Laser Ther. *2013, 22(4):255.)*

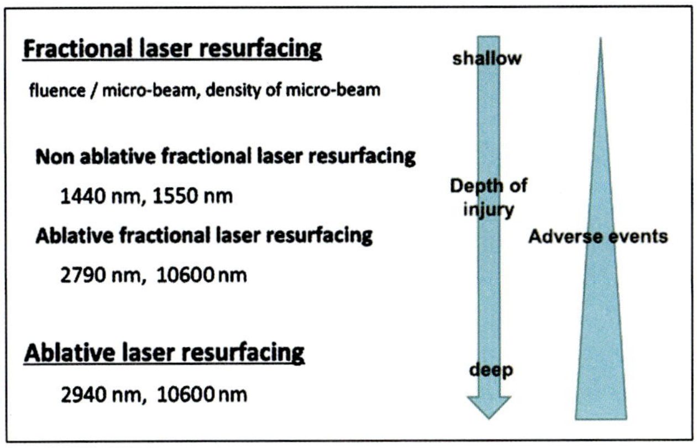

FIGURE 13-9 Resurfacing procedures and therapeutic features. *(From Ohshiro T, Ohshiro T, Sasaki K. Laser scar management technique.* Laser Ther. *2013, 22(4):255. Oshiro fractional and ablative diagram.)*

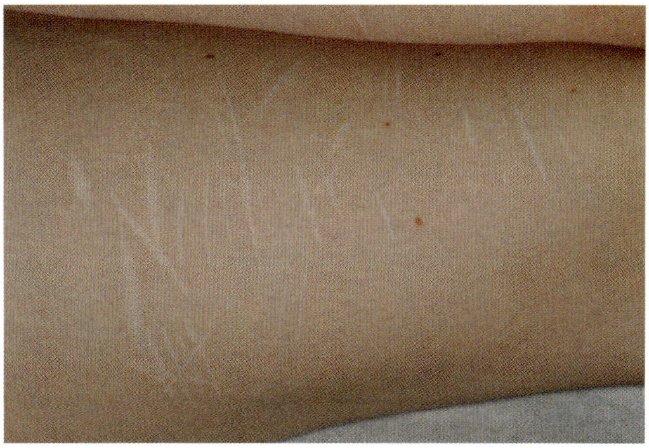

FIGURE 13-10 "Cutter" scars.

Nd:YAG, a 585- or 595-nm PDL, or intense pulsed light (IPL). Vascular lasers and IPL have been shown to help normalize a broad range of scars including hypertrophic, flat, and atrophic red scars. A reasonable question is when is the optimal time after injury to treat a red scar. Most studies have shown that 6 to 8 weeks is a safe time to treat; on the other hand, no study has proven that this interval is ideal. It depends in part on the scar origin—it might be safe to treat a linear scar upon suture removal 1 to 2 weeks after surgery, whereas treatment of a large burn wound should likely commence after the restoration of sufficient skin integrity (closer to the 6- to 8-week time point). Treatment at the time of surgery is another option for some surgical scars.

Amputation Scars

In both military and civilian practice, amputation-associated scars present an array of challenges, among them erosions and ulcerations from skin fragility and poorly fitting prostheses, excessive hair that interferes with proper fit and comfort, and erythema and atrophy/hypertrophy associated with scars regardless of the origin (see Chapter 23). A typical rehabilitation sequence, then, may involve the use of a vascular laser, fractional ablative and/or nonablative laser for scar remodeling, a hair reduction laser, and a Q-switched laser for the treatment of any traumatic tattoo. The authors have also noted that in some cases laser hair reduction has been associated with a subjective reduction in sweating. In the literature, the relationship between laser hair reduction and sweat reduction has been mixed. Some reports have indicated no change, whereas the rest of the investigators were mixed in their reports, some reporting more sweating and some less sweating.[47–50] With these scars, often the skin is thin and fragile and conservative treatment settings should be considered.

"Cutter" Scars (aka "Deliberate Self-Harm")

These scars have proven very challenging to treat. The linear pattern of the scars is conspicuous, and they often occur on the nondominant volar forearms of young women (Fig. 13-10). The loss of pigment, probably more than any other feature of the scar, makes them more noticeable. Attempts to repigment the lesions with the 308-nm excimer laser or other UV sources are often unsuccessful, and can produce a fine rim of hyperpigmentation at the edge of the narrow ellipsoid lesions.[51,52] Early red scars can be treated with a vascular laser, but once the erythema has subsided, repigmentation is best achieved with ablative fractional lasers. The authors usually start, however, with nonablative fractional lasers (nonablative fractional resurfacing, NAFR) as the treatments are better tolerated and have sometimes proved beneficial. In severe cases, skin grafts have been performed; the laser can then be applied after 6 to 8 weeks to improve the graft texture and color.

Papular Acne Scars

These focal dome-shaped scars are often associated with sebaceous hyperplasia and acne. In most cases, we use a small spot nonfractionated Er:YAG laser (1 to 2 mm) and very conservative settings to ablate the scars to a point flush with the skin. These scars are often observed on the chin and nose.

Keloid Scars

Very thick keloid scars often require a combination of interventions (see Chapters 10, and 16). Pruritus, decreased range of motion, and pain are sometimes significant, and reduction of these signs and symptoms is part of the rehabilitation process. Often intralesional steroids and 5-fluorouracil are injected over several sessions at 4- to 6-week intervals. At the same session, ablative fractional lasers can be applied immediately prior to topical application to induce remodeling and facilitate topical and/or intralesional delivery of the medication (see Chapter 14). Low-fluence Q-switched (ns) 1,064-nm Nd:YAG lasers have been used as well, where repeated pulses at 5 to 7 J per cm^2 are used to gently elevate the skin temperature for 3 to 6 minutes in a waving motion over the treatment area. Alternatively, higher fluences of long-pulsed (ms) 1,064-nm lasers (50 J per cm^2, 25 ms pulse width) with cooling have been applied with some success. In one study, treatments were carried out every month for over a year individually to thicker scars.[53]

Acne Scars

Despite the introduction of isotretinoin over 35 years ago, acne scars are ubiquitous in practice (see Chapter 17). Many classification schemes have been developed to guide diagnosis and treatment.[54] The first assessment of the scar type should identity the role of color. Early acne scars and "pseudo" scars are often red or brown in color and occur as early phenomena after inflammation. The acne lesion, particularly a deeper long-standing cystic one, leaves behind of path of destruction in the dermis much like a storm. Plewig and Kligman[55] explored the role of inflammation and its sequelae in acne lesions. Most smaller papules heal without scarring. Larger papules and nodules, especially deep-seated long-standing ones, may be associated with foreign body granulomas. Long after the clinical lesion "resolves," some inflammation may persist and scarring can occur. The nodule may result in total disintegration of the follicular structure, and the lesions are likened to volcanoes. All adnexae within a range of 10 mm can be destroyed (sweat glands, vellus follicles, sebaceous follicles, etc.). The most egregious sequela in acne is the draining sinus, which can extend over several centimeters and often leave such severe scarring that surgery may be the only option. Atrophic scars, depressed scars characterized histologically by a flattened epidermis, an increased number of vessels, and a scarcity of elastic fibers, are the most common scar type associated with inflammatory acne.

Perifollicular acne scars are typically located on the chest and neck and go by names such as postacne anetoderma-like scars and papular elastorrhexis. Histologically there is fibrosis and an absence of elastic fibers. In comparison, keloid scars are distinguished by the whorled pattern of collagen bundles and the absence of elastic fibers.

For most acne scars, a combination approach is recommended. For rolling scars, fillers and subscision can complement both fractional and nonfractional lasers. For boxcar scars, the edges can be effaced with a small spot using the fully ablative 2,940-nm Er:YAG or 10,600-nm CO_2 lasers. In the same session or in a follow-up session, ablative and nonablative fractional lasers can enhance the overall tone and texture of the skin. For red scars, IPL, PDL, and KTP lasers are used; moderate subpurpuric settings result in minimal morbidity. Sample settings for the PDL are 10 mm spot, 5 J per cm^2, and 1.5 ms pulse width. For the 532-nm KTP, we normally apply 5.5 J per cm^2 with a 3 ms pulse width and 7 mm spot. The fractional laser, particularly NAFR, can be applied immediately thereafter in the same session. Overall, ablative fractional resurfacing (AFR) achieves superior results versus NAFR (at least in terms of improvement per session); nonetheless, NAFR is applied in our facility at a ratio of over 20:1 based on practical considerations such as pain and downtime (Fig. 13-11). As an adjunct to laser treatment, newer semipermanent fillers such as polymethyl methacrylate (PMMA) outlast many of its predecessor hyaluronic acid counterparts; PMMA is at present the only tissue filler approved by the FDA for acne scars.

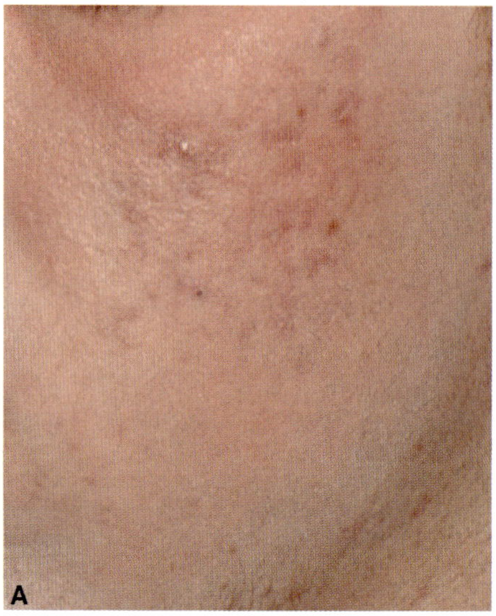

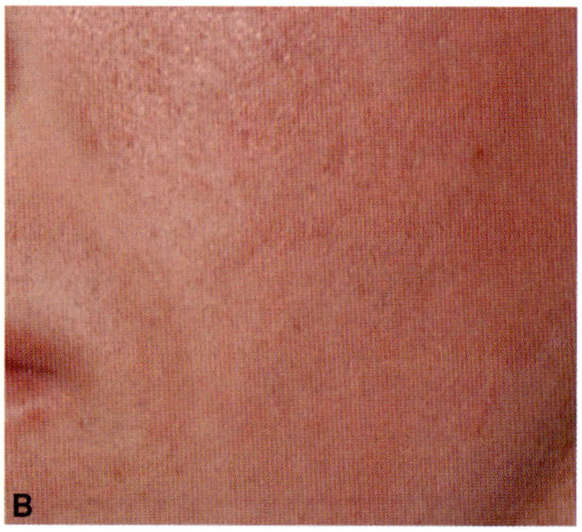

FIGURE 13-11 **A:** Pretreatment acne scarring. **B:** After three fractional nonablative treatments—50 mJ, 35% density, 1,100 μm depth, 1,550 nm, 130 μm column diameter.

Traumatic Scars with "Tattooing"

Many scars result from collisions with asphalt or debris that are delivered with such force (i.e., explosion) that the patient is tattooed from black debris in the plume or direct contact with a street surface. These black tattoos are often associated with hypertrophic scars in the same area. One of the most straightforward remedies in scar management is the use of nanosecond and picosecond pulse duration lasers to break up the pigment into even smaller particles to enhance clearance of the black discoloration. Often these "tattoos" will resolve after only one or two treatments.[56–58]

Scars with Post-Inflammatory Hyperpigmentation (PIH)

Many scars are associated with PIH. We normally do not treat PIH for at least 6 months after injury, as often time will aid in the reduction of the pigment. If one intervenes too early after the injury, more PIH might be created. For long-standing pigment we apply one of three lasers, either alone or in combination. For light-skinned patients, the Q-switched 755-nm alexandrite laser is applied with the lowest settings that achieve slight surface whitening. In darker patients, the Q-switched 1,064-nm Nd:YAG laser is used. In all patients, the fractional 1,927-nm laser can be applied in a series of treatments. The key component to success is being conservative at each treatment session.

Hypopigmented Scars

One frequent association with scars is hypopigmentation. Almost any deep scar will result in a loss of pigment. With time, some pigment restoration is observed in many cases. However, after 1 year, any remaining hypopigmentation tends to persist indefinitely. Hypopigmented scars are a particular challenge and can be recalcitrant to repigmentation efforts. The 308-nm xenon chloride (excimer) laser has been used specifically for this application. Histologically, this improvement is a result of increased melanin, melanocyte hypertrophy, and an increased number of melanocytes. The excimer laser has also been shown in a case report to improve hypopigmentation resulting from resurfacing procedures.[59] More recently, the nonablative fractionated 1,550-nm Er:fiber laser has been used for hypopigmented scars. In a pilot study, six of seven patients saw 51% to 75% improvement in scar hypopigmentation after two to four treatments.[60] Massaki et al.[61] also demonstrated improvement in hypopigmented scars using a combination of 1,550-nm Er:fiber laser, topical bimatoprost, and either tretinoin or pimecrolimus. No comparative trials have yet been published, however, that demonstrate efficacy of the laser/bimatoprost/tretinoin/pimecrolimus treatment over laser treatment alone. In a recent study, AFR was combined with topical latanoprost in a study where one-half of the patients received the combination and the other half the laser alone. After six laser sessions and twice-daily application of the drug for 24 weeks, blinded observers noted greater pigment normalization in the combination treatment group.[62]

Surgical Scars

Most linear surgical scars can potentially benefit from laser interventions, but only a small fraction are treated at all. Most will improve, to a degree, spontaneously with time. This leads to the conundrum of when, and if, a surgical scar should be treated. Nouri et al. found in a split-scar study at the time of surgery that the PDL-treated side of a scar healed less visibly than the untreated control side. Other studies have looked at "simultaneous" laser resurfacing and surgical scars and found that treated scars were less visible months after treatment.[63] However, a recent study involving a single ablative fractional laser treatment at suture removal found no differences in the treated and untreated sides.[64]

Donor site and recipient site graft scars and larger graft scars after burns are less common than surgical scars, but are also readily treatable with combinations of visible light technologies and fractional lasers. We typically evaluate surgical scars 2 to 4 months after the lesion removal, such as after Mohs surgery for skin cancer. This interval is determined somewhat arbitrarily by the timing of the surgeon's referral or when interest in scar improvement is expressed by a patient. The optimal timing for laser intervention in scar mitigation has not yet been determined. Though treatments can begin at virtually any time point after surgery, in the view of the authors, it is likely that earlier intervention may result in better ultimate outcomes. Our initial approach to a surgical scar is PDL with minimally purpuric settings, coupled with NAFR in the same session. Treatments are repeated every 4 to 8 weeks over 6 to 8 months, with repeat evaluations of the scar's response at each visit. Patients often ask about the total number of treatments at the initial presentation. We inform them that every scar treatment is an incremental step toward improvement. Normally, after four to five treatments, a pattern of scar reduction has been established and the patient and physician can plan on future treatments based on mutual goals for further scar reduction.

Combination Strategies in Scar Management

Often one can combine multiple laser technologies along with fillers, surgery, and even neuromodulators for optimal scar reduction or mitigation. Among lasers used in combination are vascular and pigment-specific lasers, often applied in tandem, with a nonablative fractional device; frequently these may all be employed at the same appointment. This three-pronged approach is one of the author's favorite go-to strategies for a red brown scar with fine textural changes.[8,65]

Some nonlaser devices have also been applied for scar management. Microneedling, where one applies a vibrating (up and down) or rolling needle array across the scar surface, creates numerous tiny nonthermal wounds to induce a cytokine milieu that promotes normalization of the skin microarchitecture.[66] The addition of platelet-rich plasma has been reported to further enhance scar reduction.[67] RF needles have also been applied to depths ranging from 0.5 to 3.5 mm, with both noninsulated and insulated needles. The pitch between the needle arrays is about 1 to 2 mm, and about 3% to 5% surface density is achieved per pass. In the case of insulated needles, the distal 300 μm of the microelectrode is exposed. Normally multiple passes are made in different planes by adjusting the depths of the needle between passes. Acne scars appear to respond particularly well to RF needles, but other types of scars have responded as well.

Although fractional lasers have been available since 2004,[24] traditional lasers have been used in a "fractional" approach as early as the 1990s, where "pinholing" was introduced with a 0.2 mm spot continuous-wave CO_2 laser. Since that time, additional studies have reported scar improvement.[68] In a recent paper, a 0.3 mm spot was applied with a traditional CO_2 laser combined with a point compression technique using a 1,540-nm laser.[69] For icepick acne scars, a similar pinhole technique has been applied.[70]

There have been few articles directly comparing ablative fractional Er:YAG and CO_2 lasers in scar management. Conventional wisdom is that CO_2 laser enjoys better hemostasis, but greater thermal damage and potentially slower healing than its erbium counterpart. In one study, fractional ablative CO_2 was compared to fractional Er:YAG in the treatment of hypertrophic scars. In this study, the CO_2 laser prevailed in final assessments using the VSS.[71] However, the study was not side-by-side and the authors conceded that the laser injuries were likely shallower and less dense on the erbium side.

A large uncontrolled study including over 130 patients was conducted in the laser treatment of burn scars. Patients received multiple sessions of combination treatments including "long-pulsed" pigment-specific lasers for hair reduction, IPL–PDL, and ablative fractional laser resurfacing to reduce surrounding hair, erythema, and normalize texture, respectively. For the CO_2 laser, a density of up to 15% was applied and the micropulse energy ranged from 15 to 90 mJ, depending on the depth of the scars (Lumenis Ultrapulse; Deep/SCAAR FX, Yokneam, Israel).[72] The typical patient received approximately three treatment sessions, and the final mean outcome was a VSS score reduction of about 5 points. In another study,[73] a fractional CO_2 laser was combined with punch elevations in the treatment of acne scarring. In this study, one side of the face was treated with the laser alone and the other with punch elevation, followed 24 hours later by the fractional CO_2 laser. Four months after two treatments, the side with the punch elevations showed greater scar reduction than the side treated with laser alone.

The treatment approach of the authors will be illustrated with a series of case examples.

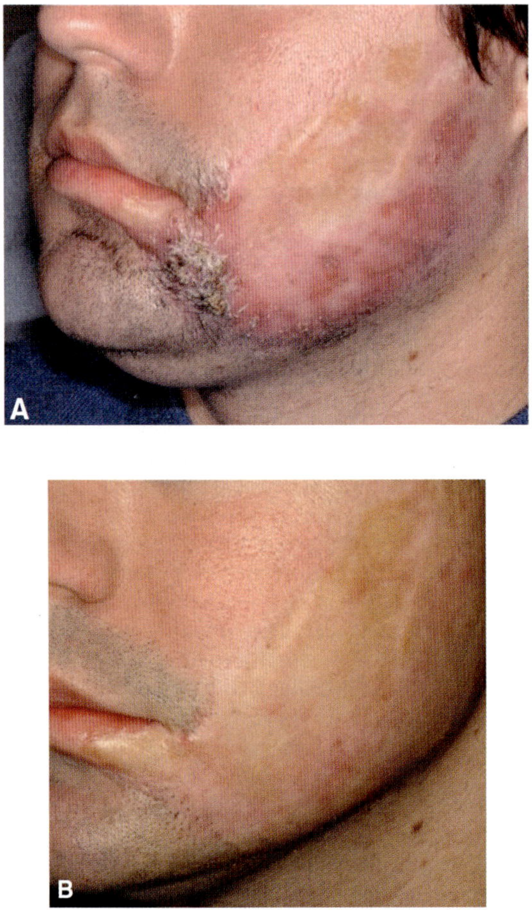

FIGURE 13-12 **A:** Pretreatment photo demonstrating a burn scar with erythema, dyspigmentation, moderate textural irregularity, and inflammation associated with ingrown hairs along the periphery. **B:** After a series of treatments including a combination of PDL, NAFR, and laser hair reduction. Typical settings were, respectively, (a) Nd:YAG—5 mm spot, 70 J per cm^2, 20 ms, contact cooling, (b) PDL 8 J per cm^2, 1.5 ms, 10 mm spot, 30 ms spray 20 ms delay DCD, and (c) fractional nonablative laser, 1550 nm, 40 mJ, 20% coverage per session. DCD = dynamic cooling device.

CASE EXAMPLES

CASE 1: A man in his 20s presented with a burn scar on the left cheek approximately 1 year after injury. On presentation, the skin showed textural changes, erythema, dyspigmentation (areas of both hyperpigmentation and hypopigmentation), and inflammation associated with ingrown hairs along the margins of the scar (Fig. 13-12A). Patients commonly present with an array of clinical findings and may benefit from a combination approach. In this case PDL (to erythematous portions of the scar), NAFR (to manage dyspigmentation and textural irregularity), and a hair reduction laser were all initiated in the first session. A reasonable treatment order would be PDL, hair reduction, and finally NAFR because the latter two may be associated with immediate skin changes including reactive erythema. Concurrent treatments should be approached with caution to minimize the risk of excessive thermal injury. For the novice operator, it may be reasonable to separate different modalities into alternating sessions. After a series of combination treatments, progressive incremental improvements are noted (Fig. 13-12B). Note that fractional laser treatments can simultaneously help improve texture and both hyperpigmentation and hypopigmentation.

CASE 2: A woman in her 20s visited a spa for a pedicure, and 1 month later developed large tender erythematous nodules on the shins. Cultures grew atypical mycobacteria. After a 1-year course of appropriate antibiotics, she presented with persistent primarily hyperpigmented scars with focal hypopigmentation and mild-to-moderate textural irregularity in the areas of inflammation (Fig. 13-13A). A series of combination Q-switched 755-nm alexandrite and NAFR sessions resulted in marked improvement (Fig. 13-13B). The alexandrite laser was applied at 3 to 5 J per cm^2, 50 ns, 4 mm spot size (two sessions 2 months apart) followed by three NAFR sessions 2 months apart (40 mJ, 1,550 nm, 30% density, 150 μm microbeam diameter).

CASE 3: A woman presented with persistent redness and hypopigmentation after surgical removal of a basal cell carcinoma on the leg (Fig. 13-14A). A series of sessions including PDL followed by NAFR resulted in a marked reduction in redness and improved homogeneity of pigmentation (Fig. 13-14B).

CASE 4: A woman in her 40s presented with cribriform scarring of the face approximately 1 year after laser resurfacing in another state (Fig. 13-15A). A combination of PDL and NAFR was applied on three occasions at 2-month intervals with minimal improvement. After a single AFR treatment, marked restoration of pigmentation and reduction in the surface skin irregularities were noted (Fig. 13-15B).

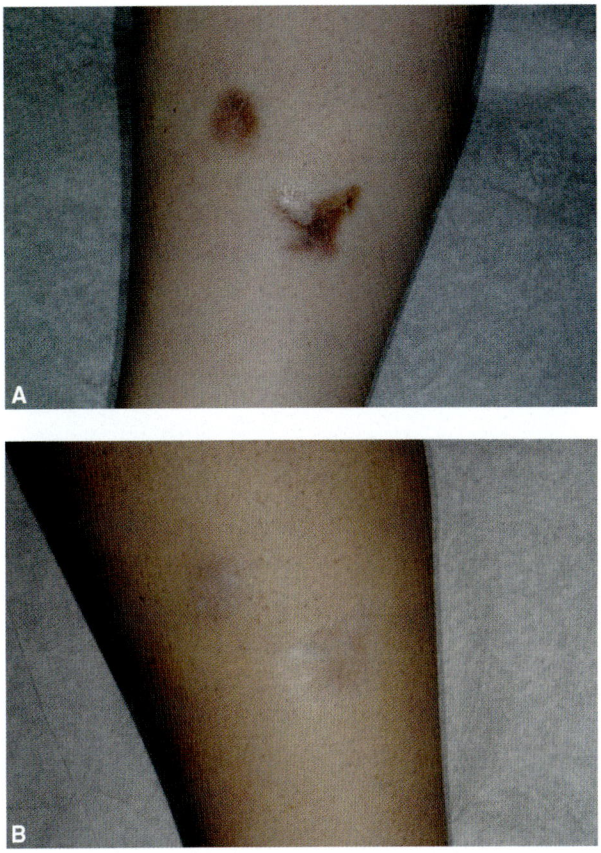

FIGURE 13-13 **A:** Hyperpigmentation and textural change after infection. **B:** After multiple treatments.

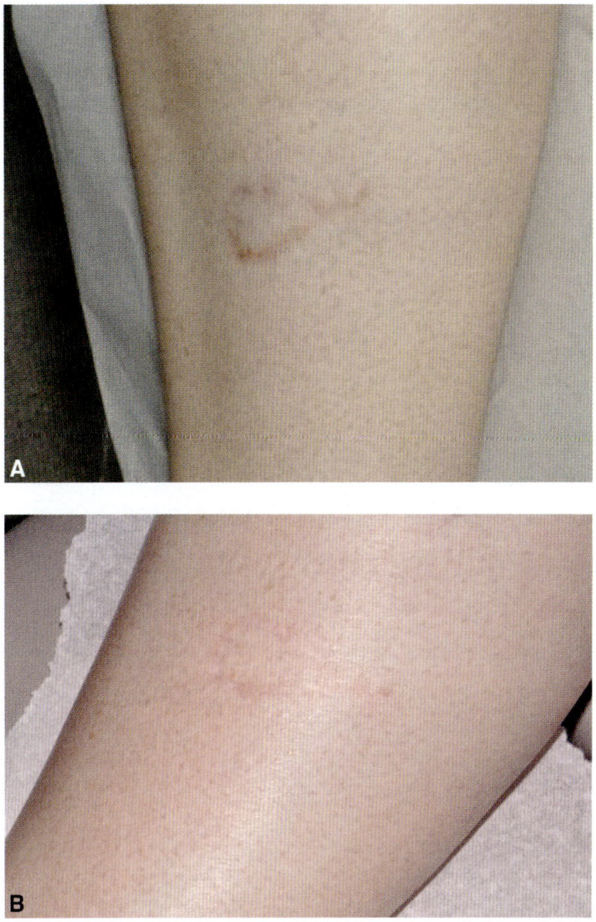

FIGURE 13-14 **A:** Erythema, textural change, and hyperpigmentation after skin cancer excision and advancement flap. **B:** After multiple treatments.

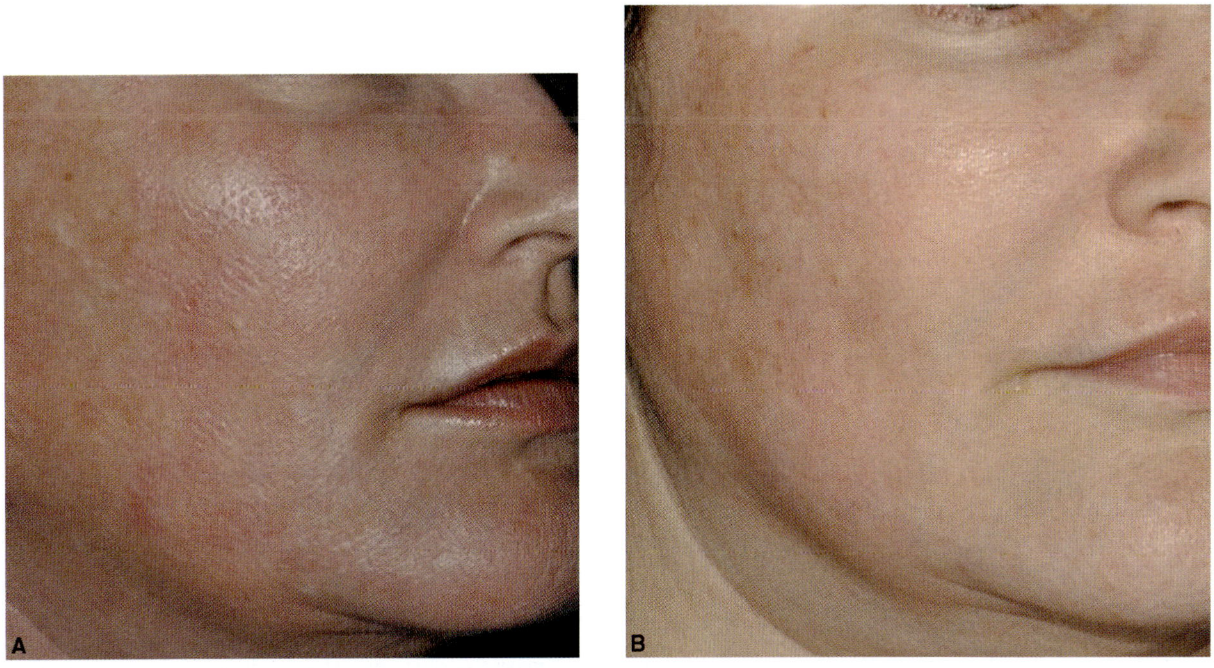

FIGURE 13-15 **A:** Cribriform scarring after resurfacing procedure. **B:** After multiple nonablative and ablative fractional laser treatments.

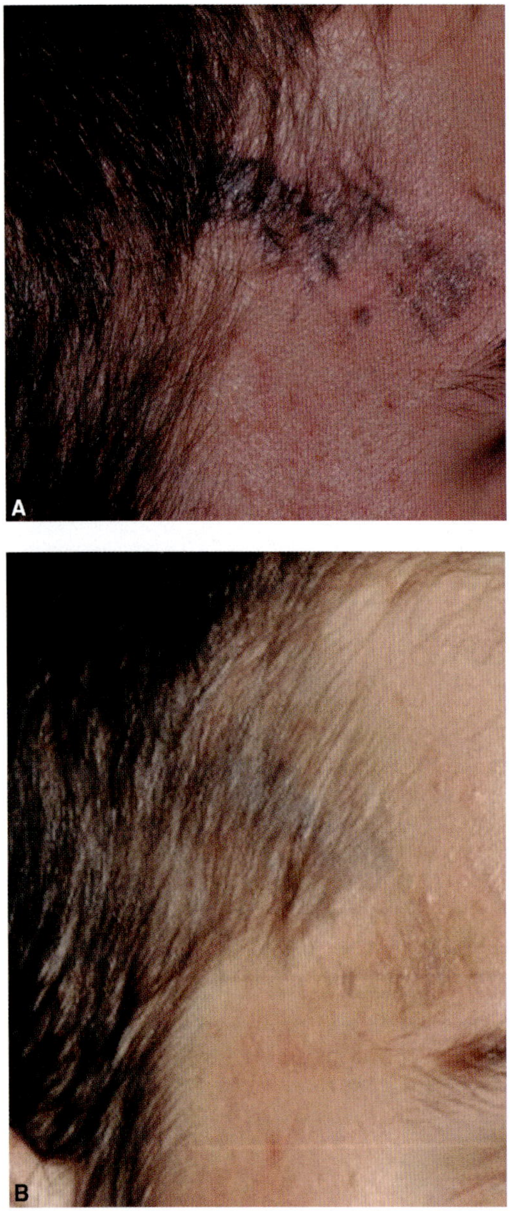

FIGURE 13-16 **A:** Traumatic scar after fall with textural change, erythema, and traumatic tattooing. **B:** After three treatments with pulsed dye laser, fractional nonablative laser, and Q-switched YAG laser.

CASE 5: A man in his 20s presented with traumatic tattooing after a motor vehicle accident (Fig. 13-16A). After two treatments with a Q-switched 1,064-nm Nd:YAG laser, there was marked reduction in the discoloration (Fig. 13-16B).

CASE 6: A man in his 20s presented with disfiguring facial scarring resulting from cystic acne (Fig. 13-17A). A series of three combination treatments including Er:YAG resurfacing, PDL, and fractional needle RF at 1-month intervals resulted in a significant interval reduction in erythema and textural improvements. Additional enhancements in erythema and texture could likely be obtained with continued treatment with PDL, fractional ablative or nonablative laser resurfacing, or fractional needle RF.

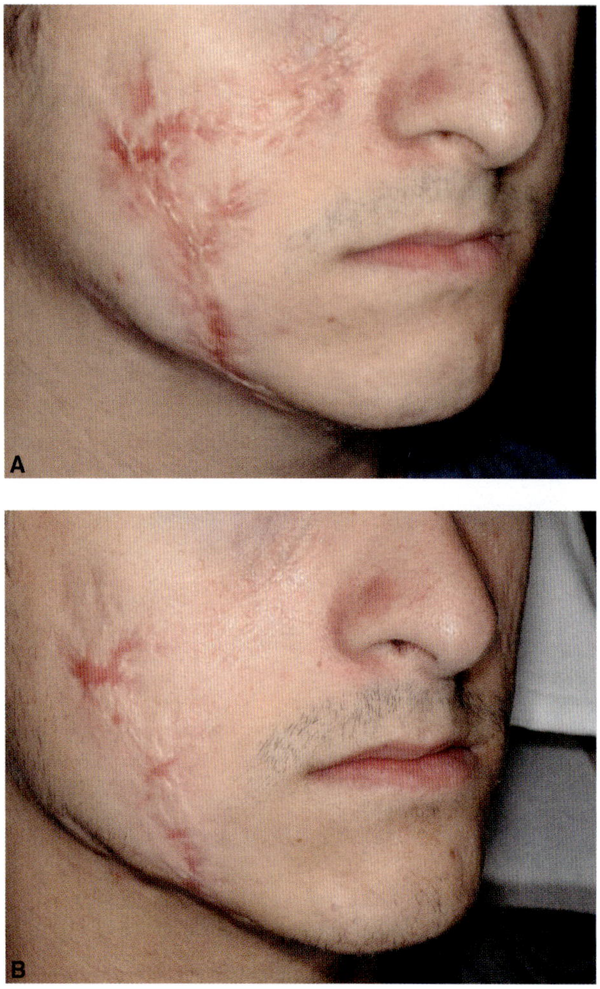

FIGURE 13-17 **A:** A man in his 20s at presentation with disfiguring acne scarring of the face. **B:** After a combination of traditional Er:YAG resurfacing, PDL, and fractional RF (three sessions 1 month apart).

REFERENCES

1. Nouri K, Rivas MP, Stevens M, et al. Comparison of the effectiveness of the pulsed dye laser 585 nm versus 595 nm in the treatment of new surgical scars. *Lasers Med Sci*. 2009;24(5):801–810.
2. Nouri K, Ballard CJ. Re: the use of pulsed dye laser for the prevention and treatment of hypertrophic scars in Chinese persons. *Dermatol Surg*. 2005;31(2):252–253; author reply 253.
3. Anderson RR. Dermatologic history of the ruby laser: the long story of short pulses. *Arch Dermatol*. 2003;139(1):70–74.
4. Murphy GF, Shepard RS, Paul BS, et al. Organelle-specific injury to melanin-containing cells in human skin by pulsed laser irradiation. *Lab Invest*. 1983;49(6):680–685.
5. Anderson RR, Parrish JA. Selective photothermolysis: precise microsurgery by selective absorption of pulsed radiation. *Science*. 1983;220(4596):524–527.
6. Anderson RR, Parrish JA. Microvasculature can be selectively damaged using dye lasers: a basic theory and experimental evidence in human skin. *Lasers Surg Med*. 1981;1(3):263–276.
7. Anderson RR, Parrish JA. The optics of human skin. *J Invest Dermatol*. 1981;77(1):13–19.
8. Ohshiro T, Ohshiro T, Sasaki K. Laser scar management technique. *Laser Ther*. 2013;22(4):255–260.
9. Anderson RR, Margolis RJ, Watenabe S, et al. Selective photothermolysis of cutaneous pigmentation by Q-switched Nd: YAG laser pulses at 1064, 532, and 355 nm. *J Invest Dermatol*. 1989;93(1):28–32.

10. Margolis RJ, Dover JS, Polla LL, et al. Visible action spectrum for melanin-specific selective photothermolysis. *Lasers Surg Med.* 1989;9(4):389–397.
11. Chan HH, Kono T. The use of lasers and intense pulsed light sources for the treatment of pigmentary lesions. *Skin Therapy Lett.* 2004;9(8):5–7.
12. Kono T, Manstein D, Chan HH, et al. Q-switched ruby versus long-pulsed dye laser delivered with compression for treatment of facial lentigines in Asians. *Lasers Surg Med.* 2006;38(2):94–97.
13. van Gemert MJ, Jacques SL, Sterenborg HJ, et al. Skin optics. *IEEE Trans Biomed Eng.* 1989;36(12):1146–1154.
14. Wang L, Jacques SL, Zheng L. MCML-Monte Carlo modeling of photon transport in multi-layered tissues. *Comput Methods Program Biomed.* 1995;47:131–146.
15. Welch AJ, Gardner CM. Monte Carlo model for determination of the role of heat generation in laser-irradiated tissue. *J Biomech Eng.* 1997;119:489–495.
16. Wanner M, Sakamoto FH, Avram MM, et al. Immediate skin responses to laser and light treatments: therapeutic endpoints: how to obtain efficacy. *J Am Acad Dermatol.* 2016;74(5):821 833.
17. Wanner M, Sakamoto FH, Avram MM, et al. Immediate skin responses to laser and light treatments: warning endpoints: how to avoid side effects. *J Am Acad Dermatol.* 2016;74(5):807–819.
18. Sommer A, Van Mierlo PL, Neumann HA, et al. Red and blue telangiectasias. Differences in oxygenation [comment]? *Dermatol Surg.* 1997;23(1):55–59.
19. Rubin IK, Farinelli WA, Doukas A, et al. Optimal wavelengths for vein-selective photothermolysis. *Lasers Surg Med.* 2012;44(2):152–157.
20. Dierickx C, Goldman MP, Fitzpatrick RE. Laser treatment of erythematous/hypertrophic and pigmented scars in 26 patients. *Plast Reconstr Surg.* 1995;95(1):84–90; discussion 91–92.
21. Kollias N, Malallah YH, al-Ajmi H, et al. Erythema and melanogenesis action spectra in heavily pigmented individuals as compared to fair-skinned Caucasians. *Photodermatol Photoimmunol Photomed.* 1996;12(5):183–188.
22. Zonios G, Bykowski J, Kollias N. Skin melanin, hemoglobin, and light scattering properties can be quantitatively assessed in vivo using diffuse reflectance spectroscopy. *J Invest Dermatol.* 2001;117(6):1452–1457.
23. Stamatas GN, Kollias N. Blood stasis contributions to the perception of skin pigmentation. *J Biomed Opt.* 2004;9(2):315–322.
24. Manstein D, Herron GS, Sink RK, et al. Fractional photothermolysis: a new concept for cutaneous remodeling using microscopic patterns of thermal injury. *Lasers Surg Med.* 2004;34(5):426–438.
25. Behroozan DS, Goldberg LH, Dai T, et al. Fractional photothermolysis for the treatment of surgical scars: a case report. *J Cosmet Laser Ther.* 2006;8(1):35–38.
26. Geronemus RG. Fractional photothermolysis: current and future applications. *Lasers Surg Med.* 2006;38(3):169–176.
27. Alexiades-Armenakas MR, Dover JS, Arndt KA. The spectrum of laser skin resurfacing: nonablative, fractional, and ablative laser resurfacing. *J Am Acad Dermatol.* 2008;58(5):719–737; quiz 738–740.
28. Cho SI, Chung BY, Choi MG, et al. Evaluation of the clinical efficacy of fractional radiofrequency microneedle treatment in acne scars and large facial pores. *Dermatol Surg.* 2012;38:1017–1024.
29. Chang M, Ma X, Ouyang T, et al. Potential molecular mechanisms involved in 5-aminolevulinic acid-based photodynamic therapy against human hypertrophic scars. *Plast Reconstr Surg.* 2015;136(4):715–727.
30. Mendoza-Garcia J, Sebastian A, Alonso-Rasgado T, et al. Ex vivo evaluation of the effect of photodynamic therapy on skin scars and striae distensae. *Photodermatol Photoimmunol Photomed.* 2015;31(5):239–251.
31. Freitas CP, Melo C, Alexandrino AM, et al. Efficacy of low-level laser therapy on scar tissue. *J Cosmet Laser Ther.* 2013;15(3):171–176.
32. Cho SB, Lee JH, Lee SH, et al. Efficacy and safety of 1064-nm Q-switched Nd:YAG laser with low fluence for keloids and hypertrophic scars. *J Eur Acad Dermatol Venereol.* 2010;24(9):1070–1074.
33. Tian WC. Savior of post-blepharoepicanthoplasty scarring: novel use of a low-fluence 1064-nm Q-switched Nd:YAG laser. *J Cosmet Laser Ther.* 2016:1–3.
34. Brauer JA, Kazlouskaya V, Alabdulrazzaq H, et al. Use of a picosecond pulse duration laser with specialized optic for treatment of facial acne scarring. *JAMA Dermatol.* 2015;151(3):278–284.
35. Driskell RR, Lichtenberger BM, Hoste E, et al. Distinct fibroblast lineages determine dermal architecture in skin development and repair. *Nature.* 2013;504(7479):277–281.
36. Verhaegen PD, van Zuijlen PP, Pennings NM, et al. Differences in collagen architecture between keloid, hypertrophic scar, normotrophic scar, and normal skin: an objective histopathological analysis. *Wound Repair Regen.* 2009;17(5):649–656.
37. Amadeu TP, Braune AS, Porto LC, et al. Fibrillin-1 and elastin are differentially expressed in hypertrophic scars and keloids. *Wound Repair Regen.* 2004;12(2):169–174.
38. Zheng P, Lavker RM, Kligman AM. Anatomy of striae. *Br J Dermatol.* 1985;112(2):185–193.
39. Orringer JS, Sachs DL, Shao Y, et al. Direct quantitative comparison of molecular responses in photodamaged human skin to fractionated and fully ablative carbon dioxide laser resurfacing. *Dermatol Surg.* 2012;38(10):1668–1677.
40. Orringer JS, Rittié L, Hamilton T, et al. Intraepidermal erbium:YAG laser resurfacing: impact on the dermal matrix. *J Am Acad Dermatol.* 2011;64(1):119–128.
41. Orringer JS, Kang S, Johnson TM, et al. Connective tissue remodeling induced by carbon dioxide laser resurfacing of photodamaged human skin. *Arch Dermatol.* 2004;140(11):1326–1332.
42. Orringer JS, Kang S, Johnson TM, et al. Tretinoin treatment before carbon dioxide laser resurfacing: a clinical and biochemical analysis. *J Am Acad Dermatol.* 2004;51(6):940–946.
43. Ozog DM, Liu A, Chaffins ML, et al. Evaluation of clinical results, histological architecture, and collagen expression following treatment of mature burn scars with a fractional carbon dioxide laser. *JAMA Dermatol.* 2013;149(1):50–57.
44. Orringer JS, Voorhees JJ, Hamilton T, et al. Dermal matrix remodeling after nonablative laser therapy. *J Am Acad Dermatol.* 2005;53(5):775–782.
45. Hantash BM, Ubeid AA, Chang H, et al. Bipolar fractional radiofrequency treatment induces neoelastogenesis and neocollagenesis. *Lasers Surg Med.* 2009;41(1):1–9.
46. Lee SJ, Jeong SY, No YA, et al. Combined treatment with botulinum toxin and 595-nm pulsed dye laser for traumatic scarring. *Ann Dermatol.* 2015;27(6):756–758.
47. Helou J, Haber R, Kechichian E, et al. A case of generalized bromhidrosis following whole-body depilatory laser. *J Cosmet Laser Ther.* 2015;17(6):318–320.
48. Helou J, Habre M, Soutou B, et al. Reversibility of hyperhidrosis post axillary depilatory laser. *Lasers Med Sci.* 2014;29(2):717–721.
49. Obeid G, Helou J, Maatouk I, et al. Depilatory laser: a potential causative factor for inguinal hyperhidrosis: report of three cases. *J Cosmet Laser Ther.* 2013;15(5):286–289.
50. Letada PR, Landers JT, Uebelhoer NS, et al. Treatment of focal axillary hyperhidrosis using a long-pulsed Nd:YAG 1064 nm laser at hair reduction settings. *J Drugs Dermatol.* 2012;11(1):59–63.
51. Goldberg DJ, Marmur ES, Schmults C, et al. Histologic and ultrastructural analysis of ultraviolet B laser and light source treatment of leukoderma in striae distensae. *Dermatol Surg.* 2005;31(4):385–387.
52. Alexiades-Armenakas MR, Bernstein LJ, Friedman PM, et al. The safety and efficacy of the 308-nm excimer laser for pigment correction of hypopigmented scars and striae alba. *Arch Dermatol.* 2004;140(8):955–960.
53. Koike S, Akaishi S, Nagashima Y, et al. Nd:YAG laser treatment for keloids and hypertrophic scars: an analysis of 102 cases. *Plast Reconstr Surg Glob Open.* 2014;2(12):e272.
54. Goodman GJ. Treatment of acne scarring. *Int J Dermatol.* 2011;50(10):1179–1194.
55. Plewig G, Kligman AM. *Acne and Rosacea*. 2nd ed. Berlin: Spriger-Verlag; 1993:726.
56. Martins A, Trindade F, Leite L. Facial scars after a road accident: combined treatment with PDL and Q-switched ND:YAG laser. *J Cosmet Laser Ther.* 2008;10(3):174–176.
57. Miles BA, Ellis E 3rd. The neodymium:YAG laser in the treatment of traumatic tattoo: a case report. *J Oral Maxillofac Surg.* 2006;64(5):850–855.
58. Chang SE, Choi JH, Moon KC, et al. Successful removal of traumatic tattoos in Asian skin with a Q-switched alexandrite laser. *Dermatol Surg.* 1998;24(12):1308–1311.
59. Raulin C, Greve B, Warncke SH, et al. Excimer laser. Treatment of iatrogenic hypopigmentation following skin resurfacing [in German]. *Hautarzt.* 2004;55(8):746–748.
60. Glaich AS, Rahman Z, Goldberg LH, et al. Fractional resurfacing for the treatment of hypopigmented scars: a pilot study. *Dermatol Surg.* 2007;33(3):289–294; discussion 293-4.
61. Massaki AB, Fabi SG, Fitzpatrick R. Repigmentation of hypopigmented scars using an erbium-doped 1,550-nm fractionated laser and topical bimatoprost. *Dermatol Surg.* 2012;38(7 Pt 1):995–1001.

62. Siadat AH, Rezaei R, Asilian A, et al. Repigmentation of hypopigmented scars using combination of fractionated carbon dioxide laser with topical latanoprost vs. fractionated carbon dioxide laser alone. *Indian J Dermatol.* 2015;60(4):364–368.
63. Grevelink JM, White VR. Concurrent use of laser skin resurfacing and punch excision in the treatment of facial acne scarring. *Dermatol Surg.* 1998;24(5):527–530.
64. Sobanko JF, Vachiramon V, Rattanaumpawan P, et al. Early postoperative single treatment ablative fractional lasing of Mohs micrographic surgery facial scars: a split-scar, evaluator-blinded study. *Lasers Surg Med.* 2015;47(1):1–5.
65. Anderson RR, Donelan MB, Hivnor C, et al. Laser treatment of traumatic scars with an emphasis on ablative fractional laser resurfacing: consensus report. *JAMA Dermatol.* 2014;150(2):187–193.
66. Sharad J. Combination of microneedling and glycolic acid peels for the treatment of acne scars in dark skin. *J Cosmet Dermatol.* 2011;10(4):317–323.
67. Asif M, Kanodia S, Singh K. Combined autologous platelet-rich plasma with microneedling verses microneedling with distilled water in the treatment of atrophic acne scars: a concurrent split-face study. *J Cosmet Dermatol.* 2016. doi:10.1111/jocd.12207.
68. Whang SW, Lee KY, Cho SB, et al. Burn scars treated by pinhole method using a carbon dioxide laser. *J Dermatol.* 2006;33(12): 869–872.
69. Ibrahim SM, Elsaie ML, Kamel MI, et al. Successful treatment of traumatic scars with combined nonablative fractional laser and pinpoint technique of standard CO_2 laser. *Dermatol Ther.* 2016;29: 52–57.
70. Lee SJ, Yeo IK, Kang JM, et al. Treatment of hypertrophic burn scars by combination laser-cision and pinhole method using a carbon dioxide laser. *Lasers Surg Med.* 2014;46(5):380–384.
71. Reinholz M, Schwaiger H, Heppt MV, et al. Comparison of two kinds of lasers in the treatment of acne scars. *Facial Plast Surg.* 2015;31(5):523–531.
72. Hultman CS, Friedstat JS, Edkins RE, et al. Laser resurfacing and remodeling of hypertrophic burn scars: the results of a large, prospective, before-after cohort study, with long-term follow-up. *Ann Surg.* 2014;260(3):519–529; discussion 529–532.
73. Faghihi G, Nouraei S, Asilian A, et al. Efficacy of punch elevation combined with fractional carbon dioxide laser resurfacing in facial atrophic acne scarring: a randomized split-face clinical study. *Indian J Dermatol.* 2015;60(5):473–478.

14 Laser-Assisted Delivery of Therapeutic Agents

JILL S. WAIBEL, ASHLEY RUDNICK, and PETER R. SHUMAKER

KEY POINTS

- The recent increase in the use of ablative fractional laser devices has fostered enthusiasm for laser-assisted delivery (LAD) of medications and other agents. LAD holds enormous promise in the management of scars and a multitude of other disorders.
- Medications and other agents have generally not been formulated specifically for this route of delivery and current use in this manner remains predominantly "off-label."
- Extensive future research is required to establish safety, efficacy, dosing, timing, combinations, and other parameters related to LAD.

Survival after severe burns and other trauma has improved dramatically in the United States and elsewhere in the developed world. New strategies are required to manage increasing numbers of patients with functionally and cosmetically debilitating scars. Multispecialty collaboration, innovative therapies, and novel combinations of existing treatments can help ensure optimal patient recovery. Ablative fractional laser-assisted delivery (LAD) of medications and other agents beyond the epidermal barrier is a prime example of one of these innovative combination strategies.

Scar rehabilitation is the attempt to restore form and function to patients. Well-established therapeutic approaches include, but are not limited to, physical therapy, compression, silicone sheeting, corticosteroids, laser therapy, and surgical revision (e.g., Z-plasty, grafts) in severe cases or those refractory to conservative measures (see Chapters 10, 12, 13, and 19). Leading the way in recent years are lasers, which are precise and effective treatment modalities to rehabilitate and consistently improve scars. Evidence for the efficacy of laser treatment alone is accumulating rapidly in the literature,[1,2] and new synergistic combinations are being explored.

Topical application of selected medications through intact skin for their local effects or for systemic absorption is routine. However, the epidermis provides an efficient barrier that limits this type of delivery to molecules of a narrow range of specific characteristics including size and fat solubility. LAD, predominantly associated with ablative fractional lasers, is a novel delivery method that enables the treating physician to uniformly distribute larger molecules and even cells through narrow channels to the desired depth in cutaneous tissue. Fractional lasers are the first platforms that allow operators to select the depth of treatment, and as long as the diameter of the channels are below a certain threshold (likely <500 μm),[1] they heal rapidly in 1 to 2 days without scarring. Thus, LAD may provide multiple advantages including delivery of larger quantities of existing topical medications to a precise depth, efficient transcutaneous delivery of large molecules previously not amenable to the transcutaneous route, and even reliable systemic administration for a broader variety of agents. With regard to scars, these channels may be used in the immediate postoperative period to deliver drugs and other substances to synergistically enhance the local therapeutic and remodeling response.

Background

Topical drug delivery is essential in the treatment of dermatologic disease. However, therapeutic benefit is often ultimately limited by the absorption of the medication through intact skin. When a drug enters and remains within the skin it is called *penetration*. This is how most topically applied drugs function to improve dermatologic disease. *Transdermal delivery* means a drug has crossed the skin barrier and entered the bloodstream. Transdermal patches have been used since the 1970s, but are limited to drugs with low molecular mass (<500 Da) and high lipophilicity and typically address dermatologic conditions for delivery of medications.[3–5] Traditional strategies to enhance topical drug delivery include chemical (solvents, surfactants), biochemical (nanoparticles, liquid synthesis inhibitors), and physical (tape stripping, sonophoresis, microneedling) methods. Chemical modifications are the most commonly utilized today and include approaches to remove or alter the stratum corneum. These have had variable success with improving drug delivery. The stratum corneum, the outermost layer, serves as the primary rate-limiting barrier for percutaneous penetration and typically only 1% to 5% of topically applied drugs are absorbed.[3] Furthermore, many medications are too large to penetrate intact skin and require either intralesional injection or systemic delivery.

LAD is an evolving modality that was first described in the literature in 2002 using full-field ablative devices.[6] Fractional ablative lasers, typically either the 10,600-nm carbon dioxide (CO_2) or the 2,940-nm erbium:yttrium aluminum garnet (Er:YAG), first emerged around 2007 and provide a novel way to create a conduit in the stratum corneum, epidermal, and dermal layers in a rapid, predictable, and controlled pattern. Both CO_2 and Er:YAG platforms are infrared lasers that target water, heating tissue rapidly to over 100°C and causing vaporization in a precise manner on a micron scale. Ablative fractional resurfacing creates narrow vertical channels of ablation surrounded by thin layers of coagulated tissue (see Chapter 13). These channels serve as access points for drug delivery and allow for transport of actives deeper into the skin. Topical drug delivery has several potential advantages over traditional oral medication. In the management of dermatologic disease, topical administration of therapies directly to the skin may limit systemic toxicity and decrease the amount of drugs required for therapeutic effects. In addition, drug degradation by first pass metabolism through the liver via the gastrointestinal system can be avoided.

Clinical Applications

LAD with ablative fractional laser pretreatment has already been reported and evaluated in animal models and clinical studies for a variety of dermatologic conditions including actinic keratosis and nonmelanoma skin cancer, cutaneous infections, inflammatory conditions, anesthetic delivery, scar management, and wound healing. Associated dermatologic drugs and other agents have included lidocaine, 5-aminolevulinic acid, methyl-5-aminolevulinate (MAL), ascorbic acid, diclofenac, ingenol mebutate, imiquimod, methotrexate, minoxidil, diphencyprone, vaccines, 5-fluorouracil (5-FU), triamcinolone acetonide (TAC), platelet-rich plasma, and poly-L-lactic acid (PLLA).[7–24] The potential applications are enormous and this incomplete list will rapidly grow much longer in the months and years to come.

Laser Selection for LAD

Ablative lasers are generally considered superior to nonablative lasers for LAD, although studies in this area are limited.[25] The general mechanism and rationale is best understood by examining immediate postprocedure histology (Fig. 14-1A and B).

Among the ablative lasers, comparative studies between CO_2 or Er:YAG platforms are lacking. CO_2 platforms are generally associated with a somewhat thicker surrounding rim of coagulated collagen around the ablative columns because of a significantly lower associated absorption coefficient for water and relatively greater degree of heat diffusion compared with Er:YAG. Does the larger coagulated rim associated with CO_2 lasers decrease absorption potential through the channel wall? Does the relative increase in bleeding associated with Er:YAG lasers interfere with the amount of drug placed into the channels? The clinical significance of these and other characteristics are not yet fully known, and future studies are required to match the optimal platform with the desired application.

Technique for Ablative Fractional LAD in Scar Management

Ablative fractional lasers are the first platforms to offer tunable depths of penetration and microcolumn density. The physician may therefore tailor depth and density settings "on the fly" to attempt to optimize treatment for the given clinical application, agent, and location. Initial data on the influence of laser channel depth and density on drug delivery has thus far been counterintuitive. It appears that topical delivery may be optimized by relatively modest energy and density settings, with diminishing returns

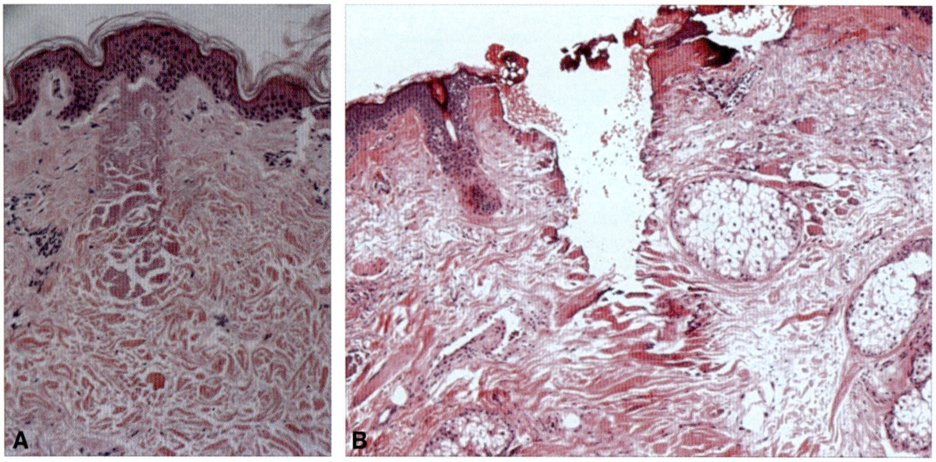

FIGURE 14-1 **A:** Histology after 1,550-nm nonablative fractional laser treatment showing dermal coagulation but no corridors. **B:** Histology after Er:YAG 2,940-nm ablative fractional laser treatment showing open channels creating a pathway for topical penetration of drugs, cells, and cosmeceuticals into the dermal compartment.

above a certain threshold. This has positive implications for the potential tolerability of LAD in the outpatient setting. Studies of the effect of laser parameters on drug delivery in the setting of scars are somewhat limited. Furthermore, the variability of epidermal and collagen thickness and vascularity in scar tissue compared to normal skin may alter these relationships and mandate future studies specifically directed toward scar management. As more is learned about how far each individual agent studied diffuses, it will allow for optimal choice of parameters. Delivery of every drug, cell, and cosmeceutical will vary somewhat based on its inherent properties such as size, diffusion coefficient, skin disease, and other factors.

Laser Parameters: Depth of Treatment

Bachhav et al.[26] used an in vitro porcine model to study the effect of Er:YAG laser pretreatment on lidocaine delivery. The authors found that greater fluences did result in greater associated channel depths. However, beyond a threshold of approximately 200 µm of penetration into the dermis, greater fluence did not result in greater lidocaine permeation at a fixed number of channels. The authors concluded that lidocaine delivery is enhanced with LAD, but the transport was independent of fluence once in the dermal compartment. This suggests that even relatively low fluences may be sufficient to enhance lidocaine delivery. In another LAD study involving lidocaine in a porcine model, Oni et al.[18] hypothesized that greater channel depth would lead to greater transdermal absorption. This experiment tested fractional ablative channels at 25, 50, 250, and 500 µm of depth. Results revealed that maximum absorption occurred at a depth of 250 µm. The authors concluded this may be due to the presence of a vascular plexus between 100 and 300 µm in depth in porcine skin. Haak et al.[7] studied the impact of laser channel depth after fractionated CO_2 laser pretreatment on the delivery of MAL in a porcine model. Test sites included laser channels ranging from 0.3 to 2.1 mm in depth. The authors found that fractional pretreatment accelerates protoporphyrin IX accumulation, but that increasing the depth of dermal penetration did not affect accumulation.

Laser Parameters: Channel Density

Bachhav et al.[26] studied the effect of channel density on permeation of topical lidocaine in an in vitro porcine model using an Er:YAG fractional ablative laser. The initial hypothesis was that by increasing the number of laser pores the overall drug delivery would increase. Densities studied included 0 (control), 150, 300, 450, 900 pores in a fixed area and stable laser fluence. There was no statistically significant difference in cumulative permeation between 450 and 900 pores at 6 hours, or 300, 450, and 900 pores at 24 hours. The authors concluded there is a threshold pore density to achieve maximum permeation, but that increasing channel density beyond this point will not improve delivery. In a study evaluating porphyrin accumulation after ablative fractional CO_2 LAD of MAL (a porphyrin precursor) in a porcine model, Haedersdal et al.[8] noted uniform delivery throughout the treated area from channels spaced approximately 3 mm apart. Haak et al.[27] evaluated the impact of laser density and molecular weight on the uptake of polyethylene glycols of increasing molecular weights from 250 to 4,000 Da. The authors found that laser pretreatment increased intra- and transcutaneous delivery, and that delivery increased with density to a point. Interestingly, densities higher than 1% resulted in decreased per-channel delivery, and larger molecules had a greater tendency toward intracutaneous retention than transcutaneous delivery. The study helped to confirm that ablative fractional treatment facilitates the uptake of both small and large molecules through the skin, and hints that laser parameters may be varied to change the distribution of molecules.

General Technique for Fractional Ablative LAD

Treatments are performed by the authors predominantly in the outpatient clinic setting, and the technique for LAD is only a modest addition to the general technique for ablative fractional laser resurfacing. Most commonly, topical anesthetic preparations are applied under occlusion for 1 hour or more prior to treatment. Forced air cooling, cold packs, local and regional anesthesia, systemic pain medications, and even sedation or general anesthesia can be used depending on factors such as patient age, area of involvement, and individual tolerance. In the view of the authors, the topical agent should ideally be applied within 2 to 3 minutes of laser treatment in a given area. Though this aspect requires further investigation, one recent study in a porcine model demonstrated the rapid formation of a fibrin plug within the ablated channel.[28] Within 5 minutes of treatment, more than 25% of the length of the channel was noted to be filled, and this increased rapidly with time. The liquid agent is applied to the treatment area and rubbed in with a gloved hand, and any excess is wiped with gauze. Delivery is likely mediated via capillary action through the channels. It should be noted that injured areas are heterogeneous, and may be a composite of hypertrophic and atrophic scar tissue. Delivery of an agent, such as corticosteroid of a particular concentration, may be desired only in specific areas. However, the agent may proceed down any open channel. Therefore, it is prudent to apply the agent judiciously and initiate laser treatment in the area where the highest concentration of agent will be applied (such as the hypertrophic portions of a scar in the case of corticosteroids).

Immediately after ablative fractional laser treatment and LAD is completed, petrolatum or a petrolatum-based ointment is applied and continued several times daily until the site is fully epithelialized, usually within 2 to 3 days.[29] Nonstick dressings are applied as needed for convenience. Patients may resume showering the following day and begin gentle daily cleansing with mild soap and water, without scrubbing. Patients are allowed to resume essentially normal activity after treatment, including physical and occupational therapy. Despite frequent treatment on the compromised skin of scars, in the experience of the authors postprocedure infection and other complications appear to be very rare. Viral prophylaxis should be considered when treating facial areas, and antibiotics may be considered for prophylaxis starting 1 day prior to treatment and continuing up to

1 week in patients considered at high risk. Antifungals may be entertained on a case-by-case basis or if patient develops localized pain or pruritus after laser treatment and a bacterial infection is not suspected. Postprocedure pain is generally minimal, so pain medication beyond baseline is not typically required. As previously discussed, optimal scar therapy requires a multidisciplinary, multimodal approach. Before, concurrent with, and after LAD therapy, the patient may be managed by a variety of specialists including surgeons, dermatologists, physical and occupational therapists, and mental health professionals.

Case Examples

Hypertrophic Scar—5-FU and TAC

TAC application immediately after fractional laser treatment takes advantage of the ablative fractional laser's ability to penetrate deeply into the hypertrophic scar to induce remodeling, and perhaps synergistically enhance collagen degradation and decrease collagen production (Fig. 14-2). Waibel et al.[21] conducted a prospective, single-arm, pilot study including 15 consecutive subjects with hypertrophic scars from burns, trauma, and surgery. Subjects were treated with three to five ablative fractional laser treatment sessions at 2- to 3-month intervals combined with immediate postoperative topical application of TAC suspension at a concentration of 10 mg per mL. Treatments were well tolerated and resulted in average overall improvement of 2.73/3.0, although the lack of control precluded a definitive determination of whether it was indeed a synergistic response. In another study, Issa et al.[30] successfully used fractional ablative radiofrequency, rather than fractional laser technology, to assist in delivery of triamcinolone for hypertrophic scars in four patients. Further research is required in this area, and multiple modalities could theoretically be used to generate fractionated wounds to promote drug delivery.

Corticosteroids do have the potential to cause several adverse effects including cutaneous atrophy, hypopigmentation, and telangiectasias. Intralesional 5-FU has been reported to be a safe and effective intralesional treatment for pathologic scars, and may provide an effective alternative for LAD in scar management.[31] Waibel and colleagues also conducted a comparative study to evaluate the efficacy of ablative fractional LAD with topically applied 5-FU versus TAC for hypertrophic scar treatment.[32] Two distinct but similar scars were each treated with either TAC suspension or 5-FU solution on the same patient. Results suggested equal efficacy of the two agents for decreasing scar height and length. However, TAC was associated with more adverse events including increased scar width and increased telangiectasias.

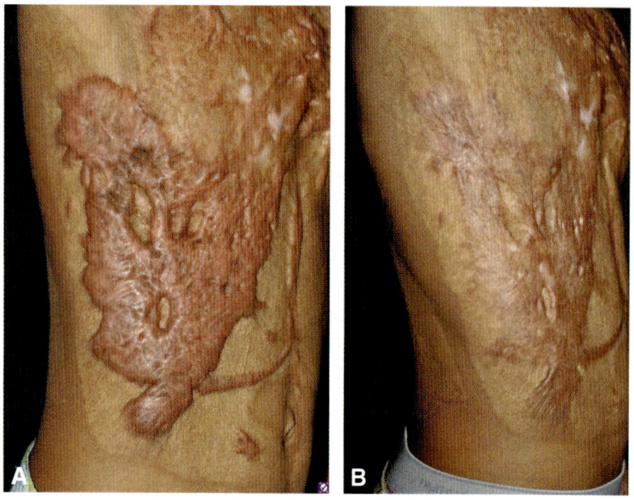

FIGURE 14-2 **A:** An 18-year-old man with Fitzpatrick skin type V with severe hypertrophic scars 4 years after a burn injury. **B:** Same patient after a total of seven ablative fractional laser treatments with an Er:YAG laser (Joule ProFractional, Sciton, Inc., Palo Alto, CA) at settings of 350 µm depth and 11% density. Immediately after each laser treatment, 10 mg per mL triamcinolone acetonide suspension was applied topically over the treatment area. Focal intralesional injections of triamcinolone acetonide 10 mg per mL were also performed in the thickest areas.

Atrophic Scar—PLLA

Atrophic scars result from a net loss of dermal and subcutaneous tissue during the healing process after trauma or inflammation. Fractional laser treatment alone has been shown to improve atrophic scars resulting from surgery and trauma.[33] However, multiple treatments are routine and results are still often suboptimal. PLLA induces neocollagenesis, and is typically injected into the subcutaneous or supraperiosteal plane for the purpose of gradual facial volume correction.[34] LAD of PLLA and potentially other tissue fillers has the potential to combine laser-induced tissue remodeling with durable neocollagenesis (Fig. 14-3).

Rkein et al.[24] conducted a prospective, uncontrolled case series of 19 patients with atrophic scars treated with a combination of ablative fractional CO_2 laser resurfacing (Lumenis UltraPulse, Deep FX, Yokneam Israel) and topically applied PLLA. A histopathologic study using fresh cadaveric tissue in advance of the clinical study showed evidence of PLLA in the ablated channels under polarized light immediately after treatment. Pulse energy settings corresponded to a treatment depth of approximately 375 to 500 µm, and the density setting was 10%. The PLLA was reconstituted at least 48 hours in advance with 6 mL sterile saline, and 2 mL 1% lidocaine with epinephrine. Photographic assessment of before and after photographs by blinded observers revealed an average overall improvement score of 2.18 on a 0 to 3 scale; 65% of the photo pairs showed an improvement score of 2.0 or above.

Hypopigmented Scar—Topical Prostaglandin (Bimatoprost and Latanoprost)

Hypopigmentation and depigmentation are common chronic problems in patients with scars resulting from surgery, inflammatory conditions, and trauma such as burns. Improving hypopigmentation has been a difficult challenge because of limited treatment options, particularly in patients with skin of color. Fractional laser treatment has been reported to improve hypopigmentation associated

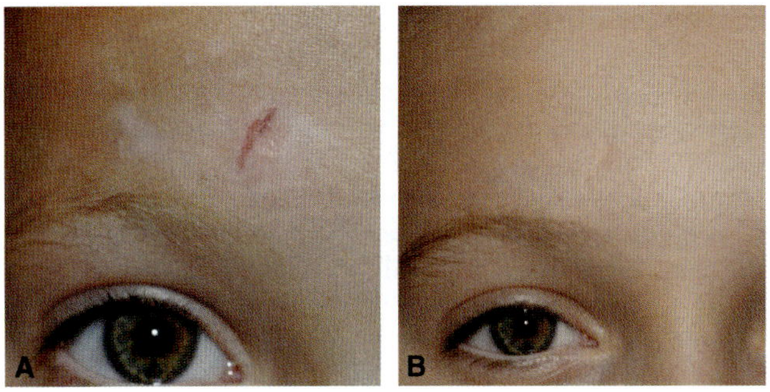

FIGURE 14-3 **A:** A 10-year-old girl with atrophic scarring 3 months after a dog bite on her right forehead. **B:** Same patient 6 months after a single fractional ablative CO_2 laser treatment (Lumenis UltraPulse, Yokneam, Israel. Deep FX: 15 mJ, 10% density) and topical laser-assisted delivery of poly-L-lactic acid (Sculptra Aesthetic, Lausanne, Switzerland, reconstituted with 8 mL sterile water and 1 mL 1% lidocaine with epinephrine at least 48 hours prior to application) immediately after laser treatment. In addition to improvement in the contour of the depressed scar, note the interval improvement in surrounding hypopigmentation.

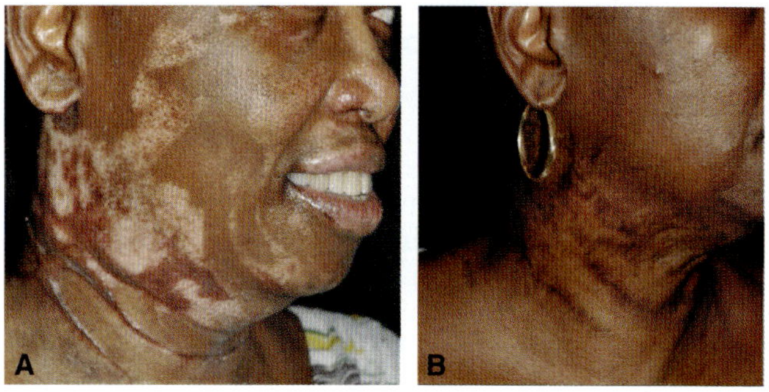

FIGURE 14-4 **A:** A 63-year-old woman with Fitzpatrick skin type V with hypertrophic scars and patchy dyspigmentation after a thermal burn. **B:** Same patient after two combination fractional ablative laser and topical bimatoprost treatments, 16 months after the initial treatment. Treatments were performed with a fractional CO_2 laser (Lumenis UltraPulse, Yokneam, Israel. Deep FX: 30 mJ, 5% density to hypertrophic areas and 15 mJ, 10% density to surrounding areas, followed by Active FX: 90 mJ, density 4 to the entire treatment area using a "painting" technique in a waving motion rather than a stamping technique to decrease the effective density of treatment) combined with topical bimatoprost (0.03%) immediately after treatment and then twice daily for 1 week. Please note that a density setting of 4 with the Active FX corresponds to nearly 100% coverage (nonfractionated) when performed in a stamping technique. This should only be considered by experienced physicians in the context of scars, especially in patients with darker skin types.

with acne and surgical scars.[33,35] The mechanism of action is hypothesized to be repopulation of melanocytes in hypopigmented areas from surrounding hair follicles and basal melanocytes, whereas fractional ablative and nonablative columns help to remove excess pigment. Although fractional lasers offer a new and promising tool for the treatment of hypopigmentation and dyspigmentation in general, results are still often disappointing.

Bimatoprost is a prostaglandin originally brought to the market to treat glaucoma, and was noted to have a side-effect profile that included periocular hyperpigmentation due to increased melanogenesis with a dose-dependent relationship. Massaki et al.[36] reported safe and effective treatment of hypopigmented scars using a combination of a series of 1,550-nm nonablative fractional laser treatments with topical bimatoprost 0.03% solution and either tretinoin or pimecrolimus. In a randomized controlled study using the prostaglandin latanoprost, Siadat et al.[37] reported a statistically significant enhancement in the repigmentation of hypopigmented scars using a combination of fractionated CO_2 laser treatment and latanoprost 0.005% compared to fractional CO_2 laser treatment alone. Because melanocytes reside in the basal layer of the epidermis, it is possible that relatively modest treatment depths may be adequate to stimulate repigmentation. Although additional research in this area is required, such treatments could potentially be well tolerated by patients, even over large areas (Fig. 14-4).

Future Applications

Percutaneous Delivery of Cells

Rodriguez-Menocal et al.[38] recently reported the first successful delivery of functional hematopoietic stem cells to distant sites in a murine model using the technique of ablative fractional Er:YAG laser pretreatment followed by the topical application of stem cell–containing external chambers. The study provides evidence that LAD is a potentially viable mechanism for the noninvasive delivery of functional cells to treat a variety of cutaneous and systemic disorders. Though this research is still in its infancy, this observation has enormous potential implications for the future of scar management and enhanced wound healing. In the area of scar management, it is conceivable that related techniques could lead to the regeneration of normal cutaneous adnexae in scarred areas, or perhaps ultimately even scarless wound healing.

Enhancing LAD

Ablative fractional laser pretreatment, as described in the preceding sections, is one of the latest and most promising of a variety of strategies used to enhance cutaneous delivery of topically applied agents. However, current LAD technique generally relies on passive uptake into the newly ablated channels. Although this has proven to increase the delivery of a variety of agents, passive uptake alone may not provide adequate access to deeper portions of the channel in part because of competing interstitial fluid and fibrin. As noted in prior discussion, increasing column depth has not been shown to lead to clear and reproducible increases in drug delivery beyond a certain threshold, though therapies such as cutaneous tumor treatment with PDT may benefit from enhanced delivery to deeper tissues. Active filling of the channels to help optimize LAD with both novel and existing adjunctive methods (e.g., pressure and sonophoresis) has thus been proposed.[25,39] Erlendsson et al.[25] investigated a standardized method to actively fill laser-generated channels by altering pressure (compressed air), vacuum, and pressure (PVP) in a porcine model. The authors found that PVP after ablative fractional laser treatment induced deeper, greater, and more rapid delivery of the test drug than conventional LAD with passive filling. Future research will be required to elaborate on the efficacy, agents, applications, and potential synergistic combinations of "active" LAD.

Limitations and Potential Safety Concerns

Fractional ablative laser treatment alone is associated with a low rate of adverse events such as infection and new or worsening scarring for scar treatment and other applications, especially in contrast to nonfractionated treatments with the same laser wavelengths [1,40] However, safety data for fractional ablative LAD are currently lacking and the concomitant risks of the drug, cosmeceutical or other agent applied to the skin must also be considered. A wide array of agents may theoretically be delivered using LAD, though these have generally not been formulated nor FDA approved for this route of delivery. Research in this area is in its infancy; with time the physiochemical properties of each drug, efficacy, safety, dosing, timing, and optimal procedural combinations and applications will begin to be elucidated. In the experience of the authors, LAD for agents such as corticosteroids, 5-FU, and cutaneous fillers for scars and aminolevulinic acid for PDT has thus far been effective and well tolerated.

A potential drawback of LAD is that fractional ablative CO_2 and Er:YAG laser systems can cost many thousands of dollars. It is not yet proven that laser-generated channels would be superior to channels with a similar diameter generated by other means (i.e., needling, etc.) for some applications. However, the efficacy of ablative fractional laser treatment alone for scars does favor additional investigation for potential synergistic effects. In the view of the authors, an appropriate amount of thermal injury likely does potentiate the response. Ablative fractional wounds are associated with a healing time of 1 to 2 days prior to reepithelialization, and an additional 1 to 2 weeks of erythema in the treatment area. The wounds also temporarily create a direct portal of entry for bacteria and other pathogens, with potential access to the circulatory system and perhaps underlying structures depending on the location and depth of treatment. Furthermore, mild to moderate discomfort is associated with the procedure itself. However, in the authors' experience the treatments are relatively safe and well tolerated in the office setting using local measures.

Because the dermal channels generate direct access to the cutaneous vascular system, there are concerns of potential systemic toxicity associated with LAD. For example, Oni et al. noted enhanced lidocaine absorption and detectable blood levels after LAD in a porcine model.[18] Potential toxicity is an especially important concept for children given their low overall body weight and high surface area to volume ratio (see Chapter 11). Furthermore, injuries such as burns may generate scars over large areas, and cutaneous absorption in these areas is already variable and difficult to predict because of the underlying changes in the integument. A systematic review of Cushing's syndrome after intralesional TAC revealed that multiple cases had been reported in the literature, and that children were at greatest risk for the complication.[41] The authors concluded that monthly doses in children should not exceed 30 mg, and advised close follow-up during treatment. It is difficult, however, to extrapolate recommendations on corticosteroid dosing for LAD based on data from the intralesional route of administration. For example, if 0.75 mL of 40 mg per mL TAC (30 mg) were rubbed onto a fractional treatment area, only a small portion would actually be absorbed into the channels; the vast majority would be taken up onto the gauze during cleanup. Furthermore, the ultimate uptake would likely depend upon variables such as the column diameter, the vehicle and concentration of the agent, and the time after treatment. Additional study is required to determine safe dosing based on the drug administered, the surface area treated, and associated laser settings such as column depth, density, and diameter.

Conclusions

Ablative fractional lasers offer a unique and promising therapeutic modality to help bypass the epidermal barrier and enhance the delivery of a variety of topically applied agents for both local and systemic effects. Many questions remain unanswered, and a great deal of additional research is required to establish the efficacy and safety of LAD for particular indications, as well as the optimal formulations, dosing, timing, and laser platform and settings. Other lines of investigation will determine appropriate adjunctive treatments to enhance LAD. Fractional laser technology itself has revolutionized scar therapy, offering unprecedented control for physicians and an excellent combination of safety and efficacy. LAD is a logical next step in the evolution of the technique, potentially opening the door to huge new advances in scar management.

Disclaimer

The views expressed in this article are those of the authors and do not necessarily reflect the official policy or position of the Department of the Navy, Department of Defense, or the United States Government. Dr. Shumaker is a military service member. This work was prepared as part of his official duties. Title 17, USC, § 105 provides that 'Copyright protection under this title is not available for any work of the United States Government.' Title 17, USC, § 101 defines a U.S. Government work as a work prepared by a military service member or employee of the U.S. Government as part of that person's official duties.

REFERENCES

1. Anderson RR, Donelan MB, Hivnor C, et al. Laser treatment of traumatic scars with an emphasis on ablative fractional laser resurfacing: Consensus report. *JAMA Dermatol.* 2014;150:187–193.
2. Waibel J, Wulkan A, Lupo M, et al. Treatment of burn scars with the 1550 nm nonablative fractional erbium laser. *Lasers Surg Med.* 2012;44:441–446.
3. Sklar L, Burnett C, Waibel J, et al. Laser assisted drug delivery: a review of an evolving technology. *Lasers Surg Med.* 2014;46:249–262.
4. Haedersdal M, Sakamoto FH, Farinelli WA, et al. Fractional CO_2 laser-assisted drug delivery. *Lasers Surg Med.* 2010;42:113–122.
5. Bloom B, Brauer J, Geronemus R. Ablative fractional resurfacing in topical drug delivery: An update and outlook. *Dermatol Surg.* 2013;39:839–848.
6. Yun PL, Tchihara R, Anderson RR. Efficacy of erbium:yttrium–aluminum–garnet laser-assisted delivery of topical anesthetic. *J Am Acad Dermatol.* 2002;47:542–547.

7. Haak CS, Farinelli WA, Tam J, et al. Fractional laser-assisted delivery of methyl aminolevulinate: impact of laser channel depth and incubation time. *Lasers Surg Med.* 2012;44:787–795.
8. Haedersdal M, Katsnelson J, Sakamoto FH, et al. Enhanced uptake and photoactivation of topical methyl aminolevulinate after fractional CO_2 laser pretreatment. *Lasers Surg Med.* 2011;43:804–813.
9. Hsiao CY, Huang CH, Hu S, et al. Fractional carbon dioxide laser treatment to enhance skin permeation of abscorbic acid 2-glucoside with minimal skin disruption. *Dermatol Surg.* 2012;38:1284–1293.
10. Marra DE, Yip D, Fincher EF, et al. Systemic toxicity from topically applied lidocaine in conjunction with fractional photothermolysis. *Arch Dermatol.* 2006;142:1024–1026.
11. Lee WR, Shen SC, Al-Suwayeh SA, et al. Laser-assisted topical drug delivery by using a low-fluence fractional laser: Imiquimod and macromolecules. *J Control Release.* 2011;153:240–248.
12. Lee WR, Pan TL, Wang PW, et al. Erbium:YAG laser enhances transdermal peptide delivery and skin vaccination. *J Control Release.* 2008;128:200–208.
13. Gomez C, Costela A, García-Moreno I, et al. Laser treatments on skin enhancing and controlling transdermal delivery of 5-fluorouracil. *Lasers Surg Med.* 2008;40:6–12.
14. Lee WR, Shen SC, Fang CL, et al. Topical delivery of methotrexate via skin pretreated with physical enhancement techniques: Low-fluence erbium:YAG laser and electroporation. *Lasers Surg Med.* 2008;40:468–476.
15. Forster B, Klein A, Szeimies RM, et al. Penetration enhancement of two topical 5-aminolaevulinic acid formulations for photodynamic therapy by erbium:YAG laser ablation of the stratum corneum: continuous versus fractional ablation. *Exp Dermatol.* 2010;19:806–812.
16. Erlendsson AM, Taudorf EH, Eriksson AH, et al. Ablative fractional laser alters biodistribution of ingenol mebutate in the skin. *Arch Dermatol Res.* 2015;307:515–522.
17. Bachhav YG, Heinrich A, Kaila YN. Using laser microporation to improve transdermal delivery of diclofenac: increasing bioavailability and the range of therapeutic applications. *Eur J Pharm Biopharm.* 2011;78:408–414.
18. Oni G, Brown SA, Kenkel JM. Can fractional lasers enhance transdermal absorption of topical lidocaine in an in vivo animal model? *Lasers Surg Med.* 2012;44:168–174.
19. Basnett A, Nguyen TA, Cannavino C, et al. Ablative fractional laser resurfacing with topical paromomycin as an adjunctive treatment for a recalcitrant cutaneous leishmaniasis wound. *Lasers Surg Med.* 2015;47(10):788–791.
20. Lee WR, Shen SC, Aljuffali IA, et al. Erbium-yttirum-aluminum-garnet laser irradiation ameliorates skin permeation and follicular delivery of antialopecia drugs. *J Pharm Sci.* 2014;103:3542–3552.
21. Waibel JS, Wulkan AJ, Shumaker PR. Treatment of hypertrophic scars using laser and laser assisted corticosteroid delivery. *Lasers Surg Med.* 2013;45:135–140.
22. Waibel JS, Mi QS, Ozog D, et al. Laser-assisted delivery of vitamin C, vitamin E, and ferulic acid formula serum decreases fractional laser post-operative recovery by increased beta fibroblast growth factor expression. *Lasers Surg Med.* 2016;48(3):238–244. doi:10.1002/lsm.22448.
23. Kim H, Gallo J. Evaluation of the effect of platelet-rich plasma on recovery after ablative fractional photothermolysis. *JAMA Facial Plast Surg.* 2015;17: 97–102.
24. Rkein A, Ozog D, Waibel JS. Treatment of atrophic scars with fractionated CO_2 laser facilitating delivery of topically applied poly-L-lactic acid. *Dermatol Surg.* 2014;40:624–631.
25. Erlendsson AM, Doukas AG, Farinelli WA, et al. Fractional laser-assisted drug delivery: active filling of laser channels with pressure and vacuum alternation. *Lasers Surg Med.* 2016;48(2):116–124. doi: 10.1002/lsm.22374.
26. Bachhav YG, Summer S, Heinrich A, et al. Effect of controlled laser microporation on drug transport kinetics into and across the skin. *J Control Release.* 2010;146:31–36.
27. Haak CS, Bhayana B, Farinelli WA, et al. The impact of treatment density and molecular weight for fractional laser assisted drug delivery. *J Control Release.* 2012;163:335–341.
28. Kositrana G, Evers M, Sajjadi A, et al. Rapid fibrin plug formation within cutaneous ablative fractional CO_2 laser lesions. *Lasers Surg Med.* 2016;48(2):125–132.
29. Banzhaf CA, Wind BS, Mogensen M, et al. Spatiotemporal closure of fractional laser-ablated channels imaged by optical coherence tomography and reflectance confocal microscopy. *Lasers Surg Med.* 2016;48(2):157–165.
30. Issa MC, Kassuga LE, Chevrand NS, et al. Topical delivery of triamcinolone via skin pretreated with ablative radiofrequency: a new method in hypertrophic scar treatment. *Int J Dermatol.* 2013;52:367–370.
31. Nanda S, Reddy BS. Intralesional 5-fluorouracil as a treatment modality of keloids. *Dermatol Surg.* 2004;30:54–56.
32. Waibel J. Treatment of hypertrophic scars using laser assisted corticosteroid delivery vs. laser assisted 5-fluorouracil delivery [Abstract]. *Am Soc Dermatol Surg.* 2013;45(3):135–140.
33. Weiss ET, Chapas A, Brightman L, et al. Successful treatment of atrophic postoperative and traumatic scarring with carbon dioxide ablative fractional resurfacing: quantitative volumetric scar improvement. *Arch Dermatol.* 2010;146:133–140.
34. Lacombe V. Sculptra: a stimulatory filler. *Facial Plast Surg.* 2009;25:95–99.
35. Tierney EP, Hanke CW. Treatment of CO_2 laser induced hypopigmentation with ablative fractional laser resurfacing: case report and review of the literature. *J Drugs Dermatol.* 2010;9:1420–1426.
36. Massaki A, Fabi S, Fitzpatrick R. Repigmentation of hypopigmented scars using an erbium-doped 1,550 nm fractionated laser and topical bimatoprost. *Dermatol Surg.* 2012;38:995–1001.
37. Siadat AH, Rezael R, Asilian A, et al. Repigmentaton of hypopigmented scars using a combination of fractionated carbon dioxide laser with topical latanoprost vs. fractionated carbon dioxide laser alone. *Ind J Dermatol.* 2015;60:364–368.
38. Rodriguez-Menocal L, Salgado M, Davis S, et al. Percutaneous bone marrow transplantation using fractional ablative Erbium:YAG laser. *PLoS One.* 2014;9(3):e93004.
39. Erlendsson AM, Anderson RR, Manstein D, et al. Developing technology: ablative fractional lasers enhance topical drug delivery. *Dermatol Surg.* 2014;40(suppl 12):S142–S146.
40. Metelitsa AI, Alster TS. Fractionated laser skin resurfacing treatment complications: a review. *Dermatol Surg.* 2010;36:299–306.
41. Fredman R, Tenenhaus M. Cushing's syndrome after intralesional triamcinolone acetonide: a systematic review of the literature and multinational survey. *Burns.* 2013;39:549–557.

15 Fat Grafting for Scar Treatment

ISAAC B. JAMES, SYDNEY R. COLEMAN, and J. PETER RUBIN

KEY POINTS

- Fat grafting is a powerful technique in scar management that functions both by replacing lost volume and remodeling tissue via its regenerative stromal constituents.
- Adipose-derived stem cells are a multipotent population of mesenchymal stem cells that are generally accepted as the primary regenerative engine of fat grafting.
- The Coleman method of fat grafting has been shown to minimize graft resorption and result in predictable and durable results. Key steps include gentle harvesting of fat to minimize tissue trauma, centrifugation to remove nonviable aqueous and oil fractions, and the injection of small volumes with each pass of the cannula to maximize dispersion and proximity to the blood supply.

Background

Fat grafting is a highly versatile, powerful technique that allows soft tissue augmentation across a wide range of defects and anatomy. Relatively recently, fat grafting has emerged as one of the most effective techniques for correcting scars in the surgeon's armamentarium. However, the idea of using fat to improve scar deformity is not new. In fact, the first published account of fat grafting by Neuber in 1893 described the treatment of a depressed facial scar.[1,2] Several others followed suit and advanced the technique, including the use of cannulas to inject fat under scars by both Hollander and Miller.[3,4] However, it was not until 100 years later, in the 1990s, that it started to become apparent that fat might provide more than just volume replacement. In the mid-1990s, Coleman[5] noticed that fat grafts were able to soften and even eliminate depressed scars in his patients. In addition to volume correction, he noted substantial rejuvenation in both injured and healthy skin. This notion was further solidified by Rigotti's pioneering work in fat grafting sites of radiation injury.[6] Volume restoration remains a pillar of fat graft efficacy, but there is clearly more to the story.

Biologic Basis for Efficacy in Scar Treatment

We now know that fat grafts improve scars by two primary functions: tissue remodeling and contour correction. Adipose-derived stem cells (ASCs) are a multipotent population of mesenchymal stem cells that reside in adipose stroma,[7,8] and are now generally accepted as the primary regenerative engine of fat grafting. Coleman's[5] processing technique of centrifuging lipoaspirate can concentrate stromal regenerative cells in the remaining graft and enhance its regenerative capacity.[9–11]

Tissue Remodeling

Biology of ASCs

Our current understanding of ASC biology suggests that they play several important roles following fat transfer.

Differentiation to Adipocytes

Even when fat is transferred with meticulous technique, a large portion of the graft dies from ischemia. ASCs from the graft replace many of these dying adipocytes, and the resulting new adipocytes account for a substantial portion of the surviving adipose tissue.[12] The initial success of cell-assisted lipotransfer lends support to the idea that the stromal regenerative cells are what drive volume retention.[13–20]

Differentiation to Other Cell Types

As a multipotent mesenchymal stem cell, ASCs are capable of differentiating into numerous tissue types when stimulated. However, the degree to which they act to replace cells other than adipocytes has not been well documented in vivo.

Paracrine Mediators

A growing body of literature suggests that ASCs direct tissue repair, remodeling, and rejuvenation primarily through complex paracrine signaling. ASCs are potent immunomodulators and mediators of angiogenesis which actively migrate to sites of injury.[21–28] Moreover, ASCs residing in the hypodermis appear to play an important role in the normal wound healing cascade.[29] When added to sites of injury acutely, ASCs improve wound neovascularization and downregulate pathways responsible for excessive scarring.[28,30,31] Animal studies of ASC and stromal vascular fraction (SVF) therapy in acute burn wounds have also demonstrated faster wound healing, enhanced CD31, increased collagen remodeling, decreased inflammation, and decreased fibroblast proliferation.[32–34] When added to established scars, ASCs reduce wound size and improve color and elasticity.[31] These acute and long-term effects appear to be mediated in a paracrine fashion by modulation of the transforming growth factor β and matrix metalloproteinase pathways.[31,35–39] This is further supported by recent work from Zhou et al.[40,41] that shows improvements in acne scars when ASC-conditioned media is added to conventional fractional carbon dioxide (CO_2) laser resurfacing. These effects are seen both in the early phase of scarring and for mature, well-established acne scars. Because processed whole fat grafts contain a substantial number of ASCs and because those stem cells are capable of migrating to sites of injury, some of the beneficial effects of ASC therapy are likely also accessible by fat grafting alone. A number of animal and human studies have confirmed this, and fat grafts processed by Coleman's technique do, in fact, elicit similar regenerative effects as ASCs.[42–46]

Contour Correction

Techniques for contour correction have evolved as fat grafting has become increasingly popular. However, the general principles of successful fat grafting are the same as when Coleman described them 30 years ago. To maximize volume retention, it is important to use very small aliquots with each pass of the cannula and to disperse fat throughout the tissue. This is particularly important in scarred wound beds that have reduced vascularity and elasticity. In areas where scars are particularly adherent, subcision can help to break fibrotic bands and allow fat to fill in the defect.

Human Clinical Data

Fat Grafting for Surgical or Traumatic Scars

Appearance

Scar appearance and contour is commonly rated using the Patient Observer Scar Assessment Score (POSAS).[47] This well-validated metric consists of both patient- and observer-reported assessments of vascularization, pigmentation, thickness, relief, pliability, and an overall score, each rated on a 10-point scale. In addition to the POSAS score, a durometer is often used as an objective measure of scar hardness (see Chapter 28).

To date, two prospective cohort studies have assessed scar appearance and contour in a nonburn population. Sardesai[42] followed 14 patients with facial scars for 1 year after subdermal fat grafting and found improved dermal elasticity, reduced scar thickness, and reduced stiffness. Klinger et al.[43] followed 20 patients for 1 year and found improvements in scar hardness by durometer as well as POSAS improvements for all measures except itch.

An observational study by Maione et al.[48] used fat grafting to treat problematic scars after limb lengthening for short-limb deformity in 36 children. After grafting, patients had better skin pliability as measured by durometer and improvement on nearly all measures of POSAS. Other case reports and smaller studies have found fat grafting to be an effective treatment for tracheostomy scars,[49] cicatricial ectropion,[50,51] and reversing atrophic alopecia in a scar across the eyebrow.[52]

Pain

Fascinating work by Huang et al.[53,54] shows at least one mechanism by which fat grafts reduce neuropathic pain in burn wounds. They found that animals receiving fat grafts following burn injury to a limb experienced less neural inflammation and apoptosis in areas associated with neuropathic pain in the spinal cord. A variety of other groups have also found improvements in pain following fat grafting. Ulrich[55] reported improved pain scores when fat grafting was conducted on 20 episiotomy scars. Fredman et al.[56] found that two sessions of fat grafting into the burn scars of seven patients with chronic, refractory neuropathic pain provided some relief to six of them, evidenced by reductions in their neuropharmacologic regimen (see Chapter 11). A number of other studies of traumatic scars and surgical scars have shown similar improvements.[42,43,49,57–59] Similarly, several other studies have shown improvements in itching.[42,43,49]

Fat Grafting in Burn Scars

To date, 11 human clinical studies have assessed the impact of fat grafting targeted specifically at burn scars.[20,43,51,60–66] Most were cohort studies, and only one had a control group. All reported some level of functional and aesthetic improvement with fat grafting. Improvements in texture, contour, color, elasticity, mobility, patient satisfaction, and softness by durometer were reported. Histology revealed improved vascularization, dermal thickening, and deposition of organized neocollagen.

Scars from Radiation Injury

Rigotti was the first to report using fat grafts to treat severe radiation injury (LENT-SOMA grade 3-4). He treated 20 consecutive patients and saw major improvements in all but one case.[6] Panettier[67] followed 61 patients with irradiated prosthetic breast reconstructions, 20 of which received multiple rounds of lipofilling. Three months after the final grafting session, he found improvements on all objective LENT-SOMA measures as well as improvements in the aesthetic rating. Akita has also reported improvement from chronic radiation injury in 10 patients when treated with ASCs.[68,69]

Keloids and Severe Hypertrophic Scars

To date, no robust trials have addressed fat grafting for the management of keloids. Klinger et al.[61] published a report of three patients with hypertrophic scars and keloids from severe burns and found improved texture, softness, thickness, and elasticity compared to their pretreatment baseline. Given the limited treatment options currently available and the relative success of ASCs in animal models of hypertrophic scarring, ongoing trials will be of great interest.

Capsular Contracture

Fat grafts have been used to treat the complications of capsular contracture since 2007 when their regenerative properties were beginning to be fully realized.[5,6,70] Missana, Yoshimura, and others have published techniques using fat grafts and cell-enriched fat grafts as a rescue procedure for capsular contracture necessitating implant removal or downsizing.[70–74] However, this phenomenon has not been studied systematically in the context of fat grafting.

Dupuytren Disease

Hovius et al.[75] recently published the first trial of fat grafting in Dupuytren disease. They placed fat grafts after percutaneous needle aponeurotomy to help prevent recurrence of contracture. They followed 50 patients for an average of 44 weeks after the procedure and found improvement in flexion contracture across multiple joints. They also noted restoration of the subcutaneous fat pads in areas where fat was placed. A total of 96% of patients were satisfied with the result. The authors report that they are currently initiating a multicenter randomized controlled trial (RCT) to validate these findings.

Scleroderma

As with keloids and severe burn contractures, scleroderma is a debilitating disease with few effective treatment options. Fat grafts have been found to improve function and quality of life in several case reports, retrospective reviews, and a case series of 20 patients receiving fat for perioral fibrosis.[76–82] Using microfat[83] and SVF injections in the face and hand, respectively, Magalon et al.[78] have found increased mobility, reduced pain, and improved quality of life. They recently completed an open label phase 1 clinical trial injecting SVF into the hands of 12 female scleroderma patients without any major adverse events.[84] Longer term RCTs will be needed to confirm these findings and to assess the capacity of fat, SVF, and/or ASCs to drive lasting improvements.

Stem Cells and Additives

Several strategies have been attempted to improve graft volume retention and thus reduce the need for repeated surgeries. Current popular strategies include the addition of ASC-rich SVF, platelet-rich plasma (PRP), and insulin. Although these techniques are still being developed, preliminary clinical data have been promising. Negenborn et al.[85] combined the results of 13 separate studies tracking volume retention by computed tomography or magnetic resonance imaging for 12 to 18 months after fat grafting for scar deformities. Fat graft alone had a mere 39% volume retention. When SVF was added, retention increased to 63%. The addition of SVF + PRP resulted in retention of 70%, and the addition of SVF + PRP + insulin resulted in a retention rate of 90%. These findings are of great interest for general fat grafting, but it remains unclear if these adjuvants have any effect on the regenerative capacity of the fat graft. PRP enhances ASC proliferation in vitro,[86] but to date, no studies have systematically assessed measures of scar remodeling when PRP is included with fat grafts. Nevertheless, improved maintenance of graft volume alone makes PRP an attractive potential adjuvant for fat grafting to scars. However, more prospective human clinical trials are needed before this is performed outside of the research setting. Many of these treatments also have regulatory issues and additional costs. Although additives could potentially reduce the future need for repeat procedures, there is currently no evidence to suggest that any of these techniques are better than standard fat grafting using Coleman's technique (see below) when it comes to tissue remodeling or long-term outcomes.

Coleman Technique

Overview

Of the clinical trials assessing the tissue remodeling aspects of fat grafts, most have employed the Coleman technique. Processing methods that employ centrifugation serve to concentrate the number of ASCs in the graft, making these techniques preferred when using fat grafting for its regenerative properties.[5,9–11] The Coleman method of fat grafting involves the gentle harvest of fat to minimize tissue trauma and cellular shearing,[87] centrifugation to remove nonviable aqueous and oil fractions,[88] and injection of small volumes with each pass of the cannula to maximize dispersion in the tissue bed and improve proximity to native blood supply.[89] Resorption is minimized and results are more predictable when these principles are followed. Scientific investigation has shown that this method yields fat grafts with high survival and normal enzymatic function.[11]

Donor Site

The ideal donor site varies based on patient preferences and on the quantity and distribution of available fat. Although differences have been observed in vitro when fat from different depots was compared, those differences have never been clearly shown to impact graft retention or tissue remodeling in vivo. Principles of preventing postliposuction deformity should be adhered to in any harvest procedure. However, in general, the medial thighs and abdomen are more at risk for wrinkling and contour deformity following liposuction, particularly when patients are thin. Experience is able to mitigate these risks, and the medial thigh can be an excellent donor site for the experienced surgeon. The love handles, lateral thighs, posterior hip, and back tend to be more forgiving. Small incisions are made to allow introduction of the harvesting cannula and are hidden in folds, creases, scars, hair-bearing areas, or stretch marks if possible. Using the same incisions, tumescent is first infiltrated into the areas planned for harvest. When cases are small and performed under local anesthesia, tumescent fluid consists of 0.5% lidocaine with 1:200,000 epinephrine. For large cases requiring general anesthesia, a tumescent solution of 0.2% lidocaine with 1:400,000 epinephrine is used instead. Ideally, the surgeon will infiltrate a volume of tumescent equal to the volume of fat planned for harvest.

Fat Harvest

Harvest of lipoaspirate is carried out manually using 10 mL syringes and a 2-hole Coleman harvesting cannula

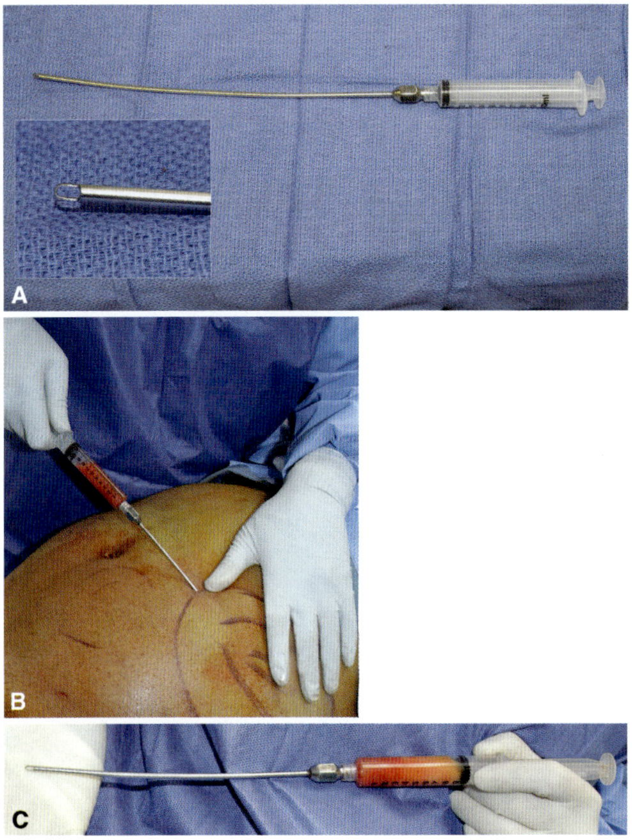

FIGURE 15-1 A 23-cm 14-G bucket handle Coleman harvesting cannula is used for harvest. The two-hole aperture of the harvesting cannula is shown in high magnification in panel (**A**). Manual harvest is carried out carefully by withdrawing the cannula slowly, about 1 cm at a time (**B**). After 9 to 10 mL of lipoaspirate has been harvested, the full syringe is swapped with an empty one (**C**).

(Fig. 15-1). Syringes are filled by slowly distracting the plunger (around 1 cm at a time) to avoid damaging adipocytes via excess negative pressure or shear. The size of the harvesting cannula should be small enough to permit passage through a 17G injection cannula but large enough to allow collection of intact fat particles.

Processing

After filling the syringe with 9 to 10 mL of lipoaspirate, the syringe is disconnected from the cannula and replaced with a new 10 mL syringe. This technique allows the harvesting cannula to remain in the adipose tissue while syringes are switched, reducing the risk of contamination. Once an adequate volume is obtained, harvesting incisions are closed with interrupted nylon suture. Lipoaspirate-filled syringes are sealed using Luer-Lok (Becton, Dickinson and Co., Franklin Lakes, NJ) caps, and sterile centrifuge sleeves are utilized to prevent contamination during centrifugation. Syringes are centrifuged at 1,286 g for 3 minutes, facilitating separation of oil and aqueous layers (Fig. 15-2A). The first syringes are likely to contain a larger fraction of aqueous tumescent and less blood than those harvested later.

After syringes are removed from the centrifuge, excess oil (Fig. 15-2B) is decanted (Fig. 15-2C). Next, the Luer-Lok cap is removed to allow the nonviable aqueous to drain out the bottom of the syringe (Fig. 15-2D). Neuro Patties or Telfa pads are utilized to wick away the remaining oil (Fig. 15-2E). Processed fat, ready to load for injection, is shown in Figure 15-2F. Figure 15-3 depicts fat after harvest (Fig. 15-3A), after centrifugation (Fig. 15-3B), and after processing by the Coleman technique (Fig. 15-3C). A good yield of fat can be obtained, but appropriate lipoaspirate volume should be taken to account for loss of volume during the process of refining the fat.

The processed fat is then loaded into 1 or 3 mL syringes depending on surgeon preference (Fig. 15-4). Fat can be transferred using a Luer-to-Luer transfer adaptor (Fig. 15-4A) or by backloading the injection syringes (Fig. 15-4B); 3 mL syringes are often utilized in larger volume sites, such as the breast, whereas 1 mL syringes are commonly preferred for grafting to small or delicate areas such as the face or hands.

Placement

Incision sites for fat placement are selected in the same fashion as harvesting sites, hiding incisions in the local anatomy whenever possible. Planned incision sites are anesthetized with 0.5% lidocaine with 1:200,000 epinephrine. A small stab incision is made just large enough to permit the passage of the injection cannula. When injecting into the face, a small amount of the 0.5% lidocaine/1:200,000 epinephrine solution can be infiltrated into the recipient bed to induce vasoconstriction prior to fat placement. This promotes constriction of damaged blood vessels and reduces the likelihood of accidental fat embolization. Postoperative bleeding is also reduced.

The goal with fat placement is to utilize the three-dimensional recipient space available to maximize contact with surrounding tissue. Combined with small injections per pass, this helps to ensure that grafted tunnels fall as close as possible to a blood supply in the recipient bed. Globules of fat >4 mm in diameter are likely to undergo central necrosis and volume loss and may result in oil cysts. The volume ratio of the fat graft relative to the size of the recipient site is also an important consideration, as grafted tunnels tend to coalesce at graft-to-recipient volume ratios above 1:4, despite best efforts at dispersion.[90]

Cannula choice is largely determined by tissue characteristics. A spatulated cannula (Fig. 15-5) may make subdermal injections or injections through scars somewhat easier. However, care should be taken as smaller or sharper cannulas are more able to puncture blood vessels. Graft injection involves gentle placement of fat parcels while withdrawing a blunt injection cannula. Blunt cannulas are less likely to puncture blood vessels, and injecting fat while withdrawing the cannula reduces the risk of injecting a column of fat into a vessel. Placement across all depths of the target area allows greater dispersion and better survival. Additionally, fat can be targeted more superficially when increased tissue remodeling is desired. In the experience of the authors, injecting fat at the dermal–hypodermal border is more likely to reduce wrinkles, decrease pore size, improve skin quality, and reduce scarring. Unfortunately, these superficial injections are at increased risk for visible contour irregularity, particularly in thin-skinned areas

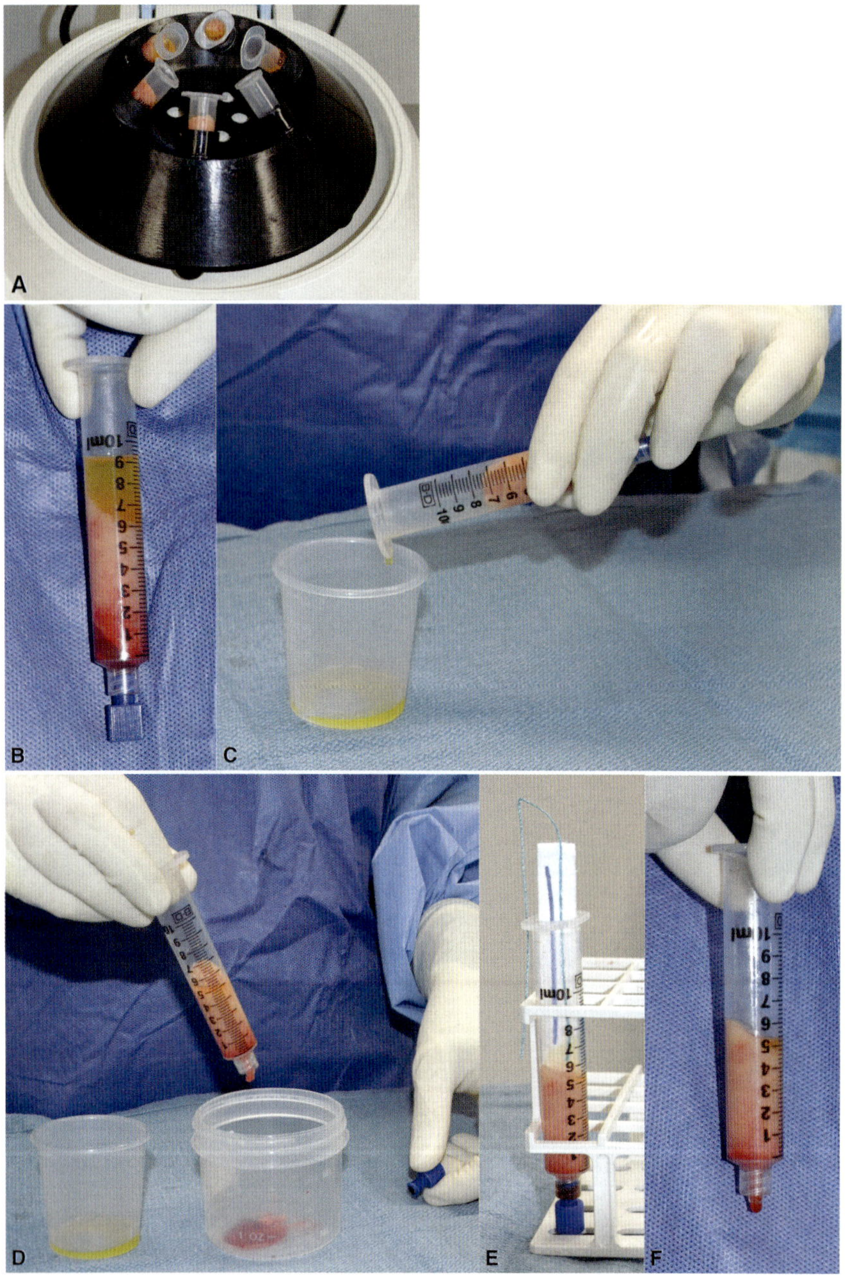

FIGURE 15-2 Once six syringes have been harvested, Luer-Lok caps are placed on the syringe to prevent leakage during centrifugation and plungers are removed. Syringes are placed into a sterile centrifuge rotor (**A**) and spun for 3 minutes at 1,286 g. After centrifugation, the fat will separate into three fractions (**B**). Oil is decanted (**C**), and the Luer-Lok cap is removed to allow drainage of aqueous (**D**). Residual oil is wicked away with a Neuro Pattie (**E**). The fat is now ready to load into 1 or 3 mL syringes for injection (**F**).

such as the eyelids. Alternatively, fat directed just above the periosteum may differentiate into bone or promote new bone formation. Injection sites are closed with a single interrupted nylon suture.

Postoperative Care

Postoperative care is dependent on the details of the procedure and anatomic location. The key concept is to provide gentle compression to the areas surrounding the recipient sites to prevent potential migration of the transplanted fat. Harvested areas are dressed with cool therapy for the first 72 hours to reduce inflammation. However, direct icing and overcooling should be avoided because low temperatures may precipitate freezing and apoptosis in the graft.

Dressings are left intact until the patient returns for a post-op visit on day 3 or 4. At this time, dressings and any sutures on the face are removed. Donor site sutures or those in higher tension areas, such as the hands, remain in place until day 5 to 7. Deep massage of recipient sites should be avoided, particularly during the first 4 weeks. However, light touch to promote lymphatic drainage can be advantageous.

Complications and Follow-Up

Most complications from fat grafting are mild and self-resolving. From an aesthetic standpoint, the most common concern is contour irregularity. However, this is avoided by careful planning and vigilance during both harvest and placement. Bruising, pigmentation, and small bumps may be present but typically resolve within 2 to

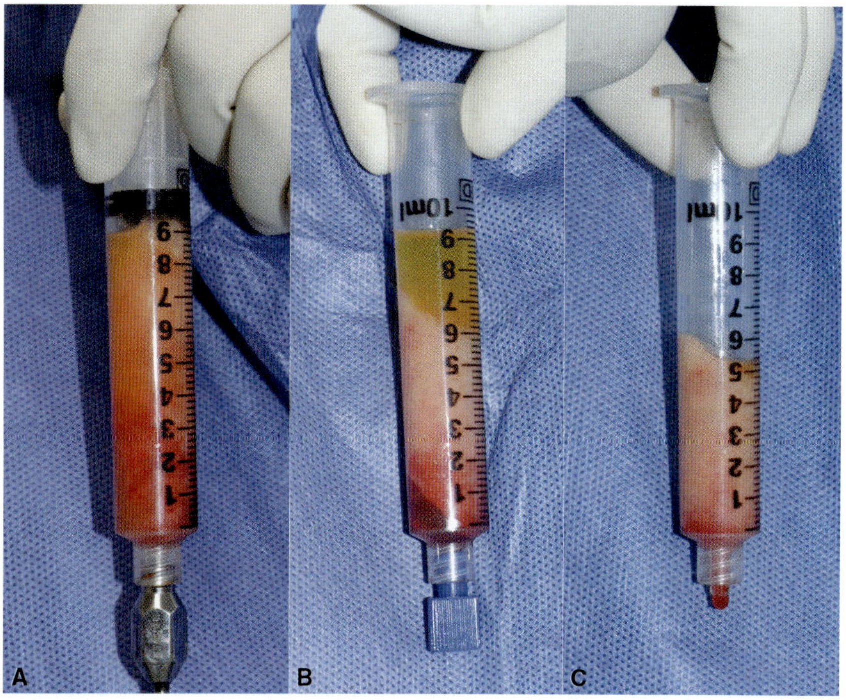

FIGURE 15-3 Each stage of the harvest and processing is shown here, from initial harvest (**A**) to postcentrifugation (**B**) to final product (**C**). Approximately 60% of the original volume remains after the fat has been concentrated.

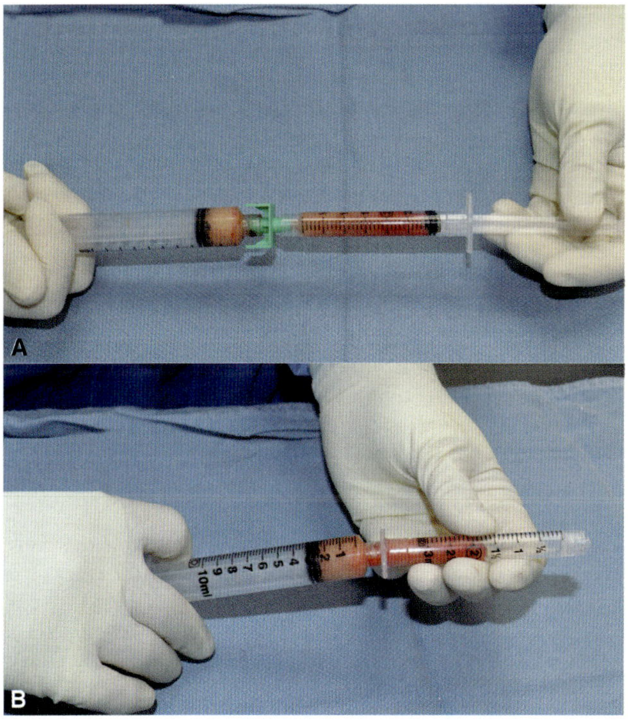

FIGURE 15-4 Processed fat can be loaded into 1 or 3 mL syringes for injection either by Luer-to-Luer transfer (**A**) or by backloading (**B**).

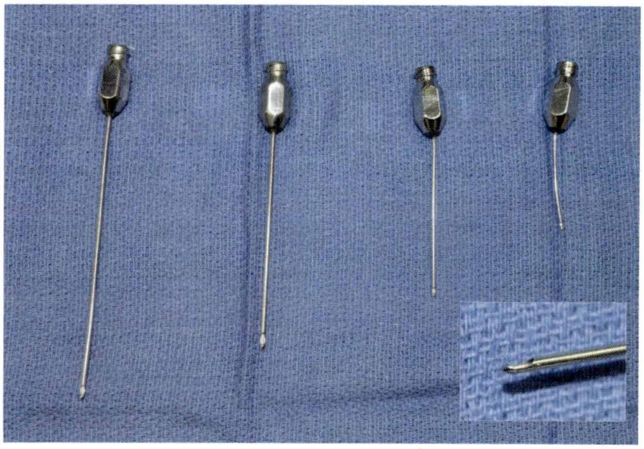

FIGURE 15-5 Different Coleman cannula lengths are available depending on the site to be injected. A spatulated tip is shown, which can be advantageous when grafting in the superficial subdermal plane or under scars.

3 weeks. Increased pigmentation lasting for several months has been reported in thin-skinned areas, such as the eyelids. Infection is also rare but can severely compromise volume retention and aesthetic outcome when it occurs. As a result, careful attention to sterile technique is critical during processing and injecting. Additionally, grafting to nonsterile areas, such as the lips or nose, is best performed only after sterile areas have been completed.

As with other facial soft tissue fillers, embolization is a rare but very serious complication. It is most often associated with the use of sharp cannulas.[91–94] The preconditions for fat embolism are well established in the orthopedic literature and include well-vascularized tissue, fragmentation of the parenchyma, and a local increase in tissue pressure.[95] Most reported cases of fat embolism to date have occurred during injection into glabellar lines, the dorsal nose, and the nasolabial fold where cannulation of the supratrochlear, dorsal nasal, or angular artery, respectively, allows retrograde transfer of fat into the ophthalmic or middle cerebral arteries, resulting in stroke or permanent blindness.[91–93,96–104] Other reports likely attributable to fat embolism include patches of skin necrosis in the region surrounding the injection. Caution is paramount when injecting fat grafts in the face, particularly around at-risk areas. Larger blunt cannulas that are introduced slowly

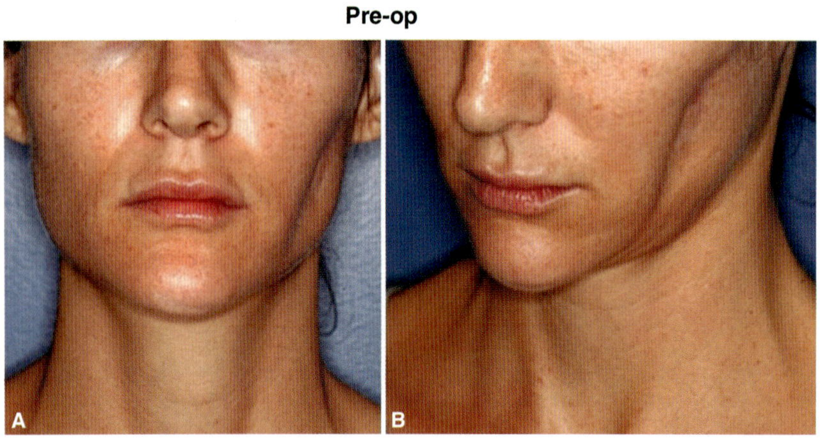

FIGURE 15-6 Patient 1 is a 35-year-old female who presented 6 months after a dog bite injury.

and gently are less likely to penetrate the arteries or their tributaries, particularly if a vasoconstrictive tumescent has been utilized. Nevertheless, if the recipient bed has substantial acute tissue injury or undermining, high local tissue pressure from overfilling the recipient bed may force fat graft into damaged arterioles and result in embolization.[105] When small aliquots of fat are injected with each pass, these elevations in tissue pressure and opportunities for embolization are minimized.[104]

Despite meticulous technique, revision procedures may be needed to manage resorption or overcorrection. If a patient gains or loses a substantial amount of weight in the postoperative period, the graft will change size accordingly. This may necessitate revision for debulking or additional grafting.[106–108] In areas with thin or delicate skin, it is very difficult to remove excess fat once placed. In these situations, it is better to undercorrect and plan to stage the filling over multiple procedures.

Representative Clinical Cases

Patient 1

Patient 1 presented at age 35, approximately 6 months after a severe dog bite injury to the left cheek necessitated excision of a "flap" of tissue. This resulted in a large soft tissue defect with darkly pigmented and retracted scarring (Fig. 15-6A and B). During her first surgery, fat was grafted to the chin and left cheek (Fig. 15-7A and B). Injections into the scar utilized a sharp 22G needle, whereas injections into the rest of the defect utilized a blunt Coleman cannula. Subcision was only partially successful because of the very retracted nature of the left cheek scar.

The patient presented 8 months after this first operation (Fig. 15-8A and B) with significant improvement in the left cheek defect but desirous of further correction. She also asked for secondary treatment of acne-related scars, and enhancement of the lips and anterior malar cheeks bilaterally (Fig. 15-9A and B). For the second surgery, placement into superficial scars was also made with a sharp 22G needle; placement outside of scars was done with blunt Coleman cannulas.

The patient presented for follow-up 4 months after her second surgery (14 months after her initial operation). She had visibly improved correction of the large soft tissue defect of the left cheek, with reduced pigmentation, as well as attractive changes in the tear troughs, anterior malar cheeks, and lips (Fig. 15-10A and B).

Patient 2

Patient 2 was a 36-year-old male who presented with severe atrophic acne scarring of the lower face, particularly in the

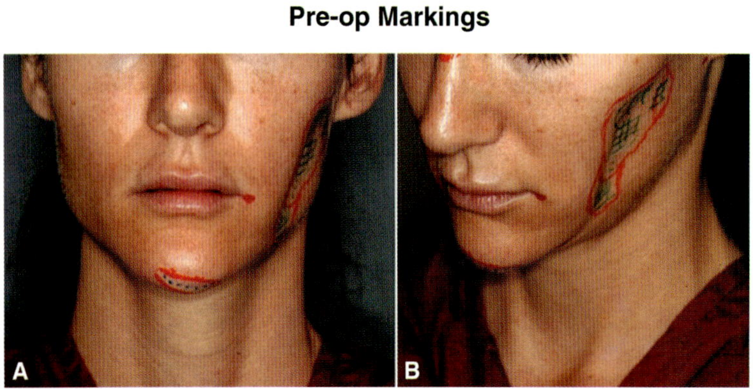

FIGURE 15-7 Preoperative markings are shown. Blue dots represent areas to receive the most placement. Green lines represent areas targeted for smaller but still significant volume change. Orange marks outline the borders of the target placement site. Red marks signify planned puncture or incision sites; 4.1 mL was placed into the left cheek defect/scars; 0.8 mL into the chin scar.

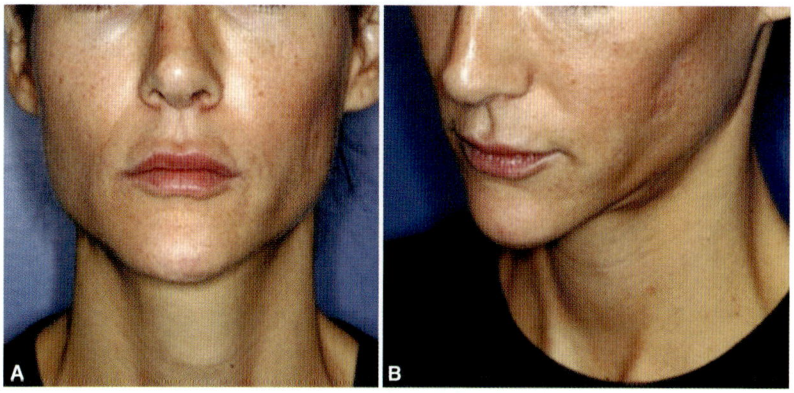

FIGURE 15-8 Eight-month postoperative views show dramatic improvements after the first procedure.

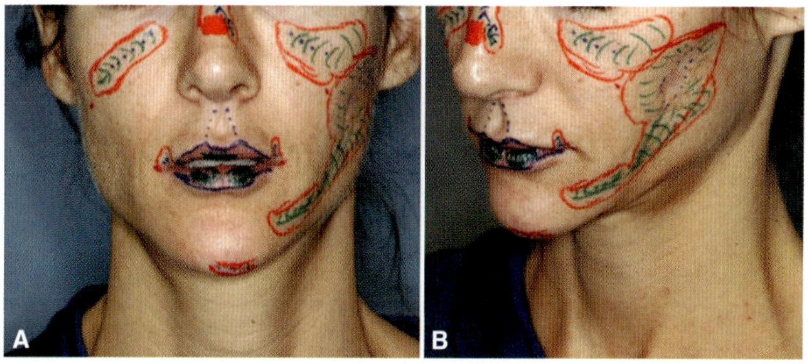

FIGURE 15-9 Presurgical markings prior to the patient's second procedure; 0.75 mL was placed into the nasal dorsum; 1.0 mL into the right anterior malar fold; 3.2 mL into the left anterior malar fold and surrounding region; 2.2 mL into the depressed scars of the left cheek; 3.0 mL superficially into the left cheek defect; 2.0 mL deeply into the left cheek defect (total of 7.0 mL into the left cheek defect); 1.3 mL into the left lower cheek "pouch" support; 0.35 mL into the chin scar; 0.25 mL into both the right and left lateral lip lines; 0.7 mL into the white roll of the upper lip; 1.3 mL into the body of the upper lip; 1.0 mL into the lower lip border; and 2.6 mL into the body of the lower lip.

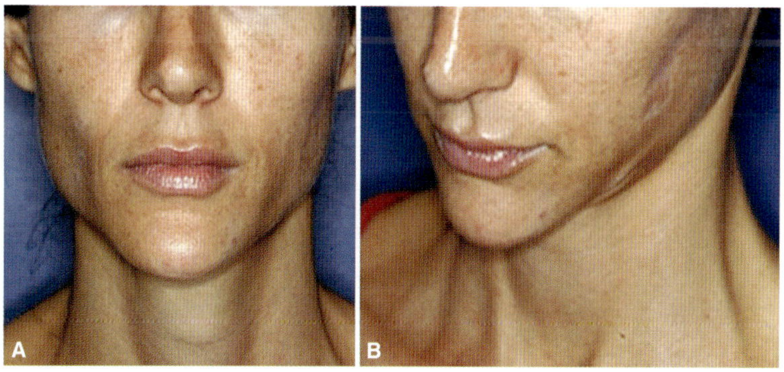

FIGURE 15-10 The patient's most recent follow-up photos were taken 14 months after initial presentation (6 months after the second procedure). Note the dramatic improvement not only in volume restoration but in skin quality.

left buccal cheek and chin areas, as well as deep subcutaneous atrophy of the malar region. Structural autologous fat was placed into bilateral anterior and lateral malar regions, the upper and local buccal cheeks, the right and left mandibular borders, and into each side of the lateral chin. A "V"-dissecting cannula was used to release the retracted scars of the cheek, allowing additional volume to be placed. A "V"-dissector was also used (always *after* fat placement) to release the other retracted scars.

The photos on the left show the patient prior to his first surgery (Fig. 15-11A–D). He had a second round of fat grafting 5 years after his first, at which time, small volumes of additional fat were added to the same areas as before. Fat was also grafted into the marionette regions and into the lips at this time. In the interim, he also underwent radiofrequency therapy (Thermage, Solta Medical, Hayward, CA) of the lower face and ultrasound therapy (Ultherapy, Ulthera, Inc., Mesa, AZ) of the lower face and neck. The photos on the right show him 15 years after his first fa• grafting surgery and 10 years after his last procedure (Fig. 15-11E–H).

There was a striking and lasting improvement in both the acne scarring and the malar atrophy. Of particular note is the dramatic correction of the scarred defects of the lower anterior buccal cheeks, particularly on the left. A total of 15 years later, at age 51, he remains quite happy with his initial corrections, but desires some minor touch-ups, primarily to the anterior mandible and chin in the near future.

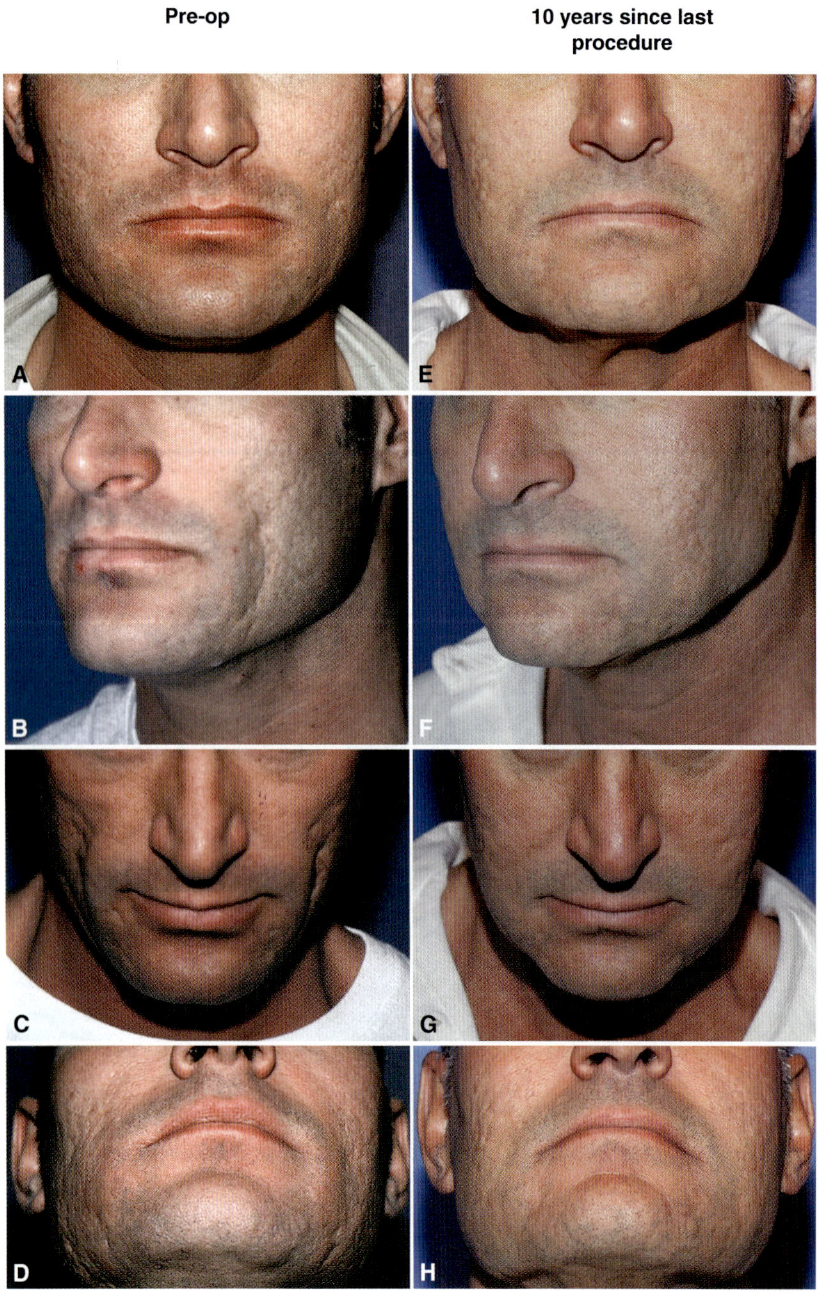

FIGURE 15-11 Patient 2 presented with depressed acne scarring of the lower face, particularly around the cheek and chin (**A–D**). A total of 2.2 mL of autologous fat graft was injected into the right anterior malar region; 1.7 mL into the left anterior malar region; 5 mL into each lateral malar region; 5 mL into each upper buccal cheek; 2 mL into each lower buccal cheek; 1.3 mL into the right mandibular border; 0.6 mL into the left mandibular border; and 1.0 mL into each side of the lateral chin. After release of retracted scars with a "V"-dissector, an additional 1.5 mL was placed into each buccal cheek. This patient also had a second fat grafting surgery 5 years after the first, at which time small volumes of additional fat were placed into the same areas, with the addition of the marionette regions (0.4 and 0.2 mL) and into the lips (upper lip, 2.8 mL; lower lip, 5.3 mL). He also underwent one round of Thermage and one of Ultherapy in the intervening years. The photos on the right were taken 15 years after his initial presentation and 10 years since his most recent procedure (**E–H**). Note the dramatic improvement in contour on the left cheek, more natural pore size, and the improved skin quality throughout the lower face.

Patient 3

Patient 3 is a 35-year-old woman who presented with subcutaneous facial atrophy, atrophic acne scarring of the cheeks and chin, and a history of Gore-Tex (W. L. Gore & Associates, Inc., Flagstaff, AZ) placement in the upper and lower lips (Fig. 15-12A–C). She desired treatment of facial lines and folds and acne scars and removal of the implants from her lips. She underwent fat grafting to the face with removal of the implants at the same time. Fat was placed into the acne scars on the right and left cheeks. A "V"-dissector was used to release scars as necessary. The lateral malar cheeks, nasolabial folds, marionette folds, and lateral chin were also enhanced bilaterally. Fat was also placed into the upper and lower lips to restore fullness. Some of the fat was placed *prior* to removing the implant, and additional fat was placed *after* removing the implant to appreciate the final contours. Experience has shown that it is often advantageous to place some fat prior to removing implants of any kind, and then (during the same operation) complete placement once the implants are removed. The patient is shown on the right at age 49, 14 years after her surgery (Fig. 15-12D–F). Note her remarkably youthful appearance, with good skin quality, beautiful, natural lips, and having retained excellent corrections in the areas of fat placement.

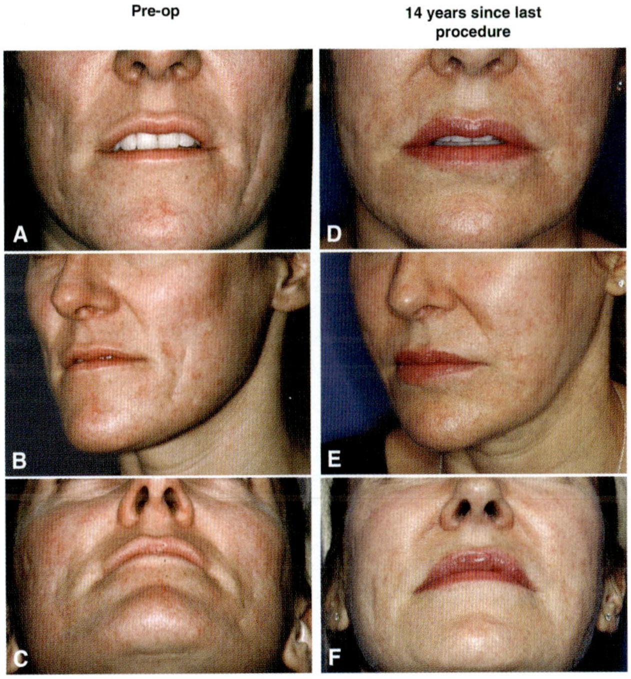

FIGURE 15-12 Patient 3 is a 35-year-old woman who presented with subcutaneous facial atrophy and acne scarring of the cheeks and chin, desiring removal of previously placed Gore-Tex from her upper and lower lips (**A–C**). A total of 8 mL of fat was placed into the acne scarring of the right cheek; 10 mL was placed on the left. A "V"-dissector was used to release some of the scars. Additionally, the lateral malar cheeks were enhanced with 4 mL on the right, and 5 mL on the left; 2.5 mL was placed into each nasolabial fold; 0.6 mL into the right marionette fold, and 0.6 mL on the left; 2 mL was placed into each side of the lateral chin; 1.4 mL was placed into the cutaneous lip. A total of 8 mL was placed into the lower lip, and 3.5 mL was placed into the upper lip. The images on the right show her 14-year follow-up (**D–F**). Note the remarkable youthful appearance and improvement in skin quality throughout. Her lips look dramatically more natural, and she generally appears younger at follow-up, despite being 14 years older.

Conclusion

Fat grafting is one of the surgeon's best tools for treating scars. It replaces lost volume and is able to remodel tissue via its regenerative stromal constituents. Most importantly, the corrections are lasting and stable. Patients often appear more youthful at long-term follow-up than at their initial presentation, despite advancing age. Although additional adjuvants may further extend the regenerative capacity of fat grafts in the future, well-controlled, long-term, blinded RCTs are needed to verify the current observations and to ensure that safety and efficacy persists over time. Meanwhile, standard fat grafting using the Coleman technique is highly effective at treating a wide range of scar locations and severities and, in the view of the authors, should be considered the gold standard for scar treatment among the methods currently available.

REFERENCES

1. Neuber G. Fettransplantation. *Chir Kongr Verhandl Dtsch Gesellsch Chir*. 1893;22:66.
2. Billings E, May JW. Historical review and present status of free fat graft autotransplantation in plastic and reconstructive surgery. *Plast Reconstr Surg*. 1989;83:368–381. doi:10.1097/00006534-198902000-00033.
3. Holländer E. Berliner klinischer. *Wochenschrift*. 1909;18.
4. Miller C. *Cannula Implants and Review of Implantation Techniques in Esthetic Surgery*. Chicago, IL: The Oak Press; 1926.
5. Coleman SR. Structural fat grafting: more than a permanent filler. *Plast Reconstr Surg*. 2006;118(3, suppl):108S–120S. doi:10.1097/01.prs.0000234610.81672.e7.
6. Rigotti G, Marchi A, Galiè M, et al. Clinical treatment of radiotherapy tissue damage by lipoaspirate transplant: a healing process mediated by adipose-derived adult stem cells. *Plast Reconstr Surg*. 2007;119(5):1409–1422; discussion 1423–1424. doi:10.1097/01.prs.0000256047.47909.71.
7. Zuk PA, Zhu M, Mizuno H, et al. Multilineage cells from human adipose tissue: implications for cell-based therapies. *Tissue Eng*. 2001;7(2):211–228. doi:10.1089/107632701300062859.
8. Zuk PA, Zhu M, Ashjian P, et al. Human adipose tissue is a source of multipotent stem cells. *Mol Biol Cell*. 2002;13(12):4279–4295. doi:10.1091/mbc.E02-02-0105.
9. Allen RJ, Canizares O, Scharf C, et al. Grading lipoaspirate: is there an optimal density for fat grafting? *Plast Reconstr Surg*. 2013;131(1):38–45. doi:10.1097/PRS.0b013e3182729cc6.
10. Coleman SR. Facial recontouring with lipostructure. *Clin Plast Surg*. 1997;24(2):347–367. http://www.ncbi.nlm.nih.gov/pubmed/9142473. Accessed November 10, 2016.
11. Pu LLQ, Coleman SR, Cui X, et al. Autologous fat grafts harvested and refined by the Coleman technique: a comparative study. *Plast Reconstr Surg*. 2008;122(3):932–937. doi:10.1097/PRS.0b013e3181811ff0.
12. Kato H, Mineda K, Eto H, et al. Degeneration, regeneration, and cicatrization after fat grafting. *Plast Reconstr Surg*. 2014;133(3):303e–313e. doi:10.1097/PRS.0000000000000066.
13. Toyserkani NM, Quaade ML, Sørensen JA. Cell-assisted lipotransfer: a systematic review of its efficacy. *Aesthet Plast Surg*. 2016;40(2):309–318. doi:10.1007/s00266-016-0613-1.
14. Matsumoto D, Sato K, Gonda K, et al. Cell-assisted lipotransfer: supportive use of human adipose-derived cells for soft tissue augmentation with lipoinjection. *Tissue Eng*. 2006;12:3375–3382. doi:10.1089/ten.2006.12.ft-274.
15. Kolle S-FT, Fischer-Nielsen A, Mathiasen AB, et al. Enrichment of autologous fat grafts with ex-vivo expanded adipose tissue-derived stem

cells for graft survival: a randomised placebo-controlled trial. *Lancet*. 2013;382(9898):1113–1120. doi:10.1016/S0140-6736(13)61410-5.
16. Koh KS, Oh TS, Kim H, et al. Clinical application of human adipose tissue-derived mesenchymal stem cells in progressive hemifacial atrophy (Parry-Romberg disease) with microfat grafting techniques using 3-dimensional computed tomography and 3-dimensional camera. *Ann Plast Surg*. 2012;69:331–337. doi:10.1097/SAP.0b013e31826239f0.
17. Gentile P, Orlandi A, Scioli MG, et al. A comparative translational study: the combined use of enhanced stromal vascular fraction and platelet-rich plasma improves fat grafting maintenance in breast reconstruction. *Stem Cells Transl Med*. 2012;1(4):341–351. doi:10.5966/sctm.2011-0065.
18. Li J, Gao J, Cha P, et al. Supplementing fat grafts with adipose stromal cells for cosmetic facial contouring. *Dermatol Surg*. 2013;39(3, Pt 1):449–456. doi:10.1111/dsu.12058.
19. Chang Q, Li J, Dong Z, et al. Quantitative volumetric analysis of progressive hemifacial atrophy corrected using stromal vascular fraction-supplemented autologous fat grafts. *Dermatologic Surg*. 2013;39(10):1465–1473. doi:10.1111/dsu.12310.
20. Gentile P, De Angelis B, Pasin M, et al. Adipose-derived stromal vascular fraction cells and platelet-rich plasma: basic and clinical evaluation for cell-based therapies in patients with scars on the face. *J Craniofac Surg*. 2014;25(1):267–272. doi:10.1097/01.scs.0000436746.21031.ba.
21. Kapur SK, Katz AJ. Review of the adipose derived stem cell secretome. *Biochimie*. 2013;95(12):2222–2228. doi:10.1016/j.biochi.2013.06.001.
22. Moon MH, Kim SY, Kim YJ, et al. Human adipose tissue-derived mesenchymal stem cells improve postnatal neovascularization in a mouse model of hindlimb ischemia. *Cell Physiol Biochem*. 2006;17(5/6):279–290. doi:10.1159/000094140.
23. Rehman J, Traktuev D, Li J, et al. Secretion of angiogenic and antiapoptotic factors by human adipose stromal cells. *Circulation*. 2004;109(10):1292–1298. doi:10.1161/01.CIR.0000121425.42966.F1.
24. Philips BJ, Marra KG, Rubin JP. Adipose stem cell-based soft tissue regeneration. *Expert Opin Biol Ther*. 2012;12(2):155–163. doi:10.1517/14712598.2012.644533.
25. Hausman GJ, Richardson RL. Adipose tissue angiogenesis. *J Anim Sci*. 2004;82(3):925–934. doi:10.1038/ijo.2010.180.
26. Planat-Benard V, Silvestre J-S, Cousin B, et al. Plasticity of human adipose lineage cells toward endothelial cells: physiological and therapeutic perspectives. *Circulation*. 2004;109(5):656–663. doi:10.1161/01.CIR.0000114522.38265.61.
27. Kolle S-FT, Oliveri RS, Glovinski PV, et al. Importance of mesenchymal stem cells in autologous fat grafting: a systematic review of existing studies. *J Plast Surg Hand Surg*. 2012;46(2):59–68. doi:10.3109/2000656X.2012.668326.
28. Seo BF, Jung S. The immunomodulatory effects of mesenchymal stem cells in prevention or treatment of excessive scars. *Stem Cells Int*. 2016;2016:1–8. doi:10.1155/2016/6937976.
29. Waterman RS, Tomchuck SL, Henkle SL, et al. A new mesenchymal stem cell (MSC) paradigm: polarization into a pro-inflammatory MSC1 or an immunosuppressive MSC2 phenotype. *PLoS One*. 2010;5(4):e10088. doi:10.1371/journal.pone.0010088.
30. Nie C, Yang D, Xu J, et al. Locally administered adipose-derived stem cells accelerate wound healing through differentiation and vasculogenesis. *Cell Transplant*. 2011;20(2):205–216. doi:10.3727/096368910X520065.
31. Yun IS, Jeon YR, Lee WJ, et al. Effect of human adipose derived stem cells on scar formation and remodeling in a pig model: a pilot study. *Dermatol Surg*. 2012;38(10):1678–1688. doi:10.1111/j.1524-4725.2012.02495.x.
32. Loder S, Peterson JR, Agarwal S, et al. Wound healing immediately post-thermal injury is improved by fat and adipose-derived stem cell isografts. *J Burn Care Res*. 2015;36(1):70–76. doi:10.1097/BCR.0000000000000160.
33. Karimi H, Soudmand A, Orouji Z. Burn wound healing with injection of Adipose-derived stem cells: a mouse model study. *Ann Burns Fire Disasters*. 2014;27(1):44–49. http://www.medbc.com/annals/review/vol_27/num_1/text/vol27n1p44.pdf. Accessed November 24, 2014.
34. Atalay S, Coruh A, Deniz K. Stromal vascular fraction improves deep partial thickness burn wound healing. *Burns*. 2014;40(7):1375–1383. doi:10.1016/j.burns.2014.01.023.
35. Spiekman M, Przybyt E, Plantinga JA, et al. Adipose tissue-derived stromal cells inhibit TGF-β1-induced differentiation of human dermal fibroblasts and keloid scar-derived fibroblasts in a paracrine fashion. *Plast Reconstr Surg*. 2014;134(4):699–712. doi:10.1097/PRS.0000000000000504.
36. Jackson WM, Nesti LJ, Tuan RS. Mesenchymal stem cell therapy for attenuation of scar formation during wound healing. *Stem Cell Res Ther*. 2012;3(3):20. doi:10.1186/scrt111.
37. Lam MT, Nauta A, Meyer NP, et al. Effective delivery of stem cells using an extracellular matrix patch results in increased cell survival and proliferation and reduced scarring in skin wound healing. *Tissue Eng Part A*. 2013;19(5/6):738–747. doi:10.1089/ten.TEA.2012.0480.
38. Zhang Q, Liu L-N, Yong Q, et al. Intralesional injection of adipose-derived stem cells reduces hypertrophic scarring in a rabbit ear model. *Stem Cell Res Ther*. 2015;6:145. doi:10.1186/s13287-015-0133-y.
39. DiMarino AM, Caplan AI, Bonfield TL. Mesenchymal stem cells in tissue repair. *Front Immunol*. 2013;4:1–9. doi:10.3389/fimmu.2013.00201.
40. Zhou B-R, Zhang T, Bin Jameel AA, et al. The efficacy of conditioned media of Adipose-derived stem cells combined with ablative carbon dioxide fractional resurfacing for atrophic acne scars and skin rejuvenation. *J Cosmet Laser Ther*. 2016;18(3):138–148. doi:10.3109/14764172.2015.1114638.
41. Zhou BR, Xu Y, Xu Y, et al. The effect of conditioned media of Adipose-derived stem cells on wound healing after ablative fractional carbon dioxide laser resurfacing. *Biomed Res Int*. 2013;2013:519129. doi:10.1155/2013/519126.
42. Sardesai MG, Moore CC. Quantitative and qualitative dermal change with microfat grafting of facial scars. *Otolaryngol—Head Neck Surg*. 2007;137(6):868–872. doi:10.1016/j.otohns.2007.08.008.
43. Klinger M, Caviggioli F, Klinger FM, et al. Autologous fat graft in scar treatment. *J Craniofac Surg*. 2013;24(5):1610–1615. doi:10.1097/SCS.0b013e3182a24548.
44. Maione L, Vinci V, Klinger M, et al. Autologous fat graft by needle: analysis of complications after 1000 patients. *Ann Plast Surg*. 2014;74(3):277–280. doi:10.1097/SAP.0000000000000050.
45. Sultan SM, Barr JS, Butala P, et al. Fat grafting accelerates revascularisation and decreases fibrosis following thermal injury. *J Plast Reconstr Aesthet Surg*. 2012;65(2):219–227. doi:10.1016/j.bjps.2011.08.046.
46. Sultan SM, Stern CS, Allen RJ, et al. Human fat grafting alleviates radiation skin damage in a murine model. *Plast Reconstr Surg*. 2011;128(2):363–372. doi:10.1097/PRS.0b013e31821e6e90.
47. Draaijers LJ, Tempelman FRH, Botman YA, et al. The patient and observer scar assessment scale: a reliable and feasible tool for scar evaluation. *Plast Reconstr Surg*. 2004;113(7):1960–1965; discussion 1966–1967. doi:10.1097/01.PRS.0000122208.16595.57.
48. Maione L, Memeo A, Pedretti L, et al. Autologous fat graft as treatment of post short stature surgical correction scars. *Injury*. 2014;45(S6):S126–S132. doi:10.1016/j.injury.2014.10.036.
49. Mazzola IC, Cantarella G, Mazzola RF. Management of tracheostomy scar by autologous fat transplantation. *J Craniofac Surg*. 2013;24(4):1361–1364. doi:10.1097/SCS.0b013e318292c1a4.
50. Tarallo M, Rizzo MI, Monarca C, et al. Optimal care for eyelid contraction after radiotherapy: case report and literature review. *J Oral Maxillofac Surg*. 2012;70(10):2459–2465. doi:10.1016/j.joms.2011.10.017.
51. Caviggioli F, Klinger F, Villani F, et al. Correction of cicatricial ectropion by autologous fat graft. *Aesthet Plast Surg*. 2008;32(3):555–557. doi:10.1007/s00266-008-9117-y.
52. Dini M, Mori A, Quattrini Li A. Eyebrow regrowth in patient with atrophic scarring alopecia treated with an autologous fat graft. *Dermatol Surg*. 2014;40(8):926–928. doi:10.1111/DSU.0000000000000051.
53. Huang SH, Wu SH, Lee SS, et al. Fat grafting in burn scar alleviates neuropathic pain via anti-inflammation effect in scar and spinal cord. *PLoS One*. 2015;10(9):1–13. doi:10.1371/journal.pone.0137563.
54. Huang S-H, Wu S-H, Chang K-P, et al. Autologous fat grafting alleviates burn-induced neuropathic pain in rats. *Plast Reconstr Surg*. 2014;133(6):1396–1405. doi:10.1097/PRS.0000000000000169.
55. Ulrich D, Ulrich F, van Doorn L, et al. Lipofilling of perineal and vaginal scars. *Plast Reconstr Surg*. 2012;129(3):593e–594e. doi:10.1097/PRS.0b013e3182419c2c.
56. Fredman R, Edkins RE, Hultman SC. Fat grafting for neuropathic pain after severe burns. *Ann Plast Surg*. 2015;77(4):491. doi:10.1097/SAP.0000000000000674.
57. Baptista C, Iniesta A, Nguyen P, et al. "Autologous fat grafting in the surgical management of painful scar: preliminary results" [in French]. *Chir Main*. 2013;32(5):329–334. doi:10.1016/j.main.2013.07.006.
58. Maione L, Vinci V, Caviggioli F, et al. Autologous fat graft in post-mastectomy pain syndrome following breast conservative surgery and radiotherapy. *Aesthet Plast Surg*. 2014;38(3):528–532. doi:10.1007/s00266-014-0311-9.
59. Caviggioli F, Maione L, Forcellini D, et al. Autologous fat graft in post-mastectomy pain syndrome. *Plast Reconstr Surg*. 2011;128(2):349–352. doi:10.1097/PRS.0b013e31821e70e7.

60. Bruno A, delli Santi G, Fasciani L, et al. Burn scar lipofilling. *J Craniofac Surg*. 2013;24(5):1806–1814. doi:10.1097/SCS.0b013e3182a148b9.
61. Klinger M, Marazzi M, Vigo D, et al. Fat injection for cases of severe burn outcomes: a new perspective of scar remodeling and reduction. *Aesthet Plast Surg*. 2008;32(3):465–469. doi:10.1007/s00266-008-9122-1.
62. Viard R, Bouguila J, Voulliaume D, et al. "Fat grafting in facial burns sequelae" [in French]. *Ann Chir Plast Esthét*. 2012;57(3):217–229. doi:10.1016/j.anplas.2011.06.003.
63. Khouri RK, Smit JM, Cardoso E, et al. Percutaneous aponeurotomy and lipofilling. *Plast Reconstr Surg*. 2013;132(5):1280–1290. doi:10.1097/PRS.0b013e3182a4c3a9.
64. Piccolo NS, Piccolo MS, Piccolo MTS. Fat grafting for treatment of burns, burn scars, and other difficult wounds. *Clin Plast Surg*. 2015;42(2):263–283. doi:10.1016/j.cps.2014.12.009.
65. Brongo S, Nicoletti GF, La Padula S, et al. Use of lipofilling for the treatment of severe burn outcomes. *Plast Reconstr Surg*. 2012;130(2):374e–376e. doi:10.1097/PRS.0b013e3182590387.
66. Caviggioli F, Villani F, Forcellini D, et al. Nipple resuscitation by lipostructure in burn sequelae and scar retraction. *Plast Reconstr Surg*. 2010;125(4):174e–176e. doi:10.1097/PRS.0b013e3181d45dee.
67. Panettiere P, Marchetti L, Accorsi D. The serial free fat transfer in irradiated prosthetic breast reconstructions. *Aesthetic Plast Surg*. 2009;33(5):695–700. doi:10.1007/s00266-009-9366-4.
68. Akita S, Yoshimoto H, Ohtsuru A, et al. Autologous adipose-derived regenerative cells are effective for chronic intractable radiation injuries. *Radiat Prot Dosimetry*. 2012;151(4):656–660. doi:10.1093/rpd/ncs176.
69. Akita S, Akino K, Hirano A, et al. Noncultured autologous adipose-derived stem cells therapy for chronic radiation injury. *Stem Cells Int*. 2010;2010:532704. doi:10.4061/2010/532704.
70. Missana MC, Laurent I, Barreau L, et al. Autologous fat transfer in reconstructive breast surgery: indications, technique and results. *Eur J Surg Oncol*. 2007;33(6):685–690. doi:10.1016/j.ejso.2006.12.002.
71. Yoshimura K, Asano Y, Aoi N, et al. Progenitor-enriched adipose tissue transplantation as rescue for breast implant complications. *Breast J*. 2010;16(2):169–175. doi:10.1111/j.1524-4741.2009.00873.x.
72. Scalise A, Bolletta E, Gioacchini M, et al. Fat transfer in periprosthetic capsule contracture in breast reconstruction. In: *Breast Reconstruction*. Vol 2. Cham, Switzerland: Springer International Publishing; 2016:1311–1323. doi:10.1007/978-3-319-18726-6_129.
73. Del Vecchio DA. "SIEF"—simultaneous implant exchange with fat. *Plast Reconstr Surg*. 2012;130(6):1187–1196. doi:10.1097/PRS.0b013e31826d9c3c.
74. Gurunluoglu R, Sacak B, Arton J. Outcomes analysis of patients undergoing autoaugmentation after breast implant removal. *Plast Reconstr Surg*. 2013;132:304–315. doi:10.1097/PRS.0b013e31829e7d9e.
75. Hovius SER, Kan HJ, Smit X, et al. Extensive percutaneous aponeurotomy and lipografting: a new treatment for dupuytren disease. *Plast Reconstr Surg*. 2011;128(1):221–228. doi:10.1097/PRS.0b013e31821741ba.
76. Barin EZ, Cinal H, Cakmak MA, et al. Treatment of linear scleroderma (en Coup de Sabre) with dermal fat grafting. *J Cutan Med Surg*. 2016;20(3):269–271. doi:10.1177/1203475415624912.
77. Roh MR, Jung JY, Chung KY. Autologous fat transplantation for depressed linear scleroderma-induced facial atrophic scars. *Dermatologic Surg*. 2008;34(12):1659–1665. doi:10.1111/j.1524-4725.2008.34343.x.
78. Magalon G, Daumas A, Sautereau N, et al. Regenerative approach to scleroderma with fat grafting. *Clin Plast Surg*. 2015;42(3):353–364. doi:10.1016/j.cps.2015.03.009.
79. Del Papa N, Caviggioli F, Sambataro D, et al. Autologous fat grafting in the treatment of fibrotic perioral changes in patients with systemic sclerosis. *Cell Transplant*. 2015;24(1):63–72. doi:10.3727/096368914X674062.
80. Lapiere JC, Aasi S, Cook B, et al. Successful correction of depressed scars of the forehead secondary to trauma and morphea en coup de sabre by en bloc autologous dermal fat graft. *Dermatol Surg*. 2000;26(8):793–797. http://www.ncbi.nlm.nih.gov/pubmed/10940068.
81. Consorti G, Tieghi R, Clauser LC. Frontal linear scleroderma. *J Craniofac Surg*. 2012;23(3):e263–e265. doi:10.1097/SCS.0b013e31824ef7e8.
82. Oh CK, Lee J, Jang BS, et al. Treatment of atrophies secondary to trilinear scleroderma en coup de sabre by autologous tissue cocktail injection. *Dermatologic Surg*. 2003;29(10):1073–1075. doi:10.1046/j.1524-4725.2003.29307.x.
83. Nguyen PSA, Desouches C, Gay AM, et al. Development of micro-injection as an innovative autologous fat graft technique: the use of adipose tissue as dermal filler. *J Plast Reconstr Aesthetic Surg*. 2012;65(12):1692–1699. doi:10.1016/j.bjps.2012.06.014.
84. Granel B, Daumas A, Jouve E, et al. Safety, tolerability and potential efficacy of injection of autologous adipose-derived stromal vascular fraction in the fingers of patients with systemic sclerosis: an open-label phase I trial. *Ann Rheum Dis*. 2014:1–8. doi:10.1136/annrheumdis-2014-205681.
85. Negenborn VL, Groen J-W, Smit JM, et al. The use of autologous fat grafting for treatment of scar tissue and scar-related conditions. *Plast Reconstr Surg*. 2016;137(1):31e–43e. doi:10.1097/PRS.0000000000001850.
86. Liao H-T, James IB, Marra K, et al. The effects of platelet-rich plasma on cell proliferation and adipogenic potential of Adipose-derived stem cells. *Tissue Eng Part A*. 2015;21(21/22):2714–2722. doi:10.1089/ten.TEA.2015.0159.
87. Coleman SR. The technique of periorbital lipoinfiltration. *Oper Tech Plast Reconstr Surg*. 1994;1(3):120–126. doi:10.1016/S1071-0949(10)80002-2.
88. Coleman S. Harvesting, refinement and transfer. In: *Structural Fat Grafting*. St. Louis, MO: Quality Medical; 2004:29–51.
89. Coleman SR. Overview of placement techniques. In: *Structural Fat Grafting*. St. Louis, MO: Quality Medical; 2004:70–71.
90. Bourne DA, James IB, Wang SS, et al. The architecture of fat grafting: what lies beneath the surface. *Plast Reconstr Surg*. 2016;137(3):1072–1079. doi:10.1097/01.prs.0000479992.10986.ad.
91. Park SW, Woo SJ, Park KH, et al. Iatrogenic retinal artery occlusion caused by cosmetic facial filler injections. *Am J Ophthalmol*. 2012;154(4):653–662. doi:10.1016/j.ajo.2012.04.019.
92. Ozturk CN, Li Y, Tung R, et al. Complications following injection of soft-tissue fillers. *Aesthetic Surg J*. 2013;33(6):862–877. doi:10.1177/1090820X13493638.
93. Li X, Du L, Lu J-J. A novel hypothesis of visual loss secondary to cosmetic facial filler injection. *Ann Plast Surg*. 2015;75(3):258–260. doi:10.1097/SAP.0000000000000572.
94. Gleeson CM, Lucas S, Langrish CJ, Barlow RJ. Acute fatal fat tissue embolism after autologous fat transfer in a patient with lupus profundus. *Dermatol Surg*. 2011; 37(1):111–115. doi:10.1111/j.1524-4725.2010.01829.x.
95. Peltier LF. Fat embolism. an appraisal of the problem. *Clin Orthop Relat Res*. 1984;(187):3–17. http://www.ncbi.nlm.nih.gov/pubmed/6378481. Accessed November 10, 2016.
96. Baumgartner RW. Middle cerebral artery occlusion AND ocular fat embolism after autologous fat injection in the face. *J Neurol*. 245(1):53–54.
97. Feinendegen DL, Baumgartner RW, Vuadens P, et al. Autologous fat injection for soft tissue augmentation in the face : a safe procedure ? 1998:163–167.
98. Egido JA, Arroyo R, Marcos A, et al. Middle cerebral artery embolism and unilateral visual loss after autologous fat injection into the glabellar area. *Stroke*. 1993;24(4):615–616. http://www.ncbi.nlm.nih.gov/pubmed/8465374. Accessed November 10, 2016.
99. Teimourian B. Blindness following fat injections. *Plast Reconstr Surg*. 1998;82(2):361.
100. Dreizen NG, Framm L. Sudden unilateral visual loss after autologous fat injection into the glabellar area. *Am J Ophthalmol*. 1989;107(1):85–87. http://www.ncbi.nlm.nih.gov/pubmed/2912125. Accessed November 10, 2016.
101. Yoon SS, Chang D IL, Chung KC. Acute fatal stroke immediately following autologous fat injection into the face Transient brainstem ischemia and recurrent syncope caused by a dural arteriovenous fistula. *Neurology*. 2003;61(8):1151–1152.
102. Danesh-Meyer HV, Savino PJ, Sergott RC. Ocular and cerebral ischemia following facial injection of autologous fat. *Arch Ophthalmol (Chicago, IL 1960)*. 2001;119(5):777–778. http://www.ncbi.nlm.nih.gov/pubmed/11346413. Accessed November 10, 2016.
103. Xing L, Almeida DRP, Belliveau MJ, et al. Ophthalmic artery occlusion secondary to fat emboli after cosmetic nasal injection of autologous fat. *Retina*. 2012;32(10):2175–2176. doi:10.1097/IAE.0b013e31826a6897.
104. Coleman SR. Avoidance of arterial occlusion from injection of soft tissue fillers. *Aesthetic Surg J*. 2002;22(6):555–557. doi:10.1067/maj.2002.129625.
105. Thaunat O, Thaler F, Loirat P, et al. Cerebral fat embolism induced by facial fat injection. *Plast Reconstr Surg*. 2004;113(7):2235–2236. doi:10.1097/01.PRS.0000123577.13397.D6.
106. Spector JA, Draper L, Aston SJ. Lower lid deformity secondary to autogenous fat transfer: a cautionary tale. *Aesthetic Plast Surg*. 2008;32(3):411–414. doi:10.1007/s00266-006-0190-9.
107. Coleman SR. Lower lid deformity secondary to autogenous fat transfer: a cautionary tale. *Aesthetic Plast Surg*. 2008;32(3):415–417. doi:10.1007/s00266-007-9007-8.
108. Miller JJ, Popp JC. Fat hypertrophy after autologous fat transfer. *Ophthal Plast Reconstr Surg*. 2002;18(3):228–231.

16 Multimodal Scar Management

REI OGAWA

KEY POINTS

- Keloids and hypertrophic scars (HSs), which result from abnormal healing of injured or irritated skin, are red, elevated scars that have an unappealing appearance and are associated with intermittent pain, persistent itching, and a sensation of contraction.
- It is possible that HSs and keloids are manifestations of the same fibroproliferative skin disorders, which are graded according to the intensity and period of inflammation and influenced by genetic, systemic, and local factors.
- Steroid injections have long been a first-line therapy; however, over the past decade, many studies have examined different approaches to the treatment and management of keloids/HSs. A multimodal approach is often required for optimal results, both in combination on the same treatment day and on alternating visits.
- Keloids and HSs are now regarded as treatable diseases. However, the therapeutic approaches still require improvement if they are to be truly successful from both a physiologic and an aesthetic perspective. This chapter will provide one expert's perspective on multimodal pathologic scar management.

Keloids and hypertrophic scars (HSs) are caused by abnormal healing of injured or irritated skin.[1] These red, elevated scars have an unappealing appearance and are associated with intermittent pain, persistent itching, and a sensation of contraction. Inflammation is continuous and local. Moreover, some keloids can discharge pus because of the presence of infected inclusion cysts. Many classical textbooks consider keloids and HSs to be completely different scar types. Clinicians define HSs as scars that do not grow beyond the boundaries of the original wound, whereas keloids spread into the surrounding normal skin. By contrast, pathologists make a histologic distinction between keloids and HSs based on the presence of thick eosinophilic (hyalinizing) collagen bundles, called "keloidal collagen," which are present in the former but absent from the latter (see Chapter 5). However, there are many cases in which a scar bears the growth and histologic features of both HSs and keloids. Indeed, it is possible that HSs and keloids are manifestations of the same fibroproliferative skin disorders,[2] which are graded according to the intensity and period of inflammation, which in turn are influenced by genetic, systemic, and local risk factors.[3]

Pathogenesis of Keloids and HSs

Various genetic, systemic, and local factors influence the quality and quantity of keloids and HSs. Genetic links to pathologic scar development may involve single-nucleotide polymorphisms (SNPs). A genome-wide association study[4] and our own research[5] show that four SNP loci in three chromosomal regions are significantly associated with keloid development in the Japanese population. There are probably many other genetic factors that are still not known.

In terms of systemic factors, adolescence and pregnancy appear to be associated with a higher risk of developing pathologic scars. It may be that sex hormones such as estrogens and androgens have vasodilatory effects that intensify inflammation and make keloids and HSs worse. According to our unpublished data, the rate of occurrence of keloids not caused by trauma suddenly increases around 10 years of age; thus, we consider that increases in the levels of sex steroids at the start of adolescence are responsible for the higher risk of pathologic scar development in adolescents, rather than increases in the likelihood of trauma. Moreover, our recent study revealed that hypertension is associated with the development of severe keloids.[6] Hypertension may damage the blood vessels, thereby increasing inflammation in scar tissue.

However, we believe that mechanical forces play a particularly important role in the pathophysiology of keloids and HSs (see Chapter 7).[7,8] Keloids show a marked preference for particular locations on the body and commonly adopt distinct site-specific shapes. The typical butterfly, crab's claw, or dumbbell shapes of keloids appear to be largely determined by the direction of the tension applied to the skin around the wound site.[7–9] Moreover, keloids usually occur at sites that are constantly or frequently subjected to tension (such as the anterior chest and scapular regions), but seldom in areas where stretching/contraction of the skin is rare (such as the parietal region or anterior lower leg), even in patients who have multiple/large keloids. In the case of the earlobe, the contribution of mechanical factors may be minor, although friction against the pillow and the weight of the keloid itself can induce keloids. Furthermore, repeated attaching and detaching of piercings may lead to repeated injury and infection, which are triggers of persistent inflammation.

Although physicians cannot (or at least find it very difficult to) control genetic and systemic factors, they can reduce the mechanical forces around keloids and HSs; this can be achieved using various surgical techniques (including Z-plasties). Moreover, anti-inflammatory treatments such as corticosteroids or anti-angiogenesis agents (which reduce the number of blood vessels) are viable clinical strategies.

Prevention of Keloids and HSs

A burn wound that heals in less than 10 days has a 4% risk of developing into a HS, whereas a burn wound that takes 21 days or more to heal has a 70% (or greater) risk of developing into a HS.[10] This means that a deep skin injury that extends to the reticular layer of dermis needs time to heal; however, if inflammation continues for a long period, then the risk of developing a pathologic scar increases. Histopathologic examination of pathologic scars reveals that the epidermis and the papillary layer of the dermis are almost normal, except for minor inflammation, but the reticular layer shows strong inflammation with an increase in the number of blood vessels and nerve and collagen fibers.[1,3]

Thus, speedy wound healing is essential to prevent the formation of pathologic scars. Keloids can arise from very small injuries or from irritated skin (e.g., acne, herpes zoster, insect bites, and skin injections). This means that special care should be taken when treating patients with a history of keloids.

Stretching of a wound risks evoking inflammation of the dermis; thus, wounds should be stabilized as soon as the exudate from the wound surface has stopped. Silicone tape is better than paper tape as its use prevents epidermal injury caused by repeated taping. Moreover, silicone tape keeps the scar surface moist. These tapes can be kept in place until they detach naturally. The patient does not need to change the tape after taking a bath/shower. In the experience of the author, patients can keep a tape in place for about 1 to 2 weeks, except in summer when perspiration can reduce tape adherence.

If the patient has a clear history of pathologic scars, then the stabilization tape should be exchanged for steroid plaster/tape at about 1 month after epithelialization. Flurandrenolide tape (Cordran tape), fludroxycortide tape (Drenison tape), and deprodone propionate tape (Eclar plaster) are available worldwide. These steroid tapes/plasters should be changed every 24 to 48 hours, and should be cut so that they just cover the wound, with minimal attachment (if any) to healthy skin (unpublished data).

Treatment of Keloids and HSs

Over the past 10 years, our understanding of the pathogenesis of keloids and HSs has increased markedly.[11] Thus, keloids and HSs are now regarded as treatable diseases. However, the available therapeutic approaches, which include surgery, radiation, corticosteroids, laser therapy, and makeup therapies, still require improvement, and combinations of these modalities may be required for optimal results.

Surgery

Surgical treatment can result in recurrence of keloids and HSs, which are then often much bigger than the original lesions. Thus, careful consideration is necessary for anything other than minor HSs. Radiation therapy after surgery markedly reduces the risk of recurrence; however, the recurrence rate can also be reduced by using particular surgical techniques; namely, subcutaneous/fascial tensile-reduction sutures, Z-plasties, and local flap transfer.

The use of subcutaneous/fascial tensile-reduction sutures relates to the fact that keloids and HSs arise from the dermis.[8] Therefore, dermal sutures do not effectively reduce tension on the dermis. To achieve this, we need to access the much deeper structures (namely, the superficial and deep fascia) and suture them (Fig. 16-1). This type of suturing will elevate the wound edges smoothly, with minimal tension on the dermis. In other words, the wound edges will naturally attach to each other. Only then should dermal and superficial sutures be used. Dermal sutures should not be used as "tension-reduction sutures." This is an important concept to prevent the formation of pathologic scars after surgery (Fig. 16-2). However, wedge excision should be the standard procedure for the earlobe[12] (Fig. 16-3), and core excision[13] should also be used for the cartilaginous part of the auricle.

Zigzag sutures, including Z-plasties, are good for releasing linear scar contractures and tension (see Chapter 12). A major benefit of Z-plasties is that segmented scars mature faster than long linear scars.[14] In particular, if a scar crosses a joint, zigzag incision and suturing is important to reduce the risk of developing pathologic scars.

In addition, various local flaps are useful for releasing scar contractures. They are also important for preventing contractures because, unlike skin grafts, local flaps expand naturally after surgery. Because skin grafting tends to generate secondary contractures that result in circular pathologic scars around the grafted skin, flap surgery is generally better for keloids. In the past, keloid reconstruction with flaps was discouraged because it was thought that the donor site could itself develop keloids. However, the development of keloids at the donor site can be prevented by multimodal therapy, which includes tension-reduction sutures and radiation therapy. Thus, flap surgery may be considered a first-line treatment when dealing with keloids.

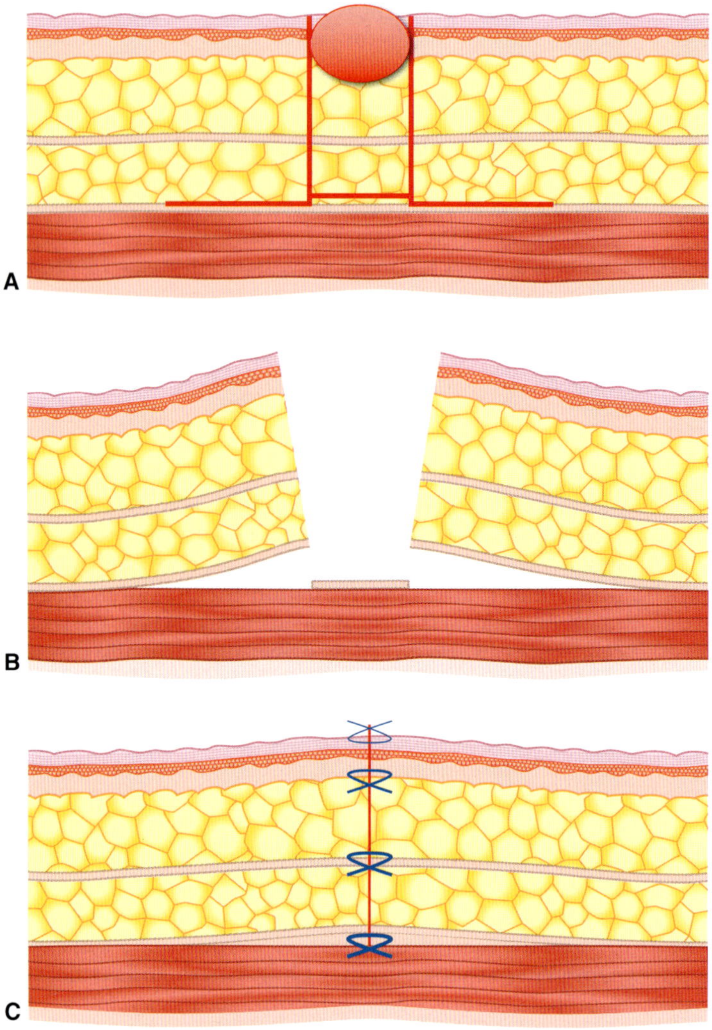

FIGURE 16-1 **Schema of the tension-reduction suture. A:** Excision of scars with fat tissue under the scars. **B:** Undermine under the deep fascia. **C:** Four-layered sutures: deep fascia, superficial fascia, dermis, and superficial layer. If deeper structures such as deep fascia and superficial fascia are sutured successfully, tension of the dermis will be kept to a minimum and the risk of pathologic scar development will decrease.

Corticosteroid Injections

Corticosteroid injections rapidly reduce the volume of a scar.[15] In general, injections are repeated monthly in severe cases. Once the entire thickness of a pathologic scar is reduced, it can be maintained using steroid tapes/plasters that patients can apply themselves (Fig. 16-4). Moreover, thinned scars can be treated effectively using 1,064-nm neodymium-doped:yttrium aluminum garnet (Nd:YAG) lasers. However, if the scar becomes flattened, it will recur if subjected to repeated tension or other types of stimulation.

The downside of corticosteroid injections includes pain (caused by the injection itself), atrophy, hypopigmentation, and difficulties associated with contraindications such as pregnancy, glaucoma, or Cushing's disease. To prevent menstrual irregularities, in the view of the author the maximum dose of triamcinolone should be 5 mg per session. This modest dose has a low rate of associated hypopigmentation, skin atrophy, or menstrual disorders in women, but it does reduce the thickness of pathologic scars when the area to be treated at each intervention is small (see Chapter 10). Lidocaine (1%) can be used to dilute the triamcinolone if used over a wide area. A narrow needle (30 G) and warming the solution can help reduce the pain associated with injection.

If side effects occur, injections should be stopped; however, there are few problems if steroid tapes/plasters are used every day by patients themselves. Children may decline injections out of fear of the procedure. However, because children have much thinner skin than adults, in the experience of the author, most cases can be treated with steroid tapes/plasters.

Corticosteroid Tapes/Plasters

Children are more sensitive to radiation than adults because their cells are actively dividing at a greater rate. Also, because they are young, the effects of radiation-induced damage may have more time to manifest themselves. Thus, radiation therapy is contraindicated in pediatric patients (less than 18 years of age). This means that, in most cases, surgery is also not indicated because surgery alone is associated with a high rate of keloid recurrence. However, if there is no alternative to surgery, steroid tapes/plasters can be used effectively to prevent the development/recurrence of pathologic scars. Moreover, children have thinner skin; therefore, steroids are very easily absorbed. Thus, children are more responsive to this type of treatment than adults. This means that steroid tapes/plasters are a reasonable

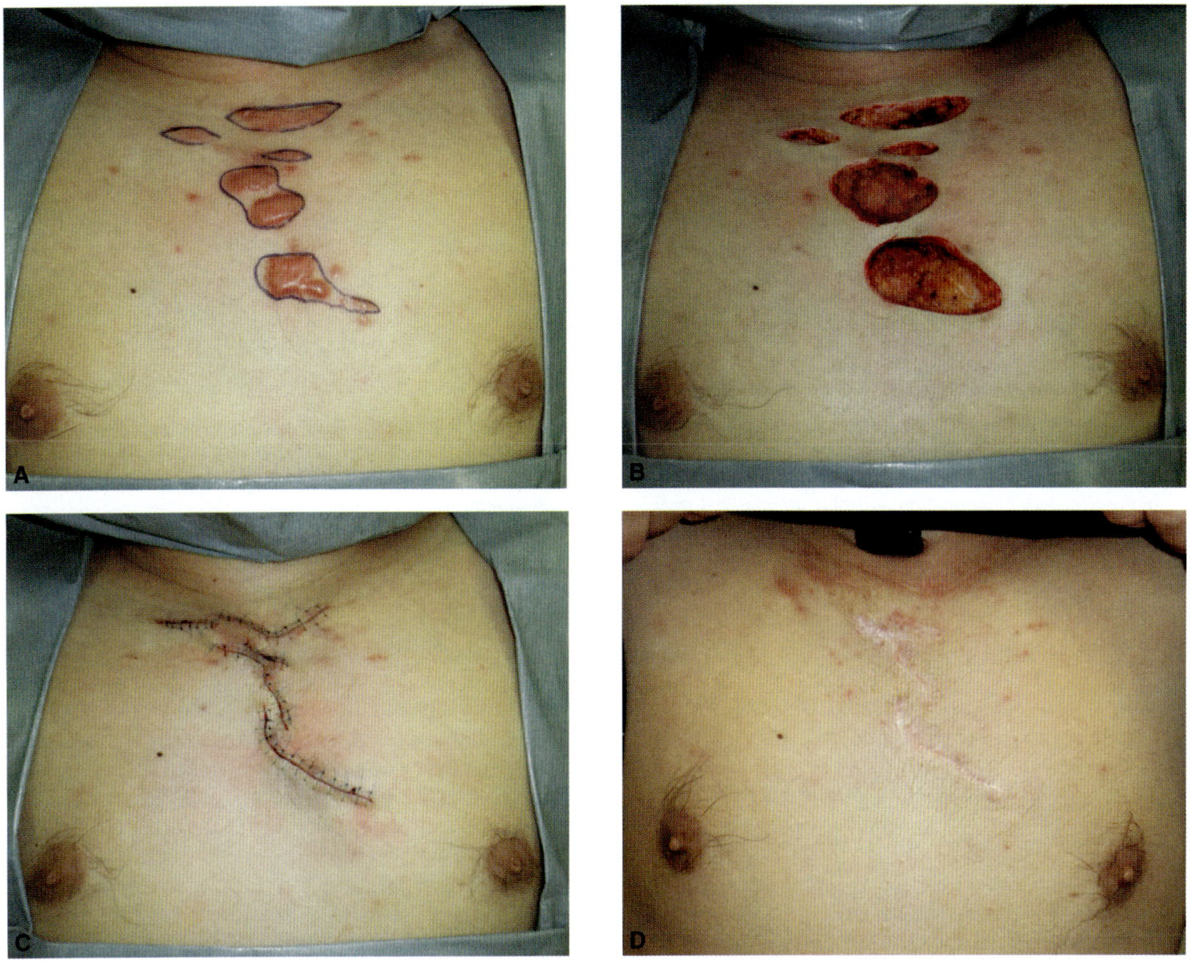

FIGURE 16-2 **A keloid on the anterior chest wall treated by surgery and radiation. A:** Preoperative view. **B**: Intraoperative view. **C:** Immediate postoperative view. **D:** Eighteen months after treatment. The patient is a 27-year-old man. All keloids were resected along with the underlying fat tissue. The deep fascia was sutured, and dermal sutures were used after confirmation that the wound edges had attached naturally. Postoperative high-dose-rate superficial brachytherapy was also used (18 Gy in three fractions for 3 days). No recurrence was noted at 18 months posttreatment.

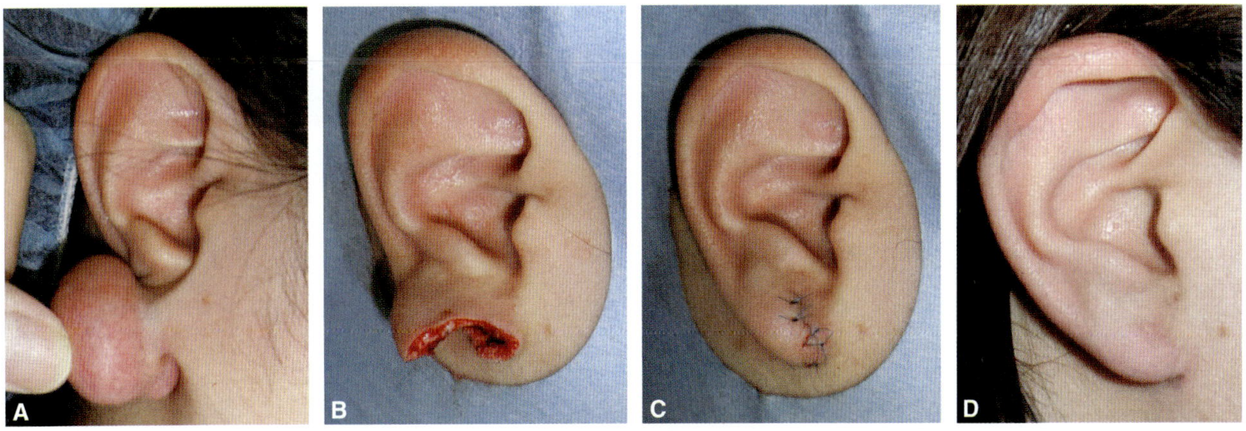

FIGURE 16-3 **Earlobe keloid treated by surgery and radiation. A:** Preoperative view. **B:** Intraoperative view. **C:** Immediate postoperative view. **D:** Eighteen months after treatment. The patient is a 26-year-old woman. The keloid was resected by wedge excision and postoperative electron beam irradiation was delivered (10 Gy in two fractions for 2 days). No recurrence was noted at 18 months posttreatment.

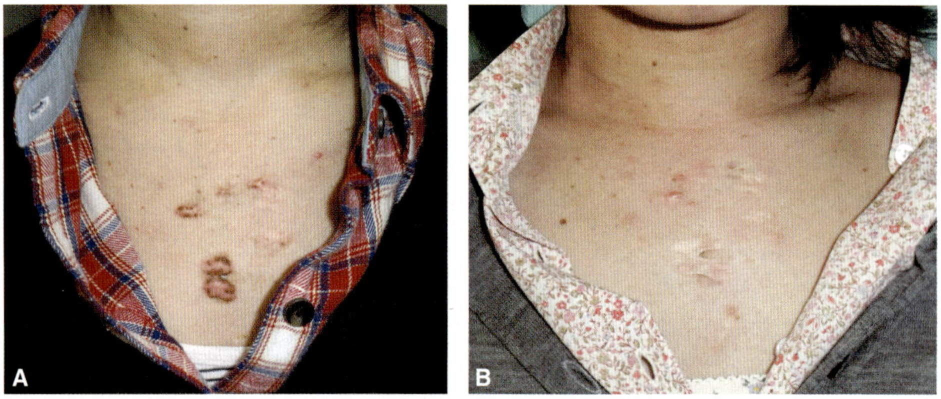

FIGURE 16-4 **Keloids on the anterior chest wall treated by a single steroid injection followed by continued use of steroid tape. A:** Pretreatment view. **B:** One year after starting the treatment. The patient is a 25-year-old woman. The patient received a single steroid injection (5 mg of 10 mg/mL triamcinolone acetonide plus 0.5 mL of 1% lidocaine with epinephrine). Fludroxycortide tape (Drenison tape) was applied everyday by the patient herself. The inflammation almost disappeared 1 year after starting treatment.

first-line therapy for keloids and HSs in all children and for minor keloids in adults (Fig. 16-5).

Interestingly, contact dermatitis, which is relatively common among adult patients who use tapes, does not tend to occur in the children in our experience. This may also be because children have thinner skin through which the steroid is easily absorbed.

Laser Therapy

The 595-nm pulsed dye laser (PDL) has long been the therapy of choice for cutaneous vascular conditions such as port wine stains; whereas PDL is effective for vascular diseases affecting the superficial layers (i.e., the epidermis and papillary layers of the dermis), it does not reach the deep dermal regions (i.e., the reticular layer of the dermis). Because 1,064-nm Nd:YAG lasers reach more deeply than PDL, they are increasingly being used to treat HSs and keloids in which the proliferating blood vessels are present mainly in the thickened reticular layer of the dermis.[16,17] Furthermore, because of decreased melanin absorption at 1,064 nm compared with 595 nm, the Nd:YAG laser may be better tolerated in darker skin types (see Chapters 13 and 18). The 1,064-nm Nd:YAG laser may act by suppressing neovascularization within pathologic scars, which is characterized by vessel overgrowth and increased numbers of nerve and collagen fibers in the reticular layer of the dermis.

This reduction in vascularity may in turn reduce cytokine or growth factor levels in the tissues; these factors promote collagen deposition. However, if these scars exist at high-tension sites, and tension is repeated on a daily basis, treatment with a 1,064-nm Nd:YAG laser may not be successful. In a previous study, we found that the response of HSs to laser treatment was significantly better than that of keloids; however, the data also suggested that if scars can be induced to mature completely, recurrence will not occur. Nevertheless, if even minor redness and induration remain, in the experience of the author scars are highly likely to recur. Thus, we need to continue to

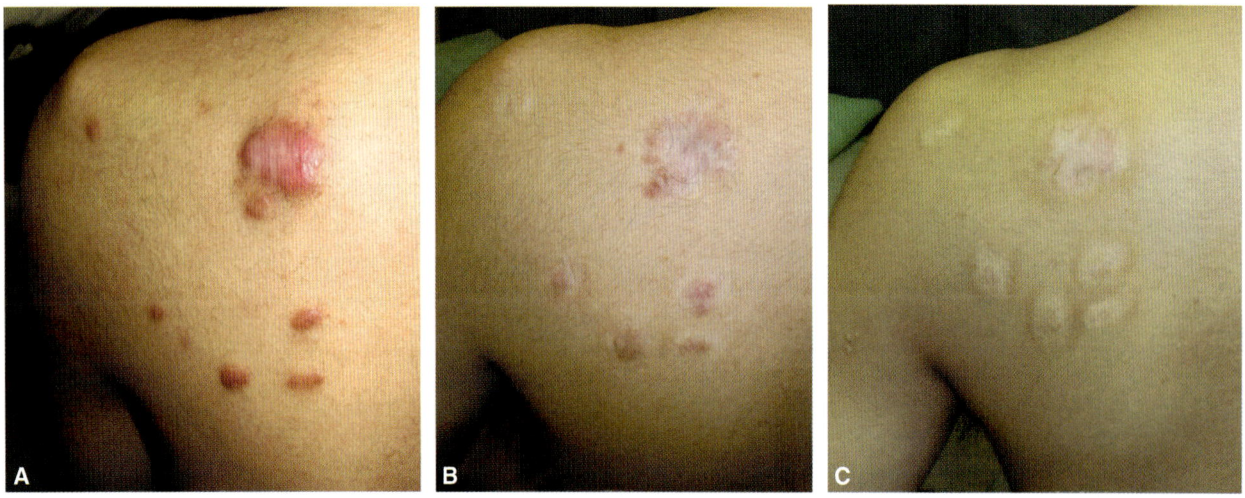

FIGURE 16-5 **Scapular keloids treated with steroid tape. A:** Pretreatment view. **B:** One year after starting treatment. **C:** Two years after starting treatment. The patient is an 18-year-old man. Fludroxycortide tape (Drenison tape) was applied everyday by the patient himself. The inflammation almost disappeared 2 years after starting treatment.

use Nd:YAG either alone or in combination with steroid tape/plaster until the redness and induration have disappeared completely.

The main energy setting used by the author for the long-pulse 1,064-nm Nd:YAG laser is 75 J per cm^2; pulse duration, 25 ms; spot size, 5 mm (Fig. 16-6). Dilated discrete capillary vessels can be treated using 150 J per cm^2; pulse duration, 25 ms; spot size, 3 mm. We have also combined PDL and Nd:YAG lasers to reduce the occurrence of multilayer vessels in keloids and HSs. We found that although this combination works, the energy delivered by each of the lasers must be reduced to avoid thermal burns. Thus, finding the correct energy setting can be more difficult in combined treatment than when using a long-pulsed Nd:YAG laser alone.

In our limited experience, fractional ablative and nonablative lasers cause more keloids and HS inflammation, even when their use is combined with the application of a steroid tape/plaster in Asian patients. Thus, we are not currently using these lasers to treat pathologic scars in this population (see Chapters 13 and 18).

Radiation Therapy

As mentioned above, the main problem with surgery for pathologic scars is recurrence. However, recurrence can be controlled using ever-improving radiation technology. In the past, superficial or orthovoltage X-rays (photons) were used.[18,19] However, the safety and efficacy of radiation therapy have improved markedly in recent years, and radiation is now used routinely as a highly effective postoperative adjuvant therapy. As a result, keloids can be treated adjunctively with high-dose-rate superficial brachytherapy (HDR-SB)[20] (Fig. 16-2) as well as electron beam radiation[21,22] (Fig. 16-3). Depending on the shape of the surgical scar, an HDR-SB applicator can be used to ensure both evenness and appropriate localization of the radiation to the wound surface. Thus, the treatment is even safer.

Our review of the literature revealed that to ensure maximum efficacy and safety, postoperative radiation therapy for keloids in adults should involve the application of 10 to 20 Gy delivered in 5 Gy fractions.[23] Use of the linear quadratic concept to calculate the biologically effective doses (BEDs) for various radiation regimens for keloid therapy revealed that when the BEDs exceeded 30 Gy, the recurrence rate was less than 10%. Moreover, the risk of secondary carcinogenesis is reduced when the BED is below 30 Gy. Thus, we propose that the maximum dose of postoperative radiation therapy for keloids is a BED of 30 Gy. A BED of 30 Gy can be obtained in several ways: a single-fraction dose of 13 Gy, two fractions of 8 Gy, three fractions of 6 Gy, or four fractions of 5 Gy. Moreover, site-dependent dose protocols for the treatment of keloids are recommended as follows: 20 Gy in four fractions over 4 days (BED = 30 Gy) for the anterior chest wall, shoulder scapular region, and suprapubic region; 10 Gy in two fractions over 2 days for the ear lobe (BED = 15 Gy); and 15 Gy in three fractions over 3 days for other sites (BED = 22.5 Gy).

A previous report stated that among 10,000 individuals between 18 and 64 years old, 670 (6.7%) will acquire skin cancer if subjected to whole-body irradiation of 1 Gy.[24] In general, skin cancer kills 1 in 500 patients. Thus, the mortality rate associated with 1 Gy of whole-body irradiation would be $6.7\% \times 1/500 = 0.0134\%$; namely, one in 7,500 people. If this reasoning is applied to earlobe keloid radiotherapy, where 0.05% of whole-body skin is irradiated with 10 Gy, the incidence of cancer associated with this treatment would be $6.7 \times 10 \times 0.05/100 = 0.0335\%$; namely, 1 in 3,000 people. The mortality rate of secondary carcinogenesis of earlobe keloid treatment would be $0.0335/500 = 0.000067\%$; namely, 1 in 1,500,000 people. We believe this can be ignored clinically if informed consent can be obtained from patients after they have been advised of the benefits and side effects of this type of treatment.

Also, we have used primary radiation therapy (radiation monotherapy) to treat older patients or patients with severe acne-related keloids. The total radiation dose in these cases is higher than that used for postoperative radiation therapy. Therefore, it is necessary to apply radiation carefully to prevent secondary radiation carcinogenesis. It is also important to obtain informed consent. However, the benefits of primary radiation therapy can be tremendous. Subjective symptoms such as pain and itching decrease immediately, and the color and thickness of the scars normalize progressively over the course of a year.

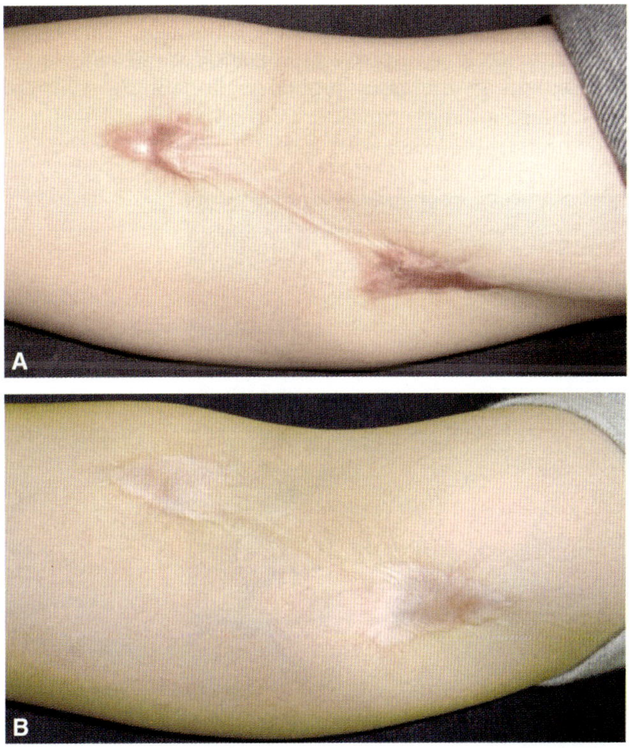

FIGURE 16-6 **Hypertrophic scars on the upper arm and forearm treated with an Nd:YAG laser. A**: Pretreatment view. **B:** Eighteen months after starting the treatment. The energy setting of the 1,064-nm Nd:YAG laser was as follows: 75 J per cm^2; pulse duration, 25 ms; spot size, 5 mm. Patients received laser therapy every month, and the inflammation almost disappeared 1½ years after starting treatment. No recurrence was observed.

Stabilization/Compression Therapy

It is difficult to treat keloids using stabilization and/or compression therapy alone; however, these therapies can improve the subjective symptoms. To limit skin stretching during healing (thereby facilitating appropriate wound stabilization), wounds or scars should be covered with a fixable material such as surgical tape, bandages, garments, silicone tape, silicone gel sheets, or polyethylene gel sheets (see Chapter 7 and Chapter 19). Indeed, we found that gel sheets have a scar tension-reducing effect; after placing the gel sheets on the scar, the tension at the edge is transferred to the edge of the gel sheet.[25] Thus, we believe such materials are effective because they reduce tension and keep the keloid surface moist. If pathologic scars occur on movable areas such as joints, a steroid tape/plaster in combination with a stabilization method such as a bandage is a good choice for personal care at home.

Makeup Therapy

Makeup therapy (rehabilitation makeup, camouflage therapy) can effectively improve the psychological status of patients with scars[26] (see Chapter 20). In our experience, the presence of noticeable scars on exposed regions of the body can inhibit patients from going out and engaging in normal social activities (see Chapter 24). A well-known makeup therapy in Japan developed by the makeup artist Ms. Reiko Kazuki, named "rehabilitation make-up," not only improves the appearance of scars, but also alleviates psychological problems because it provides patients with sufficient confidence to leave the home. This in turn helps patients to better accept their scars, after which it is no longer necessary to use makeup.

In practice, a very thin (10 μm) surface-fabricated tape (Kazuki design tape) specifically designed for rehabilitation makeup has been widely used in Japan. This tape is applied to the scars to flatten them. Next, a custom-developed foundation with a color similar to that of the patient's skin is applied on the top of the tape. The result is that the appearance of the scars is markedly improved (Fig. 16-7).

Long-Term Follow-Up

It is important that sequentially treated keloid and HS patients are followed up over the long term, and that they are appropriately educated about scar management. If patients have a tendency to develop pathologic scars, recurrent or new scars develop easily in response to minor stimulation. If these patients can be educated in self-management (including the application of steroid tape/plasters during the early stages of scar development) the appearance of these scars can be improved rapidly.

Conclusions

Plastic surgeons and dermatologists in non-Caucasian societies tend to avoid actively treating keloids because they tend to recur. Steroid injections have long been a first-line therapy. However, surgery and radiation therapy are increasingly used to successfully manage keloids and HSs. Thus, there is now sufficient evidence on which to base a standard international algorithm for treating pathologic scars. Treatments are likely to improve significantly as our knowledge of scar biology increases, higher quality clinical trials are performed, and new agents are developed (Fig. 16-8).

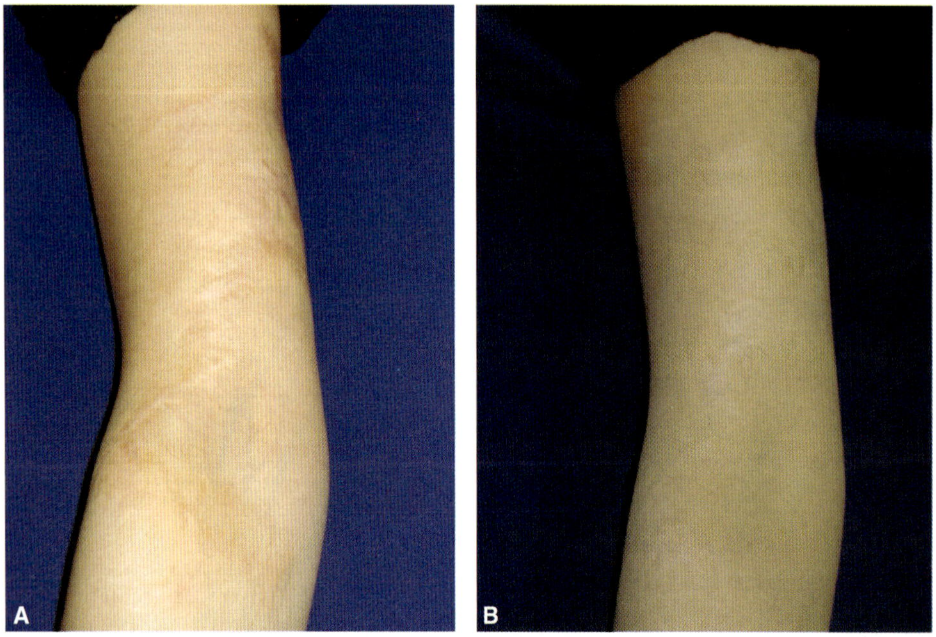

FIGURE 16-7 **Scars on the upper arm treated with rehabilitation makeup. A:** Pretreatment view. **B:** Immediately posttreatment. A very thin (10 μm) surface-fabricated tape (specifically developed for rehabilitation make-up: Kazuki design tape) was applied to the scars to flatten the surface. Next, a custom-developed foundation with a similar color to the patient's skin was applied on the top of the tape. The appearance of the scars is much improved.

Keloids

Pediatric patients

Treatment at hospital
- Steroid injection
- ✓ Nd:YAG laser
- Surgery and post-operative radiation therapy
- ✓ Surgery and post-operative steroid tape/plaster
- Radiation monotherapy

Patient self-treatment
- ✓ Steroid tape/plaster
- ✓ Stabilization/compression therapy
- ✓ Make-up therapy

Middle-age patients

Treatment at hospital
- ✓ Steroid injection
- ✓ Nd:YAG laser
- ✓ Surgery and post-operative radiation therapy
- Surgery and post-operative steroid tape/plaster
- Radiation monotherapy

Patient self-treatment
- ✓ Steroid tape/plaster
- ✓ Stabilization/compression therapy
- ✓ Make-up therapy

Elderly patients

Treatment at hospital
- ✓ Steroid injection
- ✓ Nd:YAG laser
- ✓ Surgery and post-operative radiation therapy
- ✓ Surgery and post-operative steroid tape/plaster
- ✓ Radiation monotherapy

Patient self-treatment
- ✓ Steroid tape/plaster
- ✓ Stabilization/compression therapy
- ✓ Make-up therapy

Pregnant patients

Treatment at hospital
- Steroid injection
- ✓ Nd:YAG laser
- Surgery and post-operative radiation therapy
- Surgery and post-operative steroid tape/plaster
- Radiation monotherapy

Patient self-treatment
- Steroid tape/plaster
- ✓ Stabilization/compression therapy
- ✓ Make-up therapy

A

Keloids

Patients with huge / thick keloids

Treatment at hospital
- Steroid injection
- Nd:YAG laser
- ✓ Surgery and post-operative radiation therapy
- Surgery and post-operative steroid tape/plaster
- ✓ Radiation monotherapy

Patient self-treatment
- ✓ Steroid tape/plaster
- ✓ Stabilization/compression therapy
- ✓ Make-up therapy

Patients with small / thin keloids

Treatment at hospital
- ✓ Steroid injection
- ✓ Nd:YAG laser
- Surgery and post-operative radiation therapy
- ✓ Surgery and post-operative steroid tape/plaster
- Radiation monotherapy

Patient self-treatment
- ✓ Steroid tape/plaster
- ✓ Stabilization/compression therapy
- ✓ Make-up therapy

Patients with multiple keloids

Treatment at hospital
- ✓ Steroid injection
- ✓ Nd:YAG laser
- ✓ Surgery and post-operative radiation therapy
- Surgery and post-operative steroid tape/plaster
- ✓ Radiation monotherapy

Patient self-treatment
- ✓ Steroid tape/plaster
- ✓ Stabilization/compression therapy
- ✓ Make-up therapy

Patients with single keloids

Treatment at hospital
- ✓ Steroid injection
- ✓ Nd:YAG laser
- ✓ Surgery and post-operative radiation therapy
- Surgery and post-operative steroid tape/plaster
- Radiation monotherapy

Patient self-treatment
- ✓ Steroid tape/plaster
- ✓ Stabilization/compression therapy
- ✓ Make-up therapy

B

Hypertrophic scars

General Hypertrophic scars

Treatment at hospital
- ✓ Steroid injection
- ✓ Nd:YAG laser
- ✓ Surgery alone
- ✓ Surgery and post-operative steroid tape/plaster
- Surgery and post-operative radiation therapy

Patient self-treatment
- ✓ Steroid tape/plaster
- ✓ Stabilization/compression therapy
- ✓ Make-up therapy

Hypertrophic scars with scar contracture

Treatment at hospital
- ✓ Steroid injection
- Nd:YAG laser
- ✓ Surgery alone
- ✓ Surgery and post-operative steroid tape/plaster
- Surgery and post-operative radiation therapy

Patient self-treatment
- ✓ Steroid tape/plaster
- ✓ Stabilization/compression therapy
- ✓ Make-up therapy

Recurred/ Intractable Hypertrophic scars

Treatment at hospital
- ✓ Steroid injection
- Nd:YAG laser
- Surgery alone
- Surgery and post-operative steroid tape/plaster
- ✓ Surgery and post-operative radiation therapy

Patient self-treatment
- ✓ Steroid tape/plaster
- ✓ Stabilization/compression therapy
- ✓ Make-up therapy

C

FIGURE 16-8 **Our current treatment regimen for pathologic scars. A:** Keloid treatment by age and condition. **B:** Keloid treatment by clinical findings. **C:** Hypertrophic scar treatment by clinical findings and response. In the case of keloids, treatment methods should be selected according to the age of the patient. Radiotherapy is contraindicated for pediatric patients, but it can be used for adults. Skin thickness of pediatric and elderly patients is thin; thus, a steroid tape/plaster is a good choice. Thick keloids are difficult to treat using Nd:YAG laser therapy. In the case of hypertrophic scars, recurrent scars should be treated like keloids.

REFERENCES

1. Huang C, Murphy GF, Akaishi S, et al. Keloids and hypertrophic scars: update and future directions. *Plast Reconstr Surg Glob Open*. 2013;1(4):e25.
2. Tredget EE. The molecular biology of fibroproliferative disorders of the skin: potential cytokine therapeutics. *Ann Plast Surg*. 1994;33(2):152–154.
3. Huang C, Akaishi S, Hyakusoku H, et al. Are keloid and hypertrophic scar different forms of the same disorder? A fibroproliferative skin disorder hypothesis based on keloid findings. *Int Wound J*. 2014;11(5):517–522.
4. Nakashima M, Chung S, Takahashi A, et al. A genome-wide association study identifies four susceptibility loci for keloid in the Japanese population. *Nat Genet*. 2010;42(9):768–771.
5. Ogawa R, Watanabe A, Than Naing B, et al. Associations between keloid severity and single-nucleotide polymorphisms: importance of rs8032158 as a biomarker of keloid severity. *J Invest Dermatol*. 2014;134(7):2041–2043.
6. Arima J, Huang C, Rosner B, et al. Hypertension: a systemic key to understanding local keloid severity. *Wound Repair Regen*. 2015;23(2):213–221.
7. Ogawa R. Mechanobiology of scarring. *Wound Repair Regen*. 2011;19(suppl 1):s2–s9.
8. Ogawa R, Akaishi S, Huang C, et al. Clinical applications of basic research that shows reducing skin tension could prevent and treat abnormal scarring: the importance of fascial/subcutaneous tensile reduction sutures and flap surgery for keloid and hypertrophic scar reconstruction. *J Nihon Med Sch*. 2011;78(2):68–76.
9. Akaishi S, Akimoto M, Ogawa R, et al. The relationship between keloid growth pattern and stretching tension: visual analysis using the finite element method. *Ann Plast Surg*. 2008;60(4):445–451.
10. Deitch EA, Wheelahan TM, Rose MP, et al. Hypertrophic burn scars: analysis of variables. *J Trauma*. 1983;23(10):895–898.
11. Ogawa R. The most current algorithms for the treatment and prevention of hypertrophic scars and keloids. *Plast Reconstr Surg*. 2010;125(2):557–568.
12. Ogawa R, Huang C, Akaishi S, et al. Analysis of surgical treatments for earlobe keloids: analysis of 174 lesions in 145 patients. *Plast Reconstr Surg*. 2013;132(5):818e–825e.
13. Ogawa R, Akaishi S, Dohi T, et al. Analysis of the surgical treatments of 63 keloids on the cartilaginous part of the auricle: effectiveness of the core excision method. *Plast Reconstr Surg*. 2015;135(3):868–875.
14. Ogawa R. Current keloid and hypertrophic scar treatment algorithms and our recent trials. *J Wound Technol*. 2012;15:28–29.
15. Muneuchi G, Suzuki S, Onodera M, et al. Long-term outcome of intralesional injection of triamcinolone acetonide for the treatment of keloid scars in Asian patients. *Scand J Plast Reconstr Surg Hand Surg*. 2006;40:111.
16. Akaishi S, Koike S, Dohi T, et al. Nd:YAG laser treatment of keloids and hypertrophic scars. *Eplasty*. 2012;12:e1.
17. Koike S, Akaishi S, Nagashima Y, et al. Nd:YAG laser treatment for keloids and hypertrophic scars: an analysis of 102 cases. *Plast Reconstr Surg Glob Open*. 2015;2(12):e272.
18. Levy DS, Salter MM, Roth RE. Postoperative irradiation in the prevention of keloids. *Am J Roentgenol*. 1976;127(3):509–510.
19. Enhamre A, Hammar H. Eloids with excision and postoperative X-ray irradiation. *Dermatologica*. 1983;167(2):90–93.
20. Kuribayashi S, Miyashita T, Ozawa Y, et al. Post-keloidectomy irradiation using high-dose-rate superficial brachytherapy. *J Radiat Res (Tokyo)*. 2011;52(3):365–368.
21. Ogawa R, Mitsuhashi K, Hyakusoku H, et al. Postoperative electron-beam irradiation therapy for keloids and hypertrophic scars: retrospective study of 147 cases followed for more than 18 months. *Plast Reconstr Surg*. 2003;111(2):547–553; discussion 554–555.
22. Ogawa R, Miyashita T, Hyakusoku H, et al. Postoperative radiation protocol for keloids and hypertrophic scars: statistical analysis of 370 sites followed for over 18 months. *Ann Plast Surg*. 2007;59(6): 688–691.
23. Ogawa R, Yoshitatsu S, Yoshida K, et al. Is radiation therapy for keloids acceptable? The risk of radiation-induced carcinogenesis. *Plast Reconstr Surg*. 2009;124(4):1196–1201.
24. Preston DL, Ron E, Tokuoka S, et al. Solid cancer incidence in atomic bomb survivors: 1958-1998. *Radiat Res*. 2007;168:1–64.
25. Akaishi S, Akimoto M, Hyakusoku H, et al. The tensile reduction effects of silicone gel sheeting. *Plast Reconstr Surg*. 2010;126(2): 109e–111e.
26. Kazuki, R. The role of rehabilitation makeup in modern medical care. *Jpn J Plast Reconstr Surg*. 2001;44:1029.

17 Atrophic Scar Management

JOANNA G. BOLTON, LISA A. ZALESKI-LARSEN, and MITCHEL P. GOLDMAN

KEY POINTS

- Atrophic scars are caused by a variety of inflammatory, infectious, traumatic, and individual genetic risk factors, in addition to mechanical skin stretching.
- Acne is a common disorder with a high prevalence among adolescents, and it often results in atrophic scars.
- The disfigurement from acne scarring is associated with considerable psychological distress including poor self-esteem, embarrassment, depression, anxiety, and anger. These issues may place limitations on social interactions, daily activities, and employment.
- Levels of psychosocial distress may not be accurately predicted by one's degree of disfigurement.
- Multimodal treatment regimens that combine medical, injectable, surgical, and device-based therapies are most advantageous in the treatment of atrophic acne scarring.
- Although striae distensae do not pose a health risk and are not associated with as severe psychosocial dysfunction as acne scars, they can burn, itch, and cause emotional stress.
- Multiple treatment modalities for striae distensae have been published, yet no first-line ideal therapy has emerged.
- The efficacy of multimodal regimens ("mega-combinations") is gaining popularity and is likely the future of treating atrophic scars.

Enhanced awareness of scar pathophysiology and advances in technology and applications including laser, light and energy devices, injectable, surgical and topical techniques (both alone and in combination) provide new hope to millions of patients affected by scars worldwide. The term "cosmetic" belies the enormous potential psychosocial impact of a scar on a particular individual (see Chapters 4 and 24). The primary focus of this chapter is on the aesthetic treatment of atrophic and flat scars, with particular attention to the significantly distressing conditions of acne scarring and striae. Other chapters have detailed the pathophysiology and treatment of hypertrophic and keloid scarring, and these will be discussed briefly within the context of acne scarring.

Treatment of scars to improve their cosmetic appearance has progressed significantly over the past decade.[1] The complexity of the wound-healing process dictates that a multifaceted approach is used in the minimization of scarring as well as in improving the aesthetic appearance of existing scars. With this in mind, these various facets will be discussed: (1) medical intervention—use of topical and intralesional agents that may influence the wound-healing cascade, decrease inflammation, or help remove the outer layers of skin; (2) laser, light, and energy-based interventions—use of various devices to improve the color, texture, and contour of scars and influence the wound-healing cascade; (3) soft tissue augmentation and novel approaches for transfer of material to help lift and blend scars; and (4) surgical intervention—for purposes of this chapter, defined as minor procedures that attempt to revise scars, usually in combination with other modalities (i.e., punch excision and/or grafting, subcision, dermabrasion, needling). The importance of "watchful waiting" and the "tincture of time" for optimal cosmesis cannot be overemphasized with any intervention.

The visibility of a scar depends on its width, texture, color, contrast, and flatness. Perceptions of how a scar appears is individualistic, with scars considered nearly imperceptible or normal by some being considered psychologically devastating by others. As pointed out by Tsao et al.,[2] there are basically three types of scars: (1) atrophic scars (most commonly seen in acne and postvaricella scarring), (2) exophytic scars (hypertrophic and keloid scars), and (3) flat scars, which are considered normal scars, and are frequently dyspigmented after surgery or trauma to the skin, and which gradually diminish over time with or without intervention. Although the majority of flat, hyperpigmented scars are considered "normal," they are frequently a concern of patients who seek advice and treatment for optimal cosmetic outcomes.

The authors of this chapter have chosen to include a discussion of striae, as the literature for this clinically challenging and commonly distressing condition has grown in recent years. Striae can be considered a form of atrophic scarring, resulting from various mechanisms of skin stretching. Millions of people are affected and bothered by this common condition and may seek evaluation and a discussion of treatment options.

Scar History

Assessment of scar etiology, duration, and developmental history is important. Scars less than 1 year old are normally more erythematous than are older scars, and although they may be amenable to pulsed-dye laser (PDL) and/or intense-pulsed light (IPL) treatment, the patient should be educated that a degree of spontaneous improvement is expected over the first 12 to 15 months (see Chapters 8 and 9). Generally, scars that are greater than 1 year in duration and continue to worsen or are aesthetically concerning to the patient should be considered for intervention to prevent further abnormal scar growth and to expedite improvement.

Information on prior scar treatment should be solicited at the initial evaluation. Atrophic scars that have been treated with prior dermabrasion with resultant dermal thickening may not be vaporized as readily with carbon dioxide (CO_2) laser resurfacing, possibly reducing the final clinical response.[3] On the contrary, hypertrophic and keloid scars that have only received intralesional corticosteroid injections may elicit a more robust response to subsequent laser treatment.

Systemic medication use is an important consideration. Historically, there have been concerns that patients currently taking, or with a recent history of completing, a course of oral isotretinoin are at risk for delayed reepithelialization and resultant atypical scarring from acne scar treatment. The concern stems from the medication's mechanism of action on adnexal structures, reducing or otherwise affecting the number and size of pilosebaceous glands that are essential for optimal wound healing. Historical clinical practice recommendations suggest that patients wait 6 to 12 months following discontinuation of isotretinoin therapy before undergoing resurfacing or surgical scar revision. However, these non–scientifically proven recommendations have been contradicted by recent studies. In a retrospective study ($n = 110$), patients taking oral isotretinoin (0.5 mg/kg/d) for acne or hirsutism were compared with those receiving only topical acne medications.[4] Both groups underwent invasive treatment for acne scars and/or laser hair removal.[5] Wound healing did not appear delayed nor was it associated with any adverse effects or atypical scarring in the patients taking isotretinoin. In another study, 80% of patients exhibited better than "fair" improvement and no aggravated acne scars, hypertrophic scars, or keloids following treatment with a 1,550-nm erbium-doped fiber laser to reduce acne scars while taking low-dose isotretinoin (10 mg per day) for at least 1 month.[6]

A history of immunosuppressive medications, such as chronic systemic steroids or biologic therapy, or presence of certain medical conditions, such as uncontrolled diabetes mellitus, should also give pause to major scar revision because of concerns for adverse outcomes from poor wound healing.

Acne Scars

Scar Pathogenesis

Scarring occurs as a result of damage to the skin during the healing of active acne. However, the pathogenesis remains incompletely understood. Acne can occur in any region where there is an abundance of pilosebaceous glands, especially the face, shoulders, back, and chest.[7] The risk factors for developing permanent scarring are multifactorial, including genetic predisposition, a delay or nonadherence in acne treatment, and behaviors by patients that can induce excessive inflammation and mechanical trauma to the skin, impeding the healing process and worsening outcomes (i.e., acne excoriae). Not every patient with acne develops scars, and clinically it can be difficult to predict who will. Severe disease, such as nodulocystic acne, is most likely to result in scarring, but even patients with mild acne can develop scars.[8]

The most accepted hypothesis for the pathogenesis of atrophic acne scars points to dysregulated inflammation that affects fibroblastic function, culminating in a relative collagen deficiency and tissue atrophy.[9] It has been demonstrated that acne patients prone to scarring have a particular cellular milieu different than that in those patients who do not scar.[10] A cascade of pro-inflammatory cytokines and mediators, including activator protein (AP)-1, matrix metalloproteinase (MMP)-1 (collagenase-1), and other MMPs, are overexpressed in inflammatory acne lesions, leading to prolonged inflammation, follicular rupture, and perifollicular abscess formation. The well-recognized role of MMPs in collagen matrix degradation explains the tissue atrophy characteristic of depressed scars[11] (Fig. 17-1). A study by Holland et al.[12] demonstrated that patients with a propensity to scar had a greater nonspecific inflammatory response lasting for a longer duration when compared with those patients who did not scar. This could be due to an ineffective immune response to damaged tissue and abnormal wound healing. An overzealous healing response coupled with limited collagen lysis during the remodeling phase can create a raised, firm nodule of fibrotic tissue, whereas depressions or pits may result from inadequate replacement of enzymatically degraded collagen fibers and subcutaneous fat.[13] Consequently, inflammatory acne lesions can result in permanent scars, and the longer treatment is delayed, the worse the scarring that results.

Community-based studies report acne prevalence is 90% in adolescent patients and persists into adulthood in approximately 12% to 14% of cases.[14] Acne scarring is estimated to occur in up to 95% of acne patients, and 30% may develop significant scarring.[15] Other studies have reported much lower incidences of scarring, ranging from 0.17% to 14%.[16–18] Any degree of active acne and acne scarring may have a profoundly negative impact on daily activities, social life, self-esteem, and relationships, all of which make them both common conditions for which treatment is sought or would be of benefit. It has even been noted that the ability to acquire employment in adulthood may be limited in those with acne scarring.[19] Until recently, very few studies had explored the negative impact caused by postacne scarring. Fried et al.[20] confirmed that acne scars

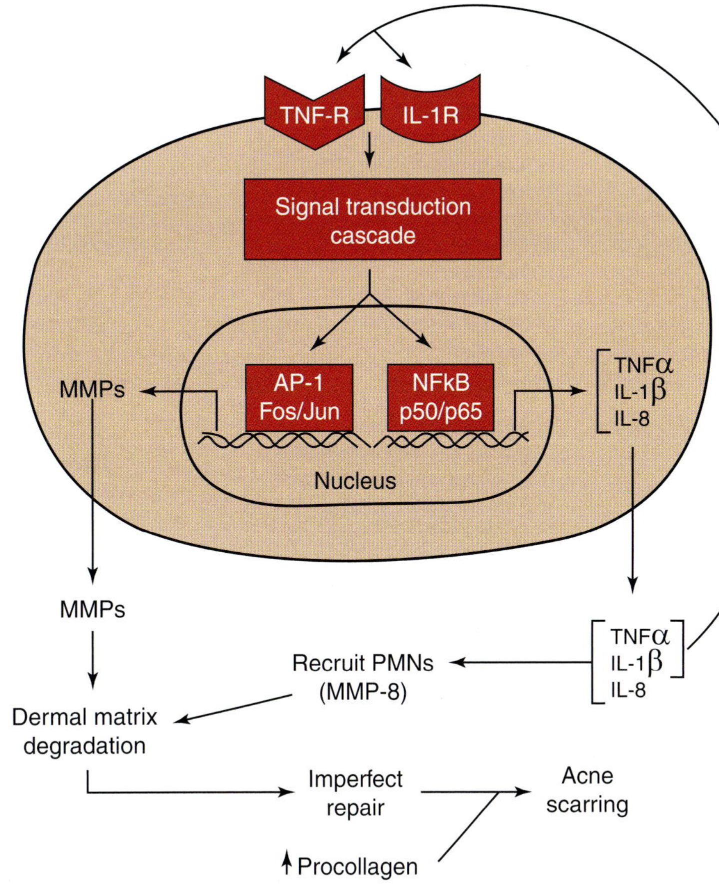

FIGURE 17-1 **Hypothetical model of the pathophysiology of inflammatory acne and dermal damage.** In inflammatory acne lesions, NF-κB signaling is activated. As a consequence, NF-κB-driven inflammatory cytokine genes (e.g., TNF-α and IL-1β) are induced. These primary cytokines will propagate the inflammatory response by acting on endothelial cells to elaborate adhesion molecules (eg, ICAM-1) to facilitate recruitment of inflammatory cells into the skin. TNF-α and IL-1β will also stimulate the production of secondary cytokines, such as IL-8, which can aid in chemotaxis of inflammatory cells. By working through their cell surface receptors, TNF-α and IL-1β not only amplify the NF-κB signaling cascade, but also activate MAP kinases to stimulate AP-1-mediated gene transcription. As a consequence of AP-1 activation (cJun induction), AP-1-driven MMPs are elaborated by resident skin cells. Along with MMP-8 and neutrophil elastase brought in by PMNs, they degrade the matrix. This is followed by matrix synthesis and repair, which is imperfect. Most of the imperfections would leave clinically undetectable deficits in the organization or composition, or both, of the extracellular matrix. However, when they occur to a significant extent throughout time, accompanied by sustained procollagen synthesis, acne scarring becomes clinically visible. *(Used with permission from Kang S, Cho S, Chung JH, et al. Inflammation and extracellular matrix degradation mediated by activated transcription factors nuclear factor-kappaB and activator protein-1 in inflammatory acne lesions in vivo.* Am J Pathol. *2005;166:1691–1699.)*

have a substantial negative impact on the overall social and functional well-being of affected individuals. In their study, an overwhelming 85.4% of subjects revealed they were unhappy looking at themselves in the mirror, with 84.4% feeling less attractive owing to their acne scars.

Although it appears that acne severity is directly proportional to the severity of the acne scarring,[15] it is important to note that levels of psychosocial distress may not be accurately predicted by one's degree of disfigurement.[21] With this in mind, it must be emphasized to patients that the most effective means of minimizing or preventing acne scarring and its associated devastating psychosocial difficulties is to treat acne early and aggressively.

Scar Classification

The nomenclature for categorizing types of acne scars has not been entirely settled in the literature.[4] Acne scars are primarily classified according to whether there is a net loss or gain of collagen in the lesion. For the purposes of practicality and ease in treatment selection, acne scars can be categorized as either "atrophic" or "hypertrophic," with "hypertrophic" including both hypertrophic and keloidal scars[10] (Table 17-1). Eighty to 90% of people with acne scars have atrophic scars compared with a minority who show hypertrophic scars and keloids.[14] Proper scar classification is important because differences in clinical subtype help guide appropriate therapeutic options on the basis of surface, depth, and three-dimensional architecture[22] (Table 17-2).

Table 17-1 Classification of Acne Scars

Scar Classification	Clinical Features
Atrophic	Loss of dermal collagen (primarily)
	Most common form of acne scarring
Ice pick (60%–70%)	Deep and narrow pitting (<2 mm)
	V-shaped, sharply demarcated epithelial tracts that extend into the dermis or subcutaneous tissue
Boxcar (20%–30%)	Round or oval depressions
	Shallow (<0.5 mm) or deep (>0.5 mm)
	1.5–4 mm diameter
	Sharply demarcated vertical edges with a wide base; do not taper to a point at base and are clinically wider at the surface than ice pick scars
Rolling (15%–25%)	Wide and shallow undulations (>4–5 mm)
	Superficial skin tethered by fibrous anchors to dermis or subcutaneous tissue, leading to shadowing and gently sloped edges that merge with normal-appearing skin
Hypertrophic	Excess collagen deposition
Hypertrophic	Pink, raised, firm papule
	Confined to the area of previous damage
Keloidal	Red to purple, firm papules and nodules
	Extend beyond original wound borders

Adapted from Gozali et al.,[23] Levy and Zeichner,[8] and Fabbrocini et al.[14]

Table 17-2 Most Common Treatment Modalities Based on Scar Type

Atrophic Scars	• Laser (ablative and nonablative; fractionated and nonfractionated) • Light therapy (i.e., IPL) • Energy therapy (i.e., RF) • Injectable dermal fillers • Autologous fat transfer • Chemical peels • Subcision • Punch techniques • Dermabrasion/microdermabrasion • Needling • Topical retinoids
Hypertrophic Scars	• Silicone gel sheeting • Intralesional corticosteroids • Cytotoxic agents: bleomycin, 5-fluorouracil • Cryosurgery • Radiotherapy • Laser (CO_2, erbium, pulsed dye)

IPL, intense-pulsed light; RF, radiofrequency; CO_2, carbon dioxide.
Adapted from Gozali et al.,[23] Levy and Zeichner,[8] and Fabbrocini et al.[14]

Table 17-3 Main Causes and Risk Factors for Developing Atrophic Scars

	Cause/Risk Factor
Inflammatory	Acne Cyst Discoid lupus erythematosus
Infective	Postvaricella
Trauma	Injury Burn Iatrogenic (surgery)
Skin stretching/striae	Pregnancy Obesity Rapid weight loss/gain Puberty/growth spurt Medications (i.e., steroids, ACTH)
Patient factors	Genetics (tendency toward atrophic scarring) Previous atrophic scars Ehlers–Danlos syndrome Primary anetoderma

Adapted from Patel L, McGrouther D, Chakrabarty K. Evaluating evidence for atrophic scarring treatment modalities. *J R Soc Med.* 2014;5(9):1–13.

In other words, treatment of acne scars must be individually directed for each patient depending on the size, type, and severity of scars present.[23] The anatomic location of the scar and the patient's skin type may also be important considerations. Clinicians may encounter scars with more than one physical characteristic, such as pigmentation or erythema, in addition to being atrophic or hypertrophic. These may be termed "hybrid" scars.[4] Various modalities, single or combined, have been used to treat acne scars. Limited efficacy and problematic side effects have made the gold standard or "home-run" treatments challenging to determine.

Atrophic Scars

Atrophic scars are dermal depressions commonly caused by collagen destruction during the course of an inflammatory skin disease, such as cystic acne or varicella,[3] though there are many causes and risk factors (Table 17-3). Histologically, atrophic scars show loss of not only collagen in the dermis but also cells in the epidermis and subcutaneous fat, all contributing to the clinical appearance of a depression of the skin.[7] Atrophic scars cause significant patient morbidity and are reported to worsen with age because of the natural lipoatrophy, which further accentuates the scars.[24]

In 2001, Jacob et al.[22] unified the previously vague terminology used to describe atrophic acne scars by proposing a classification based on width, depth, and a three-dimensional architecture of acne scars: ice pick, rolling, and boxcar scars (Fig. 17-2). Influenced extensively by Goodman,[25–27] this new classification system married scar anatomy with the available effective treatment options, facilitating precise identification of scar type with enhanced, more reproducible treatment outcomes. Ice pick scars are reported as the most prevalent subcategory at 60% to 70%, boxcar scars are second at 20% to 30%, and, finally, rolling scars at 15% to 25%.

Ice pick scars are narrow (<2 mm), deep, sharply marginated epithelial tracts that extend vertically to the deep dermis or subcutaneous tissue. With this type of scar, the opening is typically wider than the deeper infundibulum (forming a "V" shape) (Fig. 17-3). But they may also be wider at a variety of levels in the dermis so that laser ablation may actually produce a wider scar/depression. Boxcar scars are round to oval depressions with sharply demarcated vertical edges, usually wider at the surface than ice pick scars (~1.5 to 4 mm) and do not taper ("U" shape). They may be

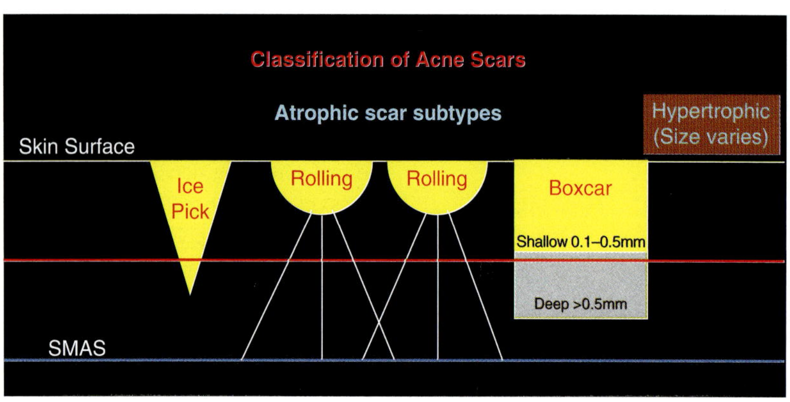

FIGURE 17-2 **Classification of acne scars.** Yellow line represents skin surface. Yellow/gray-shaded areas within scar subtypes represent loss of tissue. Brown-shaded area represents gain of tissue. Red line roughly denotes depth of ablation and resurfacing capability of the CO_2 laser. Blue line represents SMAS to which fibrous bands (*white lines*) adhere, creating rolling scars. *(Adapted by Dr. Joanna G. Bolton from Jacob CI, Dover JS, Kaminer MS. Acne scarring: a classification system and review of treatment options.* J Am Acad Dermatol. *2001;45:109–117.)*

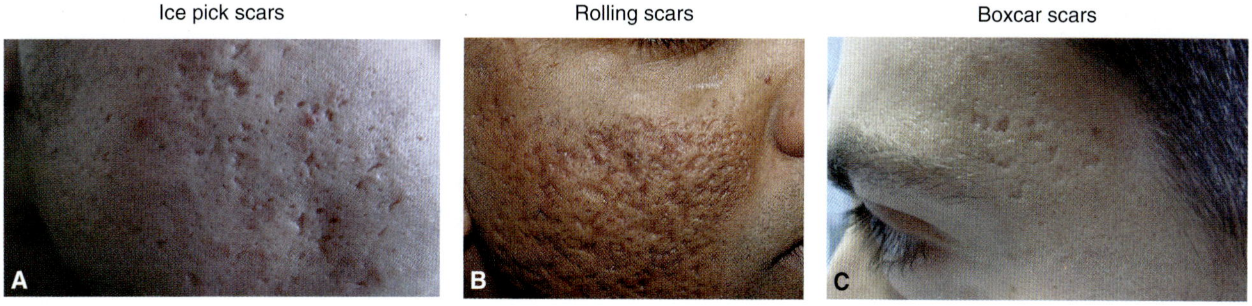

FIGURE 17-3 **Atrophic acne scars. A:** Ice pick, **B:** rolling and boxcar, **C:** boxcar. All three subcategories can be deep and coexist, making a singular clinical identification difficult. *(Photo permission granted for (**B**) by Dr. Mitchel P. Goldman, MD; (**A, C**) Copyright © 2010 Gabriella Fabbrocini et al.)*

shallow (0.1 to 0.5 mm) or deep (>0.5 mm). Shallow boxcar scars are within reach of most resurfacing treatments, but deeper boxcar scars and the tip of the infundibulum of ice pick scars are resistant to improvement in the absence of full-thickness treatment of the scar.

Rolling scars occur from dermal tethering of otherwise normal-appearing skin, usually measuring >4 mm in diameter. Abnormal fibrous bands attached to the superficial musculoaponeurotic system (SMAS) create a shadowed rolling or undulating appearance to the overlying skin ("M" shape). Although they tend to be shallow, correction of the subdermal anchoring component is required for treatment success. In general, boxcar and rolling scars are thought of as wider and more superficial than ice pick scars; however, all can be deep and intermixed on the same patient.

Hypertrophic Scars

Hypertrophic and/or keloidal scars are raised scars that present a different challenge for aesthetic treatment. Hypertrophic scars are elevated, firm erythematous scars formed at the sites of healed acneiform lesions. The result is thick, hyalinized collagen bundles consisting of fibroblasts and fibrocytes intermixed with various densities of blood vessels. Hypertrophic scars generally remain within the confines of the original integument injury and may regress without intervention over months to years. In contrast, keloids are typically reddish-purple, raised, dense and rubbery nodular scars that extend beyond the borders of the inciting wound and do not normally regress spontaneously over time. Although they can be seen in all skin types, hypertrophic scars and keloids most frequently arise at sites of moderate-to-severe acne in patients with darker skin types (Fitzpatrick III to VI) because of inherited metabolic alterations in collagen. The scars are especially likely on the chest, shoulders, and back. Controlling inflammation associated with acne is paramount in skin of color, given the higher risk for long-lasting sequelae such as distressing postinflammatory hyperpigmentation (PIH) and, in severe cases, keloids.[28] Unfortunately, undertreatment or delay in treatment of acne is common and increases the risk of hypertrophic and keloid scarring.

Further complicating matters, hypertrophic and keloid scars and the three different subtypes of atrophic scars may coexist on the same patient, making clinical differentiation between individual scars difficult and optimal treatment plans more complex. For this reason, Goodman and Baron[29–30] proposed qualitative and quantitative grading systems to help classify the level of scarring and to differentiate the clinical features. The qualitative scale, summarized in Table 17-4, is simple and universally applicable. It incorporates four

Table 17-4 Goodman and Baron Qualitative Grading Scale of Postacne Scarring

Grade	Level of disease	Characteristics
1	Macular	• Erythematous, hyper- or hypopigmented flat marks • Represent a problem of color as opposed to problems with contour and texture
2	Mild	• Mild atrophic or hypertrophic scarring that may not be obvious at social distances of 50 cm[a] or greater (i.e., mild rolling, small soft papular scars) • May be covered adequately by makeup or the normal shadow of shaved beard hair, or body hair if extrafacial, in men
3	Moderate	• Moderate atrophic or hypertrophic scarring that is obvious at social distances of 50 cm or greater (i.e. more significant rolling, shallow boxcar, mild-to-moderate hypertrophic or papular scars) • Not easily covered by makeup, or facial/body hair in men • Still able to be flattened by manual stretching of the skin (if atrophic)
4	Severe	• Severe atrophic or hypertrophic scarring that is evident at social distances greater than 50 cm (i.e. punched out deep boxcar and ice pick, gross atrophy, significant dystrophic, hypertrophic, or keloid scars) • Not easily covered by makeup, or facial/body hair in men • Not able to be flattened by manual stretching of the skin

[a]50 cm = 1 feet, 6 inches.

Adapted from Goodman GJ, Baron JA. Post acne scarring: a qualitative global scarring grading system. *Dermatol Surg*. 2006;32(12):1458–1466; Fabbrocini G, Annunziata MC, D'Arco V, et al. Acne scars: pathogenesis, classification and treatment. *Dermatol Res Pract*. 2010;2010:893080.

different grades to identify the level of postacne scarring. In those affected with mild acne, the pattern and grading is often easy to assess. However, in severe cases, different patterns are simultaneously present and may be difficult to differentiate. Their quantitative global postacne scarring assessment tool[30] is a more complex grading pattern that assigns scores on the basis of the type of scar and the number of scars present.

In summary, treatment plans for postacne scarring must be individually determined for each patient depending on the types of scars and level of disease present. The various classification systems provide tools for more effective clinical assessments and allow treatments to be tailored to the specific type of scarring noted.

Treatment Options for Acne Scars

Many treatment options are now available to help improve the cosmetic appearance of atrophic acne scarring. These include, but are not limited to, chemical peeling; laser, light, and energy-based treatments; injectable dermal fillers; autologous fat and fibroblast transplantation; subcision; punch excision techniques; dermabrasion; needling; and a variety of combination therapies. There are also promising procedures on the horizon, such as therapies with stem cells, epidermal growth factor, hair transplantation, laser-assisted delivery, and autologous platelet-rich plasma.

At the time Jacob et al.[22] published their landmark article in 2001, their four treatments of choice for acne scars were reported as punch excision, punch elevation, subcision, and laser resurfacing, with the best improvement noted when laser resurfacing followed one or all of the minor surgical interventions. Although these methods still hold significant ground in the treatment of acne scarring, over time the armamentarium of treatment techniques has expanded.[23,31–33] The pros and cons of the most common modalities are highlighted in Table 17-5.

The less common hypertrophic acne scars have a variety of treatment options, mostly similar to treatment of hypertrophic or keloidal scars resulting from any cutaneous mechanical trauma and discussed more in depth elsewhere in the text (see Chapters 10, 13, 14, and 16). Treatment options include, but are not limited to, lasers, dermabrasion, excision, cryosurgery, radiotherapy, compression with silicone sheeting, and injection of medications such as corticosteroids, bleomycin, and 5-fluorouracil. Hypertrophic scars are generally less responsive to ablative epidermal treatments like chemical peels.

It is very difficult to give clear guidelines as to which therapy is best, because the choice of treatment(s) will depend on individual patient characteristics such as skin type, type of scar, scar location, previous attempted treatments, presence of active acne, associated downtime, patient expectations with treatment, and the willingness to trial combination therapies. From the cosmetic perspective, the ultimate goal of any intervention is for improvement, not for a total cure or perfection.[31] Of utmost importance when performing aesthetic treatments is educating the patient on *realistic expectations* with the various therapies.

Table 17-5 Pros and Cons of the Most Common Treatment Modalities for Atrophic Scars

Treatment	Pros	Cons
Ablative laser therapy	Quick Can also improve wrinkling	Multiple treatments, expensive, less well tolerated, technically more involved, side effects, long downtime
Nonablative laser therapy	Quick Minimal side effects Minimal to no downtime Can also improve wrinkling	Expensive, multiple treatments (more than ablative)
Chemical peels	Quick Easier to administer More affordable	Multiple treatments, higher-strength concentrations less well tolerated but needed for better results, side effects, long downtime
Dermabrasion	Quick Minimal side effects (if administered correctly) More affordable	Multiple treatments, dubious long-term maintenance of results, posttreatment scarring and complications
Injectable dermal fillers	Quick Easy to administer Initial results in literature appear promising	Expensive, long-term efficacy unclear, repeated treatments may be needed
Autologous fat transfer	Use of patient's own fat Few side effects Good for forehead scars	Expensive, technically involved, dubious long-term maintenance of results
Subcision	Well-known and published technique More affordable Easy to utilize	Multiple treatments, significant side effects and downtime, discomfort during treatment, delay in seeing results
Tretinoin-iontophoresis	Good initial results	Technically involved procedure with special equipment, side effects, dubious long-term treatment maintenance

Adapted from Patel L, McGrouther D, Chakrabarty K. Evaluating evidence for atrophic scarring treatment modalities. *J R Soc Med.* 2014;5(9):1–13.

Table 17-6 Hierarchy of Therapy for Atrophic Acne Scars, in Descending Order of Efficacy

CO_2 ablative laser
1,450-nm diode laser/Nd:YAG laser
Long-pulsed/combined 585/1,064-nm laser
Glycolic acid/biweekly peels
Percutaneous collagen induction/TCA peels
Subcision
Autologous fat transfer
Injectables
Dermabrasion
Topical retinoids

Based on Clinical Evidence GRADE scores assigned to categorize all interventions according to their likely effectiveness based on type of study, quality, dose response, consistency of results, and significance of results. Treatments listed on the same lines were both equally effective.
Adapted from Patel L, McGrouther D, Chakrabarty K. Evaluating evidence for atrophic scarring treatment modalities. *J R Soc Med.* 2014;5(9):1–13.

Stressing postprocedure aftercare regimens, expected healing times, unpredictability with any intervention, and emphasizing the need for multiple treatment sessions spaced over many months to achieve desired appearance is essential. "Under promise, over deliver" results is a good rule of thumb.

Another consideration is out-of-pocket expense for patients. Acne scarring is the result of an inflammatory skin disease wrought with psychological impact[20]; however, treatment of these scars is often deemed "not medically necessary" and, thus, may not be covered by health insurance plans (see Chapters 4 and 25). The patient's ability to afford suggested recommendations must be considered when treatment options are offered. Because of finances, inexpensive or incomplete regimens with less demonstrated efficacy may be attempted in futility, leaving patients and physicians frustrated. Patel et al.[7] examined 41 published studies reporting treatment modalities for atrophic acne scarring and found evidence of a hierarchy favoring CO_2 ablative therapy and nonablative laser therapy as the most efficacious treatment modalities (Table 17-6), both of which come with significant expense in the hundreds to thousands of dollars.

A general review of the most common acne scar treatment modalities, including some therapies on the horizon, is provided below.

Topical Retinoids

Retinoids are vitamin A derivatives that are an important part of any aesthetic regimen with the goal to improve the appearance of facial skin. They are typically thought of as a treatment for acne vulgaris by regulating follicular hyperkeratinization and reducing inflammation. In addition, topical retinoids stimulate collagen formation, improve elastic fibers, and have been shown to increase dermal collagen synthesis. This broad range of effects explains their application in both photoaging and scars.[34–35] In fact, monotherapy with topical retinoic acid can improve acne scarring because of these mechanisms.[8] Application of tretinoin 0.05% for 4 months improved the appearance of atrophic ice pick acne scars in one study.[36] Iontophoresis has been used with tretinoin to provide increased tissue concentrations of the medication. It is a noninvasive method able to enhance transdermal drug delivery using a small electrical current applied by an iontophoretic chamber containing a similarly charged active agent and its vehicle.[37] Three-times weekly iontophoresis with tretinoin 0.025% gel was efficacious in improving acne scarring in 93% of study subjects.[38] A follow-up study to this showed the procedure was associated with a statistically significant decrease in scar depth in 94% of patients.[39] Tretinoin-iontophoresis has minimal side effects aside from erythema and stinging that are sometimes reported.[40]

Chemical Peels and CROSS Treatment

The German dermatologist P. G. Unna is credited with first discussing trichloroacetic acid (TCA) as a skin peeling agent in 1882.[14] The treatment of acne scars with chemical agents dates back to the first reported use of phenol in the 1950s.[41] There are various chemicals used to peel skin today. Peels continue to be preferred by patients because they are relatively inexpensive, noninvasive, easily obtainable, and have the added potential to simultaneously improve skin pigmentary and textural problems. The function of a chemical peel, in part, is to accelerate the normal process of exfoliation by destroying the outer damaged layers. Different agents have different depths of penetration, and therefore chemical peels can be divided into four different groups on the basis of the histologic level of necrosis that they cause.[23] The general classification of peeling agents is listed in Table 17-7.

A worrisome disadvantage of chemical peels is penetration that is often not uniform, yielding unpredictable and potentially uneven results. Furthermore, there are significant risks of PIH, milia, secondary infection, and additional scarring, especially if time of application is too long or too concentrated in a localized area. As one would expect, these risks are higher with stronger, deeper peels, such as TCA (>35%) and phenol.[42] Chemical peels should be used with caution in patients with darker skin tones (Fitzpatrick skin types IV to VI), given their inherent propensity to induce hyperpigmentation (see Chapter 18). It is recommended that superficial peeling agents be used in these patients, such as glycolic acid or Jessner solution (resorcinol, salicylic acid, and lactic acid).[43]

Of the various products, glycolic acid (in concentrations ranging from 5% to 70%) is the most commonly used peeling agent.[44–46] Since most glycolic peels are intended to be superficial, they are well tolerated with few complications and very mild postprocedure erythema and desquamation. It is an α-hydroxy acid sold over the counter in low concentrations in daily skin care products. Concentrations of 30% to 70% are generally used in chemical peels to achieve the depth needed for thinning of the stratum corneum, epidermolysis, and dispersion of basal layer melanin. The latter mechanism is the reason these peels are often employed in the treatment of melasma as well. Glycolic acid increases dermal hyaluronic acid (HA) and collagen gene expression by increasing secretion of IL-6.[47] Five sequential sessions of 70% glycolic acid every 2 weeks is suggested for best results with acne scars.[14] The superficial nature of these peels limits efficacy, and neutralization is

Table 17-7 Classification of Peeling Agents

Depth of Penetration	Histologic Level	Peeling Agents
Very superficial	Destruction of the stratum corneum without creating a wound below the stratum granulosum	• Glycolic acid, 30%–50%, brief application time (1–2 min) • Jessner's, applied in 1–3 coats • TCA 10%, applied in 1 coat
Superficial	Destruction of part or all of the epidermis, anywhere from the stratum granulosum to the basal cell layer	• Glycolic acid, 50%–70%, variable application time (2–20 min) • Jessner's, applied in 4–10 coats • TCA 10%–30%
Medium depth	Destruction of the epidermis and part or all of the papillary dermis	• Glycolic acid, 70%, variable application time (3–30 min) • TCA 35%–50% • Augmented TCA (i.e., CO_2 + TCA 35%; Jessner's + TCA 35%; glycolic acid 70% + TCA 35%)
Deep	Destruction of the epidermis and papillary dermis, extending into the reticular dermis	• Phenol 88% • Baker-Gordon phenol formula

Jessner solution preparation is made from resorcinol (14 g); salicylic acid (14 g); lactic acid (85%, 14 g); and ethanol (100 mL).
Adapted from Gozali MV, Zhou B, Luo D. Effective treatments of atrophic acne scars. *J Clin Aesth Dermatol.* 2015;8(5):33–40.

mandatory. Additionally, superficial peeling agents include Jessner solution and low-concentration (10% to 30%) TCA. Similar to light glycolic peels, they affect only the epidermis when applied correctly and are best utilized to treat only the most superficial acne scars and PIH.

Higher concentrations of TCA (35% to 50%), alone or augmented with other acids or carbon dioxide (CO_2) laser, and glycolic acid 70% applied for up to 30 minutes provide what are considered medium-depth peels, extending down to part or all of the papillary dermis. Deep chemical peels, such as TCA >50% and phenol-based peels, cause destruction extending into the reticular dermis. Medium-depth and deep peels are more effective than superficial chemical peeling agents for ice pick and deep boxcar atrophic scars, but are more commonly associated with the aforementioned higher risks.

The application of TCA to the skin causes epidermal cellular necrosis and necrosis of dermal collagen, resulting in protein denaturation (keratocoagulation) observed readily as "white frost"[23,31] (Fig. 17-4). The degree of the white frosting correlates with the depth of solution penetration. The dead cells are sloughed and the skin undergoes reepithelialization.[42] During this process, there is an increase in the production of collagen, elastin, and glycosaminoglycans.[48] The fact that TCA penetration can be easily evaluated by the color of the frost allows for easier assessment of uniformity of chemical application. Although TCA is a generally low-cost peel and may thus be favored, the associated painful stinging and burning is poorly tolerated at concentrations >25% over large areas.

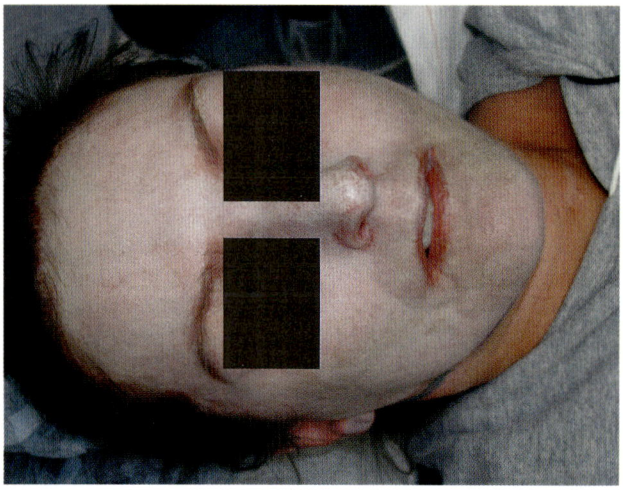

FIGURE 17-4 Patient after two coats of 30% trichloroacetic acid (TCA) with a dense white frost representing keratocoagulation. *(Photo permission granted by Joseph Niamtu, DMD.)*

Phenol peels are used infrequently because they traditionally require cardiopulmonary monitoring and intravenous hydration because of direct cardiotoxicity from phenol.[8] Commercial preparations have experimented with lower concentrations of phenol, for which monitoring and hydration are not necessary. An example is a peel that combines low concentrations of phenol (approximately 2%) and unknown proprietary concentrations of TCA, salicylic acid, retinoic acid, glycolic acid, and vitamin C (Vi Peel, Vitality Institute Medical Products, Culver City, CA) (Fig. 17-5).

While full-face peels are commonly performed, the CROSS technique (chemical reconstruction of skin scars), or dot peeling, using a high-strength TCA (65% to 100%) has been found to be a useful solo or adjunctive treatment for ice pick and small boxcar scars[24,31,49,50] (Fig. 17-6). The CROSS technique entails stretching the skin and using a fine wooden toothpick to apply TCA to the bottom of the ice pick or boxcar scar, which leads to destruction of the epithelial tract.[23] TCA is applied for a few seconds until the scar displays the characteristic white frosting.[14] Neocollagenesis ensues in the subsequent healing phase (2 to 6 weeks), filling in the depressed scar sites. Momentary mild-to-moderate burning pain is typically reported with application, but no local anesthesia or sedation is needed. On average, about 25% improvement of scars is noted with one CROSS session, with increasing efficacy reported up

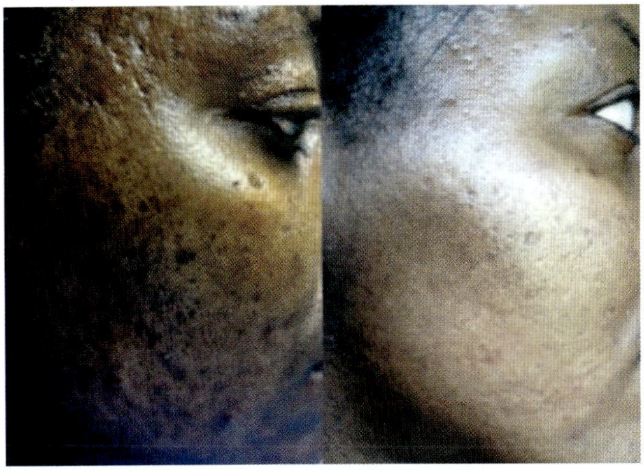

FIGURE 17-5 Acne scarring with PIH treated with a commercially available acid peel (before and after four Vi Peel treatments and a proprietary topical regimen including bleaching cream). *(Photo permission granted by Melissa McGuire, Vi Aesthetics.)*

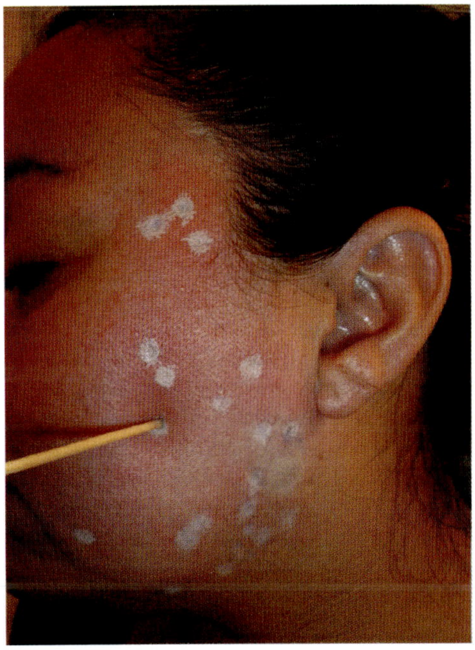

FIGURE 17-6 **CROSS technique** (chemical reconstruction of skin scars), or dot peeling, using a high-strength TCA (65% to 100%) has been found to be a useful solo or adjunctive treatment for ice pick and small boxcar scars. *(Photo permission granted by Joanna G. Bolton, MD.)*

to 70% or more after three to six treatments at intervals of 2 to 4 weeks.[51,52] Patient satisfaction was rated higher with 100% TCA versus a 65% concentration, at 94% satisfaction versus 82%, respectively, in the study by Lee et al.[52] However, Fabbrocini et al.[49] have shown that a lower TCA concentration (50%) has similar results with fewer adverse reactions. The CROSS technique has also been successful in the treatment of atrophic postvaricella (chickenpox) scarring, with over 80% of patients demonstrating moderate to marked improvement following six treatments with 70% TCA.[53]

The major advantage of the CROSS technique is that adjacent normal tissue and adnexal structures are spared, promoting more rapid healing with a lower complication rate.[51,52,54] A number of studies have demonstrated this technique can avoid postpeel scarring and reduce the risk of hyper/hypopigmentation,[55–57] making it particularly efficacious in darker skin types for which full-face, higher-strength peels are not normally recommended. However, one author (MPG) has found an unacceptable rate of hypopigmented scars in patients with Fitzpatrick skin type III to IV with this technique.

Dermabrasion/Microdermabrasion

Arguably one of the most effective but operator-dependent therapies for acne scarring is dermabrasion.[31] Dermabrasion is considered the first major advance in the treatment of acne scars.[33] Although it has largely fallen out of favor with the advent of resurfacing lasers, it remains commonly available outside dermatology offices and a basic understanding is appropriate. It is a facial resurfacing procedure that mechanically abrades damaged skin in order to promote reepithelialization and repigmentation by migration of cells to the healing surface from adjacent adnexal structures (hair follicles, sebaceous glands, and sweat ducts). Thus, the neck, chest, and back are not ideally suited for treatment because of the relative paucity of adnexal structures.[58] The wound-healing process is accompanied by new collagen formation, remodeling of structural proteins, and a smoothened appearance of scarred skin.[59] The technique completely removes the epidermis and penetrates to the level of the papillary or reticular dermis, allowing successful treatment of rolling and shallow boxcar scars. Deep boxcar and ice pick scars are not optimally treated.

Microdermabrasion, a superficial variant of dermabrasion, only removes the outer layer of the epidermis and essentially accelerates the natural process of exfoliation.[60] Because of its less aggressive nature, microdermabrasion typically produces better textural improvement of fine wrinkling and PIH, although very superficial acne scars may benefit from deeper settings. There are variable results seen with either form of treatment, and multiple sessions are usually required.

Each procedure employs different instruments with a different technical execution. Dermabrasion is accomplished by use of a high-speed brush, diamond cylinder, fraise, or manual silicone carbide sandpaper.[31] All microdermabraders include a pump that generates a stream of aluminum oxide or salt crystals with a hand piece and vacuum to remove the crystals and exfoliate the skin.[61] Unlike dermabrasion that requires local and sometimes general anesthesia because of significant pain and bleeding, microdermabrasion can be repeated at short intervals, does not require anesthesia, and is associated with a lower rate and less severe complications.[60]

Dermabrasion has many potential complications, most of which are operator and technique dependent.[8] These include prolonged erythema and healing time, eczema, milia, bacterial or viral infection, hypertrophic or keloidal scarring, unroofing of unapparent wide-based scars, telangiectases, photosensitivity (requiring strict postprocedure sun protection), treatment demarcation lines, and prolonged or permanent hyper-/hypopigmentation.[62] The pigmentary concerns are greatest for dark skin types. Postprocedural hypertrophic scarring has been reported to be a potential risk, first noted in patients undergoing dermabrasion following a recent course of oral isotretinoin therapy. This complication originally prompted the recommendation to wait 6 to 12 months for scar revision following isotretinoin use.[33,63] Despite this recommendation, there are reports of patients undergoing dermabrasion with concurrent or recent isotretinoin therapy without hypertrophic scar formation and research is ongoing.[64]

Needling

Skin needling, also called collagen induction therapy or needle dermabrasion, is a more recently employed technique for acne scars. In its simplest form for small areas, a 26G to 30G needle may be introduced into the skin to a controlled depth of about 2 to 3 mm with repeated stabs.[65] For larger areas, needling more commonly involves using a tattoo gun without pigment or a sterile roller composed of hundreds of fine, sharp needles to puncture the skin 1.5 to 2 mm to the level of the mid-dermis[13,14,32] (Fig. 17-7). Following facial skin disinfection and a topical anesthetic in place for 60 to 90 minutes, the procedure is achieved by rolling the tool until bleeding and microbruising occurs, which initiates the complex cascade of growth factors that finally results in collagen production.[23,54] The needling device is applied to the acne-scarred areas four to six times during a treatment session and should be rolled in four directions: horizontally, vertically, and diagonally left and right.[40] Results are generally appreciated after 6 weeks, but the full effect can take 3 months or more. Skin texture will continue to improve over a 12-month period, typical of skin remodeling. For best results, most patients require three to four treatments approximately 4 weeks apart.[14] The number of treatments required depends on the individual collagen response and on the desired results. Histology shows thickening of skin and a dramatic increase in new collagen and elastin fibers.

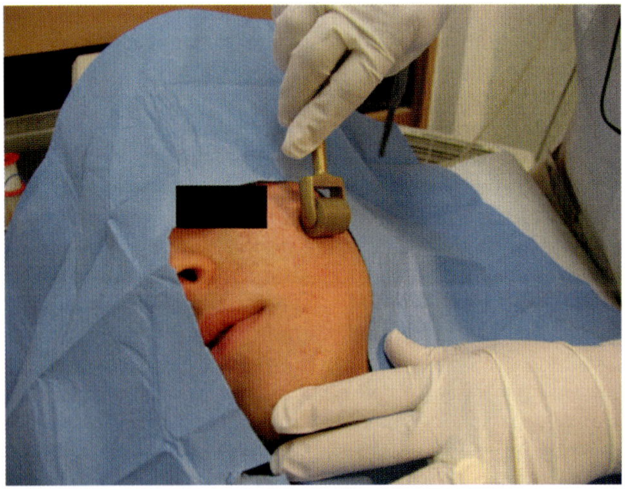

FIGURE 17-7 **Needling procedure** utilizing a sterile roller comprising hundreds of fine, sharp needles to puncture the skin 1.5 to 2 mm (level of mid-dermis). *(Copyright © 2010 Gabriella Fabbrocini et al.)*

Similar to dermabrasion, rolling and shallow boxcar acne scars are most optimally treated with needling. However, compared with dermabrasion and other resurfacing procedures such as chemical peels and laser, this technique has many advantages. Skin needling can be safely performed on all skin types with less risk of PIH, the procedure does not result in treatment demarcation lines, the recovery period is 2 to 3 days shorter than other resurfacing procedures, and needling is much less expensive for the individual patient and to incorporate into a dermatology practice.[23,66] Significant contraindications are anticoagulant therapy, bleeding disorder, active skin infection, history of injectable filler in the previous 6 months, and personal or family history of hypertrophic and keloidal scars.[40]

Subcision/Microsubcision

In the subcutaneous incisionless (subcision) technique, a specialized needle, typically a closed lumen 18G, 1½-inch with triangular cutting tip (Nokor Admix needle, Becton Dickinson & Co, Franklin Lakes, NJ), is inserted percutaneously and passed in multiple directions to release fibrotic bands in the dermis and subcutaneous tissue, similar to a "mini-scalpel"[4] (Fig. 17-8A and B). First described by Orentreich in 1995,[67] it is most useful for tethered rolling scars that have normal quality skin at the base of each scar. However, it can be helpful for any depressed scars on the face. This approach results in the scar being "released" and allows organization of blood and neocollagenesis to take place beneath the scar, helping to lift and smooth the contour.[67] It has become a first-line treatment for many isolated, moderately bound-down, atrophic scars.[68] Both Goodman[69] and Jacob et al.[22] provide excellent reviews of how to perform standard subcision following marking and administration of local anesthetic.

Microsubcision (MSUBx, Suneva Medical, Inc., San Diego, CA) is a newer technique that utilizes a standard hypodermic needle instead of a true subcision needle. Essentially, the needle is "passed back and forth" underneath a depressed scar to create a potential space, or pocket, which is then filled with a fibrin clot, or more commonly an injectable dermal filler. Both subcision and microsubcision can effectively be combined with dermal fillers, which occupy the space rather than relying solely on the created blood clot[8] (see section on tissue augmenting agents).

Advantages to subcision include being easy to perform, being inexpensive, having modest downtime, being safe for various skin types, having low rate of complications, and having remarkable and persistent improvement.[23] Complications associated with the procedure include pain, bleeding, bruising, infection, transient discoloration, possible acne exacerbation (requiring intralesional corticosteroid injection), additional, worsened, or hypertrophic scarring, and recurrence/persistence of the treated scar. It may be necessary to perform variable depths of sweeping, fanning, or lancing with the needle to disrupt the fibrous bands, and multiple treatment sessions or attempts may be required.[31] As such, the procedure must be performed judiciously to avoid damage to adjacent structures such as nerves and large vessels. Attaching a 3-mL syringe to the needle can allow for easier needle handling and better leverage.

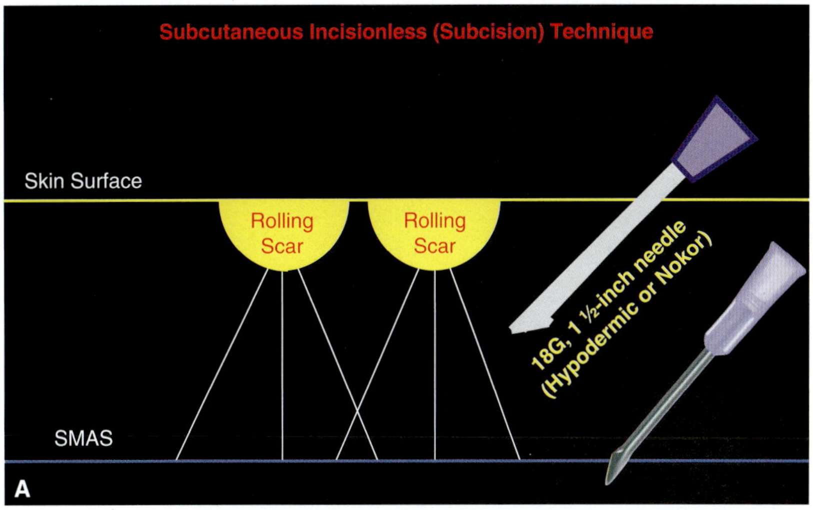

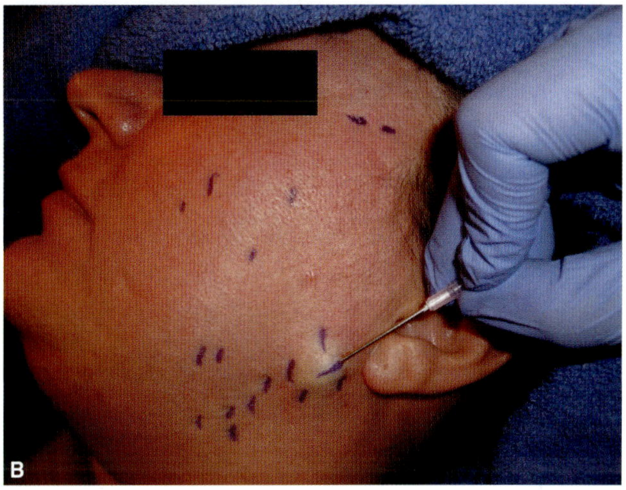

FIGURE 17-8 **A:** Schematic depicting subcision. A regular lumen, 18G, 1½-inch hypodermic needle or a triangular, solid-tipped Nokor Admix needle (*inset photo*; Becton Dickinson and Co, Franklin Lakes, NJ) may be used to undermine and separate fibrous bands (*white bands*). *Nokor needle photo is for illustration only - the level of treatment should remain above the SMAS. (Adapted by Dr. Joanna G. Bolton from Jacob CI, Dover JS, Kaminer MS. Acne scarring: a classification system and review of treatment options.* J Am Acad Dermatol. *2001;45:109–117.)* **B:** Subcision technique with Nokor needle inserted intradermally and being used to undermine a bound-down scar. Scars identified for treatment are marked preprocedure with blue ink. Piston-like motion used to release the fibrous bands; the skin is elevated to improve traction, facilitate needle motion, and avoid underlying structures. The needle may be placed on a 3-mL syringe for easier gripping and better leverage. *(Photo permission granted by Joanna G. Bolton, MD.)*

An interesting split-face study contrasted subcision on one side and a combination of subcision and nonablative laser on the other.[70] The results of the combination treatment suggested a synergistic effect between these modalities. Another study compared the effect of the 100% TCA CROSS method against subcision in treating rolling acne scars.[71] Twenty patients of skin types III and IV with bilateral rolling acnes scars received one to three sessions of the 100% TCA CROSS technique on the left side of the face and subcision for scars on the right side. The mean decrease in size and depth of scars was significantly greater for the subcision side compared with the 100% TCA CROSS. In addition, more side effects in the form of pigmentary alternation (25%) were observed with the CROSS method.

Punch Excision Techniques

Punch excision techniques are minimally invasive surgical treatments mainly indicated for ice pick or small boxcar scars. According to diameter, depth, and shape of the scar, a biopsy punch of appropriate size is used to excise the scar potentially followed by closure, elevation, or grafting.[40]

With punch excision and closure, the scar is excised and sutured (6-0 or smaller suture) after undermining, in a direction parallel to the relaxed skin tension lines. The goal is to trade a larger, deeper scar for a smaller, linear closure that will hopefully be less noticeable. If a depressed scar has a normal surface texture, punch incision to the subcutaneous tissue followed by elevation of the base and suturing to the level of surrounding skin may improve scar appearance. Retraction of the tissue occurs during the healing phase, resulting in a leveled surface.[22] Finally, in punch excision with grafting, a scar is excised and replaced with either an autologous split-thickness or full-thickness punch graft or prepackaged dermal graft material. The pre- or postauricular region or the gluteal fold are the most used donor sites for autologous grafts.[40] This is probably best for sharp-walled or deep ice pick scars, but is painstaking as often 20 or more replacement grafts are required in a single session.[23] Laser skin resurfacing with the concurrent use of punch excision techniques further improves facial acne scarring.[22,72]

Laser Treatment

Acne scar treatment with lasers varies depending on the type of scar. Ice pick scars often do not respond well to laser treatments, and in the view of the authors are better

Table 17-8 Laser Treatment of Acne Scars

Laser Treatment	Wavelength (nm)	Chromophore Target	Ablative (A) vs. Nonablative (NA)	Fractionated (F) vs. Nonfractionated (NF)
PDL	585 or 595	Blood	NA	NF
Picosecond alexandrite	755	Melanin	NA	NF
Nd:YAG	1,064	Water	NA	NF
Erbium: glass	1,500	Water	NA	F
Erbium: glass	1,540	Water	NA	F
Erbium:YAG	2,940	Water	A	NF
Erbium:YAG	2,940	Water	A	F
CO_2	10,600	Water	A	F

From Sardana[174], Ong and Bashir[88], Verhaeghe et al.[86], Leheta et al.[87], Brauer et al.[82], Koike et al.[80], Choi et al.[95], Mahmoud et al.[85], Woo et al.[89]

treated with the CROSS technique, punch techniques, and radiofrequency treatments. Shallow boxcar scars have been successfully treated with ablative and nonablative fractionated lasers in addition to subcision, dermal fillers, skin needling, radiofrequency, and/or other surgical corrections such as excision and closure, rhytidectomy, and punch-grafting techniques. Deeper boxcar scars are better treated with punch-grafting or excisional techniques and/or radiofrequency devices. Rolling acne scars have been treated with ablative and nonablative fractionated lasers in addition to dermal fillers, dermabrasion, subcision, skin needling, and/or radiofrequency devices. Hypertrophic and keloidal scars are better treated with the 585-to-595-nm PDL, 515-to-1,100-nm IPL, and ablative fractionated lasers with or without the addition of intralesional corticosteroids and/or 5% 5-fluorouracil because of the potential for a worsening of these lesions with other modalities.[73] Table 17-8 summarizes various laser treatment modalities (see Chapter 13).

Nonablative, Nonfractionated Laser Treatment of Acne Scars

The 585-to-595-nm PDL and the 532-nm Q-switched frequency-doubled neodymium–yttrium–aluminum garnet (Nd:YAG) are nonablative nonfractional lasers that target hemoglobin. Efficacy of these lasers is based on the principle of selective photothermolysis, wherein the light energy emitted is absorbed by oxygenated and deoxygenated hemoglobin, causing thermal damage of the blood vessels with resultant neocollagenesis.[74] Therefore, the 585-to-595-nm PDL or other vasculature-targeting devices such as IPL are an appropriate treatment for scars with a vascular or red component. Evidence has supported its use with keloids, hypertrophic scars, erythematous scars, and striae.[75,76]

Cannarozzo et al.[77] found the PDL to improve the vascular component of keloids and hypertrophic scars. Out of 29 patients, excellent results were seen in 49.1%, good results were seen in 25.4%, a slight improvement was seen in 20.4%, and no improvement was found in 5%. With a low side-effect profile and no downtime post procedure, the PDL is a good treatment for scars with a vascular component. Additionally, the PDL does not appear to cause progression with hypertrophic scars and keloids.

In postsurgical scars, the 595-nm PDL (Vbeam; Candela Laser Corporation; Wayland, MA) has been found to have greater improvement in epidermal appearance when compared with a 1,550-nm nonablative fractionated laser (Fraxel; Solta Medical Inc., Hayward, CA, USA), which was associated with a larger improvement in scar texture.[78] Vas et al.[79] examined 25 patients with 39 postoperative linear scars treated with three monthly split scar treatments using the 585-nm PDL and the 1,064-nm Nd:YAG (Cynergy; Cynosure Inc.; Westford, MA) compared with no treatment on the other half of the scar. The combination PDL/Nd:YAG laser treatments had superior results compared with the untreated areas.

The 1,064-nm Nd:YAG laser is a nonablative, nonfractionated laser that targets tissue water in addition to oxygenated and deoxygenated hemoglobin. Koike et al.[80] demonstrated the use of 1,064-nm Nd:YAG laser (Cutera, Brisbane, CA) to be beneficial for hypertrophic scars but not for keloidal scars. Keloidal scars recurred 6 months after treatment cessation in 4% of the abdominal scars, 25% of the scapular scars, 35.7% of the upper arm, and 52.9% of anterior chest keloids. The findings of persistent erythema or induration in keloids after treatment had the best predictive value for keloid recurrence. Because the 1,064-nm Nd:YAG laser requires high energies to thermocoagulate blood vessels because of its poor absorption by oxy- and deoxygenated hemoglobin, excessive nonspecific thermal destruction should be avoided to minimize a progression of keloidal and hypertrophic scarring.

As the face ages, acne scarring can become more prominent with increased skin laxity. Improvement of the skin laxity in turn improves acne scar appearance. The subcutaneous 1,064-nm Nd:YAG laser (Smartlipo, CynoSure, Westford, MA) has been utilized to treat acne scarring with an added benefit of skin tightening secondary to neocollagenesis.[81] This procedure is best for patients with mild skin laxity, and would likely yield better results if a combination acne treatment were completed.

Picosecond lasers emit optical pulses with a duration between 400 and 800 ps. The shorter energy pulse results in improved destruction of the target chromophore with a decrease in surrounding thermal damage. The 755-nm alexandrite picosecond laser is a nonablative nonfractionated or fractionated laser with melanin and other pigment (tattoos) as its chromophore target. Brauer et al.[82] examined 20 patients with facial acne scarring treated with the 755-nm alexandrite picosecond laser (Cynosure, Westford, MA) and found a 24.3% average improvement in appearance and texture 3 months post-treatment. Additional studies are needed to compare the cosmetic results of acne scar treatments with picosecond lasers in comparison with Q-switched and long-pulsed lasers of similar wavelength.

Nonablative Fractionated Laser Treatment of Acne Scars

Nonablative fractionated lasers produce columns of damage to the skin to enhance neocollagenesis and skin remodeling without destroying the epidermis. Geronemus treated 17 patients with ice pick, rolling, and boxcar scars with a 1,550-nm fractionated nonablative laser (NAFL, Fraxel Laser, Reliant Technology, Inc.; Mountain View, CA). A series of five treatments were given at 1-to-3-week intervals with a mean improvement of 25% to 50%. There was no posttreatment hypopigmentation, hyperpigmentation, or scarring with good results seen even in dark skin types.[83]

Sardana et al.[84] compared the efficacy of the nonablative fractionated 1,540-nm erbium-doped glass laser (StarLux-300; Lux 1,540-nm fractional hand piece; Palomar Medical Technologies; Burlington, MA) in the treatment of ice pick, boxcar, and rolling acne scars. The boxcar scars responded best with an overall 52.9% improvement, rolling scars improved 43.1%, and ice pick scars improved 25.9%. Ice pick acne scars appeared to be more effectively treated with the CROSS technique, punch techniques, and radiofrequency treatments. Fractionated nonablative treatment success with boxcar and rolling acne scars may improve when combined with other treatments.[73]

Mahmound utilized the 1,550-nm Er:YAG laser (Fraxel SR1500; Fraxel; Solta Medical Inc., Hayward, CA, USA) in the treatment of acne scars in skin types IV and VI. A significant improvement was noted after five monthly treatments with no difference found between fluences of 10 and 40 mJ. However, the pain level was significantly higher in darker skin with resultant PIH.[85]

Hypertrophic scars have also been treated with nonablative fractionated lasers. Verhaeghe et al.[86] found the nonablative fractionated 1,540-nm laser (StarLux-300; Lux 1,540-nm fractional hand piece; Palomar Medical Technologies; Burlington, MA) produced no immediate change in the treatment of hypertrophic scars, but a small improvement was slowly noted over 3 months. The combination of laser-assisted drug delivery of 5% 5-fluorouracil or triamcinolone acetonide suspension immediately after laser treatment may help to improve the outcome. Although nonablative lasers do not produce as high of a transdermal delivery of drugs compared to ablative lasers, there is an improvement over cutaneous application alone.

Combination treatments with lasers (i.e., "multimodal therapy") are proving effective as acne scar treatment. Leheta et al.[87] found a combination of the nonablative fractionated 1,540-nm laser (StarLux-300; Lux 1,540-nm fractional hand piece; Palomar Medical Technologies; Burlington, MA) with 20% trichloroacetic acid (TCA) improved atrophic acne scars by 78.27% compared with the 1,540-nm laser alone at 61.83% and TCA alone at 59.79%. Additional studies are needed to validate the long-term efficacy of nonablative fractionated lasers in acne scar treatment and to determine the best combination treatments.

Ong et al.[88] completed a review of over 26 studies utilizing ablative and nonablative fractionated lasers in the treatment of acne scars. Ablative fractionated laser treatment was found on average to have erythema for 3 to 14 days that resolved in 12 weeks. Approximately 92.3% of the patients developed PIH that lasted up to 6 months and had postoperative pain rated 5.90 to 8.10/10. Nonablative fractional laser treatment typically had erythema for 1 to 3 days that resolved in 1 week. Of the patients, 13% developed PIH that lasted up to 1 week and postoperatively had 3.90 to 5.66/10 pain. The severity of side effects is greater with ablative compared with nonablative lasers, but treatment outcomes were typically better with more aggressive therapy.

The authors of this chapter have had success treating facial scars resulting from chickenpox, similar in appearance to atrophic acne scars, with a 1,565-nm laser (ResurFX, Lumenis Ltd., Yokneam, Israel) (Fig. 17-9).

Nonfractionated Ablative Laser Treatment of Acne Scars

The 2,940-nm Er:YAG laser is an ablative laser for skin resurfacing and can be used at a variety of pulse duration and energy levels to produce different effects on the skin. The short-pulsed Er:YAG uses 500-µs pulses of ablation. The variable-pulsed Er:YAG uses short pulses of ablation and longer pulses of 1 to 10 ms to induce greater nonspecific thermal damage. The dual-mode Er:YAG laser uses short ablative pulses of high fluence and coagulative long pulses of a low fluence. Woo et al.[89] compared the short-pulsed, variable-pulsed, and dual-mode Er:YAG lasers (Sciton Inc.; Palo Alto, CA) in the treatment of ice pick, boxcar, and rolling acne scars in 158 patients. Shallow boxcar and ice pick scars were successfully treated with all three types of the Er:YAG laser. Rolling and deep boxcar scars benefitted from the increased thermal effect of the longer pulse duration for a successful treatment outcome.

Similarly, Jeong et al.[90] treated 35 patients of skin types III to V with pitted facial acne scars with the long-pulsed Er:YAG laser (Lumenis Ltd.; Yokneam, Israel) and found 36% (10/35) had excellent results, 57% (16/35) had good results, and 7% (2/35) had fair results with an overall average improvement of 71%. Ablative nonfractionated lasers, depending on fluence, number of passes, and technique, may induce prolonged erythema and delayed-onset dyspigmentation and scarring. Fractionated lasers have a lower rate of these side effects and have mostly replaced ablative nonfractionated lasers in the treatment of acne scarring, but with a resultant decrease in overall efficacy.

Fractionated Ablative Laser Treatment of Acne Scars

Given the dermal involvement of atrophic acne scars, treatment modalities that provide an effect on dermal remodeling tend to give better results. Fractionated ablative lasers can produce a deeper dermal effect and have been shown to give the best cosmetic results for acne scars with the lowest side-effect profile. Side effects with fractionated ablative lasers most commonly include erythema and dyspigmentation. However, the length and severity of these side effects is less than ablative nonfractionated lasers.[91]

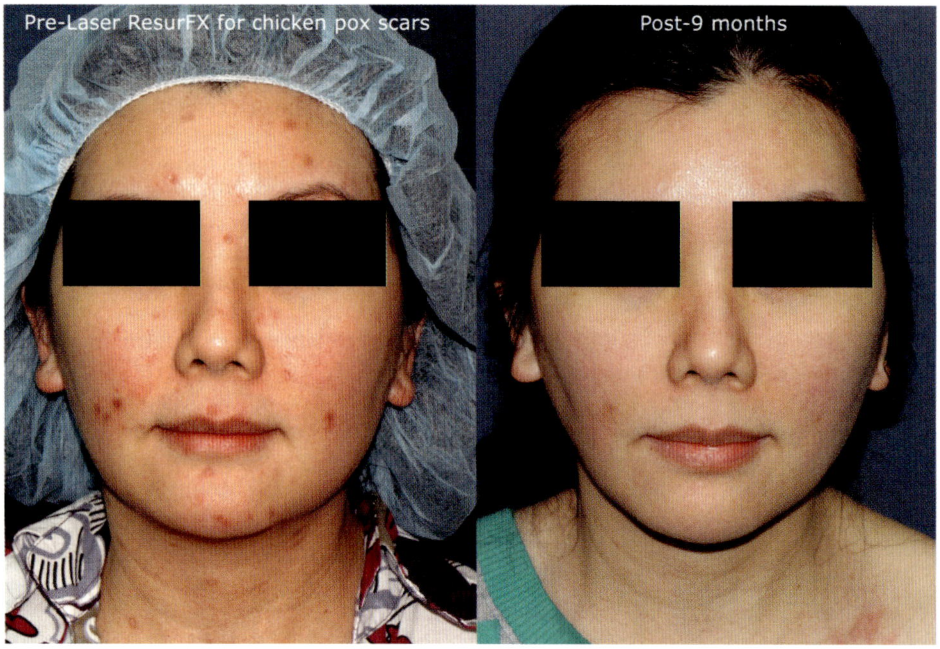

FIGURE 17-9 Pre- and postresurfacing treatment of chicken pox scars with a nonablative fractionated 1,565-nm laser (ResurFX, Lumenis). *(Photo permission granted by Mitchel P. Goldman, MD.)*

Cho et al.[92] evaluated 20 Korean patients with atrophic acne scars treated with a single session with the fractionated ablative 10,600-nm CO_2 laser (UltraPulse Encore Deep FX; Lumenis Inc.; Santa Clara, CA). Three months postprocedure, 5% (1/20) had a >75% improvement, 45% (9/20) had a 51% to 75% improvement, 35% (7/20) had a 26% to 50% improvement, and 15% (3/20) had minimal to no improvement noted. The main side effects included scaling, crusting, erythema, edema, oozing, and hyperpigmentation that lasted approximately 6 days. Although nonablative lasers have a lower side-effect profile, more treatment sessions are needed to achieve results comparable with ablative lasers. The authors concluded that the fractionated ablative CO_2 laser offers a method of acne scar treatment that can improve the appearance with less treatment time.

Walia et al.[93] utilized the high-energy pulsed CO_2 laser (Coherent; Santa Clara, CA) to treat atrophic acne scars in 60 patients and found an average improvement in appearance of 69% at 1 month that increased to 75% at 18 months posttreatment. Because of the continued improvement of the scars up to 18 months after treatment, a longer postoperative interval between treatments that is closer to 12 to 18 months may be warranted in order to capture the full benefit from the prior treatment.

Yuan et al.[94] compared different settings with the fractionated CO_2 laser (UltraPulse Encore Deep FX; Lumenis Inc., Santa Clara, CA) in the treatment of 20 Asian patients with facial acne scars. The settings were varied including pulse energies ranging from 10 to 20 mJ and densities from 10% to 20%. All laser settings produced good results. However, higher rates of adverse effects (prolonged erythema and PIH) were seen with higher density and pulse energy.

Choi et al.[95] compared the fractionated ablative 2,490-nm Er:YAG (Sciton Inc., Palo Alto, CA) and 10,600-nm CO_2 lasers (UltraPulse Encore, Lumenis Inc., Santa Clara, CA) in the treatment of acne scars in 13 patients. A 28.2% improvement was noted with a single treatment with the Er:YAG and a 49.8% improvement with the CO_2 laser. The CO_2 fractionated ablative laser was considered to be a safe, effective treatment for acne scars with a particular improvement in the pliability of the scars. Atrophic scars seem to respond better to ablative fractionated CO_2 lasers. Authors Lupton and Alster caution against the use of fully ablative lasers with keloids and hypertrophic scars as there is a theoretical risk for progression or recurrence.[75,76]

Radiofrequency Devices

With an increased interest in treatments that yield fewer side effects and less downtime, radiofrequency (RF) devices are an emerging option for improving acne scars. RF technology is used worldwide in aesthetic medicine not only for acne scar revision but for cellulite reduction, treatment of hypertrophic scars and keloids, rosacea, inflammatory acne, and most commonly, tissue tightening to improve skin laxity and reduce wrinkles.[96] RF is nonionizing electromagnetic radiation with a frequency range between 3 and 300 GHz.[23] The treatments work by passing a current through the dermis at a preset depth to produce small, pyramid-shaped zones of thermal injury that, in turn, stimulate dermal remodeling to produce new collagen and soften scar defects.[97] Of significant potential advantage, patients of variable skin types can be treated more confidently because the technology is not a chromophore-based intervention, theoretically reducing the risk of PIH and other complications.

RF devices are generally mono/unipolar or bipolar. A monopolar device requires use of a remotely placed grounding pad and uses a single contact location for the area of origin. Electric current is delivered and diminishes as it flows toward the pad. A bipolar device has two local

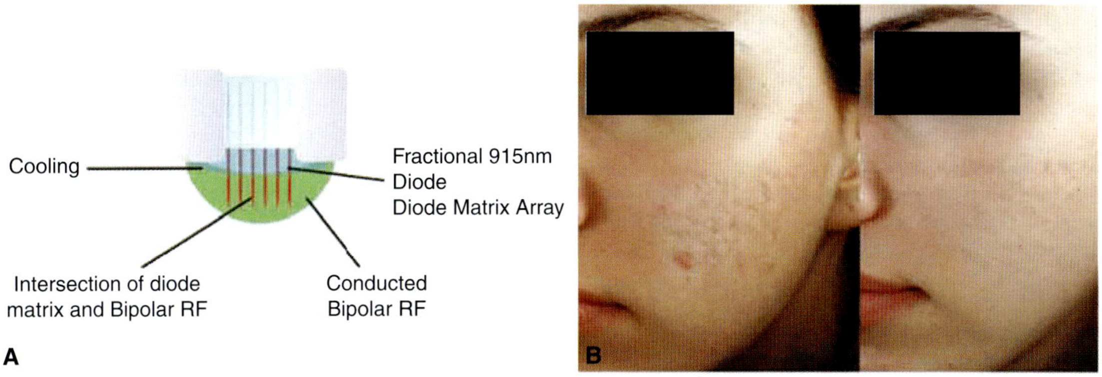

FIGURE 17-10 **Sublative fractional bipolar RF. A:** Schematic of combination bipolar matrix array and bipolar RF. The intersection of the two modalities creates thermal bands at 1.5 mm into the dermis, causing collagen contraction. *(Image courtesy of Syneron Medical LTD.)* **B:** Hispanic study patient before and 1 month after three treatments of fractional bipolar RF and DLRF (diode laser/bipolar RF). *(Image courtesy of Amy Taub, MD.)*

electrodes between which current flows. Because there is no path of current through the body, a grounding pad is not required.[98] A study investigating the use of nonablative RF for the treatment of moderate-to-severe acne (scar-preventative treatment) noted, as an incidental result, that there was qualitative improvement in underlying scarring,[99] prompting additional investigation.

More recently, fractionated bipolar RF, based on the principle of "sublative rejuvenation," which causes low epidermal disruption with high dermal remodeling, has been introduced to improve the efficacy and reduce the side effects normally associated with ablative fractionated lasers for acne scar treatment.[100–102] Unlike fractionated ablative laser treatments, which can disrupt up to 10% to 70% of the epidermis, the sublative rejuvenation technique affects only up to 5% of the epidermis with each pass, confining most of the effect to the dermis.[102] This translates into minimal downtime for patients and makes it an optimal choice for darker skin. In two similar studies, the combination of a diode laser (915-nm) and fractionated bipolar RF (DLRF handpiece Matrix IR) followed by a fractionated sublative bipolar RF handpiece (Matrix RF, Matrix eLaser, Syneron, Irvine, CA) has been reported as a safe and statistically effective combined modality for the treatment of both superficial and deep acne scars in skin types II–V[103,104] (Fig. 17-10). In Taub and Garretson's[103] study, acne scars improved significantly 1 month after three treatments and improvement persisted for at least 12 weeks after the fifth treatment, with improvement not affected by skin type. Adverse effects were limited to transient crust formation, erythema, and edema, all of which resolved within 1 to 4 days. Peterson et al.[104] showed improvement of acne scarring, skin texture, and pigmentation in more than 60% of study subjects with five monthly treatments. Rolling and boxcar scars improved more dramatically than ice pick scars.

Another new technique pairs fractionated bipolar RF with needling. In a study performed in South Korea, a minimally invasive fractionated RF microneedle (FRM) device (INTRAcel, Jeisys, Seoul, Korea) showed improvement in the grade of acne scars and size of large pores in more than 70% of patients.[105] Skin surface roughness, dermal density, and microscopic and composite images also improved. With FRM, temperatures high enough for coagulation are induced at a specific level ranging from approximately 0.5 to 3.5 mm, depending on the selected microneedle. There is also a physical effect of stretching by the microneedle on the fibroblasts, which leads to further neocollagenesis.

The efficacy of a relatively new high-intensity focused RF device with insulated microneedles (Infini, Lutronic Inc., Fremont, CA) was evaluated in a small case series.[106] This novel system delivers energy through an array of 49 insulated microneedles with a total spot size of 10 × 10 mm. The depth of penetration can be controlled from 0.5 to 3.5 mm, similar to the Korean device, with the depth of the thermal delivery adjusted before each of the three passes per treatment. Each patient had three to four treatments, depending on severity of acne scars. Controlling the depth of the needle penetration during each pass allows for the creation of a latticework of focal RF injuries, thus customizing the treatment for the depth of the acne scars.[106] In theory, having insulated needles (except for the treatment tip) ensures maximum thermal injury zones in the target zone while allowing for little to no long-term damage to the epidermis. Significant improvement of acne scars was noted in all subjects, with patient downtime reported as usually no more than 4 to 8 hours. Because radiofrequency energy is not specifically absorbed by melanin and this new technology allows delivery through an array of insulated microneedles at precise depths that spare the epidermis, there is the ability to treat the full spectrum of skin types with potentially less downtime than ablative and nonablative fractionated lasers.

A recent retrospective review demonstrated that out of all RF modalities, microneedle bipolar RF and fractionated bipolar RF treatments offer the best results for acne scarring.[97] An improvement of 25% to 75% can be expected after three to four treatment sessions using one to two passes per session with an RF device. Treatment results are optimal approximately 3 months after final treatment. It is reasonable to theorize an overlap exists between the skin tightening and rejuvenation properties of RF and its beneficial effects on acne scars on the basis of its documented improvements in wrinkled and sagging skin.[107] Still, additional studies are needed to evaluate the treatment of acne scarring with RF technology and to determine what modality is best for specific scar subtypes.

Plasma skin regeneration (PSR) is another form of RF that has been shown to improve acne scars by resurfacing the skin, but the literature for this method is scant and reported complication rates are high.[108–113] Plasma pulses are created by passing ultrahigh radiofrequency energy through inert nitrogen gas, leading to stripping of electrons and formation of ionized gas.[31] The energy is then directed to the patient's skin surface by the handpiece to stimulate a thermal effect. PSR, similar to other RF techniques and unlike lasers or IPL sources, is not chromophore dependent.[68] It does not vaporize tissue but leaves a layer of intact, denatured epidermis, which may act as a natural dressing favoring accelerated wound healing. Reepithelialization completes in about 1 week with shedding of the destroyed epidermis. Roughly 10 days after treatment, fibroblasts depositing new collagen and elastin fibers can be seen.[23] Histology from patients that received PSR suggests continued collagen production, reduction of elastosis, and progressive skin rejuvenation beyond 1 year after treatment.[111] However, in a recent review 36 out of 65 PSR cases (55%) were complicated by infection, with postprocedure scarring being the second most common complication (15%).[113] The infection rate from PSR was higher than in any of the multiple other forms of cosmetic laser and energy treatments reviewed. Despite these findings, there is continued pursuit to improve PSR.

To compare the efficacy and safety of a novel monopolar fractionated microplasma RF device versus a fractionated CO_2 laser in the treatment of atrophic acne scars in Asian skin, Zhang et al.[114] performed a randomized, split-face, evaluator-blinded prospective study with 33 patients each receiving three treatment sessions every 6 to 12 weeks. With this RF technology, a combined ablative and thermal effect is produced as multiple RF plasma microdischarges are created in a gap between the applicator and the skin surface. When the applicator is a certain distance from the skin, the electromagnetic RF energy excites a grid of microsparks that cause mild epidermal ablation and perforate the dermis superficially.[114] Once the handpiece contacts the skin, it creates monopolar RF effects. In the study, both modalities showed improvement of the acne scars. However, on the RF-treated sides postprocedure crusting and erythema cleared in half the time as compared with the CO_2-treated sides (crusting 5.7 vs. 10.2 days; erythema 6.8 vs. 12.3 days) and PIH was not seen (0% vs. 36%), which might make it a better choice for patients with darker skin. Of note, pain was reported as slightly higher on RF sides (5.9 vs. 4.3/10), but was not too severe and lasted for just minutes.

Intense-Pulsed Light

IPL devices emit a wide range of wavelengths from their source that can be precisely narrowed using filters and are thus considered "energy devices" as opposed to a true laser. IPL is considered a good option for acne vulgaris treatment (40% to 60% improvement with IPL alone) and has shown even better results when combined with photodynamic therapy (PDT) (60% to 80% improvement with IPL + PDT).[115] With this in mind, along with studies that revealed post-IPL histologic increases in papillary dermal fibrosis and numbers of dermal fibroblasts,[116] IPL has been trialed in the cosmetic treatment of macular and superficial atrophic acne scarring with benefit noted (Fig. 17-11). As well, IPL has shown efficacy in some studies for reducing hypertrophic acne scars because of its ability to target the vasculature. Although both IPL and PDL produced comparable results in split scar studies, IPL offers a therapeutic alternative to the gold-standard PDL for the treatment of hypertrophic scars since it minimizes the development of posttreatment purpura.[117] A common complication of IPL treatments are resultant burns,[113] underscoring the importance of appropriate selections of wavelength (filter), energy, pulse duration, and cooling.

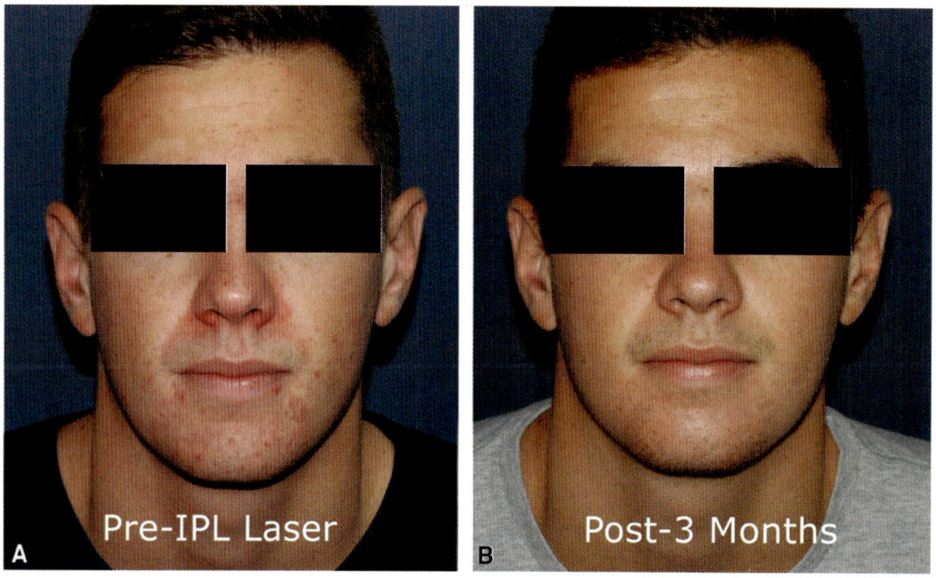

FIGURE 17-11 Patient treated with IPL for macular and superficial acne scarring. **A:** Baseline. **B:** 3 months posttreatment. *(Photo permission granted by Mitchel P. Goldman, MD.)*

Tissue Augmenting Agents

Injectable Dermal Fillers

Injectable dermal fillers offer an important nonsurgical technique to correct acne scars and improve skin texture. They are commonly used in conjunction with other "lifting" procedures—such as subcision and punch elevation—and in combined regimens that may also include laser and energy devices. Lifting procedures try to draw the base of a deep scar toward the surface and smooth out the skin.[4] Fillers may be used to treat any depressed acne scar but are particularly helpful for deep, rolling scars, which become even more apparent with facial skin aging. They can even work for scars with discrete edges and, arguably, should be considered a first-line approach for atrophic acne scars. When combining fillers with treatments such as laser or peels, the clinician must bear in mind that the fillers may have already elicited a local inflammatory response that may exacerbate the same response from the peel or laser.[118]

An ideal filler material should be hypoallergenic and safe, be well tolerated with few adverse side effects, be painless and easy to inject, be effective, be inexpensive, and offer durable, long-lasting results. Although some are close to ideal, none of the treatments available meet all of the criteria completely. With this in mind, there are a variety of newer and older autologous, nonautologous, biologic, and nonbiologic tissue augmentation agents that have been used for atrophic scar contour correction. Older agents, now less favored because of high incidence of side effects, include bovine collagen, silicone, autologous fibroblasts (Isolagen), donated cadaveric human skin (Alloderm), gelatin matrix implant (Fibrel), and polymethylmethacrylate (Artecoll). Perhaps the most frequently used agent currently is HA[26] based on safety profile, ease of use, and availability. However, poly-L-lactic acid (PLLA), calcium hydroxyapatite (CHA), a rebranded bovine collagen admixed with polymethylmethacrylate (PMMA), and autologous fat and fibroblasts are all current options as well.[31] New substances are constantly being created or tried for use in augmentation of scars. Selected agents are highlighted below.

HA is a hydrophilic, linear polysaccharide that occurs naturally in the body's connective tissue, offering reduced risk of immunogenicity and hypersensitivity without the need for skin testing. Injection of commercially available cross-linked HA stimulates collagen synthesis and partially restores dermal matrix components, proposed to result from mechanical stretching of the dermis that leads to activation of dermal fibroblasts.[8] HAs do not require an initial overcorrection, in contrast to collagen, for example, because there is less water loss after injection. Long-term improvements can be seen after one to three treatments. Although the correction is temporary, the duration of effect for acne scars is roughly a year or more.[31] Side effects potentially include erythema, edema, bruising, inflammation, delayed reactions, infection, pain, milia or acne, and rare reports of necrosis.[119]

An interesting needleless pressure injection system for introducing HA into acne scars over multiple sessions has had good results with minimal downtime, pain, or side effects.[120] The machine (Enerjet, PerfAction, Inc., Rehovot, Israel) is capable of pneumatically accelerating a carrier fluid jet containing high-mass molecules of HA. The accelerated jet penetrates the epidermis through a tiny entry point and spreads the HA laterally in all directions once it reaches the dermis, filling an area of 10 × 10 cm.[68] Controlled microinjury to the dermal layer is produced, which initiates the wound-healing process and neocollagenesis, a favorable secondary effect.[121] Patel et al.[120] concluded that pneumatic jet volumetric remodeling (JVR) technology to deliver HA to the tissue is an effective and safe method for improving acne scars, even in patients with dark skin types. As an emerging technique, JVR is expected to be studied in additional clinical trials.

Volumizing fillers, such as PLLA (Sculptra, Galderma Laboratories, Bridgewater, NJ) and CHA (Radiesse, Merz Aesthetics, Raleigh, NC), can be delivered to areas where laxity of skin or deep tissue atrophy is accentuating the appearance of acne scars.[50] Injectable PLLA is a biocompatible and biodegradable synthetic polymer that elicits long-lasting endogenous stimulation of fibroblasts and, subsequently, collagen.[122] PLLA has a duration of effect of 2 years or more with serial treatments, distinguishing itself from injectable collagens that last 2 to 4 months and injectable HAs that last 3 to 12 months.[123] It does not require skin testing. Initially approved for the treatment of HIV lipoatrophy, PLLA received its cosmetic approval for facial volume restoration from the FDA in 2009. Patients often require multiple treatments with PLLA for maximum improvement, and injections can occur at 1-month intervals.[8] Clinical trials and several case reports have documented improvement in facial atrophic acne scars after treatments with PLLA.[122–125] One case report found significant improvement of atrophic acne scars after several PLLA injections despite previous failure of calcium hydroxylapatite (CHA) and HA injections.[125] In a recently published phase II study utilizing three camera systems, Sapra et al.[123] set out to determine how well the collagen builder PLLA could correct rolling (or "hill and valley") acne scars. Researchers injected PLLA over three to four treatments at 4-week intervals. The percentage of patients with "much to excellent" improvement based on photographic comparison assessments ranged from 45.5% to 68.2%. Subject treatment satisfaction scores increased steadily by 44% during the study, with all completing the treatment course. One patient experienced a palpable, nonvisible nodule. Side effects of PLLA are possibly worsened by factors such as excess injection of material, inadequate duration between injections, low dilution, dilution time less than 24 hours, and superficial injection, but these can be minimized using appropriate injection technique.[126]

CHA is a semipermanent dermal filler composed of 25-to-45-μm-diameter calcium hydroxyapatite microspheres in a moldable hydrogel vehicle. The hydrogel provides immediate volume correction, but is degraded over time. Similar to the mechanism of action of PLLA, the CHA microspheres stimulate fibroblast production of collagen, which grows over the CHA scaffold deposited in the skin.[8] Improvement in appearance can occur after a single injection, with results maintained for 12 to 16 months. There is little inflammation, minimal side-effect profile, and no requirement for allergy testing.[31]

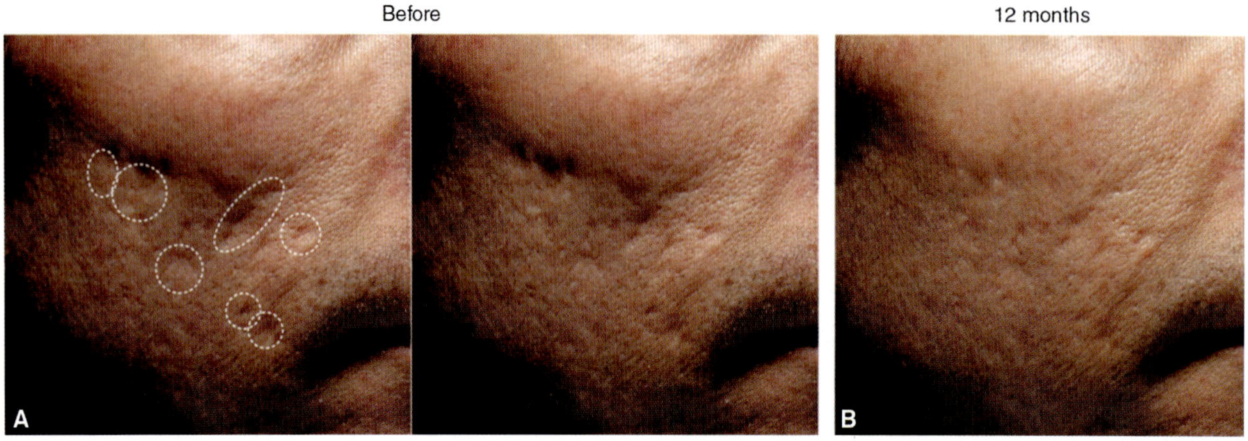

FIGURE 17-12 Patient treated with nonresorbable polymethylmethacrylate filler (Bellafill). **A:** Baseline—only circled scars were treated. **B:** 12 months posttreatment. *(Photo reprint from Suneva Medical, Inc.)*

In 2015, the FDA approved a bovine collagen solution (80%) with nonresorbable PMMA microspheres (20%) and 0.3% lidocaine (Bellafill, Suneva Medical, Inc., San Diego, CA) for the correction of moderate-to-severe, atrophic, distensible facial acne scars on the cheek in patients over the age of 21 years[127] (Fig. 17-12). Originally introduced as Artefill for correction of nasolabial folds in 2006, the collagen in the solution provides immediate volume and lift below scars while the PMMA microspheres remain in place and create a matrix that supports collagen production in the dermis for lasting improvement. Thus, it permanently provides supportive scaffolding and helps normalize reflective optics (reflection/refraction) of the skin surface by reducing shadowing of the base of the scar.[4] Now relabeled as Bellafill, it represents the first dermal filler in the United States specifically FDA approved for the treatment of acne scars. Only very small amounts are needed, typically 0.1 to 0.2 mL per scar per treatment session, and correcting to optimal surface contour or slightly undercorrecting is recommended. If a site is overfilled, the excess filler should be squeezed or "milked out," or if need be, punch excised, to prevent a palpable nodule. Treated sites should be gently massaged for 2 minutes each morning and night for 1 to 2 weeks to help maintain even distribution of the microspheres. Of note, product labeling recommends intradermal skin testing and observation for 28 days to assure there is no sensitivity to bovine collagen or lidocaine.

Two instrumental studies were involved with the FDA-approval of Bellafill. In a single-center, open-label, pilot study (n = 14 patients, 57 scars), atrophic acne scars were subjected to subcision and then the PMMA filler was injected into the scar bases. At 8 months, investigators rated 96% of atrophic acne scars had improved.[128] No adverse events were reported. In a double-blind, multicenter study of 147 patients with at least four moderate-to-severe atrophic facial acne scars, patients were randomized for an injection of Bellafill or saline, with a second injection 4 weeks later, if needed. The majority of patients in the active-treatment group and some in the control group (64% vs. 33%, respectively) achieved the primary endpoint, a 2-point improvement on the 4-point validated acne scar rating scale in ≥50% of scars at 6 months.[129] There were no significant differences in results between sexes, skin type, or age of patients. The fear of using a nonbiodegradable product has been an expressed concern by treating physicians because it represents a permanent treatment with a risk of permanent complications. Clinical trial safety data from a 5-year study as well as the pivotal acne scar study referenced above confirm the low adverse event occurrence across more than 1,500 subjects.[4]

Autologous Fat Transplantation

Autologous fat transplantation may be suitable for the treatment of severely depressed scars or scars with abnormal contours in which there is a loss of subcutaneous fat.[130] Fat is close to the ideal augmentation material in that it is cheap, readily available, and has a low incidence of side effects as it is incapable of being rejected or causing allergic reaction. However, it must be anticipated that the deformity is initially overcorrected and will need refining (see Chapter 15).[118] The technique consists of two phases: procurement of the graft and placement of the graft.[14] The grafts are placed in small aliquots in multiple tunnels to allow maximal access to blood supply. Subcision is an important step before fat transplant to ensure fibrous bands do not impede the fat injections from normalizing the contours of the skin. Most acne-scarred patients achieve maximum results about 3 months after the procedure.[23]

Autologous Fibroblast Transplantation

Azficel-T (LaViv, Fibrocell Technologies, Inc., Exton, PA) is an autologous cellular product consisting of collagen-producing fibroblast cells that are harvested from skin biopsies behind the ear. The fibroblasts from the tissue samples are cultured and allowed to multiply so they can be injected to treat appropriate dermal targets. The manufacturing process takes 11 to 22 weeks after receipt of the patient's biopsy samples. Although FDA approved in 2011 solely for improvement of the appearance of moderate-to-severe nasolabial fold wrinkles, it is commonly used off-label to treat other areas of the face, including atrophic acne and posttraumatic or surgical scars (Fig. 17-13). A randomized, double-blind, placebo-controlled clinical trial involving 99 patients was performed to compare the efficacy and safety of treatment

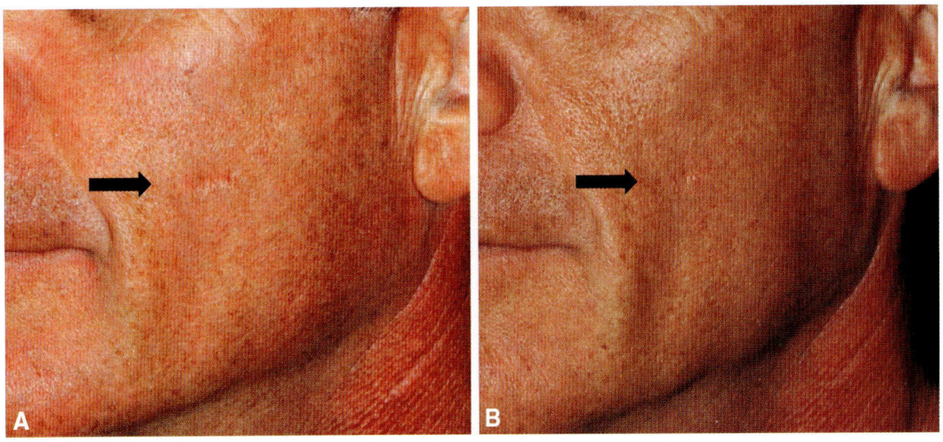

FIGURE 17-13 A 60-year-old man with left cheek atrophic scar following a cycling accident. Photos before (**A**) and 2 years following three treatments with azficel-T (LaViv) (**B**). *(Photo permission granted by Mitchel P. Goldman, MD.)*

of depressed, distensible acne scars using autologous fibroblasts. Three sessions of autologous fibroblast injection was associated with significantly greater treatment success than a vehicle control for the subject (43% vs. 18%), evaluator (59% vs. 42%), and independent photographic viewer's assessment of acne scarring 1 to 4 months after the last treatment.[131] The treatments were well tolerated, without permanent adverse effects.

A single vial of azficel-T contains approximately 18 million autologous fibroblasts in a 1.2-mL suspension, sufficient to administer 1 mL of product.[132] The recommended treatment regimen is three treatment sessions, administering up to two vials (2 mL) per session at 3-to-6-week intervals. Treatment benefit has been demonstrated for at least 9 to 12 months,[133] with anecdotal evidence of long-lasting efficacy beyond 2 years. This option comes with high expense, making it prohibitive for the majority of patients. However, similar to fat transplantation, it offers an autologous therapy for those unable or unwilling to consider a synthetic filler.

In today's increasingly cost-conscious health care market, the expense of dermal fillers may pose a substantial obstacle, especially since these products are usually combined with other procedures when treating acne scars. Even when patients are prepared to pay out of pocket, they may think the cost is prohibitively high, leading to reluctance.[4] Reaffirming the value in this kind of treatment to improve self-esteem and quality of life should be emphasized. Long-lasting or permanent dermal fillers (PLLA, PMMA, fat, fibroblasts) offer durability and longevity, and possibly a permanent solution that will not need repetitive treatments over time, reducing overall costs.

Visible papules or nodules may occur with the use of any filler, particularly PLLA, and may occur if the injection is too superficial or the volume of dilution is too low.[134] Intravascular injection of filler or compression of vascular lumens are rare adverse events, but do occur and can lead to tissue necrosis.[135] If blanching during injection or mottled pigmentation of skin is noted postinjection, a warm compress and a filler reversal, such as hyaluronidase for an HA filler, should be considered. With respect to injection of filler for acne scars, there are not typically vessels larger than 0.5 mm present in the depressed areas, making the risk of tissue necrosis less worrisome.

Innovative Therapies: Laser-Assisted Delivery, Autologous Platelet-Rich Plasma, Hair Transplantation, Epidermal Growth Factor, and Stem Cell Therapy

Over the past 20 years, there has been a revolution in the number of techniques that can be used for the treatment of postacne scarring, as highlighted thus far in the chapter. A few additional new and innovative therapies that deserve mention are laser-assisted drug delivery, autologous platelet-rich plasma, hair transplantation, epidermal growth factor, and stem cell therapy.

Laser-Assisted Delivery

Laser-assisted drug delivery is a new application for the use of fractionated lasers as a method to increase the transdermal delivery of topical medications (see Chapter 14). Waibel et al.[136] utilized the fractionated ablative CO_2 laser (UltraPulse, Lumenis, Inc., Yokneam, Israel) to treat hypertrophic scars with an immediate postlaser treatment topical application of triamcinolone acetonide suspension over the treatment site. The 15 patients had an average improvement of 2.73 on a scale of 0 to 3. The level of scar hypertrophy improved an average of 2.76 on a scale of 0 to 3, texture was improved an average of 2.84, and dyschromia was improved an average of 2.36 with one treatment. There was no rebound hypertrophy noted posttreatment. Larger additional split scar studies are needed to fully assess the safety and efficacy.

Rkein et al.[137] used an ablative fractionated CO_2 laser (UltraPulse, Lumenis Ltd., Yokneam, Israel) to treat atrophic scars with an immediate posttreatment application of PLLA. Three months postprocedure, 95% of the 19 patients had at least a 33% improvement from baseline in their atrophic scars. Split scar studies are needed to determine if the laser-assisted delivery of PLLA produces a statistically significantly improvement over ablative fractionated CO_2

laser alone. Also, the effects of PLLA typically require two to four treatments in order to obtain the desired level of neocollagenesis. A single laser-assisted delivery of PLLA may be inadequate to fully assess the potential of this application.

Autologous Platelet-Rich Plasma

Autologous platelet-rich plasma (PRP) is a relatively new modality that can be used to improve the healing of wounds created by ablative fractional resurfacing.[138–142] It has also been compared against CROSS with 100% trichloroacetic acid (TCA) and in combination with skin needling.[143,144] PRP is a highly concentrated autologous solution of plasma prepared by centrifuging a patient's own blood and has been used for various dermatologic conditions. The plasma contains four to seven times the baseline concentration of human platelets.[145] The platelets contained in a PRP specimen are purported to release numerous growth factors, including epidermal growth factor, platelet-derived growth factor, transforming growth factor β, and vascular endothelial growth factor. In turn, these growth factors are very useful to accelerate wound healing and tissue repair. A comprehensive review of PRP was published by Leo et al.[142] that explains the preparation of PRP, its components, subtypes, and range of dermatologic applications.

In separate studies, patients receiving PRP after treatment with Er:YAG-fractionated laser or CO_2-fractionated laser showed significant improvements in the overall clinical appearance of facial acne scars compared with controls, and experienced shorter durations of posttreatment edema and erythema.[139,140] The comparative efficacy and safety of intradermally injected PRP (ID-PRP) and topical PRP preparations was evaluated in another study.[141] Thirty patients were randomized into two split-face study groups. The first group received fractionated CO_2 laser (FCO_2) and ID-PRP or FCO_2 and placebo (intradermal saline). The second group received either FCO_2 and ID-PRP or FCO_2 with topical PRP. Following three monthly treatments with follow-up assessment at 6 months, both the topical and ID-PRP-treated groups had shorter recovery times and demonstrated significant improvements in clinical appearance of acne scars compared with the control group that received FCO_2 with placebo. There were no significant differences between the topical and ID-PRP treatment groups, but the topical PRP was better tolerated.[141,142] Additionally, a study by Na et al.[138] revealed topical PRP following FCO_2 to the inner arms resulted in marked reductions in posttreatment erythema, melanin index, and transepidermal water loss. Furthermore, this study was unique in that it obtained biopsies from the PRP-treated areas that revealed thicker collagen bundles than those from the control areas.[138]

Fabbrocini et al.[144] have proposed the combined use of skin needling and topical PRP. Its application on the skin immediately before the treatment with a microneedling device showed that the combined use of skin needling and PRP is more effective in improving acne scars than skin needling alone. In another study of 45 patients with atrophic acne scars randomly assigned to three equal groups, Nofal et al.[143] evaluated the efficacy and safety of ID-PRP (0.1 to 0.3 mL injected into each scar treated) versus 100% TCA CROSS versus a combined skin needling plus topical PRP. Needling was accomplished with a rolling device consisting of 192 needles, each 2 mm long, followed by topical application of 0.5 to 1.0 mL of PRP at each treated scar. Each patient received three treatment sessions at 2-week intervals. All patients completed the study, and all three groups showed statistically highly significant improvement in the degree of acne scars after treatment. There was no difference in efficacy or pain between the groups, and no major adverse effects were observed. Interestingly, this was the first study to use ID-PRP alone for treatment of acne scars in one of the groups. The results indicate ID-PRP is a new and promising modality for the treatment of atrophic acne scars with minimal risk of hyperpigmentation or scarring (Fig. 17-14). Further trials to evaluate the efficacy of ID-PRP injection alone in a larger number of patients with acne scars, and in association with other techniques such as TCA, fractional laser, needling, and subcision are suggested.

In conclusion, topically applied and injected PRP appears to improve recovery after cosmetic treatments for acne scars, and there is early evidence ID-PRP may represent a novel stand-alone intervention. The superiority of the combination of fractionated laser with PRP is clearly evident in several aspects, including the rapidity and degree of

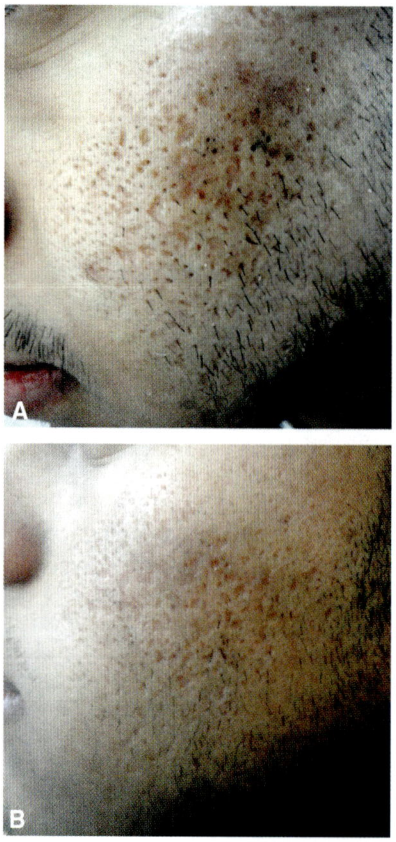

FIGURE 17-14 **Intradermal platelet-rich plasma.** A man with grade IV acne scars. **A:** Before treatment. **B:** Excellent response 2 months after the last session. *(Used with permission from Ahmad Nofal, MD, Dermatology Department, Faculty of Medicine, Zagazig University.)*

improvement of acne scars, fewer side effects, and shorter downtime.[23] With the fact that acne scars remain clinically challenging and psychologically devastating, future studies are warranted to expand on these promising benefits of PRP.

Hair Transplantation

Sarangal et al.[146] described the first successful hair transplantation into multiple large atrophic, alopecic rolling and boxcar acne scars in the beard distribution of a 24-year-old man. He underwent subcision procedures before the hair transplantation with little improvement. Because there was complete loss of hair from the scars, making them more visible as compared with the surrounding normal beard, the idea for hair transplantation was considered in an attempt to camouflage the sites. Follicular units were extracted from the submandibular and submental beard, instead of scalp, so that the texture, color, and thickness of transplanted hairs would be congruous. There was almost 80% graft uptake, making the large acne scars less visible and more aesthetically acceptable. The donor areas showed negligible scarring. It is important to ensure the patient does not have a tendency to keloid, particularly in darker skin types in this relatively high-risk site. The authors concluded that hair transplantation for acne scars in the beard area in men can be a successful, efficient, and relatively inexpensive technique that can be performed in a single setting with minimal postprocedure side effects.

Epidermal Growth Factor

In a pilot study, Seidel and Moy[9] have recently reported the efficacy of topically applied epidermal growth factor (EGF) serum in reducing the appearance of atrophic acne scars. Eight patients with Goodman and Baron grade II to IV acne scars followed a standardized regimen of twice-daily application of EGF serum to scarred areas over 12 weeks. On final self-assessment, all but one patient reported "good" to "excellent" improvement in their scars compared with baseline. The mean time at which improvement was first perceived was 7.5 weeks. Seventy-five percent of patients who received alternative treatments in prior years self-reported EGF serum to be more efficacious. At the end of the trial, 50% of patients demonstrated improvement in investigator global assessment, and 25% of patients demonstrated an improvement in Goodman and Baron grade. There were no reports of adverse reactions or side effects during the trial. The stimulatory effect that EGF has on fibroblasts likely underlies the improvements in acne scarring. Whereas resurfacing procedures rely on epidermal and dermal injury to trigger its release, direct topical application of EGF serum offers the effects of EGF without the associated discomfort and downtime. It is hypothesized that the production of new collagen from stimulated fibroblasts, which replaces the residual fragmented fibers resulting from inflammatory acne lesions, thickens the dermis and combats tissue atrophy.[9] Future studies with a larger number of patients comparing improvement between EGF serum and vehicle alone are planned.

Stem Cell Therapy

Stem cell therapy appears promising for the treatment of atrophic acne scars. The role of epidermal and adipose stem cells in contributing to homeostatic maintenance of the skin and wound repair has been well acknowledged for many years.[147,148] So much, in fact, that stem cell therapy has emerged as a promising new approach for almost every medical problem.[149] Stem cells demonstrate two defining features, namely self-renewal and multipotency, which are instrumental for renewal, regeneration, and repair.[150] In other words, stem cells have the ability to renew themselves as well as differentiate into specialized cell types.[151] This makes them particularly helpful when trying to heal or create new tissue to fill in a defect, as is present in atrophic acne scars. The traditional concept of stem cell therapy comprises the isolation of stem cells from patients, propagation and differentiation in vitro, and subsequent reinjection of autologous cells into the patient.[23] An alternate approach that could be easier includes local activation and recruitment of endogenous stem cells to the site of the defect for new tissue regeneration. An example is the topical application of an agent after laser resurfacing. This may occur in response to certain agents, still under investigation, that can promote proliferation and differentiation of stem cells.[149] With respect to wound healing, Yun et al.[148] were able to demonstrate that adipose-derived stem cells decrease the activity of mast cells and inhibit the action of transforming growth factor-β3-mediated fibroblast suppression, in addition to positively stimulating scar remodeling through greater expression of MMP-1. These actions resulted in smaller scar sizes, improved color, and better flexibility of the skin. Ongoing research should continue to shed light on the mechanisms through which stem cell therapy may help improve existing scars and the wound-healing process.

Multimodal Therapy for Acne Scars

Patients most frequently will require a multimodal approach for optimal scar treatment (see Chapter 16), as one must address scar type, color, tone, texture, tightness, and volume to improve appearance of acne scars, or scars resulting from other mechanisms such as trauma, surgery, or infection. For example, the use of a vascular laser for red scars; fillers for depressed, distensible scars; punch excision of ice pick scars; and ablative and nonablative fractional lasers for boxcar scars.[4] Figure 17-15 demonstrates the successful treatment of a skin type IV patient with active acne and acne scars utilizing a combination of laser, light sources, and topical and oral medications. Staging combination therapy must be personalized to meet a patient's individual needs, types of scars present, skin type, age, budget, timeline, risk tolerance, treatment expectations, and psychological impact. For example, for a patient without significant atrophy, a chemical peel or laser/energy-based therapy may be performed first, with fillers following if needed. If there is significant atrophy and tethering, a surgical procedure, such as subcision combined with filler may be the initial approach, followed by a resurfacing procedure. It would appear that a triple combination therapy (i.e., CROSS, subcision, and fractionated laser) is a safe and very effective approach for a variety of atrophic acne scars.[14,152] In most cases for all skin types, a dermal filler plus resurfacing will provide better results than either procedure alone.

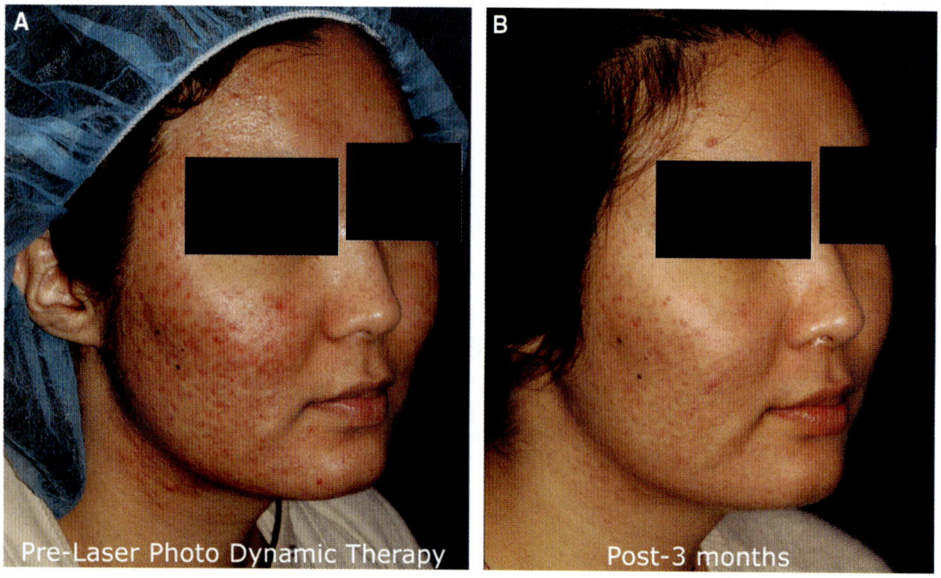

FIGURE 17-15 Combination treatment for acne scar treatment. A 22-year-old skin type IV patient with active acne and numerous erythematous and atrophic acne scars. **A:** Baseline. **B:** 3 months status-post combination PDT utilizing red and blue-light sources, PDL, and use of spironolactone and topical benzoyl peroxide. *(Photo permission granted by Sabrina Guillen Fabi, MD.)*

Striae

Striae distensae, or stretch marks, are a common disfiguring "scar" that manifests as epidermal and dermal atrophy. Although striae do not pose a health risk, they can burn, itch, and cause emotional stress due to cosmetic concerns.[153] Striae are 2.5 times more common in women and tend to occur in areas of increased fat content such as the thighs, hips, abdomen, and breasts.[154] Striae have been associated with many factors including pregnancy, growth spurts, obesity, rapid weight gain or loss, rapid muscle growth, long-term systemic or topical steroid use, prolonged adrenocorticotropic (ACTH) hormone therapy, Cushing syndrome, Marfan syndrome, and diabetes mellitus (Table 17-9).[155]

Striae evolve from an early stage, called *striae rubra*, where the lesions are characteristically flat and pink with widening, lengthening, and deepening to a purple color over time.[154] *Striae alba* is the clinical end stage, appearing as atrophic white depressed scars. Additional types of striae have been reported to include striae nigrae and striae caerulea, which are seen in darker skin types with increased melanization.[156]

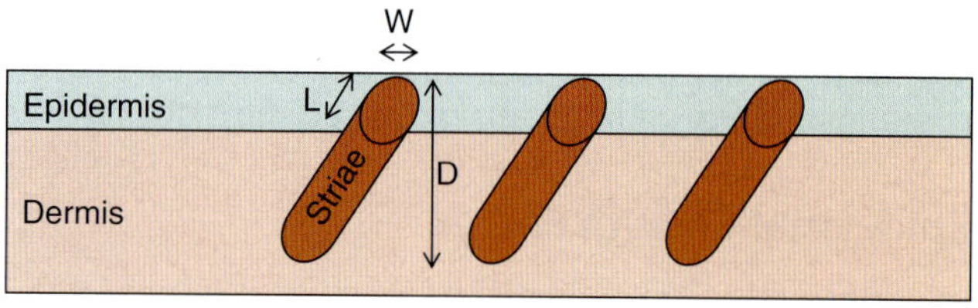

FIGURE 17-16 A three-dimensional demonstration of striae distensae. Treatment of the scar should address all three dimensions. L, length; W, width; and D, depth. *(Adapted from Sardana K. Lasers for treating striae: an emergent need for better evidence.* Indian J Dermatol Venereol Leprol. *2014;80:392–394.)*

Striae are histologically identical to atrophic scars with a flattening of the rete ridges and a loss of collagen and elastin. Collagen bands in the upper reticular dermis are stretched and aligned parallel to the surface of the skin (Fig. 17-16).[157–159]

The pathogenesis of striae is multifactorial (Table 17-10). Striae tend to appear in skin with a combination of rigid cross-linked collagen and "elastic" unlinked collagen permitting a stretch and a slight intradermal rupture. The cross-linkage of collagen is important with the stretch of the skin, and

Table 17-9 Causes of Striae Distensae

Pregnancy
Growth spurts
Obesity
Quick or excessive weight gain
Quick or excessive weight loss
Muscle hypertrophy
Genetic factors
Diabetes mellitus
Long-term systemic or topical steroid use
Prolonged adrenocorticotrophic (ACTH) hormone therapy

From Chang AL, Agredano YZ, Kimball AB. Risk factors associated with striae gravidarum. *J Am Acad Dermatol.* 2004;51:881–885.

Table 17-10 Pathogenesis of Striae Distensae

Mechanical stretching of the skin
Normal growth
Increased steroid hormones (Cushing syndrome), steroid therapy has a catabolic effect on fibroblasts[164]
Infection with a striatoxin[165]
Immunosuppressive states (HIV, pregnancy-induced hypertension, tuberculosis, typhoid)[161]
Chronic Liver disease
Genetic factors–Ehlers–Danlos syndrome[166], Marfan syndrome[167], pseudoxanthoma elasticum[168]

From Kogoj[165], Stevanovic[164], Elsaie et al.[161], Castrow and Ritche[166], Pinkus et al.[167], Neldner[168].

the unlinked collagen is important for the elasticity of the skin. A combination of these factors has been postulated to be involved with the development of striae.[160] Mechanical stretching of the skin may result in a higher predictability of developing striae.[161] Normal growth in adolescence[162] is associated with striae owing to rapid growth and a simulation of the hypothalamic–pituitary–adrenal axis.[163] An increase in steroid hormones such as in Cushing syndrome or topical or systemic steroid therapy can result in catabolic effects on fibroblasts leading to striae[164] Kogoj et al.[161] speculated that infections leading to the release of striatoxin can damage dermal tissues resulting in striae, but no specific microbial agent was identified.[165] Various immunosuppressive states such as infections with HIV, tuberculosis, and typhoid can also be associated with striae.

A multitude of genetic factors are likely involved with the development of striae. Ehlers–Danlos syndrome,[166] Marfan syndrome,[167] and pseudoxanthoma elasticum (PXE)[168] can affect collagen and elastin properties and ultimately result in striae. Striae found in unusual areas (other than the buttock, thigh, breast, or hip) are found to be more prominent in patients with Marfan syndrome (MS) and may be a good diagnostic criterion.[169] Additionally, the presence of striae atrophicae has been found to be an external predictive marker for the risk of aortic dissection in MS.[170]

Abnormal fibroblastic function may also lead to the development of striae. Lee et al.[159] found an altered fibroblast metabolism in patients with striae and a decreased expression of collagen, elastin, and fibronectin genes. It has also been proposed that certain patients are predisposed to the development of striae through a dormant phenotype of dermal fibroblasts. Fibroblasts in lesional and nonlesional skin in patients with striae are found to have slower growth, migration, and proliferation compared with patients without striae. Additionally, less elastin, collagen 1, fibrillin 1, and fibronectin are also seen in patients with striae.[171]

Striae may also be a marker for internal disease. Kurt et al.[172] completed a study of 488 women who had undergone gynecologic surgery and divided them into symptomatic pelvic organ prolapse (POP) and nonsymptomatic POP groups. The presence and number of striae increased the risk of POP by 1.29-fold and 1.19-fold, respectively.

Striae on the breast may occur after cosmetic augmentation because of rapid expansion and stretching of the skin in genetically predisposed patients. A retrospective study evaluating 549 patients with breast augmentation found a 3.1% incidence of breast striae postaugmentation. The risk of striae after breast augmentation was 14.38 times more likely in those who were nulliparous, 9.24 times more likely if their last menstrual period was >14 days before surgery, 6.11 times more likely with a history of striae, and 3.3 times more likely if they were younger than 25 years of age.[173] Timing breast augmentation around the menstrual cycle may thus minimize the risk of developing breast striae. Additionally, women with multiple risk factors for the development of striae should be counseled on their elevated risk.

Treatment of Striae

Multiple treatment modalities for striae have been published, with no single ideal therapy. Treatment results have been most favorable in earlier stages, especially with erythematous striae.[154] There are two main targets of striae treatment. The first is the increased vascularity, and the second is the depressed scar itself.[174] Both aspects may require treatment to obtain a cosmetically appealing result.

Topical Treatment

Multiple topical treatments have been studied in an attempt to prevent striae, with none demonstrating uniform efficacy (Table 17-11). Bitter almond oil combined with massage helped to decrease the incidence of striae in one study,[175] though cocoa butter has not been shown to prevent striae.[176] Onion extract cream with *Centella asiatica* and HA has been shown to improve the overall appearance, texture, color, and softness compared with untreated skin.[177]

The topical treatment of striae has been shown to improve clinical appearance over time but does not cause complete resolution. Ash et al.[178] evaluated 10 skin type I to V patients with striae alba, comparing topical 20% glycolic acid with 0.05% tretinoin to 20% glycolic acid and 10% L-ascorbic acid daily for 12 weeks. Both treatments were considered to be safe and effective, increasing epidermal thickness and improving the appearance of striae. The 20% glycolic acid and 0.05% tretinoin combination was found to increase elastin content within striae.

Topical tretinoin has been shown to restore collagen I and antagonize the induction of matrix-degrading enzymes caused by UV radiation or stretching of the skin.[179,180] Tretinoin induces a multitude of transcriptional changes in more than 93 genes, resulting in numerous clinical effects.[181] Kang et al.[182] found a significant improvement of striae rubra after 6 months of daily tretinoin 0.1% cream. Conversely, Pribanich et al.[183] found no improvement of striae rubra or alba with a low-dose 0.025% tretinoin after 8 months of daily use. The lower dose of tretinoin decreased the topical irritation but also decreased efficacy. Tretinoin can improve the appearance of striae rubra but has not been shown to improve striae alba.[184]

Dermabrasion

Dermabrasion is a procedure wherein the top layers of the skin are mechanically abraded, allowing new skin to replace the older damaged skin. A comparison of tretinoin 0.05% applied daily compared with a superficial localized dermabrasion revealed similar results in striae improvement.

Table 17-11 Topical Treatments for Striae

Tretinoin
Glycolic acid
Ascorbic acid
5-Aminolevulinic acid (5-ALA)
Methylaminolevulinate (MAL)
Bitter almond oil
Cocoa butter
Onion extract cream with *Centella asiatica* and hyaluronic acid (HA)

From Griffiths et al.,[179] Fisher et al.,[180] Kang,[184] Pribanich et al.,[183] Hexsel et al.,[185] Ash et al.,[178] Mendoza-Garcia et al.,[191] Timur Tashan and Kafkasli,[175] Osman et al.,[176] Draelos et al.,[177].

However, dermabrasion was found to have fewer side effects and better patient adherence.[185] Tretinoin requires nightly application and compliance can decrease due to symptoms of irritation and erythema. Dermabrasion as a single procedure eliminates the variability of compliance. Additional studies are needed to fully determine the superior treatment.

Needling Therapy

Needling therapy was originally developed for transdermal drug delivery but was later found to improve the appearance of scars through the induction of neocollagenesis.[186] Park et al.[187] completed a study that evaluated 16 Korean patients with striae rubra and alba who received three disk microneedle therapy (DTS roller, DTS-MG, Inc., Seoul, Korea) at 4-week intervals. In all, 43.8% (7/16) of the patients showed excellent improvement and 56.2% (9/16) patients had minimal to moderate improvement. Side effects included erythema, mild pain, and spotty bleeding that were reported as tolerable. Overall, microneedling is an easy-to-perform option that is considered to be safe and effective in the treatment of striae.[188]

Intense-Pulsed Light

IPL is a nonlaser, nonablative, noncoherent filtered flashlamp that can emit broadband visible light between 515 and 1,200 nm. Various cutoff filters can be placed to eliminate light below a desired wavelength. Hernandez-Perez et al.[189] evaluated the response of striae alba in 15 women of skin types III–IV to five IPL treatment sessions using a 645-nm cutoff filter (VascuLight Plus, Lumenis, Yoknaem, Israel) at 2-week intervals. The overall number and size of the stretch marks improved along with the general appearance. Shokeir et al.[190] compared the 656-nm cutoff filter IPL (Medical Bio Care, Gothenburg, Sweden) to the 585-nm PDL (Cynosure, Chelmsford, MA) in the treatment of striae rubra and alba in skin types III and IV. Striae rubra responded better than striae alba. The PDL had a larger enhancement of collagen I compared with the IPL. However, both the PDL and IPL enhanced collagen stimulation. Caution is warranted with the use of IPL in skin types V and VI, with the risk of a minimal clinical effects and development of dyspigmentation.

Photodynamic Therapy

Photodynamic therapy (PDT) was originally FDA approved for the treatment of actinic keratosis, but it has been shown to induce a reorganization of the matrix in both hypertrophic and keloidal scars. PDT involves the placement of 5-aminolevulinic acid (ALA) or methylaminolevulinate (MAL) onto a treatment area for 1 to 24 hours before a red- or blue-light treatment. ALA and MAL are transformed into porphyrins in the skin and accumulate in sebaceous glands, epidermal, and neoplastic cells. Mendoza-Garcia et al.[191] applied ALA or MAL in combination with the red light at 635 nm to treat striae alba. Matrix metalloproteinase 3 (MMP-3) and tropoelastin (ELN) were both increased post PDT compared with normal skin in an ex vivo study. There was no statistical difference between 5-ALA- and MAL-treated skin. Additional studies are needed to fully evaluate the effectiveness of PDT in the treatment of striae.

Nonablative Laser

The targeted narrow-band UVB laser has proven to be successful in the treatment of various leukodermas including vitiligo, hypopigmented scars, and striae alba. Approximately 80% improvement in hypopigmentation associated with striae alba has been noted with use of the 308-nm Excimer laser (XeCl Excimer, Xtrac PhotoMedex, Radnor, PA) with an average of 8.4 treatments.[192] The Excimer laser and a similar narrow-band UVB 311 to 313-nm laser (ReLume, Lumenis, Santa Clara, CA) were both shown to increase melanocyte number and melanin content in leukodermic striae. A temporary increase in collagen was noted after the laser treatment, but was not permanent.[193]

The PDL is most effective for treating striae rubra at low energy densities. Striae alba, however, has not been successfully treated with the PDL because of the lack of chromophore.[194,195] Caution should be used in skin types V and VI because of the high risk of postinflammatory pigmentation with minimal clinical effects.[196] The 10-mm spot size has been associated with greater improvements than the 5- and 7-mm spot sizes, likely because of a relative increase in photon penetration with the larger spot size.

The 1,064-nm Nd:YAG is a nonablative laser targeting water as well as oxygenated and deoxygenated hemoglobin. Goldman et al.[197] examined 22 patients of skin type II to VI with striae rubra treated with the 1,064-nm long-pulsed Nd:YAG laser (Smartepil, DERA, Firenze, Italy) and found excellent improvement in 55% on patient assessment and excellent improvement in 40% on physician assessment. Gungor et al.[198] examined 20 patients with skin type II to V with striae alba and found histologic improvement of the striae but without associated clinical improvement. The 1,064-nm laser appears to be best for treating early striae rubra.

The 1,450-nm diode is a nonablative laser with water as its chromophore target. Tay et al.[199] treated 11 Asian patients of skin types III, V, and VI with striae rubra and alba with the 1,450-nm diode laser (Smoothbeam, Candela Corp, Wayland, MA). PIH was significant, and no clinical improvement of the striae was noted. The 1,450-nm diode laser is not recommended in darker skin types, and additional studies are needed to examine the effectiveness in lighter skin types.

The 1,320-nm laser is also a nonablative laser with water as its chromophore target. Goldman et al.[200] utilized the 1,320-nm CoolTouch II laser (Cool Touch Inc.; Roseville, CA) to treat 15 patients with striae rubra and alba in skin types I to IV. After four monthly treatments, 2/15 had no improvement, 5/15 had <25% improvement, and 8/15 had a 25%-to-50% improvement, with an average improvement of 30% (Figs. 17-17 and 17-18). The improvement was not related to the age of the striae, and the lesions continued to improve months after the treatment. All of the patients experienced minimal erythema that resolved within an hour, 4/15 had erythematous papules that resolved within 4 days, and 2/15 had vesicles with no scarring. Additional studies are needed to find the optimal wavelength laser for the treatment of striae.

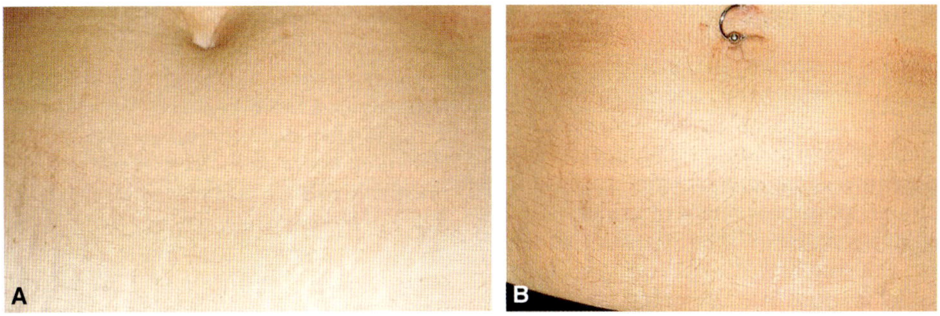

FIGURE 17-17 **A:** Striae alba on the abdomen before treatment. **B:** A 50% improvement of the striae alba was noted after four treatments with the CoolTouch 1,320-nm laser *(From Goldman MP, Rostan EF: Treatment of striae distensae with a 1320 nm dynamic cooling laser. J Eur Acad Dermatol Venereol. 2000;14(suppl 1):52).*

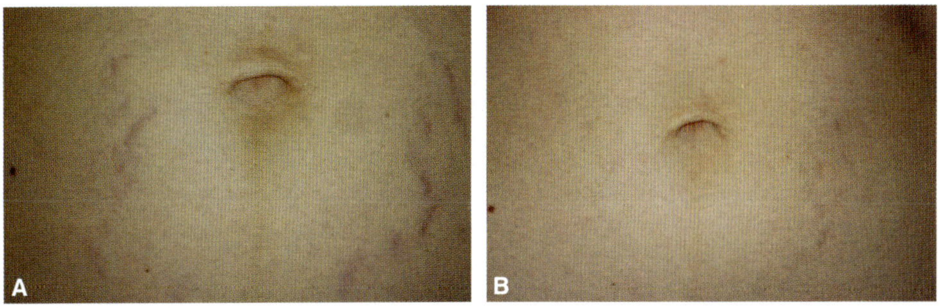

FIGURE 17-18 **A:** Striae rubra before treatment. **B:** Striae rubra after four monthly treatments with the CoolTouch 1,320-nm laser at a 5-month postprocedure follow-up. *(From Goldman MP, Rostan EF. Treatment of striae distensae with a 1320 nm dynamic cooling laser. J Eur Acad Dermatol Venereol. 2000;14(suppl 1):52.)*

Ablative Laser

The 10,600-nm CO_2 laser in full-field mode completely ablates the epidermis and superficial dermis, with tissue water as its target chromophore. Hypopigmentation, PIH, and a visible line of demarcation of treated and untreated skin are the main potential side effects. Nouri et al.[201] treated four patients with skin type IV–VI with striae alba with the nonfractionated CO_2 laser (Coherent, Santa Clara, CA) and PDL (Cynosure, Bedford, MA). The short-pulsed CO_2 laser test sites showed persistent erythema in skin types IV and V and PIH with minimal striae alba improvement. The PDL demonstrated no improvement in striae alba and induced PIH in type VI skin.

Nonablative Fractionated Laser

Fractionated lasers produce small columns of thermal damage in the skin to induce neocollagenesis, most commonly with water as the target chromophore. Angelis et al.[202] completed a study evaluating 51 patients with striae rubra and alba treated with the 1,540-nm Er:glass fractionated nonablative laser (Lux1540, Palomar Medical Technologies, Inc., Burlington, MA) and found a 50%-to-75% improvement at least 3 months after two to four treatments. Malekzad et al.[203] completed a study of 10 patients with striae alba treated with the 1,540-nm fractionated nonablative laser (Star Lux 500, Palomar Medical Technologies, Inc., Burlington, MA) and found that 3 months after the fourth monthly treatment a noticeable improvement was found compared with baseline.

Bak et al.[204] treated 22 skin type IV Asian patients with striae rubra and alba with the 1,500-nm Fraxel SR fractionated nonablative laser (Fraxel, Solta Medical Inc., Hayward, CA). In all, 27% (6/22) had good to excellent clinical improvement and 63% (16/22) showed various degrees of improvement at 1 month after a single treatment. The full remodeling process with neocollagenesis may not have fully developed at the 1-month follow-up, warranting additional studies to examine the long-term effects.

Additionally, Scotland et al.[205] examined 20 patients with striae rubra and alba in skin types I–IV treated with the 1,550-nm erbium-doped fiber-fractionated nonablative laser (Fraxel Re:Store, Solta Medical Inc., Hayward, CA). After six treatments at 2-to-3-week intervals, overall striae improvement was noted in 26% to 50% of the patients 3 months after the third treatment, with texture having the greatest level of improvement. Overall, the 1,550- and 1,500-nm lasers appear to be effective in improving texture in patients with striae alba without significant side effects.

Clementoni et al.[206] utilized the 1,565-nm ResurFX (Lumenis, Inc., Yokneam, Israel) laser in the treatment of 12 patients with striae rubra and alba and found a 51%-to-75% overall improvement, a 91.7% volume of depression improvement, and an 83.3% color improvement. The nonablative fractionated 1,500-, 1,540-, 1,550-, and 1,565-nm lasers appear to improve the appearance of striae alba but additional comparative studies are needed.

Ablative Fractionated Lasers

The rejuvenating effects of ablative fractionated lasers have been well documented. However, their use for striae is still under examination. The 2,940-nm Er:YAG-fractionated ablative laser is commonly used to improve the appearance of photodamaged skin. However, studies on striae are lacking. Gauglitz et al.[207] found an improvement of axillary striae rubra with the combination of the PDL (Syneron Candela, Irvine, CA) and the 2,940-nm Er:YAG-fractionated ablative laser (Sciton Inc., Palo Alto, CA). Additional studies are needed to examine the effect of the Er:YAG in striae alba because the PDL laser alone has been shown to improve striae rubra.

The fractionated 10,600-nm CO_2 laser has also been studied in treating striae. Lee et al.[208] treated 77 patients with striae alba with a fractionated CO_2 laser (UltraPulse DeepFX, Lumenis, Inc. Yokneam, Israel). Three months after a single treatment, the results were graded on a scale of 1 to 4 with 7.4% (2/27) at a grade IV improvement, 51.9% (14/27) at grade III, 33.3% (9/27) at grade II, and 7.4% (2/27) at grade I improvement. Naeini et al.[209] examined 88 patients with striae alba with a split study comparing the fractionated ablative CO_2 laser and the nonablative PDL. The combination of the CO_2 laser and PDL had a better improvement than either treatment alone. A combination of therapies may provide the largest benefit by targeting different aspects of the striae. Overall, the fractionated ablative CO_2 laser can clinically improve striae, but it has the potential adverse effect of prolonged hyperpigmentation. Table 17-12 reviews the reported laser and light-based treatments for striae.

Radiofrequency Devices

Radiofrequency (RF) energy devices provide high-frequency alternating electrical currents that heat dermal tissue, resulting in neocollagenesis, neoelastogenesis, and skin tightening. RF devices can be used in all skin types and allow for different depths of penetration to target various tissues. Several studies have found an improvement of both striae rubra and alba with the use of monopolar and tripolar RF (Table 17-13).

Radiofrequency can now be subclassified into fractionated, nonfractionated, ablative, and nonablative. Additionally, minimally ablative radiofrequency devices using microneedles that can be noninsulated (heat over the entire length of the needle) or insulated (heating at the tip of the needle) have been developed.[210] Ryu et al.[211] found a combination of the fractionated CO_2 laser (CICU2, ilooda, Suwon, South Korea) and a noninsulated fractionated microneedle RF device (Secret, ilooda) is a safe and effective treatment of striae rubra and alba. Thirty patients were treated with the fractionated CO_2 laser alone, the microneedle RF alone, or a combination. Examined with a global improvement scale of 1 to 4 (1 = 0% to 30%, 2 = 30% to 50%, 3 = 51% to 80%, 4 = >81% improvement), there was an improvement of 2.2 points in the fractionated CO_2 laser group, an improvement of 1.8 points with the microneedle RF device, and an improvement of 3.4 points in the combination group. Additional studies are needed to fully delineate which device is more beneficial and if increasing the number of treatments increases improvement.

Nonablative nonfractionated RF devices have also been studied for the treatment of striae. Dover et al.[212] found an improvement in length and width of striae in 14/16 patients who had been treated six times with a bipolar RF device (Venus Freeze, Venus Concept, Toronto, Ontario, Canada). Manusakia et al.[213] reported that 6 weeks post radiofrequency (TriPollar, Pollogen Ltd., Tel Aviv, Israel) treatment of striae, 23% (4/17) were satisfied and 65% (11/17) were very satisfied. Suh et al.[214] combined the insulated monopolar Thermage (Thermage, ThermaCool TC, Thermage Inc., Hayward, CA) with the PDL and found 89.2% of patients had a “good” to “very good” overall improvement, and 59.4% of patients had “good” and “very good” elasticity improvement. A combination of treatment modalities may provide enhanced efficacy in the treatment of striae.

Table 17-12 Laser and Light-Based Treatment of Striae

Laser/Light Treatment	Wavelength (nm)	Chromophore Target	Ablative (A) vs. Nonablative (NA)	Fractionated (F) vs. Nonfractionated (NF)
Excimer	308	Protein	NA	NF
UVB laser	311–313	Protein	NA	NF
Red light PDT	635	Blood	NA	NF
PDL	585	Blood	NA	NF
IPL (nonlaser)	515–1,200	Blood	NA	NF
Nd:YAG long pulsed	1064	Water	NA	NF
CoolTouch	1,320	Water	NA	NF
Diode	1,450	Water	NA	NF
Erbium: glass	1,540	Water	NA	F
ResurFX	1,565	Water	NA	F
Er:YAG	2,940	Water	A	F
CO_2 short pulsed	10,600	Water	A	NF
CO_2	10,600	Water	A	F

From Goldberg et al.,[192,193] Hernandez-Perez et al.,[189] Shokeir et al.,[190] Nehal et al.,[194] Jimenez et al.,[196] McDaniel et al.,[195] Goldman et al.,[197] Gungor et al.,[198] Tay et al.,[199] Alves et al. 2015,[218] Malekzad et al.,[203] Angelis et al.,[202] Tretti Clementon et al.,[206] Gauglitz et al.,[207] Bak et al.,[204] Stotland et al.,[205] Lee et al.,[208] Naeini et al.,[209] Nouri et al.,[201] Mendoza-Garcia et al.,[191] Goldman et al.[200]

Table 17-13 Radiofrequency Treatment of Striae

Radiofrequency Device	Polarity	Application	Ablative (A) vs. Nonablative (NA)	Fractionated (F) vs. Nonfractionated (NF)
TriPollar (Apollo, Pollogen Ltd., Tel Aviv, Israel)[213]	Tripolar	Topical noninvasive	NA	NF
Venus Freeze[212]	Bipolar	Topical noninvasive	NA	NF
Thermage[214]	Unipolar	Topical noninvasive	NA	NF
Microneedle RF (Secret; ilooda)[211]	Unipolar	Fractionated grid needle pattern	A	F
Pixel Roller; In-motion tip[216]	Unipolar	Fractionated grid needle pattern	A	F

ThermiTight (Thermi, Irving, TX) is a monopolar RF device that is used percutaneously to produce a slow heating of the tissues with resultant skin tightening. ThermiTight has not been studied as a treatment for striae but is a possible future treatment to decrease the three-dimensional aspect of these scars.[215]

Radiofrequency and Ultrasound-Assisted Drug Delivery

Issa et al.[216] demonstrated the improvement of striae alba with the combination of fractionated ablative radiofrequency (Pixel Roller, in-motion tip) and acoustic pressure ultrasound (Legao System—Alma Lasers Ltd.) with the delivery of retinoic acid 0.05%. Radiofrequency treatment alone did not result in overall improvement of striae. Laser-assisted drug delivery is another approach to combined treatments that may prove more effective than either treatment alone.

Striae—Conclusion

Striae distensae is a difficult entity to treat on the basis of the 3-dimentional aspect of the scar, the varying pathogenesis, and limitations of light-based therapies for darker skin types. Currently, a good treatment outcome is considered to be an improvement in the clinical appearance but not a complete resolution. The PDL laser has a good efficacy for striae rubra but is not effective for striae alba, and it is not recommended in darker skin types. Fractionated laser therapy appears to have the largest improvement in striae alba and is safe in all skin types. Algorithms with a combination of treatments are likely going to be the mainstay of treatment in the future.

Yet another approach to treatment may be the reseeding of striae with autologous fibroblasts injected into the dermal atrophic scar. LAVIV (Fibrocell Science, Inc., Exton, PA), as previously mentioned in the acne scar section, is an FDA-approved treatment for improving volume loss in the nasolabial fold. Autologous fibroblast implantation has also been found to improve the appearance of atrophic acne scars.[217] It is proposed that autologous implantation into atrophic striae followed by fibroblastic stimulation through the use of transepidermal growth factors and/or nonablative fractionated or confluent lasers may provide optimal improvement.

Summary

None of the currently available treatments has emerged as first-line to achieve complete resolution of atrophic acne scars or striae, but with each year new medical, injectable, surgical and device-based therapies—used alone or in combination—are reported in this pursuit. The efficacy of combined regimens ("mega-combinations") is gaining popularity and is likely the future of treating these conditions to achieve optimal cosmesis. Whether treating acne scars or striae, patient tolerance is an undeniably important component of treatment satisfaction. Guidelines are necessary, and are constantly evolving, to quantify the benefits, to establish the duration of effects, to review cost-effectiveness, and to evaluate the psychological improvement and quality of life for patients using the various treatment modalities.

REFERENCES

1. Fitzpatrick RE. Treatment of scars. In: Goldman MP, ed. *Lasers and Energy Devices for the Skin*. 2nd ed. Boca Raton, FL: CRC Press; 2013.
2. Tsao SS, Dover JS, Arndt KA, et al. Scar management: keloid, hypertrophic, atrophic, and acne scars. *Semin Cutan Med Surg*. 2002;21:46–75.
3. Alster TS, Railan D. Laser scar revision. In: Goldman MP, ed. *Cutaneous and Cosmetic Laser Surgery*. Philadelphia, PA: Mosby Elsevier; 2006.
4. Werschler WP, Herdener RS, Ross EV, et al. Treating acne scars: what's new? Consensus for the experts. *J Clin Aesthet Dermatol*. 2015;8(8):s2–S8.
5. Chandrashekar BS, Varsha DV, Vasanth DV, et al. Safety of performing invasive acne scar treatment and laser hair removal in patients on oral isotretinoin: a retrospective study of 110 patients. *Int J Dermatol*. 2014;53(10):1281–1285.
6. Yoon JH, Park EJ, Kwon IH, et al. Concomitant use of an infrared fractional laser with low-dose isotretinoin for the treatment of acne and acne scars. *J Dermatolog Treat*. 2014;25(2):142–146.
7. Patel L, McGrouther D, Chakrabarty K. Evaluating evidence for atrophic scarring treatment modalities. *J R Soc Med*. 2014;5(9):1–13.
8. Levy LL, Zeichner JA. Management of acne scarring. Part II: a comparative review of non-laser based, minimally invasive approaches. *Am J Clin Dermatol*. 2012;13(5):331–340.
9. Seidel R, Moy RL. Improvement in atrophic acne scars using topical synthetic epidermal growth factor (EGF) serum: a pilot study. *J Drugs Dermatol*. 2015;14(9):1005–1010.
10. Sobanko JF, Alster TS. Management of Acne Scarring, Part I: a comparative review of laser surgical approaches. *Am J Clin Dermatol*. 2012;13(5):319–330.
11. Kang S, Cho S, Chung JH, et al. Inflammation and extracellular matrix degradation mediated by activated transcription factors nuclear factor-kappaB and activator protein-1 in inflammatory acne lesions in vivo. *Am J Pathol*. 2005;166:1691–1699.
12. Holland DB, Jeremy AH, Roberts SG, et al. Inflammation in acne scarring: a comparison of the responses in lesions from patients prone and not prone to scar. *Br J Dermatol*. 2004;150(1): 73–81.

13. Fife D. Practical evaluation and management of atrophic acne scars: tips for the general dermatologist. *J Clin Aesthet Dermatol.* 2011;4:50–57.
14. Fabbrocini G, Annunziata MC, D'Arco V, et al. Acne scars: pathogenesis, classification and treatment. *Dermatol Res Pract.* 2010;2010:893080.
15. Layton AM, Henderson CA, Cunliffe WJ. A clinic evaluation of acne scarring and its incidence. *Clin Exp Dermatol.* 1994;41(4):577–580.
16. Cunliffe WJ, Gould DJ. Prevalence of facial acne vulgaris in late adolescence and in adults. *Br Med J.* 1979;1:1109–1110.
17. Johnson MT, Roberts J. *Skin Conditions and Related Need for Medical Care Among Persons 1–74 Years, United States, 1971–1974* (series 11, no. 212). Washington, DC: US Department of Health, Education and Welfare, Vital and Health Statistics; 1978.
18. Goulden V, Stable GI, Cunliffe WJ. Prevalence of facial acne in adults. *J Am Acad Dermatol.* 1999;41:577–580.
19. Cunliffe WJ. Unemployment and acne. *Br J Dermatol.* 1986;115:386.
20. Fried RG, Werschler P, Berson D, et al. The psychosocial impact of post-acne scarring. *Dermatologist.* 2015;23(9):24–29.
21. Rumsey N, Clarke A, White P. Exploring the psychosocial concerns of outpatients with disfiguring conditions. *J Wound Care.* 2003;12:247–252.
22. Jacob CI, Dover JS, Kaminer MS. Acne scarring: a classification system and review of treatment options. *J Am Acad Dermatol.* 2001;45:109–117.
23. Gozali MV, Zhou B, Luo D. Effective treatments of atrophic acne scars. *J Clin Aesth Dermatol.* 2015;8(5):33–40.
24. O'Daniel GT. Multimodal management of atrophic acne scarring in the aging face. *Aesthetic Plast Surg.* 2011;35:1143–1150.
25. Goodman, GJ. Postacne scarring: a review of its pathophysiology and treatment. *Dermatol Surg.* 2000;26(9):857–871.
26. Goodman, GJ. Management of post-acne scarring: what are the options for treatment? *Am J Clin Dermatol.* 2000;1(1):3–17.
27. Goodman, GJ. Post-acne scarring: a short review of its pathophysiology. *Austral J Derm.* 2001;42:84–90.
28. Alexis AF. Acne vulgaris in skin of color: understanding nuances and optimizing treatment outcomes. *J Drugs Dermatol.* 2014;13(6):s61–s65.
29. Goodman GJ, Baron JA. Post acne scarring: a qualitative global scarring grading system. *Dermatol Surg.* 2006;32(12):1458–1466.
30. Goodman GJ, Baron JA. Post acne scarring: a quantitative global scarring grading system. *J Cosmet Dermatol.* 2006;5(1):48–52.
31. Rivera A. Acne scarring: a review and current treatment modalities. *J Am Acad Dermatol.* 2008;59:659–676.
32. Goodman GJ, Baron JA. The management of post acne scarring. *Dermatol Surg.* 2007;33:1175–1188.
33. Goodman G. Post acne scarring: a review. *J Cosmet Laser Ther.* 2003;5:77–95.
34. Schiltz JR, Lanigan J, Nabial W, et al. Retinoic acid induces cyclic changes in epidermal thickness and dermal collagen and glycosaminoglycan biosynthesis rates. *J Invest Dermatol.* 1986;87(5):663–667.
35. Varani J, Perone P, Griffiths CE, et al. All-trans retinoic acid (RA) stimulates events in organ-cultured human skin that underlie repair: adult skin from sun-protected and sun-exposed sites responds in an identical manner to RA while neonatal foreskin responds differently. *J Clin Invest.* 1994;94(5):1747–1756.
36. Harris DW, Buckley CC, Ostlere LS, et al. Topical retinoic acid in the treatment of fine acne scarring. *Br J Dermatol.* 1991;125(1):81–82.
37. Dhote V, Bhatnagar, Mishra PK, et al. Iontophoresis: a potential emergence of a transdermal drug delivery system. *Sci Pharm.* 2012;80:1–28.
38. Schmidt JB, Binder M, Macheiner W, et al. New treatment of atrophic acne scars by iontophoresis with estriol and tretinoin. *Int J Dermatol.* 1995;34(1):53–57.
39. Schmidt JB, Donath P, Hannes J, et al. Tretinoin-iontophoresis in atrophic acne scars. *Int J Dermatol.* 1999;38(2):149–153.
40. Fabbrocini G, De Vita V, Cozzolino A, et al. The management of atrophic acne scars: overview and new tools. *J Clin Exp Dermatol Res.* 2012;s5:1–7.
41. Mackee GM, Karp FL. The treatment of post-acne scars with phenol. *Br J Dermatol.* 1952;64(12):456–459.
42. Collins PS. Trichloroacetic acid peels revisited. *J Dermatol Surg Oncol.* 1989;15(9):933–940.
43. Grimes PE. Management of hyperpigmentation in darker racial ethnic groups. *Semin Cutan Med Surg.* 2009;28(2):77–85.
44. Clark E, Scerri L. Superficial and medium-depth chemical peels. *J Clin Dermatol.* 2008;26:209–218.
45. Landau M. Chemical peels. *Clin Dermatol.* 2007;26:200–208.
46. Starling J, Karimpour DJ. Nonlaser superficial resurfacing techniques: superficial chemical peel and microdermabrasion. In: Tosti A, ed. *Evidence-Based Procedural Dermatology.* New York, NY: Springer; 2012:301–316.
47. Bernstein EF, Lee J, Brown DB, et al. Glycolic acid treatment increases type 1 collagen mRNA and hyaluronic acid content of human skin. *Dermatol Surg.* 2001;27(5):429–433.
48. Brody HJ. Variations and comparisons in medium-depth chemical peeling. *J Dermatol Surg Oncol.* 1989;15(9):953–963.
49. Fabbrocini G, Cacciapuoti S, Fardella N, et al. CROSS technique: chemical reconstruction of skin scar method. *Dermatol Ther.* 2008;21:S29–S32.
50. Fife D, Zachary CB. Combining techniques for treating acne scars. *Curr Dermatol Rep.* 2012;1:82–88.
51. Khunger N. Facial peels. In: Giuseppe MASaAD, ed. *Cosmetic Surgery.* Berlin: Springer; 2013:147–166.
52. Lee JB, Chung WG, Kwahck H, et al. Focal treatment of acne scars with trichloroacetic acid: chemical reconstruction of skin scars method. *Dermatol Surg.* 2002;28:1017–1021.
53. Barikbin B, Saadat N, Akbari Z, et al. Focal high-concentration trichloroacetic acid peeling for treatment of atrophic facial chickenpox scars: an open-label study. *Dermatol Surg.* 2012;38:1662–1667.
54. Leheta T, El Tawdy A, Abdel Hay R, et al. Percutaneous collagen induction versus full-concentration trichloroacetic acid in the treatment of atrophic acne scars. *Dermatol Surg.* 2011;37:207–216.
55. Al-Waiz MM, Al-Sharqi AI. Medium-depth chemical peels in the treatment of acne scars in dark-skinned individual. *Dermatol Surg.* 2002;28(11):383–387.
56. Yug A, Lane JE, Howard MS, et al. Histologic study of depressed acne scars treated with serial high-concentration (95%) trichloroacetic acid. *Dermatol Surg.* 2006;32(8):985–990; discussion 990.
57. Khunger N, Bhardwaj D, Khunger M. Evaluation of CROSS technique with 100% TCA in the management of ice pick acne scars in darker skin types. *J Cosmet Dermatol.* 2011;10:51–57.
58. Orentreich D, Orentreich N. Acne scar revision update. *Dermatol Clin.* 1987;5:359–368.
59. Frank W. Therapeutic dermabrasion: back to the future. *Arch Dermatol.* 1994;130(9):1187–1189.
60. Fernandes M, Pinheiro NM, Crema VO, et al. Effects of microdermabrasion on skin rejuvenation. *J Cosmet Laser Ther.* 2014;16:26–31.
61. Shpall R, Beddingfield III FC, Watson D, et al. Microdermabrasion: a review. *Facial Plast Surg.* 2004;20(1):47–50.
62. Roenigk HH Jr. Dermabrasion: state of the art. *J Dermatol Surg Oncol.* 1985;11:306–314.
63. Katz BE, MacFarlane DF. Atypical facial scarring after isotretinoin therapy in a patient with previous dermabrasion. *J Am Acad Dermatol.* 1994;30:852–853.
64. Bagatin E, dos Santos Guadanhim LR, Yarak S, et al. Dermabrasion for acne scars during treatment with oral isotretinoin. *Dermatol Surg.* 2010;36(4):483–489.
65. Goodman GJ. Treating scars: addressing surface, volume, and movement to optimize results. Part 1: mild grades of scarring. *Dermatol Surg.* 2012;38:1302–1309.
66. Dogra S, Yadav S, Sarangal R. Microneedling for acne scars in Asian skin types: an effective low cost treatment modality. *J Cosmet Dermatol.* 2014;13(3):180–187.
67. Orentreich D, Orentreich N. Subcutaneous incisionless (subcision) surgery for the correction of depressed scars and wrinkles. *Dermatol Surg.* 1995;21:543–549.
68. Goodman GJ. Treating Scars: addressing surface, volume, and movement to expedite optimal results. Part 2: more-severe grades of scarring. *Dermatol Surg.* 2012;38:1310–1321.
69. Goodman GJ. Therapeutic undermining of scars (Subcision®). *Austral J Dermatol.* 2001;42:114–117.
70. Fulchiero GJ Jr, Parham-Vetter PC, Obagi S. Subcision and 1320-nm Nd:YAG nonablative laser resurfacing for the treatment of acne scars: a simultaneous split-face single patient trial. *Dermatol Surg.* 2004;30:1356–1359.
71. Ramadan SA, El-Komy MH, Bassiouny DA, et al. Subcision versus 100% trichloroacetic acid in the treatment of rolling acne scars. *Dermatol Surg.* 2011;37(5):626–633.
72. Grevelink JM, White VR. Concurrent use of laser skin resurfacing and punch excision in the treatment of facial acne scarring. *Dermatol Surg.* 1998;24(5):527–530.
73. Lanoue J, Goldenberg G. Acne scarring: a review of cosmetic therapies. *Cutis.* 2015;95(5):276–281.
74. Bouzari N, Davis SC, Nouri K. Laser treatment of keloids and hypertrophic scars. *Int J Dermatol.* 2007;46(1):80–88.
75. Lupton JR, Alster TS. Laser scar revision. *Dermatol Clin.* 2002;20(1):55–65.

76. Alster TS. Laser treatment of hypertrophic scars, keloids, and striae. *Dermatol Clin*. 1997;15(3):419–429.
77. Cannarozzo G, Sannino M, Tamburi F, et al. Flash-lamp pulsed-dye laser treatment of keloids: results of an observational study. *Photomed Laser Surg*. 2015;33(5):274–277.
78. Ha JM, Kim HS, Cho EB, et al. Comparison of the effectiveness of nonablative fractional laser versus pulsed-dye laser in thyroidectomy scar prevention. *Ann Dermatol*. 2014;26(5):615–620.
79. Vas K, Gaal M, Varga E, et al. Effects of the combined PDL/Nd:YAG laser on surgical scars: vascularity and collagen changes evaluated by in vivo confocal microscopy. *Biomed Res Int*. 2014;2014:204532.
80. Koike S, Akaishi S, Nagashima Y, et al. Nd:YAG laser treatment for keloids and hypertrophic scars: an analysis of 102 cases. *Plast Reconstr Surg Glob Open*. 2015;2(12):e272.
81. Gentile RD. Combined laser treatment of actinic sun damage and acne scarring. *Facial Plast Surg Clin North Am*. 2012;20(2):187–200.
82. Brauer JA, Kazlouskaya V, Alabdulrazzq H, et al. Use of a picosecond pulse duration laser with specialized optic for treatment of facial acne scarring. *JAMA Dermatol*. 2015;151(3):278–284.
83. Geronemus R. Fractional photothermolysis: current and future applications. *Lasers Surg Med*. 2006;38:169–176.
84. Sardana K, Manjhi M, Garg VK, et al. Which type of atrophic acne scar (icepick, boxcar, or rolling) responds to nonablative fractional laser therapy? *Dermatol Surg*. 2014;40:288–300.
85. Mahmoud BH, Srivastava D, Janiga JJ, et al. Safety and efficacy of erbium-doped yttrium aluminum garnet fractionated laser for treatment of acne scars in Type IV to VI skin. *Dermatol Surg*. 2010; 36:602.
86. Verhaeghe E, Onegenae K, Bostoen J, et al. Nonablative fractional laser resurfacing for the treatment of hypertrophic scars: a randomized controlled trial. *Dermatol Surg*. 2013;39:426–434.
87. Leheta TM, Abdel Hay RM, Hegazy RA, et al. Do combined alternating sessions of 1540 nm nonablative fractional laser and percutaneous collagen induction with trichloroacetic acid 20% show better results than each individual modality in the treatment of atrophic acne scars? A randomized controlled trial. *J Dermatol Treat*. 2014;25(2):137–141.
88. Ong MW, Bashir SJ. Fractional laser resurfacing for acne scars: a review. *Br J Dermatol*. 2012;166(6):1160–1169.
89. Woo SH, Park JH, Kye YC. Resurfacing of different types of facial acne scar with short-pulsed, variable-pulsed, and dual-mode Er:YAG laser. *Dermatol Surg*. 2004;30(4, Pt 1):488–493.
90. Jeong JT, Kye YC. Resurfacing of pitted facial acne scars with a long-pulsed Er:YAG laser. *Dermatol Surg*. 2001;27(2):107–110.
91. Tierney EP. Treatment of acne scarring using a dual-spot-size ablative fractionated carbon dioxide laser review of the literature. *Dermatol Surg*. 2011;37:945–961.
92. Cho SB, Lee SJ, Kang JM, et al. The efficacy and safety of 10,600-nm carbon dioxide fractional laser for acne scars in Asian patients. *Dermatol Surg*. 2009;35:1955–1961.
93. Walia S, Alster TS. Prolonged clinical and histologic effects from CO_2 laser resurfacing of atrophic acne scars. *Dermatol Surg*. 1999;25(12):926–930.
94. Yuan XH, Zhong SX, Li SS, et al. Comparison study of fractional carbon dioxide laser resurfacing using different fluences and densities for acne scars in Asians: a randomized split-face trial. *Dermatol Surg*. 2014;40:545–552.
95. Choi JE, Oh GN, Kim JY, et al. Ablative fractional laser treatment for hypertrophic scars: comparison between Er:YAG and CO_2 fractional lasers. *J Dermatolog Treat*. 2014;25(4):299–303.
96. Krueger N, Sadick NS. New-generation radiofrequency technology. *Cutis*. 2013;91(1):39–46.
97. Simmons BJ, Griffith RD, Falto-Aizpurua LA, et al. Use of radiofrequency in cosmetic dermatology: focus on nonablative treatment of acne scars. *Clin Cosmet Investig Dermatol*. 2014;7:335–339.
98. Alster TS, Lupton JR. Nonablative cutaneous remodeling using radiofrequency devices. *Clin Dermatol*. 2007;25:487–491.
99. Ruis-Esparza J, Gomez JB. Nonablative radiofrequency for active acne vulgaris: the use of deep dermal heat in the treatment of moderate to severe acne vulgaris (thermotherapy): a report of 22 patients. *Dermatol Surg*. 2003:29:333–339.
100. Rongsaard N, Rummaneethorn P. Comparison of a fractional bipolar radiofrequency device and a fractional erbium-doped glass 1,550-nm device for the treatment of atrophic acne scars: a randomized split-face clinical study. *Dermatol Surg*. 2014;40:14–21.
101. Kim JE, Lee HW, Kim JK, et al. Objective evaluation of the clinical efficacy and fractional radiofrequency treatment for acne scars and enlarged pores in Asian skin. *Dermatol Surg*. 2014;40:988–995.
102. Brightman L, Goldman MP, Taub AF. Sublative rejuvenation: experience with a new fractional radiofrequency system for skin rejuvenation and repair. *J Drugs Dermatol*. 2009;8(11, suppl):s9–S13.
103. Taub AF, Garretson CB. Treatment of acne scars of skin types II to V by sublative fractional bipolar radiofrequency and bipolar radiofrequency combined with diode laser. *J Clin Aesthet Dermatol*. 2011;4(10):18–27.
104. Peterson JD, Palm MD, Kiripolsky MG, et al. Evaluation of the effect of fractional laser with radiofrequency and fractionated radiofrequency on the improvement in acne scars. *Dermatol Surg*. 2011;37:1260–1267.
105. Cho SI, Chung BY, Choi MG, et al. Evaluation of clinical efficacy of fractional radiofrequency microneedle treatment in acne scars and large facial pores. *Dermatol Surg*. 2012;38:1017–1024.
106. Ibrahimi OA, Weiss RA, Weiss MA, et al. Treatment of acne scars with high intensity focused radio frequency. *J Drugs Dermatol*. 2015;14(9):1065–1068.
107. Akita H, Sasaki R, Yokoyama Y, et al. The clinical experience and efficacy of bipolar radiofrequency with fractional photothermolysis for aged Asian skin. *Exp Dermatol*. 2014;23(suppl 1):37–42.
108. Bogle AB, Arndt KA, Dover JS. Plasma skin regeneration technology. *J Drugs Dermatol*. 2007;6:1110–1112.
109. Potter MJ, Harrison R, Ramsden A, et al. Facial acne and fine lines: transforming patient outcomes with plasma skin regeneration. *Ann Plast Surg*. 2007;58:608–613.
110. Gonzalez MJ, Sturgill WH, Ross EV, et al. Treatment of acne scars using the plasma skin regeneration (PSR) system. *Lasers Surg Med*. 2008;40:124–127.
111. Foster KW, Moy RL, Fincher EF. Advances in plasma skin regeneration. *J Cosmet Dermatol*. 2008;7:169–179.
112. Kono T, Groff WF, Sakurai H, et al. Treatment of traumatic scars using plasma skin regeneration (PSR) system. *Lasers Surg Med*. 2009;41:128–130.
113. Zelickson Z, Schram S, Zelickson B. Complications in cosmetic laser surgery: a review of 494 food and drug administration manufacturer and user facility device experience reports. *Dermatol Surg*. 2014;40:378–382.
114. Zhang Z, Fei Y, Chen X, et al. Comparison of a fractional microplasma radiofrequency technology and carbon dioxide fractional laser for the treatment of atrophic acne scars: a randomized split-face clinical study. *Dermatol Surg*. 2013;39:559–566.
115. Wat H, Wu DC, Rao J, et al. Application of intense pulsed light in the treatment of dermatologic disease: a systematic review. *Dermatol Surg*. 2014;40:359–377.
116. Goldberg DJ. New collagen formation after dermal remodeling with an intense pulsed-light source. *J Cut Laser Ther*. 2000;2:59–61.
117. Bellew SG, Weiss MA, Weiss RA. Comparison of intense pulsed light to 595-nm long-pulsed pulsed dye laser for treatment of hypertrophic surgical scars: a pilot study. *J Drugs Dermatol*. 2005;4:448–452.
118. Jemec G, Jemec B. Acne: treatment of scars. *Clin Dermatol*. 2004;22:434–438.
119. Bisaccia E, Saap L, Kadry R, et al. Non-invasive procedures in cosmetic dermatology. *Skin Aging*. 2007;15:38–40.
120. Patel T, Tevet O. Effective treatment of acne scars using a pneumatic injection of hyaluronic acid. *J Drugs Dermatol*. 2015;14(1):74–76.
121. Kim BJ, Yoo KH, Kim MN. Successful treatment of depressed scars of the forehead secondary to herpes zoster using subdermal minimal surgery technology. *Dermatol Surg*. 2009;35(9):1439–1440.
122. Sadove R. Injectable poly-L lactic acid: a novel sculpting agent for the treatment of dermal fat atrophy after severe acne. *Aesthet Plastic Surg*. 2009;33:113–116.
123. Sapra S, Stewart J, Mraud K, et al. A Canadian study of the use of poly-L-lactic acid dermal implant for the treatment of hill and valley acne scarring. *Dermatol Surg*. 2015;41(5):587–594.
124. Beer K. A single-center, open-label study on the use of injectable poly-L-lactic acid for the treatment of moderate to severe scarring from acne or varicella. *Dermatol Surg*. 2007;33(s2):s159–s167.
125. Sadick NS, Palmisano L. Case study involving use of injectable poly-L-lactic acid (PLLA) for acne scars. *J Dermatol Treat*. 2009;20(5):302–307.
126. Goldman MP. Cosmetic use of poly-L-lactic acid: my technique for success and minimizing complications. *Dermatol Surg*. 2011;37:688–693.

127. Anonymous. Bellafill for acne scars. *Med Lett Drugs Ther*. 2015;57(1471):93–94.
128. Epstein RE, Spencer JM. Correction of atrophic scars with artefill: an open-label pilot study. *J Drugs Dermatol*. 2014;71(1):77–83.
129. Karnik J, Baumann L, Bruce S, et al. A double-blind, randomized, multicenter, controlled trial of suspended polymethylmethacrylate microspheres for the correction of atrophic facial acne scars. *J Am Acad Dermatol*. 2014;71(1):77–83.
130. Cooper JS, Lee BT. Treatment of facial scarring: lasers, filler, and nonoperative techniques. *Facial Plast Surg*. 2009;25(5):311–315.
131. Munavalli GS, Smith S, Maslowski JM, et al. Successful treatment of depressed, distensible acne scars using autologous fibroblasts: a multi-site, prospective, double blind, placebo-controlled clinical trial. *Dermatol Surg*. 2013;39:1126–1136.
132. LaViv® (azficel-T), Fibrocell Technologies, Inc., Exton, PA, package insert. http://www.fda.gov/downloads/BiologicsBloodVaccines/CellularGeneTherapyProducts/ApprovedProducts/UCM260489.pdf. Accessed September 21, 2015.
133. Weiss RA, Weiss MA, Beasley KL, et al. Autologous cultured fibroblast injection for facial contour deformities: a prospective, placebo-controlled, phase III clinical trial. *Dermatol Surg*. 2007;33:263–268.
134. Cox SE. Clinical experience with filler complications. *Dermatol Surg*. 2009;35(suppl 2):1661–1666.
135. Cohen J. Understanding, avoiding, and managing dermal filler complications. *Dermatol Surg*. 2008;34(suppl 1):s92–s99.
136. Waibel JS, Wulkan AJ, Shumaker PR. Treatment of hypertrophic scars using laser and laser assisted corticosteroid delivery. *Lasers Surg Med*. 2013;45(3):135–140.
137. Rkein A, Ozog D, Waibel JS, et al. Treatment of atrophic scars with fractionated CO_2 laser facilitating delivery of topically applied poly-L-lactic acid. *Dermatol Surg*. 2014;40:624–631.
138. Na JI, Choi JW, Choi HR, et al. Rapid healing and reduced erythema after ablative fractional carbon dioxide laser resurfacing combined with the application of autologous platelet-rich plasma. *Dermatol Surg*. 2011;37:463–468.
139. Lee JW, Kim BJ, Kim MN, et al. The efficacy of autologous platelet rich plasma combined with ablative carbon dioxide fractional resurfacing for acne scars: a simultaneous split-face trial. *Dermatol Surg*. 2011;37:931–938.
140. Zhu JT, Xuan M, Zhang YN, et al. The efficacy of autologous platelet-rich plasma combined with erbium fractional laser therapy for facial acne scars. *Mol Med Rep*. 2013;8:233–237.
141. Gawdat HI, Hegazy RA, Fawzy MM, et al. Autologous platelet rich plasma: topical versus intradermal after fractional ablative carbon dioxide laser treatment of atrophic acne scars. *Dermatol Surg*. 2014;40:152–161.
142. Leo MS, Kumar AS, Kirit R, et al. Systematic review of the use of platelet-rich plasma in aesthetic dermatology. *J Cosmet Dermatol*. 2015;14(4):315–323.
143. Nofal E, Helmy A, Nofal A, et al. Platelet-rich plasma versus CROSS technique with 100% trichloroacetic acid versus combined skin needling and platelet-rich plasma in the treatment of atrophic acne scars: a comparative study. *Dermatol Surg*. 2014;40:864–873.
144. Fabbrocini G, De Vita V, Pastore F, et al. Combined use of skin needling and platelet-rich plasma in acne scarring treatment. *Cosmet Dermatol*. 2011;24:177–183.
145. Marx RE. Platelet-rich plasma (PRP): what is PRP and what is not PRP? *Implant Dent*. 2001;10:225–228.
146. Sarangal R, Yadav S, Dogra S. Hair transplant for acne scars: an innovative approach. *J Cosmet Dermatol*. 2012;11:158–161.
147. Senoo M. Epidermal stem cells in homeostasis and wound repair of the skin. *Adv Wound Care*. 2013;273–282.
148. Yun IS, Jeon YR, Lee WJ, et al. Effect of human derived stem cells on scar formation and remodeling in a pig model: a pilot study. *Dermatol Surg*. 2012;38:1678–1688.
149. El-Hadidy MR, El-Hadidy AR, Bhaa A, et al. Role of epidermal stem cells in repair of partial-thickness burn injury after using Moist Exposed Burn Ointment (MEBO®) histological and immunohistochemical study. *Tissue Cell*. 2014;46(2):144–151.
150. Shen Y, Dai L, Li X, et al. Epidermal stem cells cultured on collagen-modified chitin membrane induce in situ tissue regeneration of full-thickness skin defects in mice. *PLoS One*. 2014;9:1–14.
151. Oni G, Lequeux C, Cho MJ, et al. Transdermal delivery of adipocyte-derived stem cells using a fractional ablative laser. *Aesthet Surg J*. 2013;33:109–116.
152. Kang WH, Kim YJ, Pyo WS, et al. Atrophic acne scar treatment using triple combination therapy: dot peeling, subcision and fractional laser. *J Cosmet Laser Ther*. 2009;11:212–215.
153. Liu L, Ma H, Li Y. Interventions for the treatment of stretch marks: a systematic review. *Cutis*. 2014;94:66–72.
154. Sarnoff DS. Therapeutic update on the treatment of striae distensae. *J Drugs Dermatol*. 2015;14(1):11–12.
155. Chang AL, Agredano YZ, Kimball AB. Risk factors associated with striae gravidarum. *J Am Acad Dermatol*. 2004;51:881–885.
156. Hermanns JF, Pierard GE. High-resolution epiluminescence colorimetry of striae distensae. *J Eur Acad Dermatol Venereol*. 2006;20:282–287.
157. Salter SA, Kimball AB. Striae gravidarum. *Clin Dermatol*. 2006;24:97–100.
158. Watson RE, Parry EJ, Humphries JD, et al. Fibrillin microfibrils are reduced in skin exhibiting striae distensae. *Br J Dermatol*. 1998;138:931–937.
159. Lee KS, Ro YJ, Jang SI, et al. Decreased expression of collagen and fibronectin genes in striae distensae tissue. *Clin Exp Dermatol*. 1994;19(4):285–288.
160. Shuster S. The cause of striae distensae. *Acta Derm Venereol Suppl (Stockh)*. 1979;59(85):161–169.
161. Elsaie ML, Baumann LS, Elsaaiee LT. Striae distensae (stretch marks) and different modalities of therapy: an update. *Dermatol Surg*. 2009;35:563–573.
162. Ammar NM, Rao B, Schwartz RA, et al. Adolescent striae. *Cutis*. 2000;65:69–70.
163. Sisson, WR. Colored striae in adolescent children. *J Pediatr*. 1954;45:520–530.
164. Stevanovic DV. Corticosteroid induced atrophy of the skin with telangiectasia: a clinical and experimental study. *Br J Dermatol*. 1972;87:548–556.
165. Kogoj F. Seitrag Zur Atiologie und pathogense de stria cutis distensae. *Arch Dermatol Syphiliol*. 1925;149:667.
166. Castrow FF 2nd, Ritchie EB. Nonatrophic striae symmetrica in Ehlers-Danlos syndrome. *Arch Dermatol*. 1968;98:494–495.
167. Pinkus H, Keech MK, Mehregan AH. Histopathology of striae distensae, with special reference to striae and wound healing in the Marfan syndrome. *J Invest Dermatol*. 1966;46:283–292.
168. Neldner KH. Pseudoxanthoma elasticum. *Clin Dermatol*. 1988;6:83–92.
169. Ledoux M, Beauchet A, Fermanian C, et al. A case-controlled study of cutaneous signs in adult patients with Marfan disease: diagnostic value of striae. *J Am Acad Dermatol*. 2011;64(2):290–295.
170. Bence A, Benke K, Szilveszter B, et al. Possible extracardiac predictors of aortic dissection in Marfan syndrome. *BMC Cardiovasc Disord*. 2014;14:47.
171. Mitts TF, Jimenez F, Hinek A. Skin biopsy analysis reveals predisposition to stretch mark formation. *Aesthet Surg J*. 2005;25(6):593–600.
172. Kurt S, Toz E, Canda MT, et al. Can striae be used as a marker for the prediction of pelvic organ prolapse? *Eur J Obstet Gynecol Reprod Biol*. 2014;180:116–119.
173. Tsai TL, Castillo AC, Moliver CL. Breast striae after cosmetic augmentation. *Aesthet Surg J*. 2014;34(7):1050–1058.
174. Sardana K. Lasers for treating striae: an emergent need for better evidence. *Indian J Dermatol Venereol Leprol*. 2014;80:392–394.
175. Timur Tashan S, Kafkasli A. The effect of bitter almond oil and massaging on striae gravidarum in primiparous women. *J Clin Nurs*. 2012;21(11/12):1570–1576.
176. Osman H, Usta IM, Rubeiz N, et al. Cocoa butter lotion for prevention of striae gravidarum: a double-blind, randomized and placebo-controlled trial. *Br J Obstet Gynaecol*. 2008;115(9):1138–1142.
177. Draelos ZD, Gold MH, Kaur M, et al. Evaluation of an onion extract, centella asiatica, and hyaluronic acid cream in the appearance of striae rubra. *Skinmed*. 2010;8(2):80–86.
178. Ash K, Lord J, Zukowski M, et al. Comparison of topical therapy for striae alba (20% glycolic acid/0.05% tretinoin versus 20% glycolic acid/10% L-ascorbic acid). *Dermatol Surg*. 1998;24(8):849–856.
179. Griffiths CEM, Russman AN, Majmudar G, et al. Restoration of collagen formation in photodamaged human skin by tretinoin (retinoic acid). *N Engl J Med*. 1993;329:530–535.
180. Fisher GJ, Datta S, Talwar HS, et al. Molecular basis of sun-induced premature skin aging and retinoid antagonism. *Nature*. 1996;379:335–339.
181. Gillbro JM, Al-Bader T, Westman M, et al. Transcriptional changes in organoculture of full-thickness human skin following topical application of all-trans retinoic acid. *Int J Cosmet Sci*. 2014;36(3):253–261.
182. Kang S, Kim KJ, Griffiths CE, et al. Tropical tretinoin (retinoic acid) improves early stretch marks. *Arch Dermatol*. 1996;132:519–526.

183. Pribanich S, Simpson FG, Held B, et al. Low-dose tretinoin dos not improve striae distensae: a double-blinded, placebo-controlled study. *Cutis*. 1994;54(2):121–124.
184. Kang S. Topical tretinoin therapy for management of early striae. *J Am Acad Dermatol*. 1998;38:S90–S92.
185. Hexsel D, Soirefmann M, Porto MD, et al. Superficial dermabrasion versus topical tretinoin on early striae distensae: a randomized, pilot study. *Dermatol Surg*. 2014;40:537–544.
186. Camirand A, Doucet J. Needle dermabrasion. *Aesthet Plast Surg*. 1997;21:48–51.
187. Park KY, Kim HK, Kim SE, et al. Treatment of striae distensae using needling therapy: a pilot study. *Dermatol Surg*. 2012;38:1823–1828.
188. Aust M, Walezko N. Acne scars in striae distensae: effective treatment with medical skin needling. *Hautarzt*. 2015;66(10):748–52.
189. Hernandez-Perez E, Colombo-Charrier E, Valencia-Ibiett E. Intense pulsed light in the treatment of striae distensae. *Dermatol Surg*. 2002;28(12):1124–1130.
190. Shokeir H, El Bedewi A, Sayed S, et al. Efficacy of pulsed dye laser versus intense pulsed light in the treatment of striae distensae. *Dermatol Surg*. 2014;40(6):632–640.
191. Mendoza-Garcia J, Sebastian A, Alonso-Rasgado T, et al. Ex vivo evaluation of the effect of photodynamic therapy on skin scars and striae distensae. *Photodermatol Photoimmunol Photomed*. 2015;31(5):239–251.
192. Goldberg DJ, Marmur ES, Hussain M. 308 nm Excimer laser treatment of mature hypopigmented striae. *Dermatol Surg*. 2003:29:596–599.
193. Goldberg DJ, Marmur ES, Schmults C, et al. Histologic and ultrastructural analysis of ultraviolet B laser and light source treatment of leukoderma in striae distensae. *Dermatol Surg*. 2005;31:385–387.
194. Nehal KS, Lichtenstein DA, Kamino H, et al. Treatment of mature striae with the pulsed dye laser. *J Cutaneous Laser Ther*. 1999;1: 41–44.
195. McDaniel DH, Ash K, Sukowski M. Treatment of stretch marks with the 585-nm flashlamp-pumped pulsed dye laser. *Dermatol Surg*. 1996;22:332–337.
196. Jimenez GP, Flores F, Berman B, et al. Treatment of striae rubra and striae alba with the 585-nm pulsed-dye laser. *Dermatol Surg*. 2003;29:362–365.
197. Goldman A, Rossato F, Priati C. Stretch marks: treatment using the 1064-nm Nd:YAG Laser. *Dermatol Surg*. 2008;34:686–692.
198. Gungor S, Sayilgan T, Gokdemir G, et al. Evaluation of an ablative and non-ablative laser procedure in the treatment of striae distensae. *Indian J Dermatol Venereol Leprol*. 2014;80(5):409–412.
199. Tay Y-K, Kwok C, Tan E. Non-ablative 1,450-nm diode laser treatment of striae distensae. *Lasers Surg Med*. 2006;38:196–199.
200. Goldman MP, Rostan EF. Treatment of striae distensae with a 1320nm dynamic cooling laser. *J Eur Acad Dermatol Venereol*. 2000;14(suppl 1):52.
201. Nouri K, Romagosa R, Chartier T, et al. Comparison of the 585 nm pulse dye laser and the short pulsed CO_2 laser in the treatment of striae distensae in skin types IV and VI. *Dermatol Surg*. 1999;25(5):368–370.
202. Angelis F, Kolesnikova L, Renato F, et al. Fractional non-ablative 1540-nm laser treatment of striae distensae in Fitzpatrick skin types II to IV: clinical and histological results. *Aesthet Surg J*. 2011;31(4):411–449.
203. Malekzad F, Shakoei S, Ayatollahi A, et al. The safety and efficacy of the 1540 nm non-ablative fractional XD probe of star lux 500 device in the treatment of striae alba: before-after study. *J Lasers Med Sci*. 2014;5(4):194–198.
204. Bak H, Kim BJ, Lee JW, et al. Treatment of striae distensae with fractional photothermolysis. *Dermatol Surg*. 2009;35:1215–1220.
205. Stotland M, Chapas AM, Brightman L, et al. The safety and efficacy of fractional photothermolysis for the correction of striae distensae. *J Drugs Dermatol*. 2008;7(9):857–861.
206. Tretti Clementoni M, Lavagno R. A novel 1565 nm non-ablative fractional device for stretch marks: a preliminary report. *J Cosmet Laser Ther*. 2015;17(3):148–155.
207. Gauglitz GG, Reinholtz M, Kaudewitz P, et al. Treatment of striae distensae using an ablative Erbium:YAG fractional laser versus a 585-nm pulsed-dye laser. *J Cosmet Laser Ther*. 2014;16(3):117–119.
208. Lee SE, Kim JH, Lee SJ, et al. Treatment of Striae distensae using an ablative 10,600-nm carbon dioxide fractional laser: a retrospective review of 27 participants. *Dermatol Surg*. 2010;36:1683–1690.
209. Naeini FF, Nikyar Z, Mokhtari F, et al. Comparison of the fractional CO_2 laser and the combined use of a pulsed dye laser with fractional CO_2 laser in striae alba treatment. *Adv Biomed Res*. 2014;3:184.
210. Naouri M, Mazer JM. Non-insulated microneedle fractional radiofrequency for the treatment of scars and photoaging. *J Eur Acad Dermatol Venereol*. 2016;30(3):499–502.
211. Ryu HW, Kim SA, Jung HR, et al. Clinical improvement of striae distensae in Korean patients using a combination of fractionated microneedle radiofrequency and fractional carbon dioxide laser. *Dermatol Surg*. 2013;39:1452–1458.
212. Dover JS, Rothaus K, Gold MH. Evaluation of safety and patient subjective efficacy of using radiofrequency and pulsed magnetic fields for the treatment of striae (stretch marks). *J Clin Aesthet Dermatol*. 2014;7(9):30–33.
213. Manusakiatti W, Boonthaweeyuwat E, Varothai S. Treatment of striae distensae with a tripolar radiofrequency device: a pilot study. *J Dermatolog Treat*. 2009;20(6):359–364.
214. Suh DH, Change KY, Son HC, et al. Radiofrequency and 585-nm pulsed dye laser treatment of striae distensae: a report of 37 Asian patients. *Dermatol Surg*. 2007;33:29–34.
215. Key DJ. Integration of thermal imaging with subsurface radiofrequency thermistor heating for the purpose of skin tightening and contour improvement: a retrospective review of clinical efficacy. *J Drugs Dermatol*. 2014;13(12):1485–1489.
216. Issa MC, de Britto Pereira Kassuga LE, Chevrand NS, et al. Transepidermal retinoic acid delivery using ablative fractional radiofrequency associated with acoustic pressure ultrasound for stretch marks treatment. *Lasers Surg Med*. 2013;45(2):81–88.
217. Weiss RA. Autologous cell therapy: will it replace dermal fillers? *Facial Plast Surg Clin North Am*. 2013;21(2):299–304.
218. Alves Ro, Boin MF, Crocco EI. Striae after topicalcorticosteroid: treatment with nonablative fractional laser 1540nm. *J CosmetLaser Ther*. 2015;17(3):143-147.

18 Scar Management in Skin of Color

CHI KEUNG YEUNG and HENRY HIN LEE CHAN

KEY POINTS

- Scar management in patients with skin of color requires a varying set of considerations compared to patients without substantial constitutive pigmentation. Hyperpigmentation and hypopigmentation may both be more prominent at initial presentation, pathologic scars are more common, and the tendency toward hyperpigmentation following various treatment interventions must be more thoroughly accounted for.
- Scar appearance can be improved with repeated sessions of minimally invasive modalities such as the vasculature-targeting pulsed dye laser and fractional resurfacing technology to induce collagen remodeling.
- Intralesional corticosteroid combined with 5-fluorouracil remains a mainstay in the treatment of hypertrophic scars and keloids in skin of color.
- Early intervention with fractional laser devices appears to improve the appearance and function of atrophic and hypertrophic scars. A lower density of microscopic treatment zones is preferred for skin of color to minimize the risk of postinflammatory hyperpigmentation.
- Different subtypes of scars require varying combinations of treatment modalities, preferably at an early stage of scar formation. Darker skin tones require lower treatment densities and greater attention to epidermal cooling for optimal laser efficacy and safety.

Scars are a common reason for consultation in clinicians' offices. They develop during the normal wound-healing response when connective tissue replaces lost tissue in the dermis or deeper planes because of injury or various inflammatory conditions. Frequent causes of scars include surgery, burns and other trauma, acne, body piercing, tattoos, and infections. Scars frequently lead to unfavorable cosmetic outcomes with associated symptoms such as pruritus and contractures that may impair limb function. "Skin of color," also referred to as ethnic skin, describes individuals with greater constitutive pigmentation, including those of African, Asian, Hispanic, Native American, Middle Eastern, and Pacific Island backgrounds with Fitzpatrick skin types III to VI based on the assessment of the burning and tanning histories of each individual (Table 18-1). The current system may have limitations as little data have been reported on skin responses for populations with dark skin color. Skin of color carries a higher risk of keloid and hypertrophic scar formation, and postinflammatory hyperpigmentation (PIH) of atrophic scars also poses a significant potential cosmetic impact.

There are a multitude of treatment modalities described for scar management, but standard treatment protocols are lacking because of a paucity of controlled therapeutic studies, especially in skin of color. The importance of ultraviolet protection (including sun avoidance and sunscreen use in the early period after wounding) to prevent scar hyperpigmentation and postlaser PIH cannot be overemphasized. PIH is most prominent in the skin of color and can be observed in scars and after laser treatment. Inflammation induced by sun exposure or injury is often accompanied by pigmentary alteration in darker skin types.

Apart from the cross-talk between keratinocytes and melanocytes in the control of melanocyte function, increasing evidence has highlighted the critical role played by the interactions between mesenchymal and epithelial cells mediated through the release of fibroblast-derived growth factors. In particular, keratinocyte growth factor (KGF), in combination with interleukin (IL)-1α, induces melanin deposition in vitro and hyperpigmented lesions in vivo. Furthermore, a moderate increase of KGF and induction of its receptor have been shown in sun-damaged lesions, suggesting the involvement of this growth factor in the onset of the hyperpigmentation.[1] The risk of PIH appears to be related to the degree of disruption of the dermoepidermal junction (DEJ) during laser resurfacing, and the subsequent inflammation at the DEJ with pigmentary incontinence (analogous to the interface dermatitis in lichen planus).

Currently available therapies include topical medications and intralesional injections, silicone-based sheets, compression therapy, cryotherapy, radiation, surgical revision, and laser therapy (see Chapter 10).[2] A variety of lasers can be applied based on different scar subtypes in darker skin provided that

Table 18-1 Fitzpatrick's Classification of Skin Phototypes

Phototype	Basic Skin Color	Response to Sun Exposure
I	Pale white	Burns easily; does not tan
II	White	Burns easily; tans with difficulty
III	White	May burn initially but tans easily
IV	Light brown/olive	Hardly burns; tans easily
V	Brown	Usually does not burn; tans easily
VI	Black	Does not burn; becomes darker

From Fitzpatrick TB. The validity and practicality of sun-reactive skin types I through VI. *Arch Dermatol.* 1988;124:869–871.

appropriate treatment parameters and cooling methods are used[3] (see Chapter 13). Most treatments carry a higher risk of adverse effects in this population, such as the propensity to develop pathologic scars and pigmentary alteration, owing to higher melanin content in the epidermis. In general, darker skin tones require lower fluences, greater attention to epidermal cooling when using pulsed dye laser (PDL), and lower treatment densities when using fractional lasers for optimal efficacy and safety (Table 18-2).

Table 18-2 Minimizing the Risk of PIH Associated with Laser Treatment in Skin of Color

- Ensure adequate sun protection in the pre- and postoperative periods
- Pretreatment with topical bleaching agents is not effective
- When using fractional lasers, decrease treatment density and the number of passes in each session, and increase the number of sessions and interval between treatments (at least 4–6 wk)
- Ensure adequate epidermal cooling; when using a pulsed dye laser, settings of 40 ms dynamic cooling spray and 20 ms delay are recommended
- Topical corticosteroid use is recommended if significant and persistent erythema is observed after laser treatment

Types of Scars

Proper recognition and classification of scars is essential for selecting the optimal treatment modalities (see Chapter 5). Scars present with various morphologies and are generally classified into hypertrophic and atrophic subtypes. Keloids and hypertrophic scars result from excessive fibrotic tissue formation, and occur less frequently than atrophic scars on the face. Atrophic acne scars are further classified into ice-pick, rolling, shallow, and deep boxcar scars, and are the result of compromised collagen production and increased degradation during the natural wound-healing process following inflammation or injury, which leads to surface undulations[4] (see Chapter 17) (Fig. 18-1).

Pathologic scars (hypertrophic scars and keloids) result from an aberrant wound-healing response and are seen in ethnic skin at rates ranging from 3- to 18-fold higher than in Caucasians. The incidence of keloids is 4.5% to 16% in skin of color, including African and Hispanic populations, especially in the second and third decades of life.[3] Predisposing factors include location (particularly on jaw line, upper chest, sternal area, shoulder, upper back, and earlobe), race, family history, and past history of tendency to scar. Differences in scar characteristics between skin of color and Caucasian skin include an increased risk of hypertrophic scars and keloids with PIH. In addition, prolonged erythema, pigmentary alteration, hypertrophic scarring, and longer recovery period are more likely to occur in darker skin types (Fig. 18-2).

Hypertrophic scars differ from keloids in a number of ways. Hypertrophic scars are pink scars that are confined within the borders of the original wound, and they tend to improve over time. Keloids often form nodules and plaques of deep red color that extend beyond the original wound border with claw-like projections. The lesions may occur months or even years following injury, and they tend to enlarge and recur over time despite treatment. The lesions are disfiguring and are frequently associated with pain and pruritus. Histopathologically, keloids are composed of thick, disorganized collagen fibers with abundant mucoid matrix, whereas hypertrophic scars are comprised of more organized parallel collagen fibers within scanty mucoid matrix[5] (see Chapter 5).

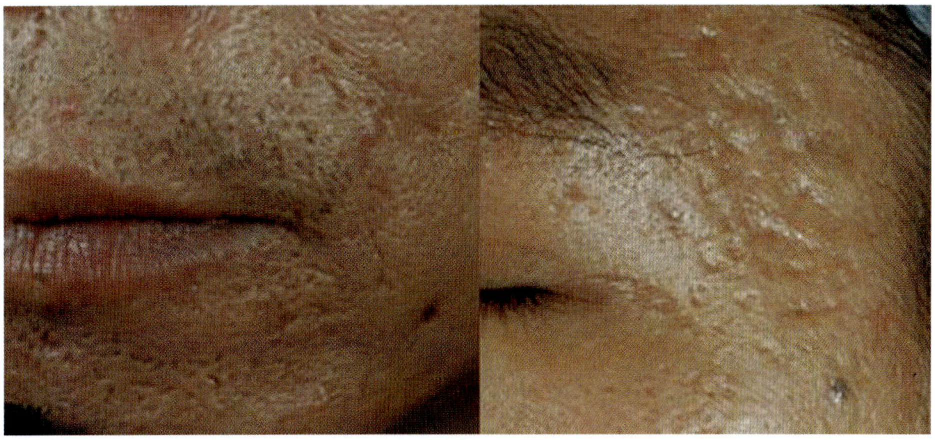

FIGURE 18-1 **Left:** Icepick scars with a sharp, demarcated V-shaped configuration reaching to the deep dermis. **Right:** Rolling scars with broad ill-defined superficial depressions of the skin.

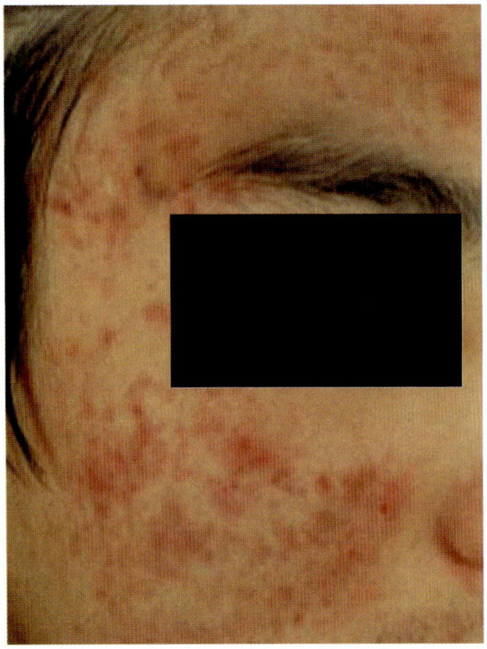

FIGURE 18-2 Postinflammatory hyperpigmentation on right temporal and malar areas associated with active inflammatory acne in a Chinese man.

Atrophic facial scarring is a common long-term complication of moderate to severe acne, and patients with inflammatory acne should be counseled early that they have a significant risk of scar development. Every effort should be made to treat the inflammatory lesions and prevent this long-lasting complication. Acne scars can have substantial cosmetic and psychological effects, particularly in adolescence and young adulthood. Concerns about PIH and scarring are one of the main motivational factors that lead patients to seek treatment for acne.[6] The precise prevalence of acne scarring is unknown. One community-based study reported the presence of acne scars in 14% of women and 11% of men aged 25 to 58 years.[7] Most patients presented with macular atrophic or ice-pick scars. Other studies reported that between 30% and 95% of patients with acne developed some form of associated scarring, and a higher incidence of scarring on the trunk was observed in men.[8]

Pathophysiology of Scarring

The exact mechanism of scar formation has not been fully elucidated (see Chapter 6). Inflammatory acne lesions often lead to atrophic scarring, and the formation of acne scars of various morphologies depends on the degree, depth, and duration of inflammation and on the extent of tissue damage.[9] Acne scars are the result of a suboptimal wound-healing process that involves inflammation, granulation tissue formation with fibroplasia and new vessel formation during the proliferative phase, and wound contracture and tissue remodeling.[10]

Wound healing involves a stepwise process consisting of multiple overlapping phases including inflammation, proliferation, and remodeling. Tumor necrosis factor β and IL-6 appear to play a role in the scarring process.[2] Under normal circumstances, the immature scar passes into the final maturation phase, with degradation of the extracellular matrix and transformation of the immature type III collagen of early wound into mature type I collagen. The delicate balance of synthesis and degradation of different scar components is tightly regulated by a number of molecules, particularly epidermal growth factor, TGF-β, matrix metalloproteinases (MMPs), and basic fibroblast growth factor. The delay in regression of angiogenesis also contributes to persistent erythema in incipient pathologic scars.[11] Deep scars are more liable to occur when the destruction of subcutaneous fat is involved in the inflammatory process, because the enzymatic activity and inflammatory mediators also destroy the deeper tissue.

It is not clear why some wounds heal to become atrophic scars whereas others become hypertrophic. An abnormal healing response with persistent collagen production, unbalanced production of collagen type I relative to that of collagen type III, abnormal expression of a variety of growth factors, and dysregulation of the extracellular matrix have all been implicated in the formation of keloids, which tend to occur in families with a racial predisposition for dark skin. TGF-β is overproduced in keloids with a loss of feedback control during the production of collagen and the extracellular matrix.[12] Hypertrophic scars are primarily composed of well-organized bundles of type III collagen, whereas keloids contain disorganized type I and III collagen bundles. Fibroblasts in keloids have a greater number of growth factor receptors and thus an increased sensitivity to growth factor stimulation, particularly platelet-derived growth factor and TGF-β.[13] The use of topical agents such as retinoids to treat acne may help to modulate the course of wound healing and prevent acne scar formation.[14]

Prevention and Minimization of Pathologic Scars

For those patients with a family or personal history of pathologic scarring after surgery or injury, elective invasive procedures of the skin are best avoided. This is especially true over high-risk areas such as the chest, shoulders, beard area, and earlobes. The current trend is early intervention after surgery to modulate scar formation (Table 18-3) (see Chapters 8 and 9). Optimization of the wound-healing

Table 18-3 Prevention of Keloid and Hypertrophic Scars in Skin of Color

- Avoid invasive procedures to high-risk areas, such as upper torso
- Employ occlusive dressings or topical silicone-based material
- Consider early postoperative use of potent topical corticosteroids, such as clobetasol propionate 0.05%, to scars on limbs and fusidic acid/betamethasone cream to areas prone to develop folliculitis
- Modulate wound healing by early use of the pulsed dye laser 2 weeks after surgery, or when stitches are removed. Doses are usually subpurpuric: 595 nm, pulse width 450 μs, 4.75–5.25 J/cm^2, spot size 12 mm, 10% overlap, 2–3 passes, DCD 40/20 ms
- Early intralesional corticosteroid plus 5-FU injection if pathologic scars start to develop

response with early interventions such as a vascular-specific 595-nm PDL and the use of occlusive dressings may help minimize the development of hypertrophic scars or keloids. A reduction of the pigmentation and vascularity of newly revised surgical scars has been demonstrated by the application of silicone gel sheeting daily for 3 months after surgery in Asian patients.[15] Topical silicone gel has also been shown to minimize the formation of hypertrophic scars in the early postoperative period after sternotomy in Asian patients.[16] Intervention with laser treatment within the first weeks of the scar remodeling process after suture removal has been shown to ultimately reduce the amount of scar tissue formed.[17] Early postoperative intralesional injection of 2 mg per mL triamcinolone acetonide combined with PDL treatment using subpurpuric settings has also been shown to minimize the development of hypertrophic scars after thyroidectomy in Asian patients.[18] In the experience of the authors, scars earlier in the remodeling process seem to respond better and required fewer treatment sessions than more mature scars, indicating that proactive laser intervention may better modulate the wound-healing response. To prevent keloid or hypertrophic scar formation, scars should always be reevaluated 4 to 8 weeks after surgery to determine if further scar therapeutic interventions are needed. Intralesional injection of corticosteroid plus 5-fluorouracil (5-FU) should be considered once scar thickness increases, indicating the development of pathologic scars.

Patients who have nodulocystic acne with intense visible inflammation are more liable to develop scarring, particularly when there is a delay in the effective treatment of the problem. In contrast, scarring may occur early regardless of the severity of the acne. Thus, the early treatment of acne is of paramount importance to reduce the risk of scarring. Retinoids have been shown to reduce the inflammation in acne by the inhibition of leukocyte migration in the skin, and oral isotretinoin reduces the expression of MMP-9 and MMP-13 in the sebum of acne patients. This may prevent acne scar formation by normalizing the balance of MMPs and tissue inhibitors.[19] In the practice of the authors, intervention with lasers can be considered 6 months after completion of isotretinoin therapy for acne.

Treatment of Hypertrophic Scars and Keloids

Pathologic scars including hypertrophic scars and keloids are difficult to treat because of their persistent and recurrent nature. Hypertrophic scars are associated with a better prognosis and tend to improve somewhat with time. Treatments including intralesional corticosteroids and 5-FU, cryotherapy, pressure therapy, silicone gels or sheets, laser therapy, and radiotherapy have all been previously described in the literature[12] (see Chapters 10 and 13). However, treatment results are not consistent and frequently disappointing. Furthermore, treatment-related complications such as atrophy and dyspigmentation are especially problematic in skin of color. Ultimately, the selected treatment course depends on a variety of factors such as patient expectations and needs, scar classification, constitutive skin pigmentation, procedural pain, treatment cost, number of visits, and potential downtime and adverse effects, particularly PIH risk in skin of color (Table 18-4). Scar location, functional disturbance resulting from scar contractures, and their overall psychosocial impact are important points to consider so that the treatment objective can match the patients' expectations (see Chapter 18).

Table 18-4 Factors to be Considered in the Choice of Treatment Modalities

- Patients' expectations regarding treatment endpoints such as cosmetic outcome and symptomatic relief
- Psychosocial impact and functional disturbance
- Scar types, size, and location
- Skin phototypes
- Tolerance to procedural discomfort
- Estimated number of treatment sessions and duration
- Cost and downtime
- Adverse effects (e.g., PIH and chance of recurrence)

The application of silicone-based gel sheeting up to 12 hours per day for 2 to 6 months' duration is a well-established and well-tolerated choice for hypertrophic scars and is used widely in clinical practice for prophylaxis of pathologic scars.[20] Although surgical intervention for keloids is tempting, particularly for the seemingly ubiquitous earlobe keloid, surgery should be approached with extreme caution and not without a management plan beginning immediately after surgery. This is due to an extremely high relapse rate of at least 50% after surgical excision and difficulty in predicting the treatment course. Additional management options for keloids, either alone or as adjuncts to surgical excision, include pressure therapy, intralesional corticosteroids and 5-FU, and radiotherapy. In general, multiple treatment sessions and many months, even years, may be required for significant improvements in pathologic scar appearance and symptoms. The treatment aims are cosmetic improvement, relief of symptoms such as pain and itch, and mitigation of scar contractures that limit limb movement. In the experience of the authors, it takes an average of 3 years to achieve treatment goals for pathologic scars on the face. Intralesional corticosteroid plus 5-FU injection every 4 to 6 weeks remains the mainstay of treatment in the early stage. The injection interval can be gradually spaced out to every 2 to 3 months depending on the response. It is more cost-effective to initiate PDL to improve telangiectasias and scar erythema at later stages of management, when the scars are almost flattened. The appearance and texture of scars can then be further improved by fractional laser resurfacing.

Lesional factors affecting the treatment response include the age of the scar, color (hyperpigmentation or hypopigmentation), location, and lesional stability (active growth). In general, younger scars respond better to treatment. Less invasive, safer, and simpler interventions with minimal side effects are generally preferred in ethnic skin. A palliative approach can be adopted with the aim of improving pliability, reducing scar volume, erythema, and dyspigmentation, and to relieve symptoms such as pain and itch. It is also imperative to communicate with the patient adequately to educate them on the course of treatment and the expected response and risk.

Scar origin does not seem to be as important as morphology when developing a treatment plan. The standard treatment for keloids and hypertrophic scars resulting from acne is similar to that of other excessive scarring that results from trauma and surgery. Intralesional corticosteroids decrease collagen synthesis and inhibit fibroblast proliferation.[21] PDL therapy has been shown to downregulate the expression of TGF-β and upregulate MMP-13, which results in reduced fibroblast proliferation and collagen type III deposition.[22] Laser therapy improves erythema and vascularity as well as scar texture and elevation. Radiotherapy is reserved for recalcitrant keloids; it penetrates into the dermis and inhibits fibroblast proliferation effectively. However, its usefulness is limited by its considerable adverse effects, which include mottled dyspigmentation, radiation dermatitis, and a low risk of carcinogenesis.[14] A combination of the various treatment modalities is often adopted to achieve the optimal cosmetic results (see Chapter 16).

Intralesional Injection

Corticosteroids (such as triamcinolone acetonide suspension at doses of 10 to 40 mg per mL) and antitumor agents such as 5-FU and bleomycin can be injected directly into the pathologic scars, either alone or in combination. Hyperpigmentation is a major side effect of intralesional bleomycin in darker skin types, affecting 71.4% of patients in one study.[23] Corticosteroids can inhibit TGF-β, can decrease fibroblast proliferation, and have vasoconstrictive effects. Common side effects associated with intralesional corticosteroids include injection site pain, local skin atrophy, telangiectasia, and hypopigmentation. Iatrogenic Cushing's syndrome following repeated corticosteroid injections for keloids has been reported.[24] 5-FU, as a potent inhibitor of TGF-β/SMAD signaling, is capable of blocking TGF-β-induced, SMAD-driven upregulation of α2 type I collagen (COL1A2) gene expression in a c-Jun N-terminal kinase (JNK)-dependent manner.[25] 5-FU is contraindicated in pregnant and pediatric patients. Injections are performed with a 30-gauge needle every 4 to 8 weeks; injection site pain can be ameliorated with a cooling agent or the use of topical anesthesia. Clinical improvement of keloidal and hypertrophic sternotomy scars after treatment with intralesional corticosteroid alone or combined with 5-FU, 5-FU alone, and PDL appeared comparable, though intralesional corticosteroid with or without 5-FU achieved faster resolution and greater improvement of induration of scars than PDL in a randomized controlled study.[26] In the experience of the authors, multimodal treatments combining intralesional corticosteroid with 5-FU and laser treatment sessions can reduce the number of treatments to reach treatment goals compared to either modality alone (Table 18-5).

Table 18-5 Technique for Intralesional Injection of Corticosteroid and 5-FU

- Diprospan suspension (5 mg of betamethasone and 2 mg of betamethasone as sodium phosphate) mixed with 5-FU (conc. 50 mg/mL) in a ratio of 7:3, 6:4, 1:1, 1:9 for intralesional injection, tapering corticosteroid dose in later treatment stages
- Use 1-mL syringe and 30-G needle to reduce injection pain
- Clean the injection site with alcohol pad
- Reduce pain by ethyl chloride spray immediately before injection
- Inject no more than 1 mL per session depending on lesion size; avoid superficial injections
- Apply antibiotic (fusidic acid) cream followed by a bandage to cover the injection site
- Inject every 4–6 wk initially, then gradually taper to every 2–3 mo depending on improvement of symptoms and scar appearance

Laser Therapy

Pulsed Dye Laser

The selective thermal effects of lasers have been used to treat scars since the early 1980s. PDL treatment has been consistently shown to be useful for hypertrophic scars with various pulse durations and the use of dynamic cooling for epidermal protection and for improving scar texture, redness, thickness, and pliability[27,28] (Fig. 18-3). Though the exact mechanism remains to be elucidated, injury to the vasculature induced by PDL and other devices that target hemoglobin results in a gradual and cumulative collagen remodeling response. Hypertrophic scars have been shown to improve by over 50% after three laser treatments in Asian patients.[29] Keloids are more resistant to laser treatment owing to their lower density of vessels compared to hypertrophic scars, among other factors. Moreover, increased epidermal melanin (resulting in the less effective targeting of the vasculature and greater risk of postlaser dyspigmentation) and hyperactive fibroblasts that lead to increased risk of pathologic scars render laser treatment of scars more difficult in the skin of color. Thus, more judicious settings and additional treatment sessions are often required. Concomitant use of PDL and injection therapy with corticosteroids and 5-FU seems most effective in reducing erythema and improving scar texture in this population[12,26] (Table 18-6). In the experience of the authors, PDL should be used before each injection session so as to avoid reduced laser energy absorption due to blanching induced by repeated steroid injection. There is inadequate evidence to support the use of intense pulsed light for the treatment of keloids and hypertrophic scars at this time.

Regarding laser parameters for treatment of scars, use of subpurpuric doses of PDL for erythematous scars is the trend. Use of more modest fluences and higher dynamic cooling settings are preferred in treating scars in darker skin types to minimize the risk of PIH and epidermal injury. Modest improvements in pruritus and erythema, but not thickness and hardness, were demonstrated in a controlled study in Chinese patients using suprapurpuric dosing of a 585-nm PDL with pulse duration of 1.5 ms.[27] In the view of the authors, this combination cannot be considered as the standard of practice for the treatment of hypertrophic surgical scars, especially on the chest, in Asian skin. For the PDL of 595-nm wavelength (Vbeam Perfecta, Syneron Candela, Wayland, MA) to treat scars, the authors employ fluences ranging from 4.75 to 5.25 J per cm^2 (spot size 12 mm, pulse duration 450 μs, 10% overlap, 1 to 3 passes).

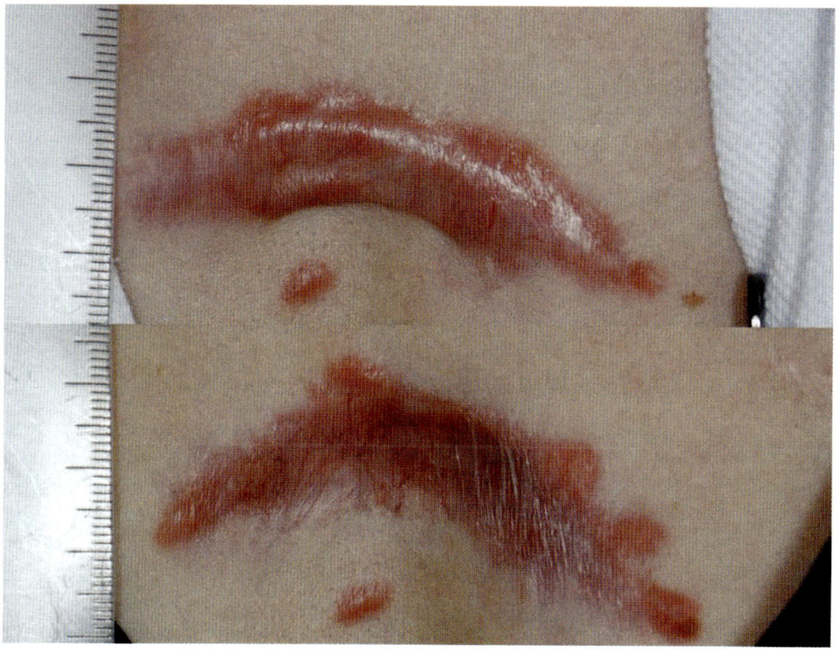

FIGURE 18-3 Improvement of keloids on presternal area treated with PDL and intralesional corticosteroid plus 5-FU. **Top:** Before treatment. **Bottom:** After treatment.

Table 18-6 Combined Injection and Laser Treatment Modalities for Hypertrophic Scars and Keloids

- Intralesional injection of corticosteroid plus 5-FU in early stages every 4–6 wk, with gradual reduction of steroid to 5-FU ratio
- Introduce subpurpuric PDL (595 nm, 450 μs, 12 mm spot size, 4.75–5.25 J/cm^2, 1–3 passes) for diffuse scar erythema before each injection every 2–3 mo when scars are almost flat at later stages of treatment
- PDL is effective for clearing telangiectasias associated with repeated steroid injection using parameters: 595 nm, 10 ms, 10 × 3mm spot size, 13 J per cm^2 in multiple passes as required

Table 18-7 Use of Pulsed Dye Laser with Dynamic Cooling for the Treatment of Pathologic Scars in Skin of Color

- PDL of 595 nm wavelength (Vbeam Perfecta, Syneron Candela, Wayland, MA) to treat scars: fluences ranging from 4.75–5.25 J/cm^2 (spot size 12 mm, pulse duration 450 μs, 10% overlap, 1–3 pass). DCD settings: 40 ms duration and 20 ms delay; every 4–6 wk
- Telangiectasia associated with corticosteroid injection needs multiple sessions of PDL (pulse duration 10 ms, fluence 13 J/cm^2, spot size 3 × 10 mm, DCD 40/20, multiple passes until vessel constriction) every 4–6 wk
- Intralesional injection of corticosteroid plus 5-FU after laser treatment to prevent proliferation of scar tissue

Epidermal Cooling

Darker skin patients have more epidermal melanin that can act as a competing target chromophore for laser emissions, thus causing an increased risk of adverse effects when using PDL (and other platforms emitting visible light) and reduced effective laser energy reaching the dermis. Epidermal cooling in conjunction with laser treatment can be useful in improving clinical efficacy and patient tolerance by diminishing the pain and swelling associated with the procedure, and reducing the incidence of adverse effects with higher laser settings. Although a variety of contact cooling approaches have been attempted including the application of ice packs/cubes or a chilled sapphire window, none has proven entirely satisfactory for a better therapeutic outcome.[30] This is largely due to the fact that contact cooling methods are nonselective, and cool not only the epidermis but also the targeted lesional blood vessels. Hence, overcooling potentially reduces the effectiveness of laser treatment. In another cooling method, cryogen spray cooling (CSC), cryogen spurts are sprayed onto the lesions through an electronically controlled nozzle positioned approximately 3 cm from the skin surface. Cryogen spurt durations (approximately 30 to 40 ms) and the delay between cryogen delivery and laser irradiation (approximately 20 ms) are controlled with a programmable digital delay generator. These parameters are adjusted based on fluences, skin type, and the treatment location. Higher settings of the dynamic cooling device (DCD), such as 40 ms spray duration and 20 ms delay, are optimal for skin phototypes of III and IV for epidermal protection. However, higher fluences should be used cautiously in the skin of color even with PDL-CSC treatment. As melanin can act as a competing target chromophore for incoming laser light, a high epidermal melanin content can overwhelm the protective effect of CSC. For distinct telangiectasias associated with corticosteroid injection, multiple sessions of PDL (pulse duration 10 ms, fluence 13 J per cm^2, spot size 3 × 10 mm, DCD 40/20) can be performed every 4 to 6 weeks (Table 18-7).

Patients are instructed to keep the area trauma free and apply a topical antibacterial ointment (mupirocin) continuously if any scaling or crusting develops after laser treatment. For postoperative pain, relief is usually achieved with ice

Table 18-8 Fractional Lasers for Scar Treatment in Darker Skin Types

- Treatment density is more significant than fluence in determining the risk of PIH
- PIH risk is reduced at lower treatment densities (e.g., 10% cumulative coverage) compared to higher treatment densities (e.g., 20% cumulative coverage) with a 1,550-nm erbium-doped fiber fractional laser
- The risk of acne flare is reduced using a lower density (10%) compared to a higher density (20%) approach
- Beware of cutaneous herpes simplex reactivation, especially in the perioral area. Prophylactic antivirals may be indicated
- More treatment sessions are necessary using a low-density approach to achieve the same therapeutic goals

packs, cooling soaks, or the application of emollients such as Aquaphor ointment. Oral analgesics (acetaminophen, celecoxib) can be given for significant pain. Patients are cautioned to avoid excessive sun exposure. Daily application of sunscreen with a sun protection factor of 30 or more is suggested. Sun protection is recommended for at least 3 months after treatment to prevent hyperpigmentation.

In one study, utilizing a 595-nm PDL with a short pulse width of 0.45 ms was more effective in decreasing scar size and improving scar pliability than that of 40 ms.[31] The clinical end point is mild redness or faint purpura of the scar area. The occurrence of dark purpura resulting from high fluences is to be avoided owing to the risk of its persistence in pigmented skin. Overly aggressive treatment manifest by significant purpura can also increase the risk of scar reactivation. The fluence should be reduced for the subsequent treatment if crusting, blistering, or excessive purpura develops that may increase the risk of PIH. For patients with darker skin, a lower fluence should be used.

For scar mitigation after surgery, PDL is best performed as soon as possible after stitch removal.[32] Side effects of PDL include purpura lasting up to 10 days, hyperpigmentation, and (rarely) blistering with oozing. Sun protection and bleaching cream such as hydroquinone cream may be used if PIH develops.

Fractional Lasers

Nonablative fractional photothermolysis at monthly intervals is a promising modality for the treatment of hypertrophic and burn scars with improvement in texture, dyschromia, and thickness.[33–35] Skin color influences the ultimate outcome after fractional laser treatment for scars, and adverse effects such as prolonged erythema and pigmentary changes are more common in ethnic skin. Lower laser fluences and treatment densities should be used to treat patients with darker skin types. As a result of more conservative treatment, more treatments may be necessary to achieve the desired results.[3] In the experience of the authors, treatment density is more significant than fluence in determining the risk of PIH in Asian skin[36] (Table 18-8). Furthermore, sun protection is of paramount importance after laser treatment to minimize the risk of PIH.

Hypertrophic burn scars produce significant morbidity, including disfigurement, pain, and contracture. Multiple sessions of fractional ablative laser therapy hold promise for the management of hypertrophic burn scars (Fig. 18-4). Special considerations should be given to ablative fractional laser treatment in darker skin types with regard to the risk of PIH. The rate of PIH after laser treatment correlates with the degree of inflammation and the extent of DEJ disruption.[37] A recent study of fractional ablative CO_2 laser treatment in Asians yielded PIH rates of 55.5%

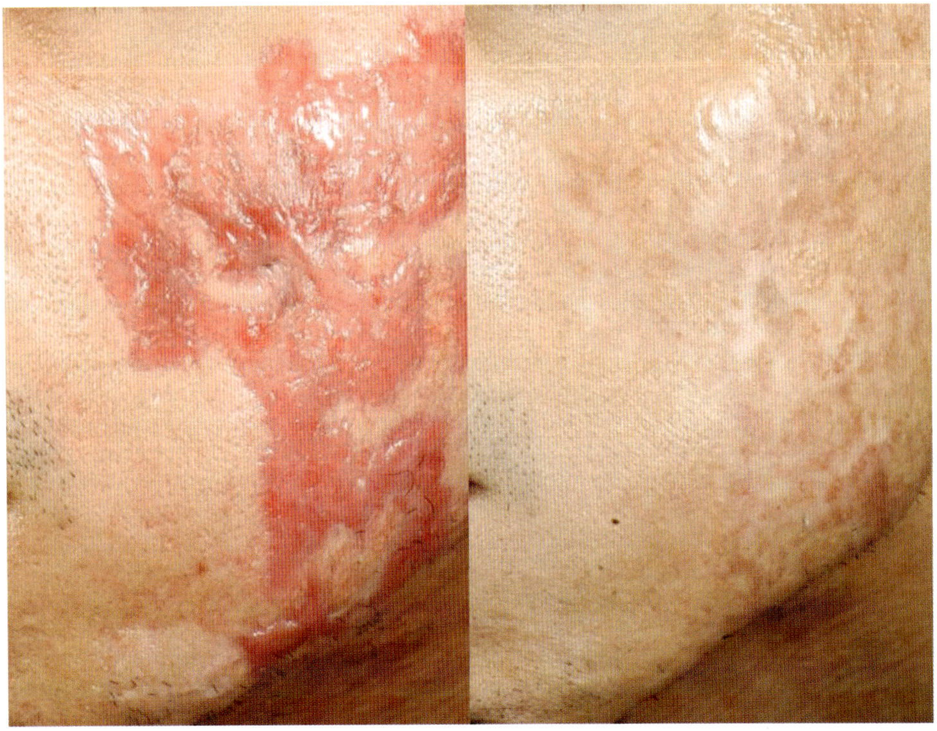

FIGURE 18-4 Burn injury on left cheek before **(left)** and after **(right)** a series of initial intralesional corticosteroid plus 5-FU injections followed by PDL in the intermediate stage, and finally repeated nonablative fractional 1,550-nm laser and ablative fractional CO_2 laser treatments.

and 37.5% at 1 and 3 months of follow-up, respectively.[38] The relatively high rates of PIH were probably due to aggressive treatment parameters for optimal clinical efficacy, leading to increased inflammation in that study. In a prospective, before–after cohort study in burn patients with hypertrophic scars, treatment including an ablative fractional CO_2 laser was shown to significantly improve both the signs and symptoms of hypertrophic burn scars, as measured by objective and subjective instruments.[39] Additional studies are required to confirm the usefulness of ablative and nonablative fractional laser treatment to improve scar appearance and function, to determine appropriate dosing and timing, and to compare efficacy.[40]

Treatment of Atrophic Scars

Atrophic scars are frequently dyspigmented or erythematous depressions in the skin related to local depletion of dermal collagen (and potentially fat) following inflammatory destructive processes such as acne, trauma, and surgery. The treatment of atrophic scarring is a challenge to clinicians because the common long-term consequences and outcomes of initial skin injury are variable and depend on the type and extent of the insult (see Chapter 17). A variety of different treatment modalities including chemical peels, surgical techniques such as subcision and punch excision, mechanical and laser dermabrasion, and tissue augmentation with fillers have been used in various combinations for atrophic scars. There are a lack of randomized controlled prospective studies with universally accepted methods to evaluate long-term treatment effects of acne scars. Device-based treatment options for atrophic scars include nonablative laser treatments, ablative and nonablative fractional laser resurfacing, full-field ablative laser resurfacing, and fractional radiofrequency (RF). The results of the above techniques aim to induce neocollagenesis and remodeling, but are less predictable in darker skin color with a variable risk of PIH that may last for several months. These options need to be discussed with individual patients with regard to their respective risks and benefits prior to the start of any type of treatment regime.

Multiple modalities are often combined to optimize the treatment outcome based on different scar types (Fig. 18-1).[17] Because the apex of ice-pick scars often extend beyond the effective depth of most resurfacing tools, a punch excision can be performed prior to the resurfacing procedure. Tethering to the subcutis by fibrous adhesions in rolling acne scars can be released using a subcision technique. Fractional technologies are largely replacing various resurfacing techniques, including chemical peels and full-field laser ablation, for the improvement of shallow boxcar scars. Soft tissue fillers that were initially used for facial contouring and volume augmentation can be used to correct atrophic acne scars. Common temporary fillers including hyaluronic acid (e.g., Restylane, Juvederm) appear to offer transient relief in the treatment of boxcar scars.

The nonselective absorption of water and the deeper penetration of the mid-infrared lasers lead to a bulk tissue heating effect with subsequent dermal remodeling. These nonablative lasers, such as the 1,320-nm neodymium:yttrium–aluminum–garnet (Nd:YAG) laser, have the putative advantages of a minimal recovery time and a relatively low risk of adverse effects. Although the long wavelength of the mid-infrared laser is expected to be of advantage in darker skin, the risk of PIH after the use of a 1,450-nm diode laser with dynamic cooling for acne scars is significant in Asian patients (Fig. 18-5). The total duration of 40 to 60 ms for the cryogen spray probably contributes to the high PIH rate of 39% in Asian patients.[41]

Fractional Technologies for Scars

Although the 10,600-nm CO_2 and 2,940-nm erbium-doped YAG(Er:YAG) laser systems can be used in traditional full-field ablative mode to effectively treat facial scarring, their use may be associated with a prolonged recovery period and high risk of hyper- or hypopigmentation in skin of color.[42] For this reason, the use of fractional nonablative/ablative laser resurfacing has become the mainstay of treatment for atrophic scars in this population. Fractional technology permits the use of high fluences to attain deeper penetration depths with the promise of a reduced risk of complications. Fractional lasers are used to induce zones of microscopic injury (microscopic treatment zones [MTZs]) based on the heating of tissue water. These create discrete areas of tissue coagulation (nonablative) or vaporization

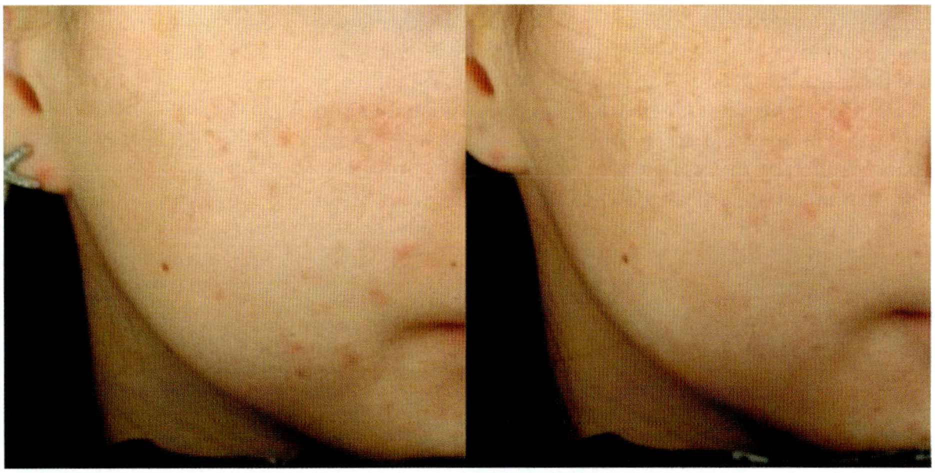

FIGURE 18-5 **Left:** The right cheek before treatment. **Right:** postinflammatory hyperpigmentation on the cheek 4 weeks after the first treatment with a 1,450-nm diode laser for acne scars.

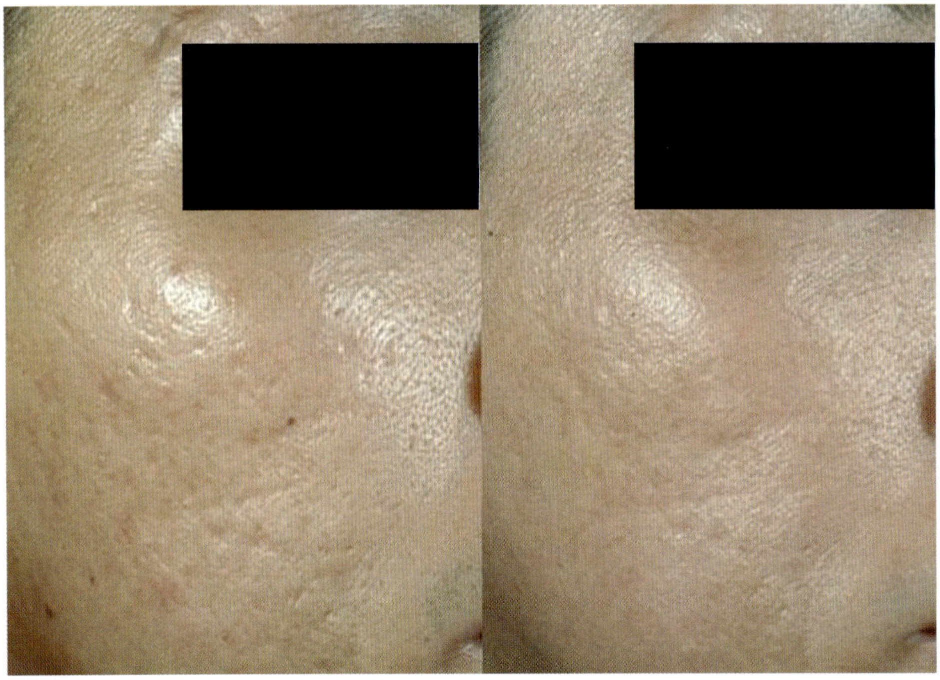

FIGURE 18-6 Acne scars on right face before **(left)** and 1 month posteighth nonablative fractional resurfacing treatment **(right)**.

(ablative) from tens to hundreds of microns in diameter surrounded by normal viable tissue. The adjacent viable tissue allows the rapid lateral migration of keratinocytes, leading to the complete reepithelialization of the epidermis within 24 hours. Hence, skin remodeling can be achieved with a minimal risk of complications (such as infection, dyspigmentation, and additional scarring) and a high degree of efficacy. During each treatment session, a variable proportion of the skin is treated, the extent of which is primarily determined by the density settings of the device and the number of passes. Depending on the particular characteristics of each device, approximately 16% to 32% of the skin surface is targeted per treatment session. In addition, the depth of collagen remodeling that is associated with the use of fractional resurfacing can be deeper than the conventional aggressive laser resurfacing procedure (up to thousands of microns compared with hundreds).[43] Fractional techniques therefore appear to be more efficient and result in faster recovery than nonablative resurfacing and full-field ablative skin resurfacing.[44]

One of the most common nonablative fractional lasers is the 1,550-nm erbium-doped fiber laser. Despite the above discussion, they are not equally safe and effective for all skin types, and patients with skin of color can have a significant risk of PIH. The percentage of skin directly affected by the fractional laser is related to the total MTZ density, which is determined by multiplying the MTZ density per pass by the total number of passes. The selection of energy level is based on the desired depth of penetration, which corresponds to the depth of the acne scars. Treatment densities and fluence can be adjusted according to the extent of acne scarring, its anatomical location, and skin tone. The energy and the MTZ density may be limited by patient discomfort, and the additional use of an air-cooling system may lead to greater patient tolerance.[45]

An early study evaluated the effect of three treatments using a nonablative fractional laser at monthly intervals for mild to moderate atrophic acne scars in 53 patients. Clinical improvement ranged from 51% to 75% in 90% of the subjects.[46] The device improved the appearance of scars by 51% to 75% in patients with Fitzpatrick skin type III and IV,[36] with the risk of PIH ranging from 6% to 18% depending on the fluence and density used (Fig. 18-6). The side effects were mild and consisted of temporary erythema, edema, and minimal scab formation. Acneiform eruptions are the most common condition exacerbated by fractional laser treatment. Higher density settings seem to be more strongly associated with postprocedure edema, erythema, and hyperpigmentation than higher fluence settings in these zones.[37] Nonablative fractional resurfacing can be used safely in skin of color by reducing the number of passes and the total treatment density to reduce the risk of PIH (Table 18-9). Clinical efficacy could be maintained by increasing the total number of treatment sessions.

Ablative fractional Er:YAG and CO_2 lasers seem to provide comparable results in the resurfacing of atrophic acne scars in Asians, with less pain induced by the Er:YAG laser[47] (Fig. 18-7). Adverse effects, particularly PIH, are more evident in patients treated with ablative fractional CO_2 laser resurfacing at higher densities or fluences for

Table 18-9 Minimizing PIH with the Use of Nonablative Fractional Resurfacing for Atrophic Scars in Darker Skin Types

- Reduce the number of passes in the treatment area
- Decrease total treatment density by approximately 50%
- Maintain treatment efficacy by increasing number of treatment sessions from approximately 4 to 8 at 1–3 mo intervals
- Fluences are proportional to scar depth and need not be reduced in skin of color
- Effective sun protection by sunscreen of SPF 50 or above and avoidance of sun before and after laser treatment
- Use a bleaching agent, such as hydroquinone 4%, only if PIH develops. Preventive treatment is generally not effective

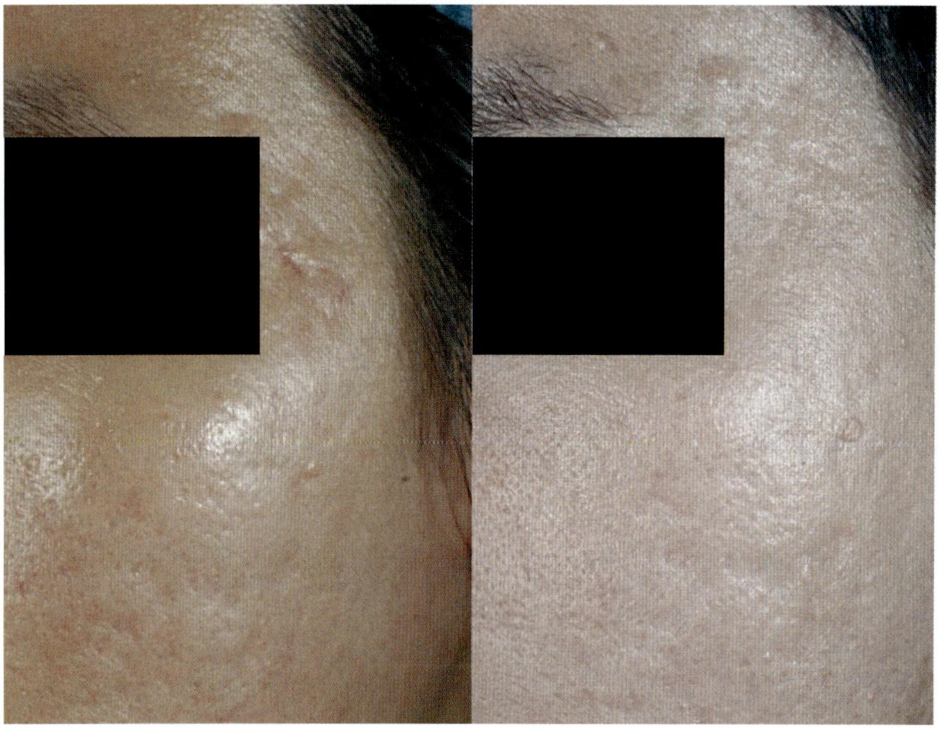

FIGURE 18-7 Improvement of atrophic acne scars on left temporal and malar area after series of three nonablative fractional 1,550 nm laser and two fractional ablative CO_2 laser treatments. **Left:** Before treatment. **Right:** After treatment.

acne scars in Asians.[48] It is particularly important to use lower treatment density when thickened or contracted traumatic scars are treated by fractional lasers. Superficial scarring may be more amenable to treatment with a fractional nonablative device than ice-pick and deep acne scars. Deeper penetration depths are available to ablative fractional devices such as CO_2 or Er:YAG lasers. It remains to be fully elucidated whether the increased penetration depth of ablative devices correlates with increased efficacy for various indications, but skin dimpling lasting for months may occasionally develop (Fig. 18-8). Ablative fractional treatment was better at reducing surgical scar hardness, whereas nonablative fractional treatment was superior for lightening color in one study.[49] PDL may also be used to target the telangiectatic component of atrophic scars after the course of fractional treatment. Sequential use of PDL plus injection therapy and then fractional technology is more likely to give superior results for hypertrophic scars and keloids.

Other Fractional Devices

The major limitation of fractional laser ablation for acne scars in more heavily pigmented skin types is a relatively lower level of safety, and perhaps a lower level of efficacy because more conservative treatment is often required. RF devices can also deliver energy in a fractional form to achieve selective heating of the deep dermis while protecting the overlying epidermis to initiate a wound-healing response. The minimization of the epidermal disruption by the use of these devices may reduce the potential for PIH in skin of color.[50] Fractional RF can also be used for acne scars using a sublative approach with relative sparing of epidermis, in

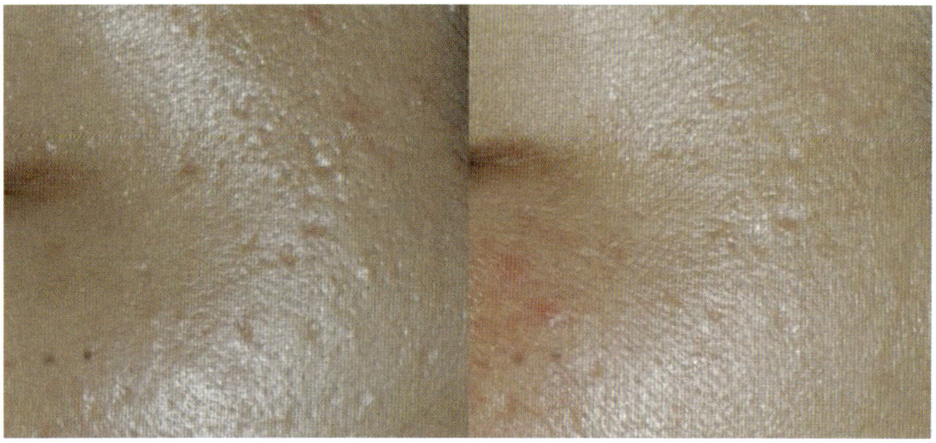

FIGURE 18-8 Fractional CO_2 laser treatment for acne scars on left malar area. **Left:** Before treatment. **Right:** 1 month posttreatment, complicated by mild dimpling of skin.

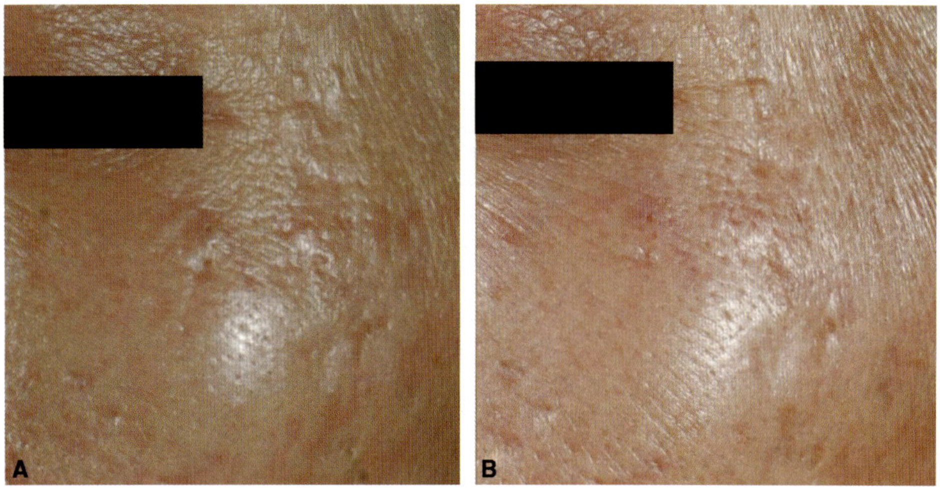

FIGURE 18-9 **A:** Atrophic acne scars on left cheek before treatment. **B:** Improvement in acne scars is seen 3 months after five sessions of combined treatments with fractional RF and fractional laser with RF.

principle further reducing the risk of PIH in Asians. The combination device of a fractionated mid-infrared diode laser and RF energy with a built-in contact cooler has been used to successfully treat wrinkles and acne scarring.[51] A combination of fractional bipolar RF and a fractional diode laser plus RF energy can be used to improve acne scars by the enhancement of collagen production in the scar indentation and by causing ablation and resurfacing of the scar edges[50] (Fig. 18-9). In the experience of the authors, the efficacy of fractional RF for atrophic acne scars is modest compared with fractional laser as a result of the lower inflammatory reaction and subsequent healing response. Thus, fractional RF can be considered in patients who want treatments of lower PIH risk and less downtime with redness and edema. An alternative approach with potentially less adverse effects is the use of a picosecond pulse width laser alternating with fractional RF every 4 to 6 weeks to enhance the effectiveness.

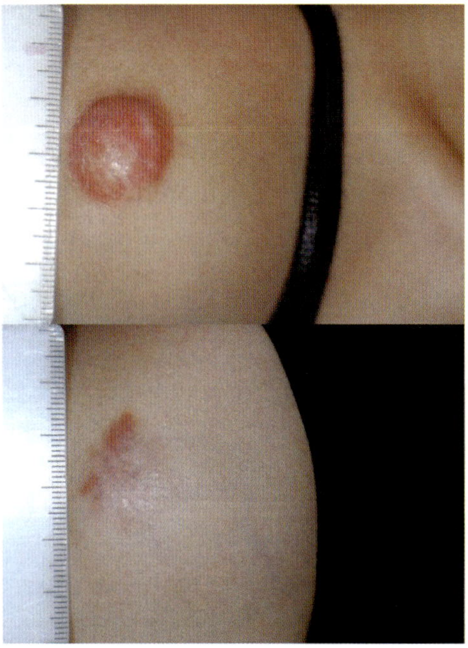

FIGURE 18-10 Improvement of keloid with hyperpigmentation on right shoulder in terms of volume, redness, and pigmentation after a series of PDL, picosecond laser using microlens array (0.71 J per cm^2, 10 Hz, 6 mm, 4 passes), and intralesional corticosteroid plus 5-FU. **Top:** Before treatment. **Bottom:** After treatment.

Picosecond pulse duration devices such as the 755-nm alexandrite laser with diffractive microlens array have emerged as a new option in the treatment of facial acne scarring. The short pulses induce plasma formation with effects that appear to be similar to fractional laser technology. A recent study of 20 subjects with Fitzpatrick skin types I through V and atrophic facial acne scarring was performed.[52] Patients received six treatments with a 755-nm picosecond laser with a spot size of 6 mm, fluence of 0.71 J per cm^2, frequency of 5 Hz, and pulse width of 750 ps. The mean pain score was low with high patient satisfaction and corresponding histologic improvements. A three-dimensional analysis revealed a mean 24.3% improvement in scar volume, maintained at 1 (24.0%) and 3 (27.2%) months after treatment. The same 755-nm picosecond laser with specialized optics may also be used for three to four passes to improve PIH resulting from scars and prior therapy (Fig. 18-10). Apart from the commonly used Q-switched Nd:YAG 1,064-nm laser to treat scar pigmentation or PIH after scar management intervention, 1,064-nm picosecond lasers are now being tested to improve PIH.

Minimizing PIH Following the Use of Fractional Devices

PIH is the most significant adverse effect of fractional laser therapy in skin of color.[53] As noted previously, the rate of PIH after fractional laser treatment correlates with the degree of inflammation at the DEJ and the extent of DEJ disruption.[37] Although some clinicians pretreat patients with topical bleaching agents and retinoic or glycolic acid compounds before laser resurfacing to help prevent PIH, no studies have demonstrated any reduction in the rate of PIH with this practice.[54] Besides, prolonged use of topical bleaching agents may induce issues such as contact dermatitis and exogenous ochronosis. Avoidance of sun exposure and consistent use of sunblock creams is the most critical measure to prevent PIH before and after laser surfacing.

Our group reported a PIH rate of 18.2% among Asian patients treated with approximately four sessions of nonablative fractional resurfacing with a 1,550-nm erbium-doped fiber laser and a mean total treatment density of 442.5 MTZ per cm^2.[36] However, the risk of PIH was lowered to 6.0% when the total treatment densities were reduced to 210.5 MTZ per cm^2 by decreasing the number of passes from eight to four. Although both the energy and density of fractional resurfacing appear to influence the generation of PIH in pigmented skin types, treatment density seems to be of particular importance.[55] This implies that the adverse effects of nonablative fractional resurfacing can be markedly reduced by lowering the density of resurfacing, whereas clinical efficacy can be maintained by increasing the total number of treatment sessions.

A study of fractional ablative CO_2 laser treatment in Asian patients by the authors yielded PIH rates of 55.5% and 37.5% at 1 and 3 months of follow-up, respectively.[38] The relatively high rates of PIH in this study were probably due to aggressive treatment parameters (Fraxel Re:pair, Solta Medical, Hayward, CA, energy 60 to 70 mJ, 4 passes, treatment level 8 to 11, skin surface coverage 35% to 40%) for optimal clinical efficacy, leading to adequate inflammation and healing response. A split-face study comparing nonablative and ablative fractional laser treatment for acne scarring showed similar effectiveness after one treatment for acne scars in Asians, with a PIH rate of approximately 10%.[56] The observed lower rate of PIH might be related to the lower treatment energy and densities used in that study. Mild PIH was reported in another Asian study in 92% of the subjects or 51% of treatment sessions after three sessions of fractional CO_2 resurfacing laser for acne scars. PIH was completely resolved in an average of 5 weeks after the final laser treatment.[57] In contrast, the risk of PIH in another study after fractional CO_2 laser treatment predominantly in patients with Fitzpatrick skin types I to II was 1.2%.[58] Another split-face study comparing fractional CO_2 laser and Er:YAG lasers for acne scars in Asian patients showed PIH rates of 35% and 50% at the Er:YAG and CO_2 laser sites, respectively.[47] The difference in the rate of PIH was not statistically significant, although there was a trend toward a higher incidence of PIH associated with the fractional CO_2 laser treatment compared to the fractional Er:YAG laser treatment. Complete resolution of the PIH was noted within 6 weeks using hydroquinone 4% cream once daily.

In addition to the underlying constitutive pigmentation, the presence of a suntan 2 weeks before or after laser procedures is also a risk factor for PIH. The use of epidermal cooling such as with a forced air device during the procedure may decrease the incidence of postprocedural dyschromia. The short-term use of prophylactic systemic corticosteroids (prednisolone 10 mg daily for 3 days) has been suggested to reduce postlaser inflammatory reactions and subsequent PIH caused by the disrupted epidermal barrier.[59] However, the risk of side effects of a short course of systemic corticosteroids for this indication has not been adequately evaluated in clinical studies. Alternatively, local wet wrap therapy with the application of a moderately potent topical corticosteroid (diluted mometasone 0.1% ointment) under a wet occlusive dressing to the facial treatment area can be used to reduce risk of PIH in patients with significant inflammatory response immediately after fractional laser, followed by a 3-day course of mometasone 0.1% cream twice daily (Table 18-10).

Table 18-10 Methods to Reduce PIH Following Fractional Laser Resurfacing

- Treat at lower density with more treatment sessions
- Use a forced air-cooling device during the procedure
- Suntan avoidance and diligent sunscreen use 2 wk before and 3 mo after laser treatment
- Wet wrap with diluted topical corticosteroid ointment with occlusive dressing right after treatment, if excessive erythema and swelling develop
- Combined topical hydroquinone 4%, mometasone furoate 0.1%, and azelaic acid 20% cream daily for 4–6 wk if PIH develops

For the treatment of PIH resulting from laser therapy, combined topical hydroquinone 4%, mometasone furoate 0.1%, and azelaic acid 20% cream daily can be used for 4 to 6 weeks. The hydroquinone component of this topical regime can increase to 6% if no irritation develops upon review 4 weeks later. It can alternate with Triluma cream (fluocinolone acetonide 0.01%, hydroquinone 4%, and tretinoin 0.05%) 4 weeks later if patients can tolerate this combined approach. Patients are advised to stop topical bleaching treatment if erythema, scaling, or symptoms of irritation develop to avoid aggravation of cutaneous inflammation. Cutaneous atrophy resulting from topical corticosteroid use should be monitored closely with serial photographic assessment. Consistent use of sunblock creams and sun avoidance is also important. A Q-switched (nanosecond pulse range) Nd-YAG 1,064-nm laser can be considered for PIH after laser treatment in skin of color using spot size 8 mm, 3.1 J per cm^2, 10 Hz, 3 to 5 passes. A picosecond range 1,064-nm Nd-YAG laser (Picoway, Syneron Candela, MA) can also be effective to treat PIH at settings of 0.9 J per cm^2, large spot size, 3 passes. Induction of erythema should be avoided when using these lasers to treat PIH (Table 18-11).

Table 18-11 Treatment of PIH After Laser Therapy

- 3 days of mometasone 0.1% cream twice daily to reduce inflammation if significant erythema develops after laser treatment
- Consider combined topical hydroquinone 4%, mometasone furoate 0.1%, and azelaic acid 20% cream daily if early signs of PIH develop
- Step up to hydroquinone 6%, mometasone furoate 0.1%, and azelaic acid 20% cream for persistent PIH if no irritation upon follow-up at 4 wk
- Alternate with fluocinolone acetonide 0.01%, hydroquinone 4%, and tretinoin 0.05% (Triluma cream) daily for persistent PIH if no irritation upon follow-up at 4 wk
- Strict sun protection with avoidance and use of sun block
- Consider laser therapy for developing PIH with a Q-switched (nanosecond) 1,064-nm Nd-YAG, spot size 8 mm, 3.1 J/cm^2, 3–5 passes, 10 Hz or a (picosecond) 1,064-nm, 0.9 J/cm^2, 3 passes, large spot size

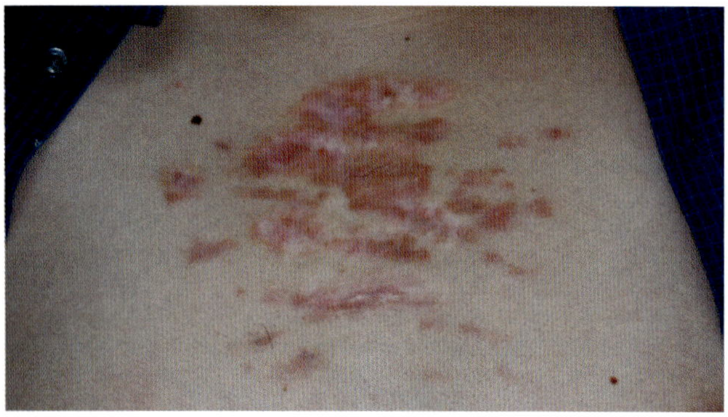

FIGURE 18-11 Treatment of keloids on anterior chest by cryotherapy was complicated by prolonged hypopigmentation.

Miscellaneous Therapies

Cryotherapy use for keloids in Asian and other patients with darker skin types carries a high risk of dyspigmentation, especially prolonged hypopigmentation. It is known that melanocytes are more sensitive to cryotherapy in comparison with other cutaneous cell components such as keratinocytes, fibroblasts, and endothelial cells. Cryotherapy induces intracellular ice formation and irreversible damage to the melanocytes. For this reason intralesional cryotherapy with relative sparing of epidermal melanocytes is preferred if this treatment method is chosen to reduce the hypopigmentation rate[60] (Fig. 18-11). The usefulness of surgical excision is limited by high rate of recurrence unless it is followed by adjunctive treatments such as radiotherapy. Other adjunctive treatments such as interferon and imiquimod 5% cream are lacking in long-term studies of effectiveness and are themselves associated with pigmentary changes. Topical retinoid alone is generally not effective in improving scars in ethnic skin, although it may provide some benefit for the management of PIH.

Conclusion

Hypertrophic scars and keloids are more likely to develop in skin of color (Table 18-12). The use of PDL during the early stages of scar formation may help lower the incidence of severe hypertrophic scars and keloids. For existing hypertrophic scars and keloids, PDL in combination with intralesional corticosteroid and 5-FU appears to be most effective. The risk of postinflammatory pigmentary alternation needs to be considered in the treatment of scars in darker skin with its higher melanin content. Lower laser parameters with higher epidermal cooling levels are generally safer and preferred when lasers are used to treat scars. The fractional nonablative and ablative lasers will continue to play an increasingly important role in treating a range of scar types including atrophic acne scars and hypertrophic burn scars. Picosecond lasers and RF devices are among the promising emerging modalities in scar management.

Table 18-12 Synopsis of Scar Management in Skin of Color

- Pathologic scars with PIH commonly complicate treatments in skin of color
- Early use of PDL helps prevent pathologic scars
- A combination of PDL and intralesional injections remains a mainstay of treatment
- Lower fluences and adequate cooling allow safe use of PDL and other lasers
- Decreased treatment density and skin coverage in fractional resurfacing are the key to reduce PIH

REFERENCES

1. Cardinali G, Kovacs D, Picardo M. Mechanisms underlying post-inflammatory hyperpigmentation: lessons from solar lentigo. *Ann Dermatol Venereol*. 2012;139(suppl 4):S148–S152.
2. Reish RG, Eriksson E. Scars: a review of emerging and currently available therapies. *Plast Reconstr Surg*. 2008;122(4):1068–1078.
3. Alster T, Zaulyanov L. Laser scar revision: a review. *Dermatol Surg*. 2007;33(2):131–140.
4. Sriprachya-anunt S, Marchell NL, Fitzpatrick RE, et al. Facial resurfacing in patients with Fitzpatrick skin type IV. *Lasers Surg Med*. 2002;30(2):86–92.
5. Slemp AE, Kirschner RE. Keloids and scars: a review of keloids and scars, their pathogenesis, risk factors, and management. *Curr Opin Pediatr*. 2006;18:396–402.
6. Taylor SC, Cook-Bolden F, Rahman Z, et al. Acne vulgaris in skin of color. *J Am Acad Dermatol*. 2002;46(2):S98–S106.
7. Goulden V, Stables GI, Cunliffe WJ. Prevalence of facial acne in adults. *J Am Acad Dermatol*. 1999;41(4):577–580.
8. Del Rosso JQ, Bikowski JB, Baum E, et al. A closer look at truncal acne vulgaris: prevalence, severity, and clinical significance. *J Drugs Dermatol*. 2007;6(6):597–600.
9. Rivera AE. Acne scarring: a review and current treatment modalities. *J Am Acad Dermatol*. 2008;59(4):659–676.
10. Goodman GJ. Management of post-acne scarring. What are the options for treatment? *Am J Clin Dermatol*. 2000;1(1):3–17.
11. Connolly KL, Chaffins M, Ozog D. Vascular patterns in mature hypertrophic burn scars treated with fractional CO_2 laser. *Lasers Surg Med*. 2014;46(8):597–600.
12. Wolfram D, Tzankov A, Pülzl P, et al. Hypertrophic scars and keloids—a review of their pathophysiology, risk factors, and therapeutic management. *Dermatol Surg*. 2009;35(2):171–181.
13. Al-Attar A, Mess S, Thomassen JM, et al. Keloid pathogenesis and treatment. *Plast Reconstr Surg*. 2006;117(1):286–300.
14. Ogawa R, Yoshitatsu S, Yoshida K, et al. Is radiation therapy for keloids acceptable? The risk of radiation-induced carcinogenesis. *Plast Reconstr Surg*. 2009;124(4):1196–1201.
15. Rhee S-H, Koh S-H, Lee D-W, et al. Aesthetic effect of silicone gel on surgical scars in Asians. *J Craniofac Surg*. 2010;21(3):706–710.
16. Chan KY, Lau CL, Adeeb SM, et al. A randomized, placebo-controlled, double-blind, prospective clinical trial of silicone gel in prevention of hypertrophic scar development in median sternotomy wound. *Plast Reconstr Surg*. 2005;116(4):1013–1020.
17. Lee Y. Combination treatment of surgical, post-traumatic and post-herpetic scars with ablative lasers followed by fractional laser and non-ablative laser in Asians. *Lasers Surg Med*. 2009;41(2):131–140.
18. Ryu H-W, Cho J-H, Lee K-S, et al. Prevention of thyroidectomy scars in Korean patients using a new combination of intralesional injection of low-dose steroid and pulsed dye laser starting within 4 weeks of suture removal. *Dermatol Surg*. 2014;40(5):562–568.
19. Thiboutot D, Gollnick H, Bettoli V, et al. New insights into the management of acne: an update from the Global Alliance to Improve Outcomes in Acne group. *J Am Acad Dermatol*. 2009;60(5):S1–S50.
20. Gold MH, McGuire M, Mustoe TA, et al. Updated international clinical recommendations on scar management. Part 2: algorithms for scar prevention and treatment. *Dermatol Surg*. 2014;40(8):825–831.
21. Tosti A, De Padova MP, Beer KR. *Acne Scars: Classification and Treatment*. London: Informa Healthcare; 2010.
22. Kuo Y-R, Wu W-S, Jeng S-F, et al. Suppressed TGF-β1 expression is correlated with up-regulation of matrix metalloproteinase-13 in keloid regression after flashlamp pulsed-dye laser treatment. *Lasers Surg Med*. 2005;36(1):38–42.

23. Payapvipapong K, Niumpradit N, Piriyanand C, et al. The treatment of keloids and hypertrophic scars with intralesional bleomycin in skin of color. *J Cosmet Dermatol.* 2015;14(1):83–90.
24. Fredman R, Tenenhaus M. Cushing's syndrome after intralesional triamcinolone acetonide: a systematic review of the literature and multinational survey. *Burns.* 2013;39(4):549–557.
25. Wendling J, Marchand A, Mauviel A, et al. 5-fluorouracil blocks transforming growth factor-beta-induced alpha 2 type I collagen gene (COL1A2) expression in human fibroblasts via c-Jun NH2-terminal kinase/activator protein-1 activation. *Mol Pharmacol.* 2003;64(3):707–713.
26. Manuskiatti W, Fitzpatrick RE. Treatment response of keloidal and hypertrophic sternotomy scars: comparison among intralesional corticosteroid, 5-fluorouracil, and 585-nm flashlamp-pumped pulsed-dye laser treatments. *Arch Dermatol.* 2002;138(9):1149–1155.
27. Chan HH, Wong DS, Ho WS, et al. The use of pulsed dye laser for the prevention and treatment of hypertrophic scars in Chinese persons. *Dermatol Surg.* 2004;30(7):987–994.
28. Sobanko JF, Alster TS. Laser treatment for improvement and minimization of facial scars. *Facial Plast Surg Clin North Am.* 2011;19(3):527–542.
29. Kono T, Ercocen AR, Nakazawa H, et al. The flashlamp-pumped pulsed dye laser (585 nm) treatment of hypertrophic scars in Asians. *Ann Plast Surg.* 2003;51(4):366–371.
30. Chiu CH, Chan HH, Ho WS, et al. Prospective study of pulsed dye laser in conjunction with cryogen spray cooling for treatment of port wine stains in Chinese patients. *Dermatol Surg.* 2003;29(9):909–915.
31. Manuskiatti W, Wanitphakdeedecha R, Fitzpatrick RE. Effect of pulse width of a 595-nm flashlamp-pumped pulsed dye laser on the treatment response of keloidal and hypertrophic sternotomy scars. *Dermatol Surg.* 2007;33(2):152–161.
32. Nouri K, Jimenez GP, Harrison-Balestra C, et al. 585-nm pulsed dye laser in the treatment of surgical scars starting on the suture removal day. *Dermatol Surg.* 2003;29(1):65–73.
33. Verhaeghe E, Ongenae K, Bostoen J, et al. Nonablative fractional laser resurfacing for the treatment of hypertrophic scars: a randomized controlled trial. *Dermatol Surg.* 2013;39(3 Pt 1):426–434.
34. Waibel J, Wulkan AJ, Lupo M, et al. Treatment of burn scars with the 1,550 nm nonablative fractional erbium laser. *Lasers Surg Med.* 2012;44(6):441–446.
35. Haedersdal M, Moreau KE, Beyer DM, et al. Fractional nonablative 1540 nm laser resurfacing for thermal burn scars: a randomized controlled trial. *Lasers Surg Med.* 2009;41(3):189–195.
36. Chan NPY, Ho SGY, Yeung CK, et al. The use of non-ablative fractional resurfacing in Asian acne scar patients. *Lasers Surg Med.* 2010;42(10):710–715.
37. Chan HH, Manstein D, Yu CS, et al. The prevalence and risk factors of post-inflammatory hyperpigmentation after fractional resurfacing in Asians. *Lasers Surg Med.* 2007;39(5):381–385.
38. Chan NPY, Ho SGY, Yeung CK, et al. Fractional ablative carbon dioxide laser resurfacing for skin rejuvenation and acne scars in Asians. *Lasers Surg Med.* 2010;42(9):615–623.
39. Hultman CS, Friedstat JS, Edkins RE, et al. Laser resurfacing and remodeling of hypertrophic burn scars: the results of a large, prospective, before-after cohort study, with long-term follow-up. *Ann Surg.* 2014;260(3):519–529.
40. Sobanko JF, Vachiramon V, Rattanaumpawan P, et al. Early postoperative single treatment ablative fractional lasing of Mohs micrographic surgery facial scars: a split-scar, evaluator-blinded study. *Lasers Surg Med.* 2015;47(1):1–5.
41. Chua SH, Ang P, Khoo LSW, et al. Nonablative 1450-nm diode laser in the treatment of facial atrophic acne scars in type IV to V Asian skin: a prospective clinical study. *Dermatol Surg.* 2004;30(10):1287–1291.
42. Tay YK, Kwok C. Minimally ablative erbium:YAG laser resurfacing of facial atrophic acne scars in Asian skin: a pilot study. *Dermatol Surg.* 2008;34(5):681–685.
43. Manstein D, Herron GS, Sink RK, et al. Fractional photothermolysis: a new concept for cutaneous remodeling using microscopic patterns of thermal injury. *Lasers Surg Med.* 2004;34(5):426–438.
44. Jih M, Kimyaiasadi A. Fractional photothermolysis: a review and update. *Semin Cutan Med Surg.* 2008;27(1):63–71.
45. Fisher GH, Geronemus RG. Short-term side effects of fractional photothermolysis. *Dermatol Surg.* 2005;31:1245–1249.
46. Alster TS, Tanzi EL, Lazarus M. The use of fractional laser photothermolysis for the treatment of atrophic scars. *Dermatol Surg.* 2007;33(3):295–299.
47. Manuskiatti W, Iamphonrat T, Wanitphakdeedecha R, et al. Comparison of fractional erbium-doped yttrium aluminum garnet and carbon dioxide lasers in resurfacing of atrophic acne scars in Asians. *Dermatol Surg.* 2013;39(1, Pt 1):111–120.
48. Yuan XH, Zhong SX, Li SS. Comparison study of fractional carbon dioxide laser resurfacing using different fluences and densities for acne scars in Asians: a randomized split-face trial. *Dermatol Surg.* 2014;40(5):545–552.
49. Shin JU, Gantsetseg D, Jung JY, et al. Comparison of non-ablative and ablative fractional laser treatments in a postoperative scar study. *Lasers Surg Med.* 2014;46(10):741–749.
50. Yeung CK, Chan NPY, Shek SYN, et al. Evaluation of combined fractional radiofrequency and fractional laser treatment for acne scars in Asians. *Lasers Surg Med.* 2012;44(8):622–630.
51. Kim S. The dual treatment of acne vulgaris using two kinds of ELOST (electro optical synergy) system: a simultaneous split-face trial. *J Cosmet Laser Ther.* 2008;10(4):213–216.
52. Brauer JA, Kazlouskaya V, Alabdulrazzaq H, et al. Use of a picosecond pulse duration laser with specialized optic for treatment of facial acne scarring. *JAMA Dermatol.* 2015;151(3):278–284.
53. Davis EC, Callender VD. Postinflammatory hyperpigmentation: a review of the epidemiology, clinical features, and treatment options in skin of color. *J Clin Aesthet Dermatol.* 2010;3(7):20–31.
54. West TB, Alster TS. Effect of pretreatment on the incidence of hyperpigmentation following cutaneous CO2 laser resurfacing. *Dermatol Surg.* 1999;25(1):15–17.
55. Kono T, Chan HH, Groff WF, et al. Prospective direct comparison study of fractional resurfacing using different fluences and densities for skin rejuvenation in Asians. *Lasers Surg Med.* 2007;39(4):311–314.
56. Cho SB, Lee SJ, Cho S, et al. Non-ablative 1550-nm erbium-glass and ablative 10 600-nm carbon dioxide fractional lasers for acne scars: a randomized split-face study with blinded response evaluation. *J Eur Acad Dermatol Venereol.* 2010;24(8):921–925.
57. Manuskiatti W, Triwongwaranat D, Varothai S, et al. Efficacy and safety of a carbon-dioxide ablative fractional resurfacing device for treatment of atrophic acne scars in Asians. *J Am Acad Dermatol.* 2010;63(2):274–283.
58. Shamsaldeen O, Peterson JD, Goldman MP. The adverse events of deep fractional CO_2: a retrospective study of 490 treatments in 374 patients. *Lasers Surg Med.* 2011;43(6):453–456.
59. Cho SB, Lee SJ, Kang JM, et al. Combined fractional laser treatment with 1550-nm erbium glass and 10,600-nm carbon dioxide lasers. *J Dermatolog Treat.* 2010;21(4):221–223.
60. van Leeuwen MC, van der Wal MB, Bulstra AE, et al. Intralesional cryotherapy for treatment of keloid scars: a prospective study. *Plast Reconstr Surg.* 2015;135(2):580–589.

19 Rehabilitative Burn Scar Management

MICHAEL A. SERGHIOU and JONATHAN NISZCZAK

KEY POINTS

- A comprehensive program of rehabilitation is essential in the recovery of the burn patient.
- Hypertrophic scar formation is one of the most prominent sequelae of burn injury; this chapter emphasizes the role of rehabilitation in managing hypertrophic scars that have the potential to limit function and result in catastrophic cosmetic outcomes for the burn survivor.
- Focus in this chapter is placed on (a) the formation of hypertrophic scar; (b) scar assessment; (c) scar management to include pressure therapy, inserts, massage, and heat modalities; (d) orthotics; and (e) exercise.

Scar Formation

Wounds normally heal by forming scar to replace the injured or destroyed tissues at the injury site. This replacement scar tissue is much more restrictive than normal skin tissue, and often leads to complications in both functional movements and aesthetic appearance. Stedman[1] defined *scar* as the fibrous tissue that replaces normal tissues that have been destroyed by an injury or disease. Historically, the earliest references to scarring are provided by Linares who credits the first full medical description of scars to Petz in 1790 (see Chapter 1).[2]

As the burn wound begins to heal or after skin grafting operations have been completed, scars begin to form. In general, the longer a wound remains open the higher the chances are for the development of hypertrophic scars (see Chapter 6).[3,4] From a morphologic perspective, the two pathologic scar types (hypertrophic and keloid) differ in that keloid scars are mainly composed of thick type III collagen fibers with associated cyclooxygenase (COX)-2 overexpression, whereas hypertrophic scars are mainly composed of thin type I collagen fibers with a COX-1 overexpression (see Chapter 5).[5] These two scar types differ in their timing of formation in that keloids tend to develop later in the healing process. Also, hypertrophic scars remain within the wound margins, whereas keloids proliferate outside of the wound margins.

Scar Hypertrophy

Scar hypertrophy has a prevalence of over 65% after burn injury.[6] Factors that may contribute to the development of hypertrophic scars include: wound infection, the patient's genetic makeup, repeatedly harvested donor sites, the patient's age, chronic inflammation, location of the injury, and skin tension (see Chapter 7).[7] An overgrowth of scar tissue is classified as hypertrophic or keloidal, both of which may be considered dermatoproliferative disorders of the skin.[8] Hypertrophic scars are typically characterized as raised, red, rigid, painful, pruritic and may restrict joint motion or skin mobility *within* the confines of the burn.[9] In contrast, keloid scars extend *beyond* the margins of the original injury advancing into the surrounding soft tissue and are somewhat less contractile in form (Fig. 19-1).[9] Hypertrophic scars are not cosmetically appealing and can have a negative impact on a patient's self-esteem and body image.[10] Generally, the deeper the burn injury, the longer the inflammatory wound process, or the longer a wound remains unhealed, the greater the potential for formation of hypertrophic scars (see Chapters 6, 8, and 9).[3,4,11] Burn scar contractures may occur because of the effect of myofibroblasts and free actin in the scar.[12] Contractures are characterized as either *intrinsic* (loss of tissue in the injured area with subsequent distortion of the involved anatomic part) or *extrinsic* (loss of tissue is at a distance from the affected area, but the distorted structures are not injured themselves).[13] As the wound heals, collagen fibers are deposited to bridge the wound, forming an immature (active) scar.[14–16] Extensive study with well-defined, randomized controlled trials is lacking in understanding hypertrophic scar development in part because of the limited consensus on an adequate animal model of abnormal scarring.[8] However, progress continues to be made in understanding and potentially unlocking the scar development cascade, including the signal mediator transforming growth factor β, the overproduction of extracellular matrix, and keratinocyte signal expression research.[17–19]

Scar Assessment

It is critically important for a burn rehabilitation specialist to assess the burn scar carefully before initiating

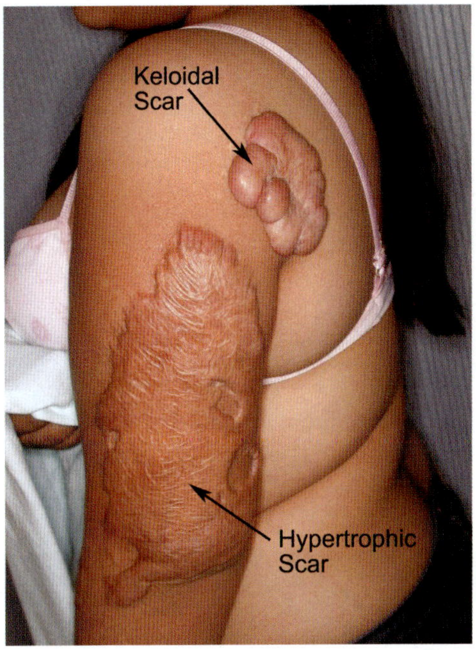

FIGURE 19-1 Hypertrophic scar and keloid scar.

management (see Chapter 28). Burn scar assessment, even though time consuming, is vital in the rehabilitative process as it relates to functional and cosmetic outcomes. Several scar assessment tools and scales have been developed to quantify the burn scar and can be used to determine the effectiveness of scar management protocols and track outcomes in rehabilitation. Some of these scar assessment devices are objective (provide quantitative measurements of scar parameters/characteristics) and some are more subjective (provide qualitative measurement of the scar and are observer dependent). Individual tools designed to assess the burn scar specifically address various scar parameters including pliability (Pneumatonometer,[20,21] Cutometer,[22,23] Tonometer,[24,25] and Extensometer[26]), firmness (Durometer[27]), color (Chromameter, DermaSpectrometer, Mexameter, and Colorimeter[28]), thickness (Ultrasound scanners[23,29-31]), tissue perfusion (Laser Doppler imaging [LDI][32–35]), and three-dimensional topography.[32,36,37] These tools are considered more objective in assessing the burn scar, although their validity and reliability in assessing all scar types have been questioned.

Several scar assessment scales have been developed to provide a more comprehensive way to assess the burn scar. The Vancouver Burn Scar Assessment (VBSA) developed by Sullivan et al.[38] in the 1990s is currently the most frequently utilized burn scar assessment scale, even though it was originally developed over 25 years ago. The VBSA subjectively assesses physical scar parameters that relate to the healing and maturation of scars. These include scar pigmentation, vascularity, pliability, and height.[39] Through the years other authors have attempted to improve upon the original VBSA, with some success highlighted in the publications of Baryza and Nedelec.[40–42] The VBSA is considered to be subjective and it is utilized to track the maturation progress of small linear scars within an individual, rather than between individuals. Other prominent scar assessment scales include the Patient and Observer Scar Assessment (POSAS) and the Manchester Scar Scale (MSS). Fearmonti et al.[43] have described and compared various scar scales and individual scar assessment tools highlighting their limitations. To date, a comprehensive, reliable, and valid burn scar assessment that looks into all scar parameters relevant to burn rehabilitation remains elusive.[44] Individual scar assessment tools that assess single scar parameters may in some cases show some validity and reliability. However, they are generally expensive and their use in burn rehabilitation is often impractical.[43,45]

Rehabilitative Management of Scars

Despite significant improvements in medicine in recent years, hypertrophic scars remain very problematic and are difficult to manage. Improvements in medical life-saving procedures have improved the survivability of extensive total body surface area (TBSA) burns, so it is imperative that rehabilitative techniques also advance to achieve optimal functional and aesthetic outcomes. To that extent, it is imperative that scar management should be a continual process that is reviewed during every aspect of wound maturation. The best treatment for scars is to prevent their appearance, so vigilance is key. Even though the mechanism of scar maturation is not yet fully understood, clinically most rehabilitation specialists treat hypertrophic scars through combinations of the following modalities—pressure therapy, exercise/range of motion (ROM), inserts, splints, massage, heat modalities, and silicones.

Pressure Garment Therapy

Pressure therapy has long been utilized to manage scars that are red, thick, and elevated and are widespread in nature. Pressure therapy, which should be instituted early on in the burn scar maturation process, is by far the most widely used and recognized modality. Means of pressure therapy include pressure garments, inserts, and conforming orthotics. The first medical reference to describe the use of pressure for the treatment of immature scars was written by Johnson in 1678 referencing the work of Ambroise Paré in the 16th century.[2] Other important historical events described by Linares include the use of elastic bandages in 1860, pressure provided by plaster casting in 1881, and the use of traction to treat scars in 1902. Linares' historical review also includes descriptions of Nason's work in 1942 in which he observed that pressure exerted onto the injured skin by undergarment elastic produced ischemia, which in turn stopped the overproduction of scar tissue.[2,46]

The use of pressure in effectively depressing scars was well documented by Silverstein and Larson in the 1970s; their observations and studies led to the development of pressure garments that today appear to be the "gold standard" in managing developing scars. When an active scar is compressed it blanches, which indicates decreased blood flow in the area.[47] Although the mechanism of action of pressure garments has not been fully elucidated, it has been hypothesized that less blood leads to decreased oxygenation in the tissues, which in turns leads to decreased collagen production, establishing a balance between collagen synthesis and collagen breakdown (lysis). When a balance in the production and breakdown of collagen is reached, the resultant scar appears flatter.[48] Kealey et al.[49] conducted a prospective randomized study to investigate the efficacy of pressure garments in patients who survived burn injuries. In this study, patients were randomly assigned to receive either pressure garments or no pressure garments. Assessment of scar maturity included use of the VBSA. The results of this study revealed no significant differences between the two groups when age, body surface area burned, length of hospital stay, or time to wound maturation were compared. Other studies have reported problems related to lack of adherence due to the application schedule, discomfort, blistering, ulceration or scar breakdown, swelling of extremities, and skeletal and dental deformity due to excessive pressures. These issues can lead to significant side effects, poor compliance, and even permanent deformity.[46,47,49–54]

On the other hand, studies have also reported the benefits of pressure garments.[55–57] Several excellent reviews on the efficacy, or lack of efficacy, of pressure garments in the management of hypertrophic burn scars have appeared recently in the literature.[58,59] One reason for the absence of strong, undisputed evidence in the efficacy of pressure garments is that garments must be worn continuously for at least 23 hours a day, making adherence difficult to measure.[2,52,59] Furthermore, the optimal therapeutic pressure required to depress hypertrophic scars is not yet known.[52,60–62] The debate regarding the effectiveness of pressure garments continues to this date. Until more definitive evidence is gathered to support the use of pressure garments or prove them ineffective in managing scars, pressure therapy in the form of elastic garments will continue to be a standard component of scar management. It should be noted that all pressure garment studies conducted thus far do not include the examination of burns over joints, nor do they include burns of the hands, neck, and face. It would be unethical to withhold pressure treatment on a patient's face or the other body surfaces mentioned above just to confirm if pressure works or not.[46]

As long as the scars are active they may be influenced by pressure therapy. However, not all burn scars require pressure. Patients with burn wounds that heal within 7 to 14 days frequently do not need pressure therapy. Those patients whose wounds heal within 14 to 21 days are closely monitored for pressure therapy needs, and may be advised to use pressure garments prophylactically. A wound that heals after 21 days will generally require the use of pressure garments.[48] The correct amount of pressure required to suppress hypertrophic scar formation has not yet been determined. Pressure of as little as 10 mm Hg may be effective in remodeling the scar tissue over time. Pressures over 40 mm Hg, however, may be destructive to tissues and cause paresthesias.[47] Traditional forms of pressure therapy include the use of elastic bandages directly applied on the newly healed skin, or on top of the burn dressings. The use of conforming thermoplastics along with elastic bandages (Fig. 19-2) may also be utilized as means of early pressure therapy.[63] Once the wounds are almost or completely closed, tubular elastic bandages such as Tubigrip (Mölnlycke Health Care, Göteborg, Sweden) may be utilized. These tubular elastic bandages are offered in different sizes and accommodate all anatomical circumferences (Fig. 19-3). Care should be taken in applying these tubular bandages

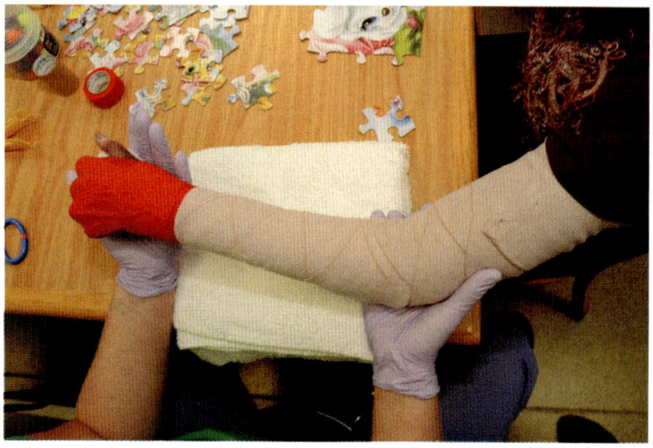

FIGURE 19-2 Elastic bandage provides approximately 10 to 12 mm Hg pressure.

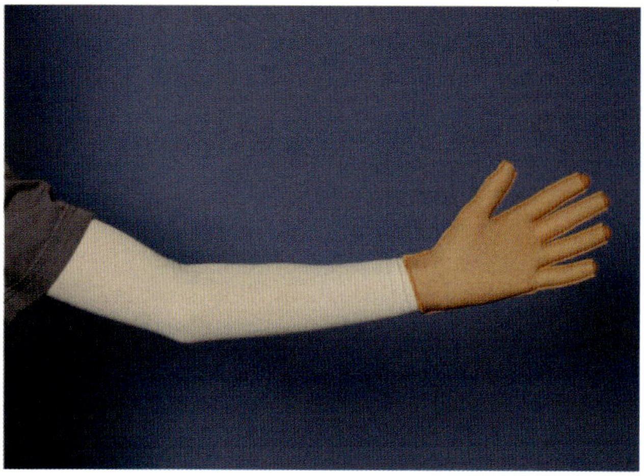

FIGURE 19-3 Tubular elastic bandage (Tubigrip) provides approximately 15 to 17 mm Hg pressure.

so that the fragile skin or the freshly applied skin grafts do not sheer, or the minimal dressing underneath is not disturbed. The burn therapist should be aware that these tubular bandages are materials made of a single elastic thread spiraling through the weave of the fabric, and disturbance of the continuous elastic by cutting holes into it will alter the pressure gradient provided by these materials. The tubular elastic bandages should be doubled over the skin surface area treated in order to provide adequate pressure.[46,64]

Early pressure application over the hand and digits can be accomplished by the use of thin, elastic, and self-adherent wraps such as Coban (3M, St. Paul, Minnesota) (Fig. 19-4). This form of pressure is excellent for adult and pediatric patients for controlling edema and aids in the early scar management of hands when the shearing forces of a glove cannot be tolerated. Small children are excellent candidates for Coban gloves versus a garment glove because of compliance issues, comprehension of instructions in assisting with the application of a custom glove, and difficulties in obtaining accurate measurements for a custom glove. Coban may be applied over the burn dressings or directly onto the healed digits. The burn therapist needs to be aware that if Coban is wrapped too tightly it may

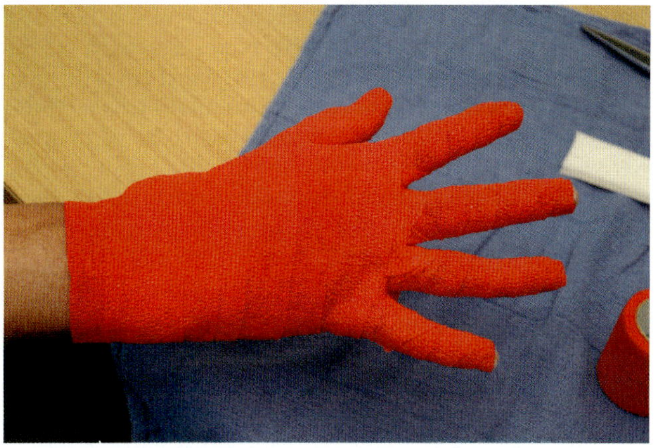

FIGURE 19-4 Self-adherent wrap (Coban) provides approximately 10 mm Hg pressure if not stretched.

deform the interosseous structures of the healing hand. However, if Coban is wrapped too loosely it may encourage swelling of the hands when used in combination with arm elastic garments.

To apply, Coban strips are precut approximately twice the length of the digits to be wrapped. Each strip is wrapped in a spiral fashion beginning at the nail bed of each digit, overlapping half of the Coban width and ending in the adjacent web space. Each fingertip needs to be exposed so that blood circulation can be monitored at all times. The Coban is stretched from 0% to 25% of the entire elasticity of each strip. Once all web spaces are covered, the rest of the hand is wrapped with Coban, extending approximately 1 inch past the wrist joint. No skin areas should be visible once the Coban glove is completed. If small hand areas remain uncovered, a small piece of Coban is stretched over the area and adheres to the rest of the Coban. When the glove is completed, the therapist should very superficially lubricate the entire glove with lotion in order to eliminate the adherent effect of the Coban and allow for the functional use of the hand. Coban should be removed on a daily basis by the therapist or the caregiver. Removal of Coban should be done carefully by cutting off or unwrapping each digit strip individually to avoid disturbing any small wound healing.[46]

The use of prefabricated interim pressure garments is widely accepted and utilized in burn rehabilitation (Fig. 19-5). These garments are available commercially by different companies and they include pieces for the entire body. Interim garments are made of softer materials and introduce the burn patient to circumferential pressure, as well as protect the newly healed skin. Another reason for using these garments prior to ordering custom-made garments is to allow for the patient's weight to stabilize (postacute hospitalization) and any remaining edema to subside. In some cases where obtaining custom-made garments on regular intervals (approximately 12 weeks) is not an option, interim garments should be the choice for long-term pressure therapy. Once the patient's weight has stabilized, edema has subsided, and the skin is able to withstand some shearing (approximately 3 to 4 weeks postwound closure), measurements are taken for the fabrication of custom-made pressure garments (Fig. 19-6). Today several companies specialize in the fabrication of these garments. Clinically, custom therapeutic pressure for the prevention, control, and correction of scar hypertrophy averages 24 to 28 mm Hg, which is approximately equal and opposing to the capillary pressure (25 mm Hg). At this pressure level, many researchers believe that scars may be altered.[46,65] In order for pressure therapy to be effective, pressure garments need to be worn at all times, day and night. They should only be removed for bathing and on occasion during exercises should they interfere with movements. Today, pressure garment companies offer multiple colors and patterns of materials. For the pediatric population, cartoon characters may be sewed on the garments to make them cosmetically appealing and improve the patients' compliance.[66] The use of facial pressure garments in children has been previously questioned as it may interfere with growth.[67,68] The authors recommend that these patients should be closely monitored for normal facial and dental development by physicians, including dental specialists.

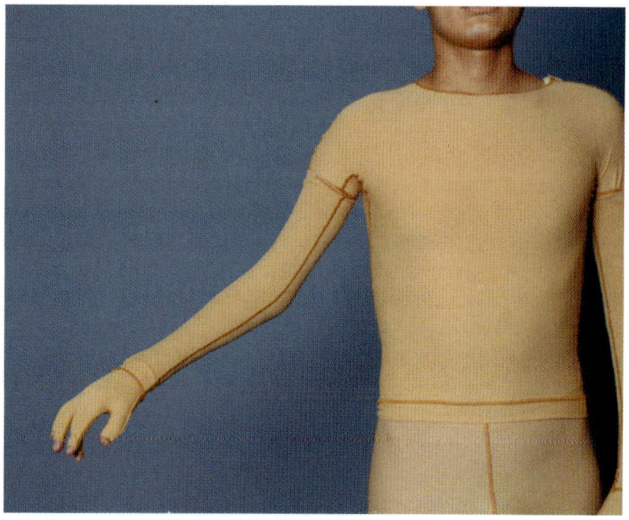

FIGURE 19-5 Interim garments provide approximately 15 to 20 mm Hg pressure.

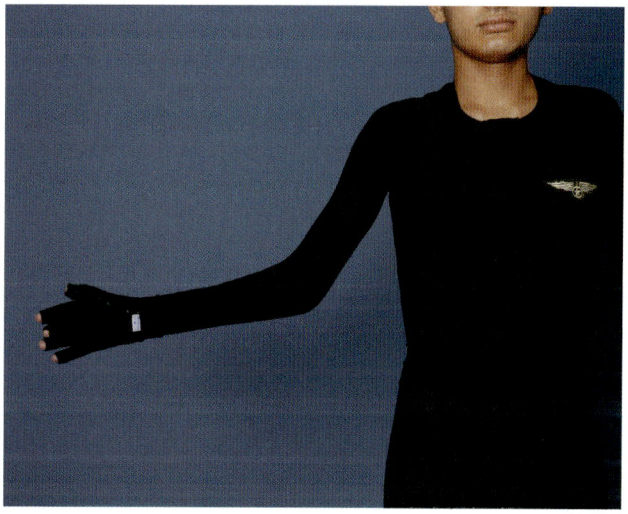

FIGURE 19-6 Custom garments provide approximately 24 to 28 mm Hg pressure.

Inserts

Inserts are various materials utilized in burn rehabilitation as an adjunct to achieving effective pressure over certain anatomical locations where it is difficult to achieve pressure with garments alone. These locations include concave body areas such as the face, neck, antecubital fossa, sternum, palm, web spaces, upper back, and arches of the feet. Laplace's law of pressure distribution guides the clinician in the application of these inserts, where pressure = tension divided by the radius of curvature. Concave areas areas have a high radius of curvature and convex surfaces have a low radius of curvature. (This equation is represented in its simplest form as $P=T/r$.) These materials come commercially prefabricated or may be custom-made by the burn therapist. Inserts come in different forms such as silicone gels, elastomers, putties mixed with a silicone catalyst, skin care silastic pads, foam, and even hard thermoplastic materials contouring to different anatomical locations. The first published use of an insert to manage contractures occurring within the web spaces of the hand was described by Quan et al.[69] The experienced burn therapist chooses the appropriate insert material best suited for the patient according to the stage of scar maturation and skin sensitivity. Generally, the initial insert is soft, thin, and elastic; later iterations may be more rigid to depress the restrictive and unyielding burn scar. Moreover, the choice of insert needs to be flexible enough to allow for joint mobility yet be rigid enough to resist the scar impacting skin surface.

Inserts need to be worn underneath pressure garments starting within a few hours of application and progressing, as tolerated, toward a 24-hour application. They should be removed frequently for cleaning (with warm water and soap), drying, and application of cornstarch to avoid maceration and skin breakdown. Patients may be allergic to certain insert materials, so the burn therapist may try different inserts until one is found to be best tolerated. In cases of scar maceration, blisters, skin breakdown, and a rash or contact dermatitis, inserts should be removed until healing occurs. Silicone, a polymer based on the element silicon, is the most widely used insert in the treatment of hypertrophic scars (Fig. 19-7). To date, the mechanism of how silicone affects the burn scar is not known. Recent investigations describe a cascade of action in the epidermal signaling mechanism, in which occlusion causes a decrease in transepidermal water loss. This serves to normalize the hydration state of the keratinocytes, which may in turn signal dermal fibroblasts to downregulate extracellular matrix production.[6,70] Clinically, silicone has been observed to hydrate the burn scar, depress the height of hypertrophic scars, prevent shrinking of fresh skin grafts, and increase the pliability of a scar, thus allowing for increases in the ROM of affected joints or affected skin creases.[46,71,72] Silicone gel and gel sheets are recommended to be used on immature scars that develop from wounds that take greater than 21 days to heal.[73] Moreover, silicone can soften the scar and improve the elasticity of the scar without pressure. However, the preferred use is in combination with pressure, especially in cases of widespread burn scarring. Patients often report that silicone is soothing to the scar and aids in pain relief. Silicone, being occlusive, may cause the collection of excessive moisture and cause skin maceration if not removed at least daily for cleaning and drying.

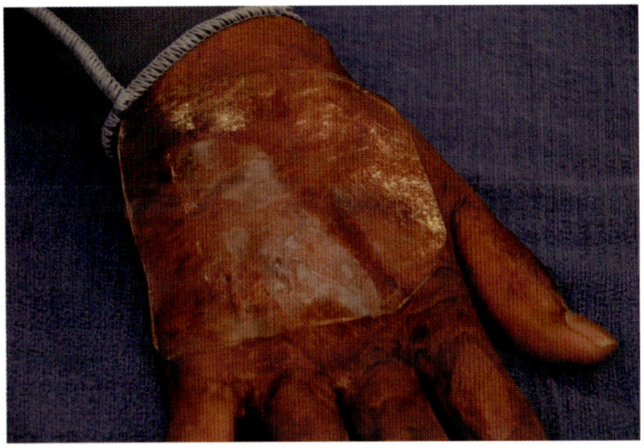

FIGURE 19-7 Clear silicone gel.

Other insert materials include liquid silicone elastomer, which when mixed with a catalyst forms a solid but elastic insert (Fig. 19-8), and various gel materials such as Medigel Z (Medical Z, Houston, Texas). The experienced therapist can create custom inserts for difficult anatomical locations such as the face and web spaces using this technique. Prosthetic Foam is a liquid-based silicone elastomer which, when mixed with a catalyst, solidifies in the form of a very pliable foam insert that works best for the palm of the hands where function needs to be preserved while pressure is applied. These foam inserts also work best for applying pressure to contoured surfaces on the face (around eyes, mouth, and nose), while protecting these sensitive areas from excessive and rigid pressure. Elastomer putties such as Otoform K/C (AliMed, Dedham, Massachusetts) or Rolyan Ezemix (Patterson Medical, Warrenville, Illinois) form semirigid but still elastic inserts (Fig. 19-9) for different areas of the body where the scar can tolerate more pressure, such as in the web spaces to prevent syndactyly.[74] Early on in scar management, a soft foam may be utilized to apply gentle pressure to the very fragile and sensitive scar tissue (Fig. 19-10).[46,74]

Burn Scar Massage

Deep partial or full-thickness burn wounds, once closed, may begin to develop scars that are red, firm, and painful. These scars begin to contract and, if they cross a joint, may cause limitations in ROM. Massage is an accepted modality in burn rehabilitation despite the fact that its benefits in scar management have not yet been fully validated. Anecdotal reports from burn rehabilitation specialists indicate that massage helps soften the burn scar and promotes tissue elasticity and extensibility. In 1999, Serghiou et al.[75] reported that massage was utilized by 96% of burn rehabilitation specialists in daily practice. In 2011, Holavanahalli et al.[76] reported that massage is included in standard burn rehabilitation protocols. Burn scar massage may be initiated by the rehabilitation therapist in an attempt to reverse contractile forces, help accelerate the scar maturation process, and maintain joint mobility. Scar massage may help soften and remodel scar tissues by freeing adherent fibrous bands, thus aiding

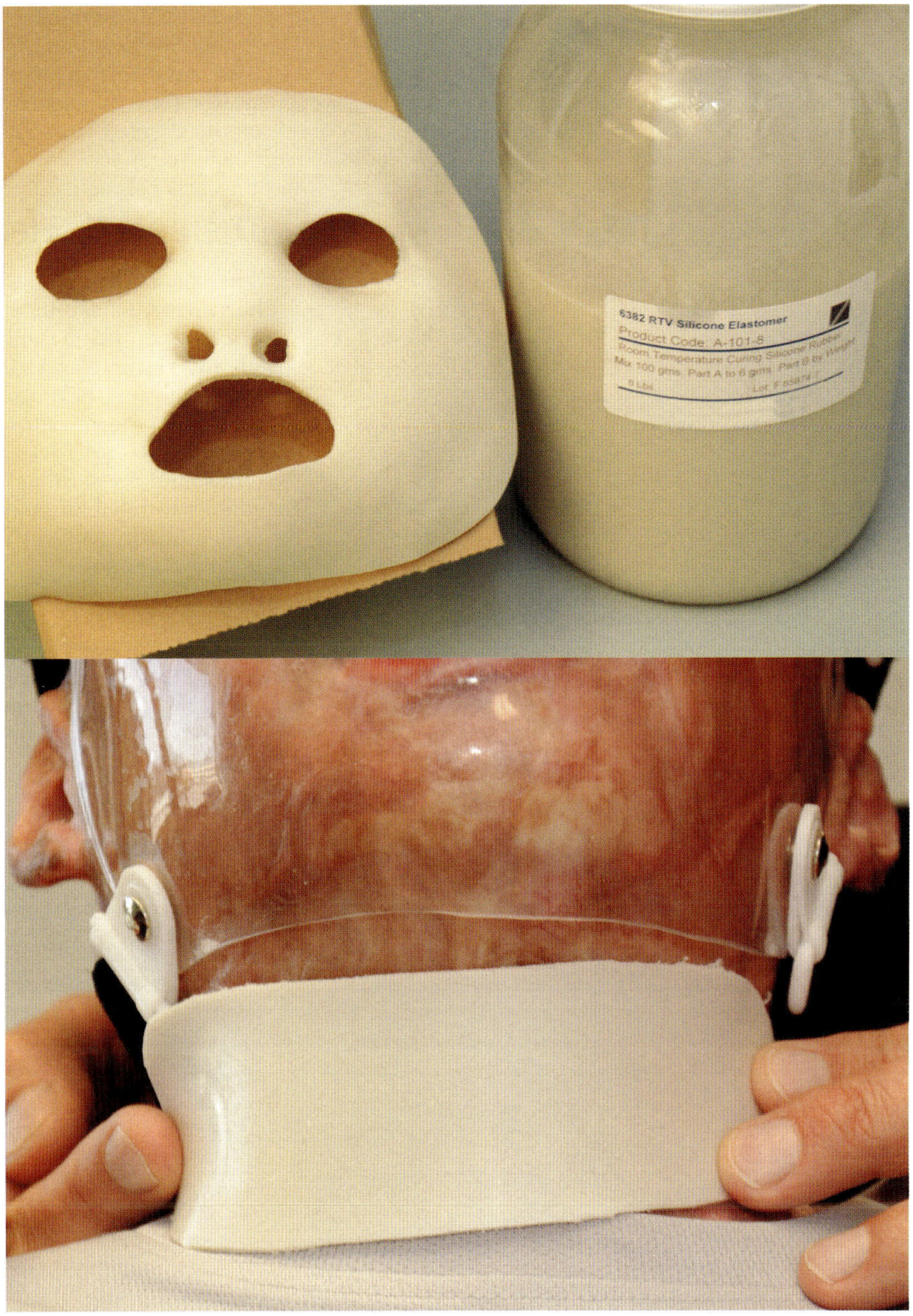

FIGURE 19-8 Silicone elastomer insert. Liquid silicone elastomer can become a semirigid insert when mixed with a silicone-based catalyst.

scar tissue in becoming more elastic and stretchy. Burn scar massage is initiated judiciously by the rehabilitation specialist who is well aware of the stages in the scar maturation process.[77]

Initially, massage applied to the fresh, painful, and fragile scar is described as gentle, stationary, and "nonfrictional." Pressure is applied to the skin until it blanches, and while pressure is exerted onto the scar, the surface area is mobilized without friction. No lubricants are utilized at this time as friction that may break down the fragile scar is avoided. As the scar matures and is able to tolerate some frictional forces, the tissue can be manipulated in rotary, parallel, and perpendicular motions, using a lubricant and applying pressure onto the skin until it blanches. As the scar progresses toward maturation, the therapist may apply progressively greater force and manipulation.[46] Clinically, massage has been found to alleviate pain and itching[78] and has also been reported to help alleviate anxiety and depression.[79] Patients and caregivers should be trained on how to perform massage and are instructed by rehabilitation specialists on how to perform it safely. Even though the exact frequency and duration of burn scar massage have not yet been scientifically determined, many therapists recommend that it should be performed three to five times daily for 5 to 10 minutes on each treated body surface area. A frequent skin assessment should be performed by

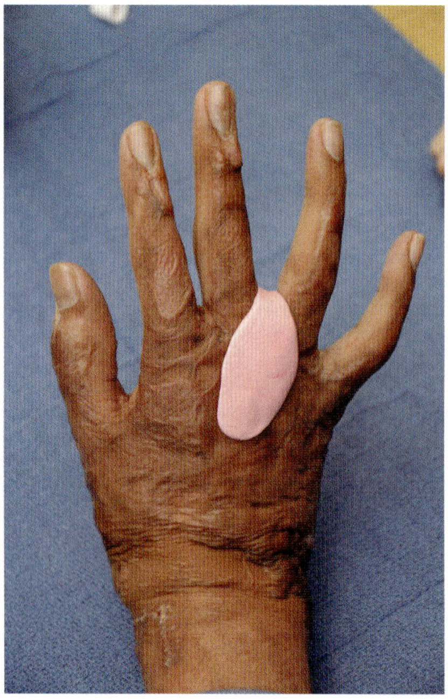

FIGURE 19-9 Silicone-based putty (Otoform K). Putty that is mixed with a silicone-based paste becomes a semirigid silicone insert.

rehabilitation specialists to ensure that the scar is mature enough to withstand pressure and friction exerted upon it. Patients and caregivers should be instructed by professionals when it is appropriate to apply more force and friction on the affected areas.[46,80]

Therapeutic Heat Modalities

Therapeutic heat is the most common modality used in burn scar management.[81] The application of heat may promote scar tissue manipulation through increased extensibility.[82] Heat relaxes tissues and makes them more pliable in preparation for mobilization, and in addition provides temporary moisture to the scar surface. Heat modalities may include hot packs, paraffin wax, fluidotherapy, and ultrasound. Even though the use of therapeutic heat as an adjunct to rehabilitation is well documented, therapeutic heat modalities are infrequently being utilized in burn rehabilitation.[83,84]

Caution should be used in the application of heat modalities on patients who have sustained a burn injury, and patients may not be able to tolerate excessive heat over areas of healed or grafted burns because of hypersensitivity.

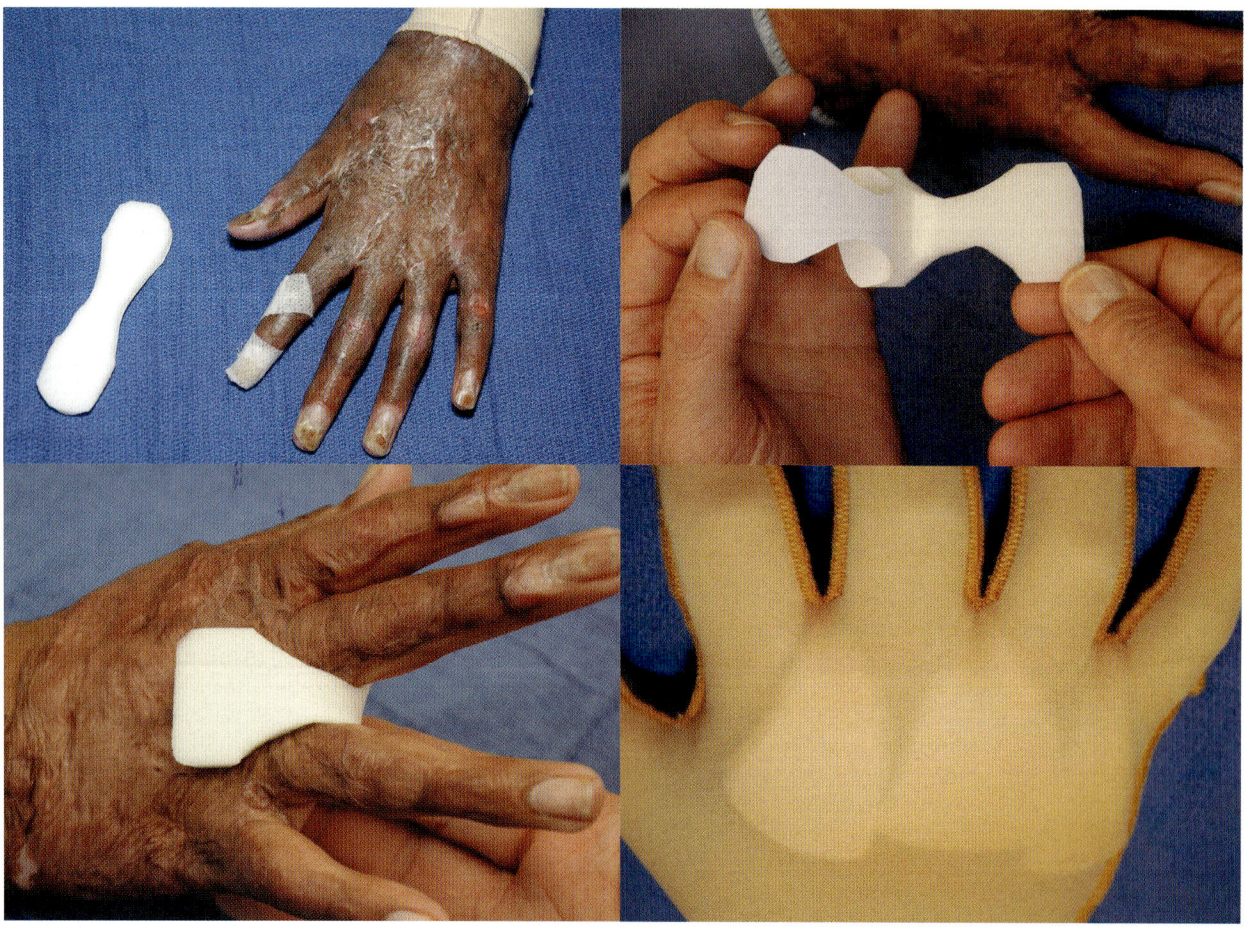

FIGURE 19-10 Silicone-lined foam (Oleeva Foam).

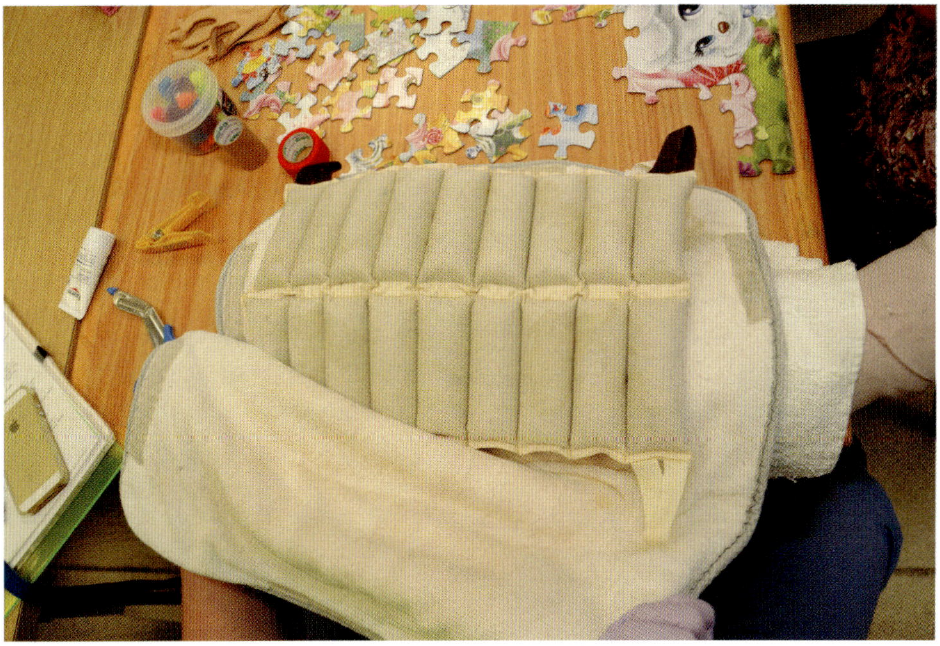

FIGURE 19-11 Hot packs help warm tissues prior to stretching and manipulation.

The temperature of paraffin wax is lessened overall in comparison to routine use (46°C to 50°C/114°F to 122°F). Conversely, patients with diminished sensation may be unable to determine if the temperature is appropriate and are at risk for further thermal injury. Although caution needs to be exercised, the use of therapeutic heat in burn patients can provide an effective method of increasing burn scar extensibility. Studies have shown that the use of therapeutic heat during a low-load prolonged stretch is an effective method for attaining rapid and lasting increases in ROM when compared to stretch alone.[85] Warren et al.[86] reported that low loads of stretch for prolonged periods of time were found to produce significantly greater residual length in rat tail tendon, especially at elevated temperatures.

Hot packs can provide superficial heat to burn scars and assist with stretching contractures. Common treatments in burn rehabilitation include the use of hot packs alone before treatment, or in conjunction with therapeutic exercise such as active ROM or prolonged stretch. Because of the shallow depth of heat penetration, hot packs may have little effect on deeper layers of scar tissue (Fig. 19-11).[82] Ultrasound has been used by rehabilitation therapists to increase temperatures within deeper tissues. Reported benefits of ultrasound in the treatment of burn scars include increased extensibility of collagen, increased blood flow, and elevation of pain thresholds[82,87] (Fig. 19-12). The combination of ultrasound and passive stretch was found to further increase tissue elongation.[82]

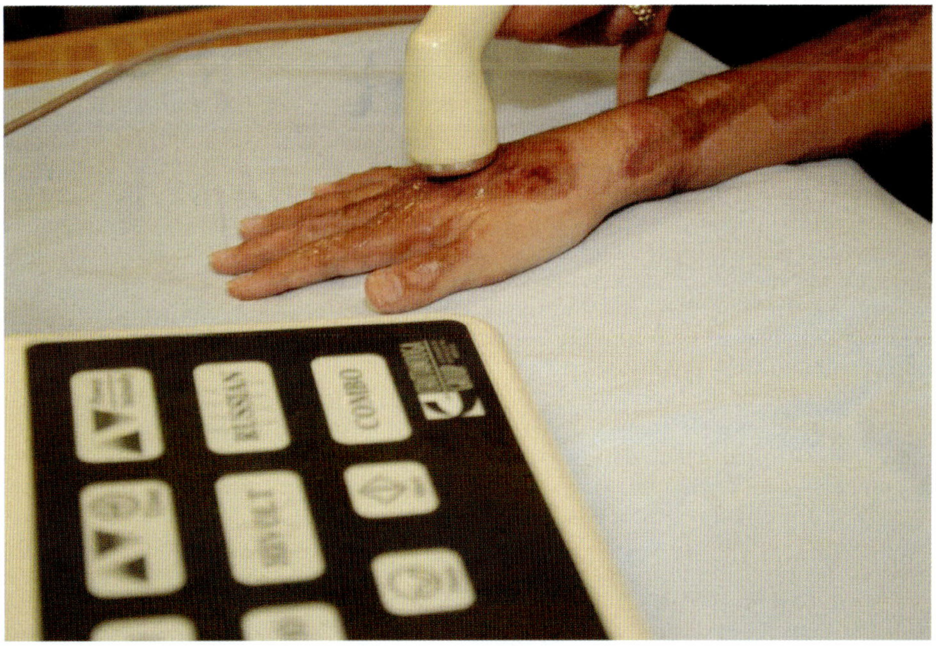

FIGURE 19-12 Ultrasound is an adjunctive modality utilized in scar management.

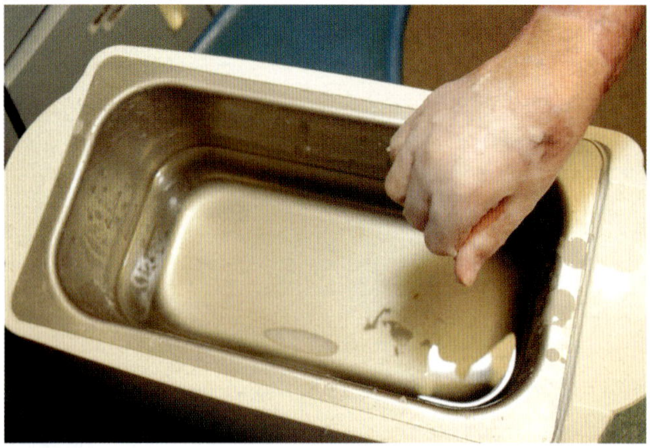

FIGURE 19-13 Paraffin wax helps warm tissues prior to stretching and manipulation.

Paraffin is an effective heat modality used most commonly for the hands or feet (Fig. 19-13). Paraffin appears to enhance the extensibility of the collagen through the associated heat, and may also be beneficial because of the softening of the scar by the mineral oil in the paraffin.[82] The use of passive stretch in conjunction with paraffin has been shown to increase joint ROM, and was found to make patient's skin noticeably softer and more pliable after use.[88] Similar to other heating modalities, paraffin has been found to increase ROM in conjunction with stretching compared to stretching alone.[89]

Orthotics/Splints

Objectives when fabricating splints and orthotics for burn patients include the prevention of scar contracture deformity, the preservation of ROM achieved in therapy or through surgical release of a contracture, and the protection of tenuous joints and other delicate structures such as tendons, vessels, nerves, skin grafts, and flaps.[90] The decision to create an orthotic for a patient with a scar contracture is based on the patient's age, level of cooperation, and three aspects particular to the burn injury itself. These include: (1) the severity of the patient's injury, (2) the patient's point of recovery in regard to the phases of wound healing, and (3) the different biomechanical principles that are associated with the rehabilitation strategy of orthotic application.[39,90] As burn survival rates have exponentially improved, the ability of the burn therapist to accurately and precisely identify the correct orthotic plan, particularly for injures involving the hand and upper extremity, is a critical rehabilitative goal to support optimal functional return and improved quality of life.[39,91,92]

The location of the burn injury is of concern, particularly if it involves skin creases overlying or adjacent to joint areas.[39] In particular skin recruitment, represented as cutaneous functional units (CFUs), contributes to the motion of specific joints prone to burn scar contracture formation. A CFU involves a field of skin that extends well beyond the near proximity of the joint itself, and utilizes up to 80% (on average) of available skin to produce specific ROM. Recent research from the work of Richard et al.[93,94] has shown that clinically CFUs are an objective measure used to substantiate patient acuity and rehabilitation staffing levels, and in the development of rehabilitation treatment plans. Additionally, this research has shown that providing increased rehabilitation time based on CFUs rather than TBSA suggested better patient outcomes for both small burns $\leq$10% (P = 0.002) and large burns >10% (P < 0.0001) (Fig. 19-14). A further consideration related to burn scar location is when the injury involves skin creases over multiple, consecutive joints. Previous work has shown that the position of an adjacent joint has an influence on skin excursion at the next joint in the series, and therapists need to consider orthotic designs that incorporate all areas of involvement.[95,96] In particular to the total hand burn, special consideration must be paid to both the first and fifth digits. Dynamic pulling forces of developing scar tissue and the multiple planes of motion within each of these digits can create significant long-term complications if not continuously monitored with precise orthotic management and carefully guided rehabilitation.[97]

A common concern regarding the fabrication of an orthosis is whether they can be used over fresh skin grafts. Generally, the area that has received a skin graft is heavily padded with dressings to absorb wound drainage and provide protection. Orthoses can be applied safely over skin grafts, particularly if the intent is to immobilize the area of injury until adherence of the graft to the wound bed is evident.[98,99] Caution should be used to avoid sheer and/or compressive stress on any grafted site. Often an orthosis may not be used because the bulk of the postoperative dressings alone can act as a block to prevent excessive joint motion. The optimal amount of time that an orthosis should be worn has yet to be determined.[39] Each patient presents a unique clinical scenario and should therefore be approached individually. Initially, adults and children should wear splints at night and, for children, during naps. Depending on the area of the body involved and the depth of injury, uncooperative patients may need to use an orthosis continuously until they are able to actively participate in the therapy regime. These patients are at high risk for developing contractures and demand a therapist's attention in regard to proper positioning, orthotic use, and exercise.

A key burn therapist axiom is: *the position of comfort is the position of contracture*—continuous and vigilant monitoring of the burn treatment intervention will help to achieve long-lasting functional recovery and positive outcomes.[97] Orthotics and splints can assume many types and forms depending on the area of the burn injury and the type and depth of the contracture. In most instances for scars impacting any part of the body below the neckline, low-temperature thermoplastics can be utilized to fabricate an orthotic/splint based on a pattern of the patient's specific body part. For other scars involving the face and neck, a high-temperature transparent thermoplastic is used to create a detailed replica of the face that is most aesthetically and functionally relevant. High-thermoplastic transparent masks were developed in 1968 by Padewski to be applied directly to the face to prevent, control, and reverse scar hypertrophy. These masks require the moulaging of the patient to create a negative facial mold—this is a technique of applying an impression material such as dental alginate or plaster to capture a copy of a patient's

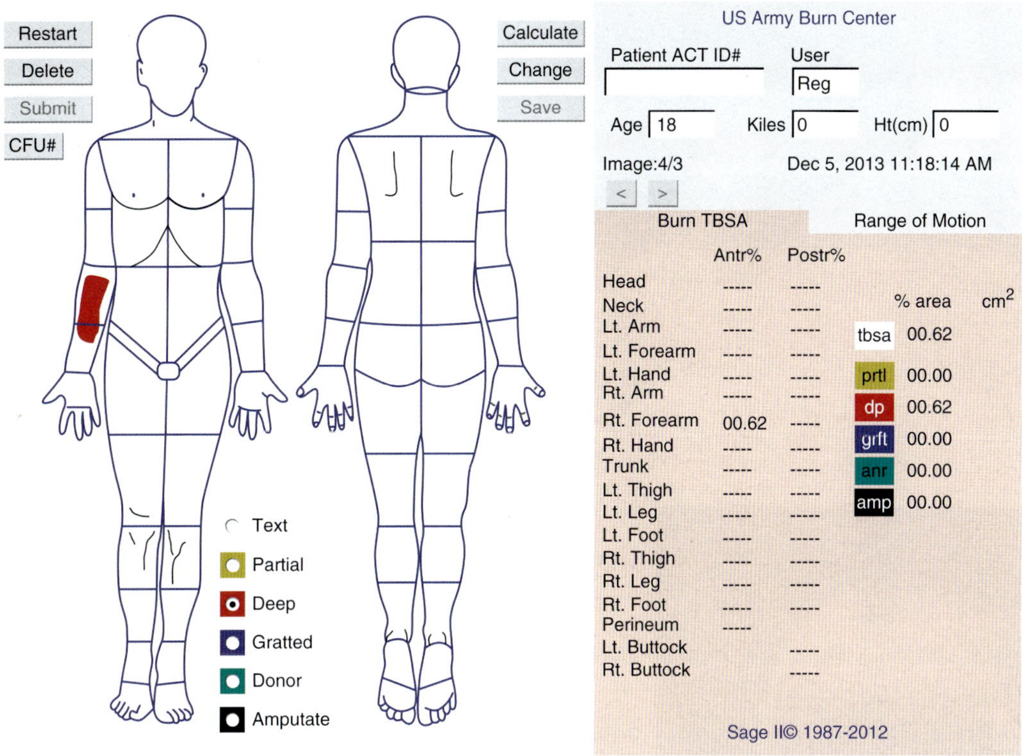

Burn Surface Areas %`s:

% TBSA	% Partial	% Deep	% Grafted	% Donor	% Amputated
0.62	0.00	0.62	0.00	0.00	0.00

CFU Area Affected %`s:

CFU#	% TBSA	% Partial	% Deep	% Grafted	% Donor	% Amputated
042000	22.32%	0.00%	22.32%	0.00%	0.00%	0.00%
042100	40.82%	0.00%	40.82%	0.00%	0.00%	0.00%
042110	24.09%	0.00%	24.09%	0.00%	0.00%	0.00%
042120	52.43%	0.00%	52.43%	0.00%	0.00%	0.00%

Legend for Numeric SAGE/CFU % TBSA

042000 = Entire anterior surface of right upper extremity
042100 = Surface of anterior right forearm alone
042110 = Anterior surface of distal right forearm CFU segment
042120 = Anterior surface of proximal right forearm CFU segment

FIGURE 19-14 Example of surface area graphic evaluation/cutaneous functional unit (SAGE/CFU) burn TBSA calculation. This is a computerized model to help determine the percentage burn within a burn body diagram based on cutaneous functional units (CFU). (*Adapted from Richard R, Jones JA, Parshley P. Hierarchical decomposition of burn body diagram based on cutaneous functional units and its utility. J Burn Care Res 2015;36:33–43.*)

face or neck (Fig. 19-15A). A positive mold of the face is then fabricated with the use of liquid plaster that is poured into the negative mold and allowed to harden prior to sculpting (Fig. 19-15B). The patient's positive facial mold is then "sculptured" in an attempt to recreate the patient's nonburned face. A high-thermoplastic material such as Uvex or W-Clear is then pulled over the positive mold in order to create the hard plastic mask. Holes for the eyes, nose, and mouth are then cut. The mask is worn under pressure garments or with an elastic strapping mechanism that provides the necessary tension to aid in decreasing scar hypertrophy (Fig. 19-15C).

Three-dimensional scanners can also be used to replace the traditional methods of face mask fabrication. Using a scanner greatly reduces patient anxiety by achieving the same accuracy as moulaging, in a fraction of the time, without physically touching the patient's face (Fig. 19-16). The scan is "sculptured" on a computer and a positive tool is manufactured out of foam off-site. The positive tool is then sent to the facility for mask fabrication. In the past, scanners were so large that facilities had to have an entire room dedicated to its use. Now they are typically small enough to fit in a portable case and are run by laptops. These newer portable scanners enable a therapist the freedom to scan patients in any setting in the hospital, including intraoperatively. In cases of significant scar hypertrophy on the face, the positive mold is "sculptured" sequentially over a period of time in order to avoid excessive pressure

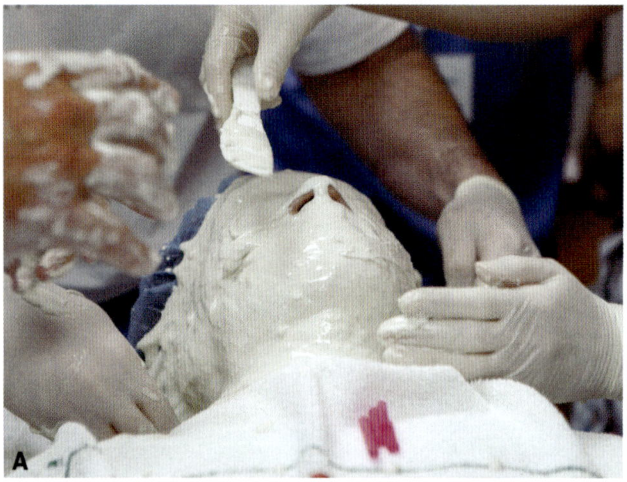

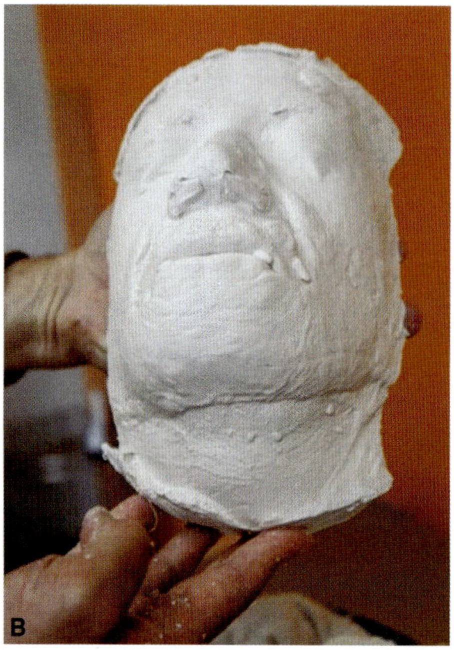

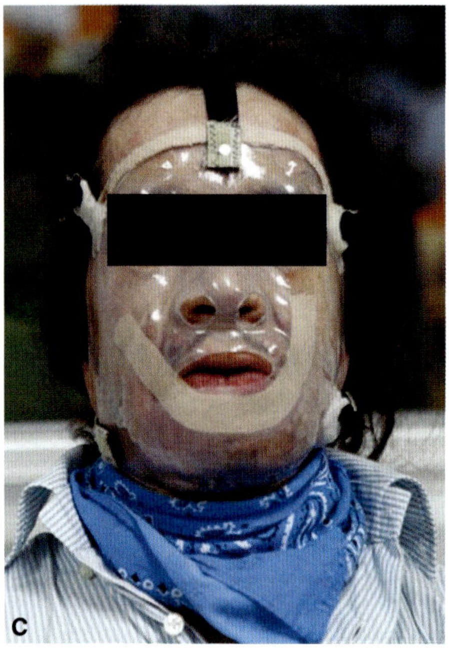

FIGURE 19-15 **A:** Negative mold fabricated utilizing dental alginate or plaster strips. **B:** Positive mold constructed out of plaster of Paris. **C:** Completed mask.

over facial scars leading to skin breakdown. A silicone elastomer face mask may be created utilizing an existing positive facial mold or by fabricating a gel mask out of large pieces of silicone or other gel materials. These soft masks are worn under facial pressure garments (Fig. 19-17). The use of the clear and silastic masks is preferred over the use of a facial garment alone as they provide conforming pressure around facial openings (eyes, nose, and mouth). Frequently, the burn therapist manufactures a clear mask to be worn during the day and the silastic mask (along with the facial garment) to be worn at night.[2,100–102] Recent research has shown that coupling silicone with the high-temperature thermoplastic produces the most effective results. Alley et al.[103] studied the effect of high-temperature silicone-lined thermoplastic face masks utilizing laser Doppler imaging to measure active superficial blood flow on the surface of the face. They demonstrated not only improved contact to the skin, but reduced blood flow measures. This research was extended further to examine the effects of wear times on blood flow after removal of these devices. It was found that after removal of a silicone-lined thermoplastic mask, approximately 30 minutes was needed for the superficial blood flow to return to baseline values as compared to the use of unlined masks.[104]

Implementing a Scar Rehabilitation Program

The management of burn scar hypertrophy includes many nonsurgical rehabilitative treatment options applied throughout the spectrum of recovery. Early and aggressive treatment may have a significant influence on ultimate scar outcome.[105,106] A combination of treatment options should be used depending on the resources available to the clinician. A scar mitigation regimen includes daily, aggressive, and continuous therapeutic interventions such as positioning, splinting, ROM exercises, scar band stretching, functional mobility, and participation in activities of daily

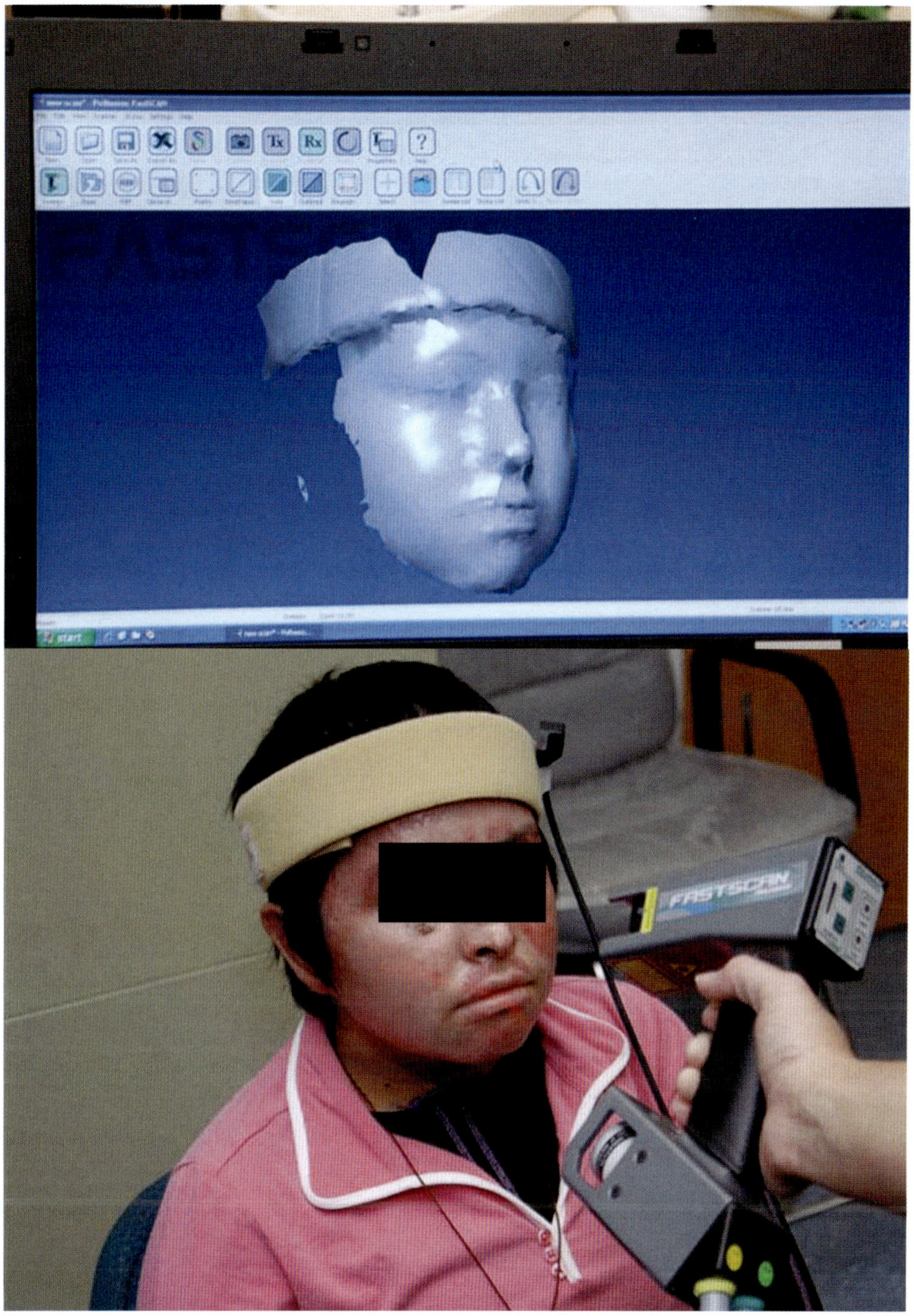

FIGURE 19-16 Scanner. (*Adapted from Parry I, Hanley C, Niszczak J, Sen S, Palmieri T, Greenhalgh D. Harnessing the transparent face orthosis for facial scar management: A comparison of methods. Burns. 2013;39:950–956.*)

living (ADLs). It is imperative that the burn rehabilitation specialist be involved in the care of the burn patient as soon as possible to ensure that these techniques are employed without prejudice and with the best intention of returning the patient to the preburn level of function by mitigating scar contracture complications. Use of casts or splints should be balanced with the patient's ability to participate actively in achieving and/or maintaining joint motion. ROM exercises, functional mobility, and ADLs are techniques for preventing contractures and can empower the patient to actively participate in their own rehabilitation. If the patient is able to maintain full ROM, then priority should be given to these activities instead of the more static interventions like splinting and casting. Immobilization places the patient at high risk for scar contracture and may also lead to restriction of underlying tissue.[107] Active ROM exercises should begin on the day of admission and continue throughout the stages of burn recovery.

Pain is often a limiting factor for performing ROM exercises and should be managed with drugs or with nonpharmacologic methods such as education, distraction, relaxation, and deep breathing (see Chapter 11). ROM may be *active*, in which the patient controls the motion independently; *active assisted*, in which the clinician assists for a portion of the motion, usually the end range; or *passive*, where the patient is entirely dependent on the clinician for movement. Once the patient is able to fully participate in their ROM exercises, additional equipment

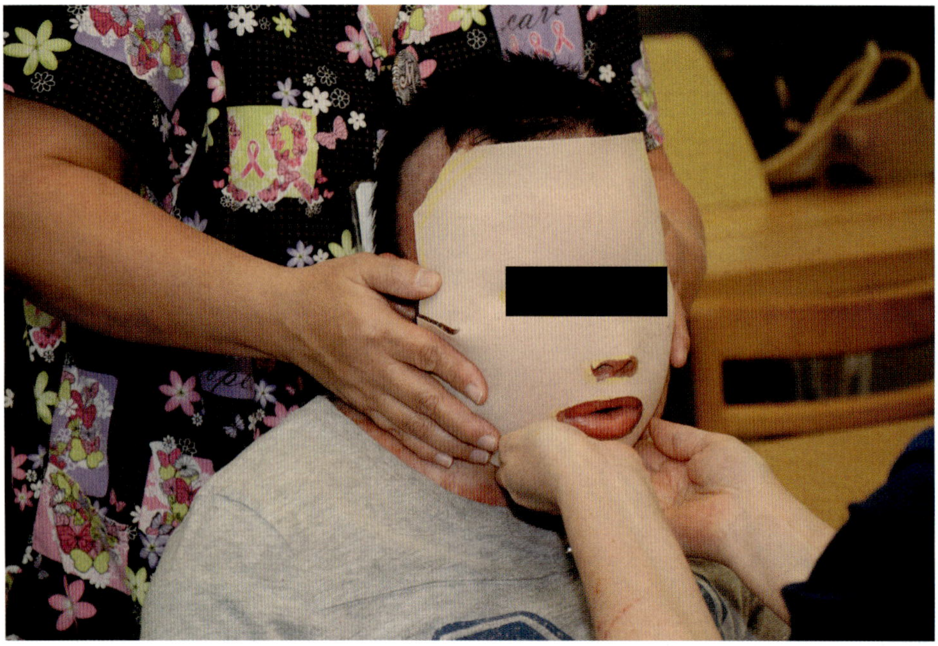

FIGURE 19-17 Gel/silicone face mask worn under a fabric pressure garment.

can be used to strengthen the muscles responsible for the motion achieved.

Immobilization and bed rest after burn injury place the patient at significant risk for complications.[108,109] When the patient is medically stable and cleared from surgical precautions, he/she should begin functional mobility. Bed mobility, transfers in and out of bed, transfers to/from a chair, and ambulation are methods of mobilizing a patient. Early mobility has been associated with improved outcome in critically ill patients.[110,111] Encouraging a patient's involvement in self-care activities during burn recovery can help restore a sense of self-worth and confidence, can be used to reinforce ROM achieved, and mitigate the effects of scar contracture.[81] ADLs such as feeding, dressing, bathing, toileting, and helping with portions of dressing change are a few of these activities. Although at first such activities may require help from a clinician or an assistive device, they provide the patient with the opportunity for functional ROM, endurance exercise, and general participation.

Early rehabilitation after burn injury is crucial to help manage scar hypertrophy and scar contracture and to help improve cosmetic and functional outcomes. Especially in the more emergent phases of the burn injury, the rehabilitation program needs to be applied prior to full wound closure to ensure that the optimal movement and function is still achievable in the latter wound and scar maturation process.[81] Despite dedicated and appropriate efforts, scar hypertrophy and contractures may still occur and surgical reconstruction may ultimately become necessary (see Chapter 12). However, additional rehabilitation following revision will be required to minimize redevelopment of hypertrophy and scar contractures.[8,16]

Burn scar management is a complicated and lengthy process. To be successful, the patient and caregivers should be committed to following the rehabilitation plan of care. Extensive training should take place addressing the use and care of pressure garments, inserts, splints, silicones, lubrication, and other therapeutic scar management procedures to be performed by the patients and their caregivers. Lubricants that do not contain perfume and other skin irritants should be selected and applied at least two to three times daily to the healing skin. Sunscreens and lubricants with a sun protection factor of at least 15 are recommended.[112] Written instructions with pictures and diagrams along with videos addressing scar management should accompany the patient home upon discharge from the hospital. Follow-up visits to the burn or rehabilitation clinic for the assessment of overall recovery to include garments, inserts, and other home therapeutic interventions are required. The therapist's knowledge, creativity, and continuing research in improving the currently existing scar management techniques may be the key to positive outcomes in functional recovery. As advances in clinical care have resulted in marked improvement in survival, the view of outcomes used to measure long-term success in burn rehabilitation must be changed. Treatment plans and interventions must emphasize restoring patients' preburn functional status while maximizing their emotional and cosmetic outcomes.[113]

REFERENCES

1. Stedman's medical dictionary, 23rd ed. Baltimore, MD: Williams and Wilkins; 1976.
2. Linares HA, Larson DL, Willis-Galstraun B. Historical notes on the use of pressure in the treatment of hypertrophic scars and keloids. *Burns*. 1993;19(2):17–21.
3. Linares HA. Hypertrophic healing: controversies and etiopathogenic review. In: Carvajal HF, Parks DH, eds. *Burns in Children: Pediatric Burn Management*. Chicago, IL: Yearbook Medical; 1988:305–323.
4. Shakespeare PG, Renterghem L. Some observations on the surface structure of collagen in hypertrophic scars. *Burns*. 1985;11:175–180.
5. Arno AI, Gauglitz GG, Barret JP, et al. Up-to-date approach to manage keloids and hypertrophic scars: a useful guide. *Burns*. 2014;40:1255–1256.
6. Bloeman MCT, Van der Veer W, Ulrich MMW, et al. Prevention and curative management of hypertrophic scar formation. *Burns*. 2009;35(4):463–475.

7. Staley M, Richard R. Scar management. In: Staley M, Richard R, eds. *Burn Care and Rehabilitation Principles and Practice*. Philadelphia, PA: F.A. Davis; 1994:380–418.
8. Gabriel V, Holavanahalli R. Burn rehabilitation. In: Braddom RL, ed. *Physical Medicine and Rehabilitation*. 4th ed. Philadelphia: Elsevier; 2011:256–298.
9. Van der Veer WM, Bloemen MCT, Ulrich MMW, et al. Potential cellular and molecular causes of hypertrophic scar formation. *Burns*. 2009; 35(1):15–29.
10. Orr DA, Reznikoff M, Smith GM. Body image, self-esteem, and depression in burn-injured adolescents and young adults. *J Burn Care Rehab* 1989;10(5):454–461.
11. Engrav LH, Garner WL, Tredget EE. Hypertrophic scar, wound contraction and hyper-hypopigmentation. *J Burn Care Res*. 2007; 28(4):593–597.
12. Junker JPE, Kratz C, Tollback A, et al. Mechanical tension stimulates the transdifferentiation of fibroblasts into myofibroblasts in human burn scars. *Burns*. 2008;34(7):942–946.
13. Donelan MB, Liao EC. Reconstruction of the head and neck. In: Herndon DN, ed. *Total Burn Care*. 4th ed. Philadelphia: Elsevier; 2013:597–615.
14. Hayakawa T, Hino M, Fuyamada H, et al. Lysyl oxidase activity in human normal skins and post-burn scars. *Clin Chim Acta*. 1976;7:245–250.
15. Hayakawa T, Hashimoto Y, Myokei Y, et al. The effects of skin grafts on the ratio of collagen types in human post-burn wound tissues. *Connect Tissue Res*. 1982;9:249–252.
16. Hawkins H, Finnerty CC. Pathophysiology of burn scar. In: Herndon DN, ed. *Total Burn Care*. 4th ed. Philadelphia, PA: Elsevier; 2013:507–514.
17. Gabriel V. Transforming growth factor-beta and angiotensin in fibrosis and burn injuries. *J Burn Care Res*. 2009;30(3):471–481.
18. Armour A, Scott PG, Tredget EE. Cellular and molecular pathology of HTS: basis for treatment. *Wound Repair Regen*. 2007;15: S6–S17.
19. Tredget E, Wang J, Jiao H, et al. Decreased fibrocytes in post-burn hypertrophic scar after treatment with interferon alpha-2b. *Wound Repair Regen*. 2008;16(2):126.
20. Spann K, Mileski WJ, Atiles L, et al. Use of a pneumatonometer in burn scar assessment. *J Burn Care Rehabil*. 1996;17:515–517.
21. Spann K, Mileski W, Atiles L, et al. The 1996 clinical research award. Use of a pneumatonometer in burn scar assessment. *J Burn Care Rehabil*. 1996;17(6 Pt 1):515–517.
22. Enomoto D, Mekkes J, Bossuyt P, et al. Quantification of cutaneous sclerosis with a skin elasticity meter in patients with generalized scleroderma. *J Am Acad Dermatol*. 1996;35:381–387.
23. Fong S, Hung L, Cheng J. The cutometer and ultrasonography in the assessment of postburn hypertrophic scar: a preliminary study. *Burns*. 1997;23(1):S12–S18.
24. Esposito G, Ziccardi P, Scioli M, et al. The use of a modified tonometer in burn scar therapy. *J Burn Care Rehabil*. 1990;11:86–90.
25. Katz SM, Frank DH, Leopold GR, et al. Objective measurement of hypertrophic burn scar: a preliminary study of tonometry and ultrasonography. *Ann Plast Surg*. 1985;14(2):121–127.
26. Clark MS. Skin tension and mobility under stress. *J Biomechanics*. 1987;20:397–406.
27. Magliaro A, Romanelli M. Skin hardness measurement in hypertrophic scars. *Wounds*. 2003;15:66–70.
28. Haudenschild DR, Nguyen B, Chen J, et al. Rho kinase-dependent CCL20 induced by dynamic compression of human chondrocytes. *Arthritis Rheum*. 2008;58:2735–2742.
29. Lau JC, Li-Tsang CW, Zheng YP. Application of tissue ultrasound palpation system (TUPS) in objective scar evaluation. *Burns*. 2005;31:445–452.
30. Hambleton J, Shakespeare PG, Pratt BJ. The progress of hypertrophic scars monitored by ultrasound measurements of thickness. *Burns*. 1992;18(4):301–307.
31. Powers PS, Sankar S, Goldgof DB, et al. Scar management: current problems and future solutions. *J Burn Care Rehab*. 1999;20:54–60.
32. Bray R, Forrester K, Leonard C, et al. Laser doppler imaging of burn scars: a comparison of wavelength and scanning methods. *Burns*. 2003;29:199–206.
33. Sarov M, Stewart AF. The best control for the specificity of RNAi. *Trends Biotechnol*. 2005;23:446–448.
34. Hosoda G, Holloway GA, Heimback DM. Laser doppler flowmetry for the early detection of hypertrophic burn scars. *J Burn Care Rehabil*. 1986;7:490–497.
35. Berry RB, Tan OT, Cooke ED, et al. Transcutaneous oxygen tension as an index of maturity in hypertrophic scars treated by compression. *Br J Plast Surg*. 1985;38:163–173.
36. Taylor B, McGrouther D, Bayat A. Use of a non-contact 3D digitizer to measure the volume of keloid scars: a useful tool for scar assessment? *J Plast Reconstr Aesthet Surg*. 2007;60:87–94.
37. Roques C, Teot L. A critical analysis of measurements used to assess and manage scars. *Int J Lower Extr Wounds*. 2007;6(4):249–253.
38. Sullivan T, Smith J, Kermode J, et al. Rating the burn scar. *J Burn Care Rehabil*. 1990;11:256–260.
39. Richard R, Baryza M, Carr J, et al. Burn rehabilitation and research: proceedings of a consensus summit. *J Burn Care Rehabil*. 2009;30(4):543–573.
40. Baryza MJ, Baryza GA. The vancouver scar scale: an administration tool and its interrater reliability. *J Burn Care Rehabil*. 1995;16(5):535–538.
41. Nedelec B, Shankowsky HA, Tredget EEJ. Burn rating the resolving hypertrophic scar: comparison of the vancouver scar scale and scar volume. *J Burn Care Rehabil*. 2000;21(3):205–212.
42. Nedelec B, Correa JA, Rachelska G, et al. Quantitative measurement of hypertrophic scar: interrater reliability and concurrent validity. *J Burn Care Res*. 2008;29(3):501–511.
43. Fearmonti R, Bond J, Erdmann D, et al. A review of scar scales and scar measuring devices. *Eplasty*. 2010;10:e43.
44. Nguyen TA, Feldstein SI, Shumaker PR, et al. A review of scar assessment scales. *Semin Cutan Med Surg*. 2015;34:28–36.
45. Forbes-Duchart L, Cooper J, Nedelec B, et al. Burn therapists' opinion on the application and essential characteristics of a burn scar outcome measure. *J Burn Care Res*. 2009;30(5):792–800.
46. Serghiou MA, Ott S, Whitehead C, et al. Comprehensive rehabilitation of the burn patient. In: Herndon DN, ed. *Total Burn Care*. 4th ed. Philadelphia, PA: Elsevier Inc; 2012:517–549.
47. Reid WH, Evans JH, Naismith RS, et al. Hypertrophic scarring and pressure therapy. *Burns Incl Therm Inj*. 1987;13(suppl):S29–S32.
48. McDonald WS, Deitch EA. Hypertrophic skin grafts in burn patients: a prospective analysis of variables. *J Trauma*. 1987;27:147–150.
49. Kealey GP, Jensen KL, Laubenthal KN, et al. Prospective randomized comparison of two types of pressure therapy garments. *J Burn Care Rehabil*. 1990;11:334–336.
50. Hubbard M, Masters IB, Williams GR, et al. Severe obstructive sleep apnoea secondary to pressure garments used in the treatment of hypertrophic burn scars. *Eur Respir J*. 2000;16:1205–1207.
51. Sawada Y. A method of recording and objective assessment of hypertrophic burn scars. *Burns*. 1994;20:76–78.
52. Cheng JC, Evans JH, Leung KS, et al. Pressure therapy in the treatment of post-burn hypertrophic scar — a critical look into its usefulness and fallacies by pressure monitoring. *Burns Incl Therm Inj*. 1984;10:154–163.
53. Leung KS, Cheng JC, Ma GF, et al. Complications of pressure therapy for post-burn hypertrophic scars. Biomechanical analysis based on 5 patients. *Burns Incl Therm Inj*. 1984;10:434–438.
54. Stewart R, Bhagwanjee AM, Mbakaza Y, et al. Pressure garment adherence in adult patients with burn injuries: an analysis of patient and clinician perceptions. *Am J Occup Ther*. 2000;54:598–606.
55. Perkins K, Davey RB, Wallis K. Current materials and techniques used in burn scar management program. *Burns Incl Therm Inj*. 1987;13:406–410.
56. Staley MJ, Richard RL. Use of pressure to treat hypertrophic burn scars. *Adv Wound Care*. 1997;10:44–46.
57. Van den Kerckhove E, Stappaerts K, Fieuws S, et al. The assessment of erythema and thickness on burn related scars during pressure garment therapy as a preventative measure for hypertrophic scarring. *Burns*. 2005;31:696–702.
58. Macintyre L, Baird M. Pressure garments for use in the treatment of hypertrophic scars — a review of the problems associated with their use. *Burns*. 2006;32:10–15.
59. Puzey G. The use of pressure garments on hypertrophic scars. *J Tissue Viability*. 2002;12:11–15.
60. Giele HP, Liddiard K, Currie K, et al. Direct measurement of cutaneous pressures generated by pressure garments. *Burns*. 1997;23: 137–141.
61. Larson DL, Abston S, Willis B, et al. Contracture and scar formation in the burn patient. *Clin Plast Surg*. 1974;1:653–656.
62. Robertson JC, Hodgson B, Druett JE, et al. Pressure therapy for hypertrophic scarring: preliminary communication. *J R Soc Med*. 1980;73:348–354.

63. Engrav LH, Nakamura DY, Dutcher KA, et al. Do splinting and pressure devices damage new grafts? *J Burn Care Rehabil.* 1983;4:107–108.
64. Rose MP, Deitch GA. The effective use of a tubular compression bandage, tubigrip, for burn scar therapy in the growing child. *J Burn Care Rehabil.* 1983;4:197–201.
65. Cheng JCY, Evans JH, Leung KS, et al. Pressure therapy in the treatment of post-burn hypertrophic scar—a critical look into its usefulness and fallacies by pressure monitoring. *Burns Incl Therm Inj.* 1984;10:154–163.
66. Thompson R, Summers S, Rampey-Dobbs R, et al. Color pressure garments vs traditional beige pressure garments: perceptions from the public. *J Burn Care Rehabil.* 1992;13:590–596.
67. Fricke NB, Omnell ML, Dutcher KA, et al. Skeletal and dental disturbances after facial burns and pressure garments use: a 4 year follow-up. *J Burn Care Rehabil.* 1999;20:239–249.
68. Fricke NB, Omnell ML, Dutcher KA, et al. Skeletal and dental disturbances in children after facial burns and pressure garments. *J Burn Care Rehabil.* 1996;17:338–345.
69. Quan PE, Rau SB, Alston DW, et al. Control of scar tissue in the finger web spaces by use of graded pressure inserts. *J Burn Care Rehabil.* 1980;1(2):27–29.
70. Mustoe TA. Evolution of silicone therapy and mechanism of action in scar management. *Aesth Plast Surg.* 2008;32:82–92.
71. Van den Kerckhove E, Stappaerts K, Boeckx W, et al. Silicones in the rehabilitation of burns: a review and overview. *Burns.* 2001;27(3):205–214.
72. Li-Tsang C, Zheng YP, Lau JC. A randomized clinical trial to study the effect of silicone gel dressing and pressure therapy on posttraumatic hypertrophic scars. *J Burn Care Res.* 2010;31(1):35–46.
73. Nedelec B, Carter A, Forbes L, et al. Practice guidelines for the application of non silicone or silicone gels and gel sheets after burn injury. *J Burn Care Res.* 2014;28(3):12–21.
74. McNee S. The use of silicone gel in the control of hypertrophic scarring. *Physiotherapy.* 1990;76:194–197.
75. Serghiou M, Walker K, Parks D. Therapeutic modalities in burn care. In: Proceedings of the American Burn Association; April 21–24, 1999; Chicago, IL. [Abstract].
76. Holavanahalli RK, Helm PA, Parry IS, et al. Select practices in management and rehabilitation of burns: a survey report. *J Burn Care Res.* 2011;32(2):210–223.
77. Niszczak J, Serghiou M. Burn scar massage. In: Proceedings of the 36th Annual Scientific Meeting of the Australian New Zealand Burn Association; October 9–12, 2012; Hobart, Tasmania.
78. Field T, Peck M, Hernandez-Reif M, et al. Postburn itching, pain, and psychological symptoms are reduced with massage therapy. *J Burn Care Rehabil.* 2000;21:189–193.
79. Field T, Peck M, Krugman BS, et al. Burn injuries benefit from massage therapy. *J Burn Care Rehabil.* 1998;19:241–244.
80. Parry I, Icaza I, Poveda SV, et al. Defining massage techniques used for burn scars. *J Burn Care Res.* Video Gallery. http://journals.lww.com/burncareresearch/pages/videogallery.aspx?videoId=5&autoPlay=false. Accessed November 17, 2016.
81. Niszczak J, Forbes L, Serghiou M. Burn rehabilitation. In: Maitin IB ed. *Current Diagnosis and Treatment Physical Medicine and Rehabilitation.* New York, NY: McGraw Hill; 2015.
82. Ward RS. The use of physical agents in burn care. In: Richard RL, Staley MJ, eds. *Burn Care and Rehabilitation Principles and Practice.* Philadelphia, PA: F.A. Davis; 1994:419–446.
83. Miles WK, Grigsby de Linde L. Remodeling of scar tissue in the burned hand. In: Hunter JM, Mackin EJ, Callahan AD, eds. *Rehabilitation of the hand.* Vol 2. 4th ed. St. Louis, CV: Mosby; 1995: 1267–1294.
84. Wood EC. *Beard's Massage: Principles and Techniques.* 2nd ed. Philadelphia, PA: WB Saunders; 1974:48–59.
85. Lentell G, Hetherington T, Eagan J, et al. The use of thermal agents to influence the effectiveness of low-load prolonged stretch. *J Orthop Sport Phys Ther.* 1992;15:200–207.
86. Warren CG, Lehmann JF, Koblanski JN. Heat and stretch procedures: an evaluation using rat tail tendon. *Arch Phys Med Rehabil.* 1976;57:122–126.
87. Ward RS, Hayes-Lundy C, Reddy R, et al. Evaluation of topical therapeutic ultrasound to improve response to physical therapy and lessen scar contracture after burn injury. *J Burn Care Rehabil.* 1994;15:74–79.
88. Head M, Helm P. Paraffin and sustained stretching in treatment of burn contractures. *Burns.* 1977;4:136–139.
89. Kowalske K, Holavanahalli R, Hynan L, et al. A randomized-controlled study of the effectiveness of paraffin and sustained stretch in treatment of burn contractures. *J Burn Care Rehabil.* 2003;24:S67.
90. Richard R, Ward RS. Splinting strategies and controversies. *J Burn Care Rehabil.* 2005;26(5):392–396.
91. Esselman PC, Thombs BD, Magyar-Russell G, et al. Burn rehabilitation: state of the science. *Am J Phys Med Rehabil.* 2006;85(4):383–413.
92. Whitehead C, Serghiou M. A 12-year comparison of common therapeutic intervention in the burn unit. *J Burn Care Res.* 2009;30(2):281–287.
93. Richard R, Jones JA, Parshley P. Hierarchical decomposition of burn body diagram based on cutaneous functional units and its utility. *J Burn Care Res.* 2015;36(1):33–43.
94. Richard R, Lester ME, Miller SF, et al. Identification of cutaneous functional units related to burn scar contracture development. *J Burn Care Res.* 2009;30(4):623–631.
95. Richard R, Ford J, Miller S, et al. Photographic measurement of volar forearm skin movement with wrist extension: the influence of elbow position. *J Burn Care Rehabil.* 1994;15:58–61.
96. Cooney MA. PT/OT Forum: splinting the pediatric patient with multiple joint involvement. *J Burn Care Rehabil.* 1984;5(3):215–217.
97. Richard RL, Niszczak J. Burn rehabilitation. In: Austin NM, Jacobs MA, eds. *Splinting the Hand and Upper Extremity: Principals and Process.* 2nd ed. Lippencott Williams and Wilkens; 2013.
98. Engrav LH, Heimbach DM, Rivara FP, et al. 12-Year within-wound study of the effectiveness of custom pressure garment therapy. *Burns.* 2010;36(7):975–998.
99. Friang J. The effects of splinting on graft take. *Proc Am Burn Assoc.* 1986;18:22.
100. Derwin-Baruch L. UVA therapists meet the challenge of scar management. *OT Week.* 1993:15–17.
101. Rivers EA, Strate RG, Solem LD. The transparent facemask. *Am J Occup Ther.* 1979;33:108–113.
102. Gallagher J, Goldfarb W, Slater H, et al. Survey of treatment modalities for the prevention and treatment of hypertrophic burn scars. *J Burn Care Rehabil.* 1990;11(2):118–120.
103. Alley RR, Van-Buendia LB, Jeng JC, et al. Laser doppler imaging of cutaneous blood flow through transparent face masks: a necessary preamble to computer-controlled rapid prototyping fabrication with submillimeter precision. *J Burn Care Res.* 2008;29(1):42–48.
104. Van-Buendia L, Allely RR, Lassiter R, et al. What's behind the mask? A look at blood flow changes with prolonged facial pressure and expression using laser doppler imaging. *J Burn Care Res.* 2010;31(3):441–447.
105. Parry I, Sen S, Palmieri T, et al. Nonsurgical scar management of the face. Does early versus late intervention affect outcome. *J Burn Care Res.* 2013;34:569–575.
106. Katz SM, Frank DH, Leopold GR, et al. Objective measurement of hypertrophic burn scar: a preliminary study of tonometry and ultrasonography. *J Burn Care Res.* 1997;8(2):171.
107. Cronin T. Effects of immobilization and mobilization on cartilaginous, bony, and soft tissue structure; review of the literature. *J Burn Care Rehabil.* 1986;7(1):54–57.
108. Schwarz RJ. Management of postburn contractures of the upper extremity. *J Burn Care Rehabil.* 2007;28:212–219.
109. LeBlanc AD, Schneider VS, Evans HJ, et al. Bone mineral loss and recovery after 17 weeks of bed rest. *J Bone Miner Res.* 1990;5: 843–850.
110. Bailey P, Thomsen GE, Spuhler VJ, et al. Early activity is feasible and safe in respiratory failure patients. *Crit Care Med.* 2007;35:139–145.
111. Morris PE, Goad A, Thompson C, et al. Early intensive care unit mobility therapy in the treatment of acute respiratory failure. *Crit Care Med.* 2008;36:2238–2243.
112. Huruitz S. The sun and sunscreen protection: recommendations for children. *J Dermatol Surg Oncol.* 1988;14(6):657–660.
113. Richard RL, Hedman T, Quick CD, et al. A clarion to recommit and reaffirm burn rehabilitation. *J Burn Care Res.* 2008;29(3):425–432.

20 Scar Camouflage

ELIZABETH ALLEN

KEY POINTS

- Camouflage can be a simple solution to complex problems.
- Topically applied products are long lasting and waterproof.
- Camouflage does not affect the skin or its structure, but does temporarily reduce the visual discoloration.
- There are various brands and potentially over 300 natural skin colors available to select an acceptable color to match the unaffected skin.

History of Skin Camouflage

There is evidence to suggest that cosmetic preparations and prostheses have been used to cover scars since antiquity.[1] The history of skin camouflage, as we know it today, began during World War II by the innovative plastic surgeon, Sir Archibald McIndoe, at the Queen Victoria Hospital, East Grinstead, West Sussex, England.[2] His patients were all Royal Air Force (RAF) aircrew with burn injuries who formed (1941) The Guinea Pigs Club (28 founding members, 649 by the end of the war), which is acknowledged as being the first patient support group founded by patients for patients. McIndoe[3] would proudly state, "It has been described as the most exclusive club in the world, but the entrance fee is something most men would not care to pay and the conditions of membership are arduous in the extreme" (see Fig. 20-1A).

McIndoe realized that scars and grafts frequently presented a different color to the surrounding skin—he could reconstruct a face, but this all too frequently resulted in a "patchwork" of skin colors. He wondered whether a topical preparation could be the solution. His first thoughts were toward Hollywood, where the Max Factor Corporation had created military camouflage for the U.S. Marines and waterproof theatrical pancake for use during Technicolor filming. He took these innovations to a colleague, Thomas Blake, and asked if the chemist could create waterproof camouflage crèmes that would mimic natural skin colors. The outcome was Veil Cover, initially with three colors (light, medium, and dark—dark being so called because it was darker than the other two) and all suitable for Fitzpatrick skin types I and II (see Fig.20-1B).

The British Association of Skin Camouflage (BASC) founder, Joyce Allsworth, was a Women's Auxiliary Air Force (WAAF) plotter at North Weald RAF Airbase during World War II and became aware of the air crew's burn injuries at East Grinstead Hospital. She felt something had to be done to improve their well-being; after the war Joyce trained as a make-up artist and returned to McIndoe and his guinea pigs. No dated record exists of the initial interactions between them and Thomas Blake, although we do know that it was her suggestion that Veil increased its color range to include mixing colors such as rose, brown, and yellow (these colors still exist to this day). Over the years, Veil has continued to revise and increase its color range, and BASC is proud to be a part of that advisory process as well as a consultant to other companies that now include skin camouflage within their brand.

Mrs. Allsworth's work was complemented by providing a comprehensive training program designed to increase the number of graduates in this specialty by training medical professionals (doctors, nurses, pharmacists, occupational therapists, and maxillofacial technicians), make-up artists, and beauty therapists. Her pioneering work has since expanded; BASC is the acknowledged major source of information and educators who train professionals to provide skin camouflage service within hospitals, clinics, and salons. BASC continues to be organized by professionals who volunteer their expertise. Although BASC-trained professionals work independently of the organization, we are proud of the part they play in helping others to *face the world, with confidence.*

The Desire to Be Accepted

We all have a great desire to be accepted by our community. In previous centuries, the majority of us would have worn the effects of life on our skin with some indifference. It would have been commonplace to see people with scars and pockmarks; given such acceptance, others would not have made disparaging comments. We might even hypothesize that people would be happy to associate with a scarred person because it indicated that, in these preantiseptic days, he or

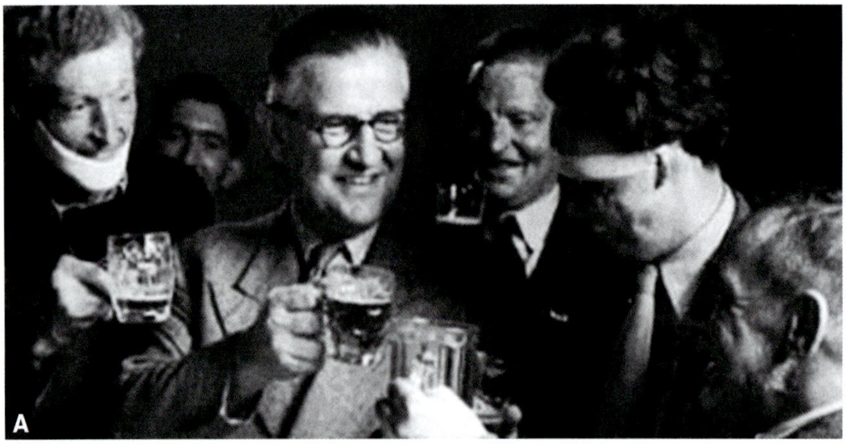

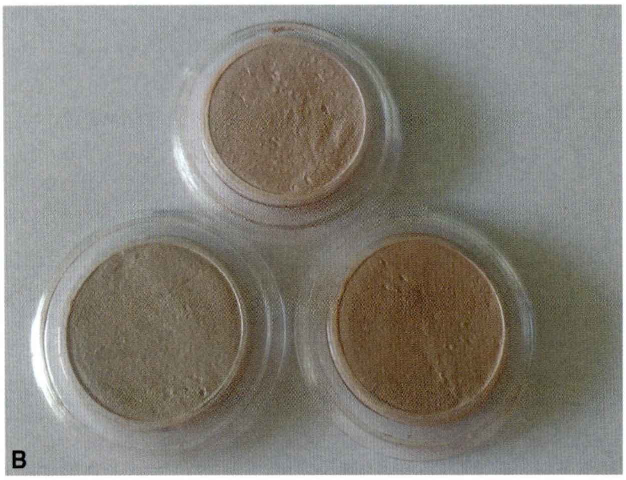

FIGURE 20-1 **A:** McIndoe with some of his guinea pigs. (© *The Guinea Pig Club.*). Photo courtesy of the Bond-McIndoe Museum, East Grinstead. **B:** Veil's three original colors. Copyright Thomas Blake Camouflage Creams, Ltd., England.

she was a survivor. Sadly, modern times have changed this all-embracing attitude as we now live in an age that makes an instant judgment based on people's outward appearance.

The 21st Century requires us to have flawless (even ageless) skin, especially on our face. Such idealism is constantly fuelled by performing arts when all too frequently a villain is depicted with facial scarring—a premise perhaps based on gangsters such as Al Capone (who when photographed hid the scars on the left side of his face, saying that they were "war wounds" rather than the result of a fight)[3]—and cartoon characters, such as Batman's The Joker. Unfortunately, such negative stereotyping[4] can only serve to promote greater anxiety in those with scars or who consider their image to be psychosocially unacceptable.

Research into keloid and hypertrophic scarring suggested that those with scar tissue 2 inches (5 cm) in length were particularly concerned, and that psychosocial inhibition was irrespective of the scar being immediately visible or hidden by clothing[5] (see Fig. 20-2).

Unfortunately, there is no collective registry to indicate how many people have a scar. Neither has any official record been kept as to the number of people who benefit from using skin camouflage over their scarring. Scars are the result of many and varied causes, including accidents, violence, and disease. We can assume that most people expect their surgical procedure will create a scar, but they may not be aware of additional problems, as when the patient was psychologically adjusted to the scar but was worried by the vascular disturbance (she requested camouflage for the veins and not the scar) (see Fig. 20-3).

It has long been acknowledged that mind and body interact upon each other; it is axiomatic that when people are distressed by some aspect of their appearance, their general health and quality of life can be adversely affected. Although there is no single accepted definition of Health-Related Quality of Life (HRQoL), there are questionnaires available for professionals to measure the impact that skin conditions have on people's well-being, such as the Dermatology Life Quality Index (DLQI)[6] and the Hospital Anxiety and Depression Score, which patients complete themselves. All evidence supports the assertion that people experience higher levels of anxiety, depression, social isolation, difficulties at school, and unemployment than those whose skin is considered to be normal.[7,8] Many people with scarring report that, at some point, they have met with rejection, name-calling, unwarranted comments, intrusive questioning, or verbal abuse. Without help, people can withdraw from employment, domestic and social-sporting activities, which may also affect the quality of life for their families. Studies into psychosocial behavior are well documented—all conclusions indicate that low self-esteem is equally devastating to men, women, and children, irrespective of religion, nationality, and skin classification group.[9–11]

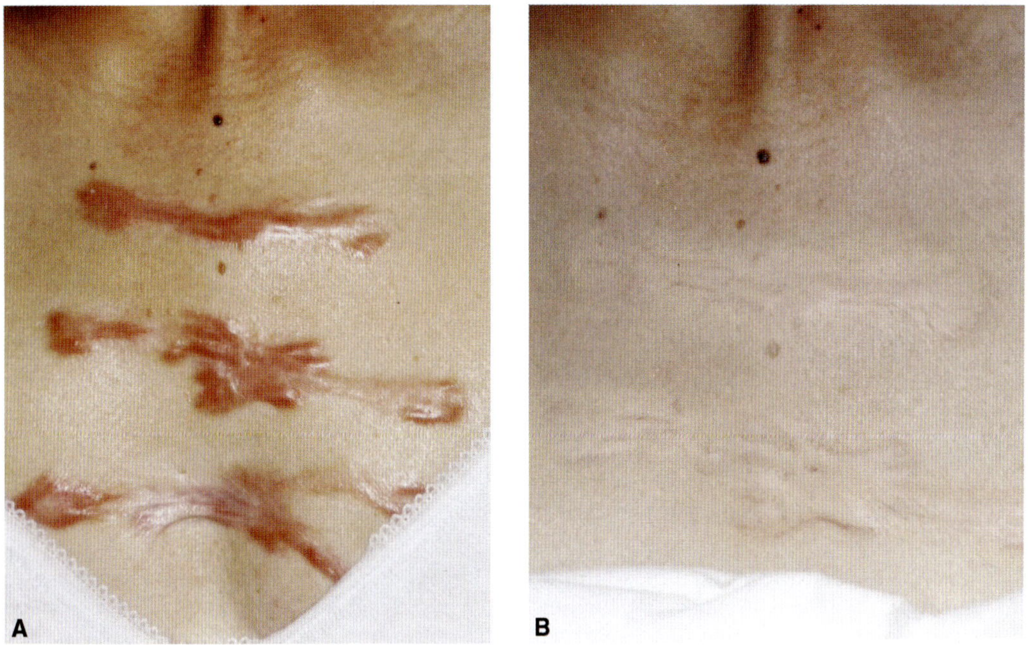

FIGURE 20-2 Camouflage applied over keloid scar to chest (cause undisclosed). *(© BASC member 1022.)*

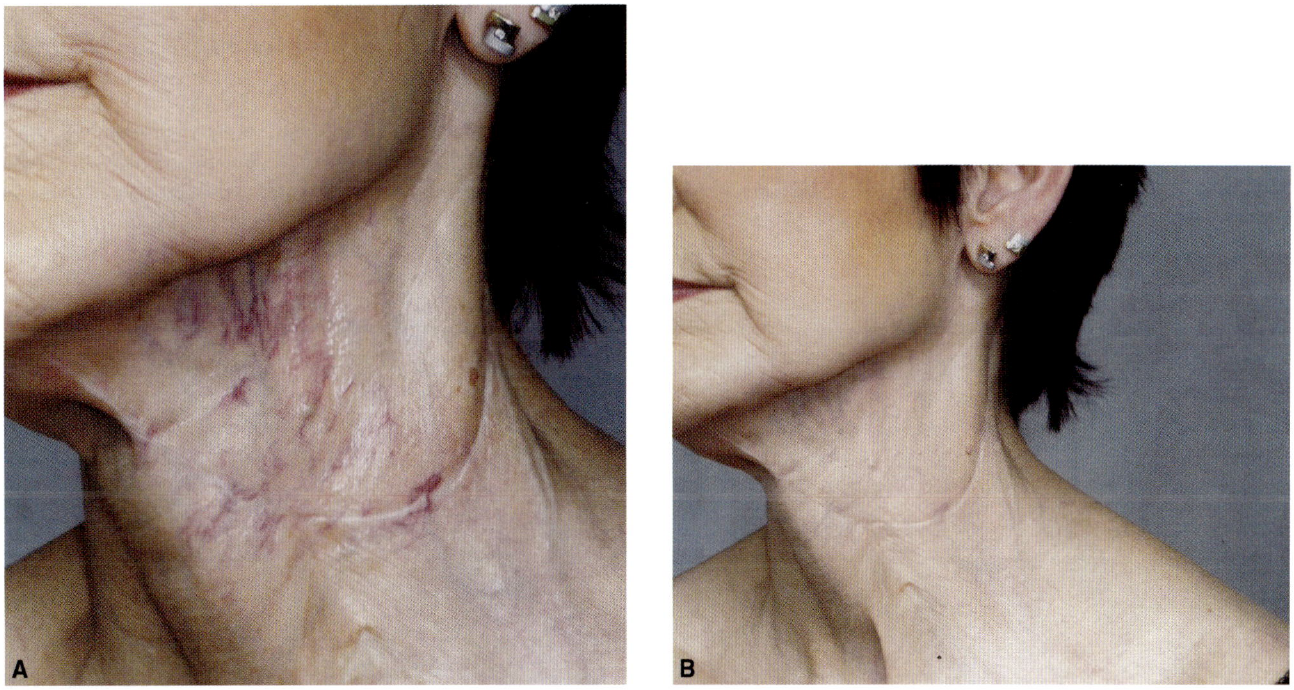

FIGURE 20-3 Camouflage used to reduce the visual effect of the residual vascular malformation following tumor removal. *(© BASC member 1022.)*

Health is a state of complete physical, mental and social well-being and not merely the absence of disease or infirmity.

—World Health Organization, Mental Health Fact Sheet No. 220, September 2010

BASC challenges the opinions of the few psychologists who consider the use of skin camouflage to be "avoidance of reality" and makes people reliant on this as a single coping strategy.[12] We consider that if using skin camouflage helps someone to feel good about him or herself, if it gives them a tool to help their confidence grow, if it helps their return to ecosocial life, then should it not be encouraged? It is also immaterial whether the camouflage is worn occasionally or frequently, for a small scar or more extensive ones (see Fig. 20-4).

Sadly, some language used by professionals can be negative and alienate the scarred person. Labels, such as "disfigured," may be a relevant medical description (especially when there is loss of a prominent facial feature, as the nose,

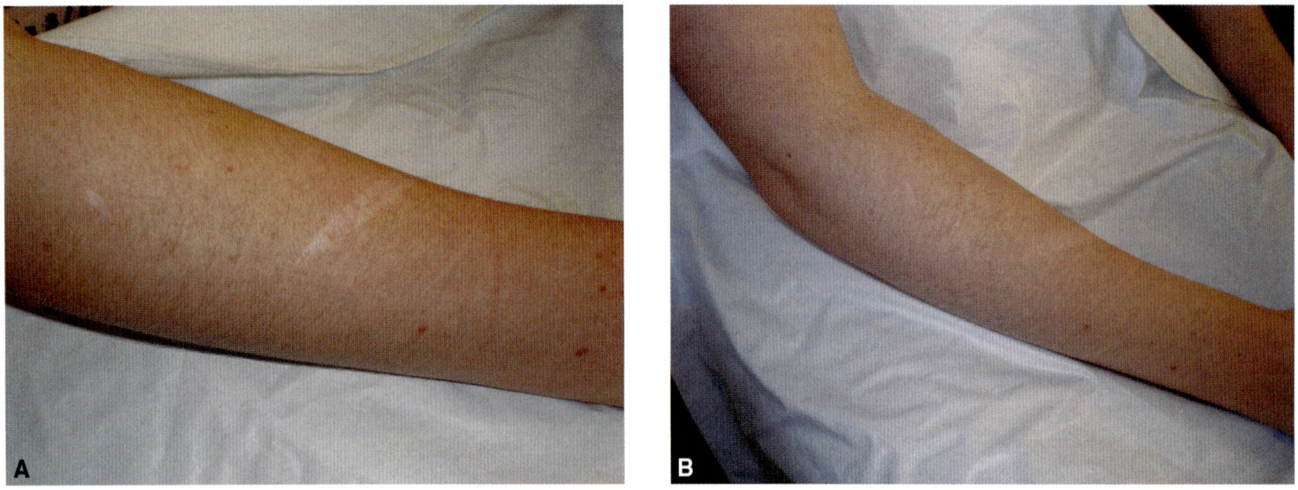

FIGURE 20-4 Before and after skin camouflage applied to small scar. *(© BASC member 2303.)*

ear, or eye), but it is a word that the scarred person may find difficult to identify with; indeed, it may create further anxiety—perhaps a tipping point that might lead to eating disorders or self-harm? (see Fig. 20-5).

Could such lack of engagement also result in the person not complying with medical procedures or treatments? To avoid these pitfalls, we strongly request that all references and language used be inclusive and empathetic to the patient. BASC totally endorses the statement made by Professor Nichola Rumsey, head of the Centre for Appearance Research, Bristol (*Daily Telegraph* newspaper, December 15, 2014):

Language is so powerful that we need to look at how it is used when talking about disfigurement. Here at the Centre, we talk of 'visible difference', which is a neutral term I would like to see used by everyone.

Skin camouflage offers a simple solution to what may be complex medical and psychological problems. From its initiation it has been accepted as a vital tool during the early stages of patients' rehabilitation and adjustment to their altered image. For others, however, wearing skin camouflage may need to be considered as a long-term process.

Without using skin camouflage to face (rosacea) and occasionally to backs of hands (psoriasis) I would be frequently asked what my medical conditions are . . . I do not think it is reasonable to be questioned on my medical history by a complete stranger in the middle of Tesco's—but the public feel it is perfectly okay to do so!

—Report of the All Party Parliamentary Group on Skin (2013 London)

Terminology used to describe skin camouflage is also crucial. Using the words "skin camouflage" does not create a psychological barrier. It is nonexclusive, whereas "cosmetics" and "make-up" can create all kinds of distress to men, children, and women who would not normally wear "make-up." For example, should the camouflage consultant suggest to a youth that "you can get some special make-up from the beauty salon," or might we engage his curiosity if we advise "would you like an appointment at the camouflage clinic?" Referring to skin camouflage as "make-up" risks trivializing its purpose and creating an association with pampering and vanity (see Fig. 20-6).

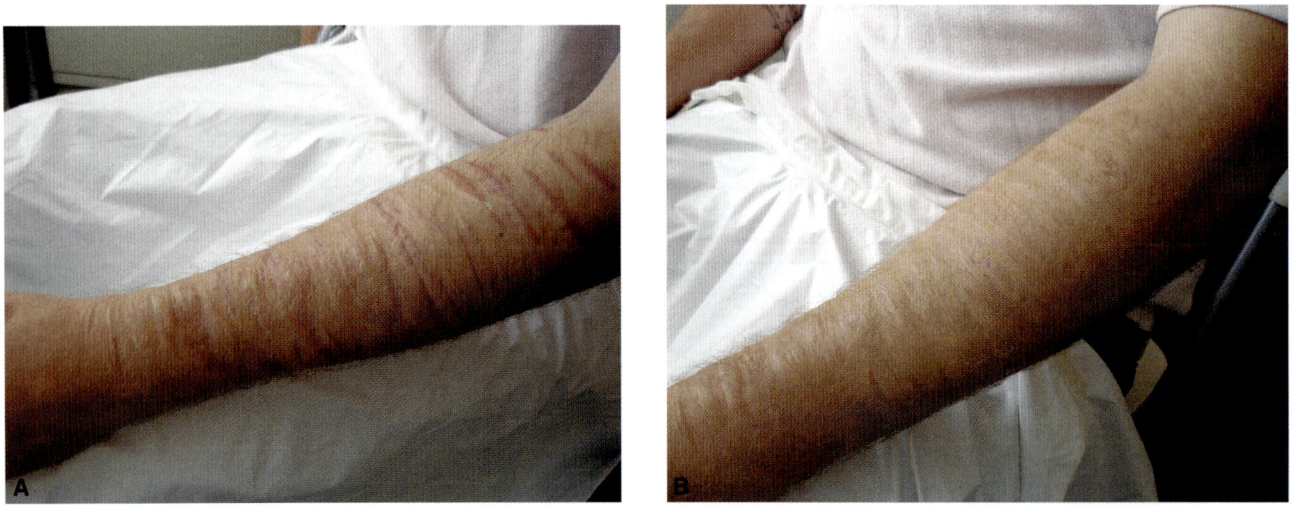

FIGURE 20-5 Before and after skin camouflage applied to multiple scars (self-harm). *(© BASC member 2303.)*

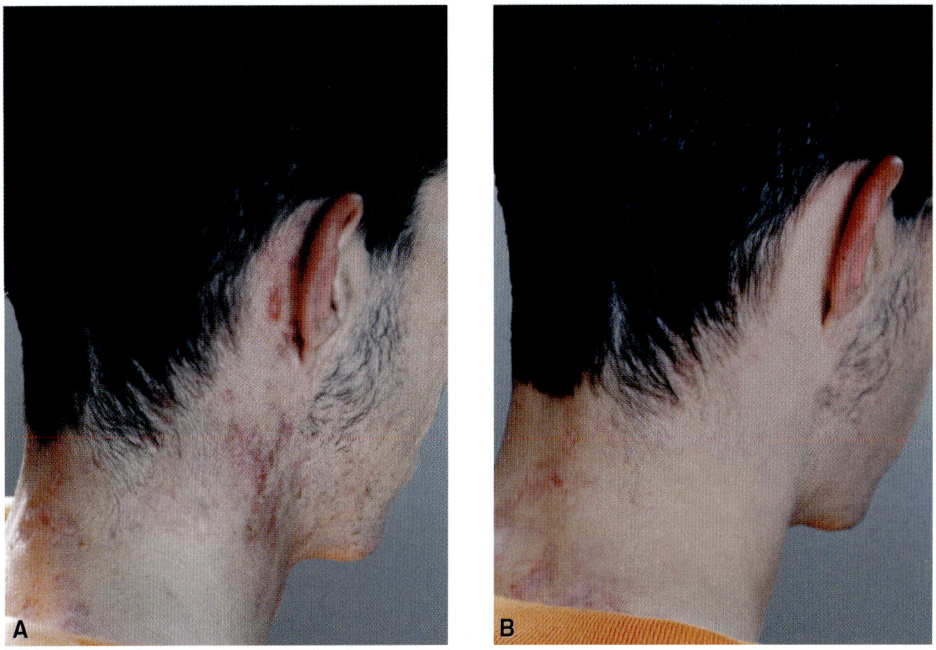

FIGURE 20-6 Camouflage after laser treatment. **A:** Immediately after laser treatment for acne scarring. **B:** After the application of camouflage. *(© BASC.)*

The psychological benefit to patients who have been taught how to successfully apply and manage their skin camouflage cannot be overemphasized. People can take advantage of a skin matching service provided by trained professionals, and with the ever-growing range of camouflage products and colors, it means that no skin group need be excluded. Skin camouflage cannot alter the texture of the skin, but the immediate visual effect does help the person regain self-confidence. Such a resolve can do much to improve their sense of well-being and assist in a return to normal social-sporting activities and employment (see Fig. 20-7).

Skin Camouflage

Initially, many people do seek help from decorative cosmetics. At base principle there would appear to be little or no difference between "corrective make-up" and "skin camouflage" as both set out to achieve the same result, which is to cover erythema, hyperpigmentation, and hypopigmentation. Although cosmetic make-up can be very effective in concealing minor discoloration, it is frequently less durable and stable than traditional skin

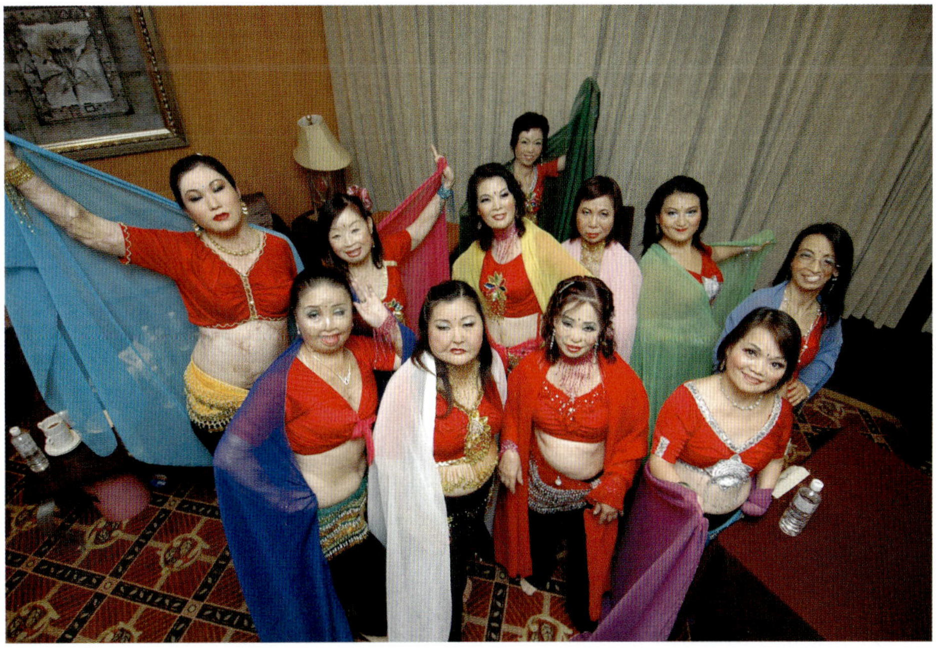

FIGURE 20-7 As part of its psychosocial rehabilitation work, the Sunshine Foundation started a belly-dancing troupe (2006) composed of ladies with burn scarring. They use skin camouflage during public performances, which highlights the self-confidence and vitality of the dancers who are comfortable with their body and passionate about their dancing. *(© Sunshine Foundation, Taiwan; BASC honorary member.)*

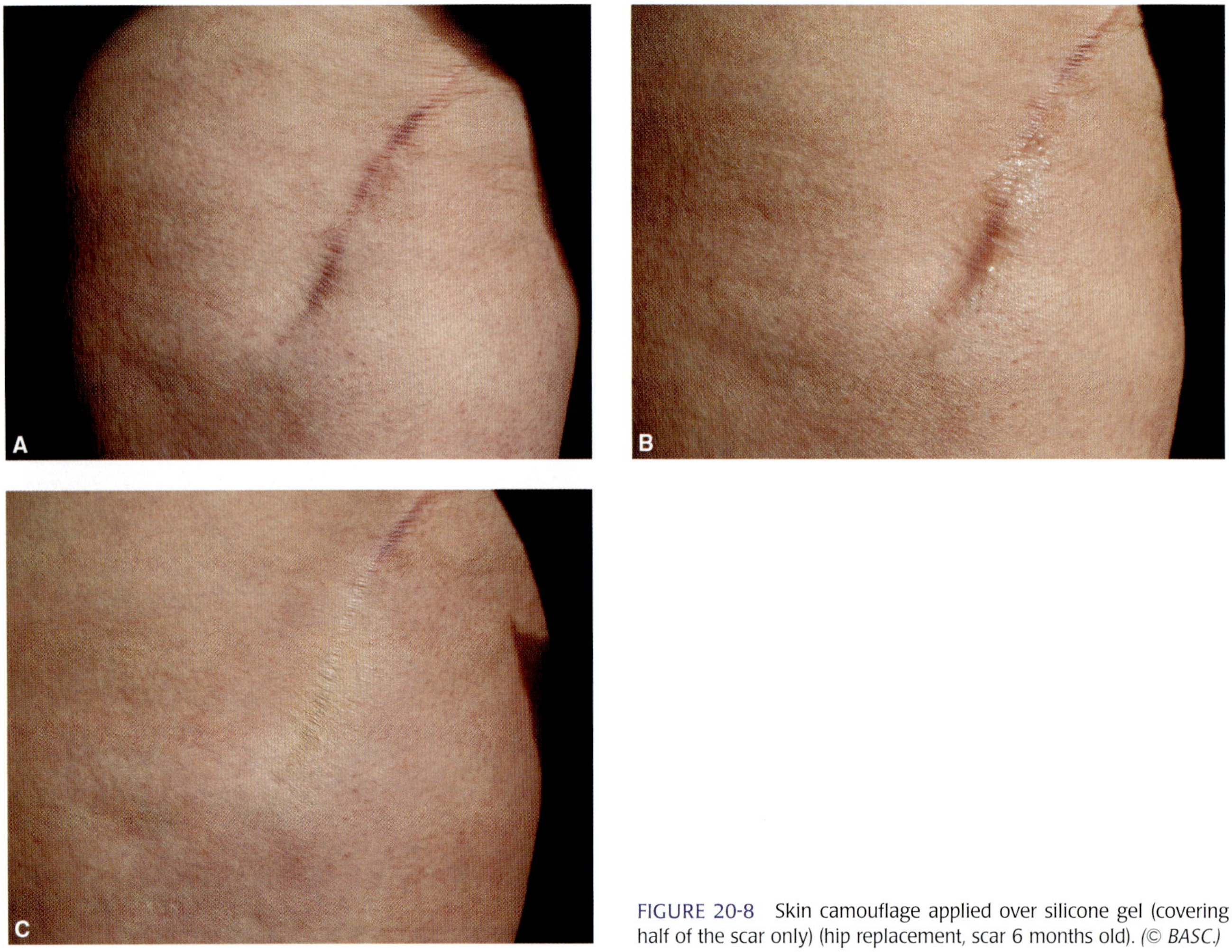

FIGURE 20-8 Skin camouflage applied over silicone gel (covering half of the scar only) (hip replacement, scar 6 months old). *(© BASC.)*

camouflage products. Skin camouflage is designed to replicate natural skin colors and differs from corrective beauty aids in that:

1. The crèmes are specially formulated to give the necessary covering power yet require only a thin application.
2. They usually last between 8 and 16 hours before the need to "touch up" or reapply.
3. The crèmes are water resistant, allowing the wearer to take part in sports or swim.
4. Make-up can be used over skin camouflage.

At the time of writing, BASC is not aware of any confirmed allergy to the products we use, but there is always the possibility that people could experience an unexpected allergic reaction to an ingredient. If this happens, we recommend the person stop using the product until a clinical patch test identifies the cause. Various camouflage brands have different ingredients. There has been no report or evidence supplied to BASC that camouflage crèmes and setting agents encourage skin conditions or are detrimental to scarring, but there should be caution when using any product that is activated and removed off the skin by alcohol because these may be too dehydrating for fragile scars, especially those on the face.

Conventionally, the scar needs to be fully "healed and sealed" before attempting use, and camouflage must never be applied over an infection or suspicious lesion. It is always recommended that people remove their skin camouflage on a daily basis to allow them to inspect their skin for changes, and apply medication, emollients, and/or sun protection. Skin camouflage can be applied over these topical preparations and also on top of silicone gel scar treatment (see Fig. 20-8). Camouflage does not adhere successfully or present convincingly over silicone sheeting.

Before You Begin

The camouflage clinic should be held in a private room, preferably with a window that will allow natural daylight without compromising confidentiality and privacy. Should this not be available, bulbs that mimic natural daylight should be used either as the room's lighting or as a portable lamp. Camouflage colors agreed under natural daylight will look acceptable in different light settings (such as candle, fluorescent, etc.), but camouflage agreed under other artificial lighting will be acceptable only under that particular lighting condition.

You will need disposable clothing protection to prevent any accidental soiling of the person's clothes and a selection of removal products. Camouflage is easily removed off the skin with soap substitutes (such as an emollient) and cosmetic pads. Care must be taken that these do not contain any sodium laureth sulfate, which is a known potential irritant, and that cosmetic wet wipes do not contain the preservatives methylisothiazolinone or methylchloroisothiazolinone because these may cause an allergic reaction. There is no need to apply a skin toner before skin camouflage. Should people be applying sun protection, it is recommended to use a broad-spectrum (UVA and UVB) sun block. This should be applied 10 minutes or so before the skin camouflage, and residue after this time should be blotted off with a cosmetic tissue.

Achieving an Acceptable Skin Match

For successful skin camouflage, the consultant needs to achieve an acceptable color to match the surrounding, unaffected skin. We all see color slightly differently. This is because as we age, the color receptor cells are not replaced; a young adult will have better color vision than a senior citizen. Consequently, the camouflage consultant must always accept the patient's choice of camouflage crème color. If a personal opinion overrides this, then it is likely that the camouflage will be considered an unacceptable skin match and the products will not be used (see Fig. 20-9).

The most economical method of removing camouflage crème from its container is to use a disposable cocktail stick. Having picked up an amount equivalent to the phosphorus on a matchstick, place the crème in your clean palm. The cocktail stick should now be used to record the color you are testing. Simply put the clean end in the palette (see Fig. 20-10).

Should the color prove unacceptable, break the stick and try another color. Using the cocktail sticks in this way also prevents you from using a rejected color twice; more importantly it will stop you from retaining the stick in your hand and the risk that you could accidentally stab the patient or yourself (see Fig. 20-11). When using products supplied in a tube, squeeze a small amount into your palm directly and make a note of color/s tested.

Putting camouflage crème into your palm also has a psychological benefit. If you placed the crème on the back of your hand, then inevitably you would create a fist. This can alarm people as it suggests you are about to punch them! Instead, an open palm is the international signal of "I mean you no harm." The suggested unaffected skin-matched camouflage is then picked up with a clean finger and the color tested on the person's scar (see Fig. 20-12). The test does not need to be larger than ½-inch (10 mm) in diameter. Incorrect trials should be immediately removed. You will need to test colors on adjacent skin should the scar begin to present erythema.

If a skin match cannot be found from your available choices, it might be necessary to mix two natural skin colors together, or to add a little of yellow or red to the skin-colored crème. The palm now becomes a convenient mixing bowl! (see Fig. 20-13).

A complementary color is sometimes needed as an undercoat when the discoloration shows through the applied skin camouflage. The complementary color theory suggests that using an opposing color will cancel this problem (see Fig. 20-14).

However, in our experience, the application of green to cancel out red results in green skin to camouflage (see Fig. 20-15)

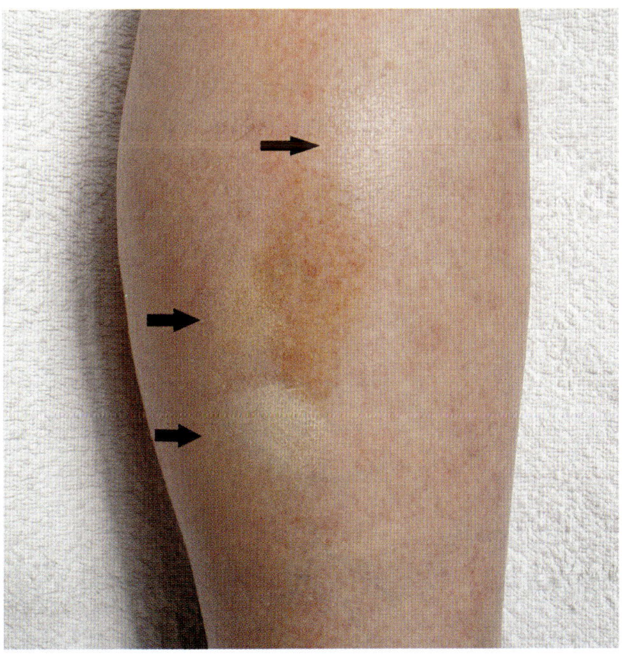

FIGURE 20-9 Three skin colors have been placed on the skin for the patient to make the final choice (café au lait mark). *(© BASC.)*

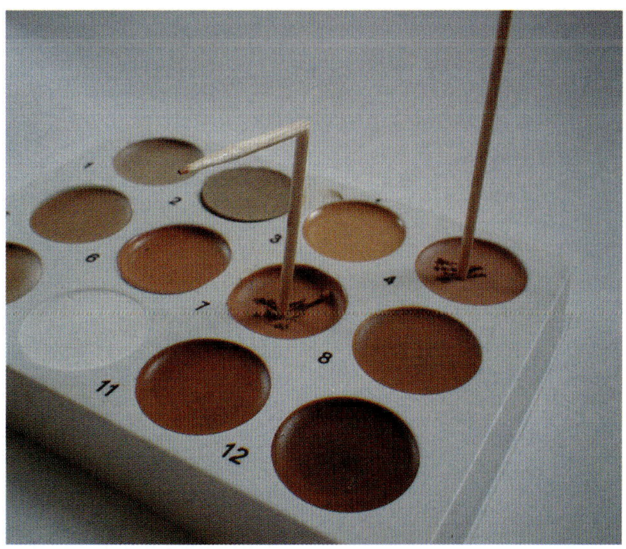

FIGURE 20-10 Return the cocktail stick to the palette, using the clean end to indicate the color tested. *(© BASC.)*

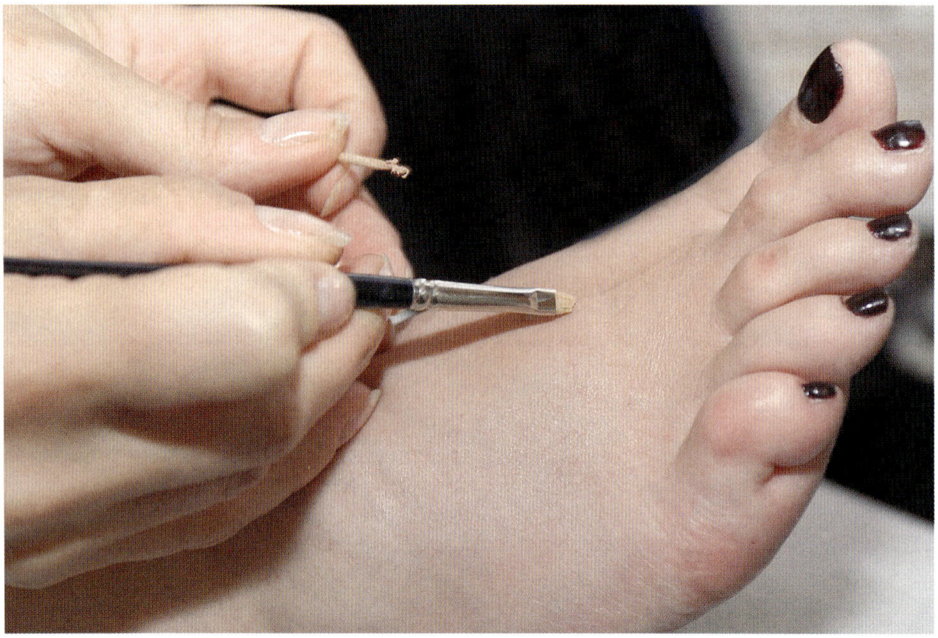

FIGURE 20-11 Risk of stabbing the person with a retained cocktail stick. (© BASC.)

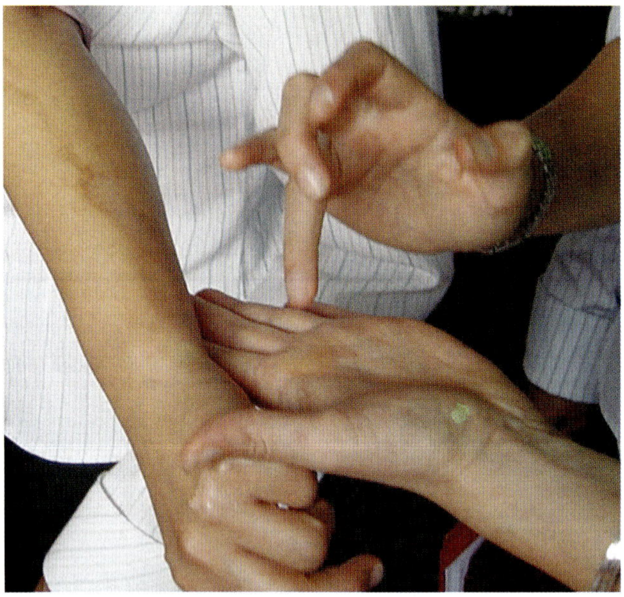

FIGURE 20-12 Transfer the camouflage from your palm to the person's scar. (© BASC.)

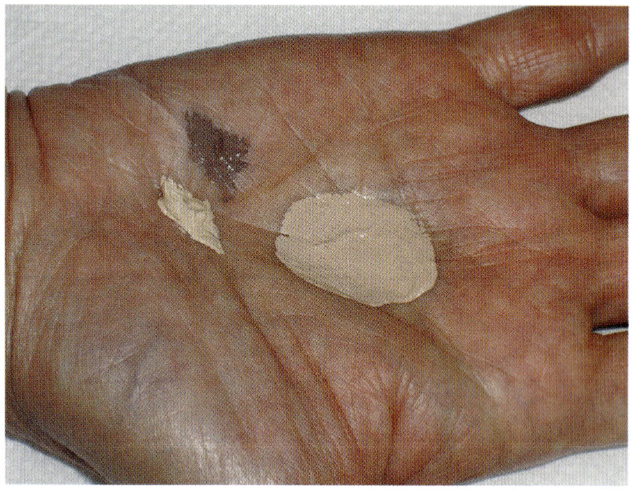

FIGURE 20-13 You will need to record the mixture ratio; in this illustration, it is 50:50. (© BASC.)

Erythema rarely requires a complementary undercoat (see Fig. 20-16), but when the scarring presents very dark brown you may need to use a complementary underneath the normal skin-matched crème. However, we would always suggest you try two layers of natural skin match first because this would prove to be the easiest option for both the person and their purse (see Fig. 20-15C).

Brown consists of red and green (which as complementary, we know, is not successful), or a mix of orange and blue. Owing to an optical illusion (red), blood appears blue through the skin; therefore, our complementary wheel now needs to consider orange as the complementary (see Fig. 20-17).

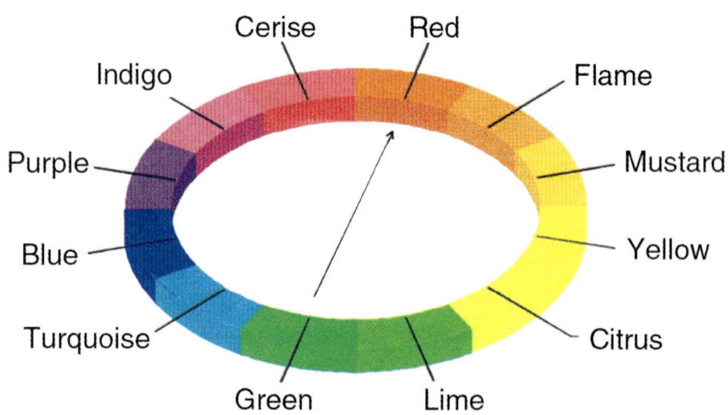

FIGURE 20-14 Green is opposite red on the complementary color theory wheel. (© BASC.)

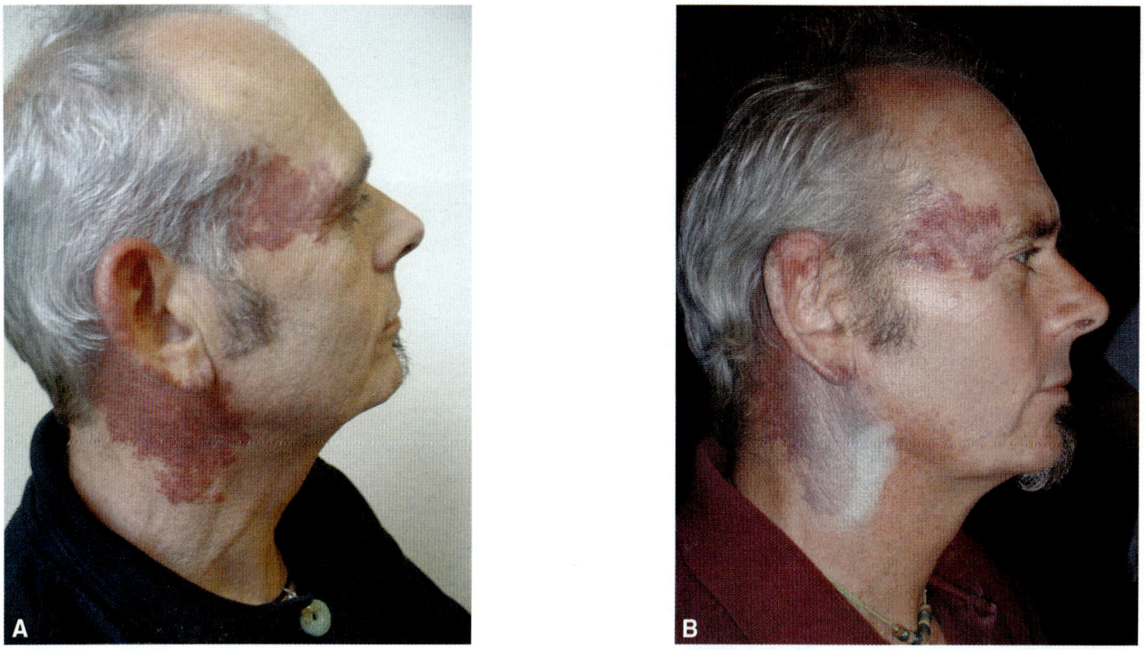

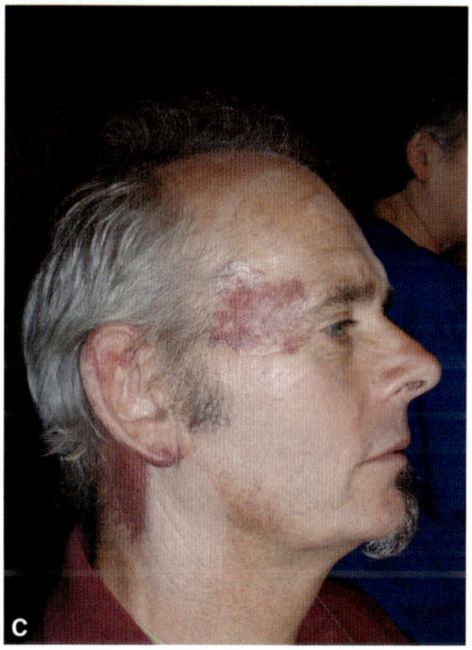

FIGURE 20-15 Camouflage applied over a port wine stain. **A:** Pot wine stain. **B:** Complementary green applied. **C:** Two layers of skin matching camouflage applied to port wine stain directly (no complementary color below). *(© BASC.)*

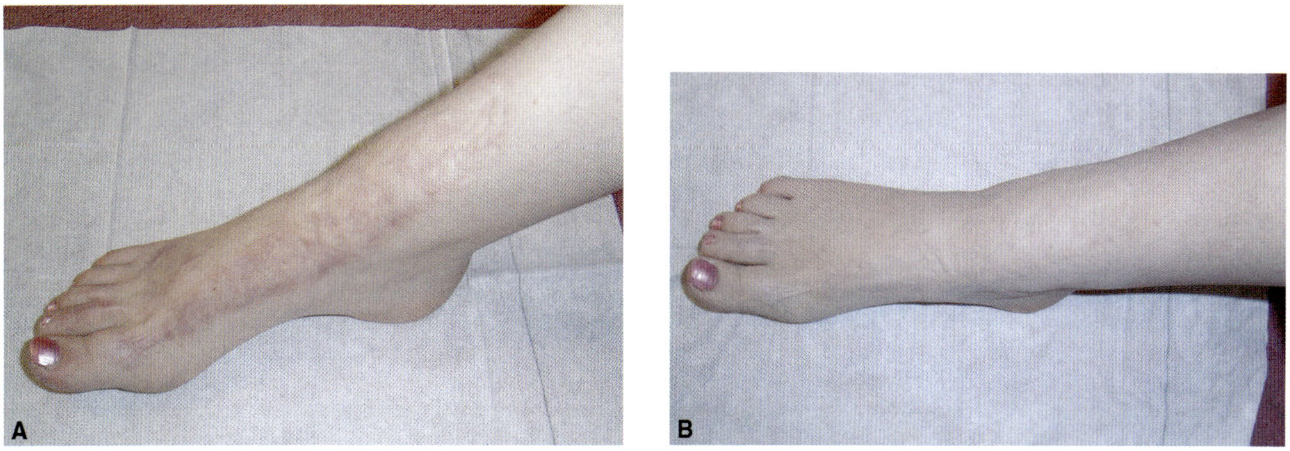

FIGURE 20-16 Only one layer of surrounding skin match was required (erythematous scarring from burn injury). *(© BASC member 2163, the Camouflage Club at the Burned Children's Club, Essex.)*

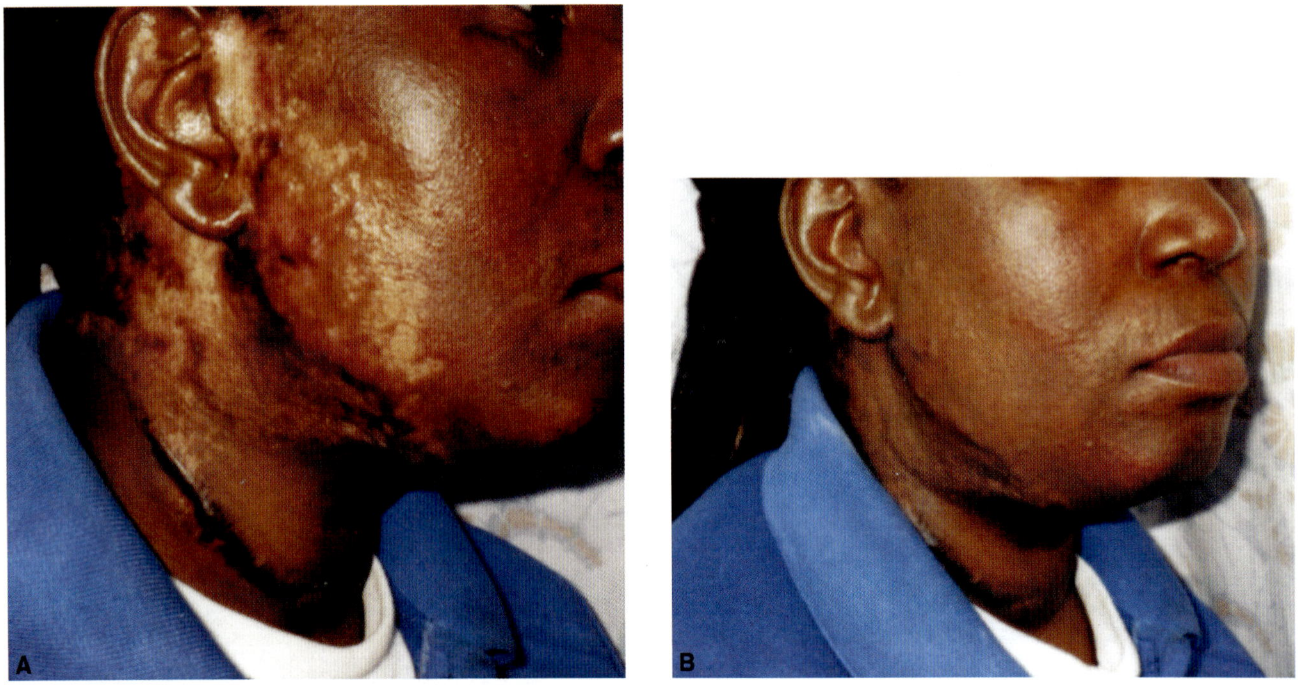

FIGURE 20-17 Lady elected not to use a complementary, preferring to use the skin match over the hyperpigmented keloid scarring *(© BASC member 1022.)*

Application Techniques

Having agreed an acceptable skin match with the person, you will then need to discuss a suitable application technique. Camouflage is applied using quick and simple techniques and should not be complicated. The more simple the routine, the more acceptable it will be to the patient.

Narrow, Linear Scar

The use of a clean cosmetic brush is recommended here, with the crème being applied in a zigzag along the scar. Then, with the ball of a clean finger tip, gently merge the crème and blend into the immediate surrounding skin. If you apply a single line of camouflage to a linear scar, it will look contrived (see Fig. 20-18).

Multiple Linear Scars

It would be too laborious for the person to employ the foregoing method to individual scars; the simplest method is for the person to swipe-wipe across the whole of the affected area (see Fig. 20-19).

Contracture and Burn Injury Scars

A gentle rubbing motion over the whole area should ensure that the camouflage crème adheres to the various skin textures (see Figs. 20-20 and 20-21).

The camouflage crème requires setting with loose powder—translucent powder will not affect the camouflage color, but tinted powders will. Apply using a traditional powder puff in a press and roll motion. Powders will create a matte finish; should this look unnatural, a fixing spray over the powder will add a slight shine.

You need to advise the person where to obtain the selected camouflage crème/s and setting products (as well as any applicators) and ensure that they know how to apply, maintain, and effectively remove their camouflage. This is particularly so where camouflage can be washed off with soap and water. This will mean the person will need to replace camouflage to the back of his or her hands when it is washed off in conformity with hygienic practices. Should the camouflage become damp owing to excessive perspiration, or wet owing to swimming or the weather, the camouflage will be stable provided the person gently blots the camouflage area dry or allows the air to naturally dry the wet skin. Camouflage should not be considered 100% rub-proof, and any minor transfer (e.g., to clothing and linens) can be easily removed with normal laundry products.

Skin camouflage consultations may take up to 1 hour. One visit is normally enough to teach the person how to apply their camouflage, how to make sure it stays on, and how to properly remove it. A second consultation may be required if there is a color change to the condition or the surrounding unaffected skin (or both).

Training Opportunities

BASC is an independent association run by dedicated professionals who volunteer their expertise. BASC is considered to be the main source of information and education material for people interested in skin camouflage. It is internationally acknowledged as the leading training authority for professionals (doctors, nurses, pharmacists, therapists, beauticians) in this specialty. Their educational

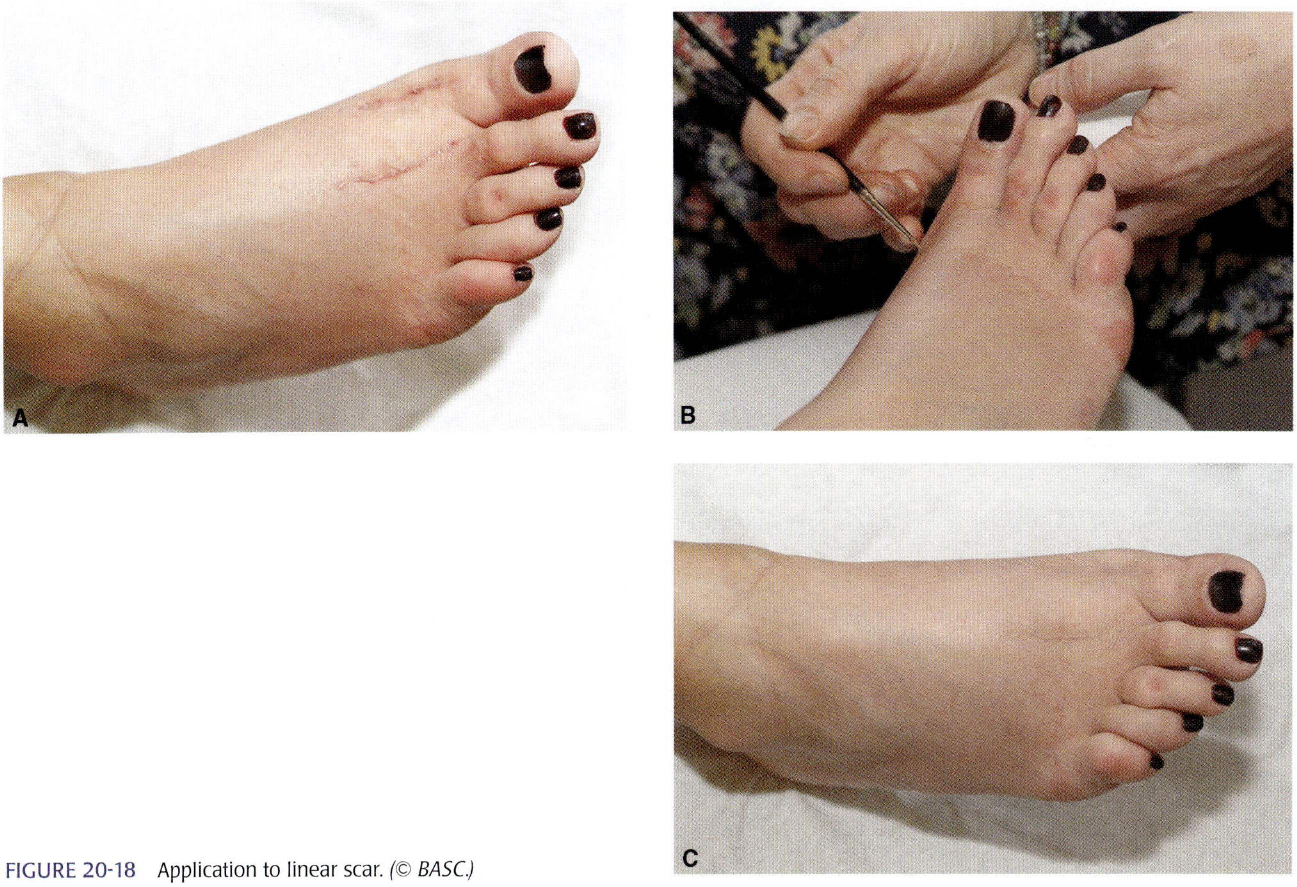

FIGURE 20-18 Application to linear scar. *(© BASC.)*

FIGURE 20-19 Application to multiple scars—outcome presents better when scarring is not atrophic or keloidal (road traffic accident). *(© BASC.)*

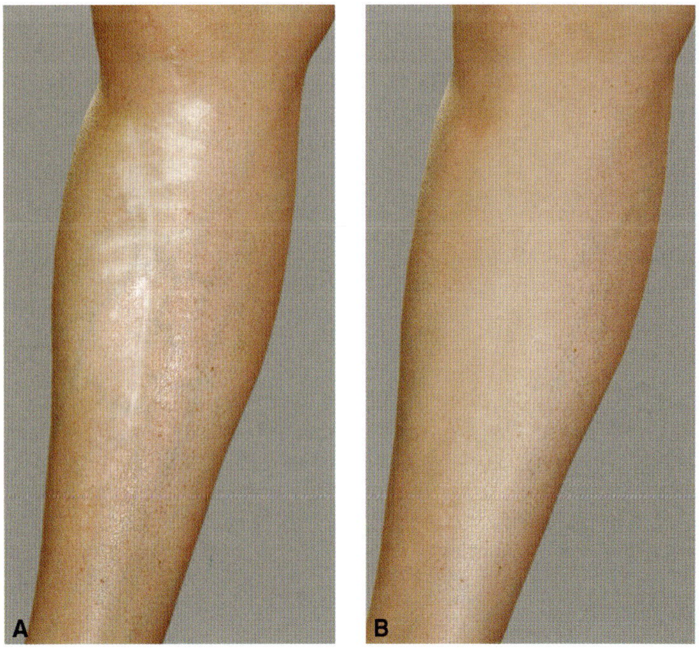

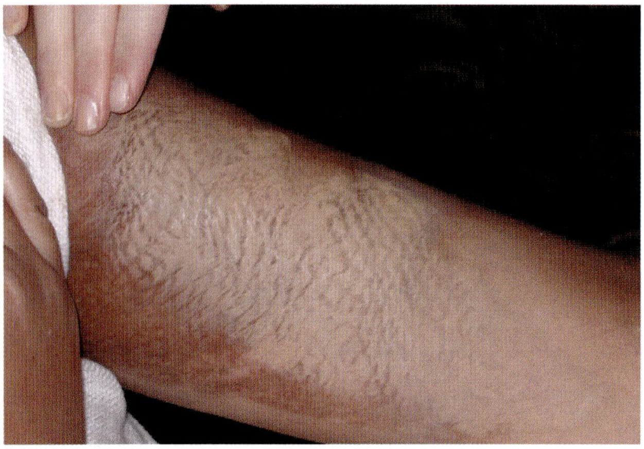

FIGURE 20-20 Application to mesh graft. *(© BASC member 1022.)*

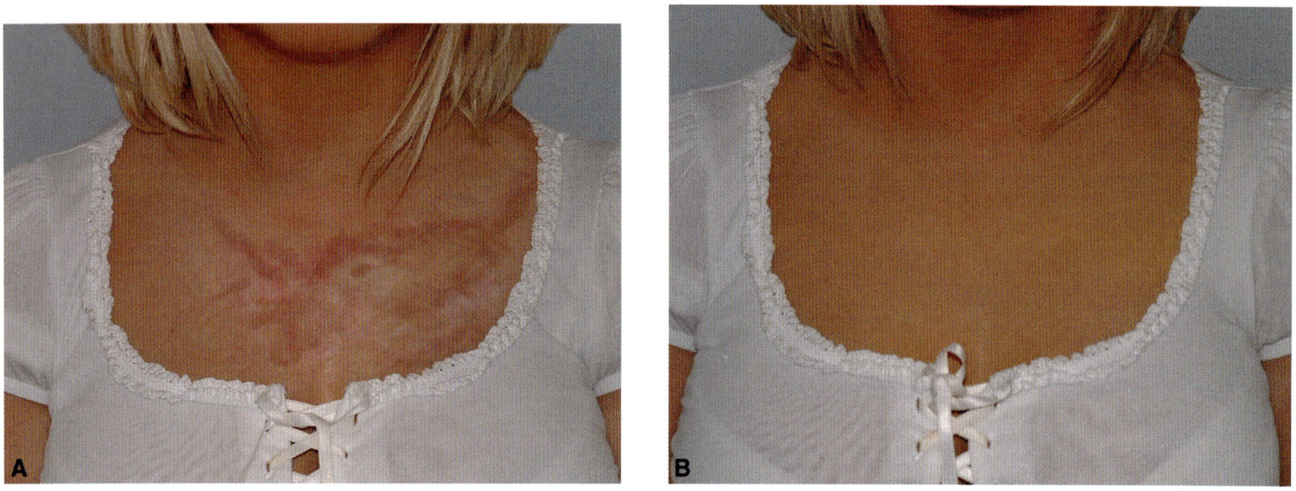

FIGURE 20-21 Application over scald injury. *(© BASC.)*

programs are monitored every year and Continuing Professional Development (CPD) accredited by the Royal College of Nursing (RCN), College of Occupational Therapists (COT), Institute of Trichologists (IoT), Institute of Maxillofacial Prosthetists and Technologists (IMPT), the Hair and Beauty Industry Authority (HABIA), and the Association of Anatomical Pathology Technology (AAPT). BASC is the specialist adviser on skin camouflage to the Confederation of International Beauty Therapy and Cosmetology (CIBTAC) who train therapists in this discipline to an exceptionally high standard.

Since 2001, BASC has worked closely with HABIA to develop industry standards (NVQ level II and III), which are then taught by colleges of further education within their awarding body's beauty therapy/make-up artistry courses.

Further information on BASC activities can be found on www.skin-camouflage.net.

REFERENCES

1. Lucas A. Perfumes and incense in ancient Egypt. *J Egypt Archaeol*, 1930;16(1/2):41–53.
2. Allen, E. *Cover the Principles and Art of Para-Medical Skin Camouflage*. Chapter 12, A Potted History of Skin Camouflage. Bloomington, IN: Authorhouse; 2010. www.skin-camouflage.net. Accessed November 19, 2016.
3. Kobler, J. *Capone, The Life and World of Al Capone*. Boston, MA: Da Capo Press; 1971:15, 36.
4. Rumsey N, Harcourt D. The psychology of appearance. *Facial Appearance and the Criminal Justice System*. Maidenhead: Open University Press; 2005:15–16.
5. Entri Research Ltd. Scar Information Service (sponsored by Smith & Nephew), December 1999.
6. Finlay AY, Khan GK. Dermatology Life Quality Index: a simple practical measure for routine clinical use. *Clin Exp Dermatol*. 1994;19:210–216.
7. All Party Parliamentary Group on Skin. *The Psychological and Social Impact of Skin Diseases on People's Lives, a report of the All Party Parliamentary Group on Skin*. London: All Party Parliamentary Group on Skin; 2013
8. Goffman E. *Stigma: Notes on the Management of Spoiled Identity*. Harmondsworth, London: Penguin Books; 1963.
9. Clarke A. *Psychol Health Med*. 1999;4(2):129–114.
10. Lansdown R, Rumsey N, Bradbury E, et al. *Visibly Different: coping with disfigurement*. London: Butterworth Heinemann; 1997.
11. Papadopoulos L, Bor R. *Psychological Approaches to Dermatology*. The British Psychological Society Books; 1997.
12. Rumsey N, Harcourt D, eds. *The Oxford Handbook of the Psychology of Appearance*. Oxford: Oxford University Press; 2012:417.

21 Medical Tattooing

DAWN CRAGG

KEY POINTS

- Can the client's expectations be met?
- Tattooing saves the daily task of applying camouflage products.
- Skin tones, including color irregularities, can be matched.
- Tattooing restores self-esteem and confidence.

History of Tattooing

Tattooing has been practiced across the globe since at least Neolithic times, as evidenced by mummified preserved skin, ancient art, and the archaeological record.[1] It was Captain James Cook, a British explorer (1796), who first coined the word 'tattoo' when describing a Polynesian practice of inlaying black pigments under the skin.[2] Traditionally associated with sailors and convicts, artistic tattoos are widespread in today's society.

History of Permanent Make-Up

Queen Cleopatra in ancient Egypt and others in India and Africa have sought permanent eye enhancement with various substances over the years. They used plant and nut pigments or ground coals (carbon) as eyeliners or eye shadows and inserted these around their eyes with fine, sharp implements. This is where permanent make-up, as we know it today, originated.

What Is Permanent Make-Up?

Permanent make-up (micropigmentation) is the implantation of colored pigments under the surface of the skin, using a very fine needle or group of needles, via a hand-held manual device or an electrically driven handpiece. This is a self-elected cosmetic procedure to *enhance* facial features such as eyebrows, eyes, and lips on normal skin.

What is Medical Tattooing?

Medical tattooing is used to *reconstruct* features such as eyebrows (lost because of alopecia) and lips (owing to cleft lip or mouth cancer), and to replace the areola following mastectomy. It may also help to reduce the perception of hypopigmentation and hyperpigmentation in scars.

Medical tattooing can cosmetically improve the scars associated with interventions such as plastic and cosmetic surgery, radiation therapy, and endoscopic surgery. Although medical tattooing will use the same products and techniques as micropigmentation, the technician will require additional training because of the nature of working on scar tissue, rather than normal skin.

The age of the scar, type, color, condition, and underlying health of the patient will affect the pigment color and technique used because all influence the outcome, as does patient compliance with aftercare. The composition of scarred skin, different types of scars, and how the scars themselves react to medical tattooing are further considerations. For example, scar tissue due to burn injury will absorb more pigment and may require several medical tattoo sessions to achieve an acceptable outcome.

After the initial treatment, the pigment will fade over time. In fair skin (Fitzpatrick skin type I and II) after the pigment has faded, the residual color will tend to be even lighter because of the need for titanium dioxide (white) to mix the color. Consequently, frequent retouches will be necessary, possibly on an annual basis.

Variegation in the skin caused by freckles and capillaries, for example, should be added on the final visit; the skin must have fully healed between appointments. Healing will take approximately 1 month on young and healthy skin. On mature skin, approximately 2 months should be allowed between treatments. Healing affects the ultimate color as it requires a layer of skin to grow over the tattooed area; therefore, the pigment will appear lighter over time.

Application Techniques

Patch testing using both glycerin-based and water-based colored pigments on several areas of a scar is paramount to determine how the skin is going to react. Scars are very unpredictable and different areas of the same scar can respond differently to the pigment. At the initial consultation, pigment can be applied topically, covered with an adhesive dressing, and left in place for 24 hours. If the area becomes irritated, the pigment should be removed immediately. In this case tattooing should not proceed.

Pigment is applied using a circular, back and forth, or hair stroke motion, depending on the area worked. Shading is applied using a flat needle and working through a very thin layer of petroleum jelly. Stippling is the application of small dots with a fine round needle. Working in natural daylight is important. If this is not possible, then daylight bulbs may be used. Work should never be attempted under artificial light. Color application should be conservative initially, and can be adjusted on subsequent visits. This is because one cannot be sure how the pigment is going to heal into the skin, and it is easier to add more color at the second appointment.

Who Can Perform Medical Tattooing and Where

It is essential that technicians are highly skilled and qualified in medical tattooing before they accept clients or patients. Because of lack of understanding of tattoo techniques, inexperienced and undertrained practitioners can cause damage to the scar, including permanent hypopigmentation. In addition, posttreatment hyperpigmentation can occur when tattooing patients with Fitzpatrick skin types IV, V, and VI. In most countries, the cosmetic tattooing industry is unregulated and without thorough training to a high standard (i.e., from a recognized training authority). Therefore expertise is potentially highly variable and insurance is difficult to obtain. A patient seeking treatment in any country can contact the Society of Permanent Cosmetic Professionals (SPCP) via their website spcp.org. They have a list of trained technicians worldwide who meet the very high standards in cosmetic and medical tattooing as required for membership.

Medical tattooing can be applied to all areas of the body, apart from the genitalia. This is because if a patient were to claim they had lost physical sensation, or if infection developed in that area, it would be nearly impossible to prove this was not caused by medical tattooing. Therefore it is unlikely to be covered on a technician's insurance. Technicians generally work from hospitals and clinics, though they may work from other premises provided that they have been inspected and licensed by their local authority.

Products Used

Good quality pigments must always be used and safety data sheets should be obtained from the distributors. For example, the author holds safety data sheets for the range of Mei-Cha Microcolors, Image, and Forever Lips pigments used for medical tattooing.

Pigments used to camouflage scars to a natural skin tone for Fitzpatrick skin types I to IV are mainly high-quality medical-grade products based on titanium dioxide. This is in contrast to pigments used in cosmetic micropigmentation, where the darker colors are more likely to have an iron oxide base. Color washes are a very important part of medical camouflage as well for blending the edges of scars or areolae.

A digital machine is preferable to alternatives because the power source is stable. Battery-operated machines are not recommended because battery power is affected by temperature and humidity. The machine must conform to the regulations of the relevant country. For example, in the United Kingdom all machines should conform to European Union regulations. The Conformite Europeene (CE) mark indicates the manufacturer's declaration that the product meets the requirements of the European Community (EC) directives.

Needles must be sterile, disposable (single use), prepackaged, color coded for easier size identification, packaged with plastic needle guard tubes, and compliant with health authority requirements.

- Single needles—should be used with great caution because of their sharpness and fineness. It is easy for an inexperienced technician to penetrate the skin too deeply, which may cause the pigment to migrate. This migration may not be visible immediately, but may be evident after a few months.
- Double needle—two single needles close together and therefore, as with the single needles, not recommended for general use.
- Triple needles—are a cluster of three; the most useful needle for creating the outline for lips and freckles.
- Flat needles—are a row of needles in a line and vary from four needles to a greater number. They are the perfect choice for eyebrow hair strokes, if used correctly, at right angles to the skin. When used this way with a sweeping motion, they are ideal for camouflaging larger areas of skin.
- Needles of five round configuration and above are best used when working over a large area of the skin. The scarred area should be approximately 2 cm^2 and above.
- Magnums—are used for shading, blending, and coloring large areas and are therefore very suitable for medical tattooing. Because of the amount of pigment that flows through, less passes are required, limiting skin damage.

Anesthetics Used in Permanent Make-Up and Medical Tattooing

Most countries have regulations regarding the use of topical anesthetics used in tattooing. Technicians should only use products that are legally available through their local pharmacy and read the full instructions for each product before use.

When is Medical Tattooing Considered Appropriate?

Medical tattooing offers a long-lasting alternative to the daily chore of applying camouflage products. The professional judgment of the client's dermatologist, consultant, or medical practitioner is required to evaluate whether techniques such as the use of laser, acids, or hydroquinone will lighten hyperpigmentation, or if medical tattooing is warranted. Tattooing is useful for cases where conventional methods are not indicated; for example, when nipple surgical reconstruction is not achievable or when a scar is relatively good quality and without erythema and would therefore not benefit from additional laser treatment.[5] Scars that will not benefit from surgical revision often present a good outcome when tattooed because of potential uneven color distribution. Hypopigmented scars generally look better with color, even if the pigment is not a perfect match. Medical tattooing can disguise scarring that results from the donor site of previous hair transplant surgery and small scars resulting from an accident or surgical procedure.

The selected color MUST be agreed with the person before proceeding. This is achieved by placing the pigment topically next to the area requiring the tattoo. Explanation must be given that initially the tattooed area will appear darker, but should settle to the selected color in approximately 4 weeks.

The design and shape of the tattoo must also be agreed before proceeding. This is most important for eyebrow and lip replacement because fashions frequently change (compare the single arched line of the 1940s eyebrow to the thicker fuller shapes that come in later), and the tattoo could become 'dated' very quickly.

Contraindications

- Either a patch (on top of the skin) or scratch (under the skin) test must be undertaken 24 hours before the planned tattooing. A 28-day patch test may be required for organic pigments. Failure to do so may invalidate insurance.
- People who are prone to hypertrophic or keloid scarring.
- Scars from burns need to be mature and completely healed prior to medical tattooing. The physician's written consent must be obtained to proceed.
- Any area of skin that has a suspicious lesion, especially indicating potential skin cancer.
- Skin types IV, V, and VI (Fitzpatrick scale) can result in hyperpigmentation.
- Scars that are less than 6 to 12 months old.
- Patients that are pregnant or breast-feeding.
- Patients with skin grafts, without prior written consent from the doctor.
- Patients with insulin-dependent diabetes, without prior written consent from the doctor.
- Patients with abnormal heart conditions, without prior written consent from the doctor.
- Patients with body dysmorphia are likely to have unrealistic expectations.
- Suntan (fake or natural).
- Some drugs may change the color of the skin; the person is advised to wait until the course of medication is completed and the physician gives permission for medical tattooing to proceed.

Cancer

Cancer patients are not contraindicated, even when undergoing chemotherapy, provided there is written medical consent from the doctor.

Vitiligo

Vitiligo patients are not contraindicated providing they have a written medical consent from their doctor or dermatologist.

Risks

The following risks must be fully explained to the person before they agree to any medical tattooing. Potential risks include:

1. Hyperpigmentation which can occur when tattooing Fitzpatrick skin types IV to VI. Hypopigmentation can be caused by incorrect insertion of the needle.
2. Successful results cannot be guaranteed.
3. Allergy to pigments. One study involving 300 people had a reported rate of adverse reactions of 10.3%. Red and black pigments were the main offenders, as well as exposure to a large range of colors. Tattoo reactions were thought to be underreported in this study as they are a common occurrence in the United States.[3]
4. Allergic reaction to topically applied anesthetic products such as lidocaine, prilocaine, and tetracaine.
5. Infection, swelling, crusting, bleeding, and nipple flattening.
6. Skin changes color according to many external and internal factors (e.g., sun and medication); an acceptable skin match on intake may later prove unacceptable.
7. The pigment will remain in the skin indefinitely, but will break down and fade with time. Tattoos that are frequently exposed to ultraviolet light will fade more quickly than those hidden by clothing.
8. Reactions to any type of tattoo can occur many years after the procedure was carried out.
9. Needles inserted too deeply can cause bleeding, migration of pigment, and damage to hair follicles.
10. Overworking the area can result in scarring.
11. Results are not instantaneous.
12. Scarred skin is unpredictable and reacts differently than undamaged skin. Results can be inconsistent across the scarred area.
13. Unrealistic expectations; scars can only be disguised, not removed.
14. Patients with body dysmorphia may have unrealistic expectations.
15. Hyperpigmentation is not resolved by tattooing a lighter color over the area, as the needle may cause further hyperpigmentation.
16. There are many color irregularities in the skin which all respond differently to tattooing. Natural excessive melanin distribution, such as freckles and lentigines, will respond differently when tattooed.
17. Anesthetics are known to blanch the skin; the choice of color may be compromised if made after their application.

In proposed new standards in the United Kingdom, all doctors carrying out cosmetic procedures will be required to fully inform patients of the risks of treatment and to give them a "cooling off" period before they commit to any procedure. They will be required to abstain from making unjustifiable claims about the results and from using promotional tactics that encourage people to make ill-considered decisions.[4]

Before and After Photographs of Medical Micropigmentation

See Figures 21-1 to 21-7. All tattooing and make-up applied by Dawn Cragg MBE. Photographs by Dawn Cragg, MBE.

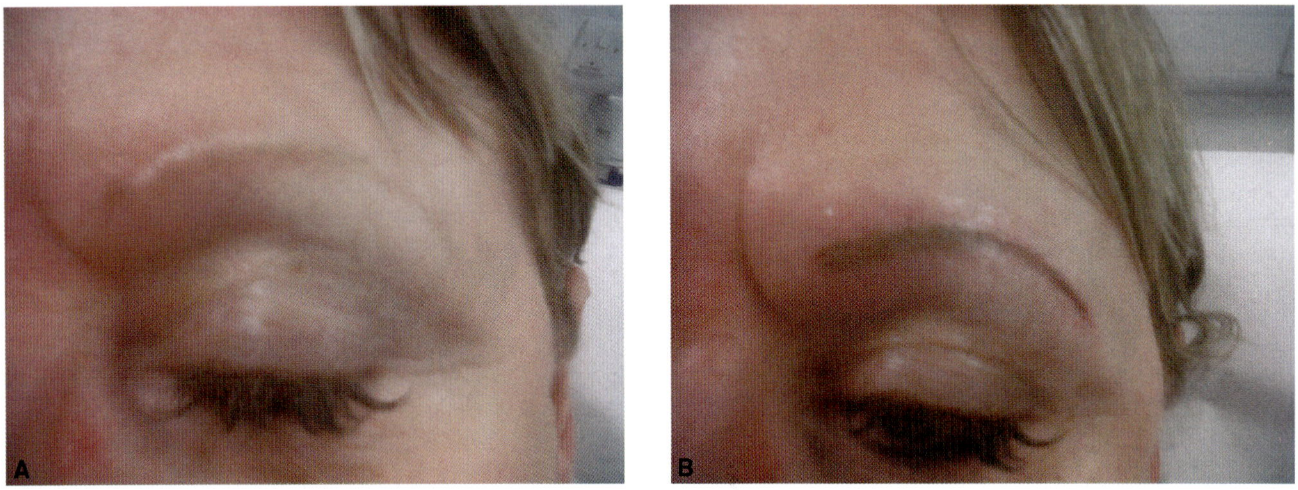

FIGURE 21-1 **A, B:** This high-profile lady had a brow lift which resulted in a scar through her eyebrow. The scar was camouflaged by "raising" the eyebrows using medical tattooing.

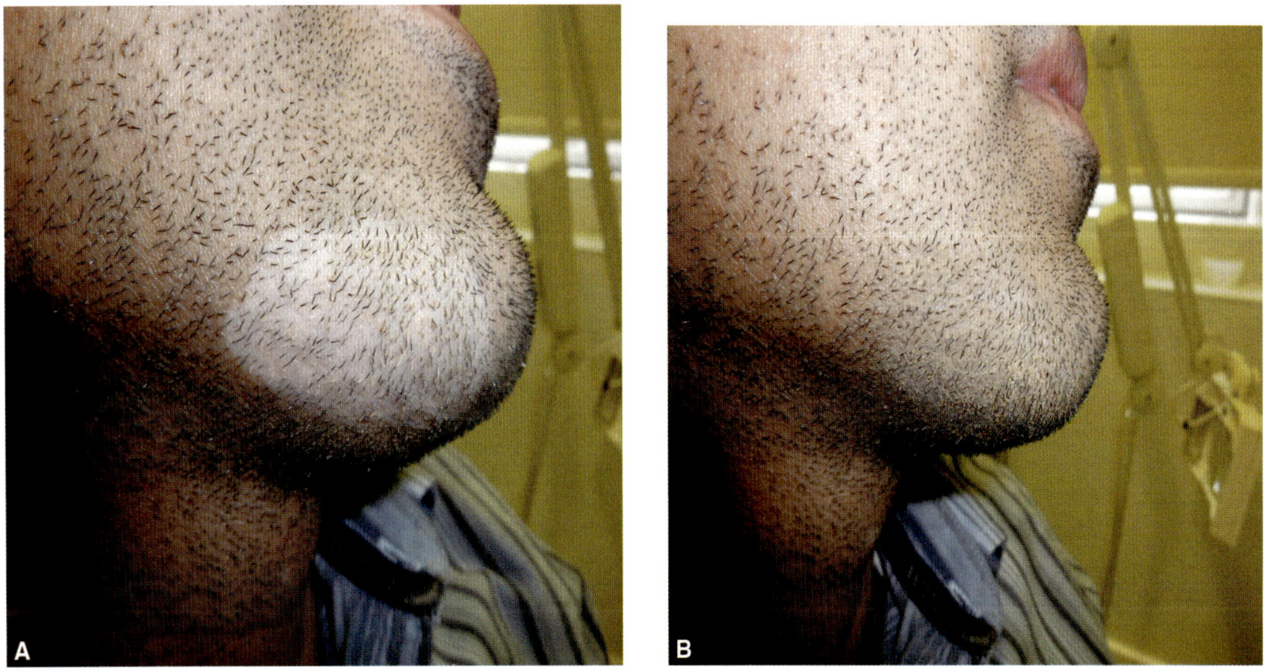

FIGURE 21-2 **A, B:** A stippling technique was used to simulate stubble on the chin and cheek areas. He later telephoned to say what a difference it has made to his life.

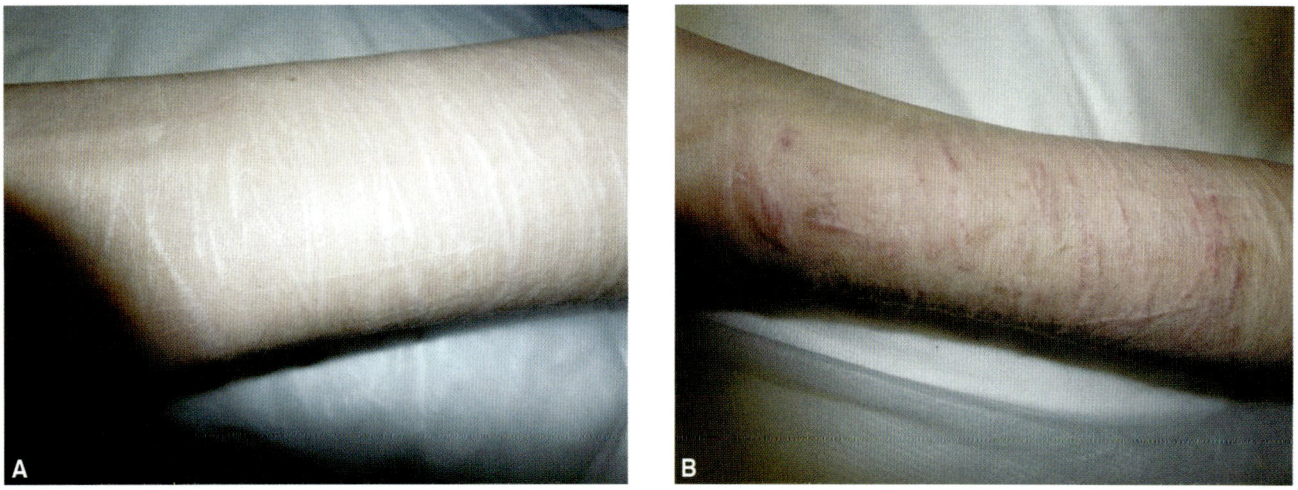

FIGURE 21-3 **A:** Hundreds of scars covered this client's arm. Psychiatric counseling is required before undertaking a self-harm patient; further self-harm over tattooing may cause adverse complications including impaired healing, infection, and tattoo pigment migration. **B:** The tattooing process causes reddening, making the scars look worse in the short term. Clients who have self-harmed must certainly go through psychological counseling before any treatment is attempted. Flashbacks to when the injuries were first inflicted can occur, and they could experience long-term psychological effects. Camouflage creams applied and removed on a daily basis are more suitable for such cases.

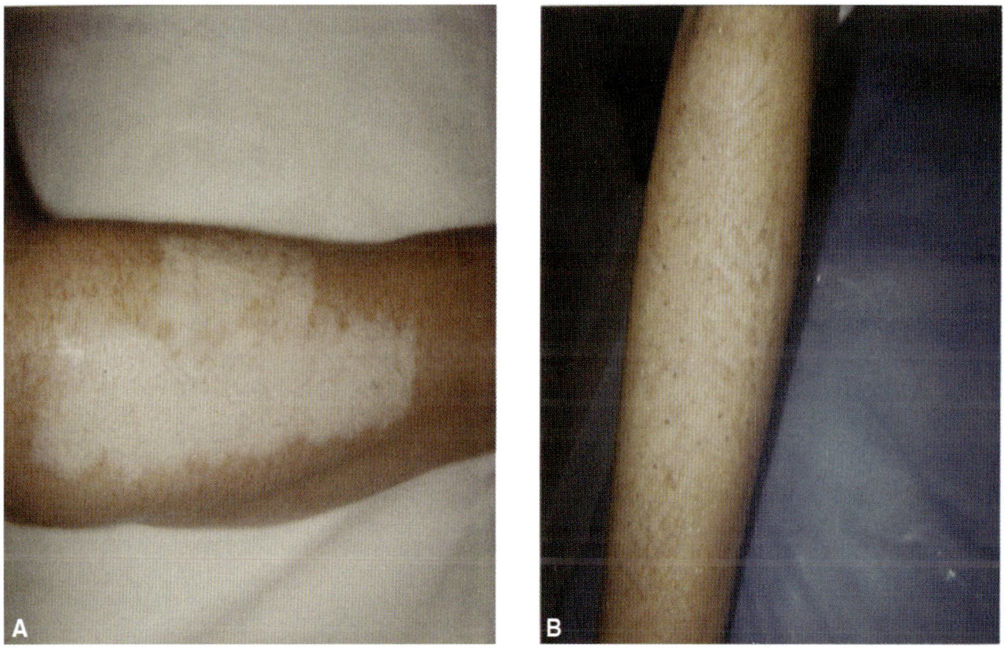

FIGURE 21-4 **A:** Scarring of the forearm was resurfaced with dermabrasion, leaving residual depigmentation. **B:** Medical tattooing was employed to resemble the natural color, including the recreation of freckles and lentigines.

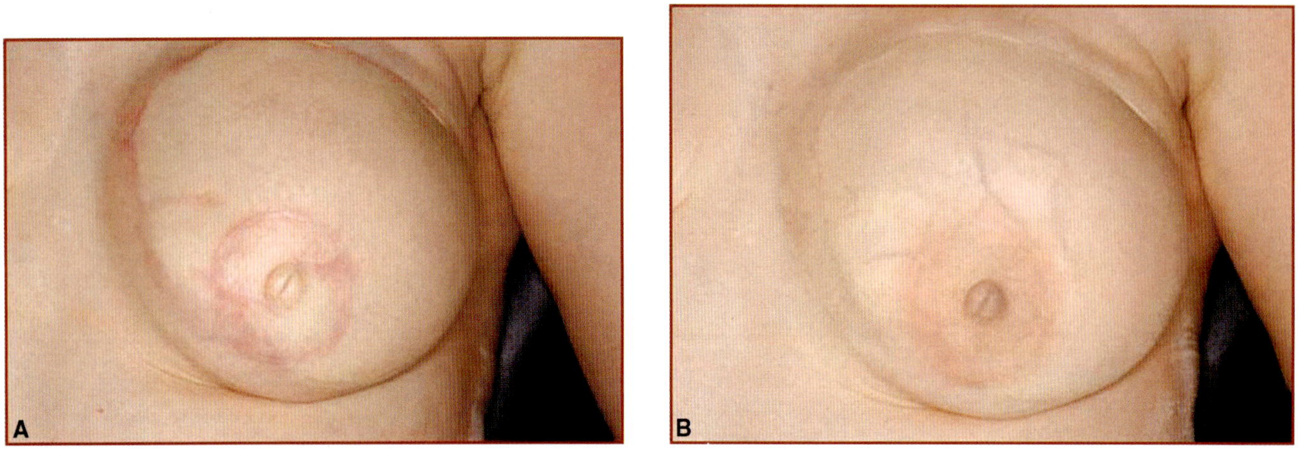

FIGURE 21-5 **A:** Artificial nipple created during reconstructive plastic surgery. **B:** The color and veining pattern were designed to match her unaffected breast.

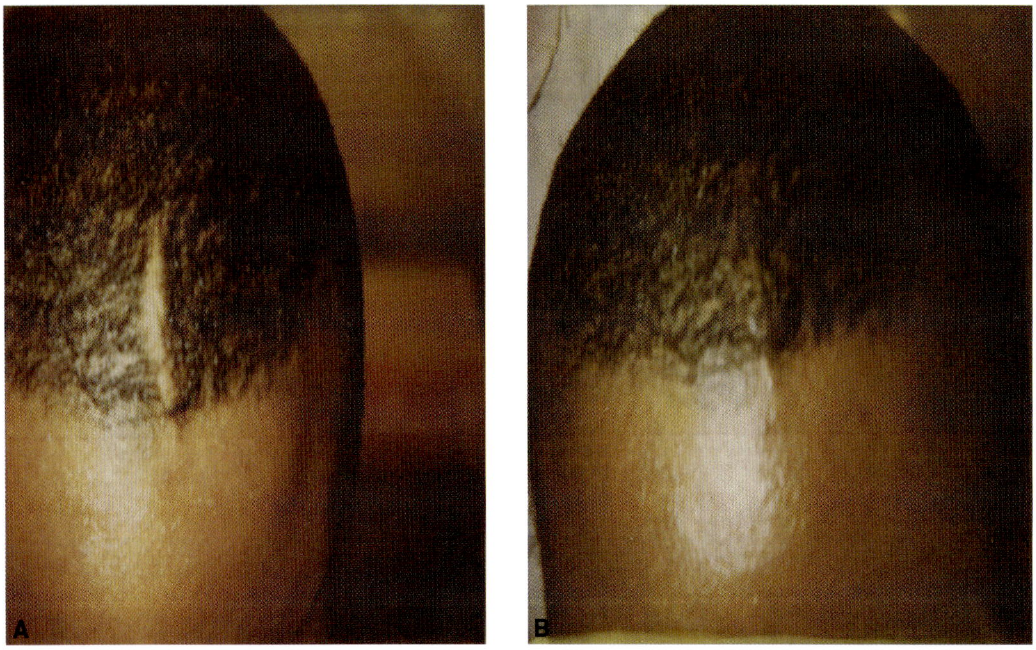

FIGURE 21-6 **A, B:** Scar on the front of his forehead. A series of dots was applied in a dark brown which matched his hair and camouflaged the scar.

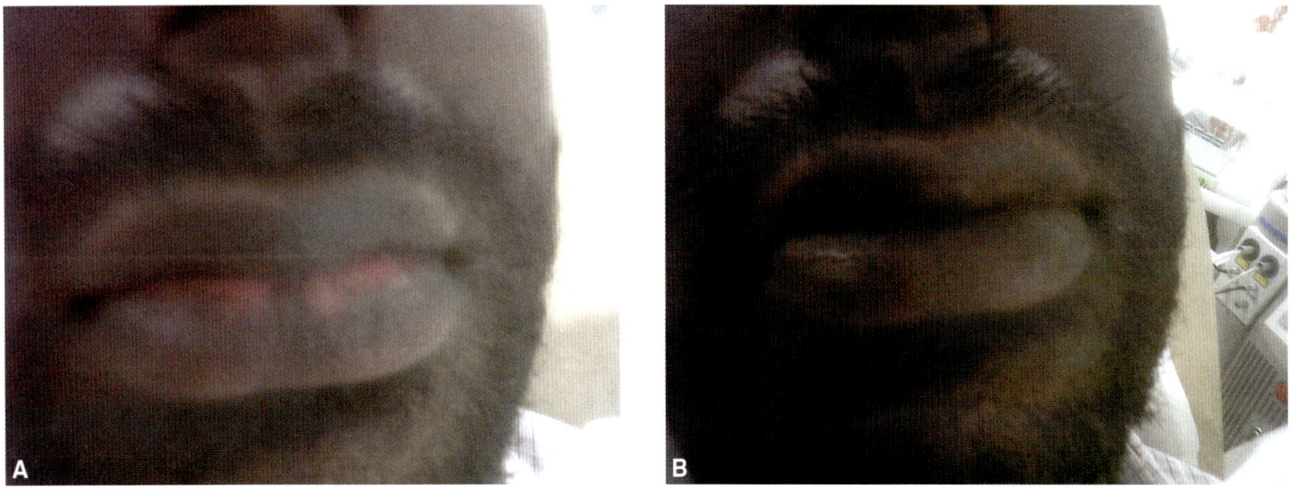

FIGURE 21-7 **A, B:** This gentleman had a habit of biting and picking the skin on his lips, which led to pigment loss caused by scarring. The affected skin was tattooed to match the surrounding unaffected skin.

REFERENCES

1. Deter-Wolf A. "The Material Culture and Middle Stone Age Origins of Ancient Tattooing." Tattoos and body modifications in antiquity. In: Proceedings of the sessions at the EAA annual meetings in The Hague and Oslo, 2010/11. *Zurich Stud Archaeol.* 2013;9:15–26.
2. Sehgal VN. *Dermatologic Surgery Made Easy.* 2nd ed. New Delhi, India: Jaypee Brothers; 2012.
3. Brady BG, Gold H, Leger EA, et al. Self-reported adverse tattoo reactions: a New York City Central Park study. *Contact Dermatitis* [Online]. 2015;73(2):91–99. http://onlinelibrary.wiley.com/doi/10.1111/cod.12425/abstract. Accessed July 14, 2015.
4. Kim EK, Chang TJ, Hong JP, et al. Use of tattooing to camouflage various scars. *Aesthet Plast Surg* [Online]. 2011;35(3):392–395. http://www.ncbi.nlm.nih.gov/pubmed/21461628. Accessed July 14, 2015.
5. General Medical Council. Give patients time to think before cosmetic procedures, doctors told. *GMC Press Release*, June 8, 2015. http://www.gmc-uk.org/news/26550.asp. Accessed July 14, 2015.

DAWN CRAGG was appointed as a Member of the Order of the British Empire (MBE) in the New Year 2010 Honors list, for outstanding achievement in the development of medical tattooing as a service to healthcare.

22 A Pediatric Perspective

ANDREW C. KRAKOWSKI and TUYET A. NGUYEN

KEY POINTS

- Although children are certainly not "just little adults," the paradigm for treating pediatric scars is mostly extrapolated directly from the adult experience.
- The adage of "use it or lose it" suggests that early intervention may be crucial when scars compromise physical, psychological, or social development.
- Emerging technologies such as ablative and nonablative fractionated lasers have revolutionized the treatment and mitigation of pediatric scars, with objective evidence supporting the case for coverage by insurance companies.
- A multimodal, multidisciplinary approach will likely prove the most successful paradigm for treating pediatric scars.
- Well-controlled, randomized, prospective studies comparing the safety and efficacy of scar treatments are lacking in the pediatric population, representing a tremendous opportunity for basic, translational, and clinical research.
- Treating even a single child's scar can improve the outlook of both the patient and the provider in ways neither of them might have ever imagined; do not be afraid to ask your pediatric patients about their scars and what they mean to them!

How Does Pediatric Skin Differ from Adult Skin?

The basic functions of the skin include serving as a barrier to the outside world (reduce fluid loss, regulate temperature, and provide protection from infection and harmful environmental agents) and as a conduit for the perception of sensations such as pain, vibration, and pressure.[1,2] Although the role of skin remains the same throughout life, pediatric skin is in some ways uniquely different from that of adult skin.

Structure

The skin of infants and children differs in several ways from that of adults in terms of structure. It has been shown that the skin of infants and children may be up to 60% thinner than that of an adult.[3] An in vivo analysis demonstrated that the thickness of the stratum corneum and suprapapillary epidermis in infants is approximately 30% and 20% less, respectively, compared to the skin of their biologic mothers.[2] Additionally, infant corneocytes and keratinocytes in the granular layer are significantly smaller than those found in adult skin, possibly representing an increased turnover rate.[2]

In the dermal layer, collagen bundles in the upper reticular dermis are not as prominent in infant skin, giving the appearance of a gradual transition between papillary and reticular dermis on histology.[4] The composition of the subcutaneous fat in infants and young children also differs from that of adults. Newborn subcutaneous fat has been found to contain a higher ratio of saturated to unsaturated fats compared to that of adults.[5] This higher proportion of saturated fats makes infants more prone to cold temperatures and panniculitis because of the higher melting point associated with saturated fats. The structure of infant skin appears to continually evolve, approaching that of adult skin around 1 year of life.[6]

Body Surface Area

Body surface area (BSA) is a measure of the surface area of the body. In infants and children, the BSA-to-volume ratio of an infant or child can reach up to five times that of an adult.[7] The difference in this ratio makes infants and children more susceptible to increased percutaneous absorption of topically applied agents, transepidermal water loss (TEWL), and skin damage leading to increased risk of toxicity and dehydration.

Decreased Barrier Function

The barrier function of the skin is dependent on the formation of the stratum corneum. In infants, decreased barrier function compared to that of adult skin has been reported. As the stratum corneum continues to develop

Table 22-1 Some Percutaneous Toxicity Risks in the Pediatric Population

Agent	Toxicity
Alcohols (topical antiseptic)	Hemorrhagic necrosis
Hexachlorophene (topical antiseptic)	Neurotoxicity
Povidone–iodine (topical antiseptic)	Hypothyroxinemia, goiter
Lidocaine–prilocaine cream (EMLA) (topical anesthetic)	Methemoglobinemia

A more exhaustive list can be found in the article by Mancini JA. Skin. *Pediatrics.* 2004;113(suppl 3). http://pediatrics.aappublications.org/content/113/Supplement_3/1114.figures-only. Accessed November 17, 2016.

during the first year of life, changes in barrier function also continue to develop during this time.[6] For example, TEWL is often used as a marker of skin barrier function. In infants, the stratum corneum contains higher water content but is also prone to increased TEWL compared to adults.[2,6] Premature infants have an even higher rate of TEWL compared to full-term infants and adults.[8] This predisposition puts infants at greater risk for dehydration and electrolyte imbalance than adults.[9]

In addition, the skin provides mechanical barrier protection by preventing the entry of foreign agents into the body. In premature infants, however, there is limited dermal to epidermal surface attachment. The fragility of premature and newborn skin leaves them more vulnerable to potential percutaneous toxicity and transepidermal infections (Table 22-1).[9]

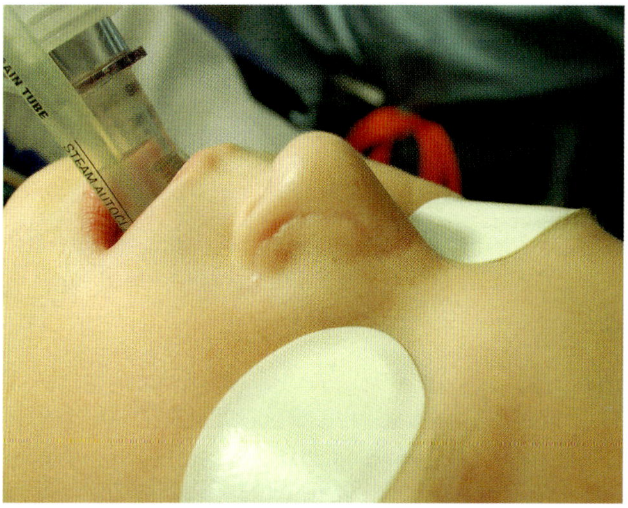

FIGURE 22-1 **Atrophic scar following flap reconstruction.** This patient suffered tissue injury and loss secondary to a motor scooter accident. Flap reconstruction successfully filled the tissue defect, but was associated with atrophy and contour irregularity at the distal aspect of the flap. *(Courtesy of Andrew C. Krakowski, MD.)*

Causes of Scars in Children

The etiology of scars in children resembles that of the adult population and can be grouped into three basic categories: trauma, burns, and medical conditions. As the medical community improves its ability to keep children alive after serious injuries, the patients are left to deal with the physical, psychosocial, and financial consequences (i.e., the so-called "survivor's paradox"), leading to significant distress for affected children, their caregivers, and providers alike.

Trauma

Unintentional injuries and trauma are one of the leading causes of morbidity in pediatric patients, and are a significant source of scarring in this population.[10] An average of 9.2 million unintentional injuries, such as car or bike accidents, occur in pediatric patients annually.[11] Mangle or friction injuries from machines such as treadmills can cause significant scarring and contractures in children.[12,13] Animal bites, such as dog bites, can also be a common source of traumatic injury, physical disability, and scarring in children (Fig. 22-1).[14–16]

Burns

Burns are another frequent source of scarring in children (Fig. 22-2). Burn injuries can arise from multiple sources in pediatric patients such as campfires, hot ash, or coals.[17,18] Electrical burns are particularly common in very young children, especially on the lips and mouth as infants and young children are more prone to oral exploration; they should also raise suspicion for neglect or nonaccidental injury.[19] However, the most frequent and preventable cause of burns in pediatric patients is scald injuries from hot liquids (Fig. 22-3).[20]

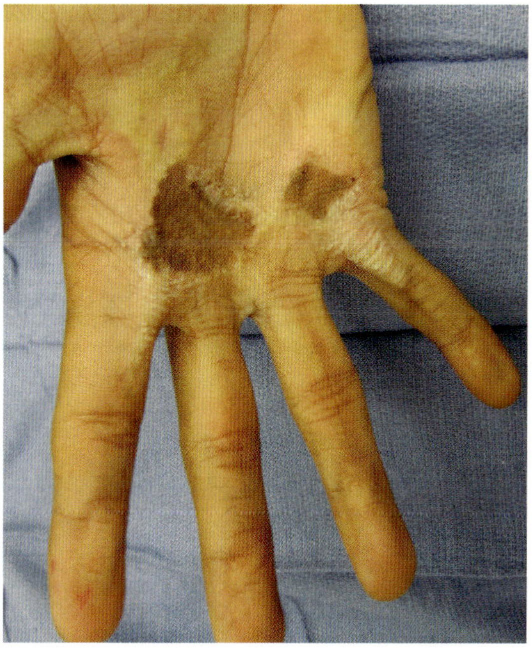

FIGURE 22-2 **Hot iron burn.** This adolescent male severely burned his hand at 1½ years of age. Split-thickness skin grafts were placed on his palm; predictably, a degree of contraction postreconstruction limited his overall function. The patient's main stated concern was that he wanted "to be able to open a jar of peanut butter" without his mother knowing. *(Courtesy of Andrew C. Krakowski, MD.)*

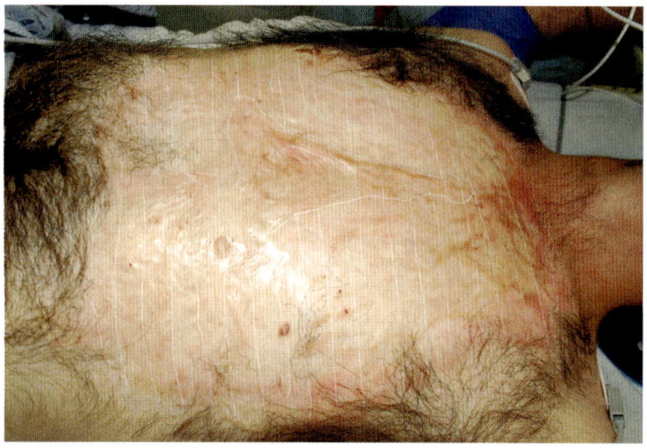

FIGURE 22-3 **Large scald burn.** This male in his 20s presented with a large burn scar secondary to a scald injury. Note the extensive area of alopecia. Objective evaluation of the scarred areas was performed using high-definition ultrasound, revealing that the majority of the "scar sheet" was approximately 1.5 mm in thickness, with focal areas up to 8 mm. A "grid" pattern was then created over the entire scar sheet using a white surgical marker to help delineate the treatment plan for ablative fractional CO2 laser resurfacing. *(Courtesy of Andrew C. Krakowski, MD.)*

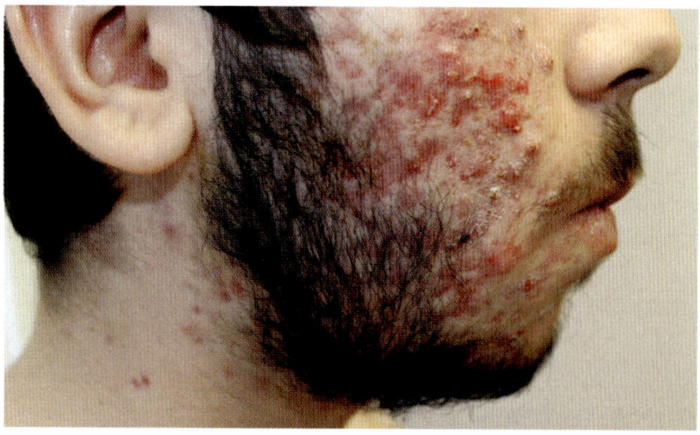

FIGURE 22-4 **Severe inflammatory acne frequently leads to atrophic scarring.** The notion that an inflammatory skin condition such as acne vulgaris, with the potential to inflict permanent physical disfigurement and psychosocial distress, is "just cosmetic" is antiquated and ignorant. A primary clinical goal of acne vulgaris management should be scar prevention; too many adolescents have been left branded with permanent reminders of missed treatment opportunities. We must evolve our thinking in order to help prevent scars before they form. Ultimately, this is the most efficacious and cost-effective scar intervention we have available today, and insurance reimbursement should reflect this reality. *(Courtesy of Andrew C. Krakowski, MD.)*

Medical Conditions

Numerous medical conditions or infections may be associated with scarring (see Chapters 3 and 17).[21–24] Acne, for example, is a frequent source of atrophic facial scars in the adolescent population; however, a larger differential diagnosis for "atrophic scars of cheeks" exists (Table 22-2; Fig. 22-4).[21,22] The treatment of childhood cancers may also be associated with scarring alopecia from radiotherapy, for example, or scarring from the placement of chest tubes, catheter lines, and medical ports.[25] Iatrogenic surgical scars obtained secondarily to the treatment of underlying medical conditions may also be a frequent source of morbidity for children (Fig. 22-5).

Multimodal, Multidisciplinary Approach

The evaluation and management of scars, like many other areas of medicine, continues to evolve. No longer is a single provider typically able to perform all facets of care required for the successful management of a patient with a complicated medical condition. Within the world of pediatric medicine, the "multidisciplinary model" has shown great promise in treating, for example, cleft lip/cleft palate and vascular malformations. The time has come for us to adopt a similar model for the care of patients with complicated scars—one that allows the complete coordination of services from specialties such as primary care (the "quarterback"), dermatology, plastic/reconstructive surgery, anesthesia, radiology, infectious disease, orthopedics, physical/occupational therapy, psychology, nutrition, and a host of ancillary support services (Figs. 22-6 and 22-7). Crucially, the patients and their caregivers must be

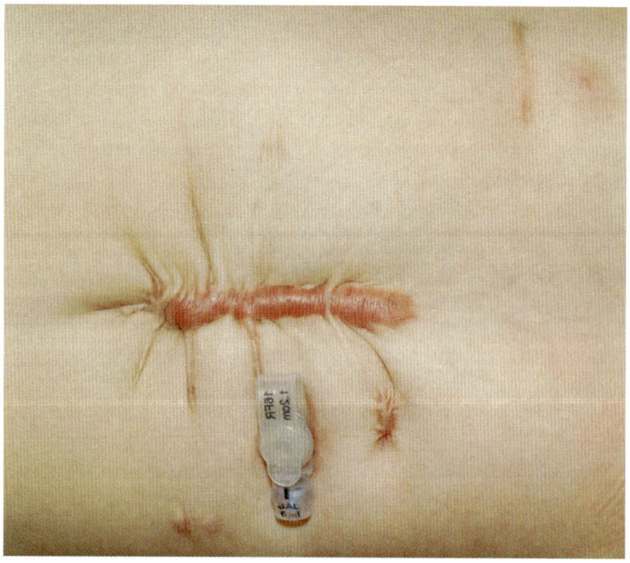

FIGURE 22-5 **Iatrogenic hypertrophic scar with scar contractures.** This infant with Rubinstein–Taybi syndrome developed a hypertrophic scar after abdominal surgery. The scar itself was pruritic and erythematous. The tension on the wound resulted in multiple "radiating" scar contractures. *(Courtesy of Andrew C. Krakowski, MD.)*

Table 22-2 Differential Diagnosis for Atrophic Scarring

Acne vulgaris
Striae distensae
Discoid lupus
Varicella
Molluscum contagiosum
Malignant atrophic papulosis (Degos disease)
Infections (especially *Staphylococcus*)
Surgery
Trauma

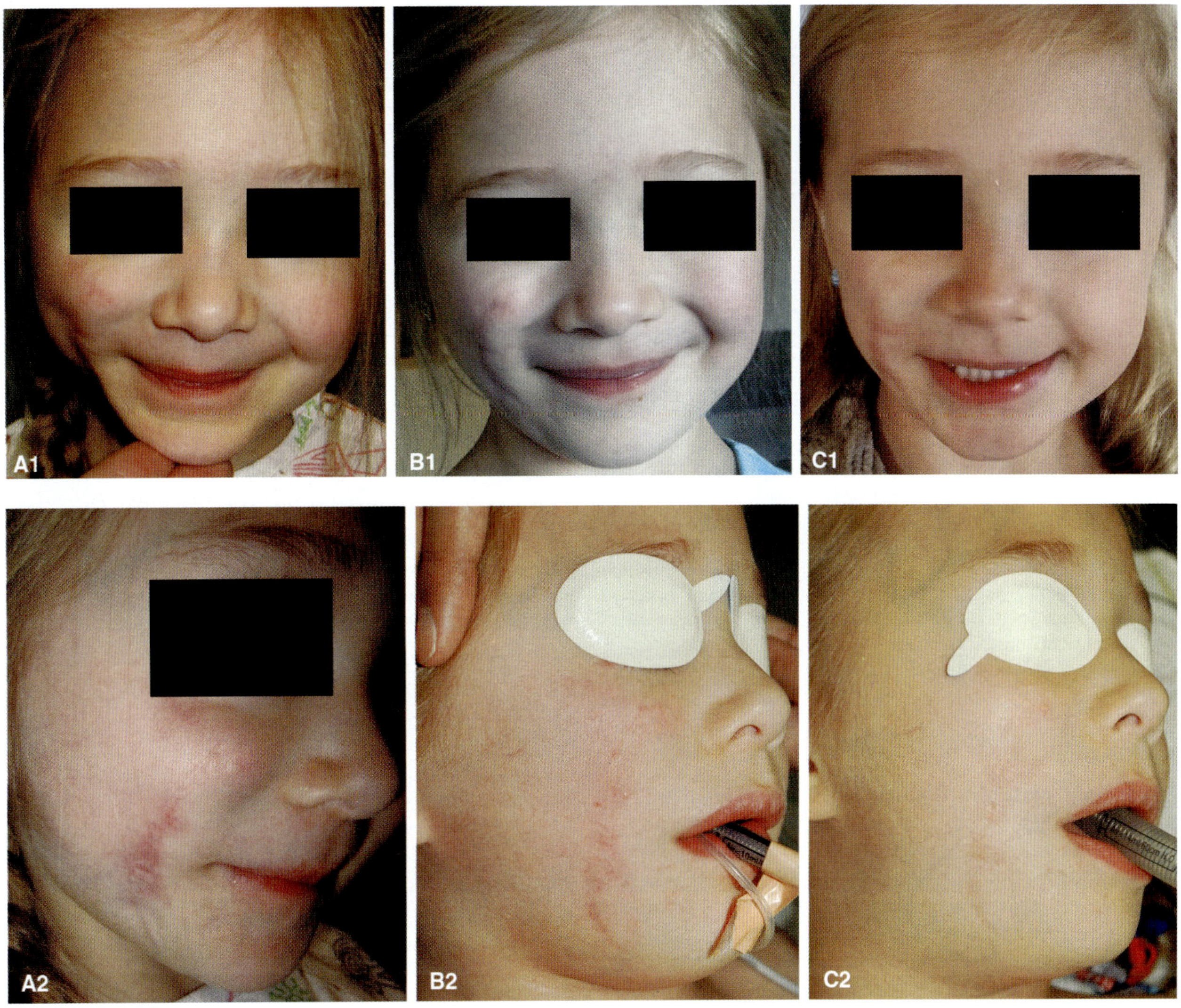

FIGURE 22-6 **Multimodal, multidisciplinary treatment of a dog bite scar on the face.** A 3-year-old girl presented with a "mixed" (i.e., atrophic and hypertrophic) scar resulting from a dog bite to the right cheek inflicted 21 months earlier. Marked erythema, irregular texture, volume loss, and scar contractures are noted (**A1, A2**). A total of nine multimodal revision procedures were performed (under general anesthesia because of her age and the extent and location of her injuries). Erythematous portions of the scar were first treated with a 595-nm pulsed dye laser (Vbeam Perfecta, Candela Corporation, Wayland, MA, USA) using a 7-mm spot size, fluence of 8 J per cm2, and 1.5-ms pulse width (clinical endpoint of minimal purpura). The entire scar sheet was then treated using an ablative microfractionated 10,600-nm CO2 laser (UltraPulse, Deep FX; Lumenis, Ltd., Yokneam, Israel) at pulse energy of 15 mJ and density of 15% in a single pass. At the time of her first laser scar revision, the patient's plastic surgery team performed autologous fat grafting (5 mL) under the depressed scar to help restore volume to her cheek. Serial pulsed dye laser treatments were repeated with fluence settings ranging from 8 to 11 J per cm2 to reach a clinical endpoint of minimal purpura. Additional ablative fractional laser resurfacing treatments were performed with pulse energies ranging from 15 to 25 mJ and corresponding treatment densities of 10% to 5%, respectively. During four early treatment sessions, the patient received triamcinolone acetonide suspension (40 mg per mL) applied topically to the areas of greatest scar hypertrophy immediately after fractional laser treatment. **B1** and **B2**: interim results approximately 10 months after her initial treatment session. **C1** and **C2**: the same patient approximately 19 months after her initial treatment. Marked improvements in scar texture, color, and facial symmetry are noted. Additional enhancements could likely be obtained with repeated interventions such as ablative and nonablative fractional resurfacing and fat grafting. *(Admani S, Gertner JW, Gosman A et al. Multidisciplinary, multimodal approach for a child with a traumatic facial scar. Semin Cutan Med Surg. 2015;34:24–27.)*

involved in the management plan from the start so that realistic expectations may be established. Payers must also be involved from the beginning, understanding that the right people performing the right treatments will yield the best, most cost-effective results.

Prevention and mitigation of scar formation are the extremely important "first steps" in the management of scars. Scars located at the shoulder, neck, presternum, and ankle are more prone to hypertrophic scars because of the high tension in these anatomical locations, and certain patients tend to be more prone to pathological scar formation or postinflammatory pigment alteration.[26] Therefore, it is imperative for health care providers to identify wounds that may be susceptible to becoming a pathological scar and take action. Selective avoidance of elective surgeries in at-risk individuals, wound closures that minimize tension, the use of proper wound dressings and wound care, optimized nutrition, and the prevention of postoperative infections can help optimize wound healing and reduce scar formation (see Chapters 8 and 9).[27]

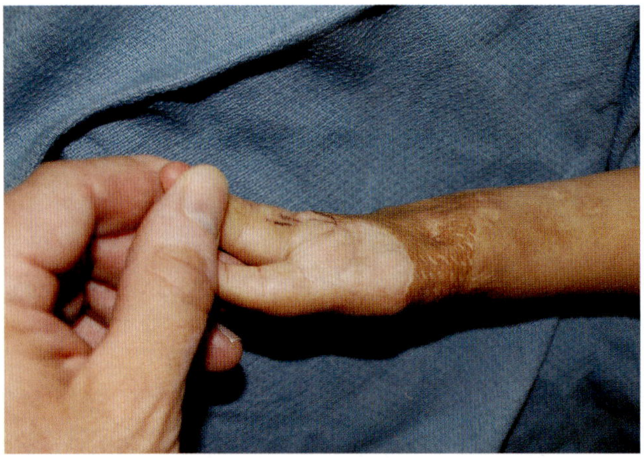

FIGURE 22-7 **Contracted split-thickness skin graft and amputation.** This 3-year-old boy survived meningococcemia but his body was left ravaged by associated necrosis. He lost several fingers and numerous split-thickness skin grafts were necessary during reconstruction. Unfortunately, many of the skin grafts contracted and caused additional functional deficits. Such a complicated presentation highlights the need for a truly specialized, multidisciplinary scar team that might include the patient's primary pediatrician (the "quarterback"); infectious disease, orthopedics, plastic surgery, dermatology, nutrition, behavior therapy, psychology specialists, and a patient advocate. *(Courtesy of Andrew C. Krakowski, MD.)*

A variety of reasonable options exist for the treatment of scars including, but not limited to, intralesional corticosteroids, silicone gel sheets, massage/pressure therapy, cryotherapy, surgical excision, and laser treatment (see Chapters 10 and 13). However, treatment is guided by the characteristics of the specific scar at a particular time point. In complex scars with an array of symptoms (e.g., anxiety, pruritus, pain, dysesthesia, etc.) and signs (e.g., hypopigmentation, erythema, functional deficit, etc.), a multimodal approach is often necessary to achieve optimal results.[16]

Why Treat?

Associated Comorbidities

The majority of scars are of little consequence for affected patients. However, findings such as erythema, dyspigmentation, pruritus, pain, hyper- or hypohidrosis, hyper- or hypotrichosis, and dysesthesias are not uncommon (Table 22-3).

Color Change

Color changes in scars can be related to pigmentary alteration or underlying vascularity (Fig. 22-8). The initial trauma and the subsequent process of wound healing and scar formation can lead to discrepancies in both the number of melanocytes and melanin density compared to normal skin.[28] This may manifest as hypopigmentation, hyperpigmentation, or commonly both. Erythema is also a common finding, especially in young scars. Although it typically fades with time, erythema may sometimes persist for years and can be an indicator of pathological scar formation.[28]

Table 22-3 Physical Scar Signs and Symptoms to Consider

- Conspicuous or subtle?
- Disruption of local cosmetic unit?
- Erythema/hypervascularity?
- Skin contracture?
- Range of motion/functional deficit?
- Dyspigmentation (hyperpigmentation/hypopigmentation/mottling)?
- Pruritus?
- Pain/tenderness?
- Dysesthesia?
- Hypertrichosis, hypotrichosis, or alopecia?
- Hyperhidrosis, hypohidrosis, or anhidrosis?
- Presence or history of infection (folliculitis, cellulitis, abscess, fasciitis, etc.) within scar area?
- Presence or history of chronic wound/chronic ulceration within scar area?
- Presence or history of lymphedema locally or regionally (suggestive of outflow obstruction)?
- Presence or history of skin cancer (i.e., Marjolin's ulcer) within scar area?

From Krakowski AC, Totri CR, Donelan MB, et al. State of the art: scar management in the pediatric and adolescent populations. *Pediatrics.* 2016;137(2):2014–2065, with permission.

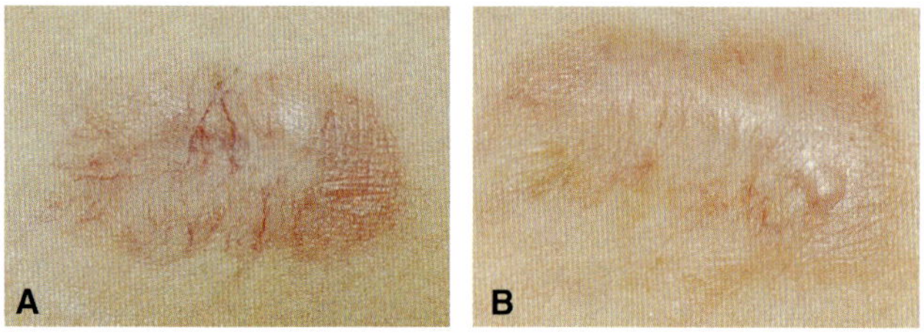

FIGURE 22-8 **Tracheostomy scar with prominent telangiectasia. A:** This adolescent female's tracheostomy scar was particularly conspicuous secondary to prominent telangiectases. **B:** A single treatment with a vascular-specific laser successfully reduced erythema and improved cosmesis, and had the overall effect of reducing the patient's anxiety levels and enhancing her ability for social interaction. *(Courtesy of Andrew C. Krakowski, MD.)*

Pruritus

Pruritus is an extremely common symptom (especially in association with hypertrophic and keloid scars), present in up to 87% of those affected.[29,30] In one study, more than 86% of patients with pruritus associated with burn scars reported the symptom as unbearable, and up to 100% of patients reported it as bothersome.[30] The cause of pruritus in scar tissue is unclear; however, localized inflammation, stimulation of small nerve fibers around the scar, and increased levels of β-endorphin are thought to contribute (see Chapter 11).[29,31]

Pain

Pain may also be a presenting symptom in existing scars. Several reports of significant and chronic pain, especially after burns, have been reported in the literature.[32,33] Even older "mature" scars can cause pain in affected patients. An editor of this textbook (ACK) has himself survived a fall through a plate glass door at the age of 7; some 36 years later, the sensation of being "stuck with an ice pick" within the deep portions of a resulting hypertrophic scar on his arm wakes him from sleep on a near-monthly basis.

Dysesthesias

Changes in sensation such as anesthesia, paresthesia, perceptions of burning or moisture, and an altered sense of touch are common findings in scar tissue. Tissue damage and the formation of scars in an area can potentially damage peripheral nerve fibers or cause nerve entrapment from aberrant collagen deposition.[29]

Hyperhidrosis/Hypohidrosis

Hyperhidrosis and hypohidrosis are fairly common findings associated with scars, as the process of wound healing can lead to abnormal tissue composition within a scar. Aberrant formation of the secretory portions of sweat glands and irregular organization of the glands have been found in scar tissue, which can lead to poor temperature regulation and hyperhidrosis or hypohidrosis. This can be particularly problematic in symptomatic patients.[34–36] Hyperhidrosis may directly interfere with proper fitting of prosthetics, the use of scar camouflage, and the application of silicone gel sheeting.

Hypertrichosis/Hypotrichosis/Alopecia

The anatomical composition of scar tissue differs from that of normal skin (see Chapter 5). The process of scar formation can frequently cause loss or disruption of hair follicles in affected areas, leading to hypotrichosis and alopecia (Fig. 22-3). Interestingly, hypertrichosis has also been reported. It has been hypothesized that this increase in hair growth is a product of increased growth factors and vascularization in healing scar tissue.[37]

Functional Compromise

Even "normal" scar formation in a particular anatomic location may lead to significant functional impairments for affected patients. Restrictive contractures and adhesions, for example, can be extremely debilitating consequences of scar formation and maturation (Fig. 22-9). These contractures occur through tightening of affected skin overlying a joint or through adhesions with underlying tissues resulting in limited range of motion.[38] Decreased ability to perform normal activities of daily living due to scar contractures can lead to significant and long-term negative consequences on a patient's overall quality of life (see Chapter 19).

Function-limiting scars can be particularly debilitating in pediatric patients where the "use it or lose it" phenomenon is a real concern because of the overlap of the patients' normal growth and development with the evolution of the scar contracture. Function-compromising scars may directly impact important developmental milestones such as development of right- or left-handedness and the formation of the concepts of self and self-worth. Therefore, it is especially important in the pediatric population to evaluate for any underlying functional compromise associated with scars, as failure to recognize these complications may lead

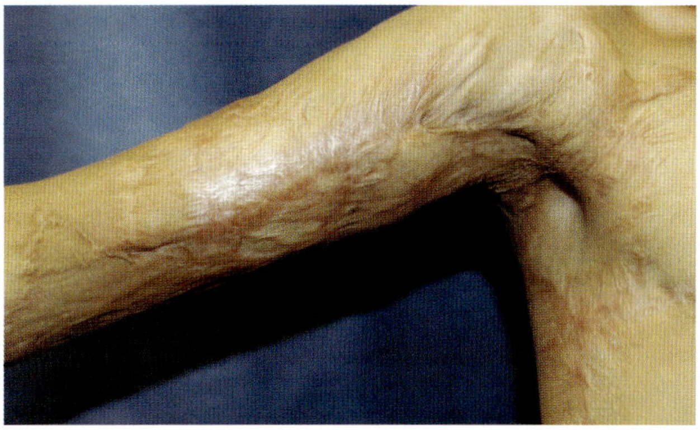

FIGURE 22-9 **Scar contracture with functional deficit.** This teenage male suffered a gasoline burn injury that resulted in a large hypertrophic scar contracture with the resulting inability to fully abduct his right arm. *(Courtesy of Andrew C. Krakowski, MD.)*

to impairment of normal development.[39] Returning affected patients as close to baseline function as possible should be the guiding principle of treatment.

Psychosocial Aspects

Scars may not only cause functional problems for a patient; they can also have significant deleterious psychosocial consequences, especially for pediatric patients (see Chapter 24). The aesthetic complications of scar formation can lead to depression, posttraumatic stress disorder, anxiety, social withdrawal, and isolation.[32,40,41] These psychosocial consequences may even be more incapacitating than the physical sequelae and, in pediatric patients, may negatively influence self-confidence, social interactions, and success in the future.[42] Despite these associations, the psychosocial consequences of scars are frequently forgotten, unrecognized, and underreported (Table 22-4).

It may be natural to assume that scar severity would correlate with psychosocial consequences for affected patients. However, the degree of distress a patient experiences does not necessarily correlate with scar origin or size.[43] Rather, more consistent predictors of psychosocial distress appear to be scar location and visibility, the patient's subjective opinion of the scar, the reaction of others to the scar, and the patient's individual personality traits.[42,44,45] Patients with visible scars often also experience significant stigmatization and discrimination from others, leading to low body image, social anxiety, and depression.[32] In children and adolescents, this stigmatization can lead to long-term consequences such as difficulty making friends and forming intimate relationships.[32] Therefore, it is pertinent for

Table 22-4 Psychosocial Scar Comorbidities to Consider

- Anxiety/stress?
- Depression?
- Posttraumatic stress disorder?
- School, work, or social performance affected?
- Overall perceived reaction of others to scar?

From Krakowski AC, Totri CR, Donelan MD, et al. State of the art: scar management in the pediatric and adolescent populations. *Pediatrics.* 2016;137(2):2014–2065, with permission.

treating physicians to assess for psychosocial comorbidities when evaluating a patient with scars and, when present, refer for early intervention.

Financial Considerations

In addition to the physical and psychosocial sequelae of scars, treatment can lead to a significant financial burden for patients and health care providers. Successful scar management, especially complex scars after extensive injury, begins with professional wound care and often requires multimodal, multisession therapy during rehabilitation. The cumulative costs of initial stabilization and wound care, topical and intralesional agents, pressure garments, conventional surgery, and other adjunctive treatments can be immense.[46–48] A study investigating the health care cost of treating chronic wounds in the United States estimated that the total annual expenditure for burn scar management is approximately $12 billion.[49] These exorbitant costs can cause a significant financial burden for affected patients and their families. Therefore, it is important to consider the financial cost when deciding on treatment plans for patients. It is also imperative that insurance companies recognize the profound importance of scar management, and partner with patients during the treatment course. Objective evidence now exists to support the notion that these treatments can improve and even fully restore functional compromise secondary to scar contractures (Fig. 22-10). As a medical community we should drive these patients to capable experts who can optimize clinical outcomes and minimize unnecessary expense.

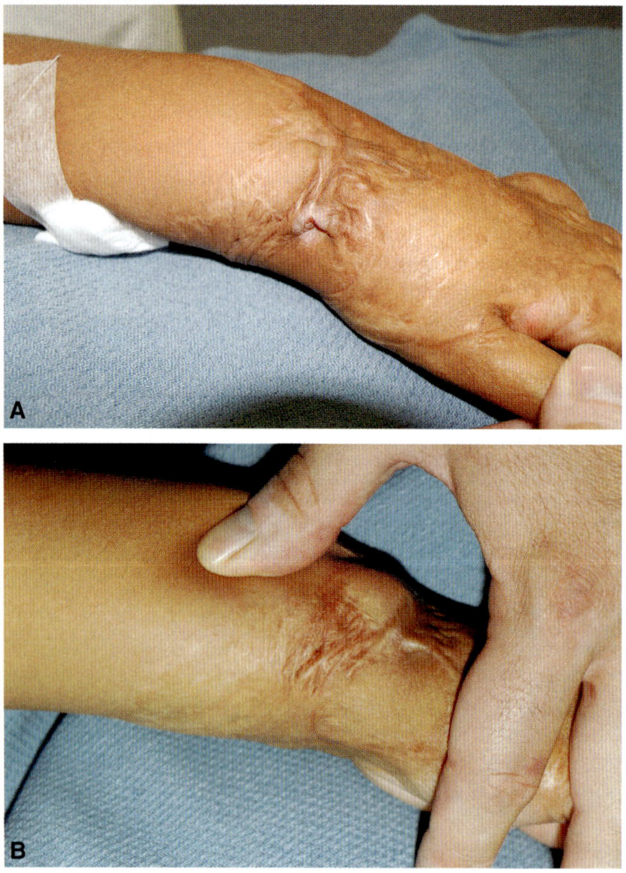

FIGURE 22-10 **Chronic wound associated with a burn scar. A:** As an infant, this 8-year-old girl had climbed into a bathtub full of hot water and liquid bleach, suffering burns to all four extremities with subsequent associated scar contractures. In one "hot spot" she developed a chronic ulcerated wound that had been present for 8 months despite ongoing traditional wound care. **B:** One treatment with an ablative, microfractionated 10,600-nm CO2 laser (UltraPulse Deep FX, Lumenis, Ltd., Yokneam, Israel) over the wound and associated contracture bands at pulse energy of 50 mJ and treatment density of 5% helped to stimulate remodeling and relieve the tension on the skin adjacent to the wound, facilitating rapid healing. *(Adapted from Krakowski AC, Diaz L, Admani S, et al. Healing of chronic wounds with adjunctive ablative fractional laser resurfacing in two pediatric patients. Lasers Surg Med. 2016;48:166–169.)*

Timing of Treatment

For decades (even centuries), the prevailing notion has been that scars should generally not be manipulated procedurally for at least 1 year after creation (i.e., until the scar has had time to "mature"). Because of recent advances in technology and minimally invasive techniques such as fractional laser resurfacing, this notion is no longer universal and requires updating to account for the potential benefits of early intervention to minimize the impact of scars as they form. The use of massage therapy and pressure garments has become fairly routine early in the course after burns to mediate scar tissue formation,[50–55] and these newer techniques could be considered in a similar (and likely more effective) vein. Additionally, some recent studies suggest early intervention may be more favorable than delayed treatment. For example, in the management of keloids, intraoperative intralesional corticosteroids may be employed to help prevent future recurrence of the lesions.[56] Newer therapies such as ablative fractional laser resurfacing (AFR) have also been effective early interventions in mediating scar tissue formation postoperatively.[50,57]

The notable exception to early treatment and prevention of scars may be conventional surgical revision. Surgical revision, such as flaps, grafts, and Z-plasties, are frequently delayed for a year or more to allow the tissue to mature and become amenable to such treatments.[51,52] However, modalities such as fractional ablative laser may be useful in mitigating scar formation and providing symptomatic relief during this waiting period.

More rigorous studies will help elucidate whether the timing of treatment has a significant impact on the ultimate quality of a scar. Certainly, the treatment of hypertrophic or keloid scars should not be patently denied because a scar is "too old" or "too mature." In the experience of the authors, older scars respond consistently to treatment. More notably, the adage of "use it or lose it" rings particularly true in a growing child; any compromise in physical, psychological, or social development should be addressed as early as possible with appropriate intervention aimed at restoring baseline function.

Procedural Management

Room Prep

When treating pediatric patients, it is important to create a comfortable and calm environment in the procedure room.

The surgical instruments should be out of sight of the child for as long as possible to minimize anxiety. Distraction tools such as tablets, music, bubbles, or interactive games may be available, and parents should be seated away from the surgical field.

Bundling Techniques

Bundling techniques can be useful as a method of restraint for procedures in a subset of pediatric patients. Bundling techniques typically utilize a bedsheet or blanket to wrap a child in a "burrito" fashion.[53] The advantage of the bundling technique is that it provides an easy, comfortable, and safe restraint without the need for significant additional hospital personnel or sedatives.[54] Bundling techniques are typically more useful with younger pediatric patients, and may not be as effective for older or larger children. However, it is a safe and effective option for patient restraint during a short procedure.

Eye Safety

Proper eye protection for the patient and all providers/parents in the room is necessary for procedures involving structures both adjacent to and distant from the eyes, particularly if lasers are employed. Several options for eye protection during pediatric procedures are available. Stick-on disposable eye shields, plastic and metal corneal protectors, and laser-specific goggles are all frequently used in dermatology.[55] Stick-on disposable shields are frequently used because of their convenience, predictable fit, and ability to protect from laser wavelengths of 190 to 11,000 nm, but have a risk of displacement during a procedure. Internal metal corneal protectors are considered one of the most effective methods of preventing adverse events from procedures near the eye, though the use of these internal eye shields can be associated with a risk of corneal abrasions.[58] Lastly, laser-specific goggles are useful in protecting the eyes from specific wavelengths, but the concern is that the goggles often do not provide a complete seal.

Skin Cleansing

The goal of cleansing the skin before a procedure is to reduce the risk of infection through the skin surface. Therefore, the degree of skin cleansing needed is dependent on the type of procedure that will be performed. For simple procedures, such as corticosteroid injections or biopsies, cleansing with 70% alcohol is usually sufficient.[59] For complex procedures, such as surgery or excisions, more extensive skin cleansing including hair clipping is usually necessary. Topical povidone–iodine and chlorhexidine are the most commonly used, and both have been shown to be effective antimicrobial agents.[59,60]

Allowing Family Members to Watch: Pluses and Minuses

For children, even simple procedures can be extremely frightening experiences. The presence of family members such as parents or siblings can often be reassuring, and several studies have shown that parental presence can reduce procedure-related anxiety in pediatric patients.[61,62] There is significant evidence that parental presence during anesthesia induction is associated with decreased anxiety, reduced need for preoperative sedatives, and improving patient compliance.[62–65] The ability to be in the room can often alleviate anxiety in the family member as well.[63] However, studies have also found a correlation between the level of parent anxiety and level of patient anxiety, and the presence of a highly anxious family member in the room may not be advantageous.[65] Therefore, the presence of family members during the procedure should probably be determined on a case-by-case basis.

Pain Management

A key aspect of scar treatment in pediatric patients is the concept of pain management. In comparison to adults, children may not be as tolerant of pain or comfortable with certain procedures. Therefore, techniques such as physical restraint or sedation with anesthesia are often necessary to perform complex procedures. For smaller procedures, however, other techniques are available to help reduce a child's fear or anxiety. Different options for pain management will be outlined below.

Distraction Techniques

Distraction is a common, simple, and effective technique that can be used for pain management in children. Distraction techniques are intended to direct a child's attention away from the painful procedure, and have been shown to reduce pain and anxiety in a number of studies.[66–68] A variety of distraction techniques are available and can be divided into active and passive; both are extremely effective in reducing pain and anxiety during pediatric procedures.[68]

Active Distraction

Active distraction techniques involve a child's active engagement in an activity during a procedure. Commonly employed active distraction techniques include toys, video games, tablets, interactive books, or visual imagery. An easy method of active distraction is controlled breathing techniques in which children are taught to blow out air, as if they were "blowing bubbles" or "blowing out a candle."[69,70] However, this method may not be appropriate for very young children. Interactive toys that engage multiple senses may be more useful in young children where other techniques may not be effective.[71] Video games and virtual reality devices have been found to be extremely effective distraction techniques.[72–74] Studies have demonstrated a statistically significant decrease in preoperative anxiety in pediatric patients while using handheld video games compared to midazolam use and baseline.[72] Recently, several studies have demonstrated that the use of tablets and smartphones helps to reduce pain, anxiety, and the need for restraints or sedation.[75,76] Lastly, interactive books, visual imagery, or engaging in conversation with the patient can be effective cognitive distractions, especially for older children.[67,77]

Passive Distraction

Passive distraction techniques, on the other hand, do not involve a child's active engagement in an activity. Passive distraction techniques are commonly used in cases where the child needs to be still for the procedure. Music, movies, and television are common examples of passive distraction methods. Music is a passive distraction technique that is often self-employed, especially by adolescent patients, and has been shown to cause a statistically significant decrease in procedural pain and anxiety for the patient and family.[78,79] Similarly movies, especially humorous movies, have been associated with increased pain tolerance during procedures.[80]

Buzzy

The Buzzy (MMJ Labs, Atlanta, GA) is a method that combines external application of cold and vibration to reduce pain sensation.[81] This method of pain control employs "gate control" theory. This theory suggests that faster A-β fibers transmitting vibration and temperature sensation can block or reduce the transmission of pain in A-δ fibers to the central nervous system, leading to an increased pain threshold.[82] Studies involving the use of the Buzzy for pain management during venipuncture, immunizations, and intravenous cannulation all demonstrated a significant decrease in pain and anxiety levels compared to baseline, with no interference on the success of a procedure.[81,83–85] In fact, one study reported that the device made the procedure easier in 81% of cases.[84]

There are few reports of complications associated with use of the Buzzy. One study by Lima-Oliveira et al.[86] suggested that it may potentially interfere with erythrocyte counts, leukocyte counts, differential, hemoglobin, and hematocrit, which may cause variations in test results. However, a follow-up study showed no significant difference between hematology test results from venipuncture using the device compared to venipuncture collected with transillumination.[83] It is unclear what the true effect of the Buzzy is on hematology results, but it is a potentially safe and effective alternative for pain management in pediatric patients receiving treatment for scars.

Topical Anesthetics

Eutectic Mixture of Local Anesthetics (EMLA)

EMLA (AstraZeneca LP, Wilmington, DE) is a eutectic mixture of lidocaine and prilocaine in a 5% emulsion preparation that is commonly used as a topical anesthetic. Studies have suggested that EMLA cream is particularly useful in the pediatric population for minor procedures such as immunizations and cryotherapy.[87–89] It may also be more useful than distraction techniques for attenuation of pain in pediatric patients.[88]

A concern about the use of EMLA, especially in pediatric patients, is the potential risk for methemoglobinemia. Since the introduction of EMLA for topical pain management, several cases of methemoglobinemia have been reported in the pediatric population.[90–93] The risk of methemoglobinemia appears to be dose dependent and is associated with a large area of application, longer application times, reduced skin barrier function, and young age.[91] The pathogenesis of methemoglobinemia in these patients is accumulation of *o*-toluidine, a metabolite of prilocaine, which leads to increased production of methemoglobin.[91] Additionally, there is a risk of developing allergic contact dermatitis with topical lidocaine use.[94] Therefore, it is important to consider this potential adverse effect when using EMLA for pain management in pediatric patients, especially if a larger surface area is to be treated.

Topical Lidocaine

LMX-4 (Ferndale Laboratories, Inc., Ferndale, MI) is a topical anesthetic cream containing 4% lidocaine, and is commonly used as a topical anesthetic for simple procedures in dermatology.[95] Studies suggest that there is no difference in the efficacy of anesthesia between LMX-4 and EMLA cream.[96] However, LMX-4 may offer several advantages. For example, it is available over the counter, which makes it more readily accessible for patients and families and may be applied at home prior to coming into the office for a procedure. Additionally, LMX-4 does not contain prilocaine, which is the component of EMLA that is associated with an increased risk of methemoglobinemia in pediatric patients.

LMX-4, like EMLA, comes with inherent risks as well. Systemic absorption of lidocaine can lead to significant adverse events such as bradycardia, hypotension, tinnitus, blurred vision, nausea, and potentially death.[97] Because of the relatively large surface-to-volume ratio of pediatric patients and decreased barrier function (particularly in infants), pediatric patients may be at increased risk for systemic absorption. One study on topical anesthetics suggested that some individuals have a higher risk for absorption for unknown reasons.[97] Additionally, there is a risk for development of allergic contact dermatitis.[94] Therefore, although LMX-4 is approved for use up to four times per day, it is important to minimize its use to only the necessary area and amount to reduce the risk of side effects.

Local Anesthetics

Local anesthetics, such as injectable lidocaine or bupivacaine solutions, are the mainstay of pain management in simple dermatologic procedures.[98] Local anesthetics are particularly useful for these simple procedures because they are readily accessible and have a rapid onset of action. Additionally, these agents are much more effective at producing sustained anesthesia and pain control compared to distraction techniques and topical agents alone. Among commonly used local anesthetics, bupivacaine has the longest duration of action, and lidocaine is associated with the least pain upon administration.[98]

Local anesthetics are generally considered very safe. However, systemic toxicity is a larger concern with injectables compared to topicals. As previously mentioned, systemic absorption of lidocaine can lead to significant adverse events such as bradycardia, hypotension, tinnitus, blurred vision, nausea, and potentially death.[97] Additionally, injectable agents such as lidocaine and bupivacaine are associated with significant pain upon administration, which may not be tolerated well in the pediatric population.[98,99] Lastly, there is a small risk of contact dermatitis with use of local anesthesia, particularly with lidocaine.[100] It is important to weigh the risks and benefits of local anesthesia when performing procedures in pediatric patients.

General Anesthesia

The use of general anesthesia has revolutionized the fields of medicine and surgery. Although most often used for complex surgeries of long duration, general anesthesia is becoming more commonly used for short periods of time during simple procedures in pediatric patients. In the United States alone, greater than one million children under the age of five undergo general anesthesia annually for a variety of reasons.[101] General anesthesia is a relatively safe modality, and offers a specific advantage in pediatric patients in whom procedure-related anxiety is common and restraints are often needed for awake procedures.

Despite its frequent use, there is still concern regarding the use of general anesthesia in pediatric patients, particularly if a patient is subjected to repeated episodes. One significant concern is the potential risk of neurotoxicity. In animal studies, there is evidence that general anesthesia may interfere with brain development, leading to apoptosis and abnormal synapses.[102] Because of this concern, several investigations into the effects of general anesthesia on the developing human brain have been performed. Most studies suggest that there is no significant neurotoxicity in pediatric patients that have undergone general anesthesia compared to controls.[102,103] One study even used functional magnetic resonance imaging to demonstrate that there was no significant difference in accuracy, response time, or activation patterns during specific tasks between children that had undergone general anesthesia and controls.[103] However, other studies suggest that children that have undergone general anesthesia multiple times have an increased risk for subsequent functional, behavioral, and emotional disturbances.[104] It is still unclear what the true risk of general anesthesia is in the pediatric population, and further research into the relationship between general anesthesia and neurodevelopment needs to be performed before definitive recommendations can be made.

Oral Sedatives

Oral medications, such as midazolam or diazepam, can be used for preprocedure sedation and anxiolysis in pediatric patients. Although not as frequently employed as other types of pain management, oral sedatives may be useful for simple procedures in pediatric patients. There is significant evidence in the pediatric dental literature demonstrating the utility of oral midazolam and diazepam. Improvements in anxiety, fear, movement, and overall behavior were seen in comparison to controls, with few reported side effects.[105–107] Side effects associated with oral sedatives are typically mild and include headache, nausea, and drowsiness. Less common but potentially more serious complications include palpitations, arrhythmias, and neurologic deficits.[108] The potential for serious side effects from the use of oral sedatives should prompt consideration for proper preprocedural and postprocedural monitoring. The pediatric dental literature has created guidelines for monitoring and management of pediatric patients undergoing oral sedation.[109] Oral midazolam or diazepam may be useful adjunctive treatments to mediate pain and anxiety in pediatric patients undergoing procedures.

Treatment Approach to Scars

Massage Therapy

One of the simplest and most readily available treatments for scars is massage therapy. It is believed to help soften scars and improve overall pliability through improvement in vascular and lymphatic drainage, scar matrix remodeling, and mediation of pain through peripheral nerves.[110–112] Although there are limited studies on the utility of massage therapy, there is some evidence demonstrating that it may be useful in improving both subjective and objective measures of scar severity.[110,113] Furthermore, massage therapy is a very safe, easy, and inexpensive technique for scar management.

Pressure Therapy

Pressure therapy is a very common treatment that utilizes specialized garments, bandages, or dressings to provide external pressure to a scar in prevention or, to improve appearance and pliability in existing scars (see Chapter 19).[114] Some studies indicate that pressure therapy may be useful for reducing scar thickness, contraction, and erythema.[114–116] One study even suggests that pressure therapy may lead to scar matrix remodeling.[117] However, others suggest that there is no significant difference in patients treated with pressure therapy and untreated controls.[118] Despite the paucity of standardized research regarding its utility, pressure therapy is still frequently used as a first-line intervention for the prevention and treatment of hypertrophic scars. Although pressure therapy is a relatively safe and potentially promising treatment, patient compliance may be an issue due to discomfort, pain, or skin changes from wearing pressure garments.[114]

Intralesional Corticosteroids

Intralesional corticosteroids are one of the most frequently used treatment options for scars, and there is a substantial body of evidence supporting their use in scar management (see Chapter 10). Studies have shown response rates of up to 100% in scars treated with intralesional corticosteroids.[119] They are useful for softening and remodeling scar tissue because of their ability to inhibit collagen production, promote collagen remodeling, and inhibit local inflammation.[120] Although intralesional corticosteroids are an effective, readily available, and inexpensive treatment option, side effects such as local skin atrophy, telangiectasias, and dyspigmentation can limit its utility for long-term treatment.[121] Significant obstacles for the use of intralesional corticosteroids in the pediatric population include the associated pain of injection, systemic absorption and hypothalamic–pituitary axis suppression, and a potential risk for toxicity in neonates from benzyl alcohol, a compound present in most injectable corticosteroid suspensions.[122,123]

Surgery

Surgical intervention remains a fundamental treatment option for scars, especially in the case of severe functional limitations or those that have failed to respond to other therapeutic options (see Chapter 12). For the treatment of large traumatic scars, surgical intervention may be considered an important part of a multimodal treatment regimen in conjunction with other less invasive treatments such as medications, pressure garments, laser scar revision, etc. When used in combination with adjunctive intralesional medications, surgical intervention may be helpful in improving a scar's bulk and reducing the risk of recurrence.[124,125] Surgical intervention, using techniques such as Z-plasty, is particularly helpful for the treatment of scar contractures with the goal of reducing tension and restoring function.[38,126] However, surgical morbidity such as pain, anesthetic requirements, additional scarring, relatively high recurrence rates, the association with treatment delay to allow for scar maturation after injury, and long postsurgical healing times need to be accounted for, especially in the pediatric population.

Pulsed Dye Laser

The 595-nm pulsed dye laser (PDL) is commonly used for treatment of vascular lesions in the skin such as port-wine stains, telangiectases, and superficial hemangiomas. It works through the principle of selective photothermolysis, using hemoglobin as the target chromophore (see Chapter 13). It has also been used frequently for the treatment of scars in adults and is particularly useful in reducing scar erythema, pruritus, and pain and in improving a scar's overall cosmetic appearance.[127–129]

The use of PDL specifically for the treatment of pediatric scars has not been examined extensively. However, it has been used frequently for the treatment of pediatric vascular lesions with minimal complications, and is therefore generally considered a safe and effective treatment modality.[130–132] The most commonly reported side effects include pain, purpura, edema, blistering, scarring, and dyspigmentation.[133] Rare cases of serious side effects such as ulceration and skin necrosis have also been reported.[134] However, because more moderate fluences are generally used for scar management, the associated risks may also be anticipated to be less frequent.[135]

Ablative Fractional Laser Resurfacing

AFR with devices such as the 10,600 nm carbon dioxide (CO_2) and 2,940 nm erbium-doped yttrium–aluminum–garnet (Er:YAG) lasers is becoming an increasingly common treatment option for various scar types. AFR works by creating narrow columns of tissue ablation and coagulation to controlled depths in a pixelated pattern between reservoirs of untreated skin. AFR offers a unique advantage for the treatment of scars over previous technology, because it offers increased and tunable depths of penetration while minimizing excessive thermal injury.[136,137] It is thought that this particular controlled thermal injury leads to decreases in transforming growth factor β, type I and III collagen deposition, increases in matrix metalloproteinase expression, and overall dermal remodeling.[138–141]

There is significant evidence demonstrating the utility of AFR for the treatment of acne, surgical, and traumatic scars.[135,142–145] Treatment with AFR has been shown to soften scars, reduce hypertrophy, and even increase functional capacity.[16,142,143,146] Additionally, AFR appears to be a relatively safe and effective procedure, with the most common reported side effects being pain, blistering, scarring, and dyspigmentation.[147,148] Although AFR has not been studied as extensively in the pediatric population, there is evidence that this therapeutic modality may be useful for the treatment of pediatric scars.[16,143,149]

Laser-Assisted Delivery

The use of topical agents is ubiquitous in dermatology. However, the utility of this treatment modality is limited by cutaneous absorption through the epidermal barrier, and agents that are large or hydrophilic can pose a significant challenge to topical delivery. Scars can add additional challenges because of the abnormal architecture and frequent dermal hypertrophy.[150] Laser-assisted delivery (LAD) is a treatment strategy that has been gaining momentum, especially for the treatment of scars (see Chapter 14). LAD uses the disruption of the skin barrier created with various ablative and nonablative fractional laser technologies to improve delivery and absorption of topically applied agents. This technology has shown considerable success in the treatment of several dermatologic disorders, including scars (Fig. 22-11).[151–156]

Although there are few studies involving the use of LAD in the pediatric population, the technique appears promising.[16,135,146] LAD may be particularly useful in hypertrophic or keloid scars, where penetration through the fibrotic tissue may be limited with topical application alone. Although few side effects related to LAD have been reported in the literature, the potential for increased systemic absorption and subsequent unintended side effects must be considered, particularly in the pediatric population.[156] Further studies are certainly required as the number of potential therapeutic agents is vast, whereas few have been studied in the context of this mode of delivery.

Q-Switched Laser for Traumatic Tattoos

A "traumatic tattoo" refers to the accidental deposition of fine foreign bodies in the skin from traumatic events such as firearms, bombs, automobile and bicycle accidents, or falls.[157] These traumatic tattoos are characterized by irregular deposition of dark particles in the superficial layer of the dermis.[157] Treatment of traumatic tattoos and removal of these particles can be challenging. In recent years, Q-switched (short-pulsed nanosecond and picosecond range) lasers, including 694-nm ruby, 755-nm alexandrite, and the 1,064-nm neodymium:YAG, have led to great strides in treating these undesired tattoos. This technique is useful because it allows destruction of the targeted chromophore (pigment) without significant heating of surrounding structures using the principle of selective photothermolysis.[158–161]

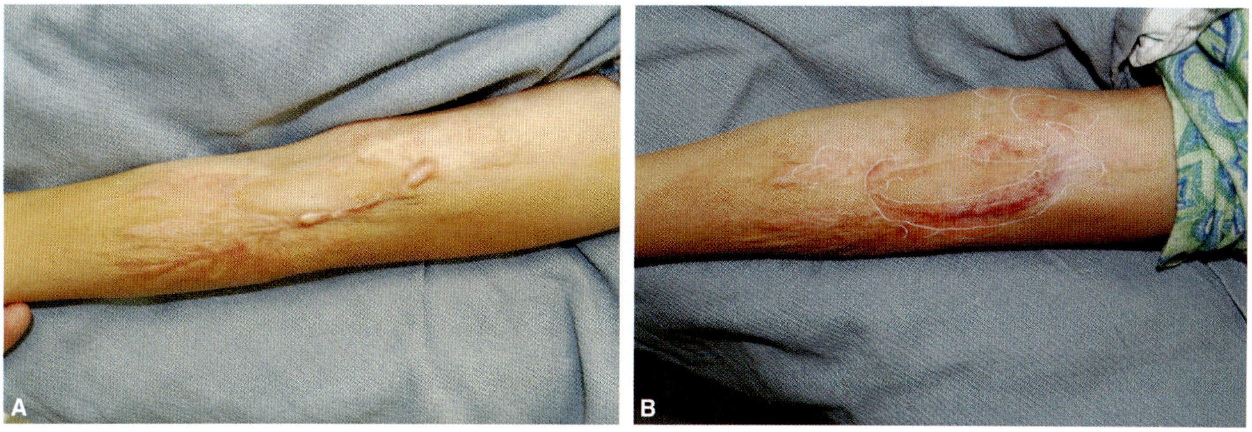

FIGURE 22-11 **Multimodal treatment of a war-related scar. A:** This 8-year-old female had been injured in an explosion 5 years prior to presentation during conflict in Iraq. Her scar was erythematous with marked contour irregularity. There were notable scar contractures present, but no clinically relevant functional deficit. To address the scar's erythema, portions of the scar were treated with a 595-nm pulsed dye laser (Vbeam Perfecta, Candela Corporation, Wayland, MA, USA) with a 7-mm spot size, fluences of 8 to 11 J per cm^2, and 1.5-ms pulse width, with a clinical endpoint of minimal purpura. Based purely on anecdotal experience, the authors chose to treat with pulsed dye laser first so that any "wheal" that resulted from subsequent modalities (i.e., ablative fractional laser resurfacing) would not act as a confounding chromophore to the pulsed dye laser. Next, the most hypertrophic portions of the patient's scar were treated using an ablative microfractionated 10,600-nm CO_2 laser (UltraPulse Deep FX, Lumenis, Ltd., Yokneam, Israel) at a pulse energy of 80 mJ and density of 3% to 5% with a single pass in a stamped pattern. The entire remaining scar sheet was then treated at a pulse energy of 20 mJ and 10% density to help improve textural irregularities and dyspigmentation. Immediately after fractional laser treatment of the hypertrophic areas, triamcinolone acetonide suspension (40 mg per mL) was applied topically to facilitate laser-assisted delivery. Additionally, intralesional injections were applied focally to the most hypertrophic portions of the scar. **B:** Same patient after 6 treatments, a total of 14 months after her first session. Several thick collagen nodules remain and will require further treatment; the overall erythema and irregular texture, however, are much-improved. *(Courtesy of Andrew C. Krakowski, MD.)*

Practice Gaps

To date, scar management in the pediatric population has mostly relied on clinical experience and anecdotal evidence extrapolated from the adult literature rather than on well-designed, prospective randomized controlled trials. The few investigations that have attempted to assess the various treatment options for symptomatic scars have yielded some promising results, but they have also had several limitations. Many of these studies do not distinguish keloids and hypertrophic scars in their clinical assessment, which can greatly confound the results and conclusions drawn from these studies. This is especially pertinent for hypertrophic scars that may spontaneously regress over time, making it difficult to determine if improvement is from direct treatment or from tincture of time. Furthermore, most of these studies have small samples sizes, lack sufficient follow-up, and do not have adequate control groups. Another difficulty has been assessing subjective qualities of scars such as pruritus, dysesthesias, and pain in a population of patients that may not be able to adequately describe them qualitatively.

Conclusion

Myriad treatment options for symptomatic scars exist, and much progress has been made in the last several years with combination therapy and a multidisciplinary team approach yielding promising clinical results. However, there is no universal consensus on what constitutes the safest and most efficacious treatment modalities within the pediatric population. Because of the high scar prevalence and the associated physical, psychological, social, and financial comorbidities, there remains a great need to enhance understanding of pediatric scar management among health care providers. Goals of therapy for any scar in this uniquely vulnerable population should be established in conjunction with the individual patient and the principle of "do no harm" in mind. Ideally, therapy should focus on relieving symptoms, improving cosmesis, reducing comorbidities, decreasing scar volume, and maximizing functional outcomes—especially in this demographic where the maxim of "use it or lose it" so crucially drives future development.

REFERENCES

1. Madison KC. Barrier function of the skin: "la raison d'être" of the epidermis. *J Invest Dermatol.* 2003;121:231–241.
2. Stamatas GN, Nikolovski J, Luedtke MA, et al. Infant skin microstructure assessed in vivo differs from adult skin in organization and at the cellular level. *Pediatr Dermatol.* 2010;27:125–131.
3. Paller AJ, Mancini AS. *Hurwitz Clinical Pediatric Dermatology*. 4 ed. New York, NY: Elsevier; 2011.
4. Vitellaro-Zuccarello L, Cappelletti S, Dal Pozzo Rossi V, et al. Stereological analysis of collagen and elastic fibers in the normal human dermis: variability with age, sex, and body region. *Anat Rec.* 1994;238:153–162.
5. Quesada-Cortés A, Campos-Muñoz L, Díaz-Díaz RM, et al. Cold panniculitis. *Dermatol Clin.* 2008;26:485–489, vii.
6. Nikolovski J, Stamatas GN, Kollias N, et al. Barrier function and water-holding and transport properties of infant stratum corneum are different from adult and continue to develop through the first year of life. *J Invest Dermatol.* 2008;128:1728–1736.
7. Thappa DM. *Clinical Pediatric Dermatology*. 1 ed. New Delhi, India: Elsevier; 2009.
8. Fluhr JW, Darlenski R, Taieb A, et al. Functional skin adaptation in infancy—almost complete but not fully competent. *Exp Dermatol.* 2010;19:483–492.
9. Shwayder T, Akland T. Neonatal skin barrier: structure, function, and disorders. *Dermatol Ther.* 2005;18:87–103.

10. Gold JI, Kant AJ, Kim SH. The impact of unintentional pediatric trauma: a review of pain, acute stress, and posttraumatic stress. *J Pediatr Nurs.* 2008;23:81–91.
11. Centers for Disease Control and Prevention. *CDC Childhood Injury Report*. Atlanta, GA: CDC; 2008.
12. Maguiña P, Palmieri TL, Greenhalgh DG. Treadmills: a preventable source of pediatric friction burn injuries. *J Burn Care Rehabil.* 2004;25:201–204.
13. Dahlin LB, Ljungberg E, Esserlind AL. Injuries of the hand and forearm in young children caused by steam roller presses in laundries. *Scand J Plast Reconstr Surg Hand Surg.* 2008;42:43–47.
14. Schalamon J, Ainoedhofer H, Singer G, et al. Analysis of dog bites in children who are younger than 17 years. *Pediatrics.* 2006;117:e374–e379.
15. Speirs J, Showery J, Abdou M, et al. Dog bites to the upper extremity in children. *J Paediatr Child Health.* 2015;51:1172–1174.
16. Admani S, Gertner JW, Grosman A, et al. Multidisciplinary, multimodal approach for a child with a traumatic facial scar. *Semin Cutan Med Surg.* 2015;34:24–27.
17. Choo KL, Fraser JF, Kimble RM. Campfire burns in children: an Australian experience. *Burns.* 2002;28:374–378.
18. Antonoff MB, Abbott AM, Rood J, et al. Pediatric burn injuries from day-old campfires: a highly morbid and preventable problem. *J Burn Care Res.* 2011;32:633–637.
19. Shinozaki F, Hayatsu Y, Komatsu Y, et al. Electrical burns of lip and mouth in children. Report of 2 cases. *Int J Oral Surg.* 1984;13:25–30.
20. Burgess JD, Kimble RM, Cameron CM, et al. Hot beverage scalds in Australian children: still simmering 10 years on. *J Burn Care Res.* 2016;37:e355–e359.
21. Antoniou C, Dessinioti C, Stratigos AJ, et al. Clinical and therapeutic approach to childhood acne: an update. *Pediatr Dermatol.* 2009;26:373–380.
22. Gozali MV, Zhou B. Effective treatments of atrophic acne scars. *J Clin Aesthet Dermatol.* 2015;8:33–40.
23. Uihlein LC, Brandling-Bennett HA, Lio PA, et al. Sweet syndrome in children. *Pediatr Dermatol.* 2012;29:38–44.
24. Krakowski AC, Admani S, Uebelhoer NS, et al. Residual scarring from hidradenitis suppurativa: fractionated CO_2 laser as a novel and noninvasive approach. *Pediatrics.* 2014;133:e248–e251.
25. Agha R, Kinahan K, Bennett CL, et al. Dermatologic challenges in cancer patients and survivors. *Oncology (Williston Park).* 2007;21:1462–1472; discussion 1473, 1476, 1481 passim.
26. Gauglitz GG, Korting HC, Pavicic T, et al. Hypertrophic scarring and keloids: pathomechanisms and current and emerging treatment strategies. *Mol Med.* 2011;17:113–125.
27. Slemp AE, Kirschner RE. Keloids and scars: a review of keloids and scars, their pathogenesis, risk factors, and management. *Curr Opin Pediatr.* 2006;18:396–402.
28. van der Wal MB, Verhaegen PD, Middelkoop E, et al. A clinimetric overview of scar assessment scales. *J Burn Care Res.* 2012;33:e79–e87.
29. Lee SS, Yosipovitch G, Chan YH, et al. Pruritus, pain, and small nerve fiber function in keloids: a controlled study. *J Am Acad Dermatol.* 2004;51:1002–1006.
30. Parnell LK, Nedelec B, Rachelska G, et al. Assessment of pruritus characteristics and impact on burn survivors. *J Burn Care Res.* 2012;33:407–418.
31. Zhu J, Cheng B, Liu H, et al. Expression of beta-endorphin in hypertrophic scar and its relationship with pruritus [in Chinese]. *Zhongguo Xiu Fu Chong Jian Wai Ke Za Zhi.* 2012;26:731–734.
32. Van Loey NE, Van Son MJ. Psychopathology and psychological problems in patients with burn scars: epidemiology and management. *Am J Clin Dermatol.* 2003;4:245–272.
33. Choi YH, Kim KM, Kim HO, et al. Clinical and histological correlation in post-burn hypertrophic scar for pain and itching sensation. *Ann Dermatol.* 2013;25:428–433.
34. Blaha J. Physiology and pathology of skin after burns and derangement of gene expression. *Acta Chir Plast.* 2006;48:127–132.
35. Meulenbelt HE, Geertzen JH, Dijkstra PU, et al. Skin problems in lower limb amputees: an overview by case reports. *J Eur Acad Dermatol Venereol.* 2007;21:147–155.
36. Fu XB, Sun TZ, Li XK, et al. Morphological and distribution characteristics of sweat glands in hypertrophic scar and their possible effects on sweat gland regeneration. *Chin Med J (Engl).* 2005;118: 186–191.
37. Gupta S, Kanwar AJ, Kumar B. Hypertrichosis surrounding scar of knee replacement surgery. *J Am Acad Dermatol.* 2004;50:802–803.
38. Motamed S, Hasanpoor SE, Moosavizadeh SM, et al. Treatment of flexion contractures following burns in extremities. *Burns.* 2006;32:1017–1021.
39. Goel A, Shrivastava P. Post-burn scars and scar contractures. *Indian J Plast Surg.* 2010;43:S63–S71.
40. Langeland W, Olff M. Psychobiology of posttraumatic stress disorder in pediatric injury patients: a review of the literature. *Neurosci Biobehav Rev.* 2008;32:161–174.
41. Gupta MA, Gupta AK. Psychiatric and psychological co-morbidity in patients with dermatologic disorders: epidemiology and management. *Am J Clin Dermatol.* 2003;4:833–842.
42. Gilboa D, Bisk L, Montag I, et al. Personality traits and psychosocial adjustment of patients with burns. *J Burn Care Rehabil.* 1999;20:340–346; discussion 338–349.
43. Nguyen TA, Feldstein SI, Shumaker PR, et al. A review of scar assessment scales. *Semin Cutan Med Surg.* 2015;34:28–36.
44. Brown BC, Moss TP, McGrouther DA, et al. Skin scar preconceptions must be challenged: importance of self-perception in skin scarring. *J Plast Reconstr Aesthet Surg.* 2010;63:1022–1029.
45. Lawrence JW, Mason ST, Schomer K, et al. Epidemiology and impact of scarring after burn injury: a systematic review of the literature. *J Burn Care Res.* 2012;33:136–146.
46. Sanchez JL, Pereperez SB, Bastida JL, et al. Cost-utility analysis applied to the treatment of burn patients in a specialized center. *Arch Surg.* 2007;142:50–57; discussion 57.
47. Pellatt RA, Williams A, Wright H, et al. The cost of a major paediatric burn. *Burns.* 2010;36:1208–1214.
48. Koljonen V, Laitila M, Rissanen AM, et al. Treatment of patients with severe burns-costs and health-related quality of life outcome. *J Burn Care Res.* 2013;34:e318–e325.
49. Sen CK, Gordillo GM, Roy S, et al. Human skin wounds: a major and snowballing threat to public health and the economy. *Wound Repair Regen.* 2009;17:763–771.
50. Lee SH, Zheng Z, Roh MR. Early postoperative treatment of surgical scars using a fractional carbon dioxide laser: a split-scar, evaluator-blinded study. *Dermatol Surg.* 2013;39:1190–1196.
51. Berman B, Bieley HC. Adjunct therapies to surgical management of keloids. *Dermatol Surg.* 1996;22:126–130.
52. Lawrence WT. In search of the optimal treatment of keloids: report of a series and a review of the literature. *Ann Plast Surg.* 1991;27:164–178.
53. Brown JC, Klein EJ. The "Superhero Cape Burrito": a simple and comfortable method of short-term procedural restraint. *J Emerg Med.* 2011;41:74–76.
54. Raskin BI. A simple pediatric restraint. *Cutis.* 2000;66:335–336.
55. Ries WR, Clymer MA, Reinisch L. Laser safety features of eye shields. *Lasers Surg Med.* 1996;18:309–315.
56. De Sousa RF, Chakravarty B, Sharma A, et al. Efficacy of triple therapy in auricular keloids. *J Cutan Aesthet Surg.* 2014;7:98–102.
57. Baca ME, Neaman KC, Rapp DA, et al. Reduction of post-surgical scarring with the use of ablative fractional CO_2 lasers: a pilot study using a porcine model. *Lasers Surg Med.* 2016. doi:10.1002/lsm.22521.
58. Ogle CA, Shim EK, Godwin JA. Use of eye shields and eye lubricants among oculoplastic and Mohs surgeons: a survey. *J Drugs Dermatol.* 2009;8:855–860.
59. Echols K, Graves M, LeBlanc KG, et al. Role of antiseptics in the prevention of surgical site infections. *Dermatol Surg.* 2015;41:667–676.
60. Dumville JC, McFarlane E, Edwards P, et al. Preoperative skin antiseptics for preventing surgical wound infections after clean surgery. *Cochrane Database Syst Rev.* 2015;(4):CD003949.
61. Powers KS, Rubenstein JS. Family presence during invasive procedures in the pediatric intensive care unit: a prospective study. *Arch Pediatr Adolesc Med.* 1999;153:955–958.
62. Gauderer MW, Lorig JL, Eastwood DW. Is there a place for parents in the operating room? *J Pediatr Surg.* 1989;24:705–706; discussion 707.
63. Astuto M, Rosano G, Rizzo G, et al. Preoperative parental information and parents' presence at induction of anaesthesia. *Minerva Anestesiol.* 2006;72:461–465.
64. Kita T, Yamamoto M. Parental presence is a useful method for smooth induction of anesthesia in children: a postoperative questionnaire survey [in Japanese]. *Masui.* 2009;58:719–723.
65. Messeri A, Caprilli S, Busoni P. Anaesthesia induction in children: a psychological evaluation of the efficiency of parents' presence. *Paediatr Anaesth.* 2004;14:551–556.
66. Sahiner NC, Bal MD. The effects of three different distraction methods on pain and anxiety in children. *J Child Health Care.* 2016;20:277–285.

67. Koller D, Goldman RD. Distraction techniques for children undergoing procedures: a critical review of pediatric research. *J Pediatr Nurs.* 2012;27:652–681.
68. Vetri Buratti C, Angelino F, Sansoni J, et al. Distraction as a technique to control pain in pediatric patients during venipuncture. A narrative review of literature. *Prof Inferm.* 2015;68:52–62.
69. French GM, Painter EC, Coury DL. Blowing away shot pain: a technique for pain management during immunization. *Pediatrics.* 1994;93:384–388.
70. Jacobs A, Price HN, Popenhagen MP. Blowing away the pain: a technique for pediatric pain management. *Pediatr Dermatol.* 2014;31:757–758.
71. Dahlquist LM, Pendley JS, Landthrip DS, et al. Distraction intervention for preschoolers undergoing intramuscular injections and subcutaneous port access. *Health Psychol.* 2002;21:94–99.
72. Patel A, Schieble T, Davidson M, et al. Distraction with a hand-held video game reduces pediatric preoperative anxiety. *Paediatr Anaesth.* 2006;16:1019–1027.
73. Minute M, Badina L, Cont G, et al. Videogame playing as distraction technique in course of venipuncture. *Pediatr Med Chir.* 2012;34:77–83.
74. Asl Aminabadi N, Erfanparast L, Sohrabi A, et al. The impact of virtual reality distraction on pain and anxiety during dental treatment in 4–6 year-old children: a randomized controlled clinical trial. *J Dent Res Dent Clin Dent Prospects.* 2012;6:117–124.
75. McQueen A, Cress C, Tothy A. Using a tablet computer during pediatric procedures: a case series and review of the "apps." *Pediatr Emerg Care.* 2012;28:712–714.
76. Low DK, Pittaway AP. The 'iPhone' induction—a novel use for the Apple iPhone. *Paediatr Anaesth.* 2008;18:573–574.
77. Kuttner L. Favorite stories: a hypnotic pain-reduction technique for children in acute pain. *Am J Clin Hypn.* 1988;30:289–295.
78. Nilsson U. The anxiety- and pain-reducing effects of music interventions: a systematic review. *AORN J.* 2008;87:780–807.
79. Klassen JA, Liang Y, Tjosvold L, et al. Music for pain and anxiety in children undergoing medical procedures: a systematic review of randomized controlled trials. *Ambul Pediatr.* 2008;8:117–128.
80. Stuber M, Hilber SD, Mintzer LL, et al. Laughter, humor and pain perception in children: a pilot study. *Evid Based Complement Alternat Med.* 2009;6:271–276.
81. Canbulat Sahiner N, Inal S, Sevim Akbay A. The effect of combined stimulation of external cold and vibration during immunization on pain and anxiety levels in children. *J Perianesth Nurs.* 2015;30:228–235.
82. Kakigi R, Shibasaki H. Mechanisms of pain relief by vibration and movement. *J Neurol Neurosurg Psychiatry.* 1992;55:282–286.
83. Baxter AL, Lawson ML. Concerns with the methodology, analysis and discussion of the Buzzy(R) and transillumination comparison article. *Blood Transfus.* 2014;12(suppl 1):s3–s5.
84. Whelan HM, Kunselman AR, Thomas NJ, et al. The impact of a locally applied vibrating device on outpatient venipuncture in children. *Clin Pediatr (Phila).* 2014;53:1189–1195.
85. Inal S, Kelleci M. Relief of pain during blood specimen collection in pediatric patients. *MCN Am J Matern Child Nurs.* 2012;37:339–345.
86. Lima-Oliveira G, Lippi G, Salvagno GL, et al. A new device to relieve venipuncture pain can affect haematology test results. *Blood Transfus.* 2014;12(suppl 1):s6–s10.
87. Lee SH, Pakdeethai J, Toh MP, et al. A double-blind, randomised, placebo-controlled trial of EMLA(R) cream (Eutectic Lidocaine/Prilocaine Cream) for analgesia prior to cryotherapy of plantar warts in adults. *Ann Acad Med Singapore.* 2014;43:511–514.
88. Basiri-Moghadam M, Kianmehr M, Pasban-Noghabi S, et al. Comparison of EMLA cream with rattles on reducing immunization pain in four months infants. *J Pak Med Assoc.* 2014;64:874–878.
89. Abuelkheir M, Alsourani D, Al-Eyadhy A, et al. EMLA(R) cream: a pain-relieving strategy for childhood vaccination. *J Int Med Res.* 2014;42:329–336.
90. Shamriz O, Cohen-Glickman I, Reif S, et al. Methemoglobinemia induced by lidocaine-prilocaine cream. *Isr Med Assoc J.* 2014;16:250–254.
91. Tran AN, Koo JY. Risk of systemic toxicity with topical lidocaine/prilocaine: a review. *J Drugs Dermatol.* 2014;13:1118–1122.
92. Raso SM, Fernandez JB, Beobide EA, et al. Methemoglobinemia and CNS toxicity after topical application of EMLA to a 4-year-old girl with molluscum contagiosum. *Pediatr Dermatol.* 2006;23:592–593.
93. Hahn IH, Hoffman RS, Nelson LS. EMLA-induced methemoglobinemia and systemic topical anesthetic toxicity. *J Emerg Med.* 2004;26:85–88.
94. To D, Kossintseva I, de Gannes G. Lidocaine contact allergy is becoming more prevalent. *Dermatol Surg.* 2014;40:1367–1372.
95. Valdovinos NC, Reddin C, Bernard C, et al. The use of topical anesthesia during intravenous catheter insertion in adults: a comparison of pain scores using LMX-4 versus placebo. *J Emerg Nurs.* 2009;35:299–304.
96. Smith DP, Gjellum M. The efficacy of LMX versus EMLA for pain relief in boys undergoing office meatotomy. *J Urol.* 2004;172:1760–1761.
97. Oni G, Brown S, Kenkel J. Comparison of five commonly-available, lidocaine-containing topical anesthetics and their effect on serum levels of lidocaine and its metabolite monoethylglycinexylidide (MEGX). *Aesthet Surg J.* 2012;32:495–503.
98. Howe NR, Williams JM. Pain of injection and duration of anesthesia for intradermal infiltration of lidocaine, bupivacaine, and etidocaine. *J Dermatol Surg Oncol.* 1994;20:459–464.
99. Osayande OO, Mahmoud AO, Bolaji BO. Comparison of topical lidocaine [2% gel] and injectable lidocaine [2% solution] for incision and curettage of chalazion in Ilorin, Nigeria. *Niger Postgrad Med J.* 2010;17:270–276.
100. Amado A, Sood A, Taylor JS. Contact allergy to lidocaine: a report of sixteen cases. *Dermatitis.* 2007;18:215–220.
101. Mann GE, Kahana M. The uncomfortable reality … We simply do not know if general anesthesia negatively impacts the neurocognitive development of our small children. *Int J Pediatr Otorhinolaryngol.* 2015;79:1379–1381.
102. Hansen TG. Anesthesia-related neurotoxicity and the developing animal brain is not a significant problem in children. *Paediatr Anaesth.* 2015;25:65–72.
103. Taghon TA, Masunga AN, Small RH, et al. A comparison of functional magnetic resonance imaging findings in children with and without a history of early exposure to general anesthesia. *Paediatr Anaesth.* 2015;25:239–246.
104. Bakri MH, Ismail EA, Ali MS, et al. Behavioral and emotional effects of repeated general anesthesia in young children. *Saudi J Anaesth.* 2015;9:161–166.
105. Tyagi P, Tyagi S, Jain A. Sedative effects of oral midazolam, intravenous midazolam and oral diazepam in the dental treatment of children. *J Clin Pediatr Dent.* 2013;37:301–305.
106. Faritus SZ, Khazaee-Koohpar M, Ziyaeifard M, et al. Oral dexmedetomidine versus midazolam as anesthetic premedication in children undergoing congenital heart surgery. *Anesth Pain Med.* 2015;5:e25032.
107. Srivastava B, Mittal N, Mittal P. Acceptability and efficacy of commercial oral preparation of midazolam for brief painful procedure: a randomized double blind clinical trial. *Int J Clin Pediatr Dent.* 2014;7:153–156.
108. Salem K, Kamranzadeh S, Kousha M, et al. Two oral midazolam preparations in pediatric dental patients: a prospective randomised clinical trial. *Int J Pediatr.* 2015;2015:349795.
109. Coté CJ, Wilson S. Guidelines for monitoring and management of pediatric patients before, during, and after sedation for diagnostic and therapeutic procedures: update 2016. *Pediatr Dent.* 2016;38:13–39.
110. Cho YS, Jeon JH, Hong A, et al. The effect of burn rehabilitation massage therapy on hypertrophic scar after burn: a randomized controlled trial. *Burns.* 2014;40:1513–1520.
111. Roques C. Massage applied to scars. *Wound Repair Regen.* 2002;10:126–128.
112. Best TM, Gharaibeh B, Huard J. Stem cells, angiogenesis and muscle healing: a potential role in massage therapies? *Postgrad Med J.* 2013;89:666–670.
113. Shin TM, Bordeaux JS. The role of massage in scar management: a literature review. *Dermatol Surg.* 2012;38:414–423.
114. Atiyeh BS, El Khatib AM, Dibo SA. Pressure garment therapy (PGT) of burn scars: evidence-based efficacy. *Ann Burns Fire Disasters.* 2013;26:205–212.
115. Kim JY, Willard JJ, Supp DM, et al. Burn scar biomechanics after pressure garment therapy. *Plast Reconstr Surg.* 2015;136:572–581.
116. Sharp PA, Pan B, Yakuboff KP, et al. Development of a best evidence statement for the use of pressure therapy for management of hypertrophic scarring. *J Burn Care Res.* 2016;37:255–264.
117. Li-Tsang CW, Feng B, Huang L, et al. A histological study on the effect of pressure therapy on the activities of myofibroblasts and keratinocytes in hypertrophic scar tissues after burn. *Burns.* 2015;41:1008–1016.
118. Anzarut A, Olson J, Singh P, et al. The effectiveness of pressure garment therapy for the prevention of abnormal scarring after burn injury: a meta-analysis. *J Plast Reconstr Aesthet Surg.* 2009;62:77–84.
119. Robles DT, Berg D. Abnormal wound healing: keloids. *Clin Dermatol.* 2007;25:26–32.

120. Krusche T, Worret WI. Mechanical properties of keloids in vivo during treatment with intralesional triamcinolone acetonide. *Arch Dermatol Res.* 1995;287:289–293.
121. Ledon JA, Savas J, Franca K, et al. Intralesional treatment for keloids and hypertrophic scars: a review. *Dermatol Surg.* 2013;39:1745–1757.
122. Fredman R, Tenenhaus M. Cushing's syndrome after intralesional triamcinolone acetonide: a systematic review of the literature and multinational survey. *Burns.* 2013;39(4):549–557.
123. Teelucksingh S, Balkaran B, Ganeshmoorthi A, et al. Prolonged childhood Cushing's syndrome secondary to intralesional triamcinolone acetonide. *Ann Trop Paediatr.* 2002;22:89–91.
124. Music EN, Engel G. Earlobe keloids: a novel and elegant surgical approach. *Dermatol Surg.* 2010;36:395–400.
125. Rosen DJ, Patel MK, Freeman K, et al. A primary protocol for the management of ear keloids: results of excision combined with intraoperative and postoperative steroid injections. *Plast Reconstr Surg.* 2007;120:1395–1400.
126. Wainwright DJ. Burn reconstruction: the problems, the techniques, and the applications. *Clin Plast Surg.* 2009;36:687–700.
127. Brewin MP, Lister TS. Prevention or treatment of hypertrophic burn scarring: a review of when and how to treat with the pulsed dye laser. *Burns.* 2014;40:797–804.
128. Garden JM, Tan OT, Kerschmann R, et al. Effect of dye laser pulse duration on selective cutaneous vascular injury. *J Invest Dermatol.* 1986;87:653–657.
129. Dierickx C, Goldman MP, Fitzpatrick RE. Laser treatment of erythematous/hypertrophic and pigmented scars in 26 patients. *Plast Reconstr Surg.* 1995;95:84–90; discussion 91–82.
130. Brightman LA, Geronemus RG, Reddy KK. Laser treatment of port-wine stains. *Clin Cosmet Investig Dermatol.* 2015;8:27–33.
131. Thajudheen CP, Jyothy K, Priyadarshini A. Treatment of port-wine stains with flash lamp pumped pulsed dye laser on Indian skin: a six year study. *J Cutan Aesthet Surg.* 2014;7:32–36.
132. Koster PH, van der Horst CM, Bossuyt PM, et al. Prediction of portwine stain clearance and required number of flashlamp pumped pulsed dye laser treatments. *Lasers Surg Med.* 2001;29:151–155.
133. Liu A, Moy RL, Ross EV, et al. Pulsed dye laser and pulsed dye laser-mediated photodynamic therapy in the treatment of dermatologic disorders. *Dermatol Surg.* 2012;38:351–366.
134. Chesnut C, Mednik S, Lask G. Hypertrophic scar treatment with intralesional triamcinolone acetonide and pulsed dye laser results in necrosis. *Cutis.* 2014;94:E12–E13.
135. Anderson RR, Donelan MB, Hivnor C, et al. Laser treatment of traumatic scars with an emphasis on ablative fractional laser resurfacing: consensus report. *JAMA Dermatol.* 2014;150:187–193.
136. Hantash BM, Bedi VP, Kapadia B, et al. In vivo histological evaluation of a novel ablative fractional resurfacing device. *Lasers Surg Med.* 2007;39:96–107.
137. Ozog DM, Liu A, Chaffins ML, et al. Evaluation of clinical results, histological architecture, and collagen expression following treatment of mature burn scars with a fractional carbon dioxide laser. *JAMA Dermatol.* 2013;149:50–57.
138. Qu L, Liu A, Zhou L, et al. Clinical and molecular effects on mature burn scars after treatment with a fractional CO(2) laser. *Lasers Surg Med.* 2012;44:517–524.
139. Orringer JS, Rittie L, Baker D, et al. Molecular mechanisms of nonablative fractionated laser resurfacing. *Br J Dermatol.* 2010;163:757–768.
140. Helbig D, Bodendorf MO, Grunewald S, et al. Immunohistochemical investigation of wound healing in response to fractional photothermolysis. *J Biomed Opt.* 2009;14:064044.
141. Xu XG, Luo YJ, Wu Y, et al. Immunohistological evaluation of skin responses after treatment using a fractional ultrapulse carbon dioxide laser on back skin. *Dermatol Surg.* 2011;37:1141–1149.
142. Hultman CS, Friedstat JS, Edkins RE, et al. Laser resurfacing and remodeling of hypertrophic burn scars: the results of a large, prospective, before-after cohort study, with long-term follow-up. *Ann Surg.* 2014;260:519–529; discussion 529–532.
143. Krakowski AC, Goldenberg A, Eichenfield LF, et al. Ablative fractional laser resurfacing helps treat restrictive pediatric scar contractures. *Pediatrics.* 2014;134:e1700–e1705.
144. Uebelhoer NS, Ross EV, Shumaker PR. Ablative fractional resurfacing for the treatment of traumatic scars and contractures. *Semin Cutan Med Surg.* 2012;31:110–120.
145. Shumaker PR, Kwan JM, Landers JT, et al. Functional improvements in traumatic scars and scar contractures using an ablative fractional laser protocol. *J Trauma Acute Care Surg.* 2012;73:S116–S121.
146. Waibel JS, Wulkan AJ, Shumaker PR. Treatment of hypertrophic scars using laser and laser assisted corticosteroid delivery. *Lasers Surg Med.* 2013;45:135–140.
147. Clayton JL, Edkins R, Cairns BA, et al. Incidence and management of adverse events after the use of laser therapies for the treatment of hypertrophic burn scars. *Ann Plast Surg.* 2013;70:500–505.
148. Hunzeker CM, Weiss ET, Geronemus RG. Fractionated CO_2 laser resurfacing: our experience with more than 2000 treatments. *Aesthet Surg J.* 2009;29:317–322.
149. Krakowski AC, Admani S, Shumaker PR, et al. Fractionated carbon dioxide laser as a novel, noninvasive treatment approach to burn scar-related nail dystrophy. *Dermatol Surg.* 2014;40:351–354.
150. Gauglitz GG. Management of keloids and hypertrophic scars: current and emerging options. *Clin Cosmet Investig Dermatol.* 2013;6:103–114.
151. Sklar LR, Burnett CT, Waibel JS, et al. Laser assisted drug delivery: a review of an evolving technology. *Lasers Surg Med.* 2014;46:249–262.
152. Yun PL, Tachihara R, Anderson RR. Efficacy of erbium:yttrium-aluminum-garnet laser-assisted delivery of topical anesthetic. *J Am Acad Dermatol.* 2002;47:542–547.
153. Lee WR, Shen SC, Al-Suwayeh SA, et al. Laser-assisted topical drug delivery by using a low-fluence fractional laser: imiquimod and macromolecules. *J Control Release.* 2011;153:240–248.
154. Lee WR, Pan TL, Wang PW, et al. Erbium:YAG laser enhances transdermal peptide delivery and skin vaccination. *J Control Release.* 2008;128:200–208.
155. Wang KH, Fang JY, Hu CH, et al. Erbium:YAG laser pretreatment accelerates the response of Bowen's disease treated by topical 5-fluorouracil. *Dermatol Surg.* 2004;30:441–445.
156. Brauer JA, Krakowski AC, Bloom BS, et al. Convergence of anatomy, technology, and therapeutics: a review of laser assisted drug delivery. *Semin Cutan Med Surg.* 2014;33:176–181.
157. Agris J. Traumatic tattooing. *J Trauma.* 1976;16:798–802.
158. Kent KM, Graber EM. Laser tattoo removal: a review. *Dermatol Surg.* 2012;38:1–13.
159. Gorouhi F, Davari P, Kashani MN, et al. Treatment of traumatic tattoo with the Q-switched Nd:YAG laser. *J Cosmet Laser Ther.* 2007;9:253–255.
160. Ashinoff R, Geronemus RG. Rapid response of traumatic and medical tattoos to treatment with the Q-switched ruby laser. *Plast Reconstr Surg.* 1993;91:841–845.
161. Cambier B, Rogge F. Traumatic tattoo: use of the variable pulsed erbium:YAG laser. *Photomed Laser Surg.* 2006;24:605–609.

23 A Perspective from Military Medicine

PETER R. SHUMAKER, THOMAS BEACHKOFSKY, ANDREW BASNETT, CARRICK BURNS, NATHAN UEBELHOER, and CHAD HIVNOR

KEY POINTS

- More than a decade of conflict and unprecedented battlefield survival rates led to an enormous influx of military personnel in need of functional and cosmetic rehabilitation.
- To adapt to the challenges posed by the number and the severity of the injuries and the high expectations for recovery of these young patients, new paradigms of coordinated multidisciplinary care emerged at multiple military centers of excellence in rehabilitation.
- Among the benefits of this type of collaborative environment are innovative approaches to care; the routine inclusion of dermatologists and their expertise in a variety of minimally invasive cutaneous procedures has enhanced ongoing rehabilitative efforts and is helping to change paradigms both within and outside the military system.
- The benefits of procedures such as ablative fractional laser resurfacing (AFR) for traumatic scars and laser hair reduction for amputees are certainly not limited to battlefield trauma, and millions of patients worldwide may benefit from these and future techniques regardless of the source of injury.

Scar management in the military setting presents many unique challenges and opportunities. Extended conflict and increased battlefield survival has left thousands of otherwise young and healthy individuals in need of long-term rehabilitation and reintegration following devastating injuries including burns, amputations, and traumatic brain injury. The need to address multiple complex medical and psychosocial issues effectively and efficiently has ushered in unprecedented levels of multidisciplinary collaboration at three military advanced rehabilitation centers of excellence including the Military Advanced Training Center (MATC) at Walter Reed National Military Medical Center in Bethesda, Maryland; the Center for the Intrepid (CFI) at Brooke Army Medical Center in San Antonio, Texas; and the Comprehensive and Complex Casualty Care Center (C5) at the Naval Medical Center San Diego. Several aspects of military medicine are conducive to collaboration and the early adoption of new innovations including a focus on mission accomplishment, ongoing experience working in cohesive multidisciplinary teams during both peacetime and conflict, and a relative lack of financial disincentives that more commonly impact civilian practice. The emergence of dermatologists as routine partners in trauma rehabilitation is a product of this environment. This chapter highlights a treatment approach and a variety of minimally invasive cutaneous procedures from the perspective of military dermatologists at two different military centers. Like so many medical advancements in history, the vast majority of the patients that may ultimately benefit from these techniques will never wear a uniform.

Unusual Aspects of Military Practice

Inherent characteristics of the wounded warrior have driven rehabilitation after major trauma to new heights, both literally and figuratively.[1] They are often young, motivated, goal oriented, and otherwise healthy and active at baseline before injury. For this cohort of recovering service personnel, simply walking or completing activities of daily living is not good enough. Patients want to return to activities as close as possible to baseline (or even higher) levels of functioning and participate in a range activities such as snowboarding, surfing, hiking, biking, swimming, and running. Others, including amputees, have returned to full duty and even deployed back to combat zones.[2] Minimally invasive procedures such as laser scar revision, laser hair reduction, and procedural sweat reduction are extremely effective adjuncts to traditional rehabilitative efforts such as physical and recreational therapy, prosthetics, mental health support, and medical and surgical management.

The psychosocial impact of a scar can vary widely from person to person depending on the size, location, symptoms, and myriad other factors. In the experience of the authors, however, the attitude of a military patient toward the presence of the scar is frequently not as uniformly negative as in nonmilitary patients. For some, the scar may be a badge of honor or a reminder of friends lost; an outward symbol of dedication and sacrifice. Although the mere presence of a scar may not always be problematic, the desire to improve functionality and reduce symptoms such as pain and itch is universal. By the time a polytrauma patient enters the clinic they may have endured numerous surgical procedures requiring general anesthesia. Many patients are grateful to have effective and minimally invasive procedures in the clinic setting. Surprisingly, they can be tolerant of temporary mild to moderate pain associated with an array of cutaneous procedures. Posttraumatic stress and anxiety are relatively common, however, and triggers such as the smell of smoke, noise, and burning pain are wisely anticipated and mitigated during treatment.

Centers of Excellence

After the entry of the United States into the conflicts in Afghanistan and Iraq in the early 2000s, the emergence of the improvised explosive device as a pervasive weapon combined with advances in battlefield resuscitation and transportation resulted in an unprecedented number of survivors with multiple severe injuries and associated sequelae including burns, amputations, disfigurement, traumatic brain injury, posttraumatic stress disorder, and loss of hearing and eyesight.[3,4] Simultaneously, an enhanced awareness of the need for higher levels of care for veterans became apparent to the American public. Thus, a highly coordinated multidisciplinary approach to rehabilitation including MATC, CFI, and C5 emerged. Additionally, other entities such as the Extremity Amputation Center of Excellence (EACE) and the Defense Centers of Excellence for Psychological Health and Traumatic Brain Injury began to collaborate through a national network to facilitate ongoing clinical care and research. The requirement for ongoing care, the need to retain skills and capacity to account for future conflicts, and the fact that coordinated care benefits patients regardless of the source of injury help ensure that these centers will have an enduring role.

Programs such as C5 operate along a similar model of multidisciplinary care on a residential or drop-in basis, as appropriate. Dedicated program staff provide active case management and patients receive coordinated care as needed through various surgical and medical specialties including but not limited to: orthopedics, neurology, dermatology, physical medicine and rehabilitation, pain management, prosthetics and gait evaluation, mental health, and physical, occupational, and recreational therapy (Fig. 23-1). Additionally, they receive other psychological and social support including pastoral care, family support groups, and career transition resources. These programs are available for all active duty patients, whether or not their injuries are combat related. However, severely injured active duty patients requiring extensive care may be assigned to a rehabilitation program as their primary duty. Often they will reside on the grounds of military medical facility to allow a consolidation of medical resources and a full-time focus on recovery. Patients have access to a broad logistics network facilitating nationwide transfer when necessary, and resources are available to bring and temporarily house patients' families near the centers. Some patients are ultimately returned to full or modified duty; others are transitioned out of active service with ongoing care coordinated to varying degrees by Veterans Administration (VA) and military treatment facilities depending on

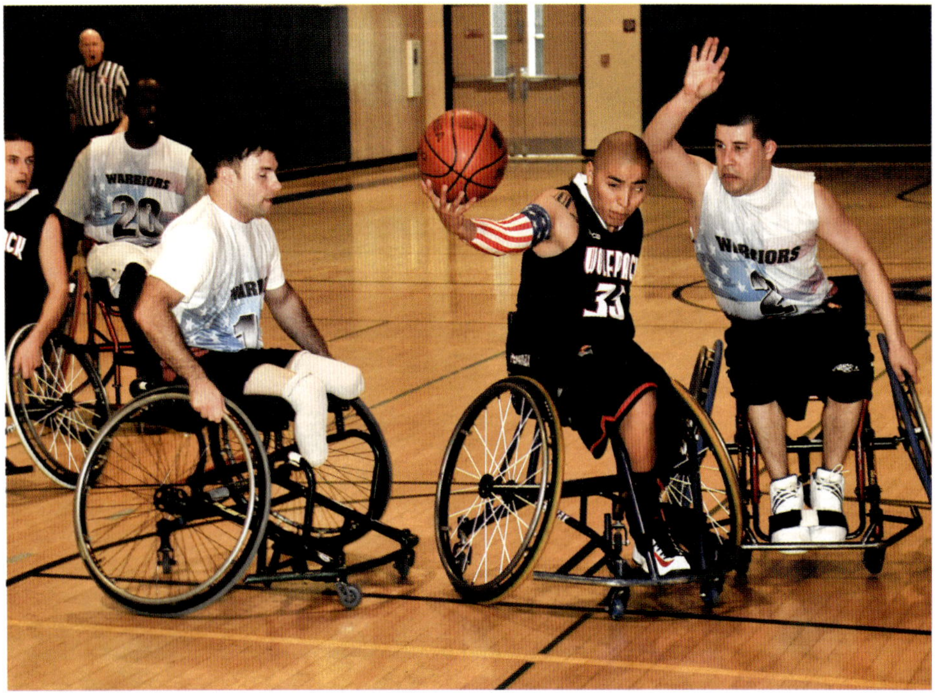

FIGURE 23-1 Retired Marine Josue Barron (#35), a member of the Naval Medical Center San Diego (NMCSD) Wolfpack wheelchair basketball team, keeps the ball away from the Fort Sam Warriors. Wolfpack is made up of 13 military and civilian members and is one of 10 teams in the West Coast Conference of the National Wheelchair Basketball Association. *(Courtesy of U.S. Navy, photo by Mass Communication Specialist Seaman Pyoung K. Yi/Released.)*

the location, spectrum of injuries, and other factors. The centers have developed resources to assist those with the transition to civilian life.

International Exchange and Humanitarian Operations

The United States regularly deploys military medical assets around the world to help build durable and effective partnerships with other nations to enhance disaster preparedness and theater security cooperation. The annual Pacific Partnership mission is an excellent example of these efforts; it is the largest multinational humanitarian assistance and disaster preparedness activity in the Indo-Asia-Pacific region. The annual mission began in 2006 following the 2004 tsunami that devastated parts of Southeast Asia. The U.S. Navy deployed assets to the international relief effort, including the hospital ship USNS Mercy. This ship, and its sister ship the USNS Comfort on the east coast of the United States, are fully capable floating hospitals with operating rooms, an intensive care unit, imaging, laboratory, pharmacy, and numerous medical specialists and support staff. The 10th iteration of Pacific Partnership was completed in 2015 and included nine partner nations and multiple nongovernmental organizations participating in activities such as direct medical and surgical care and subject matter expert exchange, public outreach, veterinary services, and engineering projects. Over the course of approximately 4 months in 2015 the Mercy traveled to Fiji, Papua New Guinea, the Philippines, and Vietnam.[5]

Among the myriad other notable activities during Pacific Partnership 2015, a multidisciplinary team consisting of dermatology, plastic surgery, orthopedics, physical therapy, and other specialties participated in direct care and high-level exchange in the management of severe scars and scar contractures resulting from burns and other trauma. This provided the team an ongoing opportunity to leverage experience gained over more than a decade treating injured service members during wartime to promote cooperation and help ease suffering in multiple corners of Southeast Asia. Combining ablative fractional laser resurfacing (AFR) with surgery and other nonsurgical modalities, numerous patients received cutting-edge treatment to help restore function and appearance during the mission (Fig. 23-2). The hospital ship provides a unique and successful platform to treat patients from a variety of settings. Performed alone or concurrently with surgery, patient follow-up extending up to 4 years from prior missions involving hundreds of patients demonstrates an excellent record of safety and efficacy, even after a single treatment (unpublished experience) (Fig. 23-3). In addition, extensive exchange with host physicians was performed to further enhance sustainable relationships.

Cutaneous Procedures in Trauma Rehabilitation

Military dermatologists have played a significant role in integrating AFR and a variety of other minimally invasive cutaneous procedures into trauma rehabilitation, whether the injuries have been sustained on or off the battlefield. A more comprehensive discussion of laser and other treatments for scars is available in other parts of the text (see Chapters 10, 12, 13 and 14). These devices and techniques are widely available in dermatology and plastic surgery offices around the world, and minor adaptations of these techniques applied regularly for aesthetic applications can help bring life-changing treatment to millions of patients worldwide. This section highlights the experience of the authors at two military centers of excellence: the Naval Medical Center San Diego and the San Antonio Military Medical Center.

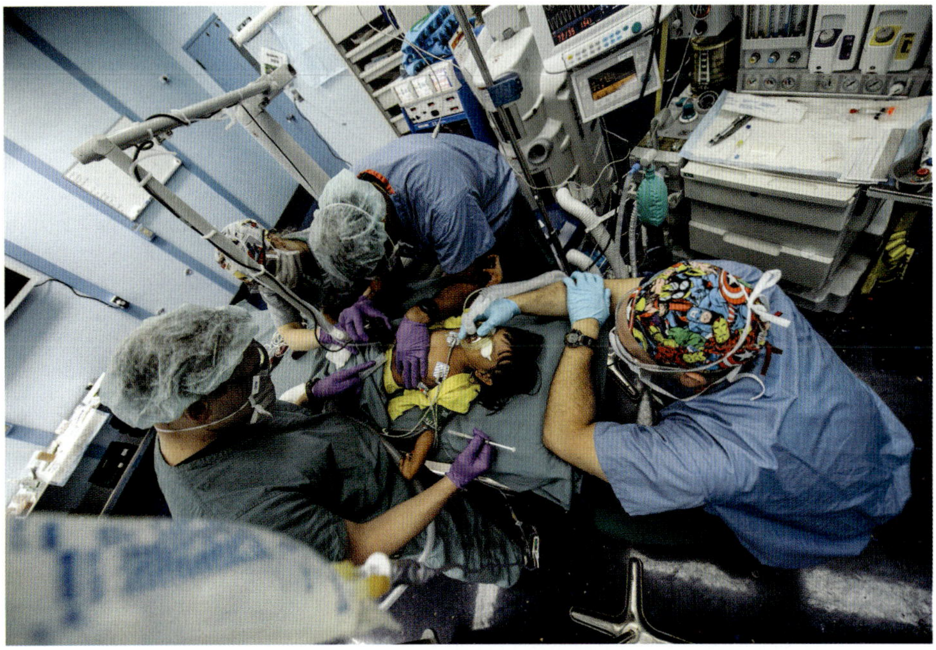

FIGURE 23-2 Service members, assigned to the hospital ship USNS Mercy (T-AH 19), perform a fractional CO_2 laser procedure on a child during Pacific Partnership 2015. *(Courtesy of U.S. Navy, photo by Petty Officer 2nd Class Mark El-Rayes/Released.)*

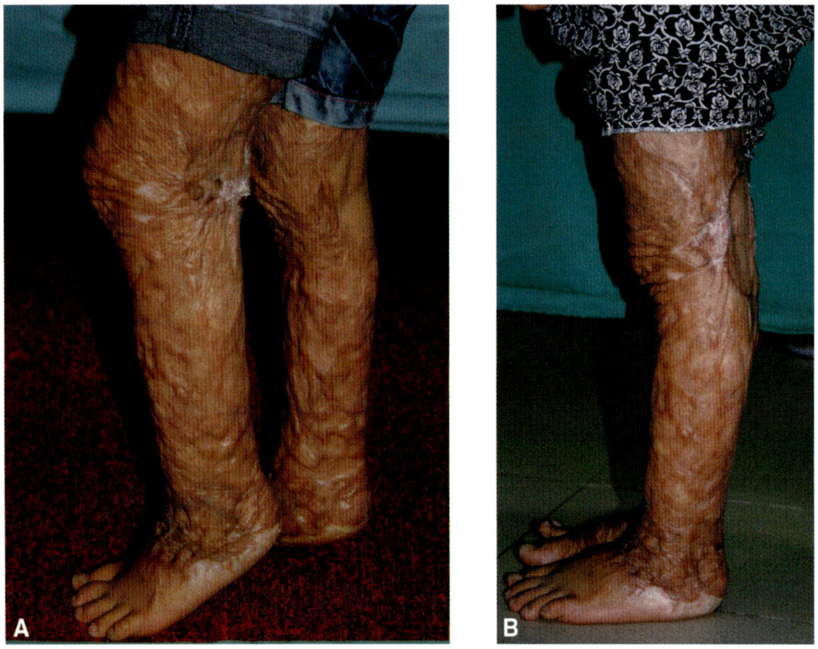

FIGURE 23-3 **A:** A 4-year-old girl approximately16 months after suffering burns over approximately 60% of her total body surface area, and approximately 12 and 4 months from her first and second ablative fractional laser treatments, respectively. Although significant interval enhancements in scar pliability and range of motion were noted, a flexion contracture at the knee and loss of pliability of the tissues surrounding the ankle precluded normal ambulation. **B:** Approximately 10 months after contracture excision, placement of a bovine collagen and glycosaminoglycan meshed bilayer dressing (INTEGRA Meshed Bilayer Wound Matrix, Integra LifeSciences Corporation, Plainsboro, NJ) and negative pressure wound therapy followed approximately 1 month later by a split-thickness skin graft. A third ablative fractional laser resurfacing procedure (Lumenis UltraPulse, Deep FX, Yokneam, Israel) was performed concurrently with contracture excision over the entire scarred area. Her range of motion had improved significantly and ambulation had largely normalized. This case demonstrates the benefits of multidisciplinary care and long-term collaboration.

Laser Scar Revision

Treatment Approach

The treatment approach to scars with lasers and light devices in the military setting has been outlined previously.[6,7] Although AFR is central to the management of debilitating scarring in the outpatient setting, it is by no means the only useful platform. A range of lasers and light devices that target the three main skin chromophores (water, hemoglobin, and melanin) are routinely used by the authors after trauma. Roughly in descending order of frequency these are: AFR, vascular lasers and light devices (such as the 595-nm pulsed dye laser [PDL]), nonablative fractional resurfacing, long-pulsed pigment-specific lasers for hair reduction, and short-pulsed (Q-switched) pigment-specific lasers for the removal of traumatic tattoos. In many instances, all of these platforms will be used concurrently or in an alternating fashion in the management of a specific patient.

Initial evaluation involves an assessment of scar erythema, degree of healing, pliability, texture, dyspigmentation, thickness, degree of contracture, and proximity to joints and free edges. Additionally, prior treatments, future surgical intervention, prosthetic use, sensitivity and pain syndromes, and the presence of posttraumatic stress should be considered when developing a treatment plan. Far from being a replacement for traditional interventions, laser treatments are most effective when complemented by ongoing multidisciplinary care including physical and occupational therapy and surgical and nonsurgical medical consultation. Because of the minimally invasive nature of laser scar revision and other related procedures, treatment can be initiated relatively early in the postinjury course. Indeed, this appears to be one of its most promising attributes. In the experience of the authors, AFR and vascular laser treatments can often safely begin within 4 to 12 weeks of severe traumatic injury and may actually help mitigate contractures and pathologic scars when performed judiciously. This is an active area of study, and future large prospective controlled trials are required to confirm these observations, as well as help refine appropriate settings, timing, and treatment combinations.

Fractional Lasers

Among the most notable advances in scar treatment in recent decades is the emergence of AFR. Manstein et al.[8] first described the concept of fractional photothermolysis in 2004, wherein emitted light in the mid-infrared (e.g., 1,540 and 1,550 nm) and far-infrared (e.g., 2,940 and 10,600 nm) range induces tissue coagulation or ablation, respectively, in a pixelated pattern through the heating of tissue water.[9] Key advancements of the technology include fractionation of the tissue injury to minimize side effects and facilitate subsequent healing, and unprecedented levels of control for the operator to determine the depth and density of treatment. In retrospect it seems this technology was tailor-made for scar revision, affording adaptable and minimally invasive treatments to be applied in the compromised and highly variable setting of scar tissue.

Fostered by the multidisciplinary environment, the rapid influx of patients with serious traumatic injuries, and relatively unfettered by billing issues (see Chapter 25), military dermatologists were among the first to elaborate on the potential for AFR to enhance functional rehabilitation in addition to aesthetic restoration.[6,7,10–12] Although the application is now beginning to expand rapidly as an emerging standard in burn centers and other venues around the world, AFR has been incorporated routinely into treatment paradigms for trauma patients in a handful of centers, including military centers of excellence, since approximately 2008.[6,13–15]

In the experience of the authors, a course of AFR is associated with consistent and significant improvements in wound healing and scar pliability, texture, and pigmentation. Furthermore, complications such as infection and worsening scarring are extremely rare when AFR is applied judiciously.[16] In virtually all cases there is at least some degree of improvement over weeks and months, although the overall impact can vary significantly from patient to patient depending on the clinical scenario. Particularly for the novice, safety is maximized by employing low treatment densities and applying treatments in alternating sessions when using multiple platforms. In the experience of the authors, AFR can be a highly effective adjunct to surgical revision for contractures when applied before, concurrent with, and after surgery.[6,7,16,17]

The interval between AFR treatments is generally at least 6 to 8 weeks to allow for adequate healing and remodeling. The majority of functional gains are usually realized in the first three to five treatments, whereas texture and dyspigmentation may continue to improve with additional ablative and nonablative fractional treatments. Contractures are usually treated with low (perhaps even the lowest) density and higher pulse energy settings (corresponding with scar thickness), whereas treatments for the enhancement of texture and dyspigmentation alone may be associated with slightly higher density and more moderate pulse energy settings. Actual treatment settings will depend on the specific platform and its associated characteristics such as microcolumn diameter, pulse duration, and available treatment depth. For ablative fractional treatments the authors favor a narrow column width (≤400 μm) and shorter pulse duration (<1 ms) to help avoid excessive thermal injury. Density settings are rarely above 10% for ablative treatments, and are frequently lower when using higher pulse energy settings.

Vascular Lasers

Erythema is a frequent finding early in the process of scar formation, and can also be a helpful indicator of persistent inflammation and an incipient pathologic scar with associated symptoms such as pain and itch. Vascular-specific lasers and light devices target hemoglobin to induce moderate vascular injury and subsequent remodeling. The 585 and 595 nm PDL is the most studied, with more than two decades of use for various scar types.[18,19] Other devices that target hemoglobin absorption peaks such as the 532 nm potassium titanyl phosphate laser and intense-pulsed light can also offer benefit.[20] In the experience of the authors, PDL and other vascular devices can be very helpful in reducing pain and itch in large erythematous traumatic scars, such as after burns. It is extremely common to use both fractional and vascular devices in the same patient in the same or alternating treatment sessions, adjusting the treatment approach during the maturation and remodeling process.

In general, moderate treatment fluences and relatively short pulse durations are used by the authors with a focus more on gradual tissue remodeling rather than tissue destruction.[16] The 595-nm PDL (Vbeam Perfecta, Syneron & Candela, Wayland, MA) is often applied with moderate fluences in the range of 7 to 9 J per cm^2 with a spot size of 7 mm and pulse duration of 1.5 ms to generate an endpoint of minimal purpura. Integration of vascular-specific devices into a scar treatment protocol is often highly desired because of its high tolerability often with minimal or no anesthesia, ability to quickly treat large areas in a single session, and consistency in reducing symptoms in parallel with erythema. Typically, vascular laser treatments are performed alone or in conjunction with other modalities such as fractional lasers and corticosteroids at 1- to 2-month intervals. Although treatment courses vary considerably, an average of four to six treatments are performed or until the desired erythema reduction endpoint is met.

CASE EXAMPLE: MULTIMODAL COSMETIC AND FUNCTIONAL RESTORATION AFTER INJURY FROM AN IMPROVISED EXPLOSIVE DEVICE

A man in his 20s suffered a traumatic full-thickness laceration of the lower face associated with an improvised explosive device (Fig. 23-4A). Initial stabilization was followed by a series of multidisciplinary reconstruction procedures involving the plastic and facial plastic surgery, oromaxillofacial surgery, and dental departments. At presentation in dermatology approximately 6 months after injury the patient was noted to have a thickened, erythematous, and tethered full-thickness scar of the right lower lip and chin (Fig. 23-4B). Significant swelling of the right lower lip and asymmetry on smiling and mouth opening was noted, with mild associated issues reported with eating and drinking. Scar hypertrophy and contracture was affecting mouth function, and likely contributed to outflow obstruction and lip edema.

A range of techniques and devices can be considered for the management of traumatic scars over time (both concurrently and in series), and each treatment is individualized at every treatment session based on the clinical findings and patient preferences. AFR is an excellent choice to help improve scar pliability and reduce tension through the induction of vigorous collagen remodeling, and can typically be initiated at early stages of rehabilitation. Erythematous scars respond well to devices targeting the vasculature, such as the 595-nm PDL. Nonablative fractional lasers are associated with minimal morbidity and can

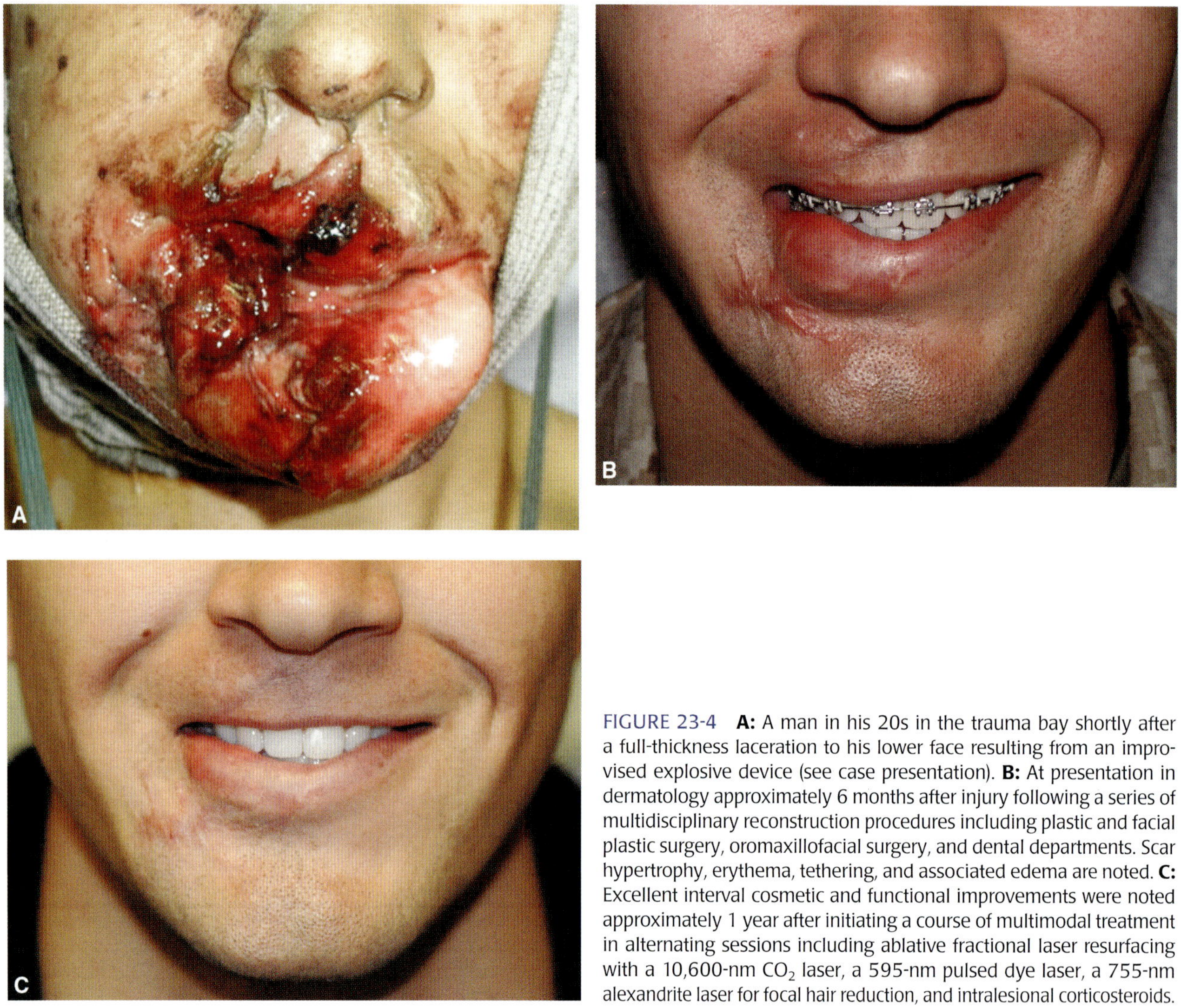

FIGURE 23-4 **A:** A man in his 20s in the trauma bay shortly after a full-thickness laceration to his lower face resulting from an improvised explosive device (see case presentation). **B:** At presentation in dermatology approximately 6 months after injury following a series of multidisciplinary reconstruction procedures including plastic and facial plastic surgery, oromaxillofacial surgery, and dental departments. Scar hypertrophy, erythema, tethering, and associated edema are noted. **C:** Excellent interval cosmetic and functional improvements were noted approximately 1 year after initiating a course of multimodal treatment in alternating sessions including ablative fractional laser resurfacing with a 10,600-nm CO_2 laser, a 595-nm pulsed dye laser, a 755-nm alexandrite laser for focal hair reduction, and intralesional corticosteroids.

also be very helpful to improve textural abnormalities and dyspigmentation. Furthermore, they can be used in mature scars without significant erythema. Corticosteroids delivered intralesionally and/or through laser-assisted delivery remain a mainstay of treatment for hypertrophic scars. Scarring in hair-bearing areas can lead to folliculitis, bundling, cosmetic issues and difficulty with shaving. Laser hair reduction can be a very helpful adjunct in these situations. Alternatively, follicular unit transplantation can help to camouflage scars in hair-bearing areas. Explosive devices and road accidents are commonly associated with traumatic tattoos; short-pulsed (nanosecond and picosecond) lasers specific for pigment, particularly at wavelengths of 755 and 1,064 nm, are very effective for improving appearance in these situations.

In this case a course of AFR with a 10,600-nm CO_2 laser (Lumenis UltraPulse, Deep FX, Yokneam, Israel) was initiated at settings of 30 to 50 mJ (depending on the estimated scar thickness—in this case lower settings were used in the periphery of the scar) and 5% density to scarred portions of both the cutaneous and mucosal lip at approximately 2- to 3-month intervals. Ablative fractional laser treatments were alternated at approximately 1- to 2-month intervals with a 595-nm PDL (Vbeam Perfecta, Syneron & Candela, Wayland, MA) using a 7 mm spot size at settings of 7 to 9 J per cm^2 and a 1.5 ms pulse width to erythematous portions of the scar. Intralesional triamcinolone acetonide suspension was applied judiciously in the early phases of treatment during each laser session at a concentration of 20 to 40 mg per mL to the thickest portions of the scar. Focal laser hair reduction was performed at the periphery of the scar because of ingrown hairs and difficulty shaving with a "long-pulsed" (millisecond) 755-nm alexandrite laser (GentleMax, Syneron & Candela, Wayland, MA) at settings appropriate for skin type. The patient noted rapid improvements in scar pliability at the beginning of his treatment course, and approximately 1 year after his initial treatment excellent improvements in cosmetic appearance and function were noted (Fig. 23-4C).

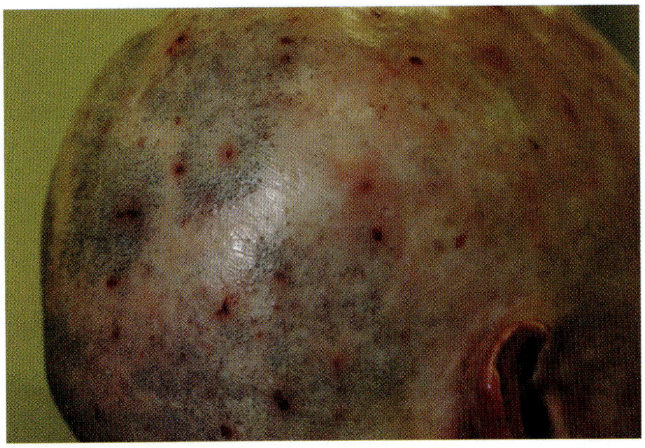

FIGURE 23-5 Following a blast injury from an improvised explosive device, patchy scarring is noted on the scalp with associated alopecia. Note the numerous erosions and ulcerations, some with terminal hairs extruding through center. After a course of laser hair removal all of the ulcerations subsided.

Scarring and Adnexal Structures (*Pilosebaceous Unit, Eccrine Glands/Ducts*)

In addition to posttraumatic fibrosis affecting limb range of motion as noted above, it is important to note that scars also impact surrounding adnexal structures such as the pilosebaceous units and eccrine glands/coils/ducts and other subcutaneous tissues. For instance, in the setting of burn scars or harvest sites for split-thickness skin grafts, functional hair follicles may result in irritation, folliculitis, abscesses, and even chronic wounds due in part to the inability of the hair to pierce through the fibrotic scar tissue (Fig. 23-5). In general, treatments in this situation are aimed at laser hair reduction combined with scar mitigation using microfractionated ablative lasers as discussed above (Fig. 23-6). Additionally, lasers are employed to remove hair relocated to unwanted areas (e.g., palms) during reconstructive procedures, and to improve the comfort and fit of prosthetic devices after extremity amputation.

Treatment protocols include the use of millisecond-range lasers with wavelengths specific to melanin absorption (most commonly 755 and 810 nm for lighter skin types and 1,064 nm for darker skin types). Additionally, the use of intense pulsed light/broadband light-emitting devices can be effective for hair removal. However, these devices require close attention to cut off filter selection and thus may not be optimal for this application, particularly in darker skin types. We have found that a series of at least six treatments at intervals of 3 to 6 weeks (depending on the treatment location) yield acceptable and reproducible results. Touch-up treatments are often necessary every 6 to 12 months to minimize regrowth.

Scarring and fibrosis of the dermis can additionally disrupt the eccrine glands and ducts. This may result in pain, pruritus, and anhidrosis (or the functional inability to perspire). It has been shown that patients with functional eccrine glands under a scar may regain the ability to sweat when treated with fractionated lasers.[21] Both excessive sweating (such as under a prosthetic liner after a lower extremity amputation) and the inability to sweat (associated with extensive traumatic scarring) are potentially important issues for many patients, and procedural interventions to both reduce and help normalize sweating may impact day-to-day quality of life. Sweat is vital for temperature regulation and heat stroke can easily occur in burn patients, particularly in areas prone to high temperatures and relative humidity such as San Antonio. In the experience of the authors, daily exercise and job function can be improved if temperature regulation is enhanced. Currently the authors utilize treatment protocols with low-density ablative microfractional laser settings of 5% to 10% with a depth of penetration equal to or close to the depth of the scar, and where the follicular or eccrine structures would reside. The exact mechanism of action is poorly understood, though recent research has shown that mesenchymal stem cells associated with eccrine glands may be important for wound healing and perhaps for sweat gland/duct regeneration.[22]

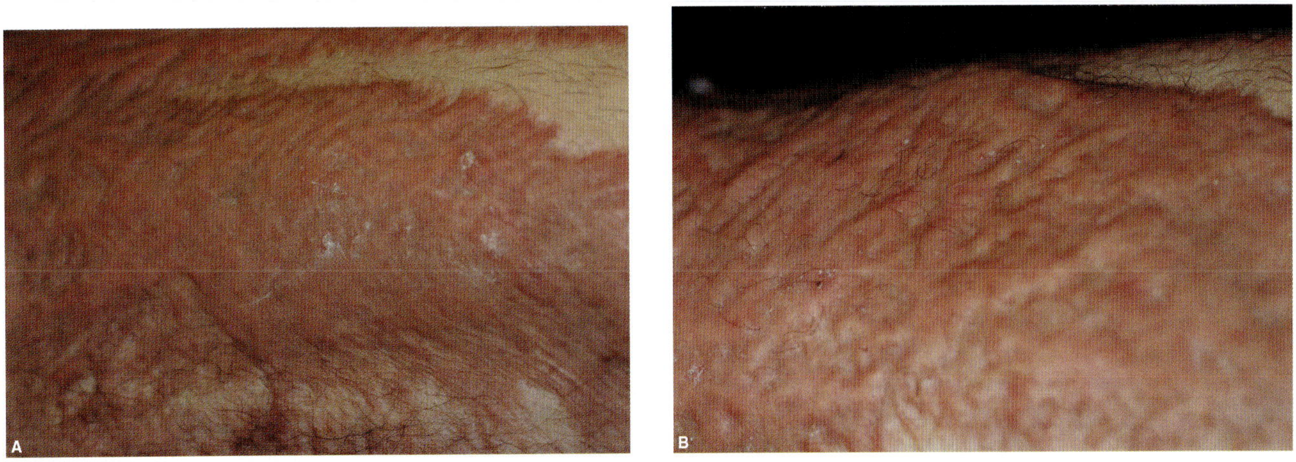

FIGURE 23-6 **A:** Donor site for split-thickness skin graft. It subsequently developed hypertrophy and was associated with significant pruritus. Note the excoriated linear streaks from scratching. **B:** Same site as (**A**) 3 months after microfractionated CO_2 laser resurfacing with obvious terminal hairs growing through the previous scar. Note the interval improvement in hypertrophy with peaks and valleys, where valleys are now the approximate thickness of normal skin.

Adjunctive Procedures in Trauma Rehabilitation

Limb amputation is relatively common among trauma patients. The partial loss of a limb creates an obvious scar on the skin, but it also predisposes patients to a range of potential dermatologic sequelae as the skin of the residual limb was not designed to accommodate weight bearing or the immersion and frictional forces associated with prosthetic use. Any member of the multidisciplinary team taking care of such patients should be mindful of such issues, and either manage them directly or refer the patient for specialty evaluation.

Phantom Limb Pain

A survey of 2,694 veteran amputees revealed 78% of these patients developed phantom limb pain (PLP).[23] As the pathophysiology of PLP is poorly understood and many treatments are associated with limited success, over 50 treatment options have been reported in the literature.[24] These include tricyclic antidepressants, sodium channel blockers, *N*-methyl-D-aspartate receptor antagonists, antiepileptics, calcitonin, opioids, lidocaine, β-blockers, capsaicin, transcutaneous electrical nerve stimulation, vibration therapy, biofeedback, electroconvulsive therapy, hypnosis, stump revision, and neurectomy.[25] Within the last decade new treatment options with encouraging results have been reported in the literature. A number of reports describe improvement following the injection of botulinum toxin types A and B; they are employed in a variety of dosing regimens throughout the amputated limb and/or directly into areas of increased muscle fasciculation using electromyography guidance or trigger points.[25–28] Additional large-scale studies are required to further evaluate the potential of this promising treatment modality.

Hyperhidrosis

Prosthetic devices can be invaluable in improving the functionality and overall quality of life for amputees. However, accommodations are required and studies have reported that 25% to 50% of these patients will report chronic skin problems, 37% to 43% will be bothered by odors coming from their prosthetic, and as many as 70% will be bothered by excessive sweating.[29,30] Specific dermatologic issues include, but are not limited to, distal stasis with edema and verrucous hyperplasia, skin breakdown, folliculitis, bacterial and fungal infections, and irritant and allergic contact dermatitis.[31–33] Occlusion and excessive sweating in and around the areas of prosthetic use can exacerbate these problems.

The use of a Minor starch iodine test has been successfully reported in multiple studies to identify areas of hyperhidrosis.[31,34,35] However, it is important to note that not all patients that report being bothered by excessive sweating may show increased focal hyperhidrosis using this testing modality.[27] Regardless, hyperhidrosis of the stump within the socket and/or the accumulation of sweat that has descended from the proximal stump into the socket may result in maceration of the distal residual limb. Additionally, excessive accumulation of perspiration has been reported to predispose to seal compromise, precipitating prosthetic leg disengagement during mid stride and recurrent falls for a patient.[35]

A recent review by Lezanski et al.[36] summarized the results of seven case series over the past 12 years evaluating the treatment of prosthesis-related hyperhidrosis with botulinum toxin A or B. It was noted that reduced perspiration was reported with the diffuse injection of onabotulinumtoxinA with few side effects in doses up to 500 units. Likewise, rimabotulinumtoxin B injected in doses of up to 1,750 units was found to be effective in reducing residual limb sweating. Military treatment protocols as mentioned in Gratrix et al.[35] typically include utilizing a 4 mL dilution of normal or preserved saline per 100 units of onabotulinumtoxinA (Botox, Allergan Plc, Parsipanny-Troy Hills, NJ). The areas of greatest sweat production can be targeted focally, or more commonly the entire area of the stump that is covered by the patient's prosthetic liner is treated. Although infrequently performed today and often impractical, a more objective evaluation can be done utilizing the starch iodine test. Its utility is limited by the lack of active sweating observed while patients are sitting in an (often cool) exam room without wear nor active use of their prosthetic.

Following initial treatment, if the patient reports residual focal areas of increased perspiration after several weeks it is reasonable to consider injecting additional botulinum toxin in these areas. In the experience of the authors these areas commonly include the most proximal aspect of the prosthetic liner and the most distal aspect of the residual limb. Following treatment it is the convention of the authors (TB, CH) to recommend patients stay out of their prosthetic for approximately 1 week postinjection to decrease the theoretical risk of dissemination of the toxin, though this has yet to be formally evaluated.

Folliculitis/Dermatitis

Another source of prosthesis-associated irritation includes folliculitis in the distribution of the synthetic prosthetic liner. For an amputee to place a prosthetic device on their residual limb, a rubber sleeve must first be placed onto the skin. The occlusive nature of this sleeve coupled with constant rubbing exacerbated by the accumulation of sweat can lead to a "frictional" folliculitis. This predisposes patients to infection (bacterial folliculitis and furuncle/carbuncle formation), pain, and ultimately may lead to time out of their prosthesis to allow for healing. It has been shown that laser hair reduction in the areas of sleeve coverage not only decreased the irritation associated with prosthetic use, but also decreased sweating and the patient's frustration while positively impacting the individual's comfort; the ability to exercise and work has been correlated with a statistically significant improvement in quality of life for these patients.[37,38] Anecdotally many amputees report that they are better able to achieve a seal on the prosthetic after the hair has been removed, and satisfaction with the procedure is generally very high in the experience of the authors.

The observation of decreased perspiration in areas treated with laser hair removal has been reported relatively recently.[37,39,40] The mechanism of action still remains to be elucidated, as the hair follicle and the eccrine gland are distinct structures within the integument. Approved procedural treatments for focal axillary hyperhidrosis (e.g., microwave technology, miraDry, Miramar Labs, Santa Clara, CA) also hold promise for excessive sweating in amputees, though there is significant room for additional research in this area.[41]

Traumatic Tattoo

Traumatic tattooing can occur from many mechanisms of injury sustained both on and off the battlefield. Frequent examples include asphalt and dirt from motorcycle injuries ("road rash"—Fig. 23-7) and dirt, gunpowder, and shrapnel from improvised explosive devices. These are readily treated with "short-pulsed" (Q-switched) lasers that generate pulses in the nanosecond range and, more recently, picosecond-range lasers. The most common wavelengths include 755 and 1,064 nm, sometimes in alternating sessions to treat pigment at different depths. Fewer treatments are generally required for traumatic tattoos than for professional tattoos, likely due to a smaller amount of pigment and relatively larger particle sizes.

Just as scars can be a visible and permanent reminder of negative events, traumatic tattoos can be even more obvious because of the contrast with the normal skin color. The psychological aspects of these tattoos therefore must be accounted for. For example, one patient suffered traumatic tattooing as a result of a suicide bomber; they described feeling as though part of the bomber's body was still imbedded into their skin. Thus, treating the tattoo was an important component of the patient's overall treatment plan.

Despite past reports of sparks during the treatment and bleeding from transepidermal pits,[42] the experience of the authors has been positive, with a rate of complication comparable to standard cosmetic tattoo treatment. Both ablative fractional lasers[43] and Q-switched lasers[44] have been applied individually for traumatic tattoos, and they may also be applied in combination for various tattoo types. When larger and grossly visible particles are present, excision may be required.

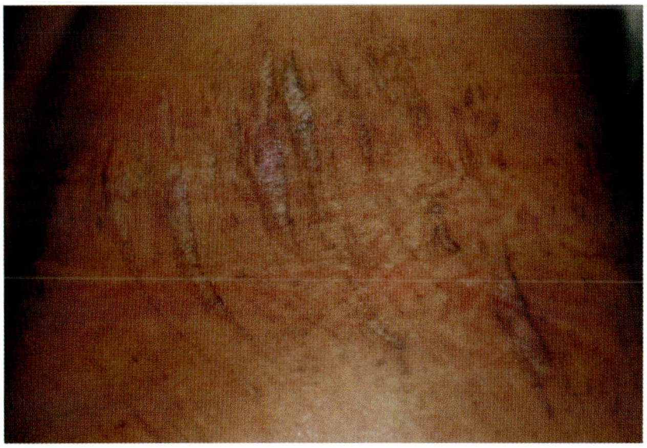

FIGURE 23-7 Textural abnormalities, dyspigmentation, and traumatic tattoo ("road rash") following a motor vehicle accident. Short-pulsed lasers specific for pigment (such as 755 and 1,064 nm) can be used for the traumatic tattoo. Ablative microfractionated lasers can help homogenize texture and color, and can also help remove pigment.

Volume Restoration

Scars are dynamic entities that must be considered in three dimensions. Trauma frequently results in volume deficits from dermal and subcutaneous tissue loss and atrophic scar formation during the healing process. Multiple treatment approaches therefore may be required for optimal volume restoration at various levels. A longer lasting synthetic filler such as poly-L-lactic acid (Sculptra, Galderma Laboratories LLP, Forth Worth, TX) can be injected subcutaneously for gradual but relatively durable correction. In addition to subcutaneous tissue filling, ablative fractional laser–assisted topical delivery of poly-L-lactic acid has been described for the treatment of dermal atrophy (see Chapter 14).[45]

Autologous fat grafting is another well-established technique in tissue augmentation that may be particularly suited for scar management by combining adipose-derived stem cell–driven tissue remodeling with direct contour restoration (see Chapter 15).[46,47] Two recent reviews highlight the potential of autologous fat grafting for the management of scars, with available reports noting consistent improvements in contour and appearance while also diminishing symptoms such as pain and itch.[48,49] However, these reviews also note the need for larger and higher quality studies to help confirm the mechanism of action, safety, and efficacy. To help facilitate the restoration of contour with tissue fillers, subcision to release tethering fibrotic chords and AFR to improve scar pliability can be applied prior to, and/or concurrent with, filler injection (Fig. 23-8).

Future Considerations

It is clear from the experience of the authors that the treatment of traumatic scarring is a multispecialty, multimodality endeavor in the context of a broader overall rehabilitative effort. Short- and medium-term goals should include enhancing our understanding of treatment modalities that are already gaining popularity. For example, despite very promising early experience, larger randomized control studies are needed to confirm the efficacy and mechanism of action of AFR for traumatic scars, and to better define the most effective laser treatment parameters, combinations, timing, imaging, and future applications. As discussed in previous sections, treatment categories reflexively dismissed as "cosmetic," such as fractional laser resurfacing, laser hair reduction, and botulinum toxin injection, may actually have significant functional impact on patients recovering from trauma. To help ensure patients both inside and outside of the military system have access to novel applications as described above, the body of evidence and the system of reimbursement must expand and adapt to our increasing knowledge (see Chapter 25).

There is great opportunity for specialties to unite in a variety of forums (such as this textbook) in a joint effort to enhance our understanding of the cellular and molecular processes involved in wound healing and ultimately scar formation, mitigation, and management. Some of this knowledge may be rooted in a better understanding of the privileged wound healing environment of the early human fetus (see Chapter 27). Importantly, increasing the rate of healing and reepithelialization after wounding can help mitigate the formation of pathologic scars.

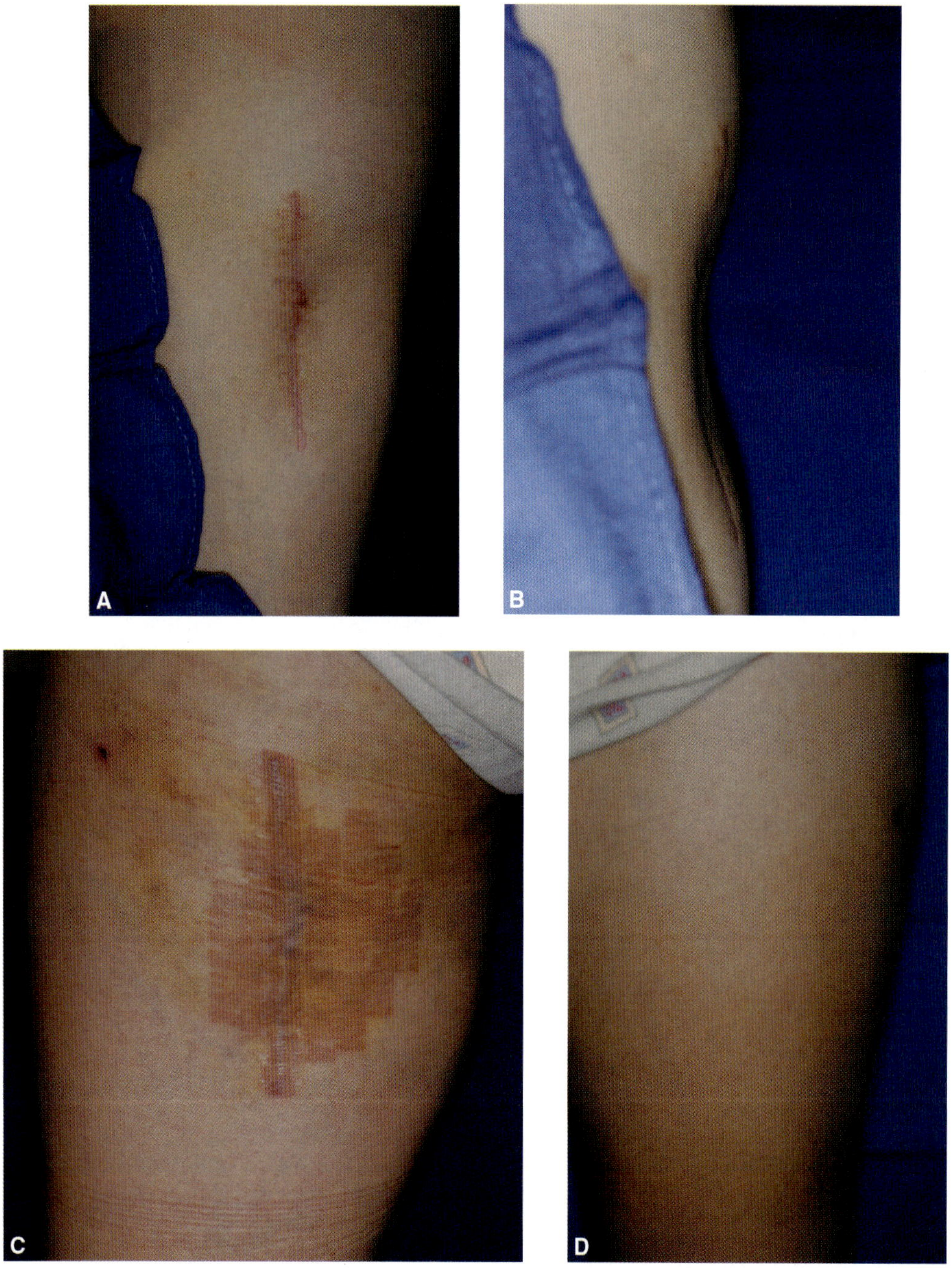

FIGURE 23-8 **A:** Side view of a gunshot exit wound on the lateral thigh of a woman in her 20s. **B:** Same site viewed from the front. Obvious contour irregularity resulted from tissue loss. Although the scar can be homogenized and softened over time with various laser types, the severe contour deficit would remain after laser treatment alone. Autologous fat grafting can be an excellent choice in these situations to help restore volume and induce a degree of scar remodeling. In the experience of the authors, pre-, post-, and concurrent treatment of the scar and surrounding area with microablative laser resurfacing can enhance the results of fat grafting by reducing tension and improving scar pliability—potentially improving the quality of the scar, the overall contour restoration of the graft, and decreasing the tendency of the graft to "doughnut" around the central tethered scar. It also highlights the benefits of combined efforts among multiple specialties. **C:** Same view as **(A)** several days after a combined treatment session including ablative fractional laser resurfacing and autologous fat grafting. **D:** Same view as (**B**) several days after a combined laser and fat grafting treatment session. Excellent early contour restoration is observed after a course of ablative fractional laser resurfacing for pretreatment of the scar combined with autologous fat grafting and concurrent laser treatment. High-quality prospective studies are required to confirm the safety and efficacy of the combined procedure. *(Photo courtesy of Trent Douglas, MD.)*

Newer technologies, with more on the horizon, such as fractional skin harvesting, fractional epidermal micrografts (CELLUTOME, Acelity, San Antonio, TX), and spray-on noncultured autologous cell suspension (ReCell, Avita Medical, Northridge, CA) can enhance wound healing after tissue loss with minimal donor site morbidity.[50–53] There has been growing technical ability to rapidly and reliably characterize the human genome in cost-efficient ways. This has spurred interest in specialized areas of genomics to include epigenomics, transcriptomics, and proteomics, combined into the study of personalized medicine. This new area of research provides us with the potential to better understand the biologic processes occurring during traumatic wounding and subsequent healing on a genetic level, with the promise of intervening to avoid pathologic scars and determining optimal adjunctive treatments.[54] Already, researchers are actively seeking out biomarkers important to epidermal stem cell regulation in relation to wound healing.[55]

Elucidation of the regional and functional characteristics of fibroblasts provides a promising foundation for novel applications, such as the induction of hair follicles and alteration of the phenotype of the skin on the residual limb in amputees to better support prosthetic devices.[56] Furthermore, multiple mechanisms are being identified by which stem cells may facilitate wound healing and minimize the impact of scarring.[57] These and future related approaches are steps on the path to the ultimate goal of scarless wound healing, and the promise of better functional and cosmetic outcomes for our patients.

Disclaimer

The views expressed in this chapter are those of the authors and do not necessarily reflect the official policy or position of the Department of Defense or the United States Government. Drs. Shumaker, Beachkofsky, Basnett, and Burns are military service members. Dr. Hivnor is a member of the U.S. Air Force Reserves. This work was prepared as part of their official duties. Title 17, USC, § 105 provides that "Copyright protection under this title is not available for any work of the United States Government." Title 17, USC, § 101 defines a U.S. Government work as a work prepared by a military service member or employee of the U.S. Government as part of that person's official duties.

REFERENCES

1. Rothbart D. Mount impossible—how a disabled veteran conquered Kilimanjaro. *GQ*, April 26, 2016.
2. Patzkowski JC, Owens JG, Blanck RV, et al. Deployment after limb salvage for high-energy lower-extremity trauma. *J Trauma Acute Care Surg*. 2012;73(2, Suppl 1):S112–S115.
3. Sheridan RL, Shumaker PR, King DR, et al. Case records of the Massachusetts General Hospital. Case 15-2014. A man in the military who was injured by an improvised explosive device in Afghanistan. *N Engl J Med*. 2014;370:1931–1940.
4. Krueger CA, Wenke JC, Ficke JR. Ten years at war: comprehensive analysis of amputation trends. *J Trauma Acute Care Surg*. 2012;73(6, Suppl 5):S438–S444.
5. Commander, U.S. Pacific Fleet. Pacific partnership 2015. http://www.cpf.navy.mil/pacific-partnership/2015/news/. Accessed May 23, 2016.
6. Uebelhoer NS, Ross EV, Shumaker PR. Ablative fractional resurfacing for the treatment of traumatic scars and contractures. *Semin Cutan Med Surg*. 2012;31:110–120.
7. Shumaker PR. Laser treatment of traumatic scars: a military perspective. *Semin Cutan Med Surg*. 2015;34:17–23.
8. Manstein DD, Herron GS, Sink RK, et al. Fractional photothermolysis: a new concept for cutaneous remodeling using microscopic patterns of thermal injury. *Lasers Surg Med*. 2004;34:426–438.
9. Hantash BM, Bedi VP, Chan KF, et al. Ex vivo histological characteristics of a novel ablative fractional resurfacing device. *Lasers Surg Med*. 2007;39:87–95.
10. Kwan JM, Wyatt M, Uebelhoer NS, et al. Functional improvement after ablative fractional laser treatment of a scar contracture. *PM R*. 2011;3:986–987.
11. Kineston D, Kwan JM, Uebelhoer NS, et al. Use of a fractional ablative 10.6 μm carbon dioxide laser in the treatment of a morphea-related contracture. *Arch Dermatol*. 2011;147:1148–1150.
12. Shumaker PR, Kwan JM, Landers JT, et al. Functional improvements in traumatic scars and scar contractures using an ablative fractional laser protocol. *J Trauma Acute Care Surg*. 2012;73(Suppl 1):S116–S121.
13. Waibel J, Beer K. Ablative fractional laser resurfacing for the treatment of a third degree burn. *J Drugs Dermatol*. 2009;8:294–297.
14. Hultman CS, Friedstat JS, Edkins RE, et al. Laser resurfacing and remodeling of hypertrophic burn scars: the results of a large, prospective, before-after cohort study, with long-term follow-up. *Ann Surg*. 2014;260:519–529.
15. Levi B, Ibrahim A, Mathews K, et al. The use of CO_2 fractional photothermolysis for the treatment of burn scars. *J Burn Care Res*. 2016;37:106–114.
16. Anderson RR, Donelan MB, Hivnor C, et al. Laser treatment of traumatic scars with an emphasis on ablative fractional laser resurfacing: consensus report. *JAMA Dermatol*. 2014;150:187–193.
17. Griffin D, Brelsford M, O'Reilly E, et al. Ablative fractional laser resurfacing: A promising adjunct to surgical reconstruction. *Mil Med*. 2016;181:e616–e620.
18. Alster TS. Improvement of erythematous and hypertrophic scars by the 585-nm flashlamp-pumped pulsed dye laser. *Ann Plast Surg*. 1994;32:186–190.
19. Parrett BM, Donelan MB. Pulsed dye laser in burn scars: current concepts and future directions. *Burns*. 2010;36:443–449.
20. Keaney TC, Tanzi E, Alster T. Comparison of 532 nm potassium titanyl phosphate laser and 595 nm pulsed dye laser in the treatment of erythematous surgical scars: a randomized, controlled, open-label study. *Dermatol Surg*. 2016;42:70–76.
21. Neiner J, Whittemore D, Hivnor C. Buried alive: functional eccrine coils buried under scar tissue? *J Am Acad Dermatol*. 2011;65:661–663.
22. Ma K, Tan Z, Zhang C, et al. Mesenchymal stem cells for sweat gland regeneration after burns: from possibility to reality. *Burns*. 2016;42:492–499.
23. Sherman R, Sherman C, Parker L. Chronic phantom and stump pain among American veterans: Results of a survey. *Pain*. 1984;18:83–95.
24. Sherman RA. Published treatments of phantom limb pain. *Am J Phys Med*. 1980;59:232–244.
25. Jin L, Kollewe K, Krampfl K, et al. Treatment of phantom limb pain with botulinum toxin type A. *Pain Med*. 2009;10:300–303.
26. Kern U, Martin C, Scheicher S, et al. Effects of botulinum toxin type B on stump pain and involuntary movement of the stump. *Am J Phys Med Rehabil*. 2004;83;396–399.
27. Kern U, Kohl M, Seifert U, et al. Botulinum toxin type B in the treatment of residual limb hyperhidrosis for lower limb amputees: A pilot study. *Am J Phys Med Rehabil*. 2011;90:321–329.
28. Charrow A, DiFazio M, Foster L, et al. Intradermal botulinum toxin type A injection effectively reduces residual limb hyperhidrosis in amputees: a case series. *Arch Phys Med Rehabil*. 2008;89:1407–1409.
29. Dillingham TR, Pezzin LE, MacKenzie EJ, et al. Use and satisfaction with prosthetic devices among persons with trauma-related amputations: a long-term outcome study. *Am J Phys Med Rehabil*. 2001;80:563–571.
30. Berke GM, Fergason J, Milani JR, et al. Comparison of satisfaction with current prosthetic care in veterans and service members from Vietnam and OIF/OEF conflicts with major traumatic limb loss. *J Rehabil Res Dev*. 2010;47:361–371.
31. García-Morales I, Pérez-Bernal A, Camacho F. Letter: Stump hyperhidrosis in a leg amputee: Treatment with botulinum toxin A. *Dermatol Surg*. 2007;33:1401–1402.

32. Yang NB, Garza LA, Foote CE, et al. High prevalence of stump dermatoses 38 years or more after amputation. *Arch Dermatol.* 2012;148:1283–1286.
33. Bulkema KE, Meyerle JH. Amputation stump: privileged harbor for infections, tumors, and immune disorders. *Clin Dermatol.* 2014;32:670–677.
34. Wollina U, Konrad H, Graefe T, et al. Botulinum toxin A for focal hyperhidrosis in leg amputees: a case report. *Acta Derm Venereol.* 2000;80:226–227.
35. Gratrix M, Hivnor C. Botulinum toxin A treatment for hyperhidrosis in patients with prosthetic limbs. *Arch Dermatol.* 2010;146:1314–1315.
36. Lezanski-Gujda A, Bingham JL, Logemann NF. Botulinum toxin: an effective treatment for prosthesis-related hyperhidrosis in patients with traumatic amputations. *Indian Dermatol Online J* 2015;6:1–3.
37. Miletta N. Improving quality of life in wounded warriors with traumatic amputations: the promising benefits of laser hair removal at the residual limb-prosthetic socket interface. In American Society of Dermatologic Surgeons Annual Meeting, San Diego, CA, November 2014.
38. Miletta NR, Kim S, Lezanski-Gujda A. et al. Improving quality of life in wounded warriors: the promising benefits of laser hair removal to the residual lower limb-prosthetic interface. *Dermatol Surg.* 2016;42(10):1182–1187.
39. Letada PR, Landers JT, Uebelhoer NS, et al. Treatment of focal axillary hyperhidrosis using a long pulsed Nd:YAG 1064 nm laser at hair reduction settings. *J Drugs Dermatol.* 2012;11:59–63.
40. Caplin D, Austin J. Clinical evaluation and quantitative analysis of axillary hyperhidrosis treated with a unique targeted laser energy delivery method with 1-year follow-up. *J Drugs Dermatol.* 2014;13: 449–456.
41. Stashak AB, Brewer JD. Management of hyperhidrosis. *Clin Cosmet Investig Dermatol.* 2014;7:285–299.
42. Fusade T, Toubel G, Grognard C, et al. Treatment of gunpowder traumatic tattoo by Q-switched Nd:YAG laser: an unusual adverse effect. *Dermatol Surg.* 2000;26:1057–1059.
43. Seitz AT, Grunewald S, Wagner JA, et al. Fractional CO_2 laser is as effective as Q-switched ruby laser for the initial treatment of a traumatic tattoo. *Cosmet Dermatol.* 2014;16;303–305.
44. Gorouhi F, Davari P, Kashani MN, et al. Treatment of traumatic tattoo with the Q-switched Nd:YAG laser. *J Cosmet Laser Ther.* 2007;9:253–255.
45. Rkein A1, Ozog D, Waibel JS. Treatment of atrophic scars with fractionated CO_2 laser facilitating delivery of topically applied poly-L-lactic acid. *Dermatol Surg.* 2014;40:624–631.
46. Coleman SR. Structural fat grafting: more than a permanent filler. *Plast Reconstr Surg.* 2006;118(3, Suppl):108S–1120S.
47. Zuk PA, Zhu M, Ashjian P, et al. Human adipose tissue is a source of multipotent stem cells. *Mol Biol Cell.* 2002;13:4279–4295.
48. Negenborn VL, Groen JW, Smit JM, et al. The use of autologous fat grafting for treatment of scar tissue and scar-related conditions: a systematic review. *Plastic Reconstr Surg.* 2016;137:31e–43e.
49. Condé-Green A, Marano AA, Lee ES, et al. Fat grafting and adipose-derived regenerative cells in burn wound healing and scarring: a systematic review of the literature. *Plast Reconstr Surg.* 2016;137:302–312.
50. Navarro FA, Stoner ML, Park CS, et al. Sprayed keratinocyte suspensions accelerate epidermal coverage in a porcine microwound model. *J Burn Care Rehabil.* 2000;21:513–518.
51. Purschke M, Asrani FA, Sabir SA, et al. Novel methods for generating fractional epidermal micrografts. *Br J Dermatol.* 2015;172:1021–1028.
52. Singh M, Nuutila K, Kruse C, et al. Challenging the conventional therapy: Emerging skin graft techniques for wound healing. *Plast Reconstr Surg.* 2015;136:524e–530e.
53. Tam J, Wang Y, Vuong LN, et al. Reconstitution of full-thickness skin by microcolumn grafting. *J Tissue Eng Regen Med.* 2016. doi:10.1002/term.2174.
54. Jones LR, Young W, Divine G, et al. Genome-wide scan for methylation profiles in keloids. *Dis Markers.* 2015;2015:943176.
55. Saldanha SN, Royston KJ, Udayakumar N, et al. Epigenetic regulation of epidermal stem cell biomarkers and their role in wound healing. *Int J Mol Sci.* 2015;17(1):16.
56. Thangapazham RL, Darling TN, Meyerle J. Alteration of skin properties with autologous dermal fibroblasts. *Int J Mol Sci.* 2014;15:8407–8427.
57. Jackson WM, Nesti LJ, Tuan RS. Concise review: clinical translation of wound healing therapies based on mesenchymal stem cells. *Stem Cells Transl Med.* 2012;1:44–50.

24 Recovery and Reintegration After Burn Injury

MARTA ROSENBERG, LAURA ROSENBERG, and WALTER MEYER III

KEY POINTS

- Recovery from a burn injury and its resulting scars can have lifelong psychological consequences.
- Perceptions about body image and scarring following burn injury can be impacted by a person's beliefs, values, family and social support, and experiences.
- Most burn survivors adapt well and achieve optimal quality of life; however, some continue to struggle emotionally and physically.
- Individuals who survive major burn injuries need to be monitored for difficulties with adjustment, trauma and stress related disorders such as posttraumatic stress disorder, and anxiety and mood disorders.
- This chapter provides information about various aspects of recovery, interventions, and relevant research that has been done in burn care. A list of resources is provided to help burn survivors during their lifelong journey to recovery for community, school and work re-entry and social support.

Survivors of burns face adjustment to various physical, health, and psychosocial changes including acceptance of visible and hidden burn scars. Several factors may impact this adjustment including one's belief system and perception of body image, perceived and actual support systems including family and friends, one's comfort in diverse social settings, health status, resilience, and preburn and postburn emotional history. This chapter provides a summary of the literature related to the impact of burns (particularly burn scars); relevant aspects related to body image and stigmatization; psychosocial and psychiatric outcomes for burn survivors; the assessment and treatment of itch, neuropathic pain, and posttraumatic stress disorder (PTSD); and postburn social reintegration.

Visible and Hidden Scars

One of the frequent consequences of burns is scarring and contractures, and both surgical and nonsurgical methods have been used to address these issues.[1] Reconstructive surgical interventions include, but are not limited to, application of skin grafts and skin flaps, release of contractures, scar reduction, tissue expanders[2] (see Chapter 12), and more recently laser treatment (see Chapter 13). Nonsurgical methods include applying pressure on the scars through the use of pressure garments and skin massage, and attendance to daily rehabilitation and exercise programs[2,3] (see Chapter 19).

Visible differences created by burn scars can lead to difficulties in physical and psychosocial functioning. Physical difficulties due to loss of function, pain, and itch are frequent and can impact daily functioning at home, work, and school and in diverse social settings. Psychosocial difficulties related to changes in appearance, difficulties accepting these changes, and difficulties with body image and self-concept may lead to social anxiety, depression, and problems with adjustment.[4–8] Both visible and hidden scars (scars in areas usually covered by clothing) may impact how a person feels and their comfort in different social situations. They often experience unwanted attention and questions about their burn scars, which may make socializing uncomfortable. They may encounter social situations in which others do not quite know how to behave around them. Some survivors may attempt to cover up their scars to avoid uncomfortable social encounters (see Chapters 20 and 21). Therefore, the availability of social skills–based programs, cognitive-behavior therapy (CBT), and support systems is crucial for assisting survivors with postburn adjustment, acceptance of burn scars, gaining self-confidence, and feeling comfortable in different social settings. Studies are needed to identify which interventions are most effective for individuals with visible differences.[8]

Body Image and Stigmatization

Body image is an individual's perception regarding physical appearance.[9] This process is influenced by personal views such as values and beliefs,[7] social and cultural experiences,[7,10,11] and appearance norms.[7] In many countries people are often exposed to information about physical attractiveness from the mass media[9,11] including magazines, television, movies, and more recently social media and individuals' interests in taking selfies. Young children's perceptions of their body image are influenced by messages they receive from their parents and family members.[10,11] School-aged children begin to observe similarities and differences between themselves and their peers, and peer acceptance becomes increasingly important as children transition to adolescence.[10,11] Body image concerns may continue throughout adult life.[7]

It is often believed burn survivors may experience body image dissatisfaction related to the changes in physical appearance due to scarring.[12–14] Some studies found a modest relationship between burn scar severity and body image.[15,16] Thombs and colleagues[17] examined body image dissatisfaction of adult burn survivors at discharge and 6 and 12 months after injury. They found that women with major burns reported greater body image concerns, and that the importance of appearance was strongly associated with body image across time. Lawrence and colleagues[18] examined the relationship between burn scar severity and body esteem of adults with burns. They found a strong relationship between scar severity and body-esteem for individuals who strongly valued their appearance. The opposite was true for individuals who rated their appearance as not important. In this study, females reported lower body-esteem with regard to appearance than males; however, males rated themselves as less attractive than others. Fauerbach and colleagues[15] studied the impact of body image dissatisfaction on quality of life for adults with major burns. They controlled for burn size, facial injury, and preburn mental and physical quality of life. Results suggested burn survivors who were dissatisfied with their appearance experienced decreased mental and physical quality of life at 2 months postinjury.

Limited research has examined body image in pediatric burn survivors. Lawrence and colleagues[16] compared body esteem of children with burns and an age-matched comparison group. No differences were found between the body esteem scores of men burn survivors and controls. However, women burn survivors reported higher body esteem than the comparison group. The authors speculated that the uniqueness of the sample, acceptance of burn scars, and social support may explain these findings.[16] Russell et al.[19] studied self-concept in young adults who sustained severe childhood burns. Burn survivors reported more difficulty on several subscales on a self-concept measure in comparison to a normative reference group. Areas of difficulty included: physical function, appearance, sexuality, moral conduct, personal values, academics and work, and identity. They reported that decreased self-concept was related to affective and anxiety disorders. Pope and colleagues[20] compared long-term psychosocial outcomes of young burn survivors to a control group of peers from school. Burn survivors, especially men, reported better body image and weight satisfaction than the control group. However, as the size of burn increased there was more dissatisfaction with appearance and lower quality of life. The development of healthy coping strategies and acceptance of burn scars may explain these findings.[20]

Outcomes

Associated Psychological and Psychiatric Difficulties

The response of the person who suffers from a major burn injury is somewhat age dependent. Children grow up knowing their bodies have scars, so they may not experience a sense of loss. They simply cannot remember looking any different. They may or may not be teased or bullied, but regardless, they will be asked hundreds of times about their scars and appearance. They face questions such as how they got injured, if it hurts, etc. Several studies have explored the nature of related psychological and psychiatric sequelae. A few studies have looked at the long-term prevalence of any psychological and psychiatric problems that might be associated with scarring. In one study of 100 young adults burned as children (14 years earlier, on average), general psychological problems were assessed using the Achenbach scales for young adults.[21] This self-report measure identifies behavioral problems such as anxiety/depression, somatic complaints, thought problems, attention problems, and aggressive and delinquent behaviors. These behaviors are further classified as internalizing or externalizing behaviors.[22] The men in this study were not different from the reference population, except in the somatic complaints related to itching and pain. These symptoms may be assumed to be related to the scarred skin. However, the women in the same group were found to have an increased number of problems compared to the reference group. They had more withdrawn behavior, thought problems, aggressive behavior, and delinquent behavior.[21] Some of this unusual behavior may be explained by the women being more concerned about their disfigurement than men.[23]

Even more unexpected and concerning is the prevalence of psychiatric disorders in this same group; approximately 50% of young adult survivors of large childhood burns met criteria for a major psychiatric disorder.[24] Women had almost twice as many psychiatric disorders (Axis 1, DSM IV) as measured by the Structured Clinical Interview as men.[24] This is true for both current and lifetime prevalence of the psychiatric disorders. Anxiety disorders were the most common, followed by affective disorders. The most common anxiety disorders were PTSD and social phobia, with any anxiety disorder being present in 30% to 37% of the young adults.[24] Other studies have also reported that the women who suffered from burn scarring often have PTSD associated with their disfiguring injuries.[25,26] There is a definite interaction between the symptoms of PTSD and the scars. A common presentation is that the scars are the major focus for many adolescent and adult burn survivors, perhaps because they are obvious and perhaps because they actually feel strange or are painful. The burn scars can be a trigger of the trauma and may complicate the person's PTSD symptoms. This somatization may also be a symptom of underlying depression. When the pain is addressed as part of the treatment of their depression and anxiety, the outcome tends to be better.[27] The medication used for the PTSD is usually a serotonin reuptake inhibitor such as fluoxetine or sertraline, but it may be a tricyclic antidepressant like amitriptyline. Amitriptyline or imipramine can be used to treat both the neuropathic pain[28] and the acute stress disorder (ASD)/PTSD.[29]

Personality disorders are more prevalent in this long-term pediatric burn survivor population, with 49% of patients achieving threshold for diagnosis. Personality disorders were more likely to occur in adults who were burned as young children compared to those burned as teenagers. It appears that the experience of recovering from a major burn injury and growing up with major scars was more likely to shape personality development. The frequency was the same in both men and women. The most common types of personality disorders were paranoid in women and antisocial in men.[30]

Thomas and colleagues[31] found that adolescent burn survivors have a significant amount of anxiety disorders. In that population the usual anxiety disorder was not PTSD, but rather agoraphobia, separation anxiety, and social phobia. In a meta-analysis study, the factors that affected outcome were the location and severity of the burn injury.[32]

Burn injury of the face and other visible areas can result in long-term psychological problems and psychiatric disorders, especially anxiety disorders. For all age groups, children and adolescents with facial burns had lower scores on psychosocial outcome measures than those without facial burns, whether the ratings were done by the parents or children.[33,34] However, variability exists in the perceptions of parents and children following burn injury. Meyer and colleagues[35] found that adolescent burn survivors and parents have similar ratings in the areas of physical and emotional health; however, adolescents in this study rated their appearance better than their parents. This may be because the adolescents felt confident about their appearance and had good family support. Robert and colleagues[36] found that adolescent survivors of large burns exhibited similar or a higher degree of self-worth as compared to peers; however, they downrated their physical appearance and athletic competence. Similar results are found for hand burns, probably because hands are often noticed more than other parts of the body.[37]

The importance of diagnosing an associated psychiatric illness cannot be overestimated. Recently, Weichman and colleagues[38] recommended some common tools to measure depression and anxiety in burn survivors, though most of these instruments are not specific to burns. The most validated ones are the following: Beck Depression Inventory-II,[39] Hospital Anxiety Depression Scale,[40] the Brief Symptom Inventory,[41] and the Achenbach Child Behavior Checklist.[42] However, the Achenbach Child Behavior Checklist is lengthy and more useful in outpatient settings.[38,42] These instruments have an associated cost and require a mental health professional to administer. Therefore, Weichman's group suggested a group of free brief scales for adults and children to screen for psychiatric complications. The Patient Health Questionnaire (PHQ-2 or 9) by Spitzer et al.[43] is both free and screens for depression. For childhood depression the Children's Depression Inventory (CDI) is recommended, even though it is not free.[44] For assessment of PTSD in adults, the PTSD Symptom Checklist—Civilian version (PCL-C) is recommended[45] and for children the UCLA PTSD Index[46] is a reasonable choice[38] (see Table 24-1).

Quality of Life

Outcomes research has focused on adjustment to the physical limitations and psychosocial changes resulting from burns for both adult and pediatric burn survivors. There is much variance in the results because of differences in methodology and the outcome measures used. Early investigations primarily used psychometric measures and clinical interviews to infer psychosocial functioning and postburn adjustment, and revealed that many burn survivors adjusted well.[47–50] Later studies used health-related quality of life measures to investigate psychosocial outcomes of burn survivors. Several studies used the Short Form 36 (SF 36), a general health survey, to assess physical and emotional functioning of pediatric burn survivors. These studies found that the majority of survivors of large burns rated their functioning similar to the general population[51,52]; however, many adult survivors continued to have physical limitations that required additional rehabilitation services[51] and continued to experience psychosocial distress.[52] Measures that examine specific behaviors have also been used. Rosenberg and colleagues[53] used the Quality of Life Questionnaire to assess specific behaviors related to quality of life with young adult pediatric burn survivors, and found that this group rated their overall quality of life slightly lower than the reference group. More recently, Murphy and colleagues[54] examined the long-term psychological distress and quality of life of young adults who were burned as children using the World Health Organization Disability Assessment Scale II (WHODAS) and the Burn Specific Health Scale—Brief (BSHS-B), and found that quality of life decreased with increased burn size and that the WHODAS reliably identified individuals with lower quality of life.

Several researchers have specifically looked at health-related quality of life in children. Landolt et al.[55] found that quality of life ratings of pediatric burn survivors were generally normal. However, lower quality of life ratings were associated with a diagnosis of PTSD. These authors also found that diminished social functioning was a primary problem,[55] which is consistent with previous research done by Blakeney and colleagues.[56] Similarly, Pope and colleagues[20] found that pediatric burn survivors rated their quality of life higher than age-matched controls, had positive feelings about their appearance, and were coping well with life changes. However, women reported poorer quality of life. Murphy and colleagues[54] found similar results when looking at long-term psychological distress and quality of life. They reported that children who were burned prior to school entry and adolescents who had not transitioned to young adulthood reported better quality of life and less disability. However, contrary to Pope's findings, they found that women reported better quality of life.[54] Stubbs and colleagues[34] examined the psychosocial impact of childhood facial burns, and found that severe facial burns that required grafts significantly impacted the quality of life ratings of teenagers and their parents.

Other studies have focused on identifying predictors of quality of life. Anzarut and colleagues[57] found that for adult survivors of large burns, the strongest predictors of physical functioning included total full thickness injury and hand function; the strongest predictors of emotional functioning included a younger age at time of injury and perceived level of social support. Similarly, Patterson et al.[58] found that both psychosocial variables (preburn psychological status and social support) and medical variables (hand burns, amputations, and days in intensive care unit) predicted the outcome for adult burn survivors. Cromes and colleagues[59] reported that less emotional distress, less pain, and greater involvement with home and social activities were predictive of better outcome among adult burn survivors. Leblebici and colleagues[60] found that having joint contractures significantly influenced burn survivors' quality of life, especially their physical functioning, and that burn size affected psychosocial outcome. Pavoni and colleagues[61] reported that in adults, quality of life was affected by psychological and physical limitations 1 year postinjury.

Research has also focused on the benefits of a comprehensive wellness and exercise program in improving physical and psychosocial functioning following burn injury. Previous work by Suman and colleagues[62–64] revealed that a comprehensive wellness and exercise program for pediatric survivors of large burns, administered 6 months postburn, significantly improved cardiopulmonary capacity, muscle mass and strength, and pulmonary function. Similarly, De Lateur and colleagues[65] reported improvements with physical functioning for adult burn survivors who participated in a structured exercise program. Additionally, Rosenberg and colleagues[66] found that parents reported significant improvements with their children's physical and psychosocial functioning following a wellness and exercise program.

As youngsters transition into adolescence, young adulthood, and adulthood, they begin to question if they can have meaningful relationships with significant others and many have questions about intimacy and sexual activity. Women may question if they can give birth given the restrictions of the burn scars and contractures. Burn survivors need to be able to openly discuss these questions with their support systems including their psychologist, psychiatrist, plastic surgeon, family, and friends. The effects of scarring on sexuality and relationships are a major concern for men and women adult burn survivors. Few studies have examined this, though a group of young adults burned as children reported normal sexual activity.[67] Both men and women reported having confidence about having sex and thinking they were sexually attractive. This did not vary much with scarring on the face and neck. However, there were exceptions. In general, women were able to find partners more readily than the men.[67] This may be because the men were too self-conscious to ask. In one group session the men stated that they were too self-conscious to approach a woman, and the women said that they did not care what the men looked like, so long as they were nice and had a good job. Men were more likely to report having no sex since the burn injury.[67] Bianchi found that men with higher sexual esteem had lower depression; however, there was no relationship between the severity of the burn and sexual esteem, depression, and preoccupation.[68]

In summary, it appears that burn survivors can adjust well to their injuries. Several factors may impact this adjustment such as the presence of strong social support and positive social reintegration, younger age at time of burn, good pain and itch management, the absence of full-thickness burns, hand and face involvement, and improved physical and psychosocial functioning through ongoing access to rehabilitation and mental health services.

Assessment and Treatment of Burn Scars

Medical Interventions

Burn scars and the graft donor sites can pose unique and chronic challenges for the physician caring for these patients. In adults, 93% of burn survivors with scars have pruritus at discharge from the hospital and 73% continue to have pruritus 2 years postburn[69] (see Chapter 11). Similar statistics are true for children.[70] Several instruments have been developed to quantify the degree of itching. For adults with burn scars, the 5D itch scale has been validated.[71] This scale is often too difficult to use in children, so Blakeney and Marvin developed The Itch Man Scale for children, which uses drawings to rate discomfort.[72] The drawings have facial expressions and red dots corresponding to the intensity of itch, which makes it easier for children to rate severity[72] (see Table 24-1). The Itch Man Scale was later validated by Morris et al.[73] Many pediatric burn survivors also experience severe itch. In the experience of the authors, itch can usually be effectively treated with diphenhydramine or hydroxyzine. The dose often has to be fairly high: diphenhydramine 1.25 mg per kg every 4 to 6 hours alternating at the 2-hour point with hydroxyzine 0.5 mg per kg. If the scar is dry it may respond to hydration. If the scar is thick it may respond to some lubrication and massage. The authors have also tried different creams such as 2% diphenhydramine, Preparation H (main ingredient is phenylephrine), EMLA (2.5% prilocaine/ 2.5% lidocaine), or 5% doxepin with some success, though the 5% doxepin cream can cause sedation if given over a large area. If these regimens are not successful, then gabapentin may be used at a starting dose of 5 to 10 mg per kg per dose given every 8 hours. This can be titrated up to 35 mg/kg/d. If there is still no reasonable response and the scar looks hyperemic and inflamed, a course of antibiotics might prove to reduce the itching. The antibiotic course is thought to reduce the total bacterial flora in the scar tissue. A commonly used regimen is sulfamethoxazole/trimethoprim and rifampin. In refractory cases, cyproheptadine (0.1 mg per kg every 6 hours) can be effective in controlling itching.

The second most common physical symptom of burn scars is pain, specifically neuropathic pain. The pain should be quantified by using a standardized scale such as the Visual Analog Scale,[74] which is more appropriate for adults, and the FACES scale[75] with children. In some patients, neuropathic pain may last for years and can be very debilitating.[76] A typical person describes this pain as a burning, stinging, or prickly feeling. Other patients describe it as a dull and constant aching. Often the pain is much worse when the patient stands, and the burned skin is stretched on the dependent extremity because of venous congestion. One burn survivor described this neuropathic pain as being bitten by hundreds of fire ants all over his legs. Another child described it as an insect walking across his skin with cleats on. Sometimes this pain is related to an associated infection in the scar. The initial treatment regimen may often include opiates.[27]

The existence of neuropathic pain is understandable in the setting of nerve regrowth and possible entrapment during the scarring process. The treatment of scar-related neuropathic pain can be topical or systemic. A common topical approach has been massage. If the area is not too large, 5% lidocaine patches can be applied every 12 hours.[77] Systemic medications include opiates (which are not as effective as amitriptyline), gabapentin, or pregabalin.[28,76] Steroid injections have also been used.[76] Schneider and colleagues[76] reported that rest, massage, compression garments, and elevation can relieve the discomfort.

Table 24-1 Summary of Instruments

Measures	Reference	Purpose	Age
Achenbach Child Behavior Checklist (CBCL)	Achenbach and Rescorla[42]	• Self-report of behavioral problems • Mental health professional administered	Children Adolescents
Patient Health Questionnaire (PHQ-2 or 9)	Spitzer et al.[43]	• Screening tool • Depressive symptoms	Adults
Children's Depression Inventory (CDI)	Kovacs[44]	• Self-report measure of depression • Mental health professional administered	Children Adolescents
Beck Depression Inventory-II (BDI-II)	Beck et al.[39]	• Self-report measure of depression • Mental health professional administered	Adults
Hospital Anxiety and Depression Scale	Zigmond and Snaith[40]	• Self-report measure of anxiety and depression • Mental health professional administered	Adults
Brief Symptom Inventory	Derogatis[41]	• Screening tool • Depression	Adults
PTSD Symptom Checklist–Civilian version (PCL-C)	Weathers et al.[45]	• Self-report measure • Screening of PTSD	Adults
UCLA PTSD Index	Pynoos et al.[46]	• Self-report measure of PTSD • Clinician administered	Children Adolescents
5D Itch Scale	Elman et al.[71]	• Self-Report Measure • Itch	Adults
Itch Man Scale	Morris et al.[73]	• Self-report measure • Itch	Children Adolescents

In dealing with burn scars, two types of psychiatric disorders are quite common: major depression and an anxiety disorder such as PTSD. These disorders must be addressed in order to help the patient deal effectively with the physical and social aspects of their scars. According to the DSM-5, major depression is characterized by at least five of the following symptoms: depressed mood most of the day every day, diminished interest or pleasure, significant weight loss, insomnia, fatigue, psychomotor agitation or retardation, feelings of worthlessness or guilt, diminished ability to concentrate, and recurrent thoughts of death.[78] In addition, the person must have clinically significant distress or impairment in social, occupational, or another area of functioning. Also, the symptoms cannot be due to substance abuse or another medical condition.[78] The most commonly effective treatment is a serotonin reuptake inhibitor such as fluoxetine or sertraline.[27] If that is ineffective then a psychiatrist should be consulted.

In DSM-5, psychiatric symptoms following a traumatic event were classified under two conditions: ASD (lasting no longer than 30 days after the initiating event) and PTSD (which can be diagnosed 30 days after the traumatic event).[78] The characteristics of the inciting traumatic event typically include the following: exposure to actual or threatened death, serious injury, or sexual violence that was experienced, witnessed, learned about, or happened to a family member.[78] Other criteria include intrusive symptoms, persistent avoidant symptoms, negative alterations in cognition and mood, and marked alternations in arousal and reactivity associated with the event. Lastly, the disturbance must cause clinically significant distress or impairment in social, occupational, or other important areas of functioning.[78] Most of the experience treating ASD and PTSD has been associated with the treatment of military personnel. Medications that are often helpful in both conditions include tricyclic antidepressants and serotonin reuptake inhibitors.[29] The safest of these is probably fluoxetine or sertraline. Some clinical trials have been done with propranolol, but it does not control the full clinical picture.[79] Psychotherapy, specifically CBT, is also extremely effective in the treatment of ASD and PTSD. Some individuals respond well to the combination of medications and CBT.

Psychosocial Interventions

Sustaining a burn injury is a traumatic event. People are often in a state of shock and disbelief, frightened, unsure about the treatment process; have concerns about their loved ones; begin to notice changes in appearance; and experience pain and anxiety. Unfamiliarity with the burn unit and pain can cause significant distress. Unmanaged pain can be a secondary trauma for the burn patient. Assessment of an individual's psychosocial needs should begin upon admission to the hospital so that interventions can be planned accordingly. Assessment for background and procedural pain, anxiety, trauma symptoms, sleep disturbance, mood, itch, and adjustment is an ongoing process. Psychological interventions such as psychotherapy for adolescents and adults and play therapy for children are an important part of the treatment plan, which addresses the burn survivors' emotional recovery. It provides a safe environment to process thoughts and feelings related to the trauma, to address concerns, and for grief work. During the recovery process, burn survivors' questions about their appearance and functional abilities become more salient.

Grief is the process of coping with loss.[80] Burn survivors may grieve the unexpected disfigurement and loss of physical abilities. Adults and children experience similar emotional reactions, but their emotional responses and ways of grieving may be different. Adults will more readily express their grief and usually talk about their thoughts and feelings. Children may be more prone to exhibit emotional liability, withdrawal, "acting out" and may express their grief through play.[81–83]

Discussion about changes in appearance is an ongoing and delicate process and is dependent on the person's readiness to address this topic. The mental health professional and family/caretakers can plan the truth-telling process and timing of the disclosure. When patients are informed about their physical changes, it is important to discuss the healing process, the things that remain the same, the areas that have changed, and the assistance the individuals will continue to receive throughout the recovery process. A plan can be made to prepare individuals to see their changes in the mirror when they are ready and wish to do so. Availability to the person's social support systems is vital in this process and can include family, friends, hospital staff, peer support from other burn survivors, spiritual advisors, etc. Bronson and Price[83] refer to this process as compassionate truth-telling. Grief work may be ongoing and continue throughout the patient's hospitalization and once they are discharged home.

Social skills–based programs, CBT, self-help materials, and support groups are beneficial in aiding with postburn adjustment. Psychotherapy can assist with identification of negative thoughts and preconceived ideas, reinforce positive thinking, and help in learning adaptive coping skills. The availability of mental health services varies at different burn centers. The psychologist, social worker, and/or child life specialist can develop treatment plans to promote stress management, improve compliance with rehabilitation and exercise programs, and provide procedural support. When working with children who exhibit behavioral problems and refuse to participate in certain procedures, it may be beneficial to discuss expectations and the reasons for the procedure, provide choices, and present tasks in a play format. For example, the use of distraction and relaxation techniques may be helpful during painful procedures such as wound care and bathing (see Chapter 22).

Use of Cosmetics

Sometimes burn survivors inquire about the use of cosmetics to cover visible burn scars on the face and body (see Chapters 20 and 21). At many facilities the use of cosmetics is addressed by mental health providers, plastic surgeons, and child life specialists. Training is done on the appropriate use and application of cosmetics. Many burn survivors report improved self-confidence and confidence in different social settings when they use cosmetics to cover up burn scars, whereas others are content without the use of cosmetics. Some burn survivors may use clothing to cover up burn scars out of discomfort of having them seen by others. Some research has been done in the areas of cosmetic concealment of burn scars. Martin and colleagues[84] examined the benefits of the use of Microskin (Microskin, New York, NY) spray as a skin camouflage for pediatric burn patients. The study patients and the wait-list patients received a 5-week trial of Microskin at two different time points and answered several psychosocial measures. Children in both groups reported psychosocial improvements after using the Microskin, and these remained at 6-month follow-up. They reported feeling happier and more confident in social settings.[84,85] A subsequent study by Maskell and colleagues[86] examined the psychological and social benefits of the use of Microskin with pediatric burn survivors across multiple sites and found similar results. Reductions with emotional symptoms and improvements in socialization were reported. Holme and colleagues[87] found significant improvements in quality of life of adults with scars and other skin conditions who attended camouflage clinic appointments 1 month postappointment. One can speculate that discussion about scar mitigation with dermatologists may be beneficial for burn survivors as well.

Social Reintegration

Community Reintegration

Community reintegration is the process of participating in diverse activities such as school, work, social, and leisure events.[88] Esselman and colleagues[88] found that burn survivors experienced difficulty after discharge with social interactions and work productivity. Burn survivors may feel apprehensive and anxious,[5] fear social rejection and stigmatization, worry about receiving limited social support,[5] and have concerns about acceptance and how others will treat them (neighbors, church, social organizations). Preparing burn survivors to return home and into the community is an ongoing process. Studies have reported that social support,[6] family acceptance,[89] and cohesive families[90–94] can facilitate the transition. Thompson and Kent recommended interventions address stereotypes regarding disfigurement and behavioral reactions.[7] In psychotherapy burn survivors can discuss their concerns and fears and explore adaptive coping strategies that can facilitate and promote positive home and community integration. Interventions that may be helpful include social skills training, cognitive-behavioral strategies, and support groups.[7,8]

Social Skills

Thompson and Kent reported that people with various kinds of disfigurement may use diverse coping strategies such as addressing people's behaviors and comments, avoidance of social situations, and covering up visible differences.[7] There are conflicting reports in the literature about children with burns and their social comfort and confidence in social situations. It is estimated that 20% to 30% of children with burns may have decreased social competence.[56] Blakeney and colleagues[95] found that children with burns experienced more difficulty with social interactions and school than the comparison group. Meyer and colleagues[96] examined adaptive behaviors of children with burns. Although parental reports suggested pediatric burn survivors had more difficulty on a measure of adaptive behaviors, the ratings of their social skills (play, leisure activities) were normal. Other studies reported children with burns were doing well socially.[90,97]

Social skills are adaptive coping strategies used to help in social situations.[7] There are existing social skills programs developed specifically for burn survivors designed to facilitate positive integration to society and improve social comfort and confidence in social situations. One program by Barbara Kammerer Quayle, available through The Phoenix Society for Burn Survivors, Inc., is the "Be Your Best" program. This program has a cognitive-behavioral component to help individuals use positive thinking and learn adaptive ways of responding to questions to increase comfort and self-confidence in diverse social settings. The author recommends individuals rehearse various responses to anticipated questions about the burn injury.[98] Another program from the United Kingdom (UK) by James Partridge ("Changing Faces," http://www.changingfaces.org.uk/Home) is designed to help individuals with facial disfigurement manage the reactions of others and feel more comfortable in social encounters. This program also emphasizes the use of positive coping skills.[99,100] These programs prepare individuals to deal with stigmatization and scarring, address negative remarks, and provide education about burn injuries. Burn survivors may benefit from rehearsing these skills in the hospital setting through use of role playing. They may then practice these skills in various social outings before they return home in order to identify problem areas and explore alternative options. Robinson and colleagues[101] reported the "Changing Faces" program facilitated socialization of adults from the UK with facial disfigurement. Blakeney and colleagues[56] investigated if the "Changing Faces" curriculum improved the social skills of adolescent burn survivors from the United States. The parents of adolescents who received social skills training perceived their teenagers as having fewer behavioral problems and exhibiting improved internalizing and externalizing behaviors.

The Phoenix Society for Burn Survivors, Inc. (http://www.phoenix-society.org)[102] organizes support groups and has an annual World Burn Congress where burn survivors and families, first responders, and burn care professionals meet to address reintegration.[102]

School Reintegration

Children with burns may experience difficulty returning to school because of physical changes in appearance, decreased mobility owing to contractures and amputations, and the need for special appliances such as masks, splints, pressure garments, and prosthetics.[103] They may require assistance returning to school to succeed academically and socially.[103] Blakeney reported children's physical limitations and changes in appearance may lead to emotional and social difficulties.[104] The use of special equipment might increase the child's apprehension about being teased, bullied, rejected by peers, and excluded from activities. The process of school reintegration can be especially difficult during the later school ages when appearance and peer approval are very important.[105] Successful school reintegration is also an essential step in achieving independent adult roles.

Many teachers and students in the traditional school system are unfamiliar with children with burns and how they can facilitate socialization upon return to the classroom. Academic performance may be affected by diminished stamina, frequent absences to attend clinic appointments, and hospital stays for surgical interventions. Collaboration between the family, school personnel, and health care professionals is important for successful reintegration[106] and to create a positive learning and social environment for children returning to school.[104] Blakeney provided the following recommendations to assist with school reintegration: (1) planning the intervention as soon as possible, (2) use of an interdisciplinary approach to educate school personnel and students in the classroom about the child's needs, (3) developing an individualized program, (4) normalizing school activities, (5) assisting the child and parents in coping, and (6) systematic follow-up.[103,104]

Several burn centers have school reentry programs that help educate school personnel and students about the child's needs, treatment, and recovery process. At many pediatric burn centers, interventions such as educational DVDs and school reentry team visits have facilitated the return to school. Before the child returns home from the hospital, the school reentry team and family plan the intervention. The program selected depends on the needs of the family and child, the school resources, and preference. The school reentry visit involves burn care professionals visiting the child's classroom, providing information about the child's burn injury and rehabilitation, promoting compassion and support for the burn survivor, and answering questions. A new program called "The Journey Back," by Clark and colleagues,[107] is a thorough program developed by The Phoenix Society for Burn Survivors, Inc. This program provides materials to assist children with burns, their family, and the school community with the reentry process. The program provides information on how to deal with public situations such as staring, intrusive questions, and explores how to deal with uncomfortable situations through the use of social skills.

Only one study has investigated the efficacy of school reintegration programs for pediatric burn survivors. Blakeney[103] examined the effectiveness of two interventions, educational videos and school visits, to assist children with burns returning to school. Children and families reported that the most problematic issue was how others reacted to them. No significant differences were found between the interventions on teacher ratings of adaptive and problematic behaviors. Other studies have examined the length of time it takes pediatric burn survivors to return to school. Staley and colleagues[108] found that children with small burns returned to school on average 1½ weeks after the injury and were successful academically. Similarly, Christiansen and colleagues[109] found that it took an average of 2 weeks for children with small burns to return to school. However, children living in rural districts took almost 1 month to get back to their academic settings. For children with large burns, returning to school may take several months after the injury, and they often receive educational services in the hospital once they are able to participate. Pidcock and colleagues[110] addressed the problem of how noncompliance with the hospital treatment program can adversely impact the process of school reintegration. Additional research is needed to identify barriers in returning to school after a burn injury and the efficacy and benefits of school reentry programs.

Return to Work

For adult burn survivors, returning to work is an essential part of community reintegration. Because of the nature and severity of the injury, individuals may encounter difficulty returning to their previous employment and may require modifications to participate in their previous jobs. Byrch and colleagues[111] reviewed studies on return to work conducted at two burn centers. They reported the average time to return to work after a burn injury was 2½ months, and that burn size was predictive of when individuals returned to work. Similarly, Quinn and colleagues[112] performed a review of studies on return to work and found that the amount of time varied widely from 1 month to 2 years postburn. They reported 66% of the adults returned to work within the first 2 years after the injury. Meyer and colleagues[21] invited young adults with childhood burns to participate in a long-term psychosocial outcome study. Sixty-five percent of the participants were employed on a part- or full-time basis.

Fauerbach and colleagues[113] identified differences between adults who were employed and unemployed at the time of the burn injury. They reported individuals who were not working were more likely to have difficulty with alcohol and substance abuse, psychiatric disorders, preburn physical impairments, and medical concerns. Several studies identified burn severity,[112,114] location of the injury,[114] amount of time in the hospital,[112,114,115] physical limitations,[113,115] pain,[116,117] psychiatric problems,[112,113,115–118] limited training opportunities,[119] and prior work history[112,114] as factors that influence when burn survivors return to work. Social support and vocational training have been identified as beneficial in assisting with work reentry.[117,119]

Camps for Burn Survivors

Social support is important in promoting healthy psychosocial adjustment after a burn injury.[120] Camps provide children with the opportunity for socialization and assist in the development of forming healthy peer relationships. The curriculum of the camp depends on the goal and type of camp. Some camps may focus on leisure and fun activities, and others promote working on psychosocial issues and rehabilitation needs.[121] Find Burn Centers & Camps | IAFF Charitable Foundations provides the following link to facilitate locating camp sites in the United States and Canada (http://www.iafffoundation.org/causes/burn-fund/find-burn-centers-camps-0.html).[122]

Studies on the benefits of burn camps suggest that they help improve self-esteem, but results have been varied.[120,123] Cox and colleagues[120] evaluated the self-esteem of adolescents with burns after they participated in focus groups at camp. They concluded the camp experience helped participants feel they belonged to a group. One study found that women perceived their self-esteem improved more than men,[124] and in another study self-esteem scores improved after camp for children who attended; however, in both studies the findings were not statistically significant. Contrary to the foregoing studies, Arnoldo and colleagues[125] reported there were no improvements on a self-esteem measure for children who went to burn camp. In a recent study, Rimmer and colleagues[126] investigated the effects of bullying on pediatric burn survivors who attended burn camp. Children took a class about bullying and answered a questionnaire regarding their experience with bullying. Several children reported bullying was problematic, especially for children with visible scars.

Conclusion

In conclusion, many burn survivors adjust well to their injuries and burn scars and go on to have productive and fulfilling lives. For those who continue to struggle with physical limitations and psychosocial difficulties, ongoing availability to rehabilitation, mental health, and medical services is vital. Social skills programs, CBT, and support groups can be beneficial and facilitate adjustment and coping as burn survivors transition through life stages.

REFERENCES

1. Kamolz LP, Huang T. Reconstruction of burn deformities: an overview. In: Herndon DN, ed. *Total Burn Care*. 4th ed. Edinburgh: Saunders Elsevier; 2012:571–580.
2. Huang T. Overview of burn reconstruction. In: Herndon DN, ed. *Total Burn Care*. 3rd ed. Edinburgh: Saunders Elsevier; 2007:674–686.
3. Celis MM, Suman OE, Huang TT, et al. Effect of a supervised exercise and physiotherapy program on surgical intervention in children with thermal injury. *J Burn Care Rehabil*. 2003;24:57–61.
4. Blakeney P, Meyer WJ. Psychological aspects of burn care. *Trauma Q*. 1994;11(2):166–179.
5. Blakeney P, Partridge J, Rumsey N. Community integration. *J Burn Care Rehabil*. 2007;28(4):598–601.
6. Orr DA, Reznikoff M, Smith GM. Body image, self-esteem, and depression in burn-injured adolescents and young adults. *J Burn Care Rehabil*. 1989;10:454–461.
7. Thompson A, Kent G. Adjusting to disfigurement: process involved in dealing with being visibly different. *Clin Psychol Rev*. 2001;21(5):663–682.
8. Bessell A, Moss TP. Evaluating the effectiveness of psychosocial interventions for individuals with visible differences: a systematic review of the empirical literature. *Body Image*. 2007;4:227–238.
9. Thompson JK, Heinberg LJ, Altabe MN, et al. *Exacting Beauty: Theory, Assessment, and Treatment of Body Image Disturbance*. Washington, DC, US: American Psychological Association; 1999.
10. Cash TF. Cognitive-behavioral perspectives on body image. In: Cash TF, Smolak L, eds. *Body Image: A Handbook of Science, Practice and Prevention*. 2nd ed. New York, NY: The Guilford Press; 2011:39–47.
11. Tiggemann M. Sociocultural perspectives on human appearance and body image. In: Cash TF, Smolak L, eds. *Body Image: A Handbook of Science, Practice and Prevention*. 2nd ed. New York, NY: The Guilford Press; 2011:12–19.
12. Blakeney P, Robert R, Meyer WJ. Psychological and social recovery of children disfigured by physical trauma: Elements of treatment supported by empirical data. *Int Rev Psychiatry*. 1998;10(3):196–200.
13. Pruzinsky T, Doctor M. Body images and pediatric burn injury. In: Tarowski KJ, ed. *Behavioral Aspects Of Pediatric Burns*. New York, NY: Plenum; 1994:169–191.
14. Lovegrove E, Rumsey N. Ignoring it doesn't make it stop: adolescents, appearance, and bullying. *Cleft Palate Craniofac J*. 2005;42(1):33–44.
15. Fauerbach JA, Heinberg LJ, Lawrence JW, et al. Effect of early body image dissatisfaction on subsequent psychological and physical adjustment after disfiguring injury. *Psychosom Med*. 2000;62(4):576–582.
16. Lawrence JW, Rosenberg LE, Fauerbach JA. Comparing the body esteem of pediatric survivors of burn injury with the body esteem of an age-matched comparison group without burns. *Rehabil Psychol*. 2007;52(4):370–379.
17. Thombs BD, Notes LD, Lawrence JW, et al. From survival to socialization: a longitudinal study of body image in survivors of severe burn injury. *J Psychosom Res*. 2008;64(2):205–212.
18. Lawrence JW, Fauerbach JA, Thombs BD. A test of the moderating role of importance of appearance in the relationship between perceived scar severity and body-esteem among adult burn survivors. *Body Image*. 2006;3(2):101–111.
19. Russell W, Robert RS, Thomas CR, et al. Self-perceptions of young adults who survived severe childhood burn injury. *J Burn Care Res*. 2013;34:394–402.
20. Pope SJ, Solomons WR, Done DJ, et al. Body image, mood and quality of life in young burn survivors. *Burns*. 2007;33:747–755.

21. Meyer WJ III, Blakeney P, Russell W, et al. Psychological problems reported by young adults who were burned as children. *J Burn Care Rehabil*. 2004;25:98–106.
22. Achenbach TM. *Manual for the Young Adult Self-Report and Young Adult Behavior Checklist*. Burlington, VT: University of Vermont Department of Psychiatry; 1997.
23. Andreasen NJ, Norris AS. Long-term adjustment and adaptation mechanisms in severely burned adults. *J Nerv Mental Dis*. 1972;154:352–362.
24. Meyer WJ, Blakeney P, Thomas CR, et al. Prevalence of major psychiatric illness in young adults who were burned as children. *Psychosom Med*. 2007;69:377–382.
25. Bission JI, Shepherd JP, Dhutia M. Psychological sequela of facial trauma. *J Trauma*. 1997;43:496–500.
26. Fukunishi I. Relationship of cosmetic disfigurement of the severity of posttraumatic stress order in burn injury or digital amputation. *Psychother Psychosom*. 1999;68:82–86.
27. Ratcliff SL, Brown A, Rosenberg L, et al. The effectiveness of a pain and anxiety protocol to treat of acute pediatric burn patient. *Burns*. 2006;32:554–562.
28. Thomas CR, Brazael BA, Rosenberg L, et al. Phantom limb pain in pediatric burn survivors. *Burns*. 2003;29:139–142.
29. Tcheung WJ, Robert R, Rosenberg L, et al. Early treatment of acute stress disorder in children with major burn injury. *Pediatr Crit Care Med*. 2005;6:676–681.
30. Thomas CR, Russell W, Robert RS, et al. Personality disorders in young adult survivors of pediatric bur injury. *J Pres Disord*. 2012;26:255–266.
31. Thomas CR, Blakeney P, Holzer CE III, et al. Psychiatric disorder in long-term adjustment of at-risk adolescent burn survivors. *J Burn Care Res*. 2009;30:458–463.
32. Noronha DO, Faust J. Identifying the variables impacting post burn psychological adjustment. *J Pediatr Psychol*. 2007;32:380–391.
33. Warner P, Stubbs TK, Kagan RJ, et al; Multi-Center Benchmarking Study Working Group. The effects of facial burns on health outcomes in children aged 5 to 18 years. *J Trauma Acute Care Surg*. 2012;73:S189–S196.
34. Stubbs TK, James LE, Daugherty MB, et al. Psychosocial impact of childhood face burns: a multicenter, prospective, longitudinal study of 390 children and adolescents. *Burns*. 2011;37:387–394.
35. Meyer WJ III, Lee AF, Kazis LE, et al; the Multi-Center Benchmarking Study Working Group. Adolescent survivors of burn injuries and their parents' perceptions of recovery outcomes: do they agree or disagree? *J Trauma Acute Care Surg*. 2012;73(3):S213–S220.
36. Robert R, Meyer W, Bishop S, et al. Disfiguring burn scars and adolescent self-esteem. *Burns*. 1999;25:581–585.
37. Palmieri TL, Nelson-Mooney K, Kagan RJ, et al; Multi-Center Benchmarking Study Working Group. Impact of hand burns on health-related quality of life in children younger than 5 years. *J Trauma Acute Care Surg*. 2012;73:S197–S204.
38. Wiechman S, Meyer W, Edelman L, et al. Psychological outcomes. *J Burn Care Res*. 2013;34(4):363–368.
39. Beck AT, Steer RA, Brown GK. *Manual for the Beck Depression Inventory-II*. San Antonio, TX: Psychological Corporation; 1996.
40. Zigmond AS, Snaith RP. The hospital anxiety and depression scale. *Acta Psychiatr Scand*. 1983;67:361–370.
41. Derogatis LR. *Brief Symptom Inventory*. Baltimore, MD: Clinical Psychometric Research; 1975.
42. Achenbach TM, Rescorla LA. *Manual for the SEBA School Age Forms & Profiles*. Burlington, VT: University of Vermont, Research Center for Children, Youth & Families; 2001.
43. Spitzer RL, Kroenke K, Williams JB. Validation and utility of a self-report version of PRIME-MD: the PHQ primary care study. Primary Care Evaluation of Mental Disorders. Patient Health Questionnaire. *JAMA*. 1999;282:1737–1744.
44. Kovacs M. *Children's Depression Inventory Manual*. North Tonawanda, NY: Multi-Health Systems, Inc.; 1992.
45. Weathers FW, Litz BT, Herman DS, et al. The PTSD checklist reliability, validity and diagnostic utility. Paper presented at: the Annual Meeting of the International Society for Traumatic Stress Studies, San Antonio, TX October, 1993.
46. Pynoos RS, Goenjian AK, Steinberg AM. A public mental health approach to the postdisaster treatment of children and adolescents. *Child Adolesc Psychiatr Clin N Am*. 1998;7:195–210, x. Review.
47. Faber A, Klasen H, Sauer E, et al. Psychological and social problems in burn patients after discharge: a follow-up study. *Scand J Plast Reconstr Surg*. 1987; 21(3):307–309.
48. Malt U. Long-term psychosocial follow-up of burned adults: review of the literature. *Burns*. 1980; 6:190–197.
49. Blakeney P, Meyer W, Moore P, et al. Psychosocial sequelae of pediatric burns involving 80% or greater total body surface area. *J Burn Care Rehabil*. 1993;14(6):684–689.
50. Blakeney P, Meyer W III, Robert R, et al. Long-term psychosocial adaptation of children who survive burns involving 80% or greater total body surface area. *J Trauma*. 1998;44:625–631.
51. Sheridan RL, Hinson MI, Liang MH, et al. Long-term outcome of children surviving massive burns. *JAMA*. 2000;283(1):69–73.
52. Baker CP, Russell WJ, Meyer W III, et al. Physical and psychologic rehabilitation outcomes for young adults burned as children. *Arch Phys Med Rehabil*. 2007;88(2):S57–S64.
53. Rosenberg M, Blakeney P, Robert R, et al. Quality of life of young adults who survived pediatric burns. *J Burn Care Res*. 2006;27:773–778.
54. Murphy ME, Holzer CE III, Richardson LM, et al. Quality of life of young adult survivors of pediatric burns using the World Health Organization Disability Assessment Scale II and Burn Specific Health Scale-Brief: a comparison. *J Burn Care Res*. 2015;36:521–533.
55. Landolt MA, Buehlmann C, Maag T, et al. Brief report: quality of life is impaired in pediatric burn survivors with posttraumatic stress disorder. *J Pediatr Psychol*. 2009;34(1):14–21.
56. Blakeney P, Thomas C, Holzer C III, et al. Efficacy of a short-term, intensive social skills training program for burned adolescents. *J Burn Care Rehabil*. 2005;26:546–555.
57. Anzarut A, Chen M, Shankowsky H, et al. Quality-of-life and outcome predictors following massive burn injury. *Plast Reconstr Surg*. 2005;116:791–797.
58. Patterson DR, Ptacek JT, Cromes F, et al. The 2000 Clinical Research Award. Describing and predicting distress and satisfaction with life for burn survivors. *J Burn Care Rehabil*. 2000;21:490–498.
59. Cromes GF, Holavanahalli R, Kowalske K, et al. Predictors of quality of life as measured by the Burn Specific Health Scale in persons with major burn injury. *J Burn Care Rehabil*. 2002;23:229–234.
60. Leblebici B, Adam M, Bagis S, et al. Quality of life after burn injury: the impact of joint contracture. *J Burn Care Res*. 2006;27:864–868.
61. Pavoni V, Gianesello L, Paparella L, et al. Outcome predictors of quality of life of severe burn patients admitted to intensive care unit. *Scand J Trauma Resusc Emerg Med*. 2010;18:1–8.
62. Suman OE, Spies RJ, Celis MM, et al. Effects of a 12-wk resistance exercise program on skeletal muscle strength in children with burn injuries. *J Appl Physiol*. 2001;91:1168–1175.
63. Suman OE, Mlcak RP, Herndon DN. Effects of exercise training on pulmonary function in children with thermal injury. *J Burn Care Rehabil*. 2002;23:288–293.
64. Suman OE, Herndon DN. Effects of cessation of a structured and supervised exercise conditioning program on lean mass and muscle strength in severely burned children. *Arch Phys Med Rehabil*. 2007; 88(12 suppl 2):S24–S29. PubMed PMID: 18036977.
65. De Lateur BJ, Magyar-Russell G, Bresnick MG, et al. Augmented exercise in the treatment of deconditioning from major burn injury. *Arch Phys Med Rehabil*. 2007; 88(12 suppl 2):S18–S23.
66. Rosenberg M, Celis MM, Meyer W III, et al. Effects of a hospital based wellness and exercise program on quality of life of children with severe burns. *Burns*. 2013;39:599–609.
67. Meyer WJ, Russell W, Thomas CR, et al. Sexual attitudes and behavior of young adults who were burned as children. *Burns*. 2011;37:215–221.
68. Bianchi TLG. Aspects of sexuality after burn injury: outcomes in men. *J Burn Care Rehabil*. 1977;18:183–186.
69. Carrougher GJ, Martinez EM, McMullen KS, et al. Pruritus in adult burn survivors: postburn prevalence and risk factors associated with increased intensity. *J Burn Care Res*. 2013;34:94–101.
70. Schneider JC, Nadler DL, Herndon DN, et al. Pruritus in pediatric burn survivors: defining the clinical course. *J Burn Care Res*. 2015;36:151–158.
71. Elman S, Hynan LS, Gabriel V, et al. The 5-D itch scale: a new measure of pruritus. *Br J Dermatol*. 2010;162:587–593.
72. Blakeney P, Marvin J. Itch Man Scale. Copyrighted by Shriners Hospitals for Children; 2000.
73. Morris V, Murphy LM, Rosenberg M, et al. Itch assessment scale for the pediatric burn survivors. *J Burn Care Res*. 2012;33:419–424.
74. Eland J. Minimizing pain associated with pre-kindergartner intra-muscular injections. *Issues Compr Pediatr Nurs*. 1981;5:361–372.
75. Whaley L, Wong D. Nursing care of infants and children. 3rd ed, St. Louis: The C.V. Mosby Company; 1987.

76. Schneider JC, Harris NL, El Sahmi A, et al. A descriptive review of neuropathic-like pain after burn injury. *J Burn Care Res*. 2006;27(4):524–528.
77. Orellana Silva M, Yañez V, Hidalgo G, et al. 5% lidocaine medicated plaster use in children with neuropathic pain from burn sequelae. *Pain Med*. 2013;14:422–429.
78. American Psychiatric Association. *Diagnostic and Statistical Manual of Mental Disorders*. 5th ed (DSM-5). Washington, DC: American Psychiatric Publishing; 2013.
79. Sharp S, Thomas C, Rosenberg L, et al. Propranolol does not reduce risk for acute stress disorder in pediatric burn trauma. *J Trauma*. 2010;68:193–197.
80. Stroebe MS, Hansson RO, StroebeW, et al. *Handbook of Bereavement Research: Consequences, Coping, and Care*. Washington, DC: American Psychological Association; 2001.
81. Kroen WC. *Helping Children Cope with the Loss of A Loved One: A Guide for Grownups*. Minneapolis, MN: Free Spirit Publishing Inc.; 1996.
82. Rando TA. *Grief, Dying, and Death: Clinical Interventions for Caregivers*. Champaign, IL: Research Press Co.; 1984.
83. Bronson M, Price S. *Grief, Loss and Healing After Burn Trauma: Helping Children*. Burn Support News: Phoenix Society for burn Survivors. 2007;4:13–15.
84. Martin G, Swannell S, Mill J, et al. Spray on skin improves psychosocial functioning in pediatric burn patients: a randomized controlled trail. *Burns*. 2008;34:498–504.
85. Lowndes L. Microskin Business Plan. Brisbane, Australia 2005. www.microskin.com.au.
86. Maskell J, Newcombe P, Martin G, et al. Psychological and psychosocial functioning of children with burn scarring using cosmetic camouflage: a multi-centre prospective randomized controlled trail. *Burns*. 2014;40:135–149.
87. Holme SA, Beattie PE, Fleming CJ. Epidemiology and health services research cosmetic camouflage advice improves quality of life. *Br J Dermatol*. 2002;147:946–949.
88. Esselman PC, Ptacek JT, Kowalske K, et al. Community integration after burn injuries. *J Burn Care Rehabil*. 2001;22:221–227.
89. Davidson TN, Bowden ML, Tholen D, et al. Social support and post-burn adjustment. *Arch Phys Med Rehabil*. 1981;62:274–278.
90. Byrne C, Love B, Browne G, et al. The social competence of children following burn injury: a study of resilience. *J Burn Care Rehabil*. 1986;7(3):247–252.
91. Le Doux J, Meyer WJ III, Blakeney PE, et al. Relationship between parental emotional states, family environment and the behavioural adjustment of pediatric burn survivors. *Burns*. 1998;24:425–432.
92. Blakeney P, Portman S, Rutan R. Family values as factors influencing long-term psychological adjustment of children after severe burn injury. *J Burn Care Rehabil*. 1990;11(5):472–475.
93. Landolt MA, Grubenmann S, Meuli M. Family impact greatest: predictors of quality of life and psychological adjustment in pediatric burn survivors. *J Trauma*. 2002;53:1146–1151.
94. Rosenberg L, Blakeney P, Thomas CR, et al. The importance of family environment for young adults burned during childhood. *Burns*. 2007;33(5):541–546.
95. Blakeney P, Meyer W, Moore P, et al. Social competence and behavioral problems of pediatric survivors of burns. *J Burn Care Rehabil*. 1993;14:65–72.
96. Meyer WJ, Blakeney P, LeDoux J, et al. Diminished adaptive behaviors among pediatric survivors of burns. *J Burn Care Rehabil*. 1995;16:511–518.
97. Moore P, Moore M, Blakeney P, et al. Competence and physical impairment of pediatric survivors of burns of more than 80% total body surface area. *J Burn Care Rehabil*. 1996;17:547–551.
98. Quayle, BK. Be your best. In: *The Journey Back*. Grand Rapids, MI: The Phoenix Society for Burn Survivors, Inc; 2006:27–35.
99. Partridge J. *Changing Faces: The Challenge of Facial Disfigurement*. London: Changing Faces; 1994.
100. Changing Faces. Available at: http://www.changingfaces.org.uk/Home.
101. Robinson E, Rumsey N, Partridge J. An evaluation of the impact of social interaction skills training for facially disfigured people. *Br J Plast Surg*. 1996;49:281–289.
102. Phoenix Society for Burn Survivors at: http://www.phoenix-society.org.
103. Blakeney P. School reintegration. *J Burn Care Rehabil*. 1995;16(2):180–187.
104. Blakeney P. School reintegration. In: Tarnowski K ed. *Behavioral Aspects of Pediatric Burns*. New York, NY: Plenum Press; 1994:217–241.
105. Sexson SB, Madan-Swain A. School reentry for the child with chronic illness. *J Learn Disabil*. 1993;26(2):115–125.
106. Sexson S, Madan-Swain A. The chronically ill child in school. *Sch Psychol Quart*. 1995;10(4):359–368.
107. Clark A, Kammerer-Quayle B, Bronson M, et al. *The Journey Back-Resources to Assist School Reentry after Burn Injury*. Grand Rapids, MI: Phoenix Society for Burn Survivors; 2006:1–159.
108. Staley M, Anderson L, Greenhalgh D, et al. Return to school as an outcome measure after a burn injury. *J Burn Care Rehabil*. 1998;20(1):91–94.
109. Christiansen M, Carrougher GJ, Engrave LH, et al. Time to school re-entry after burn injury is quite short. *J Burn Care Res*. 2007;28:478–481.
110. Pidcock FS, Fauerbach JA, Ober M, et al. The rehabilitation/school matrix: a model for accommodating the noncompliant child with severe burns. *J Burn Care Rehabil*. 2003;24:342–346.
111. Brych SB, Engrav LH, Rivara FP, et al. Time off work and return to work rates after burns: systematic review of the literature and a large two-center series. *J Burn Care Rehabil*. 2001;22:401–405.
112. Quinn T, Wasiak J, Cleland H. An examination of factors that affect return to work following burns: a systematic review of the literature. *Burns*. 2010;36:1021–1026.
113. Fauerbach JA, Engrav L, Kowalske K, et al. Barriers to employment among working-aged patients with major burn injury. *J Burn Care Rehabil*. 2001;22:26–34.
114. Hwang Y, Chen-Sea M, Chen C. Factors related to return to work and job modification after a hand burn. *J Burn Care Rehabil*. 2009;30:661–667.
115. Esselman PC, Askay SW, Carrougher GJ, et al. Barriers to return to work after burn injuries. *Arch Phys Med Rehabil*. 2007;88(2):S50–S56.
116. Schneider JC, Bassi S, Ryan CM. Barriers impacting employment after burn injury. *J Burn Care Rehabil*. 2009;30:294–300.
117. Mackey SP, Diba R, McKeown D, et al. Return to work after burns: a qualitative research study. *Burns*. 2009;35:338–342.
118. Dyster-Aas J, Kildal M, Willebrand M. Return to work and health-related quality of life after burn injury. *J Rehabil Med*. 2007;39:49–55.
119. Oster C, Kildal M, Ekselius L. Return to work after burn injury: burn-injured individuals' perception of barriers and facilitators. *J Burn Care Rehabil*. 2010;31:540–550.
120. Cox ER, Call SB, Williams NR, et al. Shedding the layers: exploring the impact of the burn camp experience on adolescents campers' body image. *J Burn Care Rehabil*. 2004;25:141–147.
121. Doctor ME. Burn camps and community aspects of burn care. *J Burn Care Rehabil*. 1992;13:68–76.
122. Find Burn Centers & Camps I IAFF Charitable Foundations: (http://www.iafffoundation.org/causes/burn-fund/find-burn-centers-camps-0.html).
123. Rimmer RB, Fornaciari GM, Foster KN, et al. Impact of a pediatric residential burn camp experience on burn survivors' perceptions of self and attitudes regarding the camp community. *J Burn Care Rehabil*. 2007;28:334–341.
124. Biggs KS, Heinrich JJ, Jekel JF, et al. The burn camp experience: variables that influence the enhancement of self-esteem. *J Burn Care Rehabil*. 1997;18:93–98.
125. Arnoldo BD, Crump D, Burris AM, et al. Self-esteem measurement before and after summer burn camp in pediatric burn patients. *J Burn Care Res*. 2006;27:786–789.
126. Rimmer RB, Foster KN, Bay CR, et al. The reported effects of bullying on burn-surviving children. *J Burn Care Res*. 2007;28:484–489.

25 Integrating Scar Management into Clinical Practice

MURAD ALAM

KEY POINTS

- In the United States, Current Procedural Terminology (CPT) codes are used to identify medical procedures, including those that may be appropriate for scar treatment. If an appropriate code is available, such as for an injection, laser, excision, or repair, this should be used.
- Often, no specific code exists for a particular scar procedure. In this case, an unlisted procedure code may have to be used in combination with appropriate documentation to support the medical necessity of a procedure, whether before the procedure is performed (preapproval) or after the fact. Code updates are indicated to parallel advances in scar management techniques, such as ablative fractional laser treatment for traumatic scars and contractures with functional and symptomatic sequelae.
- Treatment of some scars may not be considered medically necessary. For instance, atrophic acne scars may be construed as cosmetic in nature by insurers and require out-of-pocket payment by patients seeking treatment.
- Apart from acquiring technical skills and honing the clinical decision making required to treat a scar, a physician interested in scar treatment must learn to incorporate scar treatment into his or her practice in a feasible and cost-effective manner. Important pragmatic considerations include: (1) how to defray the costs of scar treatment; (2) how to promote the availability of scar treatment services; and (3) how to ensure efficient throughput of scar patients that reduces utilization of staff, space, equipment, and time.

Payment for Services: Insurance Reimbursement or Self-Pay in the United States

Although payment is not a comfortable topic, especially in the context of the emotional and physical trauma of scarring, a busy scar treatment practice must be supported by a revenue stream. Regrettably, at this point, there is no wide consensus among third-party payers that treatment of scars is medically necessary. There is also no specific CPT code for treatment of scarring that can be billed to Medicare/Medicaid or private insurers. Although it may still be possible to receive insurance reimbursement for scar treatment services, it should be made clear at the onset to patients that claims may be rejected and that they may be liable for some or all of the cost of treatment.

Governmental and Third-Party Payment

CPT Code Process

CPT codes are updated annually and are five-digit designators that describe medical procedures performed in the United States.[1,2] Code descriptors explain the procedure, and so-called code vignettes characterize how it is typically performed. CPT codes, and the definitions for each, are created, updated, and altered three times a year at face-to-face meetings of the CPT Panel, which is managed by the American Medical Association and includes members of medical specialty societies and payer groups. The CPT Panel is the voting body that decides to approve or decline so-called code change proposals (CCPs). At each CPT Panel meeting representatives of major medical professional societies called CPT Advisors who can offer testimony on behalf of particular CCPs and answer panel questions about clinical practice relevant to their specialties before the Panel votes are present. CCPs can be submitted by any interested group, including members of industry or the general public. Most successful CCPs (i.e., those that are approved by Panel vote) are supported and edited by the Advisors of the relevant specialty societies.

CPT codes for medical procedures performed by physicians are typically Category I or Category III codes. Category I codes represent routine, noninvestigational procedures. Once approved, Category I codes are sent to the Relative Value Scale Update Committee (RUC), which determines how much physician work effort and practice expense is required for completion of the procedure in question. Thereafter, the Centers for Medicare and Medicaid Services (CMS) usually accepts RUC recommendations and uses these to assign a dollar value to the code. The constituents of code value include physician work effort (i.e., the sum of preservice, intraservice, and postservice time, adjusted by the intensity of the effort), practice expense (i.e., the cost of disposable supplies, nonphysician staff time, a small fraction of the cost of durable equipment required, and other space and utilities costs), malpractice expense (i.e., a minute amount that reflects the malpractice risk per procedure), and any additional adjustments that CMS may deem appropriate. The final code values are published by the CMS each year in the Physician Fee Schedule. Private insurers usually use CMS-designated relative values, which they can adjust as they deem appropriate. For instance, a third-party insurer may price most procedures at 80% of Medicare or 120% of Medicare.

Category III codes are new procedure codes that denote experimental procedures or procedures that have not yet been widely adopted. These codes are not valued by the RUC or priced by CMS. Instead, they are "carrier priced," meaning individual insurers can choose to cover them, and if they do, they can select a payment amount. Often, procedures associated with Category III codes are redesignated with Category I codes after several years. As code utilization increases and procedures become routine, a CCP may be submitted to the Panel requesting an upgrade to Category I status. Even though Category III codes may not be paid, it is important for practitioners to submit them for consideration so that CMS can track utilization. Increased code use is often a major factor favoring eventual Category I status.

Current CPT Codes for Scar Treatment

The rule of thumb in selecting CPT codes is that if the right code does not exist, the physician provider should select the code that is the best fit. If no code is a reasonably good fit, then a code ending in -99 that designates an unspecified or miscellaneous service should be submitted, along with detailed documentation regarding the procedure and its medical necessity.

There is currently no CPT code for laser treatment of scars. Scar resurfacing, whether by nonablative or ablative lasers, does not have a specific code. Laser treatment of redness or erythema associated with scar also does not have a code, as the 17106-17018 (Table 25-1) family of laser codes are for treatment of congenital vascular disorders like port-wine stains and hemangiomas. Unless scars are part of congenital malformations or vascular proliferative lesions, these codes do not apply. There is some ambiguity because the CPT code descriptor "vascular proliferative lesion" does not specifically restrict use to lesions that are congenital or lifelong, and it may be argued that hypertrophic scars and keloids are both proliferative and mediated by a growth in underlying vascular network. The relevant local coverage

Table 25-1 Current CPT and HCPCS Codes That May Be Appropriately or Inappropriately Used for Scar Treatment

CPT Code Number	Defined Use	Appropriate Use for Scars	Inappropriate Use for Scars
17106-17108	Treatment of vascular proliferative lesions (e.g., laser)	1. Scars associated with port-wine stains and treatments for same 2. Possibly, proliferative scars and keloids, but must document	1. Nonproliferative scars (e.g., atrophic acne scars)
17110-17111	Destruction of benign lesions other than skin tags	1. May be appropriate, must explain in documentation	1. Generally inappropriate
15780-15782	Dermabrasion	1. May be appropriate, must explain in documentation 2. Unclear if these can be used for thermal dermabrasion with energy devices	1. Generally inappropriate
15788-15793	Chemical peel	1. May be appropriate, must explain in documentation	1. Generally inappropriate
11400-11446	Surgical excision	1. If medically indicated	1. If not medical indicated
12031-13153	(Postexcision) intermediate and complex repairs	1. If medically indicated	1. If not medically indicated
14000-14302	(Postexcision) adjacent tissue transfer	1. If medically indicated 2. If concurrent excision, do not code excision separately	1. If not medically indicated
11900	Injections into skin up to 7	1. If medically indicated 2. Relevant J-code for injectant coded separately	1. If not medically indicated
J3301	Triamcinolone acetonide, up to 10 mg	1. If medically indicated 2. Code with relevant CPT code	1. If not medically indicated
-99	Unlisted procedure codes	1. If no relevant code exists	1. If an appropriate procedure code already exists

determination of the Medicare contractor operating in a given region may provide additional guidance as to which ICD-10 diagnosis codes may be used with the code group 17106-17018. In general, atrophic scars, like some acne scars, would not meet the proliferation criterion, and treatment of these could not be described by these codes. Treatment of redness in a scar associated with prior surgery or previous laser treatment to treat a congenital malformation would be covered since the underlying disease process is covered.

The 17110-17111 code set is for destruction of benign lesions other than skin tags or cutaneous vascular proliferations, and a poor fit for laser treatment of scars. In some cases, vascular lesion or benign destruction codes may be used for treatment of scars, but preferably only after the insurer has been contacted and has preauthorized this usage. Alternatively, -99 category unspecified CPT codes can be submitted with a detailed explanation and procedure note detailing the need for laser scar treatment and exactly how the laser was used. Some insurers may choose to cover these claims; if they do, it will be at a price point that they deem appropriate. In practice, such miscellaneous code submissions are frequently denied, and may need to be appealed, with such appeals being labor intensive and of uncertain outcome.

Dermabrasion by any method, whether sterile sandpaper, a diamond fraise, or wire brush (including for acne scarring), can be coded as 15780-15782, depending on whether the whole face, partial face, or region other than the face is treated. Some authorities believe these codes may be the best fit for other modalities that result in skin ablation by thermal means (i.e., "thermal dermabrasion"), such as full-field ablative lasers and energy devices, given the functional similarity of such treatments to conventional dermabrasion and the lack of any more specific CPT codes for nonmechanical abrasion. Detailed documentation will be needed to clarify that the treatment is for reconstruction of functional and physical impairment, and claims may still not be approved. Chemical peels are associated with CPT codes 15788-15793 depending on the depth of the peel (epidermal or dermal) and the anatomic site (face or other). Again, insurers may summarily deny these codes and consider them cosmetic even when they are submitted with evidence that the peel was used for reconstruction of a scar causing functional impairment.

Surgical excision (CPT: 11400-11446, excision benign lesions) and reconstruction (CPT: 12031-13153, intermediate and complex repairs; 14000-14302: adjacent tissue transfer) of keloids and hypertrophic scars (ICD-10: L73.0—acne keloid; L90.5—scar conditions and fibrosis of skin; L91.0—hypertrophic scar [keloid]) may be covered by many insurers. As with all cases of scar treatment submitted for reimbursement, proper documentation is imperative. Scar revision may be considered medically necessary, and hence reimbursable, when there is documentation of significant functional impairment associated with the scar and the treatment can reasonably be expected to improve the physical functional impairment. Functional scar impairment may be related to accidental injury, disease, trauma, treatment of disease, or a congenital defect. Detailed explanations of the physical and functional impairment, its etiology, its consequences on work and home functioning, and its resistance to prior treatments may be included in documentation for preapproval (or postprocedure if preapproval was not obtained). Photographic documentation may also be provided. Once documentation is submitted, insurers may deny the claim or request additional information. Requests for additional information, whether in writing or by telecommunication, should be fulfilled promptly.

Intralesional injection of keloids and hypertrophic scars is often covered. For such injections, CPT coding includes a J-code for the material injected (e.g., J3301—triamcinolone acetonide—per 10 mg) as well as the number of injections (CPT: 11900—injections into skin up to 7).

An alternative method of drug delivery (so-called laser-assisted delivery) entails treatment of the scar with a fractional ablative or nonablative laser, followed by dripping or surface application of a medicament over the treatment field. This may accelerate absorption of the medication throughout the substance of the scar in a manner difficult to achieve even with multiple injections. Cold needling of the scar with microneedles or slightly larger needles mounted on rollers, as well as other fractional treatments like fractional radiofrequency, may also help to break up the scar or speed medication absorption. 5-fluorouracil for injection mixed with triamcinolone prior to application or injection may increase effectiveness and reduce the risk of telangiectasia associated with steroid application alone. Finally, perilesional botulinum toxin injection may help with scar prevention or remodeling, as well as reduce scar-associated itch. In general, there are no specific CPT codes for laser or energy device–mediated delivery of medications to a scar. It may be possible to use a relevant J-code for the injectant in combination with an explanatory note, or in association with an application for preapproval. Reimbursement for laser or energy device procedures may be possible, with supportive documentation, and this may differ across payers and depend on specific patient circumstances.

Denials may necessitate the need for an appeal. The treating physician will determine when reasonable efforts to pursue a claim are exhausted and the likelihood of receiving payment is slim. If a practice performs a high volume of scar revisions that result in claims submitted to a particular insurer, it may be fruitful for the treating physician to reach out to the local medical director for that insurer to communicate the importance of his or her specialized practice. Each state also has two dermatology carrier advisory committee (DermCAC) members, practicing dermatologists who volunteer their time to meet with insurer groups several times a year. The DermCAC representatives can communicate concerns about reimbursement of particular procedures (e.g., scar treatment), discuss problems with the appeals process, and advocate for payment.

Prior authorizations and appeals may reduce the likelihood of denials, but may also consume copious staff time and not be cost-effective. It may be preferable in certain instances to forego precertification, submit well-documented claims with the best-fit diagnosis and procedure codes, and hope for the best. Practice patterns and insurer reimbursement practices vary regionally, so it behooves the physician to do as is usual and customary in his or her area.

In the future, a CPT code for laser scar revision, and major scar revision in general, may become available.

Efforts are currently underway to create such a code, but the process may unfold over several years. If and when a code or code set is approved for scar treatment, procedures that meet the CPT definition will be able to be coded more accurately. Assuming the new code is a Category I code, government and private payers will reimburse the relevant code(s). Before billing such a code, practitioners will need to ensure that the procedure they performed meets the specific code definition. Not all scar treatment procedures may be covered. Approval of a relevant code set does not mean that reimbursement for specified procedures will be perceived as adequate or fair by providers. Reimbursement will be contingent on RUC valuation of the code and CMS approval and adjustments of the RUC value.

Alternative Reimbursement Methods and Self-Pay

Physicians who are performing scar treatments do not have a pecuniary motive. Scar revision procedures can be difficult, time-consuming, and frustrating for both patients and physicians. Yet both are motivated by the promise of success and the hope for symptom relief, functional improvement, and reduction of disfigurement for the patient.

The need for funding for scar procedures exists only to the extent that this funding is necessary to pay for expenses, allowing the doctor to continue his or her work. Thus, if insurance reimbursement is not forthcoming, the patient and physician may need to have a frank discussion about payment. Discounted payments, possibly in combination with payment plans, may be appropriate. Patients may be more patient and accepting once they are informed that the scar improvement process will be gradual, evolve over many treatments and follow-ups, and result in less than complete resolution. In general, even if the physician can afford to provide it, completely free care is not advisable because this may reduce the patient's commitment to the treatment process. Academic medical centers and large practices often have financial assistance offices that can estimate the patient's ability to pay out of pocket. They can then offer discounts ranging from the modest to the very large. Referring the patient to such an office can preserve the patient's dignity and allow the physician–patient relationship to remain focused solely on the medical challenges of scar treatment.

If a scar results from accidental injury, a personal injury claim may already have been adjudicated. In this case, there may be a mechanism by which the treating physician can submit a bill to an organization that is paying for the patient's medical expenses. Often, the patient will know that this is the case and be able to guide the physician in the manner in which the bill should be submitted. Although the patient may be convinced that the bill will be paid, he or she should be counseled that there is no way to definitely ascertain this prior to payment, and that he or she may be liable for unreimbursed expenses. For Medicare patients, and even for privately insured patients, it is highly advisable to complete and maintain suitable paperwork indicating that patients are aware of and accede to the fact that they will be liable for expenses deemed not medically necessary.

When scars being treated pose no functional restriction, are not associated with symptoms, are not congenital, and are small enough in scope to not be considered gravely disfiguring, then the treatment of these scars is likely considered "cosmetic" by payers rather than medically necessary. Acne scars tend to fall into this category, according to many insurers. In this case, scar treatment is self-pay and not submitted for reimbursement. Some practitioners may choose to discount their cosmetic laser fees for patients seeking treatment of scars. If the scars were created by medically necessary procedures (e.g., Mohs for skin cancer, or excision of atypical nevi) performed at the same practice, some practitioners will choose to provide heavily discounted or free laser treatment of these scars, although there is no compulsion to do so.

Facilities serving severely scarred patients, including wounded warriors and burn patients, may consider setting up a charitable venture such as a 501(c)(3) tax exempt organization that is specifically devoted to providing such services. This may allow for collection of donations that defray the cost of capital equipment purchases, supplies, and staff needed to treat numerous patients who are unable to pay or are not insured.

Promoting and Advertising Scar Removal Expertise

Having developed expertise in scar revision, a physician interested in such procedures may choose to advertise this competence. Useful strategies may include: communicating with area physicians, presenting at local and regional professional meetings, and incorporating information about scar revision in internal and external advertising, practice web sites, and social media outreach. Internal advertising (i.e., print brochures in the waiting room, video infomercials on a television, or spoken information by the check-in staff or nurse rooming them) while patients are waiting to be seen can be highly effective in communicating new areas of physician expertise, such as the advent of a scar treatment center.

It can also be useful to partner with other groups that may provide scar treatment services that a practitioner decides not to provide him- or herself. For instance, dermatologists with expertise in the use of lasers for resurfacing as well as transdermal delivery of stem cells and antimetabolites may work with a group of plastic surgeons expert in management of acute burns, skin grafts, and large surgical repairs. A multidisciplinary scar group is easier to differentiate in promotions as a premium service not otherwise widely available.

Much advertising will ultimately be word-of-mouth. Unwanted scars are ubiquitous, and satisfied patients may be the best referral source. Expertise in scar treatment is not common, likely due to the complexity and time-consuming nature of treatment combined with the modest reimbursement that ensues. Consequently, competition for patients may not be intense in most geographic areas. Low-cost advertising methods may suffice. Options may include advertising on bulletin boards or internal publications of local hospitals, schools, and houses of worship; in urban and suburban regions, advertising copy may be purchased on buses and trains carrying commuters.

Efficient In-Office Treatment of Scar Patients

Improvement of a particular scar may require different treatment modalities, with each method possibly needing to be delivered in a repeated fashion. Initial consultation visits may be prolonged, as they require discussion of complex treatment plans, patient expectations, and insurance and reimbursement issues. Prior to each treatment, adult patients may require local or regional anesthesia. Pediatric patients may benefit from sedation or general anesthesia, which may require preplanning, a consultation with anesthesiology, and a procedure in the operating room. If lasers are being used, more than one device may be needed, with this often being associated with moving the patient from room to room. Dressings and postoperative care may need to be applied after treatment, and provision made for additional wound care supplies once the patient is home. As all of this occurs in the context of modest and uncertain payment for services rendered, it is imperative to carefully control the use of resources, including staff time, space, equipment, and disposables.

To speed the preoperative consultation phase, it may be useful to have printed materials describing the treatment process in detail. Patients can peruse this in the waiting room upon arrival, or even at home prior to the appointment. Short videos can be prepared which patients can view on tablets provided by the practice. These videos can discuss treatments types and outline expected outcomes as well as posttreatment wound care and adverse events.[3]

Alternatively, patients may be invited for "shared medical appointments"[4] for consultation prior to treatment. In this approach, the treating physician collectively educates a number of patients in a classroom setting about scars, their pathophysiology, their classification, major types of therapeutic approaches, development of a treatment plan, expected outcomes, postoperative wound care, and possible adverse events. After the communal part of the education session is completed, each patient then receives a brief private consultation with the physician in which the patient's particular complaints are discussed and a treatment plan tailored to their needs. In this manner, very detailed information about scars is conveyed to patients live and directly by the physician but without the need for extreme, time-consuming redundancy. Patients may also appreciate the in-depth information that they receive, the opportunity to ask questions, and the chance to meet patients with similar problems.

Once patients are in the office to receive treatment, it is prudent to have set protocols for how these treatments are delivered. Again the goal is efficient use of time, staff, and space. If patients tend to come from far away and prefer initiating treatment immediately following the consultation, then appointments need to be spaced accordingly to avoid delays. In higher volume practices, it may be preferable to have certain half-days devoted to consultations, and other periods to treatments of specific types, such as carbon dioxide laser. This minimizes the frequency of patient stacking, whereby patients presenting for different treatment types may need to use shared resources at the same time. Additionally, segregating patient treatments by type reduces the need for staff to set up and take down rooms for different types of procedures. Flow is speeded, and inefficiency reduced, when the same types of treatments are provided in rapid succession to several patients.

Occasionally patients will have acute injuries or recent scars that need prompt resuturing, repair, or evaluation. Acute appointments should be available for such patients. Since treatment of scars can require many iterative treatments over a span of months to years, early morning, late evening, or weekend appointments may help patients get the care they need without them missing too much work.

Postoperative care can be an important part of scar management. If patients are expected to perform at-home posttreatment wound care, affix an appliance over their scar, apply or take medications, engage in any particular exercise or manipulation of the scar, or protect the healing scar from ultraviolet light; clear written and oral instructions can help. Follow-up phone calls by clinical staff and text reminders to patients' cell phones can also improve compliance.[5] Video instructions available on a web site can ensure that patients perform wound care appropriately, even in the presence of language barriers.[6]

There is a dearth of comparative effectiveness research pertaining to the treatment of scars.[7,8] Safety, effectiveness, tolerability, longevity of effect, and cumulative direct and indirect costs of different approaches to scar management have rarely been studied side by side in prospective cohort studies or randomized controlled trials. Patients would clearly benefit if optimal treatment approaches were better defined through such research. Practices that aspire to provide state-of-the-art treatment of scars may therefore consider enrolling most, if not all patients, in protocols. Research may be as innocuous and unobtrusive as a series of retrospective chart reviews or, better yet, patients may be prospectively invited to participate in treatment schemes that are approved by a local institutional Review Board. Companies that provide supplies and equipment for laser treatment may be willing to contribute resources. Participation in clinical trials could be framed as a patient benefit, with patients both benefiting directly from the treatments received and contributing to the development of improved treatment methods in the future. Enrollment in clinical trials does not preclude charging patients, with billing being appropriate as long as the treatments received are standard of care. Beyond the important scientific and patient benefits, the availability of cutting-edge clinical trials may encourage patients to select a given practice. Published investigations may also raise the stature of the practice in the eyes of medical colleagues.

Summary

Treatment of scars can be financially viable despite limitations in insurance reimbursement. The relative dearth of practitioners expert in scar treatments creates opportunities for those interested in growing such practices. Efficiency in care delivery allows patients to benefit while preserving practice feasibility for physicians. Enrolling patients in clinical trials can improve care, assist in creating better treatment paradigms, and identify practices as state-of-the-art.

REFERENCES

1. Current Procedural Terminology: Professional Edition. Chicago, IL: American Medical Association; 2016.
2. Zalla JA. CPT coding and reimbursement issues in dermatology. *Semin Cutan Med Surg*. 2005;24(3):117–123.
3. Armstrong AW, Alikhan A, Cheng LS, et al. Portable video media for presenting informed consent and wound care instructions for skin biopsies: a randomized controlled trial. *Br J Dermatol*. 2010;163(5):1014–1019.
4. Knackstedt TJ, Samie FH. Shared medical appointments for the preoperative consultation visit of Mohs micrographic surgery. *J Am Acad Dermatol*. 2015;72(2):340–344.
5. Armstrong AW, Watson AJ, Makredes M, et al. Text-message reminders to improve sunscreen use: a randomized, controlled trial using electronic monitoring. *Arch Dermatol*. 2009;145(11):1230–1236.
6. Migden M, Chavez-Frazier A, Nguyen T. The use of high definition video modules for delivery of informed consent and wound care education in the Mohs Surgery Unit. *Semin Cutan Med Surg*. 2008;27(1):89–93.
7. Alam M, Olson JM, Asgari MM. Needs assessment for cosmetic dermatologic surgery. *Dermatol Clin*. 2012;30(1):177–187.
8. Olson JM, Alam M, Asgari MM. Needs assessment for general dermatologic surgery. *Dermatol Clin*. 2012;30(1):153–166.

Prevention

SECTION V

26 Scar Treatment, Restoration, and Prevention—Beyond the Horizon?

KACHIU C. LEE and R. ROX ANDERSON

KEY POINTS

- Nature creates new tissue through three major pathways: tissue genesis, remodeling, and scarring.
- Scar mitigation and prevention after major injury relies on finding cellular and molecular strategies to guide the wound healing process toward the remodeling and regenerative pathways. Recent advances in our understanding of wound healing and scarring processes offer the promise of better treatments in the future, with several approaches demonstrating improvements in scar quality.
- The novel concept of "tissue copying" exemplifies these principles, facilitating the healing of large-scale wounds with the creation of thousands of microscopic-scale wounds that heal scarlessly through remodeling.

This book exposes the awesome human suffering that scarring can pose; it summarizes both our current understanding and how little we really know. This chapter is an attempt to synthesize many viewpoints by guessing about the future. Is suppression of scarring possible? If so, is there an underlying ability to heal by tissue regeneration or tissue remodeling? How far along are we now? What are the most promising strategies for medical, cellular, and/or surgical treatments? Are new technologies on the horizon? How far-reaching would a "cure" for scarring really be? Questions and possibilities, not answers, are the stuff of this chapter.

Scarring is a concerted response to gross injury that evolved long ago among vertebrates, but recently in the history of all living things on earth. Scarring confers a survival advantage—or at least it used to, before medical care was invented. Meanwhile, all creatures (including ourselves) can heal microwounds without scarring. Surprisingly, even scar tissue retains at least some of that ability. After micro-wounding (such as skin needling or fractional laser therapy), scars normalize to some extent (see Chapters 5 and 13). The emergence of scarring appears to be linked to the emergence of adaptive immunity, both during evolution and in an individual human fetus during its first and second trimesters (see Chapter 27). Even in adult mammals, there are many examples of tissue regeneration without scarring—all of which rein in a full-blown immune response—through systemic or local tissue mechanisms. Scars are an example of tissue with sustained inflammation. They are composed of abnormal connective tissue loaded with mast cells, inflammatory mediators, neovascularization, and lifelong hyperactive turnover of the extracellular matrix. Why? How? Thanks to the tools of molecular biology, our basic understanding of scarring has improved dramatically of late. That knowledge will eventually be the basis for specific, new molecular and cellular strategies to prevent, treat, or even fully reverse scarring.

New Wound Treatments

The missing, dead, or dying tissue of a major wound is *not* doomed to be replaced by a scar. Prevention of scarring might be as simple as making sure that appropriate, normal skin tissue replaces the major wound defect. That is the essence of full-thickness skin grafting, which immediately closes a wound, often with excellent results. Unfortunately, full-thickness grafting creates another full-thickness skin wound at the donor site, which limits this strategy to small wounds. Also, full-thickness skin grafts may or may not "take," which is equivalent to saying that they may or may not connect with the wound bed's underlying blood supply before the graft tissue dies. Even so, a successful full-thickness skin graft is nothing short of miraculous. First, it is miraculous that full-thickness skin can stay alive for days near body temperature without any blood supply (what can we do to extend that time?). Second, it is miraculous that new connections form so rapidly between vessels in the graft and vessels in the underlying wound bed (how can we enhance that process?).

For extensive wounds, split-thickness skin grafts are preferred because they can easily be expanded to cover a larger area and because the donor site eventually heals with a new epidermis formed from stem cells residing in hair follicles. Unfortunately, a disfiguring and often painful scar typically results at the donor site. As such, split-thickness skin graft donor sites are an excellent setting to test new scar prevention strategies. Unfortunately, split-thickness skin grafts are only a thin, superficial layer of epidermis and dermis—not fully functional skin. Hair follicles, sweat glands, reticular dermis, subcutaneous fat, and other deep structures are missing from split-thickness grafts. Less than a few hundred micrometers thick, split-thickness grafts can survive longer than full-thickness grafts without a blood supply. In essence, thin pieces of tissue can maintain viability by diffusion of oxygen and nutrients, until a blood supply arrives.

If the signals that initiate and sustain scarring were blocked, would regeneration take over? Does regeneration require its own specific set of signals? These questions have been answered in part. For example, members of the transforming growth factor beta (TGF-β) family of proteins have been identified as playing major roles in scar initiation. TGF-β3 in particular can promote scarless wound healing in some mammals, whereas TGF-β1 and TGF-β2 are early signals that tend to drive scar formation. Corticosteroids, which have been used for decades to control the growth of hypertrophic scars, typically increase TGF-β3 while decreasing TGF-β1 and TGF-β2.[1–4] Immediately after wounding, a sequence of cellular and molecular events occur that set forth a course of healing (see Chapter 6). In the dermis, there is a large reservoir of preformed TGFs bound to collagen, which are rapidly released and activated upon injury. An immediate medical therapy aimed at "sopping up" proscarring signals, while adding antiscarring signals, might reduce or eliminate the scarring pathway. Other potent signals derive from platelet activation, a nearly universal event after wounding. Later in the course of scar tissue formation, other growth factors from platelets appear to improve the scar. We can look forward to specific new drugs that influence the molecular pathways involved in scarring.

One fundamental goal in the field of tissue engineering is to create fully functional skin or other organs ex vivo, which can then be used for transplantation. This lofty goal amounts to mimicking or recapitulating organogenesis, without a body. For decades since the discovery that a fully differentiated epidermis could be grown from keratinocytes atop a feeder layer of cultured fibroblasts, there has been steady progress in de novo skin engineering. Autologous keratinocytes were initially used, followed by several commercial products using allogeneic cells.[5] Even though eventually replaced by the host, putting this "ersatz" allogeneic version of a split-thickness skin graft onto a clean wound bed enhances healing and, to some extent, minimizes scarring. Until tissue engineers figure out how to create full-thickness, autologous, fully functional skin in culture, this fundamental goal will remain elusive.

Another tissue engineering strategy is to seed various porous matrix materials with cells, or use the materials as a "scaffold" in the wound, into which cells can migrate, eventually remodeling into something approximating normal skin. Type I collagen, decellularized connective tissue, amniotic membrane, or other matrix materials are sometimes used now.[6,7] Placed into a clean wound, these matrices can support neovascularization and fibroblast ingrowth. A split-thickness graft is often used after vascularization has occurred to provide the epidermis. Other current strategies include mincing or dispersing cells from a conventional donor graft, then spreading or spraying them onto a clean wound, with or without culturing the cells (see Chapter 8).[8,9] These strategies appear to be an improvement over conventional skin grafting, as they can impressively expand the wound area covered. Processed fresh tissues other than skin are

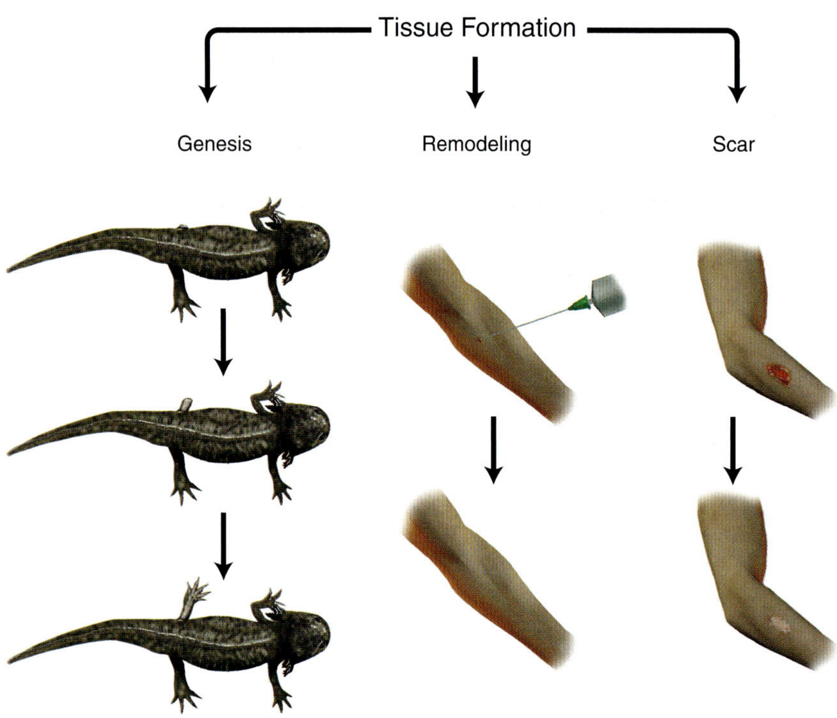

FIGURE 26-1 Nature creates new tissue by one of three distinct pathways. Some organisms, such as the axolotl, can regenerate severed limbs (Genesis). If the injury is sufficiently small (such as after venipuncture or fractional laser treatment), adult humans can heal scarlessly (Remodeling). Wounds above a threshold size in adults heal with a scar.

also helpful. With minimal processing, the stromal–vascular fraction of subcutaneous adipose tissue can be obtained from liposuction-aspirated tissue. When applied to fresh wounds, higher quality healing often occurs. In the future, when combined with appropriate matrix materials, it is conceivable that something closer to full-thickness skin or other functional tissues could be achieved.

What strategies might rapidly replace a wound with functional full-thickness skin, without creating a significant donor site wound? With support from the US Department of Defense, my laboratory group has lately been working on one we call "tissue copying," which in essence turns the problem of healing a large-scale wound by the process of scarring into that of healing thousands of microscopic-scale wounds by the process of remodeling.

Nature creates new tissue by one of three distinct pathways, each with distinctly different conditions and stimuli (see Fig. 26-1). First is *tissue genesis*—an orderly process of growth and differentiation by which the embryo develops, by which tissue regeneration occurs in some amphibians and other so-called lower animals, and by which adult deer yearly grow a brand new set of antlers. Second is *remodeling*—the orderly process of tissue growth and change within a fully formed organ. Without remodeling we would not grow, remove damaged or senescent cells, *or scarlessly repair microscopic wounds*. Third is *scarring*—a much less orderly process by which grossly missing or necrotic tissue is rapidly replaced with live scar tissue, albeit dysfunctional. Tissue copying is our attempt to use remodeling pathways, rather than scarring pathways, to heal a large wound.

What is the scale of a skin wound that can heal without scarring? For human skin, it appears to be up to about 0.5 mm. However, this question has not been studied in detail, nor have many other conditions that probably influence remodeling versus scarring after a given wound. A full-thickness surgical scalpel incision always scars; a full-thickness hypodermic needle puncture of about 25 gauge or smaller never scars. Both are wounds made by passing steel all the way through skin. We have lasers that selectively heat and destroy most of the cutaneous microvasculature, selectively destroy hair follicles, or selectively destroy tattoo pigment–laden cells throughout the entire dermis—all without causing a scar. A decade ago, when my laboratory group introduced fractional laser treatments (which turn out

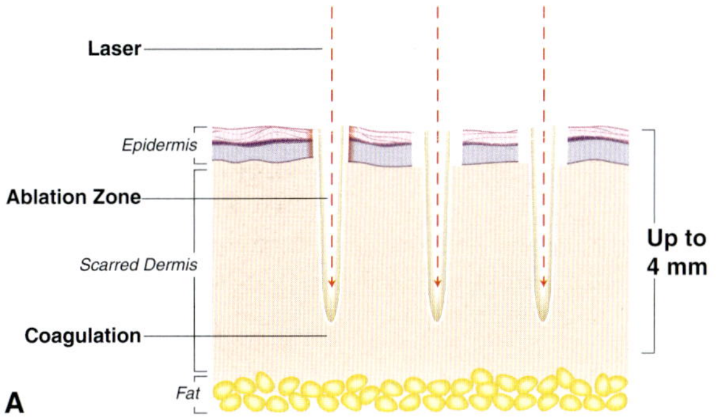

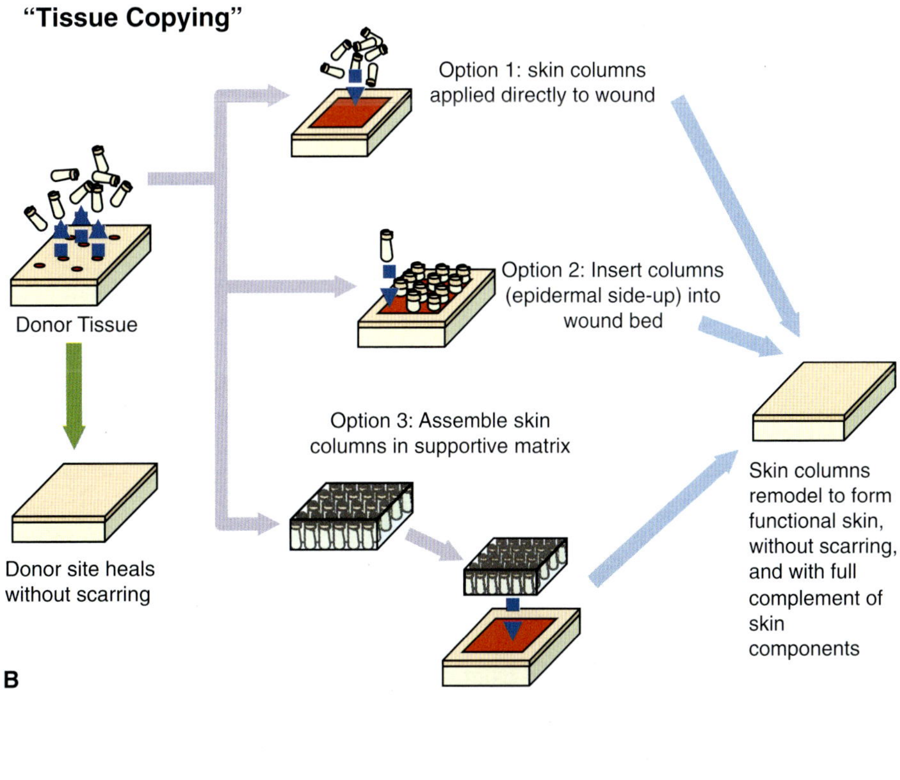

FIGURE 26-2 **A:** Diagrammatic representation of the concept of fractional photothermolysis. A small percentage of skin is ablated with penetrating microcolumns of thermal injury, and the surrounding untreated skin serves as a reservoir for expedited wound healing. **B:** Tissue copying concept. (*Figure 26-2A: Adapted from Kwan JM, Wyatt M, Uebelhoer NS, Pyo J, Shumaker PR. Functional improvement after ablative fractional laser treatment of a scar contracture. PM R. 2011;3(10):986–987.*)

to improve scars!), the same principle applied.[10,11] Fractional lasers cause thousands of narrow, deep skin burns that heal rapidly without scarring, even when a large fraction of the organ has been wounded.

The basic strategy for skin copying is to remove thousands of full-thickness, very thin columns of skin that can be used for grafting (see Fig. 26-2). Modified hypodermic needles remove a thin core of full-thickness skin, similar in size and shape to the channels made by a fractional ablative laser. As with fractional lasers, these full-thickness skin wounds heal quickly without scarring. Next, we studied how these full-thickness skin columns can be used as a graft, placing them randomly at about 10% area density on full-thickness skin wounds in swine. The wounds treated this way healed much faster than nongrafted wounds and were comparable to wounds grafted with split-thickness skin. At the skin donor site there was rapid healing, with no scarring grossly or histologically.[12] In subsequent work, we have engineered more automated, multiple-needle harvesting devices and confirmed that human skin can be "copied" this way onto immunosuppressed mice. Unlike split-thickness grafts, deep skin structures such as hair follicles and eccrine glands are transferred and there is no morbidity at the donor site. When implanted into matrix materials, the full-thickness human skin columns can remain viable for long periods of time. We surmise that this is because each small column, like a thin split-thickness graft, can live by diffusion until a blood supply is established. In some matrix materials, cells migrate out from epidermis and dermis of each column, eventually remodeling the matrix between adjacent columns (unpublished).

In the near future, we aim to integrate the following steps: rapidly harvest thousands of full-thickness skin columns from a donor site, which will subsequently heal without scarring; implant the columns right-side-up at an optimal density into an appropriate matrix material; provide a moisture barrier/dressing; and use the construct as if it were a full-thickness skin graft. Potentially, the presence of an ample "dose" of autologous full-thickness skin within a matrix material could stimulate wound healing by remodeling, rather than by scarring. Ideally, this strategy, or a similar one, could replace a wound with functional full-thickness skin with little or no scarring at either the wound or graft donor sites. Drugs, cells, and/or other tissues could conceivably also be added, and potentially, the tissue copying strategy is applicable to other organs as well.

Treatment of Scars

How nice it would be to turn scars into completely normal tissue! That capability would transform much of the practice of medicine because scarring affects almost every system of the body (see Chapter 3). Scars affect skin, fat, muscle, fascia, nerves, bone, and internal organs. After myocardial infarction, scars in the myocardium impair rhythm, valve, and pump functions. Spinal or nerve entrapment by scar tissue can be crippling. Postsurgical scarring sometimes leads to a life of pain. Fibrosis, the microscopic process that underlies scarring, also occurs from disease or toxic exposures in liver, lung, and other tissues. Again, how nice it would be to turn scars into completely normal tissue!

We are cautiously leaving an era of well-intentioned reconstructive surgery, in which hypertrophic cutaneous scars were treated as unwanted tumors. Removing scars is not a bad idea, if the subsequent rearrangement and/or skin grafts replacing the scar are well positioned and of the same skin variety and pigmentation. Unfortunately, this is often not the case for large scars. Also, unfortunately, we do not yet have a treatment that can transform scars into completely normal tissue. But, maybe it is possible. Good progress has been made with a handful of treatments that employ truly transformative medical and surgical strategies to somewhat normalize scars. This book is a great reference for that. Looking ahead, there may be wholly new approaches, with expected and unexpected synergy among the treatment strategies. As Prof. Matthias Donelan (Harvard) has noted, "All scars have a right to live" (see Chapter 12).

A deceptively simple example is the use of ablative fractional lasers or other energy-based devices in combination with locally applied or injected medications (see Chapter 14). The laser creates channels for drug delivery and dispersal, achieving orders of magnitude greater uptake than applying a topical medication to intact skin.[13] Drug-device combined treatment may also have unexpected time- and dose-dependent interactions. Drugs work by interacting with target molecules engaged in metabolic and signaling pathways; microscale injury substantially alters gene expressions. Small molecules such as corticosteroids, antimetabolites, prostaglandin modulators, and the like are already being delivered this way. Large molecules, cells, or even other nonskin tissue fragments can be delivered. A number of laboratories are exploring laser-delivered macromolecules including proteins, antiangiogenic agents, tumor necrosis factor (TNF) inhibitors, so-called biologic drugs, drug-eluting particles or polymers, small inhibitory RNAs, and oligonucleotides that stimulate or suppress specific pathways. For some molecules such as siRNA, cell membranes are a significant barrier to intracellular delivery. Electroporation and laser-initiated shock waves can permeabilize cells without necrosis. In the future, evidence-based use of devices and drugs is likely to be a winning combination for improving scars.

Simply adding stem or stem-like cells to a wound may also prove very helpful. The initial hope that stem cells would somehow miraculously differentiate into healthy new tissue has not yet been realized for wound treatment. Instead, stem cells appear to play a modulating role, regulating the immune response and the remodeling process. In a wound, tissue-resident stem cells are literally missing. In skin, hair follicles are richly endowed with epithelial stem cells. This is true even in "hairless" skin areas because of numerous vellus follicles. The stem cells create an immune-privileged "niche" by potently suppressing local cell-mediated immunity through the recruitment of regulatory T cells. Hair follicles are therefore immune privileged, and can even survive transplantation across a major histocompatibility mismatch. Scars are generally devoid of hair follicles. Could regeneration of hair follicles alone serve to settle down the chronic inflammation of a scar? Interestingly, spontaneous hair regrowth often occurs after fractional laser treatment of burn scars[14]—is the hair growth responsible for scar improvement, vice versa, or both? These questions are answerable.

The future is not what it used to be

—Paul Valery

How audacious we are, to pretend to know anything about the future! A hard-won or serendipitous discovery, by someone of whom we have never heard, could forever alter the way we approach wounds and scars. We hope so.

REFERENCES

1. Lichtman MK, Otero-Vinas M, Falanga V. Transforming growth factors beta (TGF-beta) isoforms in wound healing and fibrosis. *Wound Repair Regen*. 2016;24:215–222.
2. Penn JW, Grobbelaar AO, Rolfe KJ. The role of the TGF-beta family in wound healing, burns and scarring: a review. *Int J Burns Trauma*. 2012;2:18–28.
3. O'Kane S, Ferguson MW. Transforming growth factor r F-beta family in wound heal. *Int J Biochem Cell Biol*. 1997;29:63–78.
4. Ferguson MW, O'Kane S. Scar-free healing: from embryonic mechanisms to adult therapeutic intervention. *Philos Trans R Soc Lond B Biol Sci*. 2004;359:839–850.
5. MacNeil S. Progress and opportunities for tissue-engineered skin. *Nature*. 2007;445:874–880.
6. Hodde J. Naturally occurring scaffolds for soft tissue repair and regeneration. *Tissue Eng*. 2002;8:295–308.
7. Wilshaw SP, Kearney JN, Fisher J, et al. Production of an acellular amniotic membrane matrix for use in tissue engineering. *Tissue Eng*. 2006;12:2117–2129.
8. Wood FM, Giles N, Stevenson A, et al. Characterization of the cell suspension harvested from the dermal epidermal junction using a ReCell kit. Burns. 2012;38(1):44–51.
9. Navarro FA, Stoner ML, Park CS, et al. Sprayed keratinocyte suspensions accelerate epidermal coverage in a porcine microwound model. *J Burn Care Rehabil*. 2000;21:513–518.
10. Laubach HJ, Tannous Z, Anderson RR, et al. Skin responses to fractional photothermolysis. *Lasers Surg Med*. 2006;38:142–149.
11. Manstein D, Herron GS, Sink RK, et al. Fractional photothermolysis: a new concept for cutaneous remodeling using microscopic patterns of thermal injury. *Lasers Surg Med*. 2004;34:426–438.
12. Tam J, Wang Y, Farinelli WA, et al. Fractional skin harvesting: autologous skin grafting without donor-site morbidity. *Plast Reconstr Surg Glob Open*. 2013;1:e47.
13. Haedersdal M, Sakamoto FH, Farinelli WA, et al. Fractional CO(2) laser-assisted drug delivery. *Lasers Surg Med*. 2010;42:113–122.
14. Wu YF, Wang SH, Wu PS, et al. Enhancing hair follicle regeneration by nonablative fractional laser: assessment of irradiation parameters and tissue response. *Lasers Surg Med*. 2015;47:331–341.

27 Fetal Wound Healing

MICHAEL SUNG-MIN HU, TRIPP LEAVITT, MICHAEL T. LONGAKER, and H. PETER LORENZ

KEY POINTS

- Fetal cutaneous wounds in early gestation regenerate without the formation of a scar across mammalian species.
- Myriad differences in the extrinsic and intrinsic components of scarless fetal and scarring adult wound healing have been identified.
- Although the exact mechanism of fetal scarless wound regeneration remains unknown, recent advances in wound healing research hold promise for better understanding and recapitulating this phenomenon.

As discussed in other chapters, wound healing is a complex mechanism coordinated by multiple cell types involving numerous biologic pathways. It is highly evolved to protect against injury and infection. However, adult mammalian wound repair reproducibly results in the formation of a fibrotic scar. The resultant scar tissue quickly restores the epithelial barrier but is distinct from normal skin. Because of incomplete regeneration of the original tissue by a fibroproliferative response and an overproduction of poorly organized collagen, the resultant scar has a tensile strength that is less than 80% of its original form[1] (see Chapter 6). Scar tissue is further characterized by a flattened epidermis and loss of dermal appendages, such as hair follicles and sebaceous glands (see Chapter 5).[2] Humans are uniquely burdened with the ability to undergo pathologic scarring resulting in keloids or hypertrophic scars. These pathologic scars are characterized by an excessive deposition of collagen, sometimes extending beyond the original wound, resulting in a prominent scar often complicated by pain, itching, and/or devastating psychosocial consequences (see Chapters 9, 11, 19, and 24).[3]

However, the end result of wound healing depends on the developmental stage of the injured organism as well as the type of tissue damaged. A landmark manuscript in 1979 described that intrauterine wound healing in an early gestational human fetus does not result in scar formation.[4] Numerous studies since then have demonstrated fetal wound regeneration in early to mid-gestational fetal skin in both human and other mammalian models.[5–7] The transition from scarless wound regeneration to the postnatal scarring phenotype is dependent on gestational age and wound size, with larger wounds requiring an earlier gestational age to undergo regeneration.[3] This occurs at about 24 weeks of gestation in humans and around embryonic day 18.5 (E19) in mice (term = day 21.5 or E22).[8] Interestingly, the transition from regeneration to repair varies on the type of tissue. For example, myocardial regeneration occurs in neonatal mice until postnatal day 7.[9] In addition, oral mucosal wounds heal with little to no scar formation at an accelerated rate, even in the adult.[10–12]

Scarless fetal wound healing was initially thought to occur because of the environmental conditions; however, studies have demonstrated that the intrauterine environment is neither necessary nor sufficient for regeneration.[13] Instead, the capacity for regeneration is intrinsic to the tissue itself. Although the exact mechanisms underlying scarless fetal wound healing are yet unknown, understanding this privileged wound repair continues to be an area of investigatory interest with hopes of recapitulating this phenomenon in adult wound healing. Herein, we discuss the major differences in scarless mammalian cutaneous fetal wound healing as compared to scar-forming adult wound healing (Fig. 27-1).

Extrinsic Components of Fetal Wound Healing

To better understand the differences in wound healing capabilities in fetal and adult tissue, we classify contributions as extrinsic or intrinsic based on their relationship to the healing wound (Table 27-1). In terms of the differences between fetal and adult wound healing, extrinsic properties relate largely to the inflammatory response. The blunted inflammatory response observed in fetal wound healing tissue is understood to contribute to scarless wound healing. In this section we consider the cells that contribute to this inflammatory response, as well as the signaling molecules implicated in the process.

Inflammatory Cells

As in adult wound healing, circulating cells are recruited to the wound to initiate the inflammatory response. This

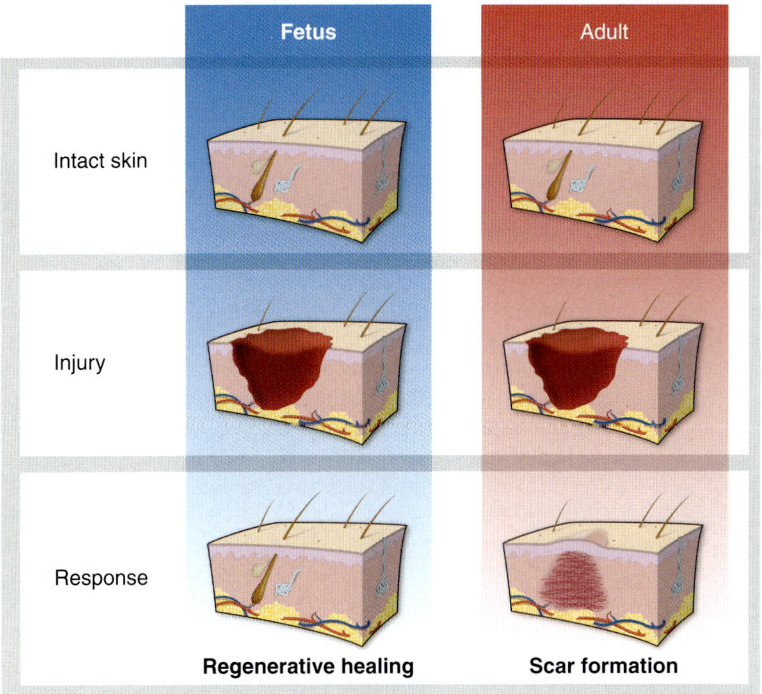

FIGURE 27-1

Table 27-1 Fetal versus Adult Wound Healing

	Fetal Healing	Adult Healing
Extrinsic Components		
Inflammatory cells	Low	High
TGF-β		
TGF-β1/2	Low	High
TGF-β3	High	Low
Interleukins		
IL-6, IL-8	Low	High
IL-10	High	Low
VEGF	Low	High
Intrinsic Components		
Rate of ECM synthesis	High	Low
Myofibroblasts	Absent	Present
Collagen		
Rate of deposition	Rapid	Delayed
Histologic pattern	Fine, reticular, large fibers	Dense, parallel, small fibers
Collagen type III:I ratio	High	Low
Cross-linking	Low	High
Hyaluronic acid		
Expression	High	Low
Receptors	High	Low
HASA	High	Low
ECM Modulators		
Fibromodulin	Increased	Decreased
Decorin	Decreased	Increased
Adhesion proteins	Rapid increase	Diminished increase
MMP:TIMP ratio	High	Low

TGF = Transforming Growth Factor; VEGF = Vascular Endothelial Growth Factor; ECM = Extracellular Matrix; HASA = Hyaluronic Acid Stimulating Activity; MMP = Matrix Metalloproteinase; TIMP = Tissue Inhibitor of Matrix Metalloproteinase

Adapted from Hu MS, Maan ZN, Wu JC, et al. Tissue engineering and regenerative repair in wound healing. *Ann Biomed Eng.* 2014;42(7):1497–1507.

sequence, beginning with neutrophils, followed by macrophages and mast cells, is maintained in fetal wound healing. It is in the magnitude and intensity of the inflammatory response that separates the privileged fetal wound from scar formation as seen in adult cutaneous wound repair.

Neutrophils

Neutrophil recruitment is usually initiated by platelet degranulation at the wound bed during initial hemostasis after wounding. It is, therefore, not surprising that the diminished inflammatory response in fetal wound healing is partly attributed to differences in platelet activity. Platelet morphology is consistent across fetal and adult tissues, but fetal platelets have been shown to produce lower levels of transforming growth factor β1 (TGF-β1) and platelet-derived growth factor.[14] They also demonstrate suboptimal aggregation in response to collagen prior to fetal transition from scarless healing to scar formation.[15] Tumor necrosis factor α (TNF-α) and interleukin-1 (IL-1) are also released during platelet degranulation. Together these molecules act as chemoattractants, directing circulating neutrophils to wounded dermal tissue. TNF-α and IL-1 also play a role in upregulating neutrophil adhesion molecules, which have been found to be much less abundant among fetal neutrophils.[16] Neutrophil migration to the fetal wound bed is limited by lower neutrophil–endothelial cell interactions secondary to attenuated adhesion molecule expression.[17,18] The absence of subpopulations of proinflammatory and anti-inflammatory neutrophils further differentiates the early stages of the fetal wound healing response from that found in adults.[19]

Macrophages

Macrophage localization to the wound bed follows neutrophil infiltration.[18] Persistent macrophage activity in wounds is thought to cause excess scar formation.[20] Studies of embryonic and fetal murine models demonstrate that macrophages are not recruited to wounds prior to gestational day 14 (E14.5), except in cases of substantial tissue damage.[21] Interestingly, fetal transition to scar formation occurs later at around E19 (term = E22).[8] Despite the potential for macrophage recruitment during this window period between E14.5 and E19, their activation remains diminished because of noticeably lower TGF-β1 levels.[22] This growth factor is in part responsible for the transition of circulating monocytes to activated macrophages. Conversely, TGF-β3 acts as a stop signal for terminal differentiation, and is at its peak concentration during the period of scarless fetal wound healing.[23,24] This favorable ratio of TGF-β1:β3 contributes to the privileged scarless wound healing phenotype.

Mast Cells

Mast cells are the third and final population to localize to the wound environment. The mast cell response is approximately halved in healing fetal tissues, and those that are recruited to the wound bed were noted to be more immature and less able to undergo degranulation. Fetal mast cells also release lower levels of inflammatory mediators including histamine, TGF-β, TNF-α, and vascular endothelial growth factor (VEGF), reducing neutrophil chemotaxis and extravasation.[25] Although mast cells were once thought to contribute to scar formation during fetal wound healing,[25] subsequent work has shown that they are not required for healing of cutaneous full-thickness excisional wounds in adult mice.[26]

Inflammatory Modulators

Regulation of inflammatory processes occurs throughout all phases of wound healing via the action of cytokines, some of which have been discussed previously. As with almost any process within the body, a balance is maintained through opposing forces. The same is true for wound healing with various cytokines acting as either agonists or antagonists to an inflammatory response. As alluded to previously, the general principle that differentiates scarless fetal wound healing from normal wound healing is that the balance is shifted in favor of an anti-inflammatory response. Key inflammatory modulators in wound healing include members of the TGF-β family, ILs, and VEGF.

Transforming Growth Factor β

Three isoforms of TGF-β exist[1,2,27] whose patterns of expression differ between adult and fetal wounds. Adult wounds demonstrate a greater quantity of TGF-β1 and TGF-β2, whereas TGF-β3 predominates in fetal wounds.[28] The finding that fetal wounds are relatively hypoxic compared to adult wounds suggests a potential role for hypoxia-inducible factor 1α in preferential TGF-β3 regulation.[29] In fact, elevated oxygen tensions have been shown to impede fetal fibroblasts.[30] TGF-β1 plays a major role in adult wound inflammation, stimulating chemotaxis in neutrophils, monocytes, and fibroblasts. The positive feedback loop generated by these infiltrating cells releasing further TGF-β1 is thus inhibited in fetal wounds, where there is a relative dearth of this proinflammatory cytokine. As mentioned previously, the TGF-β3 dominating the fetal wound response acts as a stop signal for terminal differentiation of tissue. Fetal cells at the wound bed may be held at a more immature state secondary to TGF-β3, with their less fully developed inflammatory machinery implicated in scarless healing in the fetus.

Interleukins

Similar to the TGF-β cytokine family, subtypes of ILs play antagonistic roles in the inflammatory response to acute wounding. Levels of IL-6 and IL-8, known proinflammatory signaling molecules highly expressed during adult wound healing, are diminished in the fetal wound.[18,31] IL-10, however, acts as an anti-inflammatory cytokine. Fetal wounds have been found to overexpress IL-10,[32] whereas its absence in fetal IL-10 knockout mice predisposes to scar formation that would otherwise not occur.[33] IL-10 inhibits proinflammatory expression of IL-1, IL-6, IL-8, and TNF-α[34]; it also inhibits inflammatory cell migration while allowing for normal collagen deposition and dermal architecture.[32]

Vascular Endothelial Growth Factor

VEGF is fundamental to angiogenesis in adult wound healing, but its upregulation has also been observed in association with keloid and hypertrophic scar development.[35–39] VEGF expression in fetal wound healing has been noted in some studies to be relatively tempered, resulting in fetal wounds that are less vascular than their fibrotic counterparts.[40] Our understanding of the exact role of VEGF in fetal wound healing is incomplete as results are not consistent across all studies. Colwell et al.[41] noted significant VEGF upregulation in scarless wound repair occurring in E16 fetal mice compared to scarring repair in E18. However, despite this finding, there was little difference in terms of neovascularization based on histologic findings. Beyond stimulation of angiogenesis, VEGF does act in a proinflammatory manner by increasing vascular permeability and promoting inflammatory cell infiltration of the wound bed. Antibody-mediated neutralization of VEGF resulted in up to a 75% reduction in scar width.[40] Taken together, these findings suggest that VEGF plays a multifactorial role in modulating wound healing, whether up- or downregulating scar-forming processes.

Intrinsic Components of Fetal Wound Healing

Successful wound healing and tissue regeneration is the result of complex interactions between cells at the wound bed and their surrounding environment, the extracellular matrix (ECM). No longer perceived as inert, the ECM is a dynamic network of fibrous adhesion proteins, proteoglycans, and glycosaminoglycans (GAG) critical to wound repair after injury. Cells such as fibroblasts work to synthesize the ECM around them, as well as remodel it. Though a product of these cells, the ECM in turn exerts a modulatory effect on its creators, through both molecular signals and mechanotransduction (see Chapter 7).

Extracellular Matrix

Although the muted inflammatory response seen in fetal wound healing greatly contributes to the scarless phenotype, this is only part of an even bigger picture. Within the wound bed itself, cells and tissue must be replaced or regenerated, a distinction that separates adult and fetal wound healing, respectively. In addition to cellular recruitment, the ECM must also be reestablished. Fetal wounds differ from their adult counterparts in this endeavor in terms of the subsets of cells that are recruited, their ensuing differentiation, as well as the composition, structure, and even rate of ECM formation and remodeling.

Rate of Deposition

In general terms, the formation of the ECM (and overall wound healing) is observed to occur at a faster rate in fetal tissues prior to the loss of the scarless wound healing phenotype. One reason for this observation is the unique ability of fetal fibroblasts to undergo proliferation while simultaneously secreting collagen. This is in contrast to adult fibroblasts, which necessitate delayed collagen synthesis following a separate proliferation step.[42]

Expedited ECM formation can also be partially attributed to the constituent molecules, particularly hyaluronic acid (HA). Increased levels of this GAG are associated with rapid cellular proliferation, motility, and dedifferentiation, as occurs in both adult and fetal wound healing. However, the fetal response demonstrates faster and more sustained HA deposition. Though adult wound healing also involves early HA deposition within the ECM, the initial increase is not as steep and is followed by a rapid decline.[43]

The intensity of adhesion molecule expression is another factor differentiating fetal wound healing from its adult counterpart. As mentioned previously, fetal neutrophils demonstrate relatively fewer adhesion molecules resulting in a more attenuated inflammatory response. The opposite can be said for adhesion molecules within the fetal wound ECM (such as fibronectin and tenascin), which are expressed early and to a greater extent than in adult wounds.[44] Fibronectin synthesis occurs within 4 hours of wounding during the early gestational period, whereas 12 hours is needed for its synthesis in adult wounds.[45,46] Together, rapid fibronectin and tenascin deposition stimulates early cell attachment and migration, respectively. This in turn promotes the formation of an organized wound matrix with diminished scarring.

Fibronectin and tenascin, as well as collagen, laminin, and other proteins of the fetal wound matrix, bind epidermal integrin receptors. Cass et al.[47] demonstrated that expression of these receptors by activated fetal keratinocytes near the wound edge rapidly increases during fetal healing; both the frequency of cells expressing integrin receptors and the number of receptors per cell were upregulated relative to adult wound healing. The early rise of β6-integrin receptor observed in this study was also inferred to play an important role in limiting the inflammatory response in fetal wounds. Later studies demonstrated that the prolonged expression of αvβ6 integrin with TGF-β3 was responsible for this effect, as TGF-β1 expression was also promoted by β6 integrin interactions early in scarless wound healing.[48] Overall, the delayed migration and collagen deposition observed in adult wounds is a likely instigator of scar formation.

Composition

Collagen is central to the structural integrity of the healing wound ECM. Though there are many types of collagen, type I is known to predominate in adult skin. Fetal skin differs from adult skin in that it contains more type III collagen, in addition to different cross-linking patterns (see Chapter 5). The ratio of type III to type I collagen mirrors the transition away from scarless wound healing, as type I collagen becomes more prevalent with increasing gestational age.[49–51] This finding was corroborated by analysis of procollagen levels. Murine procollagen 1α1 synthesis was decreased at mid-gestation (E15) and increased in late-gestational fibroblasts (E18); procollagen 3 expression was also diminished at the late gestational stage.[52]

As noted previously, the prevalence of HA is greater in the fetal wound matrix.[53] HA production is secondary to HA synthase activity, which is differentially regulated in fetal and adult fibroblasts via inflammatory cytokines.[54] This finding is important given the role of HA in collagen synthesis. HA has been demonstrated to upregulate type III collagen (and other noncollagen protein) deposition by fibroblasts, congruent with the greater type III:I ratio observed in the fetal dermis.[49,55] As with type III collagen, HA content within the ECM demonstrates a temporal decline beyond the late fetal period.[5]

Small leucine-rich proteoglycans (SLRPs) provide further contrasts between fetal and adult ECM. This heterogeneous group of polyanionic macromolecules, which includes decorin, biglycan, fibromodulin and lumican, covalently bind linear sulfated GAG chains (see Chapter 6). Abundant in connective tissue, these molecules interact with type I collagen to modulate fibrillogenesis and collagen turnover. Different patterns of expression are observed, with some SLRPs upregulated and others downregulated in fetal connective tissues; decorin production has been observed to increase by over 70% during the fetal transition to scar formation,[56] whereas chondroitin sulfate is present and absent in fetal and adult wounds, respectively.[45] One can infer from these findings that chondroitin sulfate is likely to be involved in scarless wound healing, whereas decorin and other sulfated GAGs are implicated more in scar formation. Fibromodulin is another proteoglycan implicated in scarless wound healing, functioning to inhibit collagen fibrillogenesis. Its induction was found to be significant prior to the ontogenetic transition to scar formation, but not in wounds made after this transition. Fibromodulin has been noted to bind and inactivate TGF-β, explaining its association with scarless wound healing.[22]

Architecture

The differences between adult and fetal wound matrices in terms of their rate of formation and biochemical/biologic composition result in structurally dissimilar extracellular matrices. Type III collagen, which predominates and is rapidly deposited in fetal wounds, is made up of finer fibers arranged in a reticular pattern akin to uninjured skin.[49] This is in contrast to the type I collagen in adult scar formation, which is arranged parallel to the skin surface in dense, parallel bundles. Fetal wounds also demonstrate less collagen cross-linking, providing for a less rigid ECM and reduced scar formation.[57]

Remodeling

Wound healing involves significant remodeling of the ECM with regard to its composition and organization; such processes are largely carried out by matrix metalloproteinases (MMPs), which in turn are regulated by tissue-derived inhibitors of metalloproteinases (TIMPs).[58,59] Compared to scar formation, scarless fetal wounds demonstrate a proclivity for MMP, rather than TIMP, expression. The environment of the fetal wound is thereby one of remodeling over collagen accumulation, a bias that is key to dictating the composition of the healing wound matrix.[60]

Mechanical Microenvironment

Within the ECM, cells are subjected to micromechanical forces which are understood to modulate cellular activity, including wound healing processes[61] (see Chapter 7). Mechanical reduction of wound tension has been demonstrated to significantly reduce scarring.[62] Conversely, tension at the wound site predisposes to scar formation, with evidence for mechanical stress via conformational ECM changes leading to fibroblast differentiation to myofibroblasts and activation of TGF-β1.[63] The extent to which fetal wound matrices may experience reduced extrinsic tension is not completely understood. However, wound closure in adult skin is attributed to myofibroblasts and wound contraction, whereas actin cables are responsible for fetal wound closure, which occurs in a purse-string fashion.[64–66] Moreover fetal fibroblasts, even when provided a stimulus such as prostaglandin E2, demonstrate relatively less contraction compared to their adult counterparts.[67]

Based on the observation of decreased tensile strength in early fetal skin, a study by Wong et al. elucidated focal adhesion kinase (FAK) as the pathway that ties mechanotransduction with fibrosis. By extracellular-related kinase (ERK), FAK activates monocyte chemoattractant protein-1 (MCP-1). The inflammatory FAK–ERK–MCP-1 pathway is associated with a number of human fibrotic disorders.[68] By knocking out or inhibiting various components of this pathway, scar formation is attenuated.[69] This work has recently translated into a stress-shielding clinical device that has been shown in two randomized controlled clinical trials to reduce scar formation.[70,71]

Fibroblasts

Fibroblast activity offers another important point of distinction between fetal and adult wound healing. Fetal fibroblasts are observed to proliferate faster[72] and produce more total collagen, with a higher proportion of type III and IV collagen, in comparison to adult fibroblasts. Fibroblast expression of the rate-limiting enzyme of collagen synthesis, prolyl hydroxylase, is demonstrably higher in early gestation as opposed to late gestation and beyond.[73]

As stated previously, collagen synthesis in fetal wound healing outpaces that of adults, a finding associated with modulation of discoid domain receptor (DDR) expression. This family of tyrosine kinases binds collagen fibers, regulating cellular proliferation, differentiation, and wound healing. In early gestational fetal fibroblasts, DDR-1 cell surface expression is increased. DDR-1 expression then proceeds to decrease with gestational age, whereas DDR-2 expression is steady throughout fetal maturation.[74] Variable presentation of DDR-1 cell surface receptors is another means by which collagen production can be regulated in a manner that leads to tissue regeneration rather than scar formation.[73]

Fetal fibroblasts also demonstrate greater numbers of HA receptors at the cell surface, as much as quadruple the quantity found in adult cells.[75] The greater HA receptor density facilitates faster fibroblast migration in fetal tissues without impeding HA production, resulting in increased cell density and accelerated wound repair. TGF-β1 also mitigates fibroblast migration secondary to its inhibition of HA synthesis, demonstrating its implications in scar formation beyond promoting an inflammatory response.[76]

The relative absence of contractile myofibroblasts in scarless wounds further differentiates the corresponding fetal and adult processes. Although fetal fibroblasts have been demonstrated to differentiate into myofibroblasts in response to TGF-β1, this response is more abrupt than in postnatal cells.[77] This coincides with the observed correlation between myofibroblast activity, contraction, and degree of scarring not seen with early gestational wound healing.[78] Furthermore, collagen fibers are oriented in the plane of the wound along the vector of myofibroblast contraction.[79,80] Their contraction may thus contribute to scar formation by distorting collagen fiber architecture.

Recent advances in developmental biology, via lineage tracing and transplantation, have allowed researchers to identify cells that contribute to scarring. Work by Dulauroy et al.[81] identified a proinflammatory subset of perivascular cells that are activated upon acute injury in muscle and dermis using transient expression of a disintegrin and metalloproteinase 12 (ADAM12). Scarring and fibrosis were decreased by ablating these cells or knocking down ADAM12. Building upon these techniques, Rinkevich et al.[82] identified a subpopulation of dermal fibroblasts, derived from Engrailed-1 (En1)-expressing progenitors, responsible for connective tissue deposition during late embryonic development and cutaneous wound healing. Using flow cytometry, dipeptidyl peptidase-4 (DPP4) was identified as a surface marker for this lineage. Inhibition of DPP4 enzymatic activity with diprotin A resulted in decreased scarring. Moreover, the authors showed that this subpopulation of fibroblasts are responsible for radiation fibrosis and melanoma–stroma formation, suggesting roles in both acute and chronic forms of fibroses (see Chapter 3). Identification, isolation, and depletion of the fibroblasts representing the cellular "culprits" of scarring hold promise for decreasing fibroses in skin and other organs.

Oral Wound Healing

As previously discussed, adult oral mucosal wound healing results in minimal scar formation resembling fetal wound healing. Like fetal repair, oral mucosa heals at an accelerated rate.[10,12,83–85] Interestingly, fibroproliferative scars, such as keloids and hypertrophic scars, rarely develop in the oral cavity.[86] In contrast to the rather extensive literature on fetal scarless wound healing, relatively few studies have investigated the privileged repair of the oral mucosal wound and the mechanisms underlying this process. Recently, several animal models of oral mucosal wound healing have provided overwhelming support of the relationship between rapid wound closure and reduced scar formation.[12,37,86,87] As in fetal scarless repair, both extrinsic and intrinsic factors of the oral mucosal wound response are thought to contribute to the scarless repair. These include saliva in the oral environment, a less robust inflammatory response, differential growth factor expression, muted angiogenesis, distinct fibroblast subpopulations, and increased capacity for ECM reorganization and remodeling.[12,36,83,87–89] Further investigation of oral mucosal wound repair promises novel insights into the mystery of fetal mammalian wound healing.

Conclusions

The past two decades have seen significant advances in wound healing. These include new technologies such as negative pressure wound therapy, skin substitutes, etc. Most recently, breakthroughs in stem cell biology and understanding fibroses (including wound repair) have been reported. With such advances, we inch toward an improved understanding of fetal mammalian wound healing and recapitulating scarless regeneration of skin.

REFERENCES

1. Gurtner GC, Werner S, Barrandon Y, et al. Wound repair and regeneration. *Nature*. 2008;453(7193):314–321.
2. Singer AJ, Clark RA. Cutaneous wound healing. *N Engl J Med*. 1999;341(10):738–746.
3. Cass DL, Bullard KM, Sylvester KG, et al. Wound size and gestational age modulate scar formation in fetal wound repair. *J Pediatr Surg*. 1997;32(3):411–415.
4. Rowlatt U. Intrauterine wound healing in a 20 week human fetus. *Virchows Arch A Pathol Anat Histol*. 1979;381(3):353–361.
5. Adzick NS, Longaker MT. Animal models for the study of fetal tissue repair. *J Surg Res*. 1991;51(3): 216–222.
6. Lorenz HP, Longaker MT, Perkocha LA, et al. Scarless wound repair: a human fetal skin model. *Development*. 1992;114(1):253–259.
7. Adzick NS, Longaker MT. Scarless fetal healing. Therapeutic implications. *Ann Surg*. 1992;215(1):3–7.
8. Colwell AS, Krummel TM, Longaker MT, et al. An in vivo mouse excisional wound model of scarless healing. *Plast Reconstr Surg*. 2006;117(7):2292–2296.
9. Aurora AB, Porrello ER, Mahmoud AI, et al. Macrophages are required for neonatal heart regeneration. *J Clin Invest*. 2014;124(3):1382–1392.
10. Sciubba JJ, Waterhouse JP, Meyer J. A fine structural comparison of the healing of incisional wounds of mucosa and skin. *J Oral Pathol*. 1978;7(4):214–227.
11. Stephens P, Davies KJ, Occleston N, et al. Skin and oral fibroblasts exhibit phenotypic differences in extracellular matrix reorganization and matrix metalloproteinase activity. *Br J Dermatol*. 2001;144(2):229–237.
12. Szpaderska AM, Zuckerman JD, DiPietro LA. Differential injury responses in oral mucosal and cutaneous wounds. *J Dent Res*. 2003;82(8):621–626.
13. Longaker MT, Whitby DJ, Ferguson MW, et al. Adult skin wounds in the fetal environment heal with scar formation. *Ann Surg*. 1994;219(1):65–72.
14. Olutoye OO, Barone EJ, Yager DR, et al. Collagen induces cytokine release by fetal platelets: implications in scarless healing. *J Pediatr Surg*. 1997;32(6):827–830.
15. Olutoye OO, Alaish SM, Carr ME Jr, et al. Aggregatory characteristics and expression of the collagen adhesion receptor in fetal porcine platelets. *J Pediatr Surg*. 1995;30(12):1649–1653.
16. Naik-Mathuria B, Gay AN, Zhu X, et al. Age-dependent recruitment of neutrophils by fetal endothelial cells: implications in scarless wound healing. *J Pediatr Surg*. 2007;42(1):166–171.
17. Olutoye OO, Zhu X, Cass DL, et al. Neutrophil recruitment by fetal porcine endothelial cells: implications in scarless fetal wound healing. *Pediatr Res*. 2005;58(6):1290–1294.
18. Satish L, Kathju S. Cellular and molecular characteristics of scarless versus fibrotic wound healing. *Dermatol Res Pract*. 2010;2010:790234.
19. Arnardottir HH, Freysdottir J, Hardardottir I. Two circulating neutrophil populations in acute inflammation in mice. *Inflamm Res*. 2012;61(9):931–939.
20. Robson MC, Barnett RA, Leitch IO, et al. Prevention and treatment of postburn scars and contracture. *World J Surg*. 1992;16(1):87–96.
21. Hopkinson-Woolley J, Hughes D, Gordon S, et al. Macrophage recruitment during limb development and wound healing in the embryonic and foetal mouse. *J Cell Sci*. 1994;107(Pt 5): 1159–1167.
22. Soo C, Hu FY, Zhang X, et al. Differential expression of fibromodulin, a transforming growth factor-beta modulator, in fetal skin development and scarless repair. *Am J Pathol*. 2000;157(2):423–433.
23. Caniggia I, Mostachfi H, Winter J, et al. Hypoxia-inducible factor-1 mediates the biological effects of oxygen on human trophoblast differentiation through TGFbeta(3). *J Clin Invest*. 2000;105(5):577–587.
24. Barrientos S, Stojadinovic O, Golinko MS, et al. Growth factors and cytokines in wound healing. *Wound Repair Regen*. 2008;16(5):585–601.
25. Wulff BC, Parent AE, Meleski MA, et al. Mast cells contribute to scar formation during fetal wound healing. *J Invest Dermatol*. 2012;132(2):458–465.
26. Nauta AC, Grova M, Montoro DT, et al. Evidence that mast cells are not required for healing of splinted cutaneous excisional wounds in mice. *PLoS One*. 2013;8(3):e59167.
27. Shih B, Garside E, McGrouther DA, et al. Molecular dissection of abnormal wound healing processes resulting in keloid disease. *Wound Repair Regen*. 2010;18(2):139–153.
28. Soo C, Beanes SR, Hu FY, et al. Ontogenetic transition in fetal wound transforming growth factor-beta regulation correlates with collagen organization. *Am J Pathol*. 2003;163(6):2459–2476.
29. Scheid A, Wenger RH, Schäffer L, et al. Physiologically low oxygen concentrations in fetal skin regulate hypoxia-inducible factor 1 and transforming growth factor-beta3. *FASEB J*. 2002;16(3):411–413.
30. Balin AK, Pratt L. Oxygen modulates the growth of skin fibroblasts. *In Vitro Cell Dev Biol Anim*. 2002;38(5):305–310.
31. Liechty KW, Adzick NS, Crombleholme TM. Diminished interleukin 6 (IL-6) production during scarless human fetal wound repair. *Cytokine*. 2000;12(6):671–676.
32. Peranteau WH, Zhang L, Muvarak N, et al. IL-10 overexpression decreases inflammatory mediators and promotes regenerative healing in an adult model of scar formation. *J Invest Dermatol*. 2008;128(7):1852–1860.
33. Liechty KW, Kim HB, Adzick NS, et al. Fetal wound repair results in scar formation in interleukin-10-deficient mice in a syngeneic murine model of scarless fetal wound repair. *J Pediatr Surg*. 2000;35(6):866–872; discussion 872-3.
34. Couper KN, Blount DG, Riley EM. IL-10: the master regulator of immunity to infection. *J Immunol*. 2008;180(9):5771–5777.
35. Amadeu T, Braune A, Mandarim-de-Lacerda C, et al. Vascularization pattern in hypertrophic scars and keloids: a stereological analysis. *Pathol Res Pract*. 2003;199(7):469–473.
36. Mak K, Manji A, Gallant-Behm C, et al. Scarless healing of oral mucosa is characterized by faster resolution of inflammation and control of myofibroblast action compared to skin wounds in the red Duroc pig model. *J Dermatol Sci*. 2009;56(3):168–180.
37. Mogili NS, Krishnaswamy VR, Jayaraman M, et al. Altered angiogenic balance in keloids: a key to therapeutic intervention. *Transl Res*. 2012;159(3):182–189.
38. van der Veer WM, Niessen FB, Ferreira JA, et al. Time course of the angiogenic response during normotrophic and hypertrophic scar formation in humans. *Wound Repair Regen*. 2011;19(3):292–301.
39. Wilgus TA. Immune cells in the healing skin wound: influential players at each stage of repair. *Pharmacol Res*. 2008;58(2):112–116.
40. Wilgus TA, Ferreira AM, Oberyszyn TM, et al. Regulation of scar formation by vascular endothelial growth factor. *Lab Invest*. 2008;88(6):579–590.

41. Colwell AS, Beanes SR, Soo C, et al. Increased angiogenesis and expression of vascular endothelial growth factor during scarless repair. *Plast Reconstr Surg*. 2005;115(1):204–212.
42. Larson BJ, Longaker MT, Lorenz HP. Scarless fetal wound healing: a basic science review. *Plast Reconstr Surg*. 2010;126(4):1172–1180.
43. Longaker MT, Chiu ES, Adzick NS, et al. Studies in fetal wound healing. V. A prolonged presence of hyaluronic acid characterizes fetal wound fluid. *Ann Surg*. 1991;213(4):292–296.
44. Whitby DJ, Longaker MT, Harrison MR, et al. Rapid epithelialisation of fetal wounds is associated with the early deposition of tenascin. *J Cell Sci*. 1991;99(Pt 3):583–586.
45. Whitby DJ, Ferguson MW. The extracellular matrix of lip wounds in fetal, neonatal and adult mice. *Development*. 1991;112(2):651–668.
46. Longaker MT, Whitby DJ, Jennings RW, et al. Fetal diaphragmatic wounds heal with scar formation. *J Surg Res*. 1991;50(4):375–385.
47. Cass DL, Bullard KM, Sylvester KG, et al. Epidermal integrin expression is upregulated rapidly in human fetal wound repair. *J Pediatr Surg*. 1998;33(2):312–316.
48. Eslami A, Gallant-Behm CL, Hart DA, et al. Expression of integrin alphavbeta6 and TGF-beta in scarless vs scar-forming wound healing. *J Histochem Cytochem*. 2009;57(6):543–557.
49. Longaker MT, Whitby DJ, Adzick NS, et al. Studies in fetal wound healing, VI. Second and early third trimester fetal wounds demonstrate rapid collagen deposition without scar formation. *J Pediatr Surg*. 1990;25(1):63–68; discussion 68-9.
50. Burd DA, Longaker MT, Adzick NS, et al. Fetal wound healing in a large animal model: the deposition of collagen is confirmed. *Br J Plast Surg*. 1990;43(5):571–577.
51. Merkel JR, DiPaolo BR, Hallock GG, et al. Type I and type III collagen content of healing wounds in fetal and adult rats. *Proc Soc Exp Biol Med*. 1988;187(4):493–497.
52. Carter R, Jain K, Sykes V, et al. Differential expression of procollagen genes between mid- and late-gestational fetal fibroblasts. *J Surg Res*. 2009;156(1):90–94.
53. Hu MS, Maan ZN, Rennert RC, et al. Tissue engineering and regenerative repair in wound healing. *Ann Biomed Eng*. 2014;42(7):1494–1507.
54. Kennedy CI, Diegelmann RF, Haynes JH, et al. Proinflammatory cytokines differentially regulate hyaluronan synthase isoforms in fetal and adult fibroblasts. *J Pediatr Surg*. 2000;35(6):874–879.
55. Mast BA, Diegelmann RF, Krummel TM, et al. Hyaluronic acid modulates proliferation, collagen and protein synthesis of cultured fetal fibroblasts. *Matrix*. 1993;13(6):441–446.
56. Beanes SR, Dang C, Soo C, et al. Down-regulation of decorin, a transforming growth factor-beta modulator, is associated with scarless fetal wound healing. *J Pediatr Surg*. 2001;36(11):1666–1671.
57. Lovvorn HN 3rd, Cheung DT, Nimni ME, et al. Relative distribution and crosslinking of collagen distinguish fetal from adult sheep wound repair. *J Pediatr Surg*. 1999;34(1):218–223.
58. Madlener M. Differential expression of matrix metalloproteinases and their physiological inhibitors in acute murine skin wounds. *Arch Dermatol Res*. 1998;290 suppl:S24–S29.
59. Parks WC. Matrix metalloproteinases in repair. *Wound Repair Regen*. 1999;7(6):423–432.
60. Dang CM, Beanes SR, Lee H, et al. Scarless fetal wounds are associated with an increased matrix metalloproteinase-to-tissue-derived inhibitor of metalloproteinase ratio. *Plast Reconstr Surg*. 2003;111(7):2273–2285.
61. Huang C, Leavitt T, Bayer LR, et al. Effect of negative pressure wound therapy on wound healing. *Curr Probl Surg*. 2014;51(7):301–331.
62. Wong VW, Beasley B, Zepeda J, et al. A Mechanomodulatory Device to Minimize Incisional Scar Formation. *Adv Wound Care (New Rochelle)*. 2013;2(4):185–194.
63. Wipff PJ, Rifkin DB, Meister JJ, et al. Myofibroblast contraction activates latent TGF-beta1 from the extracellular matrix. *J Cell Biol*. 2007;179(6):1311–1323.
64. Martin P, Lewis J. Actin cables and epidermal movement in embryonic wound healing. *Nature*. 1992;360(6400):179–183.
65. Brock J, Midwinter K, Lewis J, et al. Healing of incisional wounds in the embryonic chick wing bud: characterization of the actin purse-string and demonstration of a requirement for Rho activation. *J Cell Biol*. 1996;135(4):1097–1107.
66. Yates CC, Hebda P, Wells A. Skin wound healing and scarring: fetal wounds and regenerative restitution. *Birth Defects Res C Embryo Today*. 2012;96(4):325–333.
67. Parekh A, Sandulache VC, Singh T, et al. Prostaglandin E2 differentially regulates contraction and structural reorganization of anchored collagen gels by human adult and fetal dermal fibroblasts. *Wound Repair Regen*. 2009;17(1):88–98.
68. Wynn TA. Cellular and molecular mechanisms of fibrosis. *J Pathol*. 2008;214(2):199–210.
69. Wong VW, Rustad KC, Akaishi S, et al. Focal adhesion kinase links mechanical force to skin fibrosis via inflammatory signaling. *Nat Med*. 2012;18(1):148–152.
70. Longaker MT, Rohrich RJ, Greenberg L, et al. A randomized controlled trial of the embrace advanced scar therapy device to reduce incisional scar formation. *Plast Reconstr Surg*. 2014;134(3):536–546.
71. Lim AF, Weintraub J, Kaplan EN, et al. The embrace device significantly decreases scarring following scar revision surgery in a randomized controlled trial. *Plast Reconstr Surg*. 2014;133(2):398–405.
72. Nodder S, Martin P. Wound healing in embryos: a review. *Anat Embryol (Berl)*. 1997;195(3):215–228.
73. Bullard KM, Longaker MT, Lorenz HP. Fetal wound healing: current biology. *World J Surg*. 2003;27(1):54–61.
74. Chin GS, Lee S, Hsu M, et al. Discoidin domain receptors and their ligand, collagen, are temporally regulated in fetal rat fibroblasts in vitro. *Plast Reconstr Surg*. 2001;107(3):769–776.
75. Alaish SM, Yager D, Diegelmann RF, et al. Biology of fetal wound healing: hyaluronate receptor expression in fetal fibroblasts. *J Pediatr Surg*. 1994;29(8):1040–1043.
76. Ellis IR, Schor SL. Differential effects of TGF-beta1 on hyaluronan synthesis by fetal and adult skin fibroblasts: implications for cell migration and wound healing. *Exp Cell Res*. 1996;228(2):326–333.
77. Rolfe KJ, Richardson J, Vigor C, et al. A role for TGF-beta1-induced cellular responses during wound healing of the non-scarring early human fetus? *J Invest Dermatol*. 2007;127(11):2656–2667.
78. Estes JM, Vande Berg JS, Adzick NS, et al. Phenotypic and functional features of myofibroblasts in sheep fetal wounds. *Differentiation*. 1994;56(3):173–181.
79. Ferdman AG, Yannas IV. Scattering of light from histologic sections: a new method for the analysis of connective tissue. *J Invest Dermatol*. 1993;100(5):710–716.
80. Yannas IV. Similarities and differences between induced organ regeneration in adults and early foetal regeneration. *J R Soc Interface*. 2005;2(5):403–417.
81. Dulauroy S, Di Carlo SE, Langa F, et al. Lineage tracing and genetic ablation of ADAM12(+) perivascular cells identify a major source of profibrotic cells during acute tissue injury. *Nat Med*. 2012;18(8):1262–1270.
82. Rinkevich Y, Walmsley GG, Hu MS, et al. Skin fibrosis. Identification and isolation of a dermal lineage with intrinsic fibrogenic potential. *Science*. 2015;348(6232):aaa2151.
83. Hakkinen L, Uitto VJ, Larjava H. Cell biology of gingival wound healing. *Periodontol 2000*. 2000;24:127–152.
84. Szpaderska AM, Walsh CG, Steinberg MJ, et al. Distinct patterns of angiogenesis in oral and skin wounds. *J Dent Res*. 2005;84(4):309–314.
85. Ferguson MW, O'Kane S. Scar-free healing: from embryonic mechanisms to adult therapeutic intervention. *Philos Trans R Soc Lond B Biol Sci*. 2004;359(1445):839–850.
86. Wong JW, Gallant-Behm C, Wiebe C, et al. Wound healing in oral mucosa results in reduced scar formation as compared with skin: evidence from the red Duroc pig model and humans. *Wound Repair Regen*. 2009;17(5):717–729.
87. Schrementi ME, Ferreira AM, Zender C, et al. Site-specific production of TGF-beta in oral mucosal and cutaneous wounds. *Wound Repair Regen*. 2008;16(1):80–86.
88. Hakkinen L, Strassburger S, Kähäri VM, et al. A role for decorin in the structural organization of periodontal ligament. *Lab Invest*. 2000;80(12):1869–1880.
89. Schor SL, Ellis I, Irwin CR, et al. Subpopulations of fetal-like gingival fibroblasts: characterisation and potential significance for wound healing and the progression of periodontal disease. *Oral Dis*. 1996;2(2):155–166.

28 Clinical Scar Research: Quantitative and Qualitative Assessment of Hypertrophic Burn Scars

PAUL DIEGIDIO and C. SCOTT HULTMAN

KEY POINTS

- To familiarize researchers with some of the most common clinical scar assessment methods.
- To introduce three of the most frequently used instruments for measuring and tracking changes in scar quality: the Chroma Meter, Ultrasound, and Cutometer.
- To discuss the aspects of clinical trial design.
- To discuss current gaps in knowledge about scar treatment.
- To discuss what the ideal scar assessment tool/study would need to be included in order to address current gaps in knowledge.

When beginning a new clinical trial for burn scars, it behooves the researcher to first determine how they will assess the scar, how to incorporate subjective data (how the patient feels about the scar pre- and posttreatment), in what ways will the scar be objectively measured, and how the study design will integrate the data being collected into meaningful research. Without a predetermined series of before and after measurements, it is impossible to determine what change, beneficial or otherwise, occurred as a result of the intervention. This chapter will cover some of the most frequently used methodologies in current clinical scar research. Upon finishing this chapter, readers should be able to discuss aspects of scar research and understand the instrumentation and methodology seen in the literature. This chapter is aimed at both novice and expert scar "caretakers" who may be interested in more fully understanding the literature or potentially starting research of their own. As detailed below, ongoing research in scar care continues to advance the spectrum of our treatment modalities. However, knowledge gaps about timing of therapy initiation and ideal type, course, and length of therapy (based on scar characteristics, skin type, type of initial injury, age of scar, etc.) continue to persist. Further, most published scar scales are generally lacking in one area or another, and a comprehensive scar assessment scale does not yet exist. The challenge of mastering each individual scar measurement system may seem an arduous task, but we will attempt to give readers an edge in appreciating these topics, to avoid costly pitfalls, such as time-consuming protocol revisions, in the planning and execution of their research. Conceivably, efforts spent learning the basics in this chapter will save time, energy, and money in the long run; perhaps this is best stated or rephrased by Lewis[1]: "The longest way round is the shortest way home."

PEARL 28-1 *Clinical trial design can seem daunting at first; however, when approached in a stepwise manner and pursued with diligence and patience, it can be extremely rewarding. As food for thought, there is a discussion at the end of the chapter detailing recent advances in clinical treatment, some gaps in research that still need to be addressed, and some pointers on how to set up the "ideal" research study. Begin by identifying key points where collaborators are needed and think about how you would set up a trial like this at your own institution.*

Section 1: Clinical Scar Assessment

Currently, there are over a dozen high-quality, validated, and published scar scales. Modifications and revisions to these scales continue to produce additional versions available to researchers. In a review article by Nguyen et al.,[2] the authors assessed the Vancouver Scar Scale (VSS), a Modified Vancouver Scar Scale, Seattle Scale, Manchester Scar Scale, Hamilton Scale, Patient and Observer Scar Assessment Scale (POSAS), a Modified Patient and Observer Scar Assessment

	VSS	Modified VSS	Seattle Scale	MSS	Hamilton Scale	POSAS	Modified POSAS	MAPS	SBSES	UNC4P	VAS	DIQI
Scar description												
Type												
Age												
Surface area			●			●	●		●			
Height/thickness/ contour	●	●	●	●	●	●	●	●	●			
Anatomic location								●				
Erythema	●	●				●	●					
Pigmentation	●	●	●	●	●	●	●	●	●			
Disruption of anatomic cosmetic units												
Scar comorbidities												
Psychosocial												●
Reaction of others												●
Hypertrichosis												
Hyperhidrosis/ hypohidrosis												
Pain		●				●	●			●	●	●
Pruritus		●				●	●			●		●
Dysesthesia										●		
Infection												
lymphedema												
Chronic wound/ ulceration												
Skin cancer												
Functional impairment							●			●		●
overall appearance patient						●	●					
overall appearance observer						●	●		●			
Amenability to treatment												
Validity	●	●		●		●	●		●		●	●

FIGURE 28-1 Comparison of different parameters including currently available scar scales. DLQI, Dermatology Life Quality Index; MAPS, Matching Assessment of Scars and Photographs; MSS, Manchester Scar Scale; PSOAS, Patient and Observer Scar Assessment Scale; SBES, Stony Brook Scar Evaluation Scale; UNC4P, University of North Carolina "4P" Scar Scale; VAS, Visual Analog Scale; VSS, Vancouver Scar Scale. *(From Nguyen TA, Feldstein SI, Shumaker PR, et al. A review of scar assessment scales.* Semin Cutan Med Surg. 2015;34:28–36.*)*

Scale, Matching Assessment of Scars and Photographs, Stony Brook Scar Evaluation Scale, University of North Carolina "4P" (UNC-4P) Scar Scale, the Visual Analog Scale, and the Dermatology Life Quality Index (Fig. 28-1). This review provides a helpful comparison of the scales related to different components of these scars, functional impairment, and quality of life. In their evaluation of these scales, the authors proposed what components would constitute a comprehensive scale. However, to date, there is not a single burn scar scale that captures all of these components effectively. Our review, which follows, selects several of the most commonly used scar scales, which can be combined, so that researchers can accurately describe a hypertrophic burn scar, communicate this with their colleagues, and report data that are consistent, accurate, and reliable.

Prior to starting the discussion on each scale and what they measure, it is worth noting that most of the scales in current use combine varying degrees of subjective and objective data. The latter is generally measured by clinicians and includes parameters such as scar height, depth, discoloration, etc., on previously validated scales. There is a small but present subjective component measured by clinicians (i.e., the "overall opinion" section of Observer Scar Assessment Scale), though the vast majority of subjective information is gathered from patients. Most published literature relies on statistically significant changes in objectively measured variables, and the initial study design may focus on finding which scar scale will have the best objective data collected at the end of the study. However, overlooking the subjective portion of outcomes research would be a grave mistake. Patient care lies at the core of this research, and improving quality of life for individuals who have posttraumatic/postsurgical symptomatic scars is paramount. Pay special attention to the subjective data gathered in the following discussion on scar scales in order to genuinely understand what is being measured and, far more importantly, why.

Vancouver Scar Scale

Initially developed in 1990 as the Burn Scar Index by Sullivan et al.,[3] this scoring system has become one of the cornerstones of scar evaluation. The VSS measures the scar in four distinct ways and assigns numerical values to the individual characteristics to produce a final score that ranges from 0 to 13:

- Pigmentation
  - Normal = 0
  - Hypopigmented = 1
  - Hyperpigmented = 2
- Vascularity
  - Normal = 0
  - Pink = 1
  - Red = 2
  - Purple = 3
- Pliability
  - Normal = 0
  - Supple = 1
  - Yielding/gives way to pressure = 2
  - Firm/inflexible = 3
  - Banding with rope-like tissues that blanches with extension of the scar = 4
  - Contracture with permanent shortening of the scar causing deformity and distortion = 5
- Height
  - Normal = 0
  - <2 mm = 1
  - 2 to 5 mm = 2
  - >5 mm = 3

The normal for each category is based on the surrounding unaffected skin or contralateral skin (when available), that is, burned left forearm compared to normal right forearm.

Because of some limitations related to observer bias, the VSS has also been modified to specifically study individual populations.[4] For instance, when assessing pediatric burn patients with varying baseline skin color, Forbes-Duchart and colleagues[5] modified the Vascularity index to a 6-point scale (normal = 0, pink = 1, pink to red = 2, red = 3, red to purple = 4, purple = 5) and further printed this scale on a clear Plexiglas tool (initially developed by Baryza and Baryza[6]) to arrive at the resultant 0- to 15-point VSS that they used to evaluate their pediatric burn scar population. This new scoring system was evaluated using inter-rater reliability methodology to ensure ease of use and reproducibility, which should be done with any modification to current scoring systems, as well as validation with current literature.

Patient and Observer Scar Assessment Scale

In 2004 Draaijers et al.[7] introduced POSAS as a new, reliable tool for scar evaluation. This scale consists of the Observer Scar Assessment Scale (OSAS) and the Patient Scar Assessment Scale (PSAS), to be completed by the clinician and patient, respectively. Both of these scales use a 1- to 10-point scoring system for each variable, with 1 = normal skin and 10 = worst scar imaginable (with six variables in either PSAS or OSAS; overall scores range from 6 to 60). At the end of either scale, both the observer and the patient are asked to rank their overall opinion of the scar, as it relates to normal skin. The clinician rates six categories, each from 1 to 10, with further descriptors embedded therein that the clinician can select to delineate the specific deformity within each category against comparable normal skin:

- Vascularity
  - Pale
  - Pink
  - Red
  - Purple
  - Mixed
- Pigmentation
  - Hypopigmented
  - Hyperpigmented
  - Mixed
- Thickness
  - Thicker
  - Thinner
- Relief/irregularity
  - More relief/irregularity
  - Less relief/irregularity
  - Mixed
- Pliability
  - Supple
  - Stiff
  - Mixed
- Surface Area
  - Expansion
  - Contraction
  - Mixed
- Overall Opinion
  - Clinician subjectively rates on a scale of 1 to 10 what their opinion of this scar is.

Patients/subjects are asked to fill out the PSAS, which differs from the OSAS in that it asks subjective questions about how the patient feels about their scar, and rates them as 1 = no/normal and 10 = yes/different than normal:

- "Has the scar been painful the past few weeks?"
- "Has the scar been itching the past few weeks?"
- "Is the scar color different from the color of your normal skin at present?"
- "Is the stiffness of the scar different from your normal skin at present?"
- "Is the thickness of the scar different from your normal skin at present?"
- "Is the scar more irregular than your normal skin at present?"
- And finally, "What is your overall opinion of the scar compared to normal skin?"[8]

Patient-Reported Outcomes Information Management System

Developed by the National Institutes of Health, Patient-Reported Outcomes Information Management System (PROMIS) is "... a system of highly reliable, precise measures of patient-reported health status for physical, mental, and social well-being."[9] With a myriad of available surveys, questionnaires, scales, and rating systems available to physician-scientists, PROMIS serves as a centralized hub to measure patient endpoints using a fully integrated system that is validated and transferrable across disciplines. For example, PROMIS has been used to evaluate patient-reported pain interference, or how pain limits/interferes with an individual's physical, mental, and social well-being. Amtmann et al.[10] published a PROMIS scale developed specifically to evaluate Pain Interference (PROMIS-PI) in 2010. The authors developed a 41-item question bank that provided key information on a given patient's pain interference, which was then validated and deemed to be a good psychometric test. These questions evaluate pain interference in multiple categories such as concentration, enjoyment of life, participation in leisure activities, day-to-day activities, and family life, to name a few.

The PROMIS-PI differs from previous pain scales in that it allows researchers to evaluate pain from the patient's perspective of the degree of interference. Traditional 10-point pain scales have been somewhat limiting in differentiating the extent of lifestyle disruption that the patient experiences because of pain or, more to the point, what specifically can be addressed to provide relief from pain or to regain preinjury/presurgical function. Addressing individual issues the patient has with pain interference appears to be a step in the right direction, as previous studies have shown that simply rating the pain on a scale of 1 to 10 does not improve the quality of pain management.[11] Although using pain as the "fifth vital sign" brings this important data point to the forefront of medical records, a simple quantitative score—outside of the clinical context—does not add valuable information or assist in clinical decision-making. Additionally, from a research perspective, a validated 41-question scale that can be used to evaluate if the intervention in question provides relief from the burden of pain the patient experiences can be a useful research tool.

Short Form 36/12

The Short Form (SF)-36 is a quality of life survey initially published in 1992, followed 4 years later by an abridged version, the SF-12. This survey tests eight domains in both the full-length and 12-question version: physical functioning, role physical, bodily pain, general health, vitality, social functioning, role emotional, and mental health. The "role physical" and "role emotional" categories evaluate what physical and emotional limitations the illness has caused the individual. Two versions of the forms exist, either an acute (1-week recall) or a standard (4-week recall) version can be employed. The survey is either administered by a health care professional or self-administered by the patient. After obtaining the data, researchers split the scores into two larger components, the Physical Component Summary (PCS) and the Mental Component Summary (MCS).[12] The raw scores are then translated to a 0- to 100-point scale for ubiquity of use and ease of interpretation. The SF-12 PCS and MCS scores correlate well with the SF-36 scores, and the abridged SF-12 has been used in multiple fields since its creation.

As it relates to hypertrophic burn scars, the SF has been used in several studies to evaluate what impact scarring and disfigurement have on the subject's quality of life. The SF-12 has also been modified to be more specific for a pediatric population, when required. Notably, a study by Kinahan et al.[13] in 2012 evaluated the effects of scarring/disfigurement as a result of childhood cancer on long-term survivors' quality of life. By incorporating SF, the authors were able to better define this population and were able to find statistically significant differences that scarring had on the subject's emotional distress and quality of life. With any psychometric testing, the larger the body of available preexisting data, the more confidence one can have with these tests. That is, the researcher can be more certain that he or she is measuring what the investigator wants to measure.

Despite a large number of studies that have used the SF-36/SF-12, the literature specific to scars affecting quality of life is somewhat limited. Because of its validated content and ease of use, it is difficult to find a better alternative to measure the quality of life in any scar population, with the exception of burn scars (see below), and the SF-12 is currently employed at the authors' institution for several ongoing clinical scar assessment studies. With the current and future trials utilizing this instrument, we anticipate that the SF-36, and specifically the SF-12, will become a standard research methodology in the assessment of hypertrophic burn scars.

Burn-Specific Health Scale

Initially published in 1979 by Blades et al.[14] in an article entitled "Quality of life after major burns," the Burn-Specific Health Scale (BSHS) was a 114-item survey used to evaluate the overall health status of burn survivors. The BSHS has undergone several revisions, and currently exists in three forms worthy of discussion. The BSHS-Abbreviated (BSHS-A) consists of four main domains:

- Physical—items 1 to 20, subdivided into:
  - mobility/self-care, hand function, and role activities
- Psychological—items 21 to 50, subdivided into:
  - body image, and affective
- Social—items 51 to 65, subdivided into:
  - family/friends and sexual
- General—items 66 to 80, subdivided into:
  - pain, social sensitivity, and health

The BSHS-Revised (BSHS-R) addressed issues identified by Blalock et al.[15] who found that the original BSHS was lacking in the following areas: skin, work, treatment regimens, pain, and itching. The resultant BSHS-R had 41 items covering seven domains of postburn quality of life.

Although the BSHS-R was a much shorter version (and thought to be of more use in the clinical setting), it was followed by the BSHS-Brief (BSHS-B), which was a

40-item, 9-domain scale, scored on a 5-point scale, that combined key elements of the BSHS-R and the BSHS-A. The new domains were Heat Sensitivity, Affect, Hand Function, Treatment Regimens, Work, Sexuality, Interpersonal Relationships, Simple Abilities, and Body Image.[16] A year later, a review of the three BSHS (-A, -R, and -B) was performed to evaluate their correlation with each other, and to evaluate which subsets were best covered by these scales. Correlation was the strongest between the BSHS-R and BSHS-B ($r = 0.98$), followed by BSHS-A and BSHS-B ($r = 0.86$); the least correlated was BSHS-A and BSHS-R ($r = 0.81$). The authors also found the smallest respondent burden (i.e., the scale that was the least taxing to subjects) was either the BSHS-B or -R, due to their shorter styles. Additionally, the BSHS-R/-B had a better evaluation of heat sensitivity; and the BSHS-B and -A covered hand and sexual function better than the BSHS-R, bringing the authors to the conclusion that the BSHS-B was the most useful of the three because of both its comprehensive nature and its shorter form.[17,18]

The BSHS-B has yielded promising results since its development and introduction and can be applied to different populations with good internal consistency and validity. It has been used, for instance, in the pediatric population to contrast patients who did and did not suffer from inhalational injury in order to compare their postburn quality of life.[19] Although Rosenberg et al.[19] did not find that inhalational injury affected postburn quality of life, this publication is a good example of how this shorter, more comprehensive version of the BSHS is an effective tool for evaluating how burn scars may affect study populations.

University of North Carolina 4P

The UNC-4P has been in use at our institution since 2012 as an adjunct to the VSS and POSAS to measure the effect of laser therapy on burn scars.[20] The UNC-4P covers the patients' subjective perception of the scar to include: pruritus, pain, paresthesias, and pliability, which subjects rate on a scale of 0 (best) to 3 (worst), for a combined maximum of 12. In one of our before–after cohort studies, patients reported a mean of 6.0 on this scale prior to the start of laser therapy, and finished the study at a mean of 2.2. Although this scale has not been independently validated, it serves to capture the essence of the patients' symptoms throughout our treatment phases.

See Table 28-1 for a summary of scales and what they measure.

PEARL 28-2 *It should be noted that most of these scales exist in a state of flux between the original published scale and what is currently in use. Some have only minor modifications, whereas others have been completely revamped. If the reader is interested in a particular scale, the corresponding references are a good starting point. However, as more modern/developed scales are published, it is likely that associated usage fees will be required. A researcher on a budget may have better luck modifying the original free scale to suit their purpose, as opposed to trying to find a fee-for-use scale that needs to be modified anyway.*

Section 2: Instruments for Measurement:

In a review article by Perry et al.[22] in 2010, four key components were identified as being comprehensive in evaluating skin scars in a noninvasive, objective manner. These included color, surface area, height/depth, and pliability. The following section discusses the most common ways of measuring scars for research purposes.

Color

When evaluating all types of scars (atrophic, hypertrophic, keloid) for clinical and research purposes, one must consider color. Ongoing inflammation and neovascularization in a scar includes both aesthetic and functional considerations, as hypertrophic scars may cause pain, itching, or generalized irritation to the patient. When studying various scar conditions, the clinician and researcher must be able to make an accurate baseline assessment and determine the effect of interventions. The Chroma Meter (Minolta, Osaka, Japan) (see Figs. 28-2 and 28-3) serves this purpose and has been validated in several clinical trials involving scar research.[23] The Chroma Meter functions by emitting a white beam from a xenon lamp, which is then collected by photodetectors with preset color filters at 459, 560, and 600 nm. The Chroma Meter then gives data output in three different categories: L^* (brightness or white/black), a^* (red-green spectrum), and b^* (blue-yellow spectrum). As erythema (i.e., redness) becomes more prominent, the a^* value becomes greater, compared to darker skinned individuals who would have a higher b^* value. Someone who has very pale skin with a

Table 28-1 Summary of Scales and What They Measure

	Subjective	Objective	Quality of Life	Pediatric Version Available
VSS		X		
POSAS	X	X	X	
PROMIS-PI	X		X	
SF-36/12	X		X	X[a]
BSHS-B	X		X	X
UNC-4P	X		X	

[a] Pediatric Quality of Life Inventory[21]

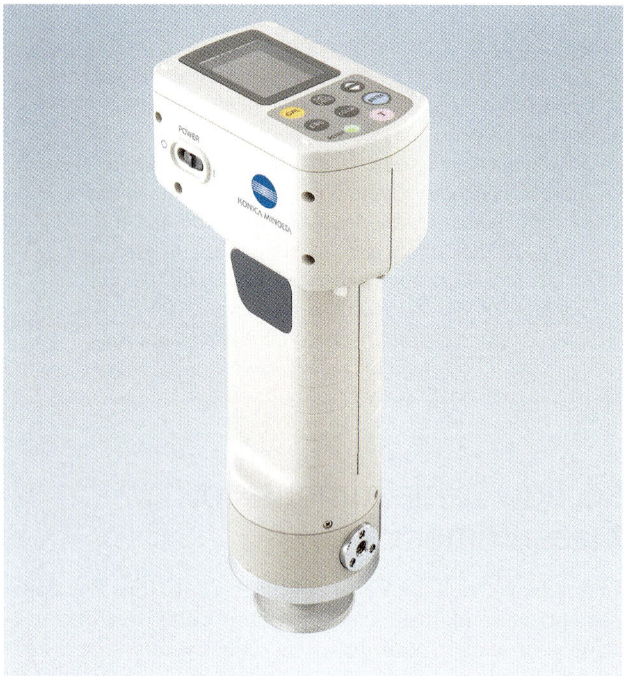

FIGURES 28-2 Chroma Meter. *(Courtesy of Konica Minolta, Inc., Osaka, Japan. All rights reserved.)*

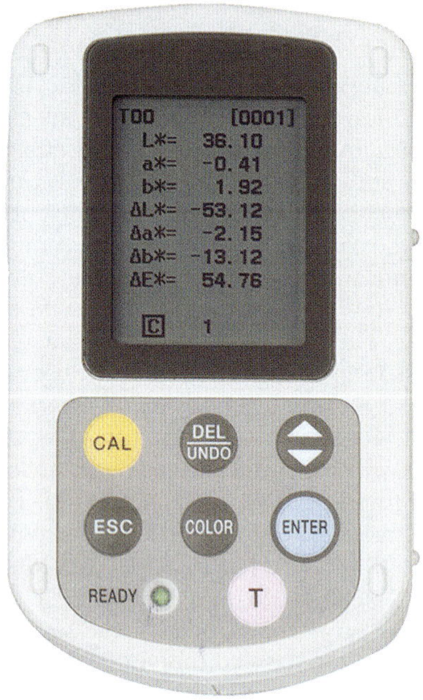

FIGURES 28-3 Chroma Meter user interface (top view). *(Courtesy of Konica Minolta, Inc., Osaka, Japan. All rights reserved.)*

large component of erythema would have a higher L^* and a^*, and someone who is dark skinned with no erythema would have a very high b^*, but lower a^* and L^*. These results are instantaneous and can be compared over the course of the research to look for statistically significant differences or overall trends. It should be noted that this instrument requires daily calibration to ensure readings fall within a predetermined standard deviation.[24]

The Chroma Meter has also been found to correlate well with the VSS vascularity scores, but it does not demonstrate statistically significant differences between normal and red coloration categories, or for hypopigmented and hyperpigmented scars, in comparison with the DermaSpectrometer.[22,25] In addition to the Chroma Meter, tools such as the Mexameter (MX18, Courage & Khazaka Electronic GmbH) and DermaSpectrometer are available to clinicians to assist in determining scar color; selection of the instrument varies from study to study based on the variables being assessed and the endpoints being measured.

Surface Area

Traditionally scar surface area calculation has been done with simple width and length measurements. However, because of the irregular nature of scars (particularly burn scars), this simplified version of determining surface area may not be accurate. Two-dimensional methods of planimetry (measuring of surface area) can involve transparency tracing, where double-layered acetate film is placed on the wound and the borders are traced. The bottom layer is discarded and the layer with the tracing imprint is then measured using manual "square counting" or by computer analysis.[22,26-28] Additional two-dimensional methods include taking photographs under standard conditions with vertical and horizontal gauging. For the more tech savvy, an Image Tool (CD Wilcox) can electronically scan the area in question and calculate the area.[25,29] One must be careful with new/fresh scars, as reports of inaccurate calculations from software due to poor border definitions have been reported.[22,30]

Three-dimensional (3-D) imaging is also becoming more available and multiple companies offer 3-D scanning and volume manipulation produce a "before and after" treatment image such as Vectra (Canfield Scientific, Fairfield, NJ) and Crisalix (Lausanne, Switzerland). The Vivid 900 3-D digitizer (Konica Minolta, UK) is another such device that has been used in keloid research for scar volume quantification.[31] The area of interest is captured, and the software calculates volume for the researchers.

Height/Depth

When trying to determine scar height/depth, ultrasound technology has by far been the most widely used in the literature, particularly the DermaScan-C (Cortex Technologies, Hadsund, Denmark) (Fig. 28-4).[22] Many companies offer skin-specific instruments; however, probes with higher frequency (choosing resolution versus penetration) in the 10 to 15 MHz rage have shallow penetration and offer adequate visualization of superficial structures. Ultrasound probes that can collect images at 20 MHz (such as the DermaScan-C) have also been able to detect subtle differences between hypertrophic scars and normal scars, as well as differences between hypertrophic scars and normal skin based on total thickness measurements.[32-34] When dealing with scars that are significantly raised above skin level, the sonographer should try their best to capture images that represent the undisturbed scar (i.e., without applying excessive force) to allow probe contact with the skin on either side. Building a bridge with the ultrasound gel, as well as using IV bags and silicone sheets as buffers, can aid the researcher in

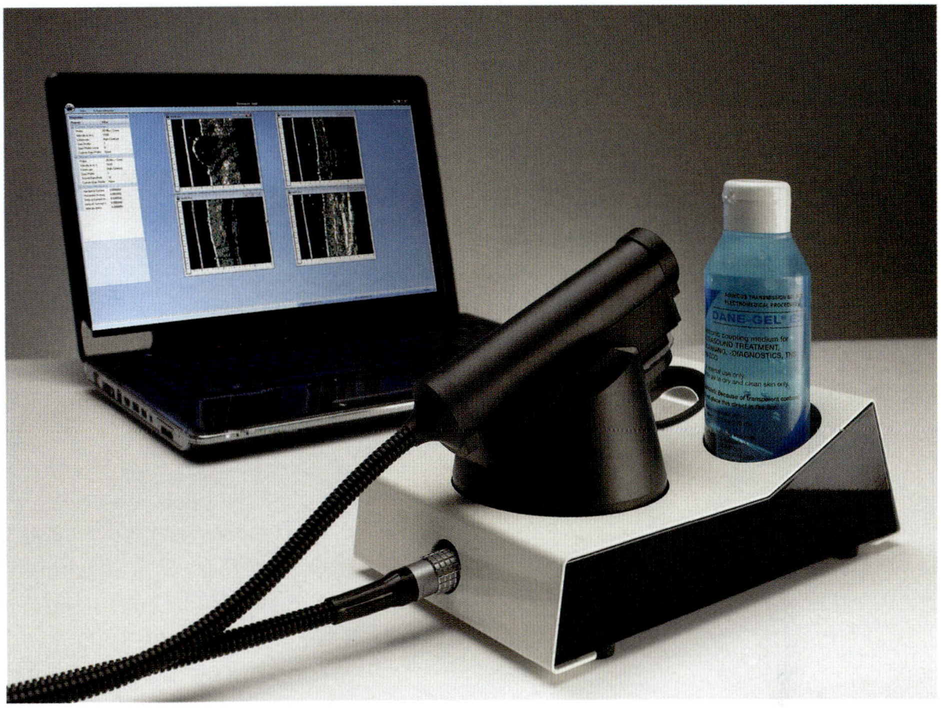

FIGURE 28-4 DermaScan-C. *(Courtesy of Cortex Technology, Hadsund, Denmark.)*

obtaining unadulterated images with good reproducibility (see Fig. 28-5A for the ultrasound bridge, and Fig. 28-5B for the corresponding image). Note how using the bridge eliminates uneven surfaces and allows for excellent images in spite of a heterogeneous scar.

Pliability

At our institution pliability is measured using the Cutometer (MPA580; Courage + Khazaka electronic GmbH, Koeln, Germany) (see Figs. 28-6 to 28-8). This device has been frequently cited in the literature as a reliable technology to measure scar pliability, and it has been shown to have good inter-/intrarater reliability and validity for hypertrophic scars.[33,35] The Cutometer has a suction probe with varying diameters (6 mm has been shown to be most efficient in measuring viscoelastic properties of the skin)[35,36] that is placed on the patients' skin. The Cutometer then applies 500 mbar of negative pressure in three rapid bursts. This stretches the area of interest and the instrument measures how quickly the skin recoils back to normal position. There are two sets of data from the Cutometer: the absolute parameters (U_a, U_e, U_f, U_r, and U_v) and the relative parameters (R_0, R_1, R_2, . . ., R_9). In scar literature, R_0, R_2, R_5, R_6, and R_7

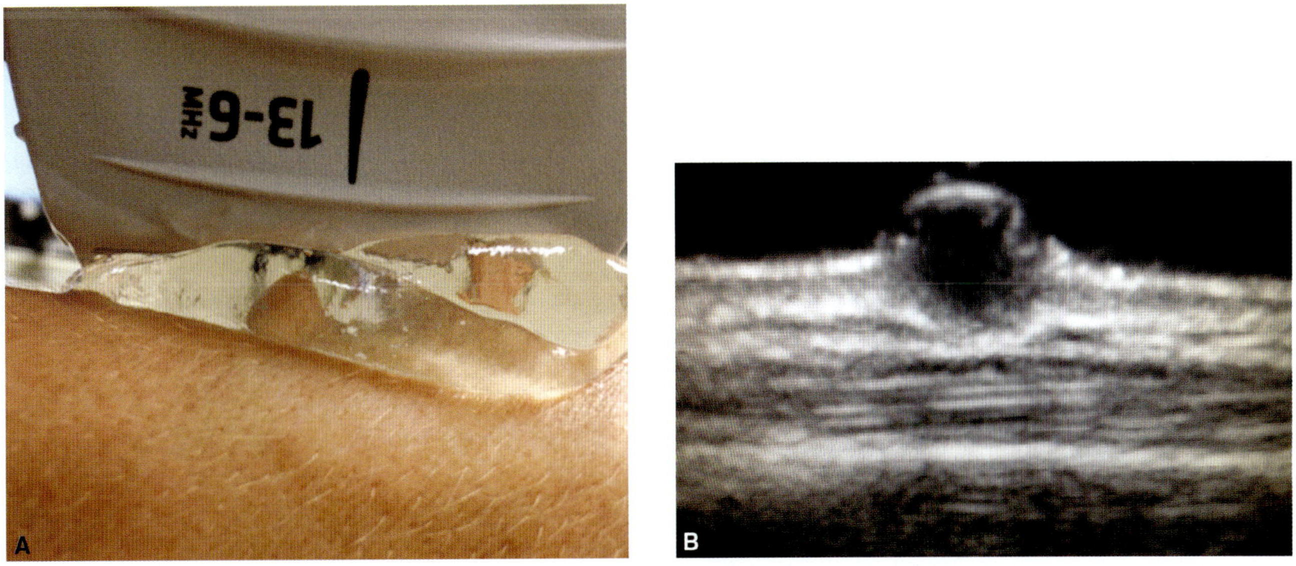

FIGURE 28-5 **A**: Ultrasound gel bridge. **B**: Corresponding clinical image.

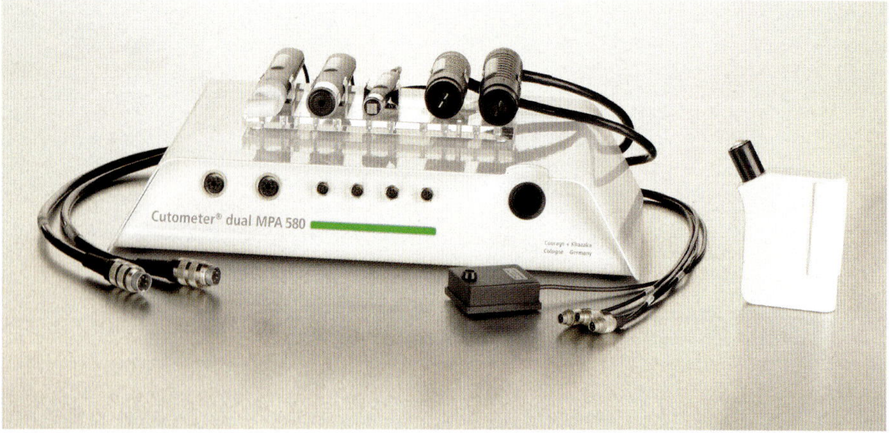

FIGURE 28-6 Cutometer base unit. *(Courtesy of Courage + Khazaka electronic GmbH, Koeln, Germany.)*

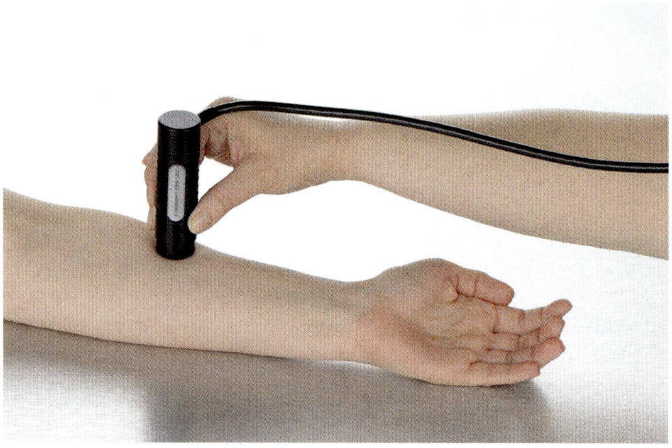

FIGURE 28-7 Cutometer application. *(Courtesy of Courage + Khazaka electronic GmbH, Koeln, Germany.)*

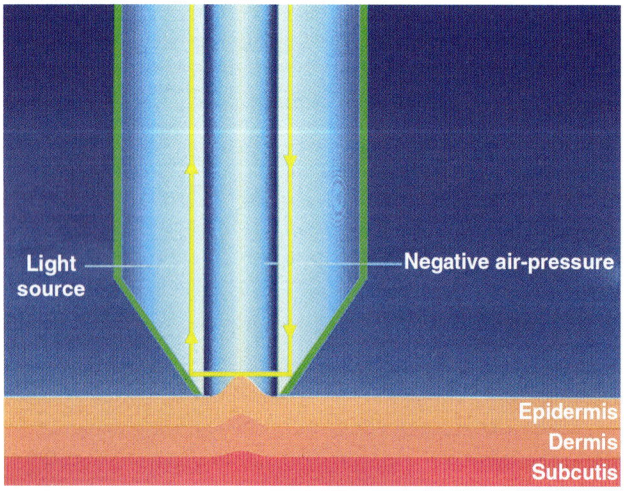

FIGURE 28-8 Cutometer probe. *(Courtesy of Courage + Khazaka electronic GmbH, Koeln, Germany.)*

have been reported on a more consistent basis.[37] These values are important as they represent the following:

- $R_0 = U_f$ = maximum deformation/extension of skin
- $R_2 = U_a/U_f$ = final retraction to maximum deformation ratio
- $R_5 = U_r/U_e$ = immediate retraction to immediate deformation ratio
- $R_6 = U_v/U_e$ = viscoelasticity to elasticity ratio
- $R_7 = U_r/U_f$ = immediate retraction to maximum deformation ratio.

See Table 28-2 for a summary of technologies and what they measure.

Section 3: Future Research and Choosing a Type of Trial

Research Structure

When initiating a new research project, we follow a basic algorithm that may seem simplistic but helps all members of the team stay on track and maintain focus. As busy clinicians at an academic medical center, we routinely teach research methods to our trainees. This involves not only mentoring new investigators, but also providing them with the intellectual and logistical capital to help them carry out and complete their projects. We follow a process of: Study Design, Find Collaborators, Obtain Funding, Get Institutional Review Board (IRB) Approval, Develop Database, Collect Data, Analyze Data, Present Data, and Publish. For interventional trials, often a Data Safety Monitoring Board (DSMB) or other institutional review will be required prior to, or as part of, the IRB process. Both the "Study Design" and "Find Collaborators" sections merit further discussion and, if done appropriately, form the backbone of a successful project.

Table 28-2 Summary of Technologies and What They Measure

Instrument Reviewed	What It Measures	Inter-/Intrarater Reliability	Validated
Chroma Meter	Color/erythema	High	Yes
Planimetry/acetate film and 3D methods	Surface area/volume	N/A	No
Ultrasound	Scar depth	High	Yes
Cutometer	Scar pliability	High	Yes

PEARL 28-3 *The design table is usually filled out as the individual components are achieved. For instance, the below example (typically a spreadsheet table; Table 28-3) is in the process of being submitted to the IRB. With multiple projects ongoing, we find it much easier to keep track of what phase the given trial is in and what the next step would be using this format.*

Study Design

Retrospective studies tend to require less forethought in their design, usually involve less work, and provide less robust data than prospective studies. Therefore, this discussion will focus on the design of prospective clinical trials. In the area of scar research, the investigator must have enough insight on the front end of trial design to avoid costly pitfalls and revision of the study design in the data collection period. For instance, when measuring scars using the above instrumentation, it is vital to consider three principles prior to submitting one's proposal to the IRB or DSMB:

1. What is the anchor spot (i.e., the physical location from which the initial and subsequent measurements will be taken)? Is this a location determined by what the patient reports is the most painful, the most contracted, the most discolored, or a more vague "worst spot" for them to choose? Clinicians may elect to choose this spot themselves as to avoid difficult-to-measure areas (e.g., spanning joints, heavily hair-bearing areas, interweb spaces); scars that are the most painful/itchy to the patient but clinically look far closer to normal skin than does another scar elsewhere; or an area that is difficult to find a control (e.g., tip of the nose, lips, etc.). Often the anchor spot location is decided during the first clinic appointment when patients discuss what bothers them the most. Clinicians can use either that same problem area or one that is close by, provided the patient agrees it is nearly as symptomatic.
2. We often will take three measurements at the problem area: the anchor spot, nearby-1, and nearby-2. This allows us to gauge the response, not only of the absolute worst spot, but also how the surrounding scarred, partially scarred, or near-normal skin is responding to treatment.
3. A measurement of normal skin should be obtained, both to see if the treatment has some overall effect on skin elasticity that is not specific to scar tissue and, more importantly, to serve as a baseline comparison of what the scar parameters should be progressing toward. We have found this to be of particular difficulty as many surgical scars tend to be midline and burn scars often involve bilateral/contralateral limbs. For anatomic regions without a contralateral area for comparison, such as those on the torso, we try to find controls that are nearby that would have similar dermal properties had the scarring not occurred. Whenever available, we use a contralateral, unaffected limb to provide baseline readings of this normal area that should be similar to an unscarred/unburned anchor spot. If one is entirely out of options because of research on an extensively scarred population, such as on burn scars that encompass >50% total body surface area, one can always resort to using population means, or getting baseline measurements from a healthy control. We have not found this to be a frequent problem, but the more tools one has in their toolbox, the more likely one is to finish the job.

To raise some additional key points in this patient population, oftentimes scar research focuses on hypertrophic scars, burn scars, keloids, and patient populations with heterogeneous injuries. Simple studies looking at postsurgical scars in a limited field are far easier to set up compared to hypertrophic burn scars where areas of interest can span the entire body and be located across different skin types, have varying scar age, contour irregularities, infections, and lymphedema, to name a few. These challenges, although not insurmountable, certainly need to be considered early in the study design, as a flawed design can lead to equivocal data/results. These data points, although somewhat difficult to study in a prospective manner, are near impossible in a retrospective design. Chart review quickly becomes inaccurate when dealing with historical data of scars across multiple skin types, hair-bearing areas, joints, etc. It has been our practice to try and avoid this type of research in favor of prospective data whenever possible to avoid these data inconsistencies.

Find Collaborators

This portion of research design cannot be overlooked when starting a clinical trial. Early discussions with statisticians, clinical and research coordinators, and departmental colleagues can be invaluable in managing the numerous design options, regulatory paperwork, and clinical throughput of the trial. It is highly suggested that the core group of researchers meet regularly and discuss aspects of the trial design at every step of the way. It would be a waste of time for the principal investigator to discuss what is being measured with the software engineer designing the database without close collaboration with a statistician, who will evaluate the data coming from the software at the end of the trial. Likewise, departmental colleagues who have experience in the field of research at a given institution can help navigate through the quagmire of institutional regulatory boards and supporting documents. It is also important to consider that this collaboration may benefit the structure of the research by bringing to light alternative research methodology that had not been previously used by your institution or in your field of study.

Table 28-3 Example of a Design Table

Design Study	Find Collaborators	Obtain Funding	Get IRB Approval	Develop Database	Collect Data	Analyze Data	Present Data	Publish
X	X	N/A	______					

PEARL 28-4 *A multidisciplinary approach to research is sometimes overlooked. Involvement of statisticians and research associates to help with portions of the study a clinician will have a more difficult time with is generally a good start. However, time should be taken to genuinely make this multidisciplinary across all points of care from the patient's perspective. The team should include burn/trauma clinicians, mental health experts, physical and occupational therapists, dermatologists, and case managers/social workers, as they may have valuable insight into some of the finer points of study design and data procurement as it relates to patient flow through the hospital and outpatient clinics.*

Sequential Multiple Assignment Randomized Trial Design

One type of trial design that has been gaining popularity in such fields as psychiatry and oncology, but not yet in surgery, has been the sequential multiple assignment randomized trial (SMART) model. Randomized controlled trials (RCTs) are limited in that one typically compares an experimental intervention with standard of care and/or a placebo. SMART trials are based on adaptive treatment strategies, where patients are entered into one treatment arm that can be changed at predetermined time or response points.[38] For example, the researcher may wish to conduct a trial in which hypertrophic burn scars receive three different treatments over time: medical management (creams, massage, compression garments, and silicone sheets), pulsed dye laser (PDL), and ablative fractional carbon dioxide laser. If the primary tailoring variable is time, then after 4 months of treatment in one arm the patient is subsequently switched to another arm. If the primary tailoring variable is response (or lack thereof), then the patient is kept in an arm until a certain result is obtained or it is determined that no response is being achieved by that specific treatment. This study design is also different from an RCT in that it does not answer a hypothesis, but rather generates a hypothesis. A large amount of prospective data can be used to individualize treatment plans, depending on baseline characteristics of the patient and the scar.

This trial design will likely be applied to multiple fields of clinical research, including scar management, in the near future. Although there will still be a role for case reports and retrospective reviews, prospective studies will be required to determine best treatment algorithms in the management of hypertrophic burn scars. In addition to cost-effectiveness studies, SMART design will allow for personalization of treatment plans in a clinical area where multiple interventions exist and results from these interventions are not consistent from patient to patient. Indeed, new methodologies in trial design may be even more important than developing new technologies for assessment of hypertrophic burn scars.[39]

Recent Advances in Scar Care

A myriad of scar treatments exist and can include topical creams, compression garments, injectables (e.g. chemotherapeutic agents, steroids, botulinum toxin), radiation (keloids), laser therapy, microneedling, and surgical excision (with or without tissue expansion), to name a few.[40] As technology continues to develop, additional modalities are sure to arise. Some of the best results at our institution are laser-centric and focus on targeting immature blood vessels in scar tissue and vaporizing scar tissue. These have been accomplished with good results to date, using the PDL and ablative fractional CO_2 laser.[20] For severe scars, one modality is often not enough and the use of multimodal treatment is required (i.e., laser therapy and steroid injections) to soften the scar and make it more pliable, followed by adjacent tissue rearrangement. No matter the success at a given institution with the therapy of choice, it will likely be replaced by newer modalities, and the physician-scientist must be willing to adapt and try new interventions in order to achieve the best possible outcome in the global sense.

The Ideal Scar Scale

The Ideal Scar Scale has yet to be created, as the comprehensive nature ranging from basic science measurements of inflammatory mediators in the scar bed to psychosocial well-being would make this an incredibly lengthy scale not applicable to most forms of research. In order to make one that is universal and applicable to most researchers, it would have to be, above all else, malleable. Nguyen et al.[2] discussed applicable variables that included the following:

- Scar type
  - Surgical, burn, acne, etc.
- Scar age
  - Time since injury, time since wound closure, time since onset versus time since last flare for acne.
- Area of involvement
  - Surface area in cm^2.
- Maximum contour irregularity
  - Maximum distance between the subcuticular-dermal border and the epidermal surface.
- Anatomic location
  - More visible scars have higher risk of posttraumatic stress disorder and poorer psychosocial outcomes.
- Erythema
  - Generally from VSS as: none, pink, red, purple.
- Dyspigmentation
  - Measured as a distinct entity and not included in erythema: hyper-, hypo-, and mixed.
- Anatomic cosmetic units
  - Distinct cosmetic units, that is, nose, lips, chin, may be less noticeable if the scar is confined to one versus spanning several.
- Psychosocial impact
  - Generally underdiagnosed and underreported, but a key element in overall well-being.
- Reaction of others to scars
  - Measuring the degree of disability due to stigmatization related to scarring and the sequelae thereof.

- Hyper-/hypotrichosis
  - Typically thought of as alopecia/hypotrichosis due to burn injury, but can manifest as hypertrichosis in rare instances.
- Hyper-/hypohidrosis
  - Due to injury to the skin or underlying nerves.
- Pain
  - A simple 10-point scale is unlikely to capture this fully and a more in-depth questionnaire such as the PROMIS would likely be needed.
- Pruritus
  - Either as a symptom in need of treatment or possibly as a heralding sign of keloid formation.
- Dysesthesia
  - Quantifying nonpain sensation such as anesthesia, burning, wetness, electric shock, and pins and needles.
- Infection
  - Recent or chronic folliculitis, cellulitis, abscesses, and fasciitis.
- Lymphedema
  - Generally not seen on current burn scars, but a potentially debilitating comorbidity in need of treatment.
- Chronic wounds
  - Due to underling tension, skin fragility, or bacteria. Potentially leading to Marjolin's ulcer if left untreated for long periods of time.
- Skin cancer
  - Generally squamous cell cancer due to chronic wounds, but basal cell and melanoma have also been reported.
- Functional impairment
  - Generally omitted from current scales with the exception of PROMIS; however, this needs to be customized to the individual study.

The above list should give the reader a sense of how comprehensive an "ideal" scar scale would need to be. Even starting with these variables one could add:

- A basic science component of biopsy and inflammatory mediator characteristics.
- Further delve into the psychosocial well-being and functional restrictions as seen in the BSHS and PROMIS.
- Pliability, as measured by a Cutometer/Elastometer.
- Objective measurements of erythema using a Chroma Meter–type device
- Depth by an ultrasound.

It would seem with all these variables, and a significant amount of detail needed in each category of interest, that we scar researchers could develop a scale similar to what breast cancer researchers have done with the BREAST-Q©.[41] This new research tool consists of several versions depending on what is being evaluated (augmentation, reconstruction, reduction, etc.), each one with multiple components related to quality of life, expectations, and even satisfaction with the treatment team. The "SCAR-Q" would need to be similarly designed, with multiple questionnaires, variable sections/subsections based on the type of scar being evaluated, and options for objective measurements based on the research question. If designed properly, like the BREAST-Q©, researchers could choose a topic and corresponding components of the "SCAR-Q," which would be entered into a searchable, analyzable database and results could be communicated across specialties in a standardized format. It is likely that astute researchers in the near future will be able to develop, implement, and validate such a scar scale.

RESEARCH DESIGN EXAMPLE

The following discussion will highlight some of the aspects of designing a research project. We will discuss some of the key points, pitfalls, and goals in order to help the reader understand, at a broad level, what is involved along the process at a typical university hospital. There will be some variance between institutions; however, the basic principles should stand.

As a new associate professor at the flagship hospital in your state, you have been tasked with developing a research project. A few recent cases of hypertrophic scar formation after panniculectomy led you to pursue an interest in postsurgical hypertrophic scar (HTS) formation. A review of the literature led you to realize that the data on incidence are fairly varied, and you would like to define this variable in your own patient population so that you will have a baseline for future research efforts.

DESIGN STUDY: Ideally prospective in nature. First, a thorough review of the literature is in order. Without first performing a literature review, you may be duplicating recent research and wasting time/effort performing a study that has already been published. Next let us decide on the patient population. Where will these patients come from? Is there a good way to recruit subjects in clinic? Would you include all panniculectomy patients so that you can see the overall incidence of HTS? Should you set early exclusion criteria to control for confounders such as known keloid formers? Will this be a clinical study with surveys, which could potentially be done at lower cost, or will there be a basic science component requiring ongoing funding? Will you be performing an intervention, and if so what is the efficacy and safety profile of this intervention compared to current treatment modalities? If you are measuring scars with newer instruments, what units do they record in, and how many patients would be required to see a meaningful difference in the intervention group?

FIND COLLABORATORS: Panniculectomy patients would typically be from the plastic surgery department, and if this is not your primary field, an early collaboration would be needed. A departmental or university employed statistician would be able to evaluate what data are being collected and determine enrollment estimates, as well as decide early on what analysis will be performed on the data at study completion. A randomization scheme could be established at this point, and knowing how much data are going to be collected on each patient at each encounter will also help determine if a research assistant(s) is/are needed to help with the process. Involvement of clinic nursing staff, social workers, and bariatric surgery staff would also give a bigger picture of patient flow and identify potential issues with study design.

OBTAIN FUNDING: By this point you should already know enrollment estimates, what intervention (if any) will be done, how the data will be collected and stored, and any associated fees for statistical services. Using these variables a rough estimate of overall cost should be calculated and funding pursued. A discussion with colleagues in your department, combined with a brief search should reveal several specialty-specific funding sources available, i.e., the Plastic Surgery Foundation grant and fellowship programs Web site.[42]

GET IRB APPROVAL: The process will vary between institutions, but fundamentally it involves submitting your proposed research project to a heterogeneous group of individuals to discuss the merit and safety of the project to ensure it falls within the governmental and ethical guidelines. This is also the point in time where you may be referred to a DSMB if an intervention is to be performed. This will ensure that the data are being reviewed and that any complications as a result of intervention are monitored.

DEVELOP DATABASE: This should generally be done with input from statistical and research personnel to ensure ease of use and accessibility. All databases should be developed, stored, and shared in accordance with the Health Insurance Portability and Accountability Act guidelines.

COLLECT DATA: This process is the most variable and can be done over a few days if retrospective surveys are employed, or may take years if a prospective trial with long-term data collection is needed.

ANALYZE DATA: This may require days to weeks based on the statistical methodology required; however, when reaching this point, it is often one of the most exciting and rewarding portions of the research as the fruits of your labor are realized.

PRESENT DATA: This should be discussed with colleagues prior to beginning research, as a goal/target meeting and corresponding journal should be selected early in the process to give the team a submission deadline to work toward. It should also be established very early who the primary author is, and who will be the presenting member of the team. We have found that this has allowed for long-term ongoing collaboration between departments and between team members of the same department.

PUBLISH DATA: As an extension of the prior point, a goal journal should have been selected at the onset of the research. It is also worth noting that a back-up journal and deadline is occasionally required and these should be kept in mind should the initial journal not be interested in publishing this work.

This work was supported in part by The UNC Center for Health Innovation at the University of North Carolina. The senior author received the 2014 Innovation Pilot Award for the project 'Novel Therapies for the Management of Hypertrophic Burn Scars: Creating an Innovative Model of Health Care Delivery, Using SMART Design to Personalize Treatment Strategies'.

REFERENCES

1. Lewis CS. *Mere Christianity*. New York: Harper Collins Publishers, 1952.
2. Nguyen TA, Feldstein SI, Shumaker PR, et al. A review of scar assessment scales. *Semin Cutan Med Surg*. 2015;34:28–36.
3. Sullivan T, Smith J, Kermode J, et al. Rating the burn scar. *J Burn Care Rehabil*. 1990;11(3):256–260.
4. Vercelli S, Ferriero G, Sartorio F, et al. How to assess postsurgical scars: A review of outcomes. *Disabil Rehabil*. 2009;31(25):2055–2063.
5. Forbes-Duchart L, Marshall S, Strock A, et al. Determination of inter-rater reliability in pediatric burn scar assessment using a modified version of the Vancouver Scar Scale. *J Burn Care Res*. 2007;28(3):460–467.
6. Baryza MJ, Baryza GA. The Vancouver scar scale: an administration tool and its interrater reliability. *J Burn Care Rehabil*. 1995;16:535–538.
7. Draaijers LJ, Tempelman FR, Botman YA, et al. The patient and observer scar assessment scale: a reliable and feasible tool for scar evaluation. *Plast Reconstr Surg*. 2004;113(7):1960–1965.
8. van de Kar AL, Corion LU, Smeulders MJ, et al. Reliable and feasible evaluation of linear scars by the Patient and Observer Scar Assessment Scale. *Plast Reconstr Surg*. 2005;116(2):514–522.
9. PROMIS. Dynamic tools to measure health outcomes from the patient perspective. In *PROMIS: overview*. http://www.nihpromis.org/about/overview. Accessed May 15, 2015.
10. Amtmann D, Cook KF, Jensen MP, et al. Development of a PROMIS item bank to measure pain interference. *Pain*. 2010;150(1):173–182.
11. Mularski RA, White-Chu F, Overbay D, et al. Measuring pain as the 5th vital sign does not improve quality of pain management. *J Gen Intern Med*. 2006;21(6):607–612.
12. Busija L, Pausenberger E, Haines TP, et al. Adult measures of general health and health-related quality of life: Medical Outcomes Study Short From 36-Item (SF-36) and Short Form 12-Item (SF-12) Heath Surveys, Nottingham Health Profile (NHP), Sickness Impact Profile (SIP), Medical Outcomes Study Short Form 6D (SF6D), Health Utilities Index Mark 3 (HUI3), Quality of Well-Being Scale (QWB), and Assessment of Quality of Life (AQoL). *Arthritis Care Res*. 2011;63(11):S383–S412.
13. Kinahan KE, Sharp LK, Seidel K, et al. Scarring, disfigurement, and quality of life in long-term survivors of childhood cancer: a report from the Childhood Cancer Survivor Study. *J Clin Oncol*. 2012;30(20):2466–2474.
14. Blades B, Mellis N, Munster AM. A burn specific health scale. *J Trauma*. 1982;22(10):872–875.
15. Blalock S, Bunker B, Moore JD, et al. The impact of burn injury: a preliminary investigation. *J Burn Care Rehabil*. 1992;13:487–492.
16. Kildal M, Andersson G, Fugl-Meyer AR, et al. Development of a brief version of the Burn Specific Health Scale (BSHS-B). *J Trauma*. 2001;51:740–746.
17. Kildal M, Andersson G, Gerdin B. Health Status in Swedish burn patients: assessment utilizing three variants of the Burn Specific Health Scale. *Burns*. 2002;28:639–645.
18. Yoder LH, Nayback AM, Gaylord K. The evolution and utility of the burn specific health scale: a systematic review. *Burns*. 2010;36:1143–1156.
19. Rosenberg M, Ramirez M, Epperson K, et al. Comparison of long-term quality of life of pediatric burn survivors with and without inhalation injury. *Burns*. 2015;41:721–726.
20. Hultman CS, Edkins RE, Lee CN, et al. Shine on: review of laser-and light-based therapies for the treatment of burn scars. *Dermatol Res Pract*. 2012;2012:243651.
21. Varni JW, Burwinkle TM, Seid M, et al. The PedsQL 4.0 as a pediatric population health measure: feasibility, reliability, and validity. *Ambul Pediatr*. 2003;3(6):329–341.
22. Perry DM, McGrouther DA, Bayat A. Current tools for noninvasive objective assessment of skin scars. *Plast Reconstr Surg*. 2010;126(3):912–923.
23. Jones HG. Clinimetrics of tristimulus colourimeters in scar assessment: a review of evidence. *J Wound Care*. 2012;21(1):30–35.
24. Van den Kerckhove E, Stappaerts K, Fieuws S, et al. The Assessment of erythema and thickness on burn related scars during pressure garment therapy as a preventive measure for hypertrophic scarring. *Burns*. 2005;31:696–702.
25. Oliveira GV, Chinkes D, Mitchell C, et al. Objective assessment of burn scar vascularity, erythema, pliability, thickness, and planimetry. *Dermatol Surg*. 2005;31:48–58.

26. van Zuijlen PP, Angeles AP, Suijker MH, et al. Reliability and accuracy of techniques for surface area measurements of wounds and scars. *Int J Low Extrem Wounds*. 2004;3:7–11.
27. Young SR, Ballard K. Wound assessment: Diagnostic and assessment applications. Part 2. In: Kitchen S, ed. *Electrotherapy: Evidence Based Practice*. London: Churchill Livingstone; 2001:308–312.
28. Mahajan AL, Tenorio X, Pepper MS, et al. Progressive tissue injury in burns is reduced by rNAPc2. *Burns*. 2006; 32:957–963.
29. de Oliveira GV, Sanford AP, Murphy KD, et al. Growth hormone effects on hypertrophic scar formation: A randomized controlled trial of 62 burned children. *Wound Repair Regen*. 2004;12:404–411.
30. van Zuijlen PP, Vloemans JF, van Trier AJ, et al. Dermal substitution in acute burns and reconstructive surgery: a subjective and objective long-term follow-up. *Plast Reconstr Surg*. 2001;108:1938–1946.
31. Taylor B, Mc- Grouther DA, Bayat A. Use of a noncontact 3D digitiser to measure the volume of keloid scars: A useful tool for scar assessment. *J Plast Reconstr Aesthet Surg*. 2007;60:87–94.
32. Nedelec B, Correa JA, Rachelska G, et al. Quantitative measurement of hypertrophic scar: intrarater reliability, sensitivity, and specificity. *J Burn Care Res*. 2008;29:489–500.
33. Timar-Banu O, Beauregard H, Tousignant J, et al. Development of noninvasive and quantitative methodologies for the assessment of chronic ulcers and scars in humans. *Wound Repair Regen*. 2001;9:123–132.
34. Nedelec B, Correa JA, Rachelska G, et al. Quantitative measurement of hypertrophic scar: interrater reliability, and concurrent validity. *J Burn Care Res*. 2008;29:501–511.
35. Barel AO, Courage W, Clarys P. Suction method for measurement of skin mechanical properties: the Cutometer. In: Serup J, ed. *Handbook for Non-Invasive Methods and the Skin*. Vol. 106. Boca Raton, FL: CRC Press, 1995:335–340.
36. Pierard GE, Nikkels-Tassoudji N, Pierard-Franchimont C. Influence of the test area on the mechanical properties of skin. *Dermatology*. 1995;191:9–15.
37. Chan HH, Wong DS, Ho WS, et al. The use of pulsed dye laser for the prevention and treatment of hypertrophic scars in Chinese persons. *Dermatol Surg*. 2004;30:987–994.
38. Collins, LM, Murphy SA, Strecher V. The Multiphase Optimization Strategy (MOST) and the Sequential Multiple Assignment Randomized Trial (SMART): new methods for more potent eHealth interventions. *Am J Prev Med*. 2007;32(5):S112–S118.
39. Almirall D, Compton SN, Gunlicks-Stoessel M, et al. Designing a pilot sequential multiple assignment randomized trial for developing an adaptive treatment strategy. *Stat Med*. 2012;31(17):1887–1902.
40. Rabello FB, Souza CD, Farina Junio JA. Update on hypertrophic scar treatment. *Clinics (Sao Paulo)*. 2014;69(8):565–573.
41. Cano SJ, Dlassen AF, Scott AM, et al. A closer look at the BREAST-Q(©). *Clin Plast Surg*. 2013;40(2)287–296.
42. The Plastic Surgery Foundation. The PSF Research Grand and Fellowship Programs. http://www.thepsf.org/research/psf-grant-funding.htm. Accessed October 20, 2015.

INDEX

Note: Page numbers followed by "f" indicate figure, and "t" indicate table.

P

Q

R

S